GOVERNORS STATE UNIVERSITY LIBRARY

3 1611 00291 9782

D1776715

A History of
THE AMERICAN MEDICAL ASSOCIATION 1847 TO 1947

BY MORRIS FISHBEIN M.D.

With THE BIOGRAPHIES OF THE PRESIDENTS OF THE ASSOCIATION BY WALTER L. BIERRING M.D.

And With HISTORIES OF THE PUBLICATIONS, COUNCILS, BUREAUS AND OTHER OFFICIAL BODIES

Philadelphia & London
W. B. SAUNDERS COMPANY

KRAUS REPRINT CO.
New York
1969

R
15
.A55
F5
1969

Copyright, 1947, by W. B. Saunders Company

Copyright under the International Copyright Union

LC Med47-46

Reprinted with the permission of the original publisher
KRAUS REPRINT CO.
A U.S. Division of Kraus-Thomson Organization Limited

Printed in U.S.A.

Introduction

AFTER HAVING CONSIDERED the subject on several previous occasions the Board of Trustees of the American Medical Association in 1929 authorized the establishment of a committee to prepare the history of the American Medical Association. During the next two years, the editor of THE JOURNAL reported to the Board of Trustees his plan for a comprehensive history of the Association, which was to include an account of the lives of its presidents and articles concerning each one of the Councils, Bureaus, publications and other activities of the Association.

When the clouds of war loomed on the horizon, the Association began to devote itself wholly to the war effort. In the years since 1941 the winning of the war has been the major objective. In the meantime, the collection of materials continued.

The Board of Trustees of the American Medical Association offer this volume as a record of its founder, its founding, its ideals and its motivations and the extent to which these have been accomplished over a period of one hundred years. The publication has been authorized by the Board of Trustees of the Association as a feature of the Centennial Celebration in 1947.

                        R. L. Sensenich, *Chairman*
                        Ernest E. Irons, *Secretary*
                        Dwight H. Murray
                        William F. Braasch
                        Louis H. Bauer
                        E. L. Henderson
                        John H. Fitzgibbon
                        James R. Miller
                        C. W. Roberts

Preface

WHEN THE AMERICAN MEDICAL ASSOCIATION developed its present building in 1929, the Board of Trustees authorized the preparation of a history of the American Medical Association and appointed a special committee to have charge of the project. The editor of THE JOURNAL made a report later in which he suggested that such a history include a general account of the history of the Association, a record of the lives of its presidents and individual reports on each of the Councils, Bureaus, official bodies and agencies of the Association.

At that time indications that the nation might soon be involved in the war led to important activities in preparedness and quite effectively halted the work on the history. However, Doctor Walter L. Bierring had agreed to prepare the lives of the presidents; and since that time he has devoted a great deal of effort and study to the preparation of the biographies which appear in this volume.

As the war neared its end and the Association began to plan for the celebration of its Centennial in 1947, attention was again directed to the desirability of preparing a history. The project was at this time turned over to the editor, who assigned to the various officers and secretaries of the individual councils the preparation of histories of such activities. Many of these have represented work carried on over several years. These reports appear in a separate section of this volume.

Attempts were made to secure an experienced historian to undertake the preparation of the history of the Association; soon it became apparent that the research and writing necessary to the project would involve intimate acquaintance with motivations and activities; the editor therefore assumed this portion of the work.

Part of the history—from 1846 through 1924—has been published serially in THE JOURNAL OF THE AMERICAN MEDICAL ASSOCIATION. The entire history through 1947 and including special chapters on the libel suits of the American Medical Association, on the life of Dr. George H. Simmons and on the indictment and trial by the United States government, occupies the first part of this book.

In the development of the history of the Association the principal sources of material have been the Transactions of the Association and the files of THE JOURNAL itself, the official proceedings of the House of Delegates, the minutes of the meetings of the Board of Trustees, the official correspondence of the Association, and the biographies of many leaders in American medicine, which the editor has been collecting for some twenty-five years.

Separate histories of THE JOURNAL and the secretary's office have not been prepared, since these activities were so completely integrated with the progress and life of the Association that it seemed unnecessary to discuss them separately.

The editor wishes to express his appreciation to Zita Wist and Marianne Pollock for many hours of work and for a great deal of help in the compilation of data and the writing of the book.

MORRIS FISHBEIN, M.D.

Chicago
May, 1947

Contents

THE FOUNDER OF
THE AMERICAN MEDICAL ASSOCIATION
By Nathan Smith Davis III, M.D.

NATHAN SMITH DAVIS, M.D., A.M., LL.D.   3

THE HISTORY OF
THE AMERICAN MEDICAL ASSOCIATION
By Morris Fishbein, M.D.

THE ORGANIZATION IS CONCEIVED	19
THE ORGANIZATION OF THE AMERICAN MEDICAL ASSOCIATION	27
A PERMANENT NATIONAL ASSOCIATION	30
THE PRINCIPLES OF MEDICAL ETHICS	35
THE FIRST ANNUAL SESSION	41
THE YEARS 1849 TO 1852	48
THE END OF THE FIRST DECADE	58
THE CIVIL WAR LOOMS	66
MEDICAL PROGRESS	71
GROWING PAINS, 1875 TO 1879	90
THE JOURNAL IS BORN	100
THE JOURNAL GAINS	119
CONFUSION AND STRIFE, 1890 TO 1894	142
THE PERMANENT SECRETARY RETIRES	167
THE REORGANIZATION, 1900 TO 1901	197
BY LEAPS AND BOUNDS, 1902 TO 1904	214
DEVELOPMENT OF THE COUNCILS	234

The Medical Trust and Oligarchy	260
The War—1915 to 1919	285
Changing Views of Sickness Insurance	318
Dr. George Henry Simmons—Editor	350
The War Against Socialized Medicine—1925 to 1929	358
Socialization Battle Intensifies—1930 to 1934	381
Compulsory Insurance and an Indictment—1935 to 1939	415
1940—New York City	452
The Century Ends	481
Dr. Olin West	493
Libel Suits of the American Medical Association	495
Indictment and Trial by the Federal Government	534

RECIPIENTS OF THE DISTINGUISHED SERVICE MEDAL
By Morris Fishbein, M.D.

Rudolph Matas, M.D.	553
James B. Herrick, M.D.	554
Chevalier Jackson, M.D.	556
James Ewing, M.D.	557
Ludvig Hektoen, M.D.	559
Elliott P. Joslin, M.D.	561
George Dock, M.D.	562
George R. Minot, M.D.	564
Anton Julius Carlson, M.D.	566

BIOGRAPHIES OF THE PRESIDENTS OF THE AMERICAN MEDICAL ASSOCIATION
By Walter L. Bierring, M.D.

The Presidents of the American Medical Association	569
Nathaniel Chapman, M.D. [first president]	573

ALEXANDER H. STEVENS, M.D. [SECOND PRESIDENT]	575
JOHN COLLINS WARREN, M.D. [THIRD PRESIDENT]	577
REUBEN DIMOND MUSSEY, M.D. [FOURTH PRESIDENT]	579
JAMES MOULTRIE, M.D. [FIFTH PRESIDENT]	581
BEVERLY R. WELLFORD, M.D. [SIXTH PRESIDENT]	583
JONATHAN KNIGHT, M.D. [SEVENTH PRESIDENT]	585
CHARLES ALEXANDER POPE, M.D. [EIGHTH PRESIDENT]	587
GEORGE BACON WOOD, M.D. [NINTH PRESIDENT]	589
ZINA PITCHER, M.D. [TENTH PRESIDENT]	591
PAUL FITZSIMMONS EVE, M.D. [ELEVENTH PRESIDENT]	593
HARVEY LINDSLY, M.D. [TWELFTH PRESIDENT]	595
HENRY MILLER, M.D. [THIRTEENTH PRESIDENT]	597
ELI IVES, M.D. [FOURTEENTH PRESIDENT]	599
ALDEN MARCH, M.D. [FIFTEENTH PRESIDENT]	601
NATHAN SMITH DAVIS, M.D. [SIXTEENTH AND SEVENTEENTH PRESIDENT]	603
DAVID HUMPHREYS STORER, M.D. [EIGHTEENTH PRESIDENT]	607
HENRY FORD ASKEW, M.D. [NINETEENTH PRESIDENT]	609
SAMUEL DAVID GROSS, M.D. [TWENTIETH PRESIDENT]	610
WILLIAM OWEN BALDWIN, M.D. [TWENTY-FIRST PRESIDENT]	614
GEORGE MENDENHALL, M.D. [TWENTY-SECOND PRESIDENT]	616
ALFRED STILLÉ, M.D. [TWENTY-THIRD PRESIDENT]	617
DAVID W. YANDELL, M.D. [TWENTY-FOURTH PRESIDENT]	619
THOMAS M. LOGAN, M.D. [TWENTY-FIFTH PRESIDENT]	621
JOSEPH MEREDITH TONER, M.D. [TWENTY-SIXTH PRESIDENT]	623
WILLIAM K. BOWLING, M.D. [TWENTY-SEVENTH PRESIDENT]	625
JAMES MARION SIMS, M.D. [TWENTY-EIGHTH PRESIDENT]	627
HENRY I. BOWDITCH, M.D. [TWENTY-NINTH PRESIDENT]	630
TOBIAS G. RICHARDSON, M.D. [THIRTIETH PRESIDENT]	632
THEOPHILUS PARVIN, M.D. [THIRTY-FIRST PRESIDENT]	634

Lewis Albert Sayre, M.D. [thirty-second president]	636
John Thompson Hodgen, M.D. [thirty-third president]	638
Joseph J. Woodward, M.D. [thirty-fourth president]	639
John Light Atlee, M.D. [thirty-fifth president]	641
Austin Flint, M.D. [thirty-sixth president]	643
Henry F. Campbell, M.D. [thirty-seventh president]	646
William Brodie, M.D. [thirty-eighth president]	648
Elisha Hall Gregory, M.D. [thirty-ninth president]	650
A. Y. P. Garnett, M.D. [fortieth president]	651
William Wirt Dawson, M.D. [forty-first president]	653
Edward Mott Moore, M.D. [forty-second president]	655
William T. Briggs, M.D. [forty-third president]	657
Henry O. Marcy, M.D. [forty-fourth president]	658
Hunter H. McGuire, M.D. [forty-fifth president]	660
James F. Hibberd, M.D. [forty-sixth president]	663
Donald MacLean, M.D. [forty-seventh president]	665
Richard Beverly Cole, M.D. [forty-eighth president]	668
Nicholas Senn, M.D. [forty-ninth president]	670
George M. Sternberg, M.D. [fiftieth president]	674
Joseph M. Mathews, M.D. [fifty-first president]	677
William W. Keen, M.D. [fifty-second president]	679
Charles Alfred Reed, M.D. [fifty-third president]	683
John Allen Wyeth, M.D. [fifty-fourth president]	685
Frank Billings, M.D. [fifty-fifth president]	688
John Herr Musser, M.D. [fifty-sixth president]	692
Lewis S. McMurtry, M.D. [fifty-seventh president]	695
William James Mayo, M.D. [fifty-eighth president]	697
Joseph Decatur Bryant, M.D. [fifty-ninth president]	702
Herbert L. Burrell, M.D. [sixtieth president]	704

WILLIAM C. GORGAS, M.D. [SIXTY-FIRST PRESIDENT]	707
WILLIAM HENRY WELCH, M.D. [SIXTY-SECOND PRESIDENT]	712
JOHN B. MURPHY, M.D. [SIXTY-THIRD PRESIDENT]	717
ABRAHAM JACOBI, M.D. [SIXTY-FOURTH PRESIDENT]	721
JOHN A. WITHERSPOON, M.D. [SIXTY-FIFTH PRESIDENT]	724
VICTOR C. VAUGHAN, M.D. [SIXTY-SIXTH PRESIDENT]	726
WILLIAM L. RODMAN, M.D. [SIXTY-SEVENTH PRESIDENT]	730
ALBERT VANDER VEER, M.D. [SIXTY-EIGHTH PRESIDENT]	733
RUPERT BLUE, M.D. [SIXTY-NINTH PRESIDENT]	735
CHARLES HORACE MAYO, M.D. [SEVENTIETH PRESIDENT]	738
ARTHUR DEAN BEVAN, M.D. [SEVENTY-FIRST PRESIDENT]	741
ALEXANDER LAMBERT, M.D. [SEVENTY-SECOND PRESIDENT]	744
WILLIAM C. BRAISTED, M.D. [SEVENTY-THIRD PRESIDENT]	748
HUBERT WORK, M.D. [SEVENTY-FOURTH PRESIDENT]	751
GEORGE E. DE SCHWEINITZ, M.D. [SEVENTY-FIFTH PRESIDENT]	754
RAY LYMAN WILBUR, M.D. [SEVENTY-SIXTH PRESIDENT]	758
WILLIAM ALLEN PUSEY, M.D. [SEVENTY-SEVENTH PRESIDENT]	762
WILLIAM D. HAGGARD, M.D. [SEVENTY-EIGHTH PRESIDENT]	766
WENDELL C. PHILLIPS, M.D. [SEVENTY-NINTH PRESIDENT]	769
JABEZ NORTH JACKSON, M.D. [EIGHTIETH PRESIDENT]	772
WILLIAM S. THAYER, M.D. [EIGHTY-FIRST PRESIDENT]	774
MALCOLM L. HARRIS, M.D. [EIGHTY-SECOND PRESIDENT]	778
WILLIAM G. MORGAN, M.D. [EIGHTY-THIRD PRESIDENT]	780
EDWARD STARR JUDD, M.D. [EIGHTY-FOURTH PRESIDENT]	782
EDWARD HENRY CARY, M.D. [EIGHTY-FIFTH PRESIDENT]	785
DEAN DEWITT LEWIS, M.D. [EIGHTY-SIXTH PRESIDENT]	788
WALTER L. BIERRING, M.D. [EIGHTY-SEVENTH PRESIDENT]	792
JAMES S. MCLESTER, M.D. [EIGHTY-EIGHTH PRESIDENT]	796
JAMES TATE MASON, M.D. [EIGHTY-NINTH PRESIDENT]	799

Charles Gordon Heyd, M.D. [ninetieth president]	801
John H. J. Upham, M.D. [ninety-first president]	803
Irvin Abell, M.D. [ninety-second president]	805
Rock Sleyster, M.D. [ninety-third president]	808
Nathan B. VanEtten, M.D. [ninety-fourth president]	810
Frank Howard Lahey, M.D. [ninety-fifth president]	813
Fred Wharton Rankin, M.D. [ninety-sixth president]	816
James Edgar Paullin, M.D. [ninety-seventh president]	819
Herman L. Kretschmer, M.D. [ninety-eighth president]	822
Roger Irving Lee, M.D. [ninety-ninth president]	824
Harrison H. Shoulders, M.D. [one hundredth president]	827
Edward L. Bortz, M.D. [hundred and first president]	829

COUNCILS AND BUREAUS OF THE AMERICAN MEDICAL ASSOCIATION

By Various Authors

The Board of Trustees *By Ernest E. Irons, M.D.*	833
Office of The Treasurer *By Josiah J. Moore, M.D.*	846
The Home of the American Medical Association *By Morris Fishbein, M.D.*	860
The Council on Pharmacy and Chemistry *By Austin Smith, M.D.*	865
The Council on Medical Education and Hospitals *By Victor Johnson, M.D., Ph.D.*	887
The Council on Physical Medicine *By Howard A. Carter*	923
The Council on Foods and Nutrition *By J. R. Wilson, M.D.*	936
The Judicial Council *By Morris Fishbein, M.D.*	948

THE COUNCIL ON INDUSTRIAL HEALTH *By Carl M. Peterson, M.D.*	961
THE COUNCIL ON MEDICAL SERVICE *By Louis H. Bauer, M.D., and George Cooley*	967
THE BUSINESS DEPARTMENT *By Thomas R. Gardiner*	979
THE BUREAU OF HEALTH EDUCATION *By W. W. Bauer, M.D., Sylvia B. Martin, and Audrey McKeever*	996
THE BUREAU OF LEGAL MEDICINE AND LEGISLATION *By J. W. Holloway, Jr.*	1010
THE BUREAU OF INVESTIGATION *By Bliss O. Halling*	1034
THE BUREAU OF INFORMATION *By M. Virginia Shuler*	1039
THE BUREAU OF EXHIBITS *By Thomas G. Hull, Ph.D.*	1042
THE BUREAU OF MEDICAL ECONOMICS *By Frank G. Dickinson, Ph.D.*	1064
THE LIBRARY OF THE AMERICAN MEDICAL ASSOCIATION *By Marjorie H. Moore*	1069
THE COMMITTEE ON SCIENTIFIC RESEARCH *By Ludvig Hektoen, M.D.*	1085
SCIENTIFIC SECTIONS OF THE AMERICAN MEDICAL ASSOCIATION *By Morris Fishbein, M.D.*	1092
WOMAN'S AUXILIARY TO THE AMERICAN MEDICAL ASSOCIATION *By Mrs. Jesse D. Hamer*	1099

PUBLICATIONS OF
THE AMERICAN MEDICAL ASSOCIATION
By Various Authors

THE ARCHIVES OF INTERNAL MEDICINE *By N. C. Gilbert, M.D.*	1111
THE AMERICAN JOURNAL OF DISEASES OF CHILDREN *By Clifford G. Grulee, M.D.*	1118
THE ARCHIVES OF OTOLARYNGOLOGY *By George M. Coates, M.D.*	1129

THE ARCHIVES OF DERMATOLOGY AND SYPHILOLOGY *By Howard Fox, M.D.*	1138
THE ARCHIVES OF NEUROLOGY AND PSYCHIATRY *By Louis Casamajor, M.D.*	1149
THE ARCHIVES OF SURGERY *By Waltman Walters, M.D., and Morris Fishbein, M.D.*	1154
THE ARCHIVES OF OPHTHALMOLOGY *By Francis H. Adler, M.D.*	1160
THE ARCHIVES OF PATHOLOGY *By Ludvig Hektoen, M.D.*	1164
THE QUARTERLY CUMULATIVE INDEX MEDICUS *By Marjorie H. Moore*	1165
THE AMERICAN MEDICAL DIRECTORY *By Frank V. Cargill*	1170
WAR MEDICINE *By Morris Fishbein, M.D.*	1180
OCCUPATIONAL MEDICINE *By Morris Fishbein, M.D.*	1183
HYGEIA, THE HEALTH MAGAZINE *By Morris Fishbein, M.D.*	1184

APPENDICES

SESSIONS AND PRESIDENTS OF THE ASSOCIATION	1189
MEMBERS OF THE BOARD OF TRUSTEES	1192
MEMBERSHIP OF THE COUNCIL ON MEDICAL EDUCATION AND HOSPITALS SINCE THE ORIGIN OF THE COUNCIL	1195
DATES IN THE HISTORY OF THE COUNCIL ON MEDICAL EDUCATION AND HOSPITALS	1198
SESSIONS AND ATTENDANCE OF THE ASSOCIATION	1200
MEMBERS OF THE JUDICIAL COUNCIL	1202

INDICES

INDEX OF PERSONS	1209
INDEX OF SUBJECTS	1219

Founder of the American Medical Association

Nathan Smith Davis, M.D.

1817-1904

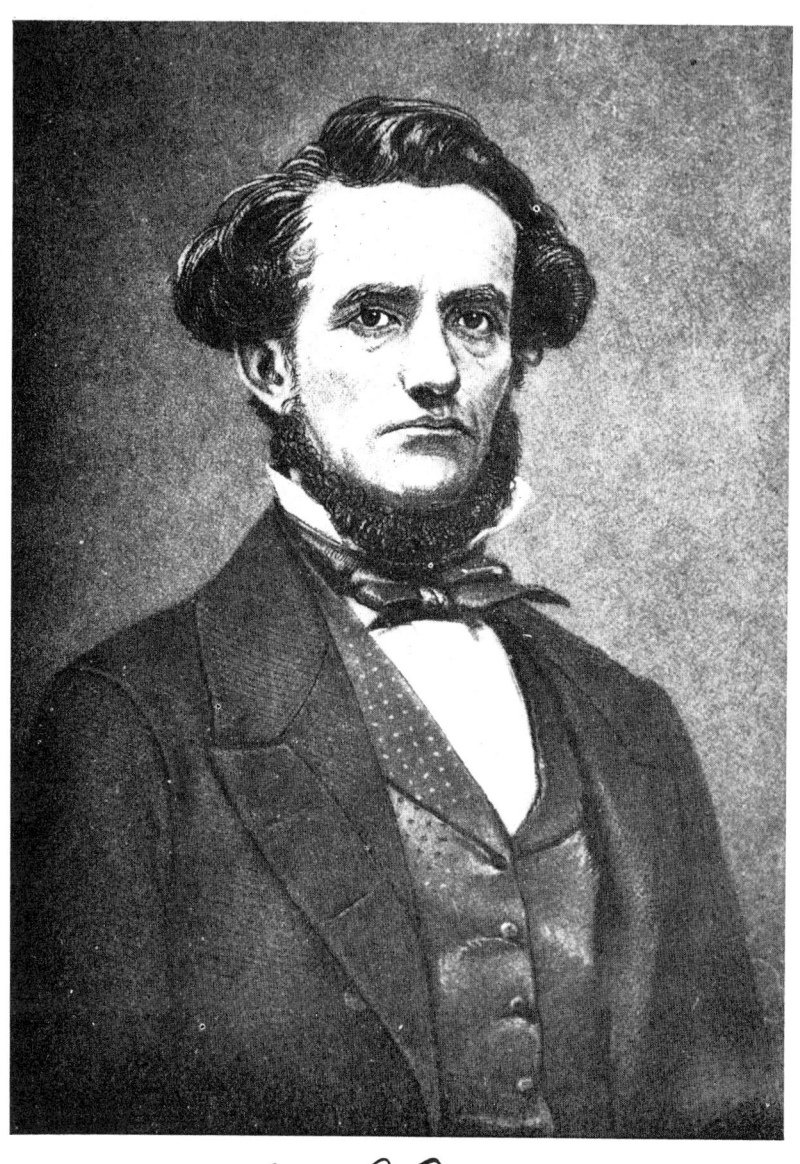

NATHAN SMITH DAVIS, M.D., A.M., LL.D.

By Nathan Smith Davis III, M.D.

IN THE SPRING OF 1833 while Nathan Smith Davis and his older brother, Stephen, were helping their father, Dow Davis, repair a rail fence, Dr. Daniel Clark of Smithville Flats, Chenango County, New York, rode by on horseback. In passing he asked if the farmer was going to make a "pill-peddler" of young Nathan. Dow Davis replied that the boy would make as good a "tin-peddler" as anything.

Apparently the family doctor knew that the sixteen year old boy had a desire for learning and an interest in natural philosophy; knew that during the previous winter, Nathan had walked two miles to and from the school in the neighboring district that he might study English grammar and natural philosophy in addition to the subjects taught in the school of his district. Possibly the doctor had loaned him the books he had been punished for reading when he should have been working on the farm.

The suggestion that he study medicine thrilled Nathan though his father's reply had been far from encouraging. Months went by during which he heard no mention of the subject. He was taken completely by surprise when, early that autumn, his father offered him his choice between remaining at home till he was ready to buy a farm and attending one six month's term at Cazenovia Seminary before commencing the study of medicine under the preceptorship of Dr. Clark. Dow Davis also agreed to help Nathan in the purchase of the farm or to give him one hundred dollars a year while he was studying medicine. Of his choice, N. S. Davis later wrote: "Of course my anxiety for better education caused me promptly to choose the latter, while the conversation showed plainly that the doctor's remark about making a 'pill-peddler' of me had been engaging his (father's) attention all summer."

Nathan Smith Davis was born January 9, 1817 in a log cabin on the farm near Greene, Chenango County, New York, which had been homesteaded and partially cleared of its original forest by his father, Dow Davis, an orphan, who had when in his early teens, run away from the cobbler to whom he had been indentured. He worked his way out to Chenango County, where he caught up with a young man he had known before named Nathan Smith who had homesteaded there and persuaded his father, Blodgett Smith, to move the rest of the family to an adjoining homestead, and start the town of Smithville Flats. Dow Davis took up a homestead in the neighboring town of Greene and married Eleanore Smith after whose favorite brother they named the youngest of their seven children— four daughters and three sons. Nathan was only seven years old when his mother died so she could not share his elation over the offer which made it possible for him to study medicine.

While at Cazenovia Seminary for the 1833-34 term, Nathan studied English grammar, chemistry, natural philosophy, algebra and Latin. The following summer he commenced the study of medicine under Dr. Clark. In return for his help in the office and in caring for the horses and doing the chores, his preceptor gave him room and board.

While the doctor was away riding horseback for long distances to visit patients, his bride frequently stayed with her parents and neglected to provide for the young student's meals. Impressed by the lack of variety and inadequacy of his diet, for one week he listed all that he had been given to eat and left the memorandum under a cap on the table in his attic room when he left to spend Sunday with his father. Dr. and Mrs. Clark inspected his room while he was away, and found the memo which caused them so much chagrin that they insisted he board elsewhere.

That he might not have to spend any of his allowance for board in Smithville Flats, he obtained permission to return home to make preparations for going to Fairfield, Herkimer County, N.Y. to attend the College of Physicians and Surgeons of Western New York. This incident was probably responsible for his changing preceptors. After his first term at Fairfield, his studies were continued under the direction of Dr. Thomas Jackson of Binghamton until he graduated on January 31, 1837.

Of his life during the three courses of lectures he attended at the Medical College of Western New York, Nathan Smith Davis later wrote: "My supply of money from home being limited, I, like many others, boarded myself, while in college, living very cheaply on roast potatoes, pudding, and milk, etc., by which I was not only able to pay my way, but saved enough to buy me a small library of books and a pocket case of instruments to commence practice with." His thesis on "Animal Temperature" in which he attempted to disprove the then prevailing doctrine concerning the union of oxygen and carbon in the lungs, was one of four read at the graduating exercises.

The following statement listing Dow Davis' contributions to his son's medical education and establishment in practice is copied from notes written and signed by Dr. Davis that were found among his papers:

N. S. DAVIS TO DOW DAVIS, DR.

1833—To board, tuition, books, etc. at Cazenovia Seminary	$ 56.07
1834—Board, clothes, books, etc. in Clark's office	33.30
Expenses to Fairfield Medical College, cash	98.38
1835—To board, tuition, clothes, etc. in Jackson's office Binghamton	84.54
To expenses at Fairfield Medical College, cash	78.82
1836—To board, clothes, books, etc. in Jackson's office	88.11
Expenses at Fairfield Medical College, Diploma, etc.	118.43
1837—To clothes, cutter, harness, saddle, horse, etc., etc. at Greene	181.42
To cash on starting to Vienna	60.00
To cash since I came to Binghamton twice	80.00
Total amount since leaving home	$879.07
Namely	
Cash $450.00	
Board, horse, clothes, etc. 429.07	

The above bill is acknowledged true and right by me.

Signed: N. S. DAVIS

Binghamton, March 3rd, 1846

While the College of Physicians and Surgeons of Western New York at Fairfield had a short life, its faculty included such well known teachers as T. Romeyn Beck, James McNaughton, John Delameter, R. D. Mussey, James Wadley and Westel Willoughby. Asked to suggest a successor for Dr. Daniel Chatfield of Vienna, New York, who was planning to retire because of ill health, the faculty recommended Dr. Davis who accepted the offer.

After a short visit with his family in Greene, Dr. N. S. Davis proceeded to Vienna and arranged to take over the practice of Dr. Chatfield and for the purchase of his property. However he soon became dissatisfied with practice in this remote town, "half agricultural and half lumber with one mail a week." "Hence," to quote Dr. Davis, "as soon as Dr. Chatfield returned with improved health, I left, which was in the latter part of July, having made a residence of only five months. My wish was then to migrate to the valley of the Mississippi, but the want of pecuniary means, even for traveling expenses, compelled me to stop in Binghamton, where I continued to practice for nearly ten years."

Here is the place to cite the first entries in his note book: "July 27th, 1837—Rented an office in the Village of Binghamton and commenced the practice of medicine, being twenty years old the January preceding on the ninth day—having graduated the winter previous at the Western Medical College of New York at Fairfield, Herkimer County.

1837—Debit			Credit
July 28th	Office Furniture, sign, etc.	$6.30	$
Aug. 29th	Postage, paper, etc.	1.21	2.59
Sep. 30th	Postage, surgical instruments, etc.	3.80	4.12
Oct. 31st	Medical Journal, stove, wood, etc.	9.91	4.25
Nov. 30th	Postage, paper, books, etc.	5.60	13.00
Dec. 30th	Postage, toll, books, etc.	2.87	15.00
		$29.69	$38.96

His short stay in Vienna was most important; while there he met Miss Anna Maria Parker, daughter of the Hon. John Parker, who was one of its leading citizens. Dr. Davis was twenty one and Miss Parker seventeen when they were married on March 5, 1838. She shared the "joys and sorrows" of his long career and died in 1908 four years after he did.

Doctor Davis joined the Broome County Medical Society Sept. 12, 1837, and for ten years was one of its most active members. While in Binghamton, he wrote articles for various medical journals with two of which he won the 1840 and 1841 essay contests of the New York State Medical Society; studied the medical botany and topography of the region; helped teach medical students by making chemical analyses and private dissections, both in human and comparative anatomy; continued the study of Latin and English; helped edit a local popular periodical; was active in a debating society and lectured at the Binghamton Academy of which he was a founder.

These activities prepared him for the important part he took in the deliberations of the New York State Medical Society when he was first seated as a delegate in 1844. He introduced one of several resolutions on medical education and licensure; was a member of the committee to which they were referred; and was elected chairman of the Committee of Correspondence for the Sixth Senatorial District. The next year Dr. Davis and Dr. M. H. Cash of Orange County introduced resolutions on medical education and licensure which expressed the views of their authors, who did not agree. The lively discussion which followed made it clear that it would be impractical for one state to try to raise standards. When it appeared that no action would be taken, Dr. Alden March privately suggested to Dr. Davis that this objection might be overcome by calling a National Medical Convention and persuading the delegates from medical colleges and institutions of the several states to act in concert. Davis of Broome County immediately introduced the following preamble and resolutions:

"Whereas, it is believed that a National Convention would be conducive to the elevation of the standard of medical education in the United States; and Whereas, there is no mode of accomplishing so desirable an object without concert of action on the part of the medical colleges, societies and institutions of all the states, therefore

"Resolved that the New York State Medical Society earnestly recommends a National Convention of delegates from medical societies and colleges of the whole Union, to convene in the City of New York, on the first Tuesday in May, in the year 1846, for the purpose of adopting some concerted action on the subject set forth in the preamble.

"Resolved, that a committee of three be appointed to carry the foregoing resolutions into effect."

Dr. Davis replied to those who considered the project "impracticable if not Utopian" because attempts to assemble a National Medical Convention had failed in 1835 and 1839, that the objectives were so important that efforts should be continued even though there were a dozen failures. The resolutions were approved and Dr. N. S. Davis of Broome County, was named chairman, Dr. James McNaughton of Albany and Dr. Peter Van Buren, Secretary of the New York State Medical Society, members of the Committee to carry them into effect. The National Medical Convention held in New York in May, 1846, proved that this twenty-nine-year-old country practitioner not only had the vision to propose such a meeting but also the ability to make it an accomplished fact.

His experience as chairman of the committee which called the meeting that led to the formation of the American Medical Association seems to have convinced the ambitious young doctor that to effectively carry on the work he had started he must move to a medical center; become a member of the faculty of a medical school; engage in research; and be connected with a medical periodical which could be used to further his objectives. Therefore in the spring of 1847, Dr. and Mrs. Davis and their daughter, Ellen Parker Davis (born in 1839), moved to New York City.

The following winter he served as Demonstrator of Anatomy in charge of the dissecting rooms and instructor in practical anatomy at the College of Physicians and Surgeons. In the spring of 1848, this thirty one year old doctor was invited to give the course in medical jurisprudence, a subject usually taught by one many years his senior. That summer his "Text Book of Agriculture" which had received an award from the New York State Agricultural Society, was published. Soon after he moved to New York City, he became assistant editor of a semi-monthly medical journal, "The Annalist," and, late in 1848, its editor and publisher.

When the National Medical Convention reconvened in the Academy of Natural Sciences of Philadelphia on May 5, 1847 to hear the reports of committees appointed at the New York meeting, almost two hundred fifty delegates from forty medical societies and twenty eight medical colleges in twenty eight states, assembled. Dr. Davis played an important part in the preparation of the report of the committee to prepare a plan for a permanent national medical society. The committee recommended the organization of a society to be called the American Medical Association, the members of which were to be delegates from state, county and local medical societies and institutions and from medical colleges. Dr. Davis' ability as a debater; his lucid statements in support of the report and in opposition especially to an amendment providing that its membership should be composed of individuals elected by the society, were largely responsible for the organization of the American Medical Association at that meeting. It approved the reports of other committees except that it referred the majority and minority reports of the committee on licensure to its Committee on Medical Education for report at the next meeting of the Association.

Dr. Davis attended forty-seven of the Association's first fifty meetings and was an "untiring, irrepressible, uncompromising and incorruptible" leader in its campaigns to elevate the standards of medical education, licensure and public health; to maintain its high ethical standards; to oppose charlatanism; to promote clinical and scientific investigation; to make available a better quality of medical service; and to establish the American Medical Association as the recognized representative organization of the medical profession of the United States.

In 1848, Dr. Davis, as chairman of the Committee on Indigenous Medical Botany stated that its purpose was the determination of the real value and actions of native plants reputed to possess medicinal properties and not, as some seemed to think, the mere listing of such plants.

In the summer of 1849, he accepted the offer of the chair of Physiology and Pathology at Rush Medical College which had added this professorship to comply with one of the recommendations of the Association. In mid August, he with his wife, daughter, Ellen, and son Frank Howard Davis (born in 1848) started on the long trek by train, barge, lake boat and stage coach, to Chicago and the Mid-West which had long attracted him. Having stopped to visit relatives in Vienna, Greene and East Bloomfield, they did not arrive in Chicago until September 12th.

Of Chicago, Dr. Davis wrote in March 1852 to Dr. S. H. French of Binghamton: "When I came here I found much to be done. We had a city of thirty thousand inhabitants, without a hospital for the sick, or an organized society to look after the poor, and without any medical society or organization whatever," and no general sewage system or water supply.

He certainly did not delay about doing something to correct this situation for in the spring of 1850 local and state medical societies were organized and that fall the Illinois General Hospital of the Great Lakes (now Mercy Hospital) was opened. Before his letter to Dr. French was written, his proposal for a general sewage system had been approved and a society for the care of the poor formed.

At the meeting of the Association in Charleston, S. C. in 1851, Dr. Davis made his most important contribution to medical science, in a paper entitled "An experimental inquiry concerning some points connected with the processes of assimilation and nutrition." This presentation which included analyses of blood entering and leaving the kidneys, gave experimental evidence which proved that alcohol lowered body temperature. This idea was so novel that the paper was not accepted for publication in the Transactions. It appeared in the Northwestern Medical and Surgical Journal which he was editing for the Rush Faculty, in which his "History of the Medical Profession, from the first settlement of the British Colonies in America to the year 1850" had appeared as a serial prior to its publication in book form in 1851.

In 1854, N. S. Davis of Illinois was elected a vice president of the Association. In a paper "On the nutritive qualities of milk, etc." presented at that meeting, he asked: "Is there not some mode by which the nutritive constituents of milk can be preserved in their purity and sweetness, and furnished to the inhabitants of cities in such quantities as to supersede the present defective and unwholesome methods of supply?" The proposal of a committee to study this problem plus that made in 1848 for one to determine the real value of indigenous plants as remedial agents may well have initiated the movement that resulted in the formation of some of the Association's Councils and in the passage of our pure food and drug laws.

His History of the American Medical Association was published in 1855. An unfinished and unpublished manuscript in Dr. Davis' handwriting continuing its history through 1869 has also been used in the preparation of this biographical sketch.

The recommendations of the Association adopted in 1847 and confirmed at many subsequent meetings had caused many schools to increase the number of professorships and some to lengthen the school term. None had had the temerity to comply with those concerning preliminary education and the grading of the curriculum. In 1858, Dr. Davis finally persuaded the Rush Faculty to approve the adoption of these changes only to have the action vetoed by the Dean, Dr. Daniel Brainard, on his return from a trip to Europe. Several of his supporters thereupon resigned from the Rush Faculty and invited Dr. Davis to join them in the founding of a new medical school, the Medical Department of Lind University (which in 1862 became the Chicago Medical College and in 1892, the Northwestern University Medical School) which, from its inception in the autumn of 1859, "boldly adopted and enforced" all of the Association's recommendations except those pertaining to preliminary education. It had raised its entrance requirements and lengthened its course to three years by 1872 when President Charles William Eliot persuaded the Harvard Medical School Faculty to adopt such a program and made that school the first to become an integral part of a University. This move by the second oldest medical school in the United States was all that was needed to start a rush by other schools to adopt the reforms though a few, among them Rush, held out for another ten or fifteen years.

The meeting of the A. M. A. planned for Chicago in 1861 was postponed because of the Civil War. In 1863, it was decided that a meeting could not again be postponed. The meeting was held in Chicago with Dr. Davis serving as chairman of the Committee on Arrangements. The Association met again in 1864 in New York. N. S. Davis of Illinois was elected President and inducted into office at its opening session.

In 1854, Dr. S. D. Gross had suggested amending the Constitution of the Association to provide for the election of officers at the end instead of at the beginning of the meetings. Dr. Davis had supported such a change when in 1858 he suggested restricting the business of the Association to the morning sessions that those in the afternoon might be used exclusively for the presentation of scientific papers and in 1859 when amendments providing for section meetings were passed. However, the changes in the Constitution providing that the newly elected officers should not assume their duties until the end of the meeting at which they were elected, were not passed until after Dr. Davis had assumed his duties as President and was presiding at the New York meeting. This resulted in his serving as President and presiding officer at both the 1864 and 1865 meetings of the Association.

Charges of disloyalty made by opponents of the changes he advocated and by enemies made by cryptic comments he had made in editorials and communications appearing in the medical press came out into the open in 1864 but were completely disproven and in no way interfered with the success of the Boston meeting in '65.

In 1867 as a member of an A. M. A. committee which called a meeting of medical college delegates, he was active in the organization of the Association of Medical Colleges and in 1869 was elected first President of the Association of Medical Editors.

At the A. M. A. meeting in 1872, Dr. Davis introduced resolutions, which were adopted, providing for the creation of the Judicial Council. He served as a member for several years during which it rendered a number of important decisions including one recommending that the delegates from the New York State Medical Society should not be seated because that Society had repudiated the Association's Code of Ethics.

The bronze medal in his honor, authorized at the Detroit meeting in 1874, was never distributed as widely as the resolutions provided and they are now quite rare. This medal was used as a model for the present Distinguished Service Medal of the Association.

His son, Frank Howard Davis, took two years of college work at the University of Michigan before entering the Chicago Medical College from which he graduated in 1872 to become his father's assistant. In 1874 he edited the second edition of his father's "Clinical Lectures on Various Important Diseases" originally published in 1873. After Dr. Frank's return from a year of study in Austria and Germany, Dr. Davis decided to take things more easily and in 1876 moved to suburban Evanston to live though he continued to practice in Chicago. This move made it possible for his younger son, Nathan Smith Davis, Jr. (born 1858), to live at home during his undergraduate days at Northwestern University from which he received an A. B. degree in 1880 and an A. M., in 1883 when he received his M. D. degree from the Chicago Medical College.

Dr. Frank Howard Davis was secretary of the Chicago Medical Society and was becoming known as a specialist in diseases of the chest when, in 1880, a urinary tract infection secondary to a traumatic perineal abscess caused his untimely death. He left a widow, a son and a daughter and a second son was born shortly after his death.

This death of his assistant made it necessary for Dr. Davis to return to Chicago to live. It also was responsible for N. S. Davis, Jr.'s decision to give up the study of biology and enter the Chicago Medical College. The early 80's were sad ones for Dr. and Mrs. Davis. In 1882, their daughter died, as did her six year old daughter. A year later her husband, Francis Henry Kales, a leading Chicago attorney, died. Dr. and Mrs. Davis made room in their home for the six orphaned grandchildren whom they brought up with the help of their son, N. S. Davis, Jr.

Extemporaneous speeches made at the 1881 and 1882 meetings of the A. M. A. are reported by those present to have demonstrated that Dr. Davis was a most accomplished orator whose command of the English language and resonant voice made it easy for him to sway his audience. In 1881 his eloquent remarks were in opposition to changes that had been proposed in the Code of Ethics. In 1882, he eloquently supported the recommendations of the committee which proposed the publication of a weekly journal in place of the annual transactions and approved of the amendments to the Constitution it outlined as necessary if the report should be approved, but he berated its members for not including resolutions to effectuate these changes. It is said that one member of the committee after another retired rather shamefacedly from the platform while he was speaking. He introduced resolutions to put into effect the recommendations of the committee. They were passed and he was elected a member of the Board of Trustees which they created, instructed to select an Editor and to proceed to publish a weekly periodical to be named THE JOURNAL OF THE AMERICAN MEDICAL ASSOCIATION.

Late in 1882, Dr. Davis resigned as Trustee to become, at 65, the first Editor of The Journal of the Association he had founded when 30 years old. The prospectus which he issued January 25, 1883 brought a satisfactory response. Volume I, No. 1 of THE JOURNAL appeared under date of July 14, 1883. THE JOURNAL was firmly established; was being printed by the Association; had a steadily increasing circulation; and was recognized as one of the leading medical periodicals of the nation when he resigned as Editor in 1888.

The first edition of his "Principles and Practice of Medicine" which appeared in 1884, was well received so that a second edition was required in 1886. This work was based on a stenographic report of his lectures at the Chicago Medical College which were famous because of the graphic descriptions of disease which he gave.

At the 1884 meeting of the A. M. A., Dr. Austin Flint, its President, was made chairman of a committee to invite the International Medical Congress to meet in Washington in 1887. The invitation was accepted. The committee, in accordance with the resolutions creating it, thereupon became a Committee on Arrangements for the Congress; increased its membership and started to work. It was severely criticized for some of its actions when the Association met in New Orleans in 1885. This resulted in a complete reorganization of the committee to give it one member from each state, territory and the District of Columbia and one each from the Army and Navy Medical Departments and the Marine Hospital Service, and made it necessary for the original committee of eight to drop the fifteen members it had added.

Dr. Davis, as Editor of the J. A. M. A. defended the Association in the acrimonious dispute which followed this action and might have made it impossible to hold the Congress. Thanks to the efforts of a few level-headed men who were determined it must be held, peace was restored. The new committee met on September 3, 1885 and nominated Austin Flint, M.D., LL.D., for President and N. S. Davis, M.D., LL.D. for Secretary-General of the Congress and continued to make arrangements for the Congress.

In January 1886, Dr. Davis had an almost complete but fortunately transient right hemiplegia following a cerebral thrombosis. He had made a complete recovery and was resuming his regular work when Dr. Flint had a cerebral hemorrhage which caused his death on March 13, 1886.

The promotion of Dr. Davis to the Presidency and nomination of John B. Hamilton as Secretary-General was approved at the A.M.A. meeting in St. Louis a few weeks later. The following August, Dr. Davis went to England as a member of a committee to invite the members of the British Medical Association meeting at Brighton, to attend the International Medical Congress of 1887. At a reception in honor of the A.M.A. delegates, he extended the invitation which was most cordially accepted by many of the most eminent physicians and surgeons of the United Kingdom.

The success of the Congress and the manner in which he presided over its sessions in Washington gave him an international reputation. When he made his second and last Trans-Atlantic trip in 1888, he again did not visit the Continent. As a private physician accompanied by a grand-daughter, he attended the Glasgow meeting of the British Medical Association and received much attention from the leaders of the British and Scotch professions.

His resignation that year after five years of service, as Editor of the J.A.M.A., marked the first step in the "Old Doctor's" second attempt to withdraw from active life. The "Young Doctor," N. S. Davis, Jr., was able to take over most of his practice though he regularly went to his office until his terminal illness. He continued his teaching program until 1892 when he became Emeritus Professor but gave the lectures on medical history at the Northwestern University Medical School through 1897 and did not become Emeritus Dean until 1898. He edited some temperance periodicals and wrote numerous articles for the medical and lay press and in 1903 published his History of Medicine, and regularly attended the meetings of the Association until he was eighty years old.

In 1890, Dr. Davis gave the annual address on "Practical Medicine" at the meeting of the Association and in 1896 at its meeting to celebrate the centennial of vaccination delivered "an address on the character of Dr. Edward Jenner and the history of his discovery of the protective value of vaccination."

In 1897 he was the only one of the four survivors of the 1847 meeting in Philadelphia at which the American Medical Association had been born, who was able to be present when it returned to celebrate its fiftieth birthday at what was called its "Jubilee Meeting." It marked the high point of his long and distinguished career. When the tumultuous applause which greeted his appearance on the platform subsided, President Nicholas Senn said: "Dr. Davis, in the name of nine thousand members of the Association I greet you and congratulate you that you have been permitted to live long enough to witness commemoration exercises of your life work, the fiftieth anniversary of your favorite child—THE AMERICAN MEDICAL ASSOCIATION."

"The ever-young man" who was eighty years old then delivered in a voice that all could hear, "A brief history of the origin of the American Medical Association, the principles on which it was organized, the object it was designated to accomplish, and how far they have been attained during the half century of its existence." The designated objectives had been attained but fortunately the principles on which it was organized set goals that can never be attained, and a virile, progressive and "ever-young" American Medical Association will in 1947 celebrate its centennial and start its second century by continuing its efforts to approach as closely as is possible to the goals set by its founders.

In 1900 he was able to contribute to the semicentennial celebrations of the Chicago and Illinois State Medical Societies, both of which were organized with his assistance. Neither of these celebrations nor the Testimonial Banquet of October 5, 1901, given in his honor under the auspices of the Chicago Medical Society could eclipse his triumph at the "Jubilee Meeting."

On June 4, 1904, after walking home from a busy day at the office, as the "young doctor" was in the East attending medical meetings, Dr. Davis had a heart attack. His grandson, John Davis Kales, M.D., who attended him until my father returned, told me that the attack was characterized by precordial pain which required chloroform and morphine for its relief, orthopnea, Cheyne-Stokes respiration, increasing weakness and on June 16 another attack of angina preceded his death. Dr. Kales felt certain that "Papa Davis," as he was called by his grandchildren, died as a result of a coronary thrombosis which developed over eighteen years after he had had a cerebral thrombosis. The funeral services were held in the home on June 19th. Six grandsons, John Davis Kales, M.D., William Robert Kales, Albert Martin Kales, Francis Henry Kales, Frank Howard Davis, II and Nathan Smith Davis, III were the active pallbearers.

When he died Nathan Smith Davis was over eighty-seven years old; had practiced his profession for sixty-seven years; and had been most happily married for over sixty-six years; was renowned as a clinician and consultant, as an organizer and administrator, as editor and author, as a citizen, as an educator and as a crusader always ready and able to defend and promote what he believed to be right and to oppose what he believed to be wrong. He was a sincere member of the Methodist Church who read his Bible every morning and always said Grace before a meal and a believer in temperance. In politics he was a Democrat and always voted the straight ticket until William Jennings Bryan became its candidate. He could not support the Democratic candidate and would not vote for a Republican so in 1896 and 1900 he voted the Prohibition ticket.

Dr. Davis was known to hundreds who had only seen him walking back and forth from his office or from Grace Methodist Episcopal Church which he attended regularly. He had never given up wearing what had been the usual costume of the medical profession when he started to practice in the 1830's and always wore a high hat, a black "claw-hammer" coat similar in cut to the full dress evening coat of to-day, with a black vest and tie, and boots with his trousers outside. His keen eyes, stern expression and characteristic stride made this recognition easy. He made every one nervous for when he took a street car in bad weather, he invariably flipped on or off before the car came to a full stop despite his age of over eighty-five years.

While his grandchildren, many of whom lived in his home from 1883 on, knew his stern expression, his abrupt manner and austere appearance they could not see how his patients could be afraid of him as many of his most devoted ones were. To them "Papa Davis" was a kindly, considerate and affectionate grandfather, who always remembered their birthdays; was always interested in hearing what they had been doing; sympathetic when they were ill or had hurt themselves. They feel that this manner was put on to make it possible to see as many patients as he did day in and day out. They know that his custom of rising at six in the winter and earlier in the summer made it possible for him to work uninterruptedly for almost two hours every morning while he was fresh from eight hours of sleep. His medical reading and some of his correspondence was taken care of during the late afternoon and evening but most of his editorial work, writing and planning of clinics and lectures, was done during those early morning hours.

In spite of his small fees, he must for many years have had a good income because so many patients paid him one or two dollars for an office call; two or three for a house call; five for a delivery or a consultation. If he had not given so generously of his money as well as of his time and skill to patients and students who were in need of help to keep the Medical College of which he was Dean for thirty-five years, among the leading schools of the United States, he might have left a large estate. When he died he had some ten thousand dollars in securities, a clear title to his home, and as memorials many institutions which, like his "favorite child" the American Medical Association, still "hold unsullied the example of his high and noble career, and perpetuate his memory during the centuries to come, by imitating his glorious example of a long life given to public service."

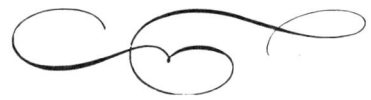

History of the American Medical Association

BY MORRIS FISHBEIN, M.D.

THE ORGANIZATION IS CONCEIVED

THE FIRST MEETING OF the American Medical Association was in May 1847 in the city of Philadelphia. The assemblage did not gather by any common impulse arising suddenly in the minds of a great number of men. The birth of the Association followed travail of many months; the pains, the jealousies and the love associated with its conception forecast the great career to be achieved by this extraordinary progeny.

A medical society was formed in New York in 1749, almost a hundred years previously. The first medical book to be published on the North American continent had been printed by the Spaniards in Mexico in 1570 and they had founded the first medical school in 1578. The only medical publication of the New England colonies in the seventeenth century was Thatcher's "Brief Rule," printed in Boston in 1677. John Shaw Billings in his notable "A Century of American Medicine" says there were at the commencement of the Revolutionary War but one medical book by an American author, three reprints and twenty pamphlets.

Before 1800 there were five good medical schools—those of the University of Pennsylvania (1765), Kings College (1764), New York, which became in 1791 the Medical Faculty of Columbia College, Harvard University (1783), the College of Philadelphia (1765) and the Medical School of Dartmouth College (1798). Small medical societies had been organized, the first in Boston in 1735 and others in New York, Philadelphia and New Haven County. State medical societies existed in New Jersey, Massachusetts, South Carolina, Delaware, New Hampshire, Connecticut and Maryland. The medical periodicals of the country were few in number and of small circulation, the first being the *Medical Repository* of New York, founded in 1797.*

---

* According to Dr. F. C. Waite:

The "New Medical Institution" the Medical Department of Rutgers College (then under the name of Queen's College) was organized in New York City in 1792. Although this suspended before 1800 it was later reorganized and continued with interruptions until 1828. It was the precursor of Geneva College which finally became the present Medical Department of Syracuse University.

Transylvania University appointed medical professors in 1799 and continued feebly

With the nineteenth century medicine began to make more progress through the development of interesting devices and new theoretical concepts. Advances made in physics and chemistry were reflected, as they are today, in medicine, but the modern scientific movement did not attain full proportions until well after the middle of the century. No doubt the discovery of anesthesia in 1846 was the most important single contribution to the advancement of medical science in those first fifty years of the nineteenth century. True, the period saw the introduction of vaccination against smallpox, the discovery of the stethoscope by Laënnec, the publication of Percival's "Code of Medical Ethics," the first ovariotomy, performed by Ephraim McDowell, the publication of the first United States Pharmacopeia (1820) and such amazing clinical contributions as Bell's description of the functions of the spinal nerve roots, Parkinson's description of paralysis agitans, Hodgkin's description of lymphadenoma, Beaumont's classic experiments on digestion, Basedow's description of toxic diffuse goiter and Oliver Wendell Holmes's essay on the contagiousness of puerperal fever. Rokitansky and Virchow had begun the fundamental studies in pathology which were to be the basis of a modern science of medicine in contrast to a century of medical art. Claude Bernard had already written a significant essay on the digestive function of the pancreas.

---

for nine years. Then after an interruption of eight years it was reorganized in 1815 and became one of the important medical colleges of the middle west up to 1851.

The correct date for Kings College is 1764 when a medical faculty was appointed. It suspended and Columbia College took its place after the war. A medical faculty was appointed in 1785 and organized with a dean, and instruction began in 1791.

Harvard Medical College dates from 1783 when instruction began. A memorandum in the archives of Harvard University signed by John Warren and Aaron Dexter says distinctly that the medical college began in 1783.

Dartmouth Medical College dates from 1797 when a medical professor was appointed. Class instruction began in 1798 and two medical degrees were conferred in course in that year.

Medical professors were appointed in 1765 in the College of Philadelphia. This institution was suspended during the war. In 1779 the charter was annuled and a new instutition organized under the name of the Medical Department of the University of the STATE OF PENNSYLVANIA. (Note the name carefully.)

The charter of the College of Philadelphia was restored in 1789 and instruction began again. In 1791 both the College of Philadelphia and the University of the State of Pennsylvania were closed and a new institution under the name of the University of Pennsylvania was chartered and began medical instruction. The University of Pennyslvania claims succession from the College of Philadelphia and dates its beginning back to 1765. It was *not* the legal successor because there were three different charters, namely: College of Philadelphia, University of the *State* of Pennsylvaia, and University of Pennsylvania. However some of the individuals that had been teaching in the two older institutions from 1789 to 1791 were included in the new University of Pennsylvania.

The Medical Department of the College of William and Mary was authorized in 1779 with only one professor and continued only two or three years.

Then came 1847. In his "History of Medicine" Fielding H. Garrison lists as the most important accomplishments of that year Helmholtz's treatise on "Conservation of Energy," the introduction by Sir James Simpson of chloroform anesthesia in obstetrics, the Semmelweis discovery of the cause of puerperal fever, the invention by Carl Ludwig of the kymograph and the founding of the Royal Academy of Sciences of Vienna and of the American Medical Association in Philadelphia.

What better source could we ask for the history of the American Medical Association from its organization up to January 1855 than Dr. Nathan Smith Davis, who, more than any other man, may be credited with being the founder of the American Medical Association? He records the incidents in his book published in 1855 in Philadelphia. At that time he said:

> Of all the voluntary social organizations in our country, none are at this time in a position to exert a wider or more permanent influence over the temporal interests of our country than the American Medical Association. This assertion may startle the mind of the professional reader and call forth a smile of incredulity, nay of contempt, from the nonprofessional; but let both patiently follow me to the end and then judge. I am aware that the details on which I am about to enter may appear to some unimportant, to others tedious and, to all of the present generation, wanting in novelty and interest; but they will appear far otherwise to those who shall come after us and live when time shall have thrown his dimming veil over all the doings of our day.

During the fifteen years between 1830 and 1845 the number of medical colleges in the United States more than doubled. There was active rivalry and competition without restraint. Because of the commercial character of these medical schools, the promoters sought by shortening of the curriculum and by the establishment of easy terms of graduation to induce great numbers of students to enter and to pay the fees. Sixteen weeks was generally adopted as the length of the college term; in some schools, it was reduced to thirteen. In New England attempts had been made to improve on this wholly inadequate curriculum. In 1835, the Faculty of the Medical College of Georgia proposed that a convention be called of delegates from all the medical colleges in the United States with a view to standardizing upward. Some of the more influential schools in the Atlantic cities, as might have been anticipated, opposed this effort. But a cry arose again in the Medical Society of the State of New York at its annual meeting in February 1839. At that time a resolution declaring that the business of teaching should be separated as far as possible from the privilege of granting diplomas was adopted by a large majority.

Following the adoption of this resolution, Dr. John McCall of Utica offered a preamble and a resolution urging a national medical convention to be held in 1840 in Philadelphia with delegates from each state medical society and each medical school in the United States. The resolution was adopted, and all the necessary steps to make it effective were taken. Then neither the societies nor the schools of other states responded to the invitation. The evil persisted, and the tension accumulated during the years that followed. In 1844 a series of resolutions were offered by Dr. Alexander Thompson of Cayuga County and N. S. Davis of Broome County attacking the abuse of the procedure by which college faculties both taught and licensed medical students and attacking as well the brief course of education leading to the receipt of a diploma. In 1845 the discussions in the state society continued; but the pattern of thinking seems to have been as stereotyped as it is now whenever improved standards are urged in any branch of education. Those who wished to set up a high standard in New York were told that students would abandon the schools of New York for those of other states where the requirements were less. The statement was made again and again that the requirements in New York were certainly as high as those of other states. At the close of the debate in 1845 Dr. Nathan Smith Davis, urged by Dr. Alden March of Albany, introduced the resolution which follows and which may be considered the first step toward the formation of the American Medical Association as we know it now:

WHEREAS, It is believed that a national convention would be conducive to the elevation of the standard of medical education in the United States; and

WHEREAS, There is no mode of accomplishing so desirable an object without concert of action on the part of the medical colleges, societies and institutions of all the states; therefore be it

Resolved, That the New York State Medical Society earnestly recommends a national convention of delegates from medical societies and colleges in the whole Union to convene in the city of New York on the first Tuesday in May in the year 1846 for the purpose of adopting some concerted action on the subject set forth in the foregoing preamble.

Resolved, That a committee of three be appointed to carry the foregoing resolution into effect.

The introduction of this resolution was followed by a discussion in which the older members of the society told how similar movements had failed in the past. Others said that the whole project was impracticable if not positively utopian. But Nathan Smith Davis persisted and urged those who agreed with him to persevere until they achieved success. The resolution was adopted; a committee consisting of Drs. Nathan Smith Davis of Binghamton, James McNaughton of Albany and Peter Van Buren, secretary of the state society, were named to make the resolution effective.

To what, then, can be ascribed the success of this resolution compared with the repeated failures of previous attempts to found a national medical society? The persistence and courage and initiative of Dr. N. S. Davis were the essential factors. Dr. Nathan Smith Davis soon after his return to Binghamton sent a copy of the preamble and resolutions to every college and medical society known to exist in the United States and to many prominent physicians in sections of the country in which such societies had not yet been formed. The proposal met with favor from societies, colleges and individuals by whom it was received except the colleges located in Philadelphia and in Boston. These schools respectfully declined to take any part in the proposed convention. The medical periodicals of the country, however, commended the holding of such a convention. Dr. Davis continued indefatigably to urge support of his project.

The New York State Medical Society in February 1846 appointed sixteen delegates to attend and accepted the invitation of the Faculty of the New York University to hold the convention in their building in May of that year. With an organizational genius equal to the best modern technics, Dr. N. S. Davis sent more communications to the medical periodicals of the country during 1845. He was aided by similar communications from Dr. Luther Ticknor, then president of the Medical Society of the State of Connecticut. Whereas Dr. Davis emphasized particularly the improvement of medical education, including higher standards of preliminary education, the quality of teaching, the qualifications required for a diploma and continuous stimulus of the medical profession, Dr. Ticknor urged quality in medical practice and graduate education and deprecated particularly the rivalry among the medical institutions and leading medical men as to who should furnish "not the most valuable and best wrought article, but who shall furnish the greatest quantity." So strong indeed were the language and the assertions of Dr. N. S. Davis that they naturally stimulated some opposition.

Professor Martyn Paine of the medical department of New York University delivered an address called "A Defense of the Medical Profession of the United States," published it and circulated it widely throughout the country. In this address he attacked the state medical society, accusing it of playing politics in its desire to extend the curriculum and said:

There is an aristocratic feature in this movement of the worst omen, however the spirit, by which it is prompted, may belong to the agrarian policy. It is oppression toward the poor for the sake of crippling the medical colleges.

This address had the strange effect of causing the Philadelphia physicians to withdraw their previous rejection of the invitation to

New York on the grounds that "the very singular address of Professor Paine" convinced them that the "convention was not designed particularly to benefit the medical schools in the city of New York." As a result, the society was convened in Philadelphia and twelve eminent physicians were appointed to attend the meeting in New York. In his book Dr. N. S. Davis philosophizes on this incident as exemplifying the necessity for frequent contacts between leaders in order to overcome distrust and bring about mutual respect. He says:

> It would be difficult to illustrate more strikingly that sleepless jealousy which pervaded more or less all our medical schools, springing into existence in rapid succession, as they had done; or the necessity of some general organization, by which the representatives of all should be brought into personal contact and intercourse, until mutual distrust should give place to mutual respect and a common object.

THE ORGANIZATIONAL MEETING

On Tuesday, May 5, 1846 the delegates and members of the medical profession from different parts of the United States assembled in the hall of the Medical Department of the New York University. Dr. Edward Delafield of New York was in the chair. Dr. William P. Buel of New York was appointed secretary. On motion a committee of one from each state represented in the convention was appointed to nominate officers for the convention. This committee unanimously agreed to propose for president Dr. Jonathan Knight of New Haven, for vice presidents Dr. John Bell of Philadelphia and Dr. Edward Delafield of New York City, and for secretaries Dr. Richard D. Arnold of Savannah, Ga., and Dr. Alfred Stillé of Philadelphia.

The Committee on Credentials reported that 119 delegates had sent credentials and that 80 of these were present at the opening of the convention. They represented medical societies and colleges from sixteen different states. No sooner had the officers been elected and conducted to their respective places than there occurred one of the most extraordinary political moves that has ever marked a medical assemblage anywhere in our country, which, incidentally, is widely known for the exciting activities of its democratic assemblages. Dr. Gunning S. Bedford, a colleague of the previously mentioned Professor Martyn Paine, arose and, after some general remarks as to the benefits of a general convention of medical men, introduced a resolution to the effect that the assemblage had failed in representation from half the United States and from a majority of the medical colleges and that therefore "this convention adjourn *sine die.*" The proposition was immediately seconded by one of his associates and naturally took the convention by surprise. There were two minutes of silence. The question was called for and a vote being taken gave 2 voting "Yes," namely Dr. Gunning S. Bedford and his colleague Dr. G. S. Pattison, and 74 "No."

Since many of the members considered the resolution an insult, motions were promptly made to withdraw the convention from the hall of New York University. This was followed by explanations and apologies by Drs. Bedford and Pattison; then the proposed withdrawal was laid on the table.

A committee of nine was appointed—headed by Dr. N. S. Davis—to bring the subject of medical education before the convention in the form of distinct proposals suitable for discussion and action and to report at the next meeting. On the following day this committee presented to the convention the following four proposals:

> First. That it is expedient for the medical profession of the United States to institute a National Medical Association.
>
> Secondly. That it is desirable that a uniform and elevated standard of requirements for the degree of M.D. should be adopted by all the medical schools in the United States.
>
> Thirdly. That is desirable that young men, before being received as students of medicine, should have acquired a suitable preliminary education.
>
> Fourthly. That it is expedient that the medical profession in the United States should be governed by the same code of medical ethics.

The committee also recommended the appointment of a committee of seven "to prepare and issue an address to the different regularly organized medical societies, and chartered medical schools in the United States, setting forth the objects of the National Medical Association, and inviting them to send delegates to the Convention to be held in Philadelphia in May 1847."

The proposals were adopted by the convention and the committees were appointed.

At this same meeting Dr. Davis tried to introduce—and received support for—a resolution to the effect that the union of the business of teaching and licensing in the same hands is wrong in principle and liable to abuse in practice. The resolution was opposed by Dr. Isaac Hays and by other members of the committee and finally was presented to the convention. Here it was fully discussed, and motions were made to lay it on the table or to refer it to various committees, but the spirited defense by Dr. N. S. Davis resulted finally in reference of the resolution to a special committee of seven, with instructions to report it at the meeting to be held in Philadelphia in May 1847.

This assemblage of physicians did not lose the opportunity to make progress toward greater efficiency in the science of medicine. On motion of Dr. John H. Griscom, committees were appointed to report on the most efficient measures for effecting a registration of births, marriages and deaths and toward the establishment of a nomenclature of diseases adapted to the United States.

Dr. N. S. Davis, looking over this epoch-making meeting in retrospect, expresses his surprise at the disparity of representation from states located equally distant from the place of meeting. New Jersey, for instance, had only two delegates, Maryland only one and Georgia only one. Indiana and Illinois had only one delegate each, so that more than half of the entire number present represented the state of New York. Eleven medical colleges were represented, which were only one third of the whole number in the United States. Again in retrospect, Nathan Smith Davis was disappointed by the absence of those to whom the medical profession had been accustomed to look as leaders in all important professional matters. He calls attention to the absence of such men as Warren, Mussey, Stevens, Chapman, Drake. Later most of these were to become quite active in the work of the medical association and some of them were elected to the presidency.

THE ORGANIZATION OF THE AMERICAN MEDICAL ASSOCIATION

THE DELEGATES TO THE National Medical Convention met in the hall of the Academy of Natural Sciences in Philadelphia on May 5, 1847. Dr. Isaac Hays, chairman of the Committee on Arrangements from the Philadelphia delegation, welcomed the delegates to the city. He told them of the gratification afforded the Philadelphia physicians in receiving the members of the convention as their guests. He then proposed the name of Dr. Jonathan Knight of Connecticut as chairman. A credentials committee was established and also a nominating committee, which was instructed to nominate four vice presidents and three secretaries. Permanent officers of the convention included as president Dr. Jonathan Knight of Connecticut; vice presidents, Dr. Alexander H. Stevens of New York, Dr. George B. Wood of Pennsylvania, Dr. A. H. Buchanan of Tennessee and Dr. John Harrison of Louisiana. The three secretaries were Dr. Richard D. Arnold of Georgia, Dr. Alfred Stillé of Pennsylvania and Dr. F. Campbell Stewart of New York.

A number of resolutions were introduced asking for places in the convention for any members of the previous convention who had not been elected to the present one, "any medical gentlemen present from states not represented" and any ex-officers of medicine from various medical schools or any professors from abroad who happened to be in Philadelphia. All these resolutions were most properly defeated. Similar technics for "stacking" conventions are examples of the notorious evils in democratic procedure.

Then Dr. Hays called for the reading of the report of the committee appointed in 1846. This report was read and ordered to be printed, as were also the reports on registration of births, marriages and deaths.

At the evening session of the same day a report was read on the requirements of the degree of M.D., another report on preliminary education and a portion of the report of the committee to prepare a code of medical ethics. Still later came the report from the committee on nomenclature of diseases and then the adjournment.

On the following day, after the convention assembled, Dr. N. S.

Davis offered a resolution for committees to record the indigenous medical botany of our country.

A controversy developed on the resolution which dealt with the union of teaching and licensing. Here majority and minority reports were presented. Then came reading of the resolutions previously introduced, with the adoption of the resolution on preliminary education. Invitations were presented to the convention for its 1848 meeting.

Just before adjournment of the morning session, the members having perhaps become somewhat prolix, Dr. Joel Hopkins of Maryland offered a resolution to the effect that "no gentleman shall be permitted to speak more than twice on the same proposition nor occupy more than fifteen minutes for speaking, without leave of the convention." This resolution was amended by changing fifteen minutes to ten minutes and then adopted.

PRELIMINARY EDUCATION

Worthy of special note was the resolution on preliminary education of the young man in the field of medicine. The resolution read as follows:

Resolved, That this Convention earnestly recommends to the members of the medical profession throughout the United States, to satisfy themselves, either by personal inquiry or written certificate of competent persons, before receiving young men into their offices as students, that they are of good moral character and that they have acquired a good English education, a knowledge of natural philosophy and the elementary mathematical sciences, including geometry and algebra, and such an acquaintance, at least, with the Latin and Greek languages as will enable them to appreciate the technical language of medicine, and read and write prescriptions.

Resolved, That this Convention also recommends to the members of the medical profession of the United States, when they have satisfied themselves that a young man possesses the qualifications specified in the preceding resolution, to give him a written certificate stating that fact, and recording also the date of his admission as a medical student, to be carried with him as a warrant for his reception into the medical college in which he may intend to pursue his studies.

Resolved, That all the medical colleges in the United States be, and they are hereby recommended and requested to require such a certificate of every student of medicine applying for matriculation; and, when publishing their annual lists of graduates, to accompany the name of the graduate with the name and residence of his preceptor, the name of the latter being clearly and distinctly presented as certifying to the qualification of preliminary education.

Some of the members in the convention opposed this resolution, urging that it would prevent many young men of limited means from entering the medical profession whose natural endowments would carry them to the highest rank, notwithstanding their inadequate preliminary preparation. The argument was answered by the statement that "Our country provides school houses and almost unlimited facilities for acquiring a knowledge of at least the ordinary branches of learning." Dr. N. S. Davis said that "young men who had not mental energy and perseverance enough to comply with the standard proposed in the resolutions, certainly had not enough to enable them to do justice to a profession as extensive, intricate and arduous as ours."

These resolutions were adopted by nearly a unanimous vote and were then reaffirmed by almost every meeting of the Association that followed. They have, in fact, constituted a guiding principle in the field of medical education in this country for a hundred years. Subsequent resolutions urged lengthening of the curriculum from four months to six months, a minimum of three entire years to be devoted to the study of medicine, a minimum age of 21 for entering the practice of medicine, at least three months devoted to dissections, at least one session of hospital practice (which, to us, would mean an internship), and a method of making certain that students actually attended lectures.

A PERMANENT NATIONAL ASSOCIATION

MOST IMPORTANT WAS THE activity of the convention which resulted in the organization of a permanent national association. The committee reported in full a constitution designed to effect such a national organization. First came resolutions from the inspired physicians who thought that they had evolved better names than the one which was ultimately chosen. Thus one name considered was "The Conventional Association of the United States," another "The Medical Association of the United States of North America." Both these proposals were lost, after which the constitution developed by the committee was offered to the convention and accepted. It included the clause "This institution shall be known and distinguished by the name and title of 'The American Medical Association.'"

This constitution wisely proposed the principle of representation by making the acting members of the Association consist of delegates from medical societies and institutions in accordance with a fixed numerical ratio.

The preamble attached to the constitution declared the purpose of the organization to be "for cultivating and advancing medical knowledge; for elevating the standard of medical education; for promoting the usefulness, honor and interests of the medical profession; for enlightening and directing public opinion in regard to the duties, responsibilities and requirements of medical men; for exciting and encouraging emulation and concert of action in the profession, and for facilitating and fostering friendly intercourse between those engaged in it."

The founding fathers urged the formation of state and local associations and so framed the constitution as to make the great majority of the members of the national association consist of delegates from permanently organized state and county medical societies throughout the nation. Thus from the very first the democratic principle prevailed.

Mindful, moreover, of the scientific aspects of the organization, committees were established on medical sciences, practical medicine, surgery, obstetrics, medical education, medical literature and publication.

The convention then resolved itself into the American Medical Association.

A committee consisting of one from each state represented was appointed to nominate officers for the ensuing year, and these were unanimously elected. The officers were:

President—Dr. Nathaniel Chapman, Pennsylvania.
Vice Presidents—Drs. Jonathan Knight, Connecticut; Alexander H. Stevens, New York; James Moultrie, South Carolina; A. H. Buchanan, Tennessee.
Secretaries—Drs. Alfred Stillé, Philadelphia; J. R. W. Dunbar, Baltimore.
Treasurer—Dr. Isaac Hays, Philadelphia.

Significant of this birth-giving meeting of May 7, 1847 were resolutions leading toward the ultimate adoption of the principles of ethics.

A resolution was offered requesting the Congress of the United States to allocate a portion of the funds of the Smithsonian Institution to uses of the American Medical Association, and that resolution was laid on the table. Dr. Austin Flint of New York presented a resolution urging the states to pass laws sanctioning and providing for the prosecution of dissections. That resolution was promptly and unanimously passed.

When Dr. Nathaniel Chapman was called to the chair, he spoke briefly but expressively:

He could find no language to express the depth of his gratitude. It had often been his good fortune during his professional life to have been complimented in the same manner, though not in the same degree. This was the most precious of all the honors he had received, as spontaneously conferred by his own brethren. He confessed his incompetence to serve the Association as he could desire. He loved his profession and should be ungrateful if he did not; whatever he possessed in this life had been bestowed by its favors; when he forgot it, or deserted it and its disciples, he remarked, with great emphasis, "may Almighty God forget and desert me." He desired that the Association should be persuaded of his ardent wishes for the cause, and that his most strenuous efforts would be unceasingly directed to advance the dignity of the profession and extend its usefulness.

QUACKERY

From the very first the American Medical Association has prosecuted its war on quackery and more than any other agency in our country can take the credit for the vast improvement that has occurred in the abolition of nostrums, secret medicines and quackery. At the session on May 7, 1847 Dr. John B. Johnson of Missouri introduced a resolution in which he pointed out that numerous and important evils result from the universal practice of allowing persons almost wholly ignorant to engage in apothecaries and still greater from the universal traffic in secret medicines. He urged that schools of pharmacy be established in the individual states and that some rule be adopted that no physician patronize a druggist or an apothecary who deals in "patent" or secret medicines.

SYSTEM OF REPRESENTATION

The convention adjourned to meet in Baltimore on the first Tuesday in May 1848. Thus ended one of the most significant assemblages in the history of our nation. This was the birth of a great organization.

Dr. Nathan Smith Davis took great pride in the fact that the principle embodied in the first constitution made the national association emanate directly from local medical organizations and institutions. This system of representation gave the organization a legitimate claim to be truly representative of the whole medical profession. Indeed the representatives were so earnest in their desire to avoid dominance by any section in the work of the organization that they also incorporated in the constitution a provision which prohibited the holding of annual meetings twice in succession in the same place.

To recapitulate, the original plan of organization as adopted in 1847 provided that "members of the American Medical Association ... should hold their appointment to membership either as delegates from local institutions, as members by invitation or as permanent members."

There were thus created three distinct classes of membership, of which the delegates constituted the bulk and the most important part. They received their appointment from "permanently organized societies, medical colleges, hospitals, lunatic asylums and other permanently organized medical institutions of good standing." Each appointment was for one year. The basis of representation was one delegate for every ten regular resident members of the medical society, two for every regularly constituted and chartered school of medicine, two for every hospital containing 100 inmates or more, and one for all permanently organized medical institutions of good standing not included in the foregoing summary. In order to admit of representation from portions of the United States not otherwise represented, provision was made for members by invitation. If a physician from sections of the country in which no medical institutions of any sort existed attended an annual session, the Association could constitute him a member by invitation for that session only. He thus became an unofficial delegate for a section that would otherwise be without representation. Thus two classes of members, both, as will be seen, of a purely temporary character and deriving their right of membership either from the organization which they represented or from the Association which invited them to a seat in its deliberations, constituted the voting membership of the American Medical Association. In order that delegates having once been members of the Association might retain some connection with it after their time as delegates had expired, it was provided that all those who had served in that capacity and such other members as might be appointed by the Association, by unanimous vote, might be made "permanent members." They were entitled to attend the meetings and to participate in the affairs of the Association without the right to vote. It was therefore recognized from the time of the first preliminary convention in 1846 that the right to vote should be limited to the duly elected and qualified delegates of local medical societies, colleges and hospitals who came bearing credentials of their election as such. Thus the American Medical Association was from the beginning a delegate body.

When its total membership reached as many as 60,000 members in the state societies, the assignment of one delegate for every ten members would have made a representative body of 6,000. This brought about ultimately the reorganization, of which more will be told later, and led finally to the formation of the House of Delegates of the American Medical Association as we know it today.

When William H. Welch was President of the Association in 1910 he called to mind the battle which took place in the originally constituted convention over the decision as to whether there should be a representative body or an organization in which the officers would themselves perpetuate the control within a small group.

"It is curious to think," said Dr. Welch, "what would have been the history of the Association had the choice not been made in favor of the more democratic representative plan."

This plan, which continued in operation for fifty-five years, was perhaps cumbersome and ineffective, but it was well suited to the conditions that existed at the time of its adoption.

Looking back at the first fifty years of life of the American Medical Association, William H. Welch noted that the founders brought into being a national organization truly representative. "Such an organization," he said, "has inherent elements of strength which secure its future even against its own blunders and still more against attacks from without. The Association has been from the beginning the great unifying force for the profession of this country, whose common interests it has been its chief endeavor to serve."

In concluding his address, William H. Welch said:

<blockquote>
Organized effort is a distinguishing mark of modern civilization. It is as essential for the advancement of science, of education, of social and industrial reform, of philanthropic endeavor as for the promotion of commerce. With the remarkable progress of medical science, especially during the last three decades, man's power to control disease has been vastly increased and the sphere of usefulness of the physician has been correspondingly widened and with advancing knowledge will continue to expand. The skill and knowledge
</blockquote>

of the physician and sanitarian have acquired a new and ever increasing importance and significance in the movements for social amelioration, for improvement of the conditions of labor and of living, for the conservation and most efficient utilization of the productive energy of the world, and for the reclamation of regions now yielding no return to civilization.

Among the organized forces for advancing the prosperity, the happiness and the well being of the people of this country, the American Medical Association has an important part to play. We are justified in the confidence that, with the united support and loyalty of the profession, this Association, broadly representative and standing for the best ideals of medical science and art and for professional and civic righteousness, will contribute a beneficent share to the working out of our national destiny.

THE PRINCIPLES OF MEDICAL ETHICS

AMONG THE RESOLUTIONS INTRODUCED in the National Medical Convention which assembled in New York in May 1846 was one which was to set a pattern of ideals for all the years that have followed. It read:

> that it is expedient that the medical profession in the United States should be governed by the same code of medical ethics, and that a committee of seven be appointed to report a code for that purpose at a meeting to be held in Philadelphia on the first Wednesday of May 1847.

The committee included Drs. John Bell, Isaac Hays and G. Emerson, Philadelphia; W. W. Morris, Dover, Del.; T. C. Dunn, Newport, R. I.; A. Clark, New York, and R. D. Arnold, Savannah, Ga. This committee presented its report on June 5, 1847 at Philadelphia.

In presenting the report Dr. Isaac Hays stated that justice required that some explanatory remarks should accompany it. The committee had examined a great number of codes of ethics adopted by different societies in the United States and found that they were all based on that of Dr. Thomas Percival and that, moreover, the phrases of this writer were preserved to a considerable extent in all of them. "Believing that language which had been so often examined and adopted must possess the greatest of merits for such a document as the present, clearness and precision, and having no ambition for the honours of authorship, the Committee which prepared this code have followed a similar course and have carefully preserved the words of Percival wherever they convey the precepts it is wished to inculcate. A few of the sections are in the words of the late Dr. Rush, and one or two sentences are from other writers." The committee said, however, that wherever it was thought that the language could be made more explicit by changing a word or even a part of a sentence, this was unhesitatingly done.

Dr. John Bell was a Philadelphia surgeon, graduated by the University of Pennsylvania in 1817. He had done good work as a writer and editor and had been associated with the production of a considerable number of books. He had also edited "Stokes' Lectures on the Theory and Practice of Physics" and Andrew Combe's "Treatise on Children." It is generally conceded that most of the work in the preparation of these principles of ethics had been done by Isaac Hays, editor of the *American Journal of the Medical Sciences* from 1827 to 1879.

Thomas Percival, from whom admittedly the committee drew extensively in preparing the first draft of the principles of ethics, was a graduate of Leyden in 1765 and was made a Fellow of the Royal Society of England in 1765 when he was 25 years old. In 1767, when he was 27 years old, Thomas Percival published a book of philosophic essays and commentaries on medical life. He conducted an extensive correspondence with John Hunter and William Withering, the latter the discoverer of the use of digitalis, and with Heberden, for whom the famous nodes are named. He was associated with Charles White, who unquestionably knew about the infectiousness of puerperal fever and who wrote important works on the subject before Semmelweis and Oliver Wendell Holmes. Thomas Percival gave much thought to the future of the medical profession. An argument started in the hospital in which he worked. This no doubt led to the codification of the principles which were the first formal code of ethics submitted to the English medical profession. In 1793 Percival was asked by the group associated with the Manchester Infirmary to draw up a series of ethical principles as a guide in the conduct of the hospital and of the infirmary. He worked three years, then drew a first draft which he circulated among his friends, including Charles White, Heberden, John Hunter and William Withering. He sent a copy also to Erasmus Darwin. All sent him their comments. Then he revised the manuscript and finally published it in 1803.

In 1823 the New York State Medical Society adopted a series of principles of ethics which were almost wholly similar to the code prepared by Thomas Percival. In 1832 the Baltimore Medical Society took Percival's series and adopted them for that society. When Isaac Hays presented the report of his committee to the convention of 1847, he too, as has already been noted, decided that little improvement could be made on the principles as set forth by Thomas Percival.

In the work "American Medical Biographies," by Howard A. Kelly and Walter L. Burrage, it is said that the name of Isaac Hays is always associated with that which is well written and worth reading in American medical literature. After graduation from the University of Pennsylvania in 1816 his father put Isaac Hays into his counting house, but one year of banking proved to be enough. Hays took up the study of medicine under Dr. Nathaniel Chapman, among the first of the presidents of the American Medical Association. In 1820 Hays took his M.D. at the University of Pennsylvania with a thesis on the subject of sympathy. Hays gained celebrity in surgery of the eye; he edited several books on diseases of the eye, physics and ornithology, and cooperated in the preparation of a dictionary of medical terms. He translated several important works of medicine from French into English and he began an American Cyclopedia of Practical Medicine and Surgery but got only as far as "A to Azygos." In 1833 he had published a work entitled "Descriptions of the Inferior Maxillary Bones of the Mastodons" and he recorded the first case of astigmatism recorded in America.

In presenting the Code of Medical Ethics to the convention, a statement was made by Dr. John Bell in which he pointed out that medical ethics comprised not only the duties but also the rights of a physician. "As it is the duty of a physician to advise, so has he a right to be attentively and respectfully listened to." His introductory statement, after emphasizing the dignity of the medical profession, calls on the physician to give of his utmost for the advancement of the public health and the sustaining of the law. He recognizes the obligation on the physician "to bear emphatic testimony against quackery in all its forms." Even as early as 1847 he recognized the dangers of insanitary food and the purveying of nostrums. He did not hesitate to condemn members of other professions, and especially ministers of the gospel, for giving "their countenance and at times direct patronage to medical empirics both by their use of nostrums and by their certificates in favor of the absurd pretentions of these impostors." He condemned also the apothecaries who lend themselves to the sale and distribution of quack medicines and nostrums. And the final portion of his address is a plea to maintain the standards of the profession by unceasing vigilance so as to prevent the introduction of those who have not been prepared by a suitable preparatory moral and intellectual training.

In a volume called "Percival's Medical Ethics," Chauncey D. Leake has analyzed the growth and development of the "Principles of Medical Ethics of the American Medical Association." The criticism was made early that the committee headed by Bell and Hays had taken its code directly from the New York State code. However, as has already been pointed out, Isaac Hays stated clearly that the code had been derived from that of Percival and thus neatly reprimanded the New York and Baltimore societies, which adopted these codes without giving credit to Percival.

From time to time after 1848, circumstances developed which made necessary reconsiderations and modifications of the Principles of Ethics. In 1852 there was serious debate over the acceptance of homeopathic doctrines by some members of the medical profession.

In 1882 delegates from the Medical Society of the State of New York presented a report which offered a simplified and brief system of medical ethics as a substitute for the national code. This was adopted. Then in June 1882, at the meeting of the American Medical Association in St. Paul, delegates from the Medical Society of the State of New York were refused admission. At that time Dr. Austin Flint wrote a commentary on the Code of Ethics in an endeavor to persuade the New York society to reenact the code of the American Medical Association. So fierce was this battle that a group was formed with the title "Society for the Prevention of the Reenactment in the State of New York of the Present Code of Ethics of the American Medical Association." The battle continued with pamphleteering, debate and discussion on both sides. At various meetings of the Medical Society of the State of New York the Code was voted in and voted out, and at one time a conservative group which found it impossible to reenact the national code in the original Medical Society of the State of New York withdrew and organized a rival New York State Medical Association.

Finally, in 1903 a special committee appointed by the American Medical Association made a report at the convention in New Orleans to which one of its members dissented. That member prepared what he considered to be a "suitable system of advisory precepts" in medical conduct. This was adopted as "The Principles of Ethics of the American Medical Association" and was considered to be much more satisfactory than the older code. Still further revisions were made in 1912.

A resolution passed by the House of Delegates of the American Medical Association in San Francisco in 1946 has called on the Judicial Council of the American Medical Association to consider again a rewriting and rephrasing of "The Principles of Medical Ethics."

The chief criticism made by Chauncey D. Leake in his consideration of the subject is the one which has been made frequently, namely that "The Principles of Medical Ethics" do not clearly differentiate actual principles of ethics from the rules of conduct and etiquette of the profession. Indeed, one rather wise commentator in the midst of the battle that was waged in New York, Dr. D. B. St. John Roosa, suggested that the only ethical offenses for which the medical profession should claim and promise to exercise discipline are "those comprehended under the commission of acts unworthy a physician and a gentleman."

The "Principles of Ethics" that now prevail emphasize first the duties of the physician to his patient. These duties include service as an ideal, patience and delicacy as highly desirable qualifications and full assumption of responsibility once a case has been undertaken. The "Principles of Ethics" emphasize that the physician is free to choose whom he will serve but point out that he should respond to any request for assistance in emergencies or whenever temperate public opinion expects the service.

The physician is told that he must be an honorable man and a gentleman and that he must conform to a high standard of morals and uphold the dignity of his profession. The solicitation of patients by an individual physician is considered unprofessional, but it is recognized that a man may conform to the customs of the community in which he lives.

Medicine has for years depended for its success on the personal relationship between physician and patient. Every article in the principle of ethics is planned to emphasize this relationship. "A pleased patient," as the "Principles of Ethics" repeatedly state, "is the best type of medical advertisement." From the very first the "Principles of Ethics" have sought to protect an uninformed public against the claims of the quack and the pretender. "It is unprofessional to promise radical cures; to boast of cures and secret methods of treatment and remedies; to exhibit certificates of skill or of success in the treatment of disease; or to employ any methods to gain the attention of the public for the purpose of obtaining patients."

Again the "Principles of Ethics" recognized the importance of having adequate consultation whenever a physician is in doubt as to what is best for his patient. "In serious illness, especially in doubtful or difficult conditions, the physician should request consultations." And, the principles continue, "In every consultation the benefit to be derived by the patient is of first importance." The "Principles of Ethics" recognize that medical diagnosis is usually paid for insufficiently in comparison with the rewards of surgical technic. "The patient should be made to realize," say the "Principles of Ethics," "that a proper fee should be paid the family physician for the service he renders in determining the surgical or medical treatment suited to the condition, and in advising concerning those best qualified to render any special service that may be required by the patient."

THE DOCTOR AND THE PUBLIC

The third phase of the principles of ethics is again a recognition of the duty of the physician to the public. He is asked to remember that he is a citizen and to aid in enforcing laws and in giving advice concerning public health. During an epidemic he must continue his labors for the alleviation of the suffering without regard to the risk of his own health or life or to financial return. He is asked to warn the public against the devices practiced and the false pretensions made by charlatans, and he is told finally that these principles do not cover all the obligations which he may have but are wholly a guide which will supplement the ordinary conduct of a gentleman and the practice of the Golden Rule. The last sentence reads "Finally, these principles are primarily for the good of the public, and their enforcement should be conducted in such a manner as shall deserve and receive the endorsement of the community."

THE FIRST ANNUAL SESSION

WHEN PRESIDENT NATHANIEL CHAPMAN opened the proceedings of the first annual meeting of the American Medical Association in Baltimore on May 2, 1848 he used strong language in telling the profession of its responsibilities. In these days when organizations throughout the nation are attempting to create popularity for themselves by the practice of what has come to be called "public relations," we hear similar indictments. The words of Dr. Chapman published about a hundred years ago resound almost as if they were of yesterday. He said:

> "This assemblage presents a spectacle of moral grandeur delightful to contemplate. Few of the kind have I ever witnessed more imposing in its aspect, and certainly none inspired by purer motives or having views of a wider range of beneficence. The profession to which we belong, once venerated on account of its antiquity—its various and profound science—its elegant literature—its polite accomplishments—its virtues—has become corrupt and degenerate to the forfeiture of its social position and, with it, of the homage it formerly received spontaneously and universally...."

Dr. Chapman then proceeded to tell the medical profession of his day what has been so frequently told to it in the years that have passed: that the medical profession always cleans its own house, that it does not need extraneous assistance in bringing about reform. Perhaps in anticipation of charges that might be made at some later date, he declined in advance to nomination for reelection to the presidency, saying "Rotation in office, I am persuaded, is the vital principle of every institution in this country. Especially do I consider it so in relation to our own association, national in its objects and constitution. Every section of the country is here represented, and equally engaged in a common cause. No monopoly of honor or privileges must be permitted to any one portion of it. I wish our conduct always to be dictated by liberality, justice and equality."

There were 195 delegates, and the Committee on Nominations was instructed to bring in the names of at least three nominees for each office. Moreover, it was required that the person elected should receive a clear majority of those voting.

The convention turned its attention to the sophistication and adulteration of drugs. Dr. A. H. Stevens of New York was elected President. Then came a number of extraordinary reports of the special committees which had been appointed in previous years. Early in the session Dr. J. C. Warren of Boston, who was first to operate on a patient under ether anesthesia in the Massachusetts General Hospital in 1847, addressed the meeting in reference to the preparation and value of chloric ether as a substitute for sulfuric ether and chloroform, whereupon Dr. F. H. Hamilton of Buffalo introduced a resolution "That, considering the present limited amount of authenticated facts in relation to the danger or safety of anesthetic agents in medicine, surgery and obstetrics, this association is not now prepared to determine upon their value or the propriety of their use, and that the subject be referred to a Special Committee who shall report at the next annual meeting." The resolution was referred to a committee and apparently not made the subject of any later report.

In addition to questions related to medical education and the publication of scientific papers, we find an interesting resolution asking the Committee on Hygiene to direct its attention to the following subjects: First, What is the influence likely to be produced by the extensive introduction of tea and coffee in the diet of persons under the age of puberty? Second, What is the influence of the substitution of the luxuries tea and coffee, as food, on the health of the laboring classes?

The reports of the committees occupy the rest of the volume of the Transactions of the American Medical Association for 1848. Volume I was printed for the Association by T. K. and P. G. Collins in Philadelphia. It contains some documents that are classic.

COMMITTEE ON MEDICAL SCIENCES

The Committee on Medical Sciences, under the chairmanship of W. T. Wragg of South Carolina, reported that it had examined all the journals published during the previous year, that there was too much literature, so that there was an embarrassment in choosing well rather than in collecting abundantly. They did not consider it desirable to limit themselves merely to contributions from America but had collected from all over the world. They then presented some fifty pages of abstracts from the medical literature of the day, dealing with a great variety of subjects.

COMMITTEE ON PRACTICAL MEDICINE

The Committee on Practical Medicine had been charged to report on the more important improvements effected in this country in the management of individual diseases and to report on the progress of epidemics. This committee also had examined the medical periodicals of the day and concluded quite widely that great discoveries are not really made in any one year. It singled out for special notice a procedure developed by Dr. Gurdon Buck of the New York Hospital which was the multiple scarification of the walls of the throat in the presence of edematous swelling or what was then called "oedematous laryngitis" in its suffocative stage. This, no doubt, was the condition from which George Washington died and would be called today either "septic sore throat" or "diphtheria."

Then came a rather prolix discussion of epidemics, with special attention to the frightful condition of emigrants coming from Europe, contrasting particularly the nutrition, cleanliness and general hygiene of the German emigrants with that of the Irish, who arrived "in most cases enfeebled from the want of sustenance, and on shipboard, destitute of supplies of wholesome food, depressed of mind, clothed in filthy garments and crowded and confined in air rendered pestiferous by the excrementitious matters eliminated from their own bodies." It called attention to the fact that thousands had perished on the voyages to the United States and Canada. From one ship, the *Virginia*, bound from Liverpool to Quebec, with 470 passengers, 158 were buried at sea.

During the year 1847, 100,000 souls left the British Isles for Canada. More than 5,000 of these died en route and another 8,000 within a few weeks after their arrival. The disease from which these people perished was typhus in its genuine form, and in some ships smallpox, dysentery and measles swelled the amount of mortality. There was much discussion of the ability to distinguish between typhus fever and typhoid fever.

As a supplement to its report the committee included the complete statement of Gurdon Buck on "Oedematous Laryngitis" together with pictures in color of the condition concerned and of the instruments especially designed by him for performing his operation.

THE COMMITTEE ON SURGERY

The Committee on Surgery was supposed to prepare a report on all the important improvements in the management of surgical diseases in America during the year, to which it succinctly replied "Neither brilliant discoveries nor any extraordinary improvements in surgery marked the past year." The committee, nevertheless, decided to make a report of progress, and the major portion of its report deals with cutting for stone and the surgical treatment of aneurysms. Dr. Daniel Brainard of Chicago had found iodine useful as a substance to be injected into infected wounds.

Then comes the report on anesthesia. Eighteen months had elapsed since the introduction of ether by Morton. A large and intelligent body of the medical community, including some of the most eminent surgeons, considered the question settled. They considered the dangers of etherization so inconsiderable as to justify its use prior to all surgical operations. Another class of surgeons wished to limit the use of anesthetics to severe operations and to discourage their general employment. A small portion of the profession objected altogether to the use of anesthetics as dangerous and harmful in their tendency.

The committee refused to take a definite stand. It did, however, offer the opinion of Dr. Henry J. Bigelow of Boston, and it took pride in the fact that anesthesia was an American contribution. At the same time the committee noted with regret that the early history of the discovery "is encumbered with angry disputes amongst rival claimants for the honor, and that attempts were made by those most intimately interested in the claim...." Much consideration is given to the claims of Horace Wells, but it is stated clearly that Wells abandoned his experiments begun in 1844, and that the first successful experiment was performed by William T. G. Morton, a dentist of Boston, on a patient from whom he extracted a tooth on Sept. 30, 1846. Dr. Henry J. Bigelow had read a paper in Boston on Nov. 3, 1846. It was published in the *Boston Medical and Surgical Journal* November 18. Within six weeks of the publication of that paper, ether had been tested and was being warmly advocated among surgeons in London. The report then lists all the various surgeons in the United States who had already used ether in surgical operations and it was noted that fatal effects following the use of chloroform had been more frequent than from ether.

Incidentally the committee reported also that it had received a number of letters about the curability of cancer and the results of operations on this class of tumors, but apparently this was too much for the committee and it made no report but merely submitted the letters to the convention.

COMMITTEE ON OBSTETRICS

The Committee on Obstetrics had the duty of preparing a report on all the important improvements in obstetric art and of the management of diseases peculiar to women and children. Obviously the matter of chief concern was the use of the anesthetics in childbirth. The committee got itself into the usual argument that labor is a physiologic or natural process and that pain should therefore be endured, but the committee attached little importance to this objection. It wisely decided that if one adopted that point of view it would be impossible even to give remedies to the parturient woman. Already anesthetic agents had been used in 2,000 cases and, as far as the committee was able to learn, without a single fatal result and few, if any, untoward results.

The committee also suggested that doctors try out chloroform on themselves as a means of dispelling their vague apprehensions in relationship to it. Indeed the committee recommended that the doctor begin with 20 to 30 drops and gradually increase the quantity to find out how to use the chloroform safely and to acquire tact and confidence in giving it to others.

There was much discussion of the relative advantages of ether and chloroform for different types of cases, chloroform being considered more convenient and ether safer, but both efficient.

To this report were appended half a dozen communications from practitioners who had used anesthetics in labor.

COMMITTEE ON MEDICAL EDUCATION

The Committee on Medical Education was charged with preparing a report on the general condition of medical education in the United States in comparison with medical education in other enlightened nations and to note particularly the quality of instruction, the number of pupils and the requirements in various states.

The committee pointed out that in most foreign countries the standard of qualifications necessary for a doctorate in medicine was higher than in the United States and that the preliminary education was broader and more thorough. As a result of the previous meeting of the American Medical Association, some medical schools had already lengthened their curriculums and added other courses of instruction. Incidentally, the committee noted that in Harvard University candidates who had not received a college education were subjected to an examination on natural philosophy and the Latin language and were required to translate *ad aperturam libri* Cicero's orations. The same practice was followed in the medical societies of Massachusetts in their examinations for licenses to practice.

The committee had already decided that there were too many doctors in the United States, the proportion being five times as great as in France. It was urged that private teachers exercise greater circumspection of students taken into their offices. The committee felt that the oversupply of doctors was largely responsible for the rise of quackery and charlatanism, and it urged that a proper medical education could be had only by spending a certain amount of time in a hospital in the actual care of patients.

COMMITTEE ON MEDICAL LITERATURE

Looking back on the perspective of one hundred years, the report of the Committee on Medical Literature, under the chairmanship of Oliver Wendell Holmes and including such distinguished men as Enoch Hale, G. C. Shattuck Jr., Daniel Drake, John Bell, Austin Flint and W. Selden, merits first place. There are some sections so clearly of the style and manner of thought of Oliver Wendell Holmes that they merit frequent quotation. There is an adequate record of the history of medical publications in the United States, with complete reports of existing medical journals.

A typical medical journal of the time is thus described:

> The first part of each number is devoted to original articles, consisting of essays, histories of epidemics and endemics, series of cases and single cases, and accounts of operations. Occasionally a more detailed and comprehensive history of some disease is introduced under the name of *monograph*, and not unfrequently extensive statistical tables are given, bearing especially upon surgical and obstetrical practice. Then follow *Reviews* or formal examinations of works recently published, usually analytical in character and having for their principal object the book rather than the general subject of which it treats. To this division succeeds a miscellaneous and heterogeneous assemblage of *bibliographical notices;* the sweepings of the critical *atelier;* the rinsings and heeltaps of the critical banquet; a necessary part of the editor's prospectus, but one which is least gratifying to minute inspection. Here the importunate friend receives his expected compliment, the dull dignitary is pacified with his scanty morsel of eulogy, the Maecenas is paid in fair words for his patronage; the book which must be noticed and has not been read is embalmed in safe epithets and inurned in accommodating generalities. Lastly, a considerable part of the number is made up of selections, either taken promiscuously from other journals and recently published works, or, in the better managed periodicals, classified so as to present a summary of the recent progress of science in its several departments.

The committee found that a great proportion of a medical journal was made up of quotations from other medical journals, so that all the medical journals were a good deal alike, since there were very few original articles published of any merit and they were found again and again repeated in the medical journals.

Following the discussions of the periodicals come discussions of the books in each of the important medical subjects and then in some half dozen pages a witty analysis of medical writings, classic in its diction and in its consideration. Special attention was paid to the so-called introductory lectures, which are really the opening statements delivered by the deans or professors in the medical schools to the incoming students. Says the report:

They must not be judged too harshly, for they are delivered to young men, who like high seasoning, and they naturally partake somewhat of the character of advertisements. Many of them are agreeable and appropriate performances, but others are open to severe comment. Turgid and extravagant attempts at eloquence, a fondness for effete Latin quotations, a parade of scholastic terms where simple ones only are called for, an inclination to adopt the cant phrases of political and literary writers, are the common faults of these productions. The physician should remember, that his style has no more occasion for pomp of oratory and glitter of epithet, than his costume for the gold lace and feathers which belong to the military chieftain. Nothing is more offensive than an attempt to tell that which should be said plainly and decently, in high flown language. It vitiates the taste of the student who listens to it or reads it, and exposes the profession to derision from those who cannot value the important truths disguised by such ill chosen finery.

COMMITTEE ON PUBLICATION

The Committee on Publication, headed by Isaac Hays, reported that it had printed 2,500 copies of the Conventions of 1846 and 1847 and they still had 800 copies left.

There is a complete list of the members who paid $3 each for membership in the Association. Then come a number of communications dealing with the ethics of the pharmaceutical profession and an exposé of the adulteration and falsification of drugs sold in the United States.

The committee, which had been supposed to ascertain the total number of doctors in the United States, reported for the states of Virginia, Delaware and Massachusetts. And finally there were two scientific papers and lists of the officers and members of the American Medical Association.

A good index completed what is even for these times an extraordinarily interesting volume.

THE YEARS 1849 TO 1852

1849
BOSTON

IN THE AMPHITHEATER OF the Massachusetts General Hospital in 1846 Dr. John Collins Warren had done the first public operation under ether anesthesia. At the meeting of the American Medical Association in 1849, held in Boston, he served as chairman of the committee of reception of the Massachusetts Medical Society; he was nominated President of the American Medical Association for the ensuing year. Whether or not there was any direct association between these facts there is, of course, no way to determine. The Association was still holding its sessions by a technic which involved the formation of special committees on such subjects as surgery, forensic medicine, indigenous botany and hygiene, but the primary interest was still the reform in medical education. The convention reiterated its approval of the resolutions on this subject adopted by the convention that met in Philadelphia in 1847. The attention of all the medical colleges was called again to the report on preliminary education. Already some agencies were endeavoring to find a substitute for clinical instruction in the hospital; a resolution was offered that the Association did not sanction or recognize college clinics as substitutes for hospital clinical instruction.

Significantly it was now agreed that state medical societies should be formed in every state in which they did not exist and that the societies should admit to their membership only those who had obtained degrees in medicine and had been licensed by a recognized licensing body.

Progress was made also in the resolution which encouraged all the schools of medicine to meet at Cincinnati before the next annual meeting of the American Medical Association and to present a plan for elevating the standard of medical education. These were the preliminary steps toward the high standard that was ultimately to prevail in the advancement of American medicine.

An innovation was the establishment of standing committees to undertake measurement of progress in each important medical field. To this resolution were appended the words "giving special attention to such as may be American." The committees included a Committee on Arrangements, Anatomy, Physiology, Materia Medica, Chemistry, Pathological Anatomy, the Principles and Practice of Medicine, of Surgery and of Obstetrics, Hygiene and Sanitary Measures, Forensic Medicine, Medical and Vital Statistics, American Medical Biography, Medical Education and Publication. These subjects of main interest were to be modified from time to time with the progress of medical science and with the advancement of knowledge in each of these specialties. Gradually anatomy, physiology, chemistry and pathology were to be directed for their scientific considerations primarily to special societies formed specifically for such purposes. Hygiene and sanitary measures, which were particularly the problem of the medical profession, were to be absorbed in the great field of public health administration. Medical and vital statistics became functions eventually of the Bureau of Census and the U. S. Public Health Service. American medical biography was to be merged gradually into the Directory of the American Medical Association. But in this formative stage each of these topics was considered of equal interest with every other; there was but one organization to give proper consideration to all of them.

Rather amusing in view of the present stage of medical education in the United States was the submission by the faculty of medicine of Harvard to the Committee on Medical Education of an elaborate defense of the limitation of the courses of medical instruction in the schools to four months—a limitation seriously opposed by the committee itself. A committee was appointed to prepare at leisure a statement of the facts and arguments which may be adduced in favor of prolonging the courses to six months.

Well in advance of their time also were resolutions indicating that the state medical associations in east Tennessee and New York had developed a series of popular lectures designed to enlighten the public mind in relation to the new position of medical men in relationship to society; it was urged that the American Medical Association recommend medical men in all associations, individually, by public lectures and otherwise, "to enlighten the public mind in regard to the duties and responsibilities of the medical profession and their just claims to the confidence of the public." Eighty years later the continuing demand for suitably informing the public caused the formation of a division of public relations in the American Medical Association.

Although but two years had passed, many members were beginning to get a little weary of the length of time required to read the annual reports. Their attention was called to the fact that the constitution merely required them to report on the progress of medicine in this country alone and only during the year of their service.

Realize too that, although the time was almost a hundred years ago, a resolution was offered requesting the Committee on Practical Medicine to inquire into the expediency of adopting the English language exclusively in the writing of prescriptions and in all directions for the composition and administration of medicines. This reform has still not reached the stage of majority approval.

These in the year 1849 were the chief interests of the American Medical Association from the point of view of its social, political and economic relationships. The reports of its special committees, however, merit at least a word because of some extraordinary interests. There was a report on the anatomy of the dodo, supposed by some to be a fictitious creation. It seemed, however, that the British *Forensic Medical and Chirurgical Review* of the previous year had published a report that this bird was not fictitious but that it was instead a massive and clumsy bird and that "we cannot form a better idea of it than by imagining a young duck or gosling enlarged to the dimensions of the swan." An investigator was convinced that there was no free hydrochloric acid in the gastric juice, and another insisted that there is nothing whatever to phrenology. Cholera was the major epidemic disease, and a gynecologist was treating dysmenorrhea by dilating the cervix of the uterus. A woman in Kentucky tried to poison her baby by giving it powdered glass, and another woman sued the doctor sixteen months after the baby was born because "he had placed hands upon her person." This action resulted from reading a book which was an attack on male obstetricians. There were extensive reports on the use of ether for anesthesia and a conclusion that all the accidents from anesthesia in the United States had resulted from the inhalation of chloroform. There had been 13 deaths from anesthesia by use of surgeons, 2 by dentists and 2 by people who had breathed chloroform for its pleasurable reactions. Typhoid raged rather widely, as did also an epidemic of streptococcic sore throat called angina, and several outbreaks of dysentery and intestinal disturbances. Cerebrospinal meningitis appeared in epidemics in a good many places, as did yellow fever.

The Committee on Surgery concerned itself also chiefly with anesthesia. Dr. J. Mason Warren had operated in a case of imperforate anus, but the progress of surgery was minute indeed. The Section on Obstetrics was chiefly concerned with misplacements of the uterus, but there was an extensive discussion on ovariotomy, which was spoken of as "this tremendous operation."

There are pages devoted to the right of the physician to use an anesthetic in labor. To this the committee wisely concluded that, "in the more severe obstetric operations, not only may anesthetics be rightfully given but they may not be rightfully withheld."

Extensive indeed was the report of the Committee on Medical Education, which offered a survey of medical education in the countries of Europe and a comparison of their education with the education offered in each of the medical schools of the United States. The continuous publication of such analyses of medical education has been one of the most potent factors in raising the standard of medical education in the United States.

The interest in public health caused the publication in the Transactions of that year of an analysis of the sanitary conditions in many of the most important cities and areas in our country. These pages constitute a source book for those interested in the progress of public health. The report from New Orleans is especially interesting in its attack on inebriety as a means of injury to the public health but more particularly in its endorsement of health education. In presenting the sanitary report of New Orleans, Dr. Edward H. Barton twice repeated the statement of Benjamin Rush that the medical profession was from twenty to thirty years ahead of the public in information in relation to health and that it required about that amount of time for the public to become sufficiently enlightened to realize the value of hygienic laws, observances and improvements.

Reports on drugs and indigenous botany occupied hundreds of pages which would be of little practical value to the physician of today with his specific synthetic chemotherapy.

One consideration for the Association was the question as to whether or not the introduction of water and gas into cities should be under the control of private agencies or municipal agencies.

As the convention came to its close, Dr. Thomas Wood presented a resolution requesting the Committee on Medical Science "to inquire into the expediency of establishing a board to analyze the quack remedies and endorsement now palmed upon the public and to publish the results of their examinations in a newspaper to be established for the purpose; and, further, to append such plain views and explanations thereto as will enlighten the public in regard to the nature and dangerous tendencies of such remedies."

1850

CINCINNATI

The year 1850 saw the convention moving as far west as Cincinnati, and an Ohio physician, Dr. Reuben D. Mussey, was chosen President.

The earlier resolutions on education had begun to bear fruit. A resolution of thanks was tendered to the faculties of the University of Pennsylvania and to the College of Physicians and Surgeons of New York and to all "other institutions which may have conformed to our recommendations." But medical education was still the most troublesome problem. One resolution demanded that young men be not admitted to medicine unless they had good moral character and had exhibited evidence of a good education. Daniel Drake amended this to demand "that the medical schools of the United States should require pupils to remain till the end of the session, whatever may be its length, except when permission may be given to depart," indicating that a good many boys who enrolled departed when the harvesting season or some other similar project demanded their presence elsewhere. Health education of the public was still a desirable object, and Dr. Austin Flint suggested that a popular address on some medical subject should be annually delivered at this Association before the citizens of the place in which the meeting is held. A few scientific papers were read, one the exhibition by Dr. Evans of Chicago, then professor of obstetrics in Rush Medical College, of a device which he called an obstetrical extractor, which he demonstrated on a manikin, and another by Nathan Smith Davis with the peculiar title "Has the Cerebellum Any Special Connection with the Sexual Propensity of Function of Generation?" This proved that there is nothing scientific about phrenology.

A resolution was passed condemning the clerical profession for "often—though, perhaps sometimes, unwarily—yielding their extensive influence in the community in giving currency to quackery and quack medicines."

Again in advance of public opinion and the times, another resolution proposed "that this Association regard it as contrary to its system of ethics for medical journals to advertise nostrums or secret remedies although their composition may have been made known to the editor."

The Association urged its support to the international copyright law. The Committee on Publications again recommended that the medical profession create its own medical literature rather than be subservient to that of England.

A group welcomed the action of the government which proposed to confer military rank on medical officers of the Army.

The meeting, being in Cincinnati, the Transactions are obviously a little less in scope and quantity than those of meetings held in the East nearer the great centers of population.

The Committee on Medical Literature called attention to the fact that a good many editors had already withdrawn to other departments of professional labor, some had tired of their ill-paid toils and thankless duties, and some had been snatched away by the hand of death. For each of these losses the committee expressed its sense of bereavement. Already there were complaints that there were too many medical journals. The committee felt that the average value would be enhanced were the quantity reduced one half. Some of the medical journals, it seemed, had been established by gentlemen connected with medical schools and for the purpose mainly of sustaining the latter. Although the journals published at a distance from great medical centers were uniformly weak, the committee thought that they ought to be encouraged since their difficulties to exist were so great. The committee felt also that "it speaks but feebly in praise of our physicians as scientific investigators, that there are but two experimental memoirs of any importance contained in the journals of the last year." Incidentally one of these dealt with the actions of poisons and the other with the nervous system of the alligator.

Indeed the annual analysis of the medical literature of the day, which had come to be a regular feature at meetings of the American Medical Association, was significant in the gradual improvement in its quality. There is an essay on the functions of the critic or reviewer which might well be an inspiring text to any one essaying that thankless task in modern times. Analyzing the books that had been published in the previous year, the committee felt that the most extensive and important was the first volume of Dr. Daniel Drake's "Treatise on Diseases of the Interior Valley of North America." Incidentally, as an appendix to the report there is a complete bibliography of original articles of interest published in American journals between May 1849 and May 1850.

There follow the usual analyses of medical literature and of medical progress in a variety of fields, with a notable essay by J. Collins Warren on the use of anesthetics. This pointed out that already in his amphitheater in the Massachusetts General Hospital more than a thousand etherizations had been done without an unfortunate result. The introduction of anesthesia had permitted surgical operations not previously possible. J. Collins Warren reported also a number of operations for the removal of cancers and other tumors.

1851

CHARLESTON, S. C.

The fourth annual meeting convened in Charleston, S. C., in 1851. Dr. Alfred Stillé, who had served as secretary of the Association and who had written the memorable report on literature of the previous year, had been compelled to tender his resignation because his health had forced him to seek relaxation abroad.

Conspicuous among those who gave direction and impetus to the work of the American Medical Association during the formative years was Dr. Alfred Stillé of Philadelphia. Dr. Stillé was the son of Swedish emigrants, a graduate of Yale University in 1832 and of the University of Pennsylvania with an A.M. in 1835, the M.D. in 1836 and the LL.D. in 1839. Following his graduation in medicine he became house physician at Blockley under W. W. Gerhard. In association with Gerhard, he is credited with being among the first to make a clear distinction between typhoid fever and typhus. The great epidemic of typhus in Philadelphia in 1836 gave him opportunity for many postmortem examinations which permitted him to make a clear distinction between the two conditions and ultimately to convince the British physicians who had refused to accept such a distinction. In 1854 he became professor of the practice of medicine in the Pennsylvania Medical College, and in 1864 he succeeded the first Dr. Pepper in the chair of medicine at the University of Pennsylvania. He was the first secretary of the American Medical Association, and he was rewarded with the presidency in 1867.

Sir William Osler knew him well, but only after Stillé had passed his seventieth year. Of him Osler wrote "He had none of those irritating features of the old doctor, who, having crawled out of the stream about his fortieth year, sits on the bank, croaking of misfortunes to come, and, with less truth than tongue, lamenting the days that have gone and the men of the past." In his valedictory address Stillé said "Only two things are essential; to live uprightly and to be wisely industrious."

The representative session was largely concerned with whether or not to admit delegates from dentistry and pharmacy into the convention, with an attempt by the Congress to repeal the law that it had passed conferring military rank on military physicians, and with continuing emphasis on the improvement of medical education.

A variety of special committees were suggested to investigate special diseases as well as epidemics. Another committee was established to receive volunteer communications and to offer a prize for the most meritorious. This year the versatile Dr. Davis read a paper on an experimental inquiry concerning the processes of assimilation and nutrition.

For those interested in budgets, the annual expenditures of the Association amounted to $1,100. Since there was a slight surplus in the treasury, some of it was made available for publishing. The prizes for the most meritorious essays came from fifty dollar gifts made by Dr. Alfred Stillé and Dr. F. G. Smith.

1852

RICHMOND, VA.

Richmond got the meeting for 1852, and in due course a Virginia physician, Dr. Beverly R. Wellford, became President. The society adopted a resolution admitting a delegate from the American Medical Society of Paris.

Dr. Austin Flint of Buffalo won the prize for the most meritorious essay out of sixteen voluntary communications. The subject of his essay was "On Variations of Pitch in Percussion and Respiratory Sounds, and Their Application to Physical Diagnosis." The essay received, incidentally, the unanimous vote of the committee.

This year the scandal in transportation of steerage passengers from Europe to the United States attracted the attention of the Association. The following resolution was introduced:

> The accumulation of passengers who are emigrants, crowded in ships coming to our shores from foreign ports, having in a great many instances numerous cases of aggravated fever, many of which prove fatal, and likewise producing similar results at the lazarettos, and even cities; the number, likewise, of sick arriving from California, and some of the South American ports, and the fact that none of these vessels are required by law to have physicians or surgeons on board, seem deserving of our attention as conservators of health, and as an act of humanity and duty on the part of the American Medical Association, to bring these facts respectfully to the consideration of Congress, and to request its legislation thereon; Be it therefore
>
> *Resolved*, That the American Medical Association do memorialize Congress to require all vessels carrying steerage passengers on the sea to have a surgeon on board.
>
> *Resolved*, Further, that a committee of this Association be appointed to draw up a memorial to Congress, making such suggestions as it may deem fit as regards the importance of this measure.

Now there arose also some complaint of doctors not connected with the faculties of the medical schools against the monopolization of practice by the teachers. A resolution was offered suggesting that "it be considered unethical to operate upon the legitimate patient of any other physician, knowing that to be such and that the possible perversion of clinics to the private emolument of those conducting them should be scrupulously guarded against."

A committee was set up to declare the contents of a medicine chest for a merchant ship and the directions that ought to go along with it.

There were new attacks on the quality of medical education and defenses by those who were for the status quo. There were amendments to the constitution and by-laws, with an interesting suggestion that the University of Virginia should be entitled to representation in the Association, notwithstanding the fact that it did not have six professors and that it did not require three years of study.

Some twenty-seven essays had been offered to the committees that were to award the prizes. There came a resolution that one prize of $250 be awarded instead of five prizes of $50 each, but another amendment that there be two prizes of $100 each prevailed.

A good many papers were read by title and offered to the publication committee.

Incidentally the resolution giving special courtesy to the University of Virginia prevailed "but only so long as the present peculiar system of instruction and examination practiced by that institution shall continue in force."

This year the income of the Association doubled but so did its expenditures, so that there was left in the treasury the sum of $56.75.

What had been going on elsewhere in the world that should perhaps have attracted more attention at the assemblages of the American Medical Association than seems to have been given?

In France, Claude Bernard was making fundamental discoveries year after year. In 1848 he had discovered the glycogenic function of the liver. In 1849 he had produced diabetes by puncture of the fourth ventricle, and in 1851 he had explained vasomotor functions of the sympathetic nerves.

In 1844 Addison had described pernicious anemia and adrenal disease. Helmholtz had measured the velocity of the nerve current, and several surgeons had operated to relieve abscess of the brain. The hypodermic syringe was invented in 1852 by Pravaz, and little was it realized how frequent would be its use at the end of one hundred years. In 1853 the Crimean war apparently stirred little interest in the meetings of the American Medical Association, but that was the war in which Florence Nightingale founded the profession of nursing. Today questions of nursing are at the very forefront of all considerations in the field of medical care.

The year 1855 saw the introduction of the laryngoscope by Manual Garcia. The Bunsen burner was invented. J. Marion Sims founded a hospital for women's diseases in New York City. Perkins developed the aniline dyes as coal tar products in 1856; from this first step came such remedies as the salicylates, aspirin and eventually arsphenamine and the sulfonamides. Then in 1857 Graefe introduced his operation for strabismus; Bouchut performed intubation of the larynx.

The operation described by J. Marion Sims in 1852 was the result of a number of discoveries beginning in 1845 which involved the development of the peculiar lateral posture known as the Sims position, the invention of the special curved speculum, the use of silver wire for sutures and of the catheter for emptying the bladder while operating on the uterus. The monumental paper of Sims was published in 1852 in the *American Journal of the Medical Sciences* in Philadelphia. It created a profound impression throughout the world. In 1853 he moved to New York, where he founded the hospital for women, which soon became the center of the best gynecologic work of its time. Such procedures were already beginning to add fame to the progress of medicine in America.

Perhaps the most significant book in these first ten years following the founding of the American Medical Association was Daniel Drake's work on "Diseases of the Interior Valley of North America." As pointed out by Fielding Garrison, this was the result of thirty years of labor based largely on personal observation. The first volume is an encyclopedia of the geography, topography, climate, plants and animals and population of the Mississippi Valley; the second volume, an account of malaria and other fevers and of the various epidemics in their relation to the geography, meteorology and topography of the area concerned. This was the first work of its kind since the treatise of Hippocrates on "Airs, Waters and Places" but went even beyond Hippocrates on its relation of epidemiology to geography. When Alfred Stillé reported on it at the meeting of the American Medical Association in 1850, Drake was greeted with prolonged and thunderous demonstrations of applause and enthusiasm such as had been seldom accorded to any American physician previously. Dr. John Shaw Billings reports that "he covered his face with his hands and wept like a child." Daniel Drake, as described by S. D. Gross, was a tall, commanding figure, simple and dignified in manner. "He was always well dressed, and around his neck he had a long gold watch-chain, which rested loosely upon his vest." He lectured with a splendid voice and with fiery eloquence.

THE END OF THE FIRST DECADE

VIEWING THE DEVELOPMENT of the American Medical Association during the first few years of its existence, Dr. Nathan Smith Davis called attention to the factor which gave force to the activities of the organization. It seemed evident to him that many members had failed to perceive clearly the true relations of the American Medical Association to the medical profession. "They seem to look upon the national organization," he said, "in the same light as a representative civil government, whose acts were laws of binding import and whose basis of representation must consequently be adjusted with the same nice care to the equality of diverse or separate interests." It seemed to be forgotten that the Association was entirely a voluntary organization the acts of which carried with them no other force than the inherent justice of the acts themselves, coupled with the *moral* weight of the body from which they emanated; and that this *moral* weight would bear a close relation to the fulness of representation from those institutions whose interests were most involved in the movements proposed.

1853
NEW YORK CITY

Several years after the preliminary meeting was held in New York in 1846, the American Medical Association met in the Bleecker Street Presbyterian Church. The chairman of the Committee of Arrangements and Reception, Dr. F. Campbell Stewart, expressed the pride of New Yorkers at the triumphant success that had followed the movement originating in their state. At this meeting thirty states and territories, the District of Columbia, the Army and Navy of the United States and the American Medical Society in Paris were represented. The attendance was 573.

A resolution from the Medical Society of Virginia urged the American Medical Association to consider the propriety of appointing some distinguished and well qualified chemist (not a practitioner of medicine) to analyze the prominent nostrums of the day as far as practical and to publish the result of such an analysis monthly in the most extensively circulated newspaper in each state in the Union represented in the Association.

LICENSURE AND EDUCATION

Again the Association indicated its interest in medical education and in epidemiology. Special committees were appointed to urge the passing of legislation for licensure of physicians in the individual states. Indeed one resolution was introduced urging that a student be not admitted to any medical school until he had graduated at some literary institution and was found to possess an English and classical education. Interesting too was a movement to compel the graduates of medical schools to take an oath to conform strictly to the code of ethics of their alma mater and to give to the faculty a right to withdraw the diploma in case the oath should be violated.

A resolution was introduced for the investigation of the value of galvanism as a therapeutic agent.

ACCOMPLISHMENTS OF THE ASSOCIATION

In the presidential address, Dr. Beverly R. Wellford of Virginia summarized in one paragraph the accomplishments of the American Medical Association in its first seven years. He was answering charges made in some quarters that the Association had as yet effected nothing. Some had affirmed that the Association had injured the profession in public estimation by exposing its deficiencies and had thus induced the patronage of homeopathy and other delusions of similar character. To this Dr. Wellford replied:

> But, gentlemen, if it be nothing to have reduced an amorphous, chaotic, professional mass to something like symmetry and order; nothing, to have awakened attention to important defects in preliminary and medical education, and, in some measure, to have removed them; nothing, to have caused the establishment and reorganization of local and State medical societies; nothing, to have caused the enactment of wholesome laws, both by the Federal and State Governments; nothing, to have produced scientific papers of acknowledged ability and erudition; nothing, to have awakened dormant talent, and elicited a vernal bloom, which promises a rich harvest of autumnal fruit; nothing, to have acquired a reputation, which renders even its membership a title of honour and distinction; is it also nothing, by unaided, intrinsic moral power, to have bound in one code of medical ethics, thousands of men in every section of this wide Union, each one free to act according to his own individual views, but yielding them in cheerful obedience to the opinions of the Association, with as much deference and submission as if it were armed with the power and the terrors of penal law? Is it nothing, unendowed with the compulsory authority of legal enactment, or the seductive influence of mileage and per diem pay, annually to convoke such an assembly, as I have now the honour to address? Gentlemen, such a congress, of such materials, and under such circumstances, presents a spectacle of moral beauty, to which the opponents of medical reform cannot be insensible. It must command their respect and admiration, even if it fail to secure their co-operation. I know not, gentlemen, what may be the effect on others of an occasion like this, but for my single self, when I thus recognize the denizen of the city and the forest; him of the frozen north and of the sunny south; him of the mountains, the rivers, and the prairies of the west, with him from the borders of the broad Atlantic bringing their various opinions and prejudices, and casting them together, as a sacrificial offering on the altar of science and professional patriotism; when I see them animated by the same honour-

able and lofty impulse, and, in fraternal harmony, uniting their efforts to attain the same grand results, I feel an honest pride in my profession and my country, and an abiding confidence, that, to such sons, the high destinies of both may be safely intrusted.

By this time Dr. N. S. Davis had begun to manifest his special interest in the medical literature of the day; he had now become chairman of the Committee on Medical Literature. He presented a report calling attention to the transactions of the individual state medical societies and the various monographs and books that had been published during the year. Much of his report dealt with his concept of the true functions of the editors of medical journals.

The prize essay was an article on "The Cell: Its Physiology, Pathology, and Philosophy; as Deduced from Original Investigations, to Which Is Added Its History and Criticism," by Waldo J. Burnett of Boston.

1854
ST. LOUIS

The President, Dr. Jonathan Knight, was unable to attend the St. Louis session in 1854; hence the address for the occasion was presented by the Vice President, Dr. Usher Parsons of Rhode Island.

The prize essay was that of Dr. Daniel Brainard of Chicago. The title was "Essay on a New Method of Treating Ununited Fractures and Certain Deformities of the Osseous System." Each of the contestants identified his essay with an appropriate quotation. Daniel Brainard chose a quotation from Ambroise Paré, which is one of the great classics of medical science:

notwithstanding all the pains that I have heretofore taken, I have reason to praise God, in that it hath pleased Him to call me to that branch of Medical practice, commonly called Surgery, which can neither be bought by gold, nor by silver, but by industry alone, and long experience.

Already some attention began to be given to pedagogics in medicine; a resolution was offered, though promptly rejected, "that the practice of professors' reading lectures to their classes, no matter with how much care selected from the musty records of antiquity, is a miserable apology for teaching, is *primâ facie* evidence of their inaptitude to instruct, and is inimical to medical progress."

Well in advance of the times also was a resolution offered by Dr. N. S. Davis calling the attention of the Association to the "great sacrifice of health and life which takes place annually, especially among children in large cities, on account of the difficulty of procuring a proper supply of pure and wholesome milk; and the great importance of devising some mode by which the nutritious constituents of the milk can be preserved in their purity and sweetness for such purposes." He exhibited to the Association a specimen of dried milk which had been placed in his hands and which was represented to be capable of preserving all the qualities of the milk perfectly for any length of time. This, it must be remembered, was in the year 1854.

At this time an announcement greeted with great pleasure was made by the local Committee on Arrangements. All the railroads, except the New York and Hudson River Railroad, had granted to the members of the American Medical Association free passage to their homes.

Another resolution urged that a committee be appointed to examine into and report on the effects of alcoholic liquors taken into the system on health and disease.

A final action failed to be taken on a resolution that the cultivation and practice of specialties in medicine and surgery are legitimate and honorable pursuits and meet the approval of the Association and that the same avenues for announcing his calling to the public that are recognized as proper to the general practitioner are open to the specialist.

On Friday morning, May 6, 1853, the day after the adjournment of the sixth annual meeting of the American Medical Association held in the city of New York, a train of the New York and New Haven Railroad passing through Norwalk, Conn., fell into the Norwalk River through an open drawbridge. Forty-four passengers of the ill-fated train were suddenly deprived of life, among them seven physicians returning from the convention. As a memorial to these physicians the convention in 1854 published a record of their medical careers.

1855

PHILADELPHIA

By 1855 the number of prize essays, which had numbered a score or more at previous meetings, had steadily diminished. Only six essays were available for consideration by the Committee on Prize Essays in 1855. Only one of these was considered worthy of notice—a paper on "Statistics of Placenta Previa" by James D. Trask of White Plains, Westchester County, N. Y.

Well in advance of the times, however, was a resolution urging the secretary of the Association to offer every facility possible to the reporters of the public press to enable them to furnish full and accurate reports of the transactions.

As an indication that the nature of man does not change, it became necessary, previous to reading a report on the "Hygrometrical

States of the Atmosphere in Various Localities, and Its Influence on Health," which was seriously interrupted by the loud conversation of members, to pass a resolution, unanimously, "that all the desultory conversation of members be done down stairs."

Realizing the importance of vital statistics, a resolution was introduced urging the Association to petition legislative bodies in the individual states to collect their vital statistics.

HOMEOPATHY VS. REGULAR MEDICINE

For the first time the battle between homeopathy and regular medicine reared its ugly head in the convention. Because the legislature of Michigan, in contravention to the charter of the University of Michigan, had put in a chair of homeopathy, a resolution was offered "That any such unnatural union as the mingling of an exclusive system, such as homeopathy, with scientific medicine in a school, setting aside all questions of its untruthfulness, cannot fail, by the destruction of union and confidence, and the production of confusion and disorder, unsettling and distracting the mind of the learners, to so far impair the usefulness of teaching as to render every school adopting such a policy unworthy of the support of the profession." This resolution was passed unanimously by the Association.

THE STATE SOCIETIES

For the first time also the authority of the national body in relation to state societies came into question; it was resolved that no state or local society should be entitled to representation in this Association which had not adopted its code of ethics, that no state or local society which had violated or discarded any article or clause should be entitled to representation and that since the State Medical Society of Ohio had violated one of the articles of the code of ethics by adopting a resolution "That it is not derogatory to medical dignity, or inconsistent with medical honor, for medical gentlemen to take out a patent right for surgical or medical instruments," therefore, be it resolved "that the secretary of this Association be directed to inform the officers of the State Medical Society of Ohio that, unless such action be rescinded, it cannot hereafter be represented in this Association."

1856

DETROIT

The "Firemen's Hall" in Detroit was the place of assemblage for the 1856 session. The number of delegates had fallen to 208, representing nineteen states, the Minnesota Territory and the United States Army.

Perhaps most significant of the considerations were those related to medical literature, urging a wider use of American articles and American medical textbooks in teaching.

The number of essays submitted for prizes had fallen still further; a resolution suggested that hereafter the money be awarded for the best essay founded on original investigations of the author.

A committee was established to classify those diseases which involved a derangement of the mental manifestations.

An expression of thanks was tendered to the Fire Department of the City of Detroit for the use of its large and commodious hall. Also it was resolved "that the urbane deportment and the elegant hospitalities of the profession and private individuals, as well as the polite attentions of citizens generally, demand of this Association a high appreciation of the cultivated manners of this city of the West, and which has tended greatly to enhance the pleasure of the session here of the delegates from abroad."

The President of the Association gloried in the progress that it had made in uniting the medical profession so that it could speak with one voice and in rallying physicians everywhere around higher standards.

AMERICAN MEDICAL LITERATURE

S. D. Gross of Louisville presented the significant report on American medical literature, analyzing the causes for its backwardness in the tradition of the original essay by Oliver Wendell Holmes. His main criticism was a lack of independence in the journalism of that day with its leaning on materials coming from abroad. He urged physicians to utilize their private and hospital practice for the study of cases which should be reported in American medical journals. And he offered as a resolution "That this Association earnestly and respectfully recommend, first, the universal adoption, whenever practicable, by our schools, of American works as textbooks for their pupils; secondly, the discontinuance of the practice of editing foreign writings; thirdly, a more independent course of the medical periodical press toward foreign productions, and a more liberal one toward American; and, fourthly, a better and more efficient employment of the facts which are continually furnished by our public institutions for the elucidation of the nature of diseases and accidents and, indirectly, for the formation of an original, a vigorous and an independent national medical literature.

"That we venerate the writings of the great medical men, past and present, of our country, and that we consider them as an important element of our professional and national glory.

"That we shall always hail with pleasure any useful or valuable works emanating from the English press, and that we shall always extend to them a cordial welcome as books of reference, to acquaint us with the progress of legitimate medicine abroad, and to enlighten us in regard to any new facts of which they may be the repositories."

Significant also was the report of the Committee on Plans for Organization of State and County Societies. It worked toward a unified organization, and it prepared the first constitution and by-laws for a state medical society.

1857
NASHVILLE

Nashville, Tenn., welcomed the doctors for the tenth annual meeting in 1857; bursts of Southern oratory reverberated in the air. Following is a paragraph from the address of welcome by Dr. C. K. Winston:

> You are the representatives of a profession distinguished alike for its antiquity, its scientific attainments and its usefulness. It constitutes the true link between science and philanthropy—science and philanthropy, moral, intellectual and physical. You come from every portion of this glorious republic—from the Kennebec to the Rio Grande—from orange groves and golden sands—from mountains clad in eternal snow and valleys smiling in perpetual verdure. You come not for purposes of self aggrandizement or personal ambition, nor yet to advance the schemes of parties or stir up the antipathies of sections. "You know no North, no South, no East, no West"; but you come as a company of philanthropists, a band of brethren, that you may pour the acquisitions of another year into a common treasury, kneel side by side at a common altar and drink the living water as it gushes from a common fountain. You have come to maintain the dignity, to elevate the ensign of a profession to which you have devoted your lives and to which you have linked your fortunes.

Protests were made against the admission of delegates from the Oglethorpe Medical College, Savannah, on the ground that the professorships had not been filled in physiology and materia medica at its sessions, but investigation revealed that all of the chairs but one had been filled and that the man was sick, so that the college was permitted to have its delegates.

Some of the committees which had regularly reported began to report that they had no report.

Now there began apparently to be some despair at the failure to progress in regulating education. Following a resolution demanding a minimum number of teachers and hours of study, an alternative resolution was offered to the effect that the Association did not have the power to control medical education and that it had most signally failed in its objective and had already introduced elements of discord. It was therefore recommended that a special committee be appointed to advise a system of medical instruction under which all medical institutions should be organized. There was great discussion but to no purpose.

A constitution for the state societies was adopted and, after hearing a number of scientific reports, the convention adjourned.

EDITORIAL OPINION OF THE ASSOCIATION

In 1855 Dr. D. M. Reese, editor of the *American Medical Gazette*, satirically minimized the work of the American Medical Association up to that time, saying:

> The conviction appears to be general, among writers, that notwithstanding the numerous reforms attempted, recommended and resolved on by repeated *"whereases"* and reiterated at every successive meeting by high-sounding resolutions, and published in each volume of the *Transactions*, yet, in *effectuating any one of these, after seven years' trial, the efforts of the Association in this regard have resulted in signal and utter failure.*

Editors of some other medical journals gave rise to sentiments of similar import. Dr. Nathan Smith Davis told them that their announcements of policy were premature. "It must be borne in mind," he said, "that our country is made up of more than thirty separate states; that the Association was, and is, not only destitute of legislative powers itself but also without access to any one legislative body possessing authority to regulate the education and interests of the profession of the whole country."

Little could any one have thought that another half century at least would be required before sufficient public opinion could be mustered within and without the medical profession to undertake a real drive for high standards in medical education.

Dr. B. Dowler, then editor of the *New Orleans Medical and Surgical Journal*, summarized the accomplishments of the first ten years of the American Medical Association in these words:

> As a social and professional *reunion* of kindred spirits and great minds, its memories afford perennial delight. It has given impetus to the progress of medical polity and science; it exercises moral suasion rather than that of authority; it has brought together a bright constellation of intellect, cemented the bonds of friendship among good men and true, and should it fail to effectuate its original and grand finality—that is, a thorough reform in medical education—it will leave a luminous track of light in the moral firmament of the Aesculapian heavens, throughout the expansions of the Republic.

THE CIVIL WAR LOOMS

1858
WASHINGTON, D. C.

THE CODE OF ETHICS was not merely window dressing; conspicuous in the session of 1858 was an apology by Dr. David M. Reese for having put on the staff of the Blockley Hospital of Philadelphia a physician who had been expelled from the American Medical Association for a violation of the Code of Ethics. The apology of Dr. Reese stirred a tempest; by the third day of the session the delegates were convened as a committee of the whole on a motion to reconsider, and Dr. Reese amended his apology by adding the words that he "regretted the action taken."

Throughout the nation there was great turmoil, for these were the years before the Civil War; but there is nothing in the discussions of the American Medical Association at that time indicating any thought that war was impending. The basic questions leading to the war were not discussed, nor is there any action indicating movement toward medical preparedness.

Most of the discussions were concerned with the reports of the committees on epidemics and on literature. American physicians had begun to take pride in their own publications. Again Austin Flint won the essay contest with a paper on "The Clinical Study of the Heart Sounds in Health and Disease."

The report on medical education was brief; the evidence indicated that standards were slowly improving. The number of scientific contributions was small.

Appended to the permanent transactions of the Association were the complete principles of Ethics, a practice that has been followed since that time.

1859
LOUISVILLE, KY.

In welcoming the members to Louisville in the following year the community took pride in informing the members of the American Medical Association of its two medical libraries containing, respectively, 4,000 and 8,000 volumes.

For the first time at the 1859 convention definite action was taken urging the legislatures of the individual states to pass laws that would control the practice of illegal abortion.

Only six essays had been submitted to the essay committee.

By this time, however, the Association had so modified its original constitution that it became necessary to issue a revision of the so-called "Plan of Organization," so that all the members could understand the various functions and technics concerned in the various committees, boards and other agencies.

Still the transactions say nothing whatever indicating that the nation was trembling on the verge of a great war.

1860
NEW HAVEN, CONN.

By the 1860 session Dr. N. S. Davis thought that a little more order ought to be introduced into the manner of the meeting. A resolution was offered that the morning meetings be devoted to the work of the Association and the afternoon sessions to the hearing of papers and discussions on scientific subjects.

The address of the President, Dr. Henry Miller, brought up openly the question of illegal abortion. On behalf of the American Medical Association, he urged action by legislatures in every state against this practice. Dr. Miller reviewed the growth of the Association and asked for renewed effort toward raising the standards of medical education.

1863
CHICAGO

The thirteenth annual meeting of the American Medical Association had been held in New Haven, Conn., in June of 1860. The next session—the fourteenth—convened in Chicago on June 2, 1863. Early in 1861 the usual notices for the regular meeting were issued. The preliminary arrangements were made. Then, according to Dr. N. S. Davis, "the sectional animosity and wickedness which had been threatening the peace of our country for several years culminated in an open, unjustifiable and monstrous rebellion." Letters were received from most of the active members of the Association asking postponement of the annual meeting. Although there was nothing in the constitution and by-laws to authorize either the officers or any one else to postpone a regular meeting, the committee finally decided to postpone until June 1862. Just about that time the battles of Belmont, Fort Donelson and Shiloh occurred; most of the members of the medical profession were needed in the prosecution of the war.

The meeting was postponed until June 1863; in February Chicago was selected as the place of meeting. Another difficulty now arose: a decision by the convention of railroad officers that there would be no further commutation of railroad fares. However, a special meeting of the railroad executives permitted them to make a commutation rate for attendance on the National Canal Convention, which was held in Chicago at the same time. The delegates to the American Medical Association were invited to sit in the National Canal Convention, where they were recorded as delegates and thereby got free tickets home.

A considerable number of delegates assembled in Bryan Hall; some of the meetings were held in the Methodist Church Block.

Apparently the Surgeon General of the Army had issued an order prohibiting the use of calomel and antimony. The American Medical Association appointed a committee to find out why. Another committee was established to see whether vaccination against smallpox should not be compulsory throughout the United States. Majority and minority reports were received on the use of calomel and antimony in the Army, and the whole subject received a most spirited discussion. A statement from the Surgeon General indicated that the use of both calomel and tartar emetic had been abused; he believed that more harm resulted from the use of both these agents than benefit from their proper administration. Many of the committee thought that this charge by the Surgeon General was entirely unwarranted. They felt that he was giving impressions and that he did not have good statistical evidence to support his opinion. Then, getting even stronger, they said that he had "committed a most grievous offense against the dignity, usefulness and humanity of our profession; that he has heaped unmerited *insult* on an intelligent, scientific and humane corps of army surgeons; that he has injured, in a most serious manner, the regular profession. We regard the order as an unwarrantable assumption of authority and a reckless attempt to cut the Gordian knot of intricate pathology by the exercise of official power." They considered his circular unwise; the withholding of ordinary medicines implied a want of confidence in the skill of physicians; they recommended that he either withdraw the circular or rewrite it.

Another resolution said that the railroads were fast becoming the great medium of land travel and that they were having many serious accidents without good medical provisions to meet them.

A long resolution called attention to the fact that the doctors in the Army were not given adequate rank and demanded that they be placed in a rank in all respects equal to and on the same footing with other officers in the service. This insufficient recognition of medical services by the line officers and the statesmen is a perennial source of dissatisfaction. When the wars end, the civilian doctors receive high praise. But proper status has never been accorded either them or doctors in the regular military services.

At this convention another fundamental action was recognition of ophthalmology as a distinct specialty in the field of medicine. Medical schools were encouraged to establish chairs in this field.

1864
NEW YORK CITY

When the Association met in New York in 1864 Dr. Nathan Smith Davis of Illinois, founder of the American Medical Association, received a reward by his election to the presidency. Apparently this nomination was not satisfactory to all; a resolution was offered to send it back to the nominating committee with the request that the committee nominate at least two persons for the presidency, to be elected by ballot. This resolution was lost and Dr. Davis was elected.

Only one resolution on the war seems to have been offered at this session, a memorial to the President of the United States respecting the necessity for the organization of an ambulance system for the U. S. Army.

More than thirty-five committees brought reports on all sorts of subjects, both scientific and political, and there were reports from the usual standing committees.

Again as the session ended there was a resolution from New York urging the President of the United States to take such action as shall cause "all medicines and medical and surgical instruments and appliances to be excluded from the list of articles called 'contraband of war,' and that such articles in any quantity may be purchased by any person in any state of the Union, and may be conveyed beyond our lines under a flag of truce" to the people in the Southern blockaded cities. Furthermore, it was resolved that "every member be requested to use all of the influence in his power in stripping this fratricidal war of some of its unnecessary horrors and thereby to inaugurate the reestablishment of more kindly feelings, and to smooth away some of the obstructions to the reconciliation of our misguided brethren." Of course there were no delegates from south of the Mason and Dixon Line at the convention. However, one physician moved promptly to lay this highly idealistic resolution on the table. Another physician moved to add the word "indefinitely." That was passed.

By this time, moreover, there had begun to be some dissatisfaction with the nominating committee which offered just one nomination for president. A resolution was offered to amend the by-laws providing for nominations from the floor. The question was raised of the right of Dr. William Thomas Green Morton to receive any vast sum for his discovery of anesthesia or for a patent on anesthesia, and the delegates voted unanimously to oppose such action.

In the *Medical and Surgical Reporter*, a weekly medical journal published in Philadelphia, the issue for Jan. 14, 1865 made a critical review of the progress of the American Medical Association. It suggested omission of proofreading by authors to hasten publication of the Transactions. The Philadelphia editor pointed out the undemocratic character of the technic of choosing delegates. A large county medical society near the place of the meeting could dominate the session. He wanted to do away with the nominating committee. And, he ended, "It is of great importance that the machinery of the Association be made as perfect as possible, for we believe that, rightly managed, it can be made to exert very great influence for good on the profession of this country and of the world."

MEDICAL PROGRESS

THE YEARS FROM 1859 to 1863 provided a short but significant list of steps in permanent medical advancement in the United States and in the world as a whole. The discovery by Pasteur of anaerobic bacteria, the mapping by Broca of the speech center in the brain, Raynaud's description of symmetric gangrene and Pasteur's detection of silkworm disease were first steps toward a sudden flowering of medical knowledge. There was no single great discovery, like anesthesia, to seize the imagination of all the world. The Civil War, which swept the United States from 1861 to 1865, was a damper on research.

The year 1865 saw the publication of Mendel's memoir on plants. In 1866 Voit established the first hygienic laboratory in Munich and Graefe described sympathetic ophthalmia. The first International Medical Congress was held at Paris in 1867 and the *American Journal of Obstetrics* was founded in the United States in 1869.

Indeed all the years up to 1876 were years of slow progress. J. Marion Sims had published his notes on uterine surgery; Esmarch introduced his first-aid bandage. There were more studies on localization of areas in the brain. Laryngology began to be demarcated as a specialty, and a laryngologic society was established in New York. As early as 1874, Paul Ehrlich introduced dried blood serums and introduced staining methods for blood cells and other tissues of the body. The name of Weir Mitchell did not appear among those interested in the American Medical Association but he had introduced his rest cure in 1875. Great Britain passed a public health act and the English Food Adulteration act in the same year, which marked also the founding of the Boston Medical Library. In fact, the year which marked the centennial of freedom in the United States also saw the founding of Johns Hopkins University and the introduction of the telephone. What would medical practice be like today without the telephone?

1865
BOSTON

The meeting of 1865 resulted in the introduction and adoption of a resolution which has had a profound effect on the quality of medical literature in the United States. Each year since then it has been sent to every physician who obtains a place on the program of the Annual Session of the American Medical Association. The resolution is a guide to the executive committees of the individual Sections of the Association in recommending papers to the Editor of THE JOURNAL. The resolution, introduced by Dr. Robert Burns, reads:

> "*Resolved*, That the several Sections of this Association be requested, in the future, to refer no papers or reports to the Committee of Publication, except such as can be fairly classed under one of the three following heads, viz: 1st. Such as may contain and establish *positively* new facts, modes of practice, or principles of real value. 2d. Such as may contain the results of well-devised original, experimental researches. 3d. Such as present so complete a review of the facts on any particular subject as to enable the writer to deduce therefrom legitimate conclusions of importance.
>
> "*Resolved*, That the several Sections be requested, in the future, to refer all such papers as may be presented to them for examination by this Association, that contain matter of more or less value, and yet cannot be fairly ranked under either of the heads mentioned in the foregoing resolution, back to their authors with the recommendation that they be published in such regular medical periodicals as said authors may select, with the privilege of placing at the head of such papers, 'Read to the   Section of the American Medical Association on the   day of   18 .'"

The Association had become active in establishing ethical considerations, particularly as related to advertising and promotion of individual physicians in the public press. Several physicians had been dropped from their local medical societies. The House of Delegates of the American Medical Association had confirmed their expulsion. At a previous session a resolution was introduced affecting Dr. Montrose A. Pallen. It was alleged that he had imperiled the lives of thousands of people in the city of New York by participating in a plot to poison the Croton reservoir by which the city is supplied with drinking water. The action followed the report of a military committee in Washington. Now a distinguished group, including more than thirty-five of the leading physicians of America, protested the previous action and asserted that the guilt of Dr. Pallen had never been established. The resolution was referred to a committee, which pointed out that this was the first time that a group before the Association had protested an action of the majority. They suggested that the evidence indicated that Dr. Montrose A. Pallen had left St. Louis early in the war in the interests of the rebellion and that the testimony pointed toward his complicity in the attempt to poison the water in the Croton reservoir. After this report was read, a telegram came from Dr. Pallen charging that the man who had testified against him had been proved the perpetrator of an infamous perjury. With this confusion of data before the meeting, the resolution was laid on the table. The following year when the committee to which the matter had been referred found that the statements on which his expulsion was based were entirely unfounded, Dr. Pallen was restored to membership. He expressed himself highly gratified by the action of the Association and thanked the members.

PRESIDENTIAL ADDRESS OF NATHAN SMITH DAVIS

Notable among the presidential addresses that had been delivered to the American Medical Association was the address by Nathan Smith Davis in 1865. He expressed the congratulations of all on the fact that the United States were again united. "The climax of human wickedness," he said, "had been reached" in the murder of the Chief Magistrate. The year had witnessed the death, too, of Drs. Jonathan Knight of New Haven, Conn., and Valentine Mott of New York.

Twenty years had passed since the first call for the formation of the American Medical Association. Dr. Davis was greatly disappointed that the meetings were now so taken up with events that proper consideration was not being given to some of the most significant interests. He said, "Whenever medical education became the theme of discussion, those more interested in the reading and discussion of papers and reports of a direct scientific and practical character were ever ready to restrict debate, refer the subject to committees or in some other way avoid what they regarded as a mere waste of time. On the other hand, if the reading of an elaborate scientific paper was commenced the author would seldom complete the first half dozen pages before the zealous advocate of educational reform would dispose of the whole subject by a motion to dispense with further reading and to refer the document directly to the Committee of Publication." The good natured lovers of good dinners and sight-seeing would always be ready to aid the other parties with their votes and to secure the acceptance of every invitation to an entertainment, an excursion or a public institution.

During the years all sorts of attempts had been made to control these difficulties by modifying the Constitution or the By-Laws. Standing committees had been abolished and committees on special subjects substituted. Papers requiring more than ten pages of manuscript were compelled to be presented in abstract, and the Committee on Arrangements had been instructed to check the evils of extravagant and costly entertainments by omitting all such from the program of arrangements.

None of these reforms had been satisfactory. "The attempt to eliminate from the program the entertainments," he said, "has resulted only in exchanging one magnificent public banquet occupying one evening for three or four private ones during the annual sessions of the Association." The Association was being criticized because its annual meetings partook more of the character of gourmandizing and sight-seeing than of grave, professional and scientific inquiry.

Nevertheless the Association had made great progress in its fundamental effort to improve medical education. Dr. Davis, therefore, proposed a plan relative to entertainments, which has been followed since that time by the American Medical Association. It is well to read the proposal in his own words:

> But the arrangements for that evening should be such as would permit the most free and cordial intercourse. A public hall should be provided in which gentlemen and ladies could mingle and promenade freely; where each could seek out his old friends and make the acquaintance of new ones; where wit, repartee, and, if need be, songs, sentiments, and speeches could be made to enliven the evening. A simple stand might be placed in some corner, where all who wished could obtain a dish of ice cream, strawberries or other fruit, and cup of coffee. But there should be neither ostentatious show, nor rich viands, nor strong drinks, for the acknowledged guardians of the public health should not, especially in their highest representative capacity, themselves publicly violate the plainest laws of hygiene.

This farsighted man made other proposals which have been effective. He recommended that each Section be authorized to choose its own officers who should prevail for a year; that each Section adopt well considered rules to govern the reading, discussion and final disposition of all reports, papers and questions that came before it; he suggested that each Section be provided with either a skilful secretary or a professional reporter who would provide a summary of all discussions on scientific questions and papers. He pointed out that results can "never be accomplished by any amount, either of good *wishes* or *fault-finding;* but by prompt, persevering, disinterested action."

1866

BALTIMORE

The first distinguished guest to appear at the meeting of the American Medical Association attended the meeting in 1866 and gave an address. He was Dr. Brown-Séquard, founder of our science of endocrinology and renowned throughout the world for his magnificent contributions in this field.

This year was notable for the majority and minority reports of the Committee on Medical Ethics dealing with specialization. The majority report listed the advantages of specialization as including minuteness in observation, acuteness in study, wideness of observation, skill in diagnosis, multiplicity of invention and superior skill in manipulation. The disadvantages were a narrowness of view, a tendency to magnify unduly the diseases which the specialty covers, a tendency to undervalue the treatment of special diseases by general practitioners, some temptation to the employment of undue measures for gaining a popular reputation and a tendency to increased fees. The advantages far outweighed the disadvantages from the point of view of the patient and of the advancement of the specialty. The committee felt that these disadvantages could be overcome if the specialist would begin as a general practitioner and gradually grow into his specialty.

The committee was especially concerned with the means by which the specialist made himself known to the community. They felt that there should be no advertising either in newspapers or medical journals.

The minority report was signed by Dr. Henry I. Bowditch. He considered that the whole tendency of modern science was toward specialism but he felt also that the Association had no business passing on the question of the advertisements unless they were evidently of a mountebank character. It was his opinion that "any Association would be better occupied in the hearing of able papers and in discussions on all subjects connected with medicine than in any movements for the mere discipline of erring members."

When these reports had been presented to the delegates they were referred to the Committee on Publication, and a motion introduced by Dr. J. Solis-Cohen of Philadelphia which suggested that these be a special order of business at the meeting in 1867 was adopted.

1867
CINCINNATI

Although N. S. Davis had remonstrated against entertainments on too lavish a scale in 1866, the convention which met in Cincinnati in 1867 had a mighty good time. The program lists a half dozen private receptions, a public reception by the physicians of Cincinnati, a steamboat excursion at the expense of the City Council, an exhibition of steam fire engines by the chief of the Fire Department, a little reception for the delegates on the closing day by the proprietors of Longworth's Wine House and an excursion to the Longview Lunatic Asylum.

There were the usual resolutions on the advancement of medical education and on the rank of medical men in the Army and Navy, with the conclusion that a committee should see the President of the United States and the Secretary of the Navy to urge adoption of the changes recommended.

Dr. Allen March of Cincinnati had been able to collect photographs of all the Presidents of the Association and it was moved that they be consigned to the archives.

As a result of action taken in a previous meeting, the delegates from the medical colleges of the country had been assembled in Cincinnati and had adopted certain principles of standardization which the American Medical Association now approved. The Association of American Medical Colleges and the Council on Medical Education now cooperate closely in maintaining standards. Again the American Medical Association urged the states to set up licensure for physicians, but a resolution asking members of the medical profession not to patronize druggists who manufactured nostrums was rejected.

At this early date there were already medical politicos who thought a great deal would be gained in the way of prestige for the American Medical Association if it could only have close contact with Washington. Indeed this argument convinced even N. S. Davis, so he offered a resolution suggesting that the next Annual Session of the American Medical Association be held in the city of Washington and that it be held there every second year thereafter. Still on the somewhat teetotalitarian and puritanic side, his resolution also suggested that whenever the Association met in Washington the Committee on Arrangements be strictly forbidden either to provide themselves or accept provision by others of any entertainment or excursion whatever. With due caution the convention amended this resolution, adopting it except that the meeting should be held in Washington until otherwise ordered and that entertainments or excursions were forbidden if they conflicted with the regular business of the body or its sections.

From Pennsylvania came a resolution urging the members of the faculty of the University of Pennsylvania and the Jefferson Medical College to join their county medical societies and participate with the rest of the medical profession in the work of the American Medical Association.

Dr. G. C. Cox, who had attended a meeting of the British Medical Association as the first delegate from the American Medical Association, indicated that he had been most graciously received by our British colleagues.

1868

WASHINGTON, D. C.

The meeting in Washington, D. C., was marked by visits to the President, the Chief Justice, the Speaker of the House of Representatives, the Army Medical Museum and the Mayor of Washington—each of whom gave receptions for the delegates. Furthermore, on Thursday night, May 7, the Capitol was lighted and the dome illuminated from 8 until 9 p. m. These multitudinous political receptions apparently minimized other features of the convention, for the volume of *Transactions* of that year is the slimmest of its generation.

The Committee on Medical Ethics had a report signed by Dr. H. I. Bowditch alone. The *Transactions* state simply:

> Dr. Bowditch had become chairman by the death of two of his colleagues. He had been unable to elicit any replies from his two other colleagues, and therefore was compelled to act in his individual capacity.

For the first time the bitter and burning question of women doctors came to the fore. Dr. Bowditch strongly advocated the recognition of regularly educated and otherwise well qualified female physicians. This resolution was made a special order of business.

As the meeting was in Washington, Senator Drake of Missouri, who visited the convention, was invited to a seat on the platform and entertained the Association with some remarks in allusion to his connection with the medical art through his father, the late Prof. Daniel Drake.

When the resolution on women doctors came to consideration, it was discussed at some length and then consideration was indefinitely postponed.

As evidence that the bitter feelings of the war had been dissipated, the Association elected as President Dr. William O. Baldwin of Alabama, who made a beautiful address in behalf of the Southern physicians. Among his concluding paragraphs was the following inspiring statement:

> For myself, and for those whom I represent, I grasp with unaffected pleasure the hand which you have so gracefully and magnanimously offered, and I hope and believe this sentiment will meet a ready response from all our brethren of the South. *Let us again be united as friends and brothers.* Ignoring past and present political differences, let us exhibit to this distracted country an example of forgiveness and toleration worthy of the emulation of a great and noble people. Let the bonds which we acknowledge here bind us in all portions of this broad land as a sacred brotherhood, engaged in a common toil, with one mind, one heart, and one purpose. Let the place annually selected for our meetings be our Mecca. There let us meet with harmony of sentiment for thorough organization, for connected and concerted action, without which no great science or art can ever attain its highest perfection. Exacting from each other only the qualifications necessary for honorable membership, let us there mingle in the sacred precincts of our humane profession, and join hands and sympathies in the strengthening influences of association and fellowship; and as we lay fresh offerings in the temple of a noble science, and build new fires on her altars, let us cherish in our hearts the ennobling sentiment of brotherly love.

Again at this meeting in Washington, the Association heard a word of praise from a President who was among the greatest of the leaders of American medicine in this country. Dr. Samuel D. Gross, who had been associated with teaching in medical schools in Louisville and in Philadelphia, urged particularly the establishment of suitable training for nurses. He said:

> I am not aware that the education of nurses has received any attention from this body; a circumstance the more surprising when we consider the great importance of the subject. It seems to me to be just as necessary to have well-trained, well-instructed nurses as to have intelligent and skilful physicians. I have long been of the opinion that there ought to be, in all the principal towns and cities of the Union, institutions for the education of men and women whose duty it is to take care of the sick, and to carry out the injunctions of the medical attendant. There is hardly one nurse, of either sex, in twenty who has a perfect appreciation of the requirements of the sick-room, or who is capable of affording the aid and comfort so necessary to a patient when oppressed by disease or injury. It does not matter what may be the skill of the medical practitioner, how assiduous or faithful he may be in the discharge of his functions, as a guardian of health and life, his efforts can be of comparatively little avail unless they are seconded by an intelligent and devoted nurse. We need in this country a million of Florence Nightingales, and at least half that number of John Howards, to aid our physicians in their strife with disease and death. Myriads of human beings perish annually, in the so-called civilized world, for the want of good nursing.

The committee which reported on the recommendations and suggestions contained in the President's address recommended the adoption of a resolution which would set forth the views of the President regarding the education of nurses and strongly recommended the establishment in all of our large cities of training schools for nurses.

1869

NEW ORLEANS

Still further demonstrating the desire for complete *rapprochement* with the Southern contingent, the convention of 1869 met in New Orleans, where they were warmly greeted by the full attendance of the Southern physicians.

At this time an Association of American Medical Editors was formed. The president, Dr. William O. Baldwin, struck a forlorn note as he viewed the accomplishments in relationship to medical education. He said:

> The plan of action you have adopted, that of endeavoring to induce forty or fifty medical colleges, with conflicting interests, to agree voluntarily upon a "uniform and elevated standard of requirements for the degree of M.D.," and adopt it in good faith, has become almost a Utopian idea, a forlorn hope. Though urged with all the force that truth could impart, and enforced with all the appealing earnestness that the gravity of the subject could inspire, yet your views and wishes have not impressed themselves on the schools to such an extent as to change their course of action. It seems to me that all hope of reform through this means must be abandoned. Nor can we expect to reach the end proposed by measures of State legislation. The obstacles here are too palpable to need enumeration. They are many, and they are unsurmountable. Almost any body of medical men may obtain a charter for a medical college in most of the States of this Union, with pretty much such regulations and privileges as they may agree upon among themselves and ask for.

I despair, therefore, of seeing this Association attain its object through any of the agencies heretofore employed. If, however, this great work *ought* to be done, it *can* be done. I believe it is within the reach of the power of this Association. But I can see no mode by which it can be accomplished, except through FEDERAL LEGISLATION.

Perhaps the most significant statement made at the 1869 convention was that of Samuel D. Gross who had been the delegate to Great Britain. Here comes the first suggestion for a weekly medical journal owned by the Association as a necessary project for the advancement of medicine in our country and the promotion of the work of the Association.

Significant also was the continuing drive toward the prohibition of alcoholic liquors. The *Transactions* contain a report of almost 100 pages on the relations of alcohol to medicine, ending with an apology because the report is not longer. The report was made by a believer in teetotalism and provides such a horrible list of mental disturbances, crimes and other reactions resulting from too much participation in the "demon rum" as to have frightened any one other than the hardy citizens who heard it.

1870
WASHINGTON, D. C.

As the delegates assembled in Washington for the Twenty-First Annual Session in 1870, there were signs of disaffection within the Association. Majority and minority reports from the Committee on Arrangements were promptly referred to the Committee on Ethics for decision. Several members took a hand in the argument. Eventually it developed that the Massachusetts Medical Society was tolerating in its midst men acknowledged to have become homeopaths and eclectics. The committee felt that the society could not be barred from the current convention because of the presence of these members but felt that unless the said society took the necessary steps to purge itself of irregular practitioners it ought not to be entitled to future representation in the American Medical Association.

There was also some disturbance over the number of delegates from the District of Columbia.

THE FOUNDING OF THE JOURNAL

Most important, however, was a resolution introduced by Dr. S. D. Gross to the effect that the Transactions should be published in a journal to be called The American Medical Association Journal, issued monthly under the supervision of a competent doctor. The resolution was referred to a committee of five for their consideration.

At this convention also a resolution was introduced urging the government of the United States to establish a national school of medicine. This resolution was referred to a committee for report the following year.

Much of the time was taken in the consideration of the right of specialists to issue cards announcing their specialties and the right of a physician not a resident of any given state to represent that state in the House of Delegates.

A committee was established to prepare a nomenclature of diseases. By this time also there was some concern over the technic of teaching residents and interns in hospitals, and the society resolved that it was not within the purview of the general management of a hospital to interfere at all with the subject of medical instruction, which belongs to the medical staff.

Far in advance of its time was a resolution requesting the editors of medical journals to refuse to notice in their journals all "patent" medicines, instruments, works of unprofessional or unscientific character, nonchartered institutions or hospitals and the cards of specialists.

ADMISSION OF NEGRO DELEGATES

A considerable division of membership of the Association arose as well over representation of the National Medical Society in the District of Columbia, the Howard Medical College, Freedman's Hospital and the Smallpox Hospital. The majority report made by N. S. Davis would have barred these institutions because of charges that had been filed against them. The minority report, headed by Dr. Alfred Stillé, recommended their admission. The majority report was sustained by a vote of 115 to 90, and these institutions were barred from membership. The nature of the charges was not at first made clear. On the next day, however, the question was again raised and a motion from Dr. G. S. Palmer of Maine demanded the reason for the barring of men from Howard University. Dr. Davis promised to give in writing the reason for the action of the majority of the committee. When Dr. Davis presented his report, it was worded to indicate that the delegates from the medical department of Howard University were barred because they were also members of the National Medical Society of the District of Columbia and that it had been brought to the attention of the Committee on Ethics that the said National Medical Society recognized and received as members medical men who were not licensed to practice. Following the presentation of this report there was further debate, after which Dr. H. R. Storer of Massachusetts offered the following statement:

Resolved, That inasmuch as it has been distinctly stated and proved that the consideration of race and color has had nothing whatsoever to do with the decision of the question of the reception of the Washington delegates, and inasmuch as charges have been distinctly made in open session today attaching the stigma of dishonor to parties implicated, which charges have not been denied by them, though present, therefore

The report of the majority of the Committee on Ethics be declared, as to all intents and purposes, unanimously adopted by the Association.

This motion passed 112 to 34.

THE LIBRARY

New at this time was the report of the librarian of the American Medical Association, who had been engaged since the last annual meeting in endeavoring to carry out the expressed wishes of the American Medical Association with regard to the formation of an American National Medical Library to be located at Washington, D. C. A circular had been sent widespread and a good many books had been received, but the Congressional Library Committee had not authorized the Library of Congress to receive the books belonging to the American Medical Association as a special deposit. Therefore a room had been fitted up in the Smithsonian Institution to house this library, and a device had been engraved for use on labels of the books belonging to this collection.

ANTICIPATING THE NEED FOR QUININE

Significant at this time was the publication of a memorial that had been sent to the Congress trying to get the Congress to plan for cultivation of the cinchona tree in the United States. When the Japanese occupied Java as one of their first steps in World War II, we realized the need for an American source of cinchona. Had it not been for the development of the synthetic quinacrine hydrochloride (atabrine) and the utilization of some cinchona from South America, we might have found ourselves in a serious state in the war against malaria.

1871

SAN FRANCISCO

Now the Association journeyed for the first time to the Pacific coast and held its meeting in May in San Francisco.

The committee to establish a journal had no report. The committee on nomenclature of diseases reported progress. The committee on medical literature had no report. The trip to the Pacific coast may have exhausted the delegates.

Now also there was introduced for the first time the concept of an organization within medicine itself to raise the standard of medical practice. A resolution proposed that the American Medical Association take measures to establish a National Academy of Medicine to which men of distinction could be elevated from the ranks and that a board of examiners function to govern entrance to this academy. This was no doubt the first step toward certifying boards for specialists.

The Massachusetts Medical Society reported that it had expelled from fellowship all those who publicly professed to practice in accordance with any exclusive dogma, whether calling themselves homeopaths, hydropaths, eclectics or what not.

From the California State Medical Society came a resolution congratulating the states of Massachusetts and California on having established departments of state medicine and urging that all the states set up departments for the prevention of disease and the correction of those agencies which injure the human race and, furthermore, that as soon as six states should set up such departments a National Health Council be formed as an auxiliary to the American Medical Association.

By this time 339 volumes including pamphlets and monographs had been collected in the Smithsonian Institution, but scarcely an American textbook had been added.

WOMEN IN MEDICINE

In his presidential address Dr. Alfred Stillé embarked on an attack on women in the medical profession, admitting their right to study medicine and to practice it but, in general, arguing that they could never qualify to eminence in the profession. Here is an example of his logic:

> Certain women seek to rival men in manly sports and occupations, and the "strong-minded" ape them assiduously in all things, even in dress. In doing so, they may command a sort of admiration such as all monstrous productions inspire, especially when they tend towards a higher type than their own. But a man with feminine traits of character, or with the frame and carriage of a female, is despised both by the sex he ostensibly belongs to, and that of which he is at once a caricature and a libel. In every department of active life man excels woman, excels her even in things for which she is esteemed most fit. In the arts of design, in painting and sculpture, no woman, albeit the artist's career has always been open to her, has ever risen far above mediocrity; while men have excelled women in not a few employments which are regarded as essentially feminine. In the art of cookery, for example, no woman ever occupied the first rank; and in more than one capital, male hairdressers and dressmakers set the fashions in which court ladies and city dames contend for the palm of beauty.

And he concluded this talk with even more bad logic:

> On the whole, then, we believe that all experience teaches that woman is characterized by a combination of distinctive qualities, of which the most striking are uncertainty of rational judgment, capriciousness of sentiment, fickleness of purpose, and indecision of action, which totally unfit her for professional pursuits. Judged by one of her own sex, the verdict is in these words: "The ignorance, the inexactness, the untrustworthiness, the

unbusiness-like ways of women, are appalling. Men are as bad as they can be, one is sometimes tempted to say; but apparently they cannot be so bad as women in these respects. Long ages of experience have, at least, educated them into a consciousness of the difference between yes and no; but women have yet to learn that they are not one and the same word. . . . They seem to lack a moral sense, or a mental perception, or whatever she faculty is which makes one capable of contracting an engagement. They do not comprehend its nature. It has for them no more binding force than a rope of sand. They break it with a serene unconsciousness that anything is broken, or that there was anything to break."

If, then, woman is unfitted by nature to become a physician, we should, when we oppose her pretensions, be acquitted of any malicious or even unkindly spirit. We may admit that she is in some sense a perfected man, and was created even a little less lower than the angels; we may admit that, guided by her affections, her judgments sometimes resemble inspirations; but in the business of life, and especially in the practice of a scientific art, it nevertheless may be true, and probably is so, that she usually displays a strange ignorance of the logic of reason, and a profound contempt for the logic of facts.

And he closed his address with a vigorous defense of the use of alcohol in medicine and an attack on those who were fighting the battle of temperance.

1872

PHILADELPHIA

The meeting of 1872 opened in Horticultural Hall but moved shortly to Presbyterian Church because people could not be heard in the original place of meeting. The sessions were largely routine on the first day, with some undistinguished papers and some routine considerations in the House of Delegates.

Then on the second day Dr. S. B. Merkel proposed to bring before the Association George Thomas, "a native of Brazil, who, although externally well formed, can move his heart about at will; and can also whirl the abdomen like a huge ball, with an undulating motion, around the umbilicus." This offer was referred to the Section on the Practice of Medicine and Obstetrics.

There was an extensive report from the committee on nomenclature of diseases, with a recommendation that it be referred for publication, but a minority report said that the matter was too important to be adopted in a hurry and suggested, rather, that extra copies be printed for circulation to the members of the medical profession so that their opinions might be ascertained.

The motion to establish a National Academy of Medicine was brought out and recommended for passage, but the motion was lost and the subject dropped.

STATE HEALTH DEPARTMENTS

The Committee on a National Health Council indicated that it had circularized thirty states with a view to getting the establishment of state health departments and that some progress was being made. However, there was already misunderstanding among the medical profession as to the significance of the term "state medicine" so that the committee said:

> As the phrase "State Medicine" is perhaps imperfectly understood by many of the profession, and is absolutely new to the general public, we wish here, parenthetically, to give an idea of what it is, quote the list of subjects which have been suggested as properly appertaining to it by a committee of the General Medical Council of Great Britain. They are: Forensic Medicine, Toxicology, Morbid Anatomy, Psychological Medicine, Laws of Evidence, Preventive Medicine, Vital and Sanitary Statistics, Medical Topography and certain portions of Engineering Science and Practice. In short, as a member of the committee well expresses it, State Medicine consists in the application of medical knowledge and skill to the benefit of communities, which is obviously a very different thing from their application to the benefit of individuals in private or curative medicine.

The concluding action of this committee was to ask that it be continued and that a special section on state medicine and public hygiene be constituted as one of the scientific sections of the Association.

The Committee on Ethics reaffirmed its previous actions relative to the refusal to admit the Freedman Hospital, the Howard University and the Academy of Medicine of Washington, D. C., to representation because some of the members of their staff were unlicensed and because one of the teachers in Howard University was a woman. The battle over the status of the physicians, the societies and the schools in the District of Columbia was fiercely fought on the floor of the convention. At the end of the extensive discussions, the report of the Committee on Ethics barring the representatives from these agencies was adopted by a large majority.

Again the delegates besought the Congress of the United States to give some attention to the cultivation of the cinchona tree, pointing out that the British and the Dutch were hard at work on this project, but apparently Congress refused to take any action.

THE PERMANENT SECRETARY

Now there arose the delicate question of the remuneration of the permanent secretary, Dr. William B. Atkinson. His duties had become more engrossing every year with the growth of the Association and his remuneration was nil. Therefore the resolution was offered that he be paid a salary of $1,000 a year in quarterly payments, and the session unanimously resolved to present him with $500 as a testimonial to his merit.

An attempt was made to get through a resolution upholding Horace Wells as the discoverer of anesthesia, and the resolution was laid on the table. As late as 1946 this question was again before the Association and again it was tabled.

WOMEN IN MEDICINE

Another resolution suggested that "whilst we admit the right of women to acquire medical education and to practice medicine and surgery in all their departments, we deem the public association of the sexes in our medical schools and at the mixed clinics of our hospitals, as impracticable, unnecessary, and derogatory to the instincts of true modesty in either sex." This resolution was also laid on the table. After a while a resolution was made to take it off the table, and after some more discussion it was indefinitely postponed.

The President of the Association, Dr. D. W. Yandell, presented a strong defense of the right of women to practice medicine but he would have limited them to certain specialties. He trusted that not many would incline to surgery, but he thought that they would be welcome visitors to many a sick chamber. "If young and handsome," he said, "I have no doubt valetudinarians of our sex would look for their morning calls as they might for angel visits, only that they would not have them 'short and far between.'" He felt that the public should really make the decision on the use of women physicians and he concluded this part of his discussion by saying:

> What the people decree in this matter is a law to which all, we and the women alike, must bow submissively. If they want women doctors, such will be found ready to meet the demand. If those now pressing forward in their studies so eagerly, find their services are not wanted, they will take down their signs, get married—if they can—or turn lecturers, or to some more lucrative employment. I hope they will never embarrass us by a personal application for seats in this Association. I could not vote for that.

1873
ST. LOUIS

Most significant of the business before the Association's meeting in 1873 was the report of the special committee to plan for better arrangements by the sections for the more rigid examination of papers offered for publication. A few of the sections were receiving maximum attendance but few listeners. A reorganization was suggested. The Committee of Publications was not doing a good job in rejecting unworthy manuscripts and was condemned for its failure to be more strict. That perhaps explains the skimpiness of the volume of Transactions for that year.

THE JUDICIAL COUNCIL

This year saw also a resolution offered by Dr. N. S. Davis for the creation of a judicial council to decide all questions of an ethical or judicial character that might arise in connection with the Association. His resolution was unanimously adopted.

From the Army came a request that the Association join its efforts to obtaining better ranks and higher promotions for the medical officers of the Army.

DISINTEREST IN NOMENCLATURE

The committee on nomenclature reported that not a single response had been received from any medical journal, and only two from physicians, to the request for the circularization of the nomenclature.

A long report dealt with the proposed salary of $1,000 a year for the permanent secretary. The committee felt that the secretary was already receiving payment of his expenses in attendance on the conventions; they felt that the revenue of the Association was inadequate to meet a salary of $1,000 a year and that, furthermore, the payment of the salary of $500 to $1,000 a year would speedily develop a number of aspirants for the position, each with his circle of friends among the members, all of whom would be quick to perceive the errors and to note the slightest tardiness or discourtesy on the part of the incumbent of the office, and that this job would be sought as a political plum. The suggestion of a salary was therefore rejected, but a motion that he be given an honorarium was approved, provided sufficient money was left in the treasury after paying the expenses of the Association.

The meeting closed with a number of resolutions condemning the alarming prevalence of ill effects of intemperance. The resolutions were either tabled or referred to committees.

1874

DETROIT

The second annual session of the Association to take place in Detroit abandoned the Fire House and moved into Hough's Detroit Theatre. Detroit had grown in the intervening years from a city of 40,000 to one of 100,000 inhabitants.

The speech of welcome was a glorification of the growth of this great industrial city and of its new city hall (erected at a cost of $600,000), from whose dome not only the city but Lake Erie was visible. The speaker boasted of the excellent sewerage system, the public school system (due chiefly to Dr. Pitcher), the public library and the police and fire departments.

THE PRINCIPLES OF ETHICS

Significant was the introduction of a report by Dr. N. S. Davis of Illinois, chairman of the Judicial Council, who had ascertained the sentiments of the physicians relative to revisions in the Principles of Ethics. It had been proposed to strike out everything having to do with the relations of the patient, the community and the public toward the members of the profession. It was felt that there ought to be more said about specialties and contract practice. After carefully reviewing the entire subject, the committee did not recommend any alteration in the Code of Ethics but desired "to express the opinion that if every medical school and society would supply each graduate as he left the school, and each member initiated into the society, with a printed copy of the Code, accompanied with the injunction that it be carefully studied, it would be productive of much good, directly to the profession and indirectly to the community." The report was unanimously adopted.

As a result of the pressure brought by the Association a bill had been introduced into the Congress relative to improved status for the medical staff of the Army. The bill had been introduced and referred to the military committee, which however had failed to take action. A resolution was therefore adopted regarding this failure to take action and sent along to the Congress.

INDEX CATALOGUE OF THE SURGEON GENERAL'S LIBRARY

Now also Dr. John Shaw Billings, assistant surgeon, United States Army, by direction of the Surgeon General forwarded to the American Medical Association a copy of the "Catalogue of the Surgeon General's Office" in three volumes. He called attention to the fact that 65,000 titles were now in the library but that this was not more than one third of what the national medical collection should contain. It was proposed to issue a new catalogue arranged according to subjects and authors. He urged physicians everywhere to send to the library files of American medical journals, transactions of medical societies, announcements of medical colleges and reports of hospitals, asylums and boards of health. "These medical pamphlets," he said, "cannot be purchased and the only prospect of obtaining them is from the garrets, closets and shelves of physicians who may have preserved them and may be willing to part with them in consideration of the object for which they are desired."

The address of the President, Dr. Joseph M. Toner, made several recommendations which stimulated action in the Association. He urged particularly the formation of a complete system of state and local medical societies and also of an international medical society.

Because the centennial of the founding of the United States was to be celebrated in Philadelphia in 1876, an invitation came from that city to hold the annual session of the American Medical Association in Philadelphia on July 4, 1876 and to invite the medical profession of the world to attend the meetings.

A resolution was passed that a suitable die for a medal be prepared with a likeness of N. S. Davis on one side and the name and date of the organization of the Association on the opposite side, with instructions that a copy be furnished to each delegate on becoming a member and also that all present as well as future members of the Association be furnished with this medal.

A motion was made to recompense the secretary with $300 for his services. On motion of J. Marion Sims of New York, this was increased to $500. The motion was seconded and adopted.

The treasurer of the Association was glad to report that "as a result of more than usual discretion on the part of the last meeting of the Association, and the more than usual care exercised in referring matter to the Committee of Publication, the volume of Transactions is of moderate size." Because of a lack of demand, there had accumulated some 2,000 volumes of previous issues of the Transactions and the treasurer moved that he be allowed to dispose of these. With this suggestion, Dr. Caspar Wister, the treasurer, offered his resignation.

A resolution was offered by Dr. Keller of Kentucky that a committee be established relative to passing proper legislation to prevent the spread of syphilis.

ADVANCES IN DIAGNOSTIC METHODS

In his presidential address Dr. Joseph Toner called attention to the beginning of laboratory and other technical methods used in the diagnosis and treatment of disease.

> The successful medical man must be fully up with the age and the times, conversant with the latest means of diagnosis, the theory of diseases and their cures. He must have tested the newest remedy, examined the most recent invention; he must have read the latest telegram. And, indeed, the genius of the profession, responding to these demands, has devised physical tests for an exact diagnosis in almost every important disease. There is scarcely a vital function the normal or diseased action of which cannot be determined with accuracy through the aid of some chemical test or mechanical device.* The improvement in this direction is still actively progressing.

---

* The dynamometer, the microscope, the ophthalmoscope, the laryngoscope, the rhinoscope, the stethoscope, the pleximeter, the endoscope, the speculum, the sphygmograph, the spirometer, the thermometer, the anesthesiometer, anesthetics, chemical examination of excretions and so on.

He called on the medical profession to urge particularly more state, county and city boards of health.

SYPHILIS

The address in surgery was delivered by S. D. Gross and was entitled "Syphilis in Its Relation to the National Health." He said that the assertion that syphilis originated in the new world and was carried back by the sailors of Columbus is without the slightest foundation in truth but, instead, that the sailors of Columbus had infected the natives. While this belief is still subject to some argument today, the vast majority of evidence inclines to the former view. His address was nevertheless a most scholarly presentation of the available knowledge of his day concerning this disease. He urged as the only possible technic for preventing its spread, the licensure of prostitution. He was a little ahead of his time in urging that people should not be allowed to marry until they could obtain a certificate showing that they did not have syphilis—but, of course, at that time there were no accurate tests of the presence of the disease such as the Wassermann and Kahn tests used today.

GROWING PAINS, 1875 TO 1879

1875
LOUISVILLE, KY.

THE SPECIAL COMMITTEE ON rank of the medical corps of the Army reported that it had used extraordinary efforts but had been unable to secure any action whatever from Congress. The Surgeon General of the Army expressed his thanks and his regret that nothing had been done; he was sanguine that in the long run the Army Medical Department would be successful if the American Medical Association would continue to take the same interest in the future as it had in the past.

Dr. J. Marion Sims was elected to the presidency of the Association.

Most important of the resolutions adopted was the determination that each year, until otherwise ordered, the President-Elect and permanent Secretary should direct an appeal in the name of the Association to the authorities of each state without a board of health, urging them to establish such boards. The Secretary was to report annually the names of states in which boards of health existed and also those which declined to establish them.

As a supplement to the annual Transactions the prize essay on "Excision of the Larger Joints of the Extremities" by H. Culbertson, M.D., was made available to the members.

1876
PHILADELPHIA

The celebration of the centennial of the United States was notably observed by the meeting in Philadelphia in 1876. The delegates were welcomed by Dr. William Pepper. He called attention to the tremendous progress that had been made by Philadelphia, which now boasted of 820,000 inhabitants and had the lowest rate of mortality of any city in the world with over half a million inhabitants. He felt that this was largely due to the lack of overcrowding in the city. Especially recommended to the delegates was a visit to the International Exposition then going on in Fairmount Park.

The President's address had dealt in part with syphilis; a motion was passed that 10,000 copies of that portion of his address be reprinted and distributed widely among the membership of the Association.

DR. SARAH HACKETT STEVENSON

At the meeting in Philadelphia in 1876, Dr. Sarah Hackett Stevenson was a delegate from the state of Illinois. She was the first woman member of the American Medical Association. When her name was called in the roll call, Dr. William Brodie of Michigan moved that the names of all female delegates be referred to the Judicial Council. This was on motion laid on the table. Dr. Stevenson, perhaps with remarkable wisdom, must have sat peculiarly quiet throughout the session since her name does not appear as a participant in the making of motions, the offering of resolutions, the discussion of any papers or the presentation of any contribution.

Sarah Hackett Stevenson was born at Buffalo Grove, Ill., Feb. 2, 1849. She graduated from the Women's Medical College of Northwestern University and in 1874 went to Europe for two years' study where she worked with Huxley and Darwin. She began to practice in Chicago in 1876 and was sent as a delegate to the annual meeting of the American Medical Association in Philadelphia during that year. She was also the first woman to serve on the staff of the Cook County Hospital.

CONDEMNATION OF CULTISM

Another resolution suggested that members of the medical profession who in any way aid or abet graduation of medical students in irregular or exclusive systems of medicine are deemed thereby to violate the spirit of ethics of the American Medical Association.

STATE BOARDS OF HEALTH

The Secretary reported that boards of health "now exist in Alabama, California, Massachusetts, Michigan, Minnesota, Virginia and Wisconsin—but eight states in all." A careful counting will reveal only seven states listed as having state boards of health. He stated further that the matter was still being urged on the legislatures of the other states.

THE PHARMACOPEIA

Significant also was a resolution introduced by Dr. E. R. Squibb urging the American Medical Association to take the whole subject of the National Pharmacopeia into consideration for a review of its management. Dr. Squibb was requested to reduce to writing his plan for the Pharmacopeia. He found that already an interval of ten years embraced so much detail that it was becoming impracticable to handle it. It was his feeling that perhaps the American Medical Association should be the proper custodian of the Pharmacopeia and that perhaps the American Medical Association should take the leadership and invite cooperation of the American Pharmaceutical Association.

ADDRESS BY DR. J. MARION SIMS

In his presidential address Dr. J. Marion Sims recalled the meeting in Philadelphia in 1872 when so much time was wasted in discussing the woman physician question and the Negro question. He asserted that the Association was a truly representative body and that if any state or county medical society should send as a delegate either a woman or a Negro, the Association was bound to receive the delegate. He felt that the creation of the Judicial Council was a great step in advance in overcoming local problems of ethics which were a great source of annoyance and danger. Dr. Sims condemned particularly the system of education in which first, second and third year students sat side by side on benches at the same time and heard the same lectures year after year. He said:

> Already Chicago moves in the right direction; but Boston now takes the lead, and inaugurates the true scholastic method of classes, and terms of study, and courses of practical instruction, now fully appreciated by such young men as are in earnest in acquiring a thorough medical training.
>
> The Harvard method, with a salaried Faculty wholly independent of fees from students, is the only plan by which we can ever hope for a medical degree of any real value.

He urged the wealthy men of the country to increase the endowments of the medical schools. In his consideration of the Code of Ethics he doubted its significance, its validity or its constitutionality. It was susceptible of being used as an agent of persecution. "Let it stand as it is," he said. "Honorable men do not need its protection; dishonest men are not influenced by its edicts."

He urged widespread publicity concerning syphilis, which he considered the great problem of the day.

J. Marion Sims was opposed to licensure of prostitution as effective in the control of venereal disease. His answer was a system of sanitary inspection and control that would enable the health officer to take charge of those with syphilis and prevent them from spreading it through the community. Boards of health ought to have power to protect the public against all contagious and infectious diseases. He said he would simply include syphilis in the great family of contagious or communicable diseases and make it subject to the same laws and regulations used for their management.

1877

CHICAGO

Dramatic indeed was the opening of the meeting of the American Medical Association in Chicago on June 5, 1877. Dr. N. S. Davis welcomed the delegates; the Transactions said "Thirty-one years ago seventy-six gentlemen met in New York, representing the medical profession in the United States. Two thirds of the members have passed away, and he now failed to recognize a single face, in the meeting today, that was present on that occasion." At that moment a hand was raised, and Dr. N. S. Davis recognized Dr. Washington L. Atlee of Philadelphia, the only physician present who was one of the original seventy-six. Only twenty-nine years had passed since the organizational meeting in New York City, and yet that twenty-nine years had seen the departure from life of many of the great leaders of the previous generation.

ADDRESS OF DR. HENRY I. BOWDITCH

The President of the Association, Dr. Henry I. Bowditch of Boston, pointed out that the American Medical Association had united the physicians of the country, ironed out local idiosyncrasies and brought together men from every section. He remembered that wine flowed freely at public and private gatherings of an earlier day and that there had been occasional disorder observable during the debates but that the Association from this disorder had cemented friendships, so that it became one of the bulwarks of the state and a help toward civilization on this continent. By 1876 he thought, however, that the American Medical Association had lost repute in the Eastern and Middle states and with some of the leaders of the Western and Southern states. This, he felt, was due to two general causes: (1) the furious discussions on points of order and the ethics of professional etiquette and (2) the consciousness that the Association had been expected to produce results in the advancement of medicine and of professional stature out of all reason. He said also that some of the meetings of the scientific sections had been used for the presentation of "papers or remarks from individuals, smitten with the *cacoethes scribendi aut loquendi*" and that they had not always had the ability or the will to check them. He also believed that the Transactions of the Association were too bulky and included now some papers that had been printed elsewhere and really constituted nothing in the way of advancement.

Another cause of disturbance was the passage of resolutions with lack of sufficient information, but which, nevertheless, compromised the entire Association. Finally, it was claimed, the Association was too democratic. Having ventured these criticisms, Dr. Bowditch offered suggestions for the improvement of the sections and for procuring scientific contributions. He praised highly the work of the Judicial Council in its settlement of questions of dispute. He urged that the social meetings include women and abandon alcoholic drinks.

He urged also, for the first time, that every member of a state medical society become a permanent member of the American Medical Association. Finally, he suggested a smaller delegation in the House of Delegates as representative of the membership.

The remainder of his address dealt with the possibility of association with the Canadian Medical Association and with the Pharmacopeia. He urged support for the Army Medical Library and Museum and of the American Medical College Association.

This address having been referred to a special committee, a report was received leading to improvement of the sections. The committee did not favor any change in the present plan of organization and considered association with the Canadian Medical Association impracticable.

The meeting in Chicago in 1877 was most impressive to Dr. Charles B. Johnson, who attended as a delegate from the Illinois State Medical Society at Champaign, Ill. The meeting was in the Palmer House and there were no elevators, so that guests climbed to the top stories. Dr. Johnson recalled seeing the venerable Dr. S. D. Gross of Philadelphia mounting the stairs laboriously. Dr. Gross stopped for a brief chat with Dr. J. Marion Sims, who had been President the year previously, and Dr. Johnson heard the renowned gynecologist say that "if he had his professional life to live over he would by hook or crook try to get more money out of it."

The address of Dr. Bowditch he remembered for a long time because of the recommendation that the American Medical Association conventions be conducted on temperance principles.

When Dr. Bowditch attended the meeting of the American Medical Association in Chicago in 1908, one of the sessions was held in a German hotel and the refreshments consisted of beer and pretzels. He tried to get a cup of coffee, but the waiter told him it could not be had. Then he asked for a glass of water. The waiter looked at him in astonishment but finally served the water.

A note from Mr. A. J. Horlick gives his father's reminiscences of the 1877 convention:

There were no arrangements for exhibits and Father with a large Gladstone bag full of samples of Horlick's Food (which later was succeeded by the product Malted Milk, which Father invented) stood in the hall and met the doctors as they came out from the meeting room and handed them samples of this Horlick's Food, which was mainly a milk modifier. Dr. Davis objected to his attempting to detail or exhibit his product to the doctors as, of course, such a thing as attending a medical convention to acquaint doctors with products was unheard of. The meeting room was, I believe, on the second floor and Father then took his bag of samples and waited outside the door at the foot of the stairs, and presented the doctors with samples as they came out.

PHARMACOPEIA VS. DISPENSATORY

In 1877 Dr. E. R. Squibb of New York presented a report on the revision of the Pharmacopeia. The underlying grievance was a personal matter between Dr. Squibb and Dr. H. C. Wood of the U. S. Dispensatory. Dr. Squibb began to read at 10 o'clock and was still reading at 11 o'clock. After another considerable period, a motion was made that Dr. Squibb be permitted to resume on Thursday at 12 noon and be given twenty minutes in which to finish his remarks. The remainder of the session was to be given to those entertaining opposite views to those of Dr. Squibb.

Intervening was a prolonged discussion on representation of homeopathic groups and the licensure of homeopathic physicians in various states.

When Dr. Squibb again began reading his address it was discovered that he could not conclude, and he was given additional time. He continued reading until the expiration of this additional time, and then, since he had not concluded, the Association proceeded to elect its officers.

Following the election by vote, a committee of five was appointed to examine the papers of Dr. Squibb and of Dr. Wood and of others and to determine the extent to which the American Medical Association should participate in the Pharmacopeia.

THE STATE BOARDS OF HEALTH

On the final day of the session, attention was called to the fact that the American Medical Association through its President and Secretary had urged the governor in every state to establish a state board of health. A resolution was passed urging the President and the Secretary of the Association to continue such an appeal year after year to the governor in every state until such state boards of health should be established. This was one of the most fundamental contributions made by the American Medical Association to the advancement of public health in the United States.

NEW SECTIONS

Now came appeals for the establishment of a new section on ophthalmology, otology and laryngology, since these specialties had assumed full stature with surgery and internal medicine.

INCREASED MILITARY MEDICAL RECOGNITION

A report was made from the committee that had urged on the Congress the establishment of better recognition of the medical staff of the U. S. Army. By this time the efforts of the committee had achieved some success. A letter from Surgeon General Joseph K. Barnes of the U. S. Army thanked the committee and expressed appreciation of the influence exerted in behalf of the medical officers of the Army by the American Medical Association.

1878

BUFFALO

Extensive reports were made by the delegates who had visited the Canadian Medical Association, the British Medical Association and the International Medical Congress of Geneva. The report from Geneva urged the possibility of developing a uniform pharmacopeia throughout the world—an ideal still sought in 1946 by the Health Organization of the United Nations.

HOMEOPATHIC PROBLEMS

The Judicial Council presented to this meeting charges against the Michigan State Medical Society for having elected as a delegate to the American Medical Association one Dr. E. L. Dunster of the University of Michigan "knowing him to be engaged in aiding and abetting the graduation of students devoted to an exclusive dogma in medicine." Nothing had been found in the Principles of Ethics which would bear directly on the charges. From time to time resolutions had been adopted referring to the practice of cultism, but these resolutions did not constitute a part of the Code of Ethics. This report was discussed freely. Finally, a motion was made asking the Judicial Council to report at a subsequent meeting a law to meet the case in question.

At the meeting of the next day, Dr. Nathan Smith Davis proposed the following addition to the Principles of Ethics:

> And hence it is considered derogatory to the interests of the public and the honor of the profession, for any physician or teacher to aid, in any way, the medical teaching or graduation of persons knowing them to be supporters and intended practitioners of some irregular and exclusive system of medicine.

ORGANIZATIONAL PROGRESS

The Buffalo meeting elected Dr. Theophilus Parvin, then of Indiana, President.

An extensive report by a committee of N. S. Davis and S. D. Gross concerned the recommendations made by the President, Henry Bowditch, in the year previously. These two leaders were not inclined to accept the suggestions of Dr. Bowditch as to changing the nature of membership in the House of Delegates. They had some alternative proposals as to the selection of papers for the sections and as to the decisions on publication of papers. Dr. Bowditch submitted for himself a minority report disagreeing with them, but the majority report was adopted.

Ultimately the ideas of Dr. Bowditch as to representation in the House of Delegates and the consideration of papers read in the sections prevailed. The improvement in general quality of the medical profession, the raising of medical standards, the organization of the state medical societies and the advancement of medical science made the suggestions wholly logical.

The committee which had been urging the establishment of state boards of health was happy to announce that three additional states had founded boards of health so that now there were nineteen in all.

RESTRAINT OF THE INSANE

Psychiatry was discussed, and a resolution was adopted that the personal restraint of the insane is an essential element in the treatment of their disease. Nevertheless it was recognized that the state had a right to surveillance or legal regulation over restraints on the insane in order to punish any abuses of the right of restraint.

The report on the Michigan State Medical Society and Dr. Dunster indicated that there was no law by which the Michigan State Medical Society could be found in conflict with medical ethics. Immediately thereafter an amendment to the Principles of Ethics was adopted as previously suggested, and this took care of the situation.

PROMOTION OF THE PUBLIC HEALTH

In his presidential address Dr. T. G. Richardson paid attention to the improvement in the sections. The most significant portion of his address dealt with the creation of the state boards of health and the prevention of illness as their proper field of activity. He urged particularly better education of the public in regard to health and spoke with scorn of the gentleman who took his 14 year old daughter out of a first class school because a human skeleton was brought into the classroom by the professor of physiology, who was going to teach the pupils a few facts in regard to respiration and circulation. Dr. Richardson opposed federal control of public hygiene, but he recognized the necessity for a federal agency to prevent the introduction of contagious and infectious diseases from abroad. The 45th Congress had taken the first action since 1799 toward enforcing public health laws. Here is the concluding paragraph from Dr. Richardson's address:

> Whatever doubts there may be as to the extent of the authority possessed by the central government, there seems to be no dispute that within the limits of each separate state resides a power which with reference to all such matters is practically supreme. It is to this power represented by the legislature and executive of each state that we must look for the enactment and enforcement of such laws as state medicine demands of a wise government, economical not less of the lives and health of its citizens than of its material resources. It is therefore upon this power that the state medical societies should concentrate all their influence, professional and social, to effect the necessary legislation. They should employ their best endeavors to have state boards of health created where these do not exist, and they should by all means secure the right of nomination for appointment upon such boards; otherwise positions which demand men of peculiar qualifications and sterling integrity will be conferred, as is too often the case, upon mere office hunters, who have no interest whatever in the matter beyond its pecuniary return.

1879

ATLANTA, GA.

Organizations fall into strange traditions of action; patterns are followed until suddenly comes realization of hazard on the path. Dr. Joseph P. Logan of Georgia, who welcomed the delegates to Atlanta on May 6, 1879, stated frankly that he had looked up the previous copies of the Transactions of the American Medical Association to discover how an address of welcome ought to be made. He decided to do a job for Atlanta which "has sprung, in little more than a decade, into a city of 40,000 people." Remember that Atlanta had been devastated by the war. "We have not, however, my friends, sat down in ignoble lamentations over our misfortunes, but have gone to work with energy and determination to rebuild and make better our desolated places." These words are the beginning of a sentence which then continues without interruption for sixteen printed lines having to do with the industries, the works and the climate of Atlanta.

THE METRIC SYSTEM

The report on the International Medical Congress pointed out that the United States Marine Hospital services had adopted the metric system, which was found to work very well, and that it had been adopted by all nations except two—the United States and England. Later in the session a resolution was adopted that the metric system be official and be used in the Transactions. The agitation regarding the metric system was to go on and on for many years; the end is not yet.

A message of congratulation was sent from the convention to Ohio which had passed a bill making possible the dissection of human bodies.

The Association was still disturbing itself as to how to get some prize essays written that would be worthy the name; now four prizes of $250 each were established for strictly original contributions to medical and surgical progress.

ETHICAL RELATIONS AND CULTISM

Especially significant was the debate on the amendment to the Principles of Ethics having to do with exclusive systems of medicine. Because the attendance in Atlanta was small, the resolution was permitted to lie over until the following year.

The representative body also heard of action taken by the section on state medicine and public hygiene in response to an address by Dr. John Shaw Billings on securing statistical data on disease and mortality.

NOTE ON PROPRIETARY MEDICINES

A resolution was offered and referred to the Judicial Council protesting the placing on the market of drugs and combinations of drugs with copyrighted names. This seems to be the first mention of the practice which bore bitter fruit for the American people for many years.

The presidential address of Dr. Theophilus Parvin declared that medicine was the queen of the sciences. He then discussed the philosophy of science and of medicine with sixty references to bibliographic material. It seems to constitute the most learned document presented up to that time as a presidential address; but it concerned itself not at all with any immediate affairs. One reads it again and again puzzling over its meaning and significance, and at last one thinks of that stanza of Omar Khayyam:

> Myself when young did eagerly frequent
> Doctor and Saint, and heard great argument
> About it and about: but evermore
> Came out by the same door wherein I went.

THE JOURNAL IS BORN

1880
NEW YORK CITY

THE SESSION OF THE American Medical Association in 1880 was to prove as the years passed among the most significant of its meetings, except perhaps that of 1847 in which it was established and that of 1901 when it was reorganized. The significance of the 1880 session lies in the fact that it gave birth to THE JOURNAL OF THE AMERICAN MEDICAL ASSOCIATION.

Until THE JOURNAL was established, the minutes of the meetings of the Association and such papers presented at its meetings as were able to survive the censorship of the Committee on Publication were printed in an annual volume of Transactions. These volumes were frequently late in their appearance, insufficiently edited and poorly published. Dr. S. D. Gross, following his visit to the meeting of the British Medical Association, had suggested that the Transactions be discontinued and that a periodical be published, to be known as the American Medical Association Journal. A resolution was passed at the meeting in Washington in 1870 but was immediately reconsidered. Nine years later Dr. S. E. Chaillé of New Orleans read a paper on more efficient organization of the Association in which he urged a change in the method of publishing the Transactions of the Association, but that suggestion was not followed. Then in his presidential address in New York in 1880 Dr. Lewis A. Sayre devoted himself to the needs of the American Medical Association and again considered the publication of the Transactions. He recognized the frequent complaints, the excessive costs, the delays in publication and the fact that the papers often had previously appeared in various medical journals of the country.

"It is very questionable," he said, "whether the mode pursued by the British Medical Association, in establishing their own journal, would not be an immense improvement on our present method. The British journal is the exclusive property of the association; and by the liberal compensation of an accomplished editor, a weekly edition is issued, instead of an annual volume."

Dr. Sayre traced the growth of the *British Medical Journal*, the decision by that organization to publish its regular journal, and the conspicuous progress that the British Medical Association had made once its journal was established. The increase in membership of the British Medical Association was definitely credited to its periodical. He pointed out not only that the British journal had become a powerful means of attracting new members to the association and of keeping them in it by maintaining their interest in connection with the association and "giving them value for their money" but that its advertising columns contributed largely to increase the funds of the British Medical Association, bringing in an income at that time of something like $25,000 a year. He pointed out that the British Medical Association had been able to carry on many activities through the profits made by its publication and that after all expenses were paid there remained an annual surplus of from $3,000 to $5,000 which had been accumulated in a reserve fund. In his consideration of the operation of the *British Medical Journal* he emphasized that not all the papers read at an annual meeting were published, but full discretion was given to the editor to publish or not according to his estimate of the importance and interest of the papers to the members at large. Indeed, Dr. Sayre said that this method included the germs of an association peculiarly adapted to American ideas. "It is essentially democratic and entirely representative. It is dependent for its success on the intelligence, union, and good will of the members. . . . Above all, it is a most successful and influential means of increasing the membership, enlarging the power and widening the basis of the association and of making it a living organism during the intervals between the annual meetings."

With unusual insight Dr. Sayre declared that "the success of the *British Medical Journal* has been largely dependent on the manner in which it has been conducted. The weekly *Journal* did little for the association until it fell into the hands of an experienced editor, whose ability is so generally recognized that there is no need to dwell upon it, and to whom a large and unfettered responsibility is left, although he remains, of course, personally responsible to the executives of the association for the right use of the power entrusted to him, as every editor does to those who appoint him. It will be necessary to find for any organ which this association may publish an editor of recognized position, whom the association would accept as its worthy officer and representative in so responsible a post, a man of literary skill, scientific knowledge and journalistic experience or, at least, journalistic instincts and tact."

This discussion, together with some reference to the metric system and to current accomplishments of American surgery, constituted most of the presidential address of Dr. Lewis A. Sayre. When the address was delivered, a vote of thanks was tendered to the President for his able address. On motion of Dr. William Brodie of Michigan a copy was requested for publication, and his recommendations were referred to a committee of five with instructions to report at the same meeting.

On the first day of the session Dr. Foster Pratt of Michigan presented a report on the suggestions that had been made at the previous session by Dr. S. E. Chaillé of Louisiana, one of which concerned the substitution of a periodical medical journal for the annual volume of Transactions. Most of the report of the Pratt committee dealt with the recommendation that the Association refuse to recognize state societies which did not provide for and encourage the organization of county societies. The Pratt committee did not favor this suggestion. Other proposals concerned the status of members of various types. One proposal urged every medical college to give a lecture or lectures to each graduating class on the importance of medical organization to the profession and the people. The committee felt that a resolution to this effect could do no harm and might do some good, but it pointed out also that the Association had delivered itself from all control of and all responsibility for medical schools and it questioned the propriety or dignity of volunteering advice where it could not compel observance.

As to the publication of a periodical, they felt "it is a consummation devoutly to be wished" and "probably a very large majority of intelligent medical men will unhesitatingly declare in favor of the periodical—*if* (and they italicize the *if*) it can be properly established and maintained." They urged patience in making progress and they expressed their belief that the "safest and surest way to attain most of the desirable ends proposed is to patiently wait the operations of the law of growth." The distinguished committee that made this report included Foster Pratt, N. S. Davis, S. D. Gross and A. N. Bell. This report, on motion of Dr. William Brodie, was accepted and ordered to be entered on the minutes.

On the third day of the session a resolution was offered by Dr. J. R. Bronson of Massachusetts requesting the appointment of a committee of five to report on the following morning on the practicability of formulating all of the proceedings in journalistic form as recommended by the President in his annual address. This resolution was unanimously adopted.

The President of the Association appointed Drs. J. R. Bronson of Massachusetts, W. W. Dawson of Ohio, W. H. Pancoast of Pennsylvania, N. C. Husted of New York and J. S. Green of New Jersey as a committee for formulating the proceedings in journalistic form.

As the session ended, Dr. J. R. Bronson, serving as chairman of the committee to consider publication of the Transactions in periodical form, made the following report:

> The committee appointed to consider the practicability of formulating all the proceedings of this Association in journalistic form find on approaching the subject that its merits are such as to warrant the belief that the medical profession as a whole, upon due consideration, will heartily endorse the radical change proposed, in that it will enable the profession aforesaid to commence to utilize at an early day the valuable contributions to the literature of this Association. The details necessarily incident to the change proposed are too important and too numerous to be compassed within the period given the committee to report. We desire, therefore, to report progress.

A motion was made to lay this on the table, but the motion was lost. Then Dr. William Brodie moved that it be accepted and the committee was continued.

At this session the Section on Practice of Medicine had a report on a diet cure of rheumatism which, it is there claimed, was successful, and a rather extensive report on the Salisbury plan in consumption by Dr. Ephraim Cutter of Boston, a method which involved removing a yeast which was supposed to cause tuberculosis from the blood and tissues by starving it out. The yeast apparently fed on starches and sugars and the diet planned to eliminate starches and sugars as much as possible.

Great progress was being made in the Section on State Medicine, which was urging the establishment of state boards of health and of a national board of health. In the membership of this section one finds such names as those of John Shaw Billings and Abraham Jacobi. Dr. John Shaw Billings traced the growth of the movement for a national board of health, recognizing the part played by the American Public Health Association and other groups.

There were proposals for the establishment of a nomenclature and for an adequate census of the population. There was a forward looking paper on the physician in education dealing with the question of the physician to the schools.

1881

RICHMOND, VA.

Early in the meeting at Richmond, Va., in 1881 a report was presented by Dr. Joseph H. Warren of Massachusetts of a trip he had taken abroad in which he referred again with great praise to the *British Medical Journal* and to its editor, Mr. Ernest Hart, who, "by his great push and enterprise, has caused the journal to outrank any other journal published by any other medical association." He pointed out that the *British Medical Journal* had brought into contact with that association the best men in the British medical profession and, he continued, "I would, Mr. President and Fellows, that the American Medical Association had, in place of its ponderous annual publication, a weekly journal published under its own immediate auspices; and I would that at its head we had an editor with a vigor equal to that of Mr. Hart, that he might, with his editorial staff, stir all the dry and moldering members into a new life, and that he might infuse into them an interest and activity equal to or even greater than that which the British Association shows today.

On the second day of the session Dr. John H. Packard of Pennsylvania read the report on journalizing the Transactions and submitted a resolution that a committee of five be appointed whose duty it should be to digest and report in detail as early as possible a plan for the publication of a weekly journal by the Association, the nomination of an editor, his salary, and the time and place of publication of such a journal. On motion of Dr. N. S. Davis this resolution was amended to leave out the nomination of the editor. Next a motion was offered that the secretary and treasurer be added to the committee and then another resolution urged that the members of the previous committee attending the session be added to the new committee. The committee appointed included Drs. John H. Packard, N. S. Davis, John Shaw Billings, Lewis A. Sayre and R. Beverly Cole, with the treasurer and the secretary.

By this time it was becoming apparent to the meeting of the American Medical Association that the system of appointing delegates from the state and county medical societies and from similar groups was not working satisfactorily. Members continued to urge the development of county medical societies as constituents of state medical societies and to suggest changes in the Constitution and By-Laws to make the Association more definitely a representative body.

The committee which had been trying to get a hearing before the Congress on better social recognition for the medical officers reported that it had arrived in Washington but found the Congress too much preoccupied with "some contested election cases to make any new enterprises probable of success." Besides, the committee had concluded that the resolution did not cover sufficient ground to include all the needed legislation and that the best thing to do was to wait for another session of the Association.

The address of the President, Dr. John T. Hodgen, dealt with the qualifications of surgeons as specialists and with various surgical contingencies.

Unusual in the printed Transactions was a paper on thumb sucking, involving the application of a cuff over the elbow to keep the child from reaching the mouth. In this astute manuscript the author said that thumb sucking is more disastrous to the child than sucking the other fingers because the thumb, once in the mouth, remains there more easily during sleep.

The report of the new committee on journalizing the Transactions, signed by Drs. Packard, Gross, Weatherby, Dunster and Gillette, considered various technics for publication of the Transactions of the Association and compared the costs of a periodical with the publication of an annual volume of transactions:

> The great aim of the movement would be to furnish the Association with an organ—an exponent of its principles, a medium of communication between it and its members, between the members themselves and between the Association and the profession at large. The columns of this journal should be open to all respectable contributors. It should be controlled by no clique, free from personalities, high in tone; discriminating, but not prejudiced; independent, but not erratic. All this—and nothing less will warrant any hope of success—implies the securing of the most able editorship. It would be necessary also to provide for the employment of one or more assistant editors, and for the payment of contributors.
>
> Beyond all doubt a weekly, properly conducted, would far better meet the requirements of the case than either a monthly or a quarterly journal; but the labor of editing it would also be much greater. Should the Association resolve to undertake this enterprise, the question of form would be a most important one.

The committee indicated that the method of collecting dues was undependable as a source of income; it felt that there must be regular annual dues. It had obtained from the treasurer of the Association a complete statement of its income and they suggested that each member receive THE JOURNAL in response to the payment of dues. The committee quoted at length from the presidential address of Dr. Sayre as to the factors which should govern the publication of a periodical and the choice of an editor, and it summarized by recommending the publication of the periodical according to the plans that had been mentioned.

1882

ST. PAUL

The first business of the Association at the meeting in St. Paul in 1882 was a battle over the admission of delegates from New York. Most of the state medical societies of the South and Middle West and that of Pennsylvania protested the admission of delegates from the state of New York. All these protests were referred to the Judicial Council. The difficulty lay in the fact that the New York State Medical Society had passed a resolution which was alleged to ignore the Code of Ethics.

The difficulties with New York had to do with the distinctions between allopathists and homeopathists.

Dr. N. S. Davis presented a resolution in behalf of the Women's National Christian Temperance Union.

Then came the report of the committee on journalizing the Transactions, which was so vital to the Association that it was made a special order for the Thursday morning session.

Resolutions continued to be offered from various states condemning any attempts to adopt unusual methods of practice. A new section had been formed, known as the Section on Dental and Oral Surgery.

The report of the committee on publication was signed by Drs. John H. Packard, N. S. Davis, L. A. Sayre, J. S. Billings, R. B. Cole, W. B. Atkinson (the secretary) and R. J. Dunglison (the treasurer). This report estimated the cost of printing THE JOURNAL at about $15,000 a year. It indicated that the annual receipts varied from $2,000 to $6,000 and it felt that changes in the plan of the organization by which the doors of the Association could be opened to all members of the state and county societies on application were imperative. According to a recent census there were some 90,000 physicians in the United States. It was thought that, if 3,000 of these should become members of the Association, the mere expenses of THE JOURNAL would be provided for. The committee also considered the methods by which the business part of the enterprise could be properly carried on. It gave thought to the possibility of selecting an experienced business manager but seemed to prefer the idea of entering into a contract with some well known and responsible publishing house to issue THE JOURNAL for it. In this connection the committee felt that it might be necessary to incorporate the Association so as to give it a substantial character. It gave thought particularly to the appointment of an editor, saying:

> Upon the selection of a suitable man will hinge, in a very great measure, the success of the whole enterprise. He must be possessed of intellectual ability, firmness, tact and judgment; free from partisanship, of high professional and moral tone, and of such standing as will enable him to attract the support and secure the influence of the best class of contributors.
>
> It is very desirable that the editor's relation to the Association should be such as to leave him, as far as may be, untrammeled, while still responsible for the due discharge of his functions; that the arrangement should be such as to make it worth while for a suitable man to accept the position and still to preserve for the Association a just and equitable control of it. There would be obvious difficulties in the way of an election by the whole body annually, and it seems to us that the matter can hardly be placed to advantage in the hands of any of the existing committees.

THE BOARD OF TRUSTEES

With extraordinary wisdom the committee proposed that there should be elected by the Association a Board of Trustees—nine in number—to serve for three year terms and that the appointment of an editor be placed in the hands of these trustees. To the editor it assigned the appointment of assistant editors and on the Board of Trustees it placed responsibility for the conduct of the financial aspects of the publication. The committee recommended that the name of the journal should be THE JOURNAL OF THE AMERICAN MEDICAL ASSOCIATION and that outside subscribers be charged $6 a year for their subscriptions. It indicated, moreover, the method by which subscribers were to be secured.

Following the presentation of this report, Dr. N. S. Davis offered some resolutions, which were seconded by Dr. William Brodie of Michigan and unanimously adopted, making effective the recommendations of the committee.

EXPERT WITNESSES

The question of expert witnesses had also begun to be agitated in the annual session of the Association. A resolution had been offered to the effect that it was "the sense of the American Medical Association that it will be conducive to justice and to the dignity of the profession if medical expert testimony can be presented to the courts without the appearance of bias or influence from either side of the case and simply as a straightforward statement of scientific facts."

PERMANENT SECRETARY AND WASHINGTON

There had apparently begun to be some agitation also against the office of permanent secretary, and a resolution was offered and set by for a year that the nominating committee hereafter annually nominate a secretary who would serve without compensation.

Dr. Davis again offered a resolution requesting that every second meeting of the Association be held in Washington.

THE JUDICIAL COUNCIL

Most of the problems before the Judicial Council related to representatives of homeopathic groups in the Association. After carefully examining the documents relating to the New York State Medical Society, the Judicial Council adopted unanimously the following opinion:

Having carefully examined the Code of Ethics adopted by the New York State Medical Society at its annual meeting in February 1882 (as furnished by the secretary of said society), the Judicial Council find in said code provisions essentially different from, and in conflict with, the Code of Ethics of this Association; and therefore, in accordance with the provisions of the Ninth By-Law of the American Medical Association, they unanimously decide that said New York State Medical Society is not entitled to representation by delegates in this Association.

The Judicial Council also dropped from membership a number of other physicians on protests from their state medical societies.

THE LIBRARY

Although little has been said in these annual summaries of the work of the Association about the library, which was slowly accumulating in Washington, the librarian reported year after year. The report for 1882 indicates that the library now contained 1,702 distinct titles with about 4,448 volumes, inclusive of pamphlets. The Association was purchasing a good many foreign periodicals and books, subscribing $50 a year to the *Index Medicus* (which needed the help) and making a great many exchanges with the foreign publications.

THE VICE PRESIDENT ACTS

This was the first meeting of the American Medical Association in which the Vice President was compelled to substitute for the president. The task was undertaken by Dr. P. O. Hooper, the First Vice President. He paid gracious tribute to Dr. N. S. Davis, to whom more than to any other one individual the American Medical Association owed its founding and its development. He praised the work of the Association and recorded its success, and he welcomed the establishment of a periodical as a landmark in its progress. Particularly did he exalt the Principles of Ethics, urging the body not to retreat, not to involve itself in a world of inconsistencies. "The broad laws of demarcation between the irregular and the true physician should never be obliterated."

THE BOARD OF TRUSTEES

On the last day of the annual session of 1882 the committee on nominations suggested the following members for the first Board of Trustees of the American Medical Association to serve three years: Drs. N. S. Davis, E. M. Moore and J. M. Toner; for two years, H. F. Campbell, J. H. Packard and L. Connor; for one year, P. O. Hooper, A. Garcelon and L. S. McMurtry. This was adopted.

1883
CLEVELAND; THE FIRST EDITOR

At the meeting in Cleveland in 1883 Dr. N. S. Davis, chairman of the Board, reported that 2,100 pledges to sustain THE JOURNAL had been received from a mailing of 40,000, thus assuring its publication. Estimates for printing had been obtained, and as the bid of a Chicago company was lowest Chicago was recommended as the place of publication. The Trustees were authorized to proceed with the publication of THE JOURNAL. Dr. N. S. Davis was then introduced to the Association as the editor-in-chief and made some remarks. A vote of thanks was tendered to Dr. Davis for his willingness to assume the burdensome duties.

The original intention was to issue the first number of THE JOURNAL on July 1, but owing to the publisher's lack of facilities for such publication the first number of THE JOURNAL did not appear until July 14, 1883. It contained in its thirty-two pages a complete transcript of the minutes of the meeting of the Association. This was a clear gain of ten months on the usual time of appearance of the Transactions. The periodical also contained a number of scientific articles, some medical news and some notes of correspondence. It was printed by A. J. Newell at 71 and 73 Randolph Street. There is a preliminary note quoting the Transactions of the Association for 1851 which reads "The American Medical Association, though formally accepting and publishing the reports of the various standing committees (and sections), holds itself wholly irresponsible for the opinions, theories or criticisms therein contained, except otherwise decided by special resolution."

The Transactions of the Association as they appear in this first issue of THE JOURNAL represent a notable advance over previous Transactions in at least two particulars. They are more complete, and the various subjects discussed are introduced with suitable headings so as to make reference easy.

The first Board of Trustees adopted certain principles which deserve repetition. For instance, the editor was asked to secure as far as practicable the services of reliable correspondents in each of the great medical centers of the country and some of those in Europe. He was asked to maintain correspondence with the secretaries or proper officers of state medical societies. He was asked to solicit "advertisements from all medical educational institutions and hospitals open for clinical instruction, from book publishers, pharmaceutists, instrument makers, and all other legitimate business interests. But all advertisements of *proprietary, trade mark*, copyrighted or patented medicines should be excluded. Neither should any advertisements be admitted with one or more names of members of the profession as indorsers, having their *official titles* or *positions* attached.

"In other words, no advertisements should be admitted which fairly contravene in letter or in spirit the principles of the national code of ethics."

A special committee was established to nominate trustees to take the place of those whose terms had expired. This committee stated that the following were selected to complete the Board: Dr. Alonzo Garcelon of Maine, Dr. P. O. Hooper of Arkansas, Dr. L. S. McMurtry of Kentucky and Dr. J. H. Hollister of Illinois.

At this session the Association took action on a resolution urging the establishment of nurses' training schools in every county in the nation. It was proposed to form a special section on psychologic medicine. A resolution to revise the Principles of Ethics was laid on the table.

The address of the President of the Association, Dr. John L. Atlee of Lancaster, Pa., was devoted largely to reminiscences of some of the distinguished teachers of the past, including Dr. Caspar Wistar, Dr. Nathaniel Chapman, Dr. Philip Syng Physick and Dr. George McClellan. He had been a classmate of Dr. Isaac Hays, editor of the *American Journal of the Medical Sciences*, and he referred to him as "one who has done more for American medical journalism than any other physician in the country."

The first issue of THE JOURNAL in which the Transactions and the address of the President are published includes also a paper on "Tonsillotomy Without Haemorrhage" by W. C. Jarvis of New York and one by Henry Gradle of Chicago on "The Treatment of Otorrhoea with Antiseptic Powders." There is another paper on plastic surgery involving restoration of a lost cheek by a flap from the shoulder, written by Dr. Edmund Andrews of Chicago. There is an editorial on the change from the Transactions to a periodical and information to the effect that an index to the Transactions of the Association from its beginning to 1883 had been prepared by the permanent secretary. There is a request for exchanges and the hope that publishers would send one copy to the Library in Washington and another to THE JOURNAL.

Rather amusing is a communication from Philadelphia telling of the excitement caused there by the appearance of the new publication. Philadelphians "hope that THE JOURNAL will be truly national in character." Interesting also is a letter to the editor from Washington, D. C., proposing the formation of an insurance company to provide benefits for widows and orphans of physicians. Some news notes with reference to transactions of various societies complete that issue.

The second issue of THE JOURNAL contains the proceedings of the American Association of Medical Editors which was held in Cleveland, June 5, 1883. Dr. N. S. Davis was the president of that organization and he delivered an address on the present status and future tendencies of the medical profession in the United States. At the conclusion of the medical editors' meeting on June 5 that association adopted a resolution recommending Dr. N. S. Davis of Chicago to the American Medical Association as being the most suitable editor for THE JOURNAL which they shortly proposed publishing. The address by Dr. Davis on the present status of the medical profession reviewed in detail the manner in which the American Medical Association came into being as a representative body interested largely in improving the standards of medical education. He was desirous that more physicians associate themselves with organizations in the states and counties. He felt the need of specific research on definite problems.

"It is this want," he said, "of definite, well devised plans of original investigation and inquiry on the one hand, and of well planned cooperative observations on the other, that has led many of the wisest and most learned among us to think that all our medical organizations, whether state or national, amount to little more than a means of making professional acquaintance, enjoying annual seasons of social intercourse with each other, highly gratifying in their nature but accomplishing little in the advancement of medical science."

He deprecated the interest in specialization, saying "In the brief period of less than fifty years we have specialties in almost every part or region in the human body." And he was concerned with the restless desire for privileges to advertise these specialties more liberally than the general code of ethics adopted by the American Medical Association would permit. He saw already a tendency to disintegrate the national organization through special interests and influences. Dr. Davis emphasized the laws that had been passed in the various states following the establishment of the American Medical Association to protect the public:

> It has appeared from the review of the past that, during the first twenty-five years of our national existence, laws were enacted in nearly all the then existing states designed to protect the people from the impositions of ignorant and designing men claiming power to heal the sick, by prohibiting unlicensed practice, etc.; but which were nearly all repealed or so amended as to render them inoperative during the next thirty years by means of popular prejudices and false representations attendant upon the rise and spread of Thompsonianism and homoeopathy; the one playing upon the mind of the masses with all the power of bold and ignorant empiricism, and the other captivating the credulous tendencies of the more fashionable circles by a mystic transcendentalism inclosed in sugar pellets. The first has died a natural death, leaving a sickly offspring bearing the name of eclectics, while the second, like some medicines, retains its name as a "trade mark," and its organization for political influence, while its once transcendental vagaries have long since practically ceased to exert an influence over the treatment of disease.

Reviewing the status of the profession, he found some 60,000 to 70,000 persons, more or less educated, engaged in the alleviation of human suffering, with many voluntary society organizations for the mutual improvement of its members, all centering in one representative national organization—the American Medical Association. He found the education of the profession in the hands of sixty or seventy independent medical schools with the influence of their rivalry perverted by the recognition of their diplomas as equivalent to a license to practice. He deprecated the long absence of any adequate laws for protecting the people from the imposition of and ignorance of medical pretenders, but he saw great gain in the establishment of national and state boards of health and regulating the laws for the practice of medicine in several of the states. These legislative tendencies, he felt, would determine the status of the profession for the next fifty years.

MEDICAL ADVERTISING

Later issues of THE JOURNAL included a Chicago letter and a Boston letter, but by the issue of July 28, 1883 there began to be some protests against the advertisements. Witness the following delightful document from Burlington, Iowa:

> *Dear Doctor:*—I have received your first number and am delighted with it as a journal; but I am not so pleased with your advertisements. Parke, Davis & Co. have bored the physicians of the Northwest sufficiently with their ready-made prescriptions. In fact, they have taken the place of Ayer's Pectoral and Humbold's Buchu and are patronized by all the quacks and all the patent medicine men in this country. Soon I presume you will advertise Warner's safe cure for kidney trouble. Now, I protest right here against the organ of the American Medical Association being the means of disseminating any such advertisements. I ask a place for this in your correspondent's column, and see if I am not indorsed by nine tenths of the physicians in the land.

PROGRESS OF THE JOURNAL

A little later there is a Cincinnati letter and it begins to be apparent that the weekly journal is serving a most useful purpose. The medical progression has found in THE JOURNAL a voice. Physicians begin to express their opinions of new discoveries and of social changes. The papers read at the sections at the meeting in Cleveland are being published within a month or two of their reading. Speeding up of report intensifies the speed of progress. There are discussions in the correspondence columns of contract practice and medical ethics, of the question of consulting with irregulars, and more and more protests against the exploitation of the medical profession by the venders of "patent" and proprietary medicines.

The issue for Oct. 27, 1883 actually contains a paper read before the American Academy of Medicine on Oct. 9, 1883. It is entitled "Is It Fair?" and it is a study of the comparative political position of the medical profession in the United States.

Toward the end of the volume there are letters from Indianapolis and from Washington, D. C. The final number for the year indicates that 3,000 or 4,000 copies are being published each week and that it has been a considerable burden on the printers. A title page and an index are provided and the editor offers to make good missing numbers to any subscriber, to any person who wants to have a complete file for the year. The editor had also arranged to secure letters from Paris, of which two were published in the volume; one was published from London.

1884
WASHINGTON, D. C.

THE JOURNAL continued on its even course. During the first months of 1884 it began to provide news of interest to the medical profession concerning bills introduced in Washington; but apparently the editor was having some difficulties in filling his pages, for he began to republish from other periodicals and he included a good many trivia in his pages. His correspondent from Burlington, Iowa, who signed himself with the initials E. H. H., continued to trouble the editor with his letters about the advertising, being now annoyed by the advertisements of medical institutions, which were apparently somewhat profuse in their descriptions of the physicians who conducted these institutions.

THE NEW YORK STATE MEDICAL SOCIETY

An important editorial appeared in the issue for Feb. 9, 1884 discussing the action relative to the New York State Medical Society that had taken place in Cleveland. The editorial asked "Was the New York State Medical Society extruded from membership in the American Medical Association, or did she take herself out by her own act?" Apparently some of the New York delegates were a little disturbed by the situation and were proposing a reconciliation. The reconciliation was to be on the basis that the Association would thereafter recognize as a delegate any licensed physician from the state which sent him.

In the issue for Feb. 23, 1884 there was a discussion of a proposed resolution from St. Louis asking the Association to deny representation to medical colleges which paraded the names of the professor in their circulars. The editor called attention to the fact that the Association had not had any representatives from medical colleges for a dozen or fifteen years. This gave the editor opportunity to discuss still further the questions raised by the representative from New York State who proposed the reconciliation. But the New

York correspondent did not take this lying down. His letter in the issue for February 23 began with the statement that the editorial confirmed his statement, "if any confirmation was needed," that the American Medical Association was in the grasp of a few men, and the writer ended with this paragraph:

> Your statements only confirm those of my former letter in showing that, however cunningly the machinery of the American Medical Association may have been devised in the interests of harmony, it certainly is not, in its plan of working, entitled to the name of "American" and must undergo material change.

By this time a writer from Buffalo had decided that the argument was sufficiently good to permit him to take a hand, and his letter also was duly published.

MEDICAL EDUCATION

The issue for April 5, 1884 had an excellent editorial on medical colleges and their endowments which ended with the significant statement that "it is not new colleges that is [sic] required but a more efficient management of old ones."

The address of the President, Dr. Austin Flint, for 1884 appeared in the issue for May 10, 1884. It was a review of the history of the Association, with increasing emphasis on the necessity for high scholarship among those who wish to be physicians, and it came to its end with the paragraph "The practical question is 'What can the Association do to promote more and more the elevation of the standard of medical education?'" He did not accept the charge that medical education in the United States was unworthy of any commendation and as contemptible when contrasted with the educational advantages of other countries. He found advantages in the American methods of teaching. He defended the medical schools against the charge of venality and deception and he set up a program for elevating the standard of medical education, utilizing the forces of the American Medical Association. Here, for the first time, is the suggestion of a standing committee on medical education designed to secure uniform action with reference to requirements for matriculation and for graduation.

THE PRINCIPLES OF ETHICS

An equal portion of Dr. Flint's address was concerned with the Code of Ethics; he discussed the new code—so called—in the state of New York which would permit consultations with all legally qualified practitioners of medicine. His argument was legalistic and he was inclined to believe that the New York code could be accepted, since that code defined an irregular practitioner as one whose practice was based on an exclusive dogma to the rejection of the accumulated experience of the profession. He emphasized that the needs of the patient are always to be the first consideration and he approved that, except in extreme emergencies, consultation with quacks, charlatans and irregular practitioners can only injure humanity.

Here we find the address of the President and also of the chairman of the Section on the Practice of Medicine appearing in THE JOURNAL at the very week of the meeting.

The editorial for May 17 was an obituary notice of S. D. Gross, followed by a report in editorial form of the thirty-fifth anniversary meeting of the American Medical Association. The meeting was held in Washington. More than 1,200 regularly registered members were present. The papers had been well chosen, and there was some condemnation of the Section on State Medicine for having only a few papers and those not especially well selected. In his address, Dr. Austin Flint had paid tribute to Dr. S. D. Gross, who had died at the very hour when the address was being delivered.

ANIMAL EXPERIMENTATION

For the first time the Association found it necessary to adopt a resolution in defense of animal experimentation. A committee of seven was appointed, to be known as the Committee on Experimental Medicine, charged with the duty of opposing, by all legitimate means, unwise or ill considered legislation. This battle against the forces of ignorance and fanaticism had gone on and on with the victory never permanently won, so that year after year in many of our states, in many of our large cities and even in the Congress of the United States it becomes necessary to defend the use of animals in experimentation for the advancement of medical science and the improvement of human health.

THE JOURNAL

The report of the Board of Trustees which appeared in this volume pointed out that the regulation relative to advertisements established at the Cleveland meeting was a wise restraint tending to elevate the dignity of THE JOURNAL but at the same time deprive it of a considerable revenue.

The publication of THE JOURNAL had brought about a remarkable increase in the income of the Association. The Association found itself with a surplus in the treasury over all expenses. In the editor's report to the Board of Trustees he pointed out that he had been compelled to reject a good deal of advertising on account of the restrictions.

Having made an excellent report, Dr. Davis had offered the Trustees his resignation. The Board, with but one dissenting voice, requested Dr. Davis to withdraw his letter of resignation. In a letter of response he was impelled "now to yield to your nearly unanimous request that I withdraw the resignation tendered" but he stated definitely that he must positively withdraw from a position involving so much labor and responsibility at the end of the next year.

A minority report was presented by Dr. John H. Packard. Dr. Packard pointed out that the Association was able to have a surplus because the editor abstained from drawing his salary and that the board was counting on his abstaining from drawing his salary for some time to come. However, this was not his chief complaint. He felt that THE JOURNAL had not, in his opinion, approached anywhere near the standard of what the organ of the associated medical profession of the United States should be. He felt that publication of THE JOURNAL in Chicago was difficult because there was not sufficient access to large libraries. He felt that contributions to its pages should be properly and liberally paid for. He did not like the printing. He thought that the resignation of Dr. Davis should be accepted and that the publication office of THE JOURNAL should be transferred to some Eastern city, preferably Washington, Philadelphia or New York. The minority report was first called for and it was laid on the table by 191 ayes to 74 noes. The majority report was then adopted.

DIFFICULTIES AND DISTURBANCES

There were other points of difference which now began to be discussed in the House of Delegates. There were many resolutions recommending changes in the Principles of Ethics. It was proposed that the Section on Ophthalmology, Otology, Laryngology and Rhinology be divided into two sections, one dealing with ophthalmology and the other with otology, laryngology and rhinology. There was even a resolution calling attention to the fact that the American Medical Association was composed of all nationalities, denominations, sects and creeds, and that many of its members were skeptics and materialists and that therefore the custom of opening the sessions of the American Medical Association with a prayer should be abolished. This motion was unanimously rejected.

Congress was urged to make proper preparations for the Medical Library and Museum. There was a resolution, well in advance of its time, asking Congress and the legislatures of the several states to label lye, a caustic potash, as poisonous. It took about fifty years for Congress to act on that one, and it required the work of Chevalier Jackson in our time to make the Congress realize the necessity.

In his editorial presenting the Transactions, Nathan Smith Davis proposed several excellent technics for registration at the annual sessions. He pointed out that the effectiveness of the sections depends on the permanence and efficiency of their secretaries and he recommended greater permanence in this office.

One is constantly amazed at the remarkable talent for organizational efficiency and the supreme qualities of leadership manifested by Nathan Smith Davis in the first forty years of the work of the American Medical Association. If ever it could be said that one man more than any other deserved credit for having inspired the necessary cooperation for advancement, for having manifested ingenuity of thought and action, for having worked with indomitable courage and energy for the advancement of an organization, that credit should go to Dr. Nathan Smith Davis.

The first issue of THE JOURNAL for June 1884 contained a paper by Leartus Connor on the "American Medical Association of the Future." He found that there had been 509 medical periodicals in the United States up to that time, of which 136 were surviving and 373 departed. He analyzed the forces which prevailed toward the inauguration of such journals and their continuance. "THE JOURNAL OF THE AMERICAN MEDICAL ASSOCIATION," he said, "is now passing through the first stages of a similar development under less favorable circumstances. Like its English brother, it has already been subjected to sharp criticism, it has had to meet the envy, jealousy and disappointed ambition of disappointed persons and localities, but we have no doubt that in the end it will surmount all these obstacles and have a future even more brilliant than its English brother."

He concluded with the suggestion of some general principles along which medical journals must move. He felt that a medical editor, like a poet, is born and not made and that he must be given freedom in his work. He was certain that the most influential medical journals would develop in the great commercial centers and that with increasing wealth and power they would be able to pay their editors such salaries that they could devote all their time to the profession of medical journalism. The medical journals of the future would be more and more separated from medical colleges, medical societies or other corporate bodies that cripple their perfect independence to work and think and speak for the great masses of the medical profession. "The advertising claims of the medical journal of the future," he said, "will have less and less influence over the utterances of the editorial pages" and, further, that the advertising columns of the best medical journals of the future "will contain a notice of nothing which shall not be free to every pharmacist to manufacture, as free as the formulas of the Pharmacopeia." He felt that the medical journals would be able to pay more for the contributions to their pages as well as to their editors. And, finally, he was convinced that experience would do most of the teaching. "The past shows," he said, "that it is impossible to persuade a man that he is unfit to run a medical journal until he has convinced himself by trying."

In the issue for June 28, 1884 N. S. Davis made some comments on the completion of his second volume. He admitted that there had been some imperfection in his work, but he was willing that the numbers issued during the last three or four months should be compared with reference to all that related to style of publication with the best weekly medical publications in this country. He was a little burned by some criticisms from the *New York Medical Journal*, which in one issue had published half a column of corrections of its own typographical errors; and he called attention to a few mistakes that he had found in the *Record*, "whose editor is so fond of criticizing others." Dr. Davis was smarting over the criticisms from the East and he said "Had either of these blunders occurred in THE JOURNAL or any other outside of 'one of the great *Eastern* cities' it would have been held up as a sample of incompetent provincial work for the next six months."

THE JOURNAL GAINS

THE YEAR 1885

ALMOST FORTY YEARS had passed since the American Medical Association had been organized at Philadelphia. In the intervening period the Johns Hopkins University had been founded; bacteria had been grown on artificial mediums; Alexander Graham Bell had introduced the telephone, for which many doctors' wives would curse him roundly in the years that were to come.

The gonococcus was discovered by Neisser in 1879, and Pasteur isolated the streptococcus and the staphylococcus in 1880. Every one of these discoveries was to be reflected within a few years in the discussions of the scientific sections of the American Medical Association.

Dr. John Shaw Billings had taken a considerable part in the work of the American Medical Association, particularly in its Section on State Medicine (which we today would call public health). In 1880 John Shaw Billings published the first volume of the *Index Catalogue*, the first attempt to index regularly the medical periodical literature of the world.

In 1880 also the American Surgical Association was founded, one of the first societies devoted exclusively to specialists. Only a few years before there had been many discussions of the rights of specialists compared with the rights of general practitioners. The economic, scientific and social aspects of specialization in medicine were to attract increasing attention and to become major subjects of medical discussion as the years rolled by.

With the discovery of bacteria and of first antiseptic and then aseptic surgery the surgeons began increasingly to invade portions of the body never before accessible. In 1881 Billroth resected the pylorus, and in the same year Czerny described vaginal excision of uterine tumors and Hahn removed a kidney. In 1882 Robert Koch discovered the tubercle bacillus.

The scientific papers read before the sections of the American Medical Association began increasingly to attempt to reconcile the newer knowledge of germs in the causation of disease with the weird and sometimes mystical classifications of disease that had characterized previous excursions by the medical profession into the problems of disease causation.

THE JOURNAL

As 1885 dawned THE JOURNAL for January 3 of that year apologized because the last issue for December of 1884 had appeared late. A single galley of proof had been tied up somewhere in the Christmas rush in the postoffice, and the list of members had taken two pages more than had been anticipated because of the increase in membership.

There was still some argument as to whether or not diphtheria was a contagious disease. Indeed, in the light of *post hoc* knowledge some of the discussions of the 1880's seem bizarre indeed. There was quite a battle over the question of whether or not a solid stethoscope would convey sound better than a hollow one.

THE JOURNAL was beginning to make its presence felt on the medical profession. The interest in the American Medical Association was increasing. Sectionalism was developing in American medicine; it was to be the source of much anguish and misunderstanding for years to come. These misunderstandings reflected in some instances the thirst for prestige and power by the publishers and editors of some of the Eastern medical journals.

Another source of disturbance was the practice of the homeopathic system and the bitterness against homeopathy manifested by such leaders as Oliver Wendell Holmes. The powers in the American Medical Association felt that the abandonment by the New York State Medical Association of principles of ethics concerned chiefly with consultations by members of the Association with physicians who adhered to peculiar medical beliefs was a direct thrust at the foundation stones of the Association itself.

In March 1885 N. S. Davis gave account of his progress with THE JOURNAL. He informed the readers that he had told the Board of Trustees that "under no circumstances" would he extend his work as editor beyond the current year. Less than two years had passed since the first number of THE JOURNAL was issued. There had been continuous growth of the membership, which had increased from 1,428 in 1875 to 3,887 in 1885. The *British Medical Journal*, cited everywhere as the foremost publication in medicine, had been founded in 1865 and had achieved by 1885 a circulation of 12,000.

In a later editorial the editor noted how greatly THE JOURNAL had aided in hastening the publication of important contributions made at the annual session and how well it had reflected the general progress of medicine in the United States. The annual income of the

American Medical Association had risen from $5,008 in 1879 to $13,017.25 in 1884 and to $18,117.25 in 1885. The Association was thus quite solvent: its income just about balanced its budget. We see later that this balancing was made possible by the failure of the editor and of some of his helpers to collect any income whatever for their work. In a final editorial on the current situation. Dr. N. S. Davis pointed out that he had been unable to employ necessary help because of inadequate funds in the treasury and that the printer had been willing to postpone some of the payment on his account. "By deferring all pay for his own services, and limiting thus the number of paid assistants, he conserved enough in the treasury to pay all publication expenses promptly and at the end of the year from the later collections received for himself a reasonable remuneration for the editorial work performed and left a surplus sufficient to pay the other current expenses of the Association."

The editor had been disturbed by the fact that members who had contributed papers, reports and addresses had failed to send them promptly to THE JOURNAL in accordance with the By-Laws. Other medical periodicals had had access to this material and they had taken away its journalistic newness by publication of abstracts before there was opportunity to publish the material in THE JOURNAL. Dr. N. S. Davis then established the policy that the address of the President of the American Medical Association should be published in the week in which he delivered it and the chairman of the individual sections would have their addresses published in THE JOURNAL each week that followed.

In the first editorial for April 1885 the editor discussed at considerable length the problems of print'ng involved in publishing THE JOURNAL. There were attempts to turn over the publication to commercial publishers and thus to take it away from its direct control by the Board of Trustees. Dr. Davis felt that it was time to fix the place of publication for a term of years and to purchase necessary printing equipment so that the composition of THE JOURNAL would be the work of the Association, although the press work could be done elsewhere. Dr. Davis urged the establishment of its own press by the Association because he felt certain that this would lead eventually to a much better publication and to complete control by the organization itself.

Another sign of growing pains was the introduction of several resolutions having to do with the membership in the Association and with membership on the nominating committee. There was naturally some objection to having members of the nominating committee nominate themselves to important offices.

THE NEW ORLEANS SESSION

The meeting in 1885 at New Orleans heard an address by the President, Dr. Henry F. Campbell of Augusta, Ga. Southern oratory rolled in resounding phrases. Thus he spoke of the passing of S. D. Gross and J. Marion Sims:

> With shining robes more honorable than any toga of office we can put upon them, with crowns more resplendent than those of earthly monarchs, and with harps and melodies more entrancing than the music of our love or the anthems of our praise, they hear no more the voice of human adulation.

However, after some pages of this florescent diction Dr. Campbell turned his attention to serious criticism. He praised the development of THE JOURNAL. He poured satire on professional testimony in the courts and on the lawyers who cross examined the medical witnesses. He urged the establishment of a section devoted to forensic medicine.

THE ARMY LIBRARY

Dr. John Shaw Billings reported the complete success of the effort to obtain an appropriation from Congress for fireproof buildings for the Army Medical Museum and Library, and he announced that the building operations would soon be commenced. The building, reported first in 1885, still stands in Washington in 1947—a veritable firetrap—holding in its bursting walls millions of books and pamphlets of incalculable value while members of the medical profession and of innumerable other agencies urge the Congress again and again to make adequate appropriation for the building of a modern structure worthy to house the treasures whose existence is threatened every moment by the inadequacy of the old building that now contains them.

THE EDITOR

The Board of Trustees announced that it had earnestly requested Dr. Davis to withdraw his resignation and to continue his relations with THE JOURNAL as its supervising editor. His sense of duty impelled him to suspend his resignation and to yield to the unanimous request of the Board to continue his editorial superintendence of THE JOURNAL until such time as a successor could be appointed.

THE BENJAMIN RUSH MONUMENT

The House of Delegates had been intent on developing funds for the monument for Benjamin Rush to be unveiled at the meeting of the International Medical Congress which would be held in 1887. Some $45,000 was needed for this purpose and it was to be collected by a maximum contribution of $1 from each subscriber; the monument would be erected in Washington. The committee called attention to the manner in which statesmen, military heroes and naval heroes had been honored with monuments as had also painters, sculptors and various scientists.

Benjamin Rush received his A.B. degree from Princeton when less than 15 years old. He studied medicine with John Redman in Philadelphia for six years and translated the aphorisms of Hippocrates from the original Greek. As a student when only 17 he had described the epidemic of yellow fever that prevailed in Philadelphia. After obtaining his degree of doctor of medicine at Edinburgh in 1766 he studied in London and in Paris and returned to the United States in 1769. He was one of the signers of the Declaration of Independence. Benjamin Rush was one of the surgeon generals in the Army of the Revolution and a member of the convention that adopted the federal Constitution, which he called "a masterpiece of human wisdom."

In 1789 he succeeded Dr. Morgan in the chair of theory and practice of medicine in the Medical College of Philadelphia. Once the federal government was established, he devoted himself wholly to his profession and to civic affairs. The only office which he accepted as a reward for his many government services was the position of president of the mint, which he held for fourteen years. He was one of the vice presidents of the American Philosophical Society; he aided in founding Dickinson College; he was president of the American Society for the Abolition of Slavery. Benjamin Rush died in 1813 at the age of 68 as a victim of an epidemic of typhus.

1886

ST. LOUIS

Early in 1886 attention was called by THE JOURNAL to the crowded character of the program of the American Medical Association. The difficulty was that the addresses of the chairmen of the sections were taking too long in some instances and not long enough in others. This agitation was to culminate in the eventual divorcement of the reading of the chairmen's addresses from the general meeting and the limitation of such addresses to the sections themselves. This divorcement, however, was another step in the tendency toward specialization, since its inevitable result was to limit the consideration of special topics to the specialists and to make impossible their delivery to the general practitioners, who might be said to need them most.

There was also some criticism of the attempts to build a program by the voluntary offering of papers. The chairmen and secretaries were urged to invite contributions from competent authorities on important subjects so that there would be at least one or two leading papers in each section and at least one or two equally qualified members to open the discussions of the papers.

One cannot but pause to marvel again at the insight and organizational ability of Nathan Smith Davis. As one views the progress and development of the American Medical Association and the elements in its activities which have obtained permanent status, one finds again and again that the concept arose in the mind of Dr. N. S. Davis, that it was presented by him so clearly and succinctly as to carry conviction and that he fought for these steps in progress with a persistence and sincerity that led inevitably to their success.

BATTLE OVER THE INTERNATIONAL CONGRESS

The jealousies of which mention has been previously made flared into public view early in 1886, when the editors of some of the Eastern medical journals denied the right of the American Medical Association to participate largely in the formation of a forthcoming International Congress of Medicine to be held in Washington. These Eastern editors endeavored to sabotage the American Medical Association's committee and tried to deter members of the profession from accepting any official positions in the preliminary organization of the congress. In an attempt to overcome this opposition, places on the national committee were offered to the most eminent of those in the opposition. The battle waged so fiercely that attempts were made to control the election of delegates to the meeting of the American Medical Association with a view to mustering a majority at the meeting in St. Louis. These efforts also failed.

Mingled with this controversy was the question of the status of the homeopathists. Apparently foreign countries had admitted homeopathists to their delegations and it was desired that homeopathists be admitted to the American delegation. Then arose the question of admitting not only homeopathists but also eclectics, physiomedical graduates, hygiotherapeutic graduates and those of some other schools. To settle the difficulty, an official announcement by the American Medical Association made it clear that any legally acknowledged practitioner would be admitted to the congress.

Much of the attack centered on Dr. John Shaw Billings, as secretary of the original committee of seven which was planning the congress. The American Medical Association called on him to explain exactly what he and his committee really did expect of the Association. The original committee of seven had been commissioned to go to Copenhagen in 1884 and to invite the International Medical Congress to meet in the United States. A somewhat satirical comment in THE JOURNAL stated that "they satisfactorily performed this office and through their spokesman promised the members a generous welcome, he pledging himself to do a variety of things without reservation (expressed, at least), as to the contingency of his not being allowed to have everything his own way."

Apparently there were a good many political appointments made to positions of distinction, and there was general resentment against these actions and attitudes.

MEDICAL ORGANIZATION

In the meantime there began to be repercussions in Philadelphia over the charge of political manipulation of its delegation to the American Medical Association. A secret caucus had been held for the nomination of delegates, and the members, having discovered this fact, began to be resentful. Some of these discussions led the editor of THE JOURNAL, Dr. N. S. Davis, to publish an editorial in the issue of Feb. 27, 1886, urging the possibility of reorganization of the American Medical Association along the lines of the British Medical Association with the fundamental principle of membership in a county and state medical society as a basis for membership in the American Medical Association. The decision to organize the American Medical Association along such lines had caused the organization of state medical societies where none existed and had caused the reorganization of state medical societies which had been allowed to die. The editor pointed out that the admission of two delegates from the faculty of each medical college and one from the staff of each hospital, lunatic asylum and dispensary not only gave these medical men a much larger number of delegates but removed from them the incentive to become members and to officiate as members in their own state medical societies. Ultimately this change in the method of organization was to be one of the most important single influences in building a strong democratic representative body.

This editorial led to an extensive correspondence objecting to the organization of the American Medical Association with branch societies as is done in Great Britain and insisting that the system whereby the state medical societies constitute the real branches of the organization was a proper one for a country such as ours. The organizational technic of N. S. Davis is nowhere better manifested than in this practice of writing an editorial to stimulate discussion in the correspondence columns, reactivating discussion by further editorials when it tended to die and thus maintaining the interest of members of the Association everywhere in the problems of its conduct.

As might be expected, however, there were certain definitely disorganizing influences which arose from this discussion. One finds an attack on a former President of the American Medical Association as being a man who did not merit the position but who was elected to it only for his political influence. There was an editorial in the *Nashville Journal of Medicine and Surgery* in February 1886 which was reprinted in the *Medical News* of Philadelphia, claiming that the American Medical Association was a body merely medico-political, full of political intrigue and trickery. There was an attack on this editorial accusing the editor of the *Nashville Journal of Medicine and Surgery* of having "the effrontery to parade such intentions before an intelligent profession." The political battle being waged in editorials and in correspondence was moving into the stage of hand-to-hand conflict at the next annual session of the American Medical Association.

SOCIAL FUNCTIONS

In April 1886 Dr. Davis was again moved to turn his attention to the social functions at the annual session. He expressed his appreciation of the meeting in Boston in 1849, when "one evening was set apart for a general social melée or promenade in a public hall for the laudable purpose of affording more direct social intercourse of members from all parts of the country. With genuine good taste the local committee provided no other refreshments than coffee, simple cakes and fruit on a side table where those who wished could partake when they pleased. But this simple and very pleasant example was quickly converted into the form of a public banquet, which each subsequent local committee of arrangements endeavored to make more magnificent and costly than their predecessors, until at New York in 1853 the banquet alone was said to have cost more than $10,000; and the next year at St. Louis its extravagance and the excesses accompanying it led to the adoption of a resolution offered by the late Professor S. D. Gross forbidding all subsequent committees of arrangements to provide any public banquet in connection with the annual meetings of the Association."

This multiplication of official functions and similar jamborees led eventually to the adoption of a general rule that each alternate meeting should be held in Washington and that the necessary expenses for halls and programs should be met by the Association.

THE ST. LOUIS SESSION

When the Association convened in St. Louis it was announced that protests had been entered against the delegates from the

Philadelphia County Medical Society, the New York Academy of Medicine, the Tri-State Medical Society, the Mississippi Valley Association and the Davidson County Medical Society, and one Tennessee doctor protested against the Tennessee State Medical Association.

The meeting in St. Louis brought an attendance of 1,100. The address of the President, Dr. William Brodie, paid tribute to the great men of the profession who had died during the year, among whom was Dr. Austin Flint. Dr. Brodie told of the effectiveness of the Association in raising the standards of medical education. He listed the prize essays as an indication of its scientific contribution. He noted the organization of special societies, of ophthalmologists, otologists, gynecologists, dermatologists, public health officers, laryngologists, surgeons and pathologists. Thus the rise of specialization had been exceedingly rapid. It was Dr. Brodie's opinion that nothing could be gained by changing the nature of the American Medical Association to resemble that of the British Medical Association with its branches. He forecast a feeble reception for the report of the committee of the ninth International Medical Congress and he pleaded with those who had fought the committee to give it their full support.

Apparently the spade work preliminary to the convention had been well done. The report of the committee was, on motion, received and adopted with enthusiasm and without an audible negative vote by the entire convention with almost a thousand delegates in the hall. Indeed the editor of THE JOURNAL was delighted to report complete harmony, whereas two months previously everyone seemed to be sharpening his knife in readiness for the conflict.

The committee on organization of the International Medical Congress in 1887 made its report suggesting the name of N. S. Davis of Chicago for president and John B. Hamilton of Washington, D. C., as secretary general. The vote was recorded as unanimous. A motion offered by a Pennsylvania delegate to reconsider this motion was laid on the table.

At this session of the Association an amendment was adopted that each section should nominate its own officers. The establishment of a section on dermatology and syphilis was approved.

The business committee, acting as a reference committee, endorsed the views of the President that all papers read in the annual session should become the exclusive property of THE JOURNAL; it asked the Judicial Council to take action against members who introduced proprietary remedies and appliances. It recommended the appointment of a committee to study reorganization of the Association. A resolution was adopted that the Association approve cremation or incineration of the dead as a sanitary necessity in all populous cities.

The meeting was notable for the presence of General William Tecumseh Sherman, who entered the room and sat on the platform during the fourth day of the session.

The Trustees reported on THE JOURNAL and then asked Dr. N. S. Davis to make an individual report. Dr. Davis expressed his dissatisfaction with the income from advertising and some defection in subscribers. These included, first, those disaffected by the New York New Code party and later the opponents to the organization for the International Medical Congress. Notwithstanding these defections there had been a total increase in members and subscribers. Dr. Davis had consented to remain as editor, and the Trustees expressed their confidence that the experiment in publishing THE JOURNAL was fully warranted and that some day it would prove that their experiment was sound.

The difficulties over delegates in this convention were thoroughly analyzed by the Judicial Council, which made its report on the final day of the session. The delegates from tristate societies were considered not entitled to admission, since the Association recognized only the state societies and the county, district and local societies affiliated with the state societies. It asked the Davidson County Medical Society in Tennessee to show up next time with some credentials which would prove its connection with the Tennessee State Medical Society. The evidence against the Mississippi Valley State Medical Society was found insufficient for consideration. The Judicial Council found also that the delegates from the Philadelphia County Medical Society had been elected by methods which were of such an irregular character that the delegates would have to be rejected. The Judicial Council authorized the return of the dues of these delegates.

When the meeting was over and the delegates had returned home, the *Medical Record* of New York published some editorial comments calculated to create the impression that this meeting of the American Medical Association was not really representative and that the action of the Judicial Council relative to the delegates from Philadelphia had started a serious split in the American Medical Association. To this the *Philadelphia Medical and Surgical Reporter* replied "It is hardly fair to speak of a split when only a few fibers are carried away; it would be more correct to say a shave or a scrape. The main body of the American Medical Association is today more united than it ever was, and it has lost the allegiance only of those who 'got mad' because they could not control." The editorial in THE JOURNAL OF THE AMERICAN MEDICAL ASSOCIATION proves that the attendance was most representative and that there was little danger that a proposed congress of American specialists "constructed from a union of half a dozen American specialist organizations could take the place of the Association."

1887
CHICAGO

In January 1887 the students of the Chicago Medical College presented N. S. Davis, in honor of his fifty years in medical practice, with an armchair and a revolving bookshelf. Such a piece of furniture as the revolving bookshelf is still found in one of the offices of the headquarters of the American Medical Association and is probably the very one which was presented to N. S. Davis at that time. In the history of medicine such gifts represent one of the finest amenities in medical relationships. In the same year Dr. J. Adams Allen, commonly known as "Uncle Allen," was presented by the students of Rush Medical College with a "tripod" consisting of a fat, chubby hand, made of solid gold. It was set on an onyx pedestal on which was inscribed:

UNCLE ALLEN'S TRIPOD

Remember these three
When we practice the art:
The condition of blood,
The nerves, and the heart.

This quotation was a verse of the college song at Rush based on some of Dr. Allen's sayings. The hand was in the position that he usually held when addressing the students.

The editorials in THE JOURNAL were increasingly devoted to scientific subjects, with less attention to problems of organization and representation. Dr. Davis was disturbed by the unsatisfactory reporting of the discussions in the sections, urging the reporters to give in greater detail the statements made by those who discussed the individual papers.

A SPECIAL ISSUE OF THE JOURNAL

As the time approached for the annual session, THE JOURNAL issued a special number in an extra large edition giving the program of the meeting and full information as to its various features. Members of the Association were requested to visit the publication office to see how well THE JOURNAL was getting along, and the members were promised four more pages of reading matter with each issue during the coming year.

As the time neared for the meeting of the Association, the members were again reminded that the business office at 65 Randolph Street was open at all times and that a clerk would be present at all times to welcome them. THE JOURNAL printing office was at 68 Wabash Avenue, only one square from the Central Music Hall, where the Association was to meet and where extra volumes of the Transactions published prior to 1883 were to be found for sale.

THE ANNUAL SESSION

The President of the Association, Dr. Elisha H. Gregory, read an address on "Cell Antagonism" which differed from every previous address in being a highly technical review of knowledge of the cell. He concluded his address by calling attention to the near approach of the International Medical Congress and by requesting all members of the American Medical Association to participate and entertain properly the numerous delegates from abroad.

The Board of Trustees reported that THE JOURNAL had been well published with the operation of its own press and that Dr. N. S. Davis had consented to continue its management. The Association now owned several fonts of type. There seemed to be a small increase in its subscription, but this was due to the fact that 524 subscribers had been added while 244 had been removed for nonpayment and for other reasons, including death.

Again attention was called by N. S. Davis to the fact that the Code controversy in New York and the battle over the International Congress had resulted in considerable damage to the Association's membership. However, these two revolts had spent their force and there had been recently increased applications for membership and renewals of subscriptions—more, in fact, than at any previous time since THE JOURNAL had been established. Dr. Davis urged again an expansion of THE JOURNAL printing office and he gave credit particularly to Dr. William G. Eggleston as assistant in editorial work and to Mr. J. Harrison White, who was both foreman and printing office and advertising manager.

CHANGES IN ORGANIZATION

Most important at this session of the Association was the report of the special committee on changes in the plan of organization and by-laws. The proposed amendments included changes in the technic of choosing members, the elimination of the nominating committee and the substitution of a general committee, the elimination of the committee on publication and the substitution of the Board of Trustees, the choice of chairmen in the individual sections by election in the sections and the new method for choosing those who were to give the annual addresses in the sections. The report of the committee was adopted. As an indication of the difference of opinion, however, a standing vote was taken on the adoption of this reorganization and the final vote was 274 for and 232 against. A roll call of the states established a committee on nominations with a representative from each state.

THE RUSH MONUMENT

An extensive report was presented by the Rush monument committee including a statement by its secretary and by its treasurer. The committee had made a very minor start on the total of $45,000 which it had started to collect. The total sum which had been sent to the treasurer was $389, and the committee had spent $143.08 on its expenses.

THE ANNUAL DINNER

As this session neared its end, several resolutions were offered which were again fundamental to the progress of the Association. One had to do with the holding of an annual dinner in which there were to be two kinds of tickets, one without wines or liquors and one with wines or liquors, so that any members of the Association could come to the dinner and not drink without feeling that he was paying for the liquor that was drunk by others. This resolution was adopted by a large majority.

THE FINANCIAL CONTROL

A resolution was offered appropriating an honorarium of $300 to the permanent secretary. To this Dr. Davis offered an amendment to the effect that the Board of Trustees be a standing committee on finance to which all propositions for the appropriation of money should be referred and reported on before final action on the same by the Association. This simple resolution, which arose out of a motion to pay a small honorarium to the permanent secretary, was probably more significant in the financial prosperity of the American Medical Association as it exists today than any other action taken up to that time.

1888

CINCINNATI

The first volume for the year 1888 indicates that THE JOURNAL was edited for the Association by N. S. Davis, assisted by William G. Eggleston and N. S. Davis, Jr.

A NATIONAL DEPARTMENT OF HEALTH

Early in the year THE JOURNAL began to agitate for a national department of health, with particular reference to a national department for the control of adulteration of foods. This, it must be remembered, was 1888. The United States does not yet have a national department of health, although it has the U. S. Public Health Service. It required the action of Theodore Roosevelt and the publication of books by Samuel Hopkins Adams called "The Great American Fraud" and by Upton Sinclair called "The Jungle" to obtain a national law that would regulate the purity of foods and drugs.

THE GENERAL MEETING

Arrangements began to be made for the next meeting of the Association in which the addresses of the chairmen would be read before the sections rather than before the general assembly. However, arrangements were made for three important addresses before the entire assembly, forecasting the modern period with the general scientific meetings, in which three complete sessions are given over to general statements reflecting the advancement of medical science.

RIGHTS OF A DOCTOR IN HIS CLINIC

The editor of THE JOURNAL was also a little annoyed because medical reporters had begun attending clinics in hospitals and selling lecture notes to Eastern medical journals. Indeed, one reporter had annoyed the editor considerably by selling three of the editor's lectures in this manner without even allowing him to see the reports as first transcribed or to read the galley proofs. A Chicago judge gave a bench opinion to the effect that such activities were illegal and that redress could be had by resort to the courts for this piracy of medical literary material.

KNOWLEDGE OF DIPHTHERIA

An editorial in the issue for March 31, 1888, pointed out that a member of the Association disagreed with the editor, who had said that diphtheria was a preventable disease. He asked the editor to explain how he would go about preventing diphtheria. The editor, after some elusive discourse on the subject, said that "diphtheria, erysipelas, cholera, yellow fever and some other diseases evidently depend on specific infections developed outside the human being and capable of being introduced into it in connection with the air we inhale or the food and drink we take. Hence our formula for the prevention of diphtheria does not consist of drugs to be obtained at the apothecaries' but of an abundance of pure air, good water, wholesome food, clean soil, and a clear personality." In the light of modern use of antidiphtheria toxoid, this formula can be viewed only with praise for its sincerity. Just a few weeks passed until the editor had to write on the subject again. A member had suggested that probably isolation and disinfection should have been mentioned. Here the editor did a brilliant piece of open field running by pointing out that any family that was as clean as he had proposed would have nothing to isolate or disinfect. It was his idea that isolation and disinfection are performed only after infection has already occurred and that therefore they have little to do with the prevention of infection.

DRESS REFORM

About this time a prominent German professor became convinced that gallstones and tight lacing had a definite relationship. The editor of THE JOURNAL rather doubted that there was a true causal relationship but he was inclined to think that perhaps it was just frequent coincidence. He pointed out that the tight lacing goes on during the day and is loosened up at night. However, he felt that persistent tight lacing could cause a change in the configuration and that probably after all some cases of gallstones and perhaps also cancers of the gallbladder were due to tight lacing. Incidentally, a few pathologists had found the liver completely deformed by the tight stays of the corset of that day. It is not surprising then to find that Dr. Helen L. Betts of Boston read a paper before the Gynecological Society of Boston in December 1887 on the dress of woman and its relationship to the etiology and treatment of pelvic disease. Dr. Betts was an ardent advocate of dress reform. She wanted women to get rid of all the clinging garments with which their bodies were enveloped and she wanted them to get some exercise and outdoor life similar to that permitted to boys. She attributed congestion of the internal organs of women to their clothing and their habits. She cited a case from her own practice in which she felt that this was the primary trouble:

> The first, clearest indication seemed to remove the superincumbent pressure; so, as usual, I examined her mode of dress. You will be interested from a professional standpoint to know what this patient wore. I examined her at her home, so she had on simply her indoor garments. There were knit and muslin drawers, flannel and muslin underskirts, hoopskirt and bustle, then a muslin and a dress skirt, seven bands; fourteen thicknesses were buttoned closely about the corset, and, not long before, her physician, having noticed that she wore her garters about her legs, said he feared they would interfere with circulation and advised that she should put an elastic band about the waist and fasten the stockings to this! I asked if her clothes were not oppressive. She said she thought she wore very light clothing but had noticed at night a purple crease about the waist where the bands came about the corset and wondered if that could keep her from gaining strength. With all this weight and compression this poor woman was waiting to get well,

wondering why she could not stand, that her limbs ached and prickled, and why she could not walk without getting so tired. Neither physician nor specialist had spoken of her mode of dress.

And Dr. Betts went further by pointing out that the men doctors simply did not know about these things because the men themselves had never submitted to that kind of clothing.

THE CINCINNATI MEETING

The meeting in Cincinnati heard an address by Dr. A. P. Y. Garnett which was a fine analysis of the medical education of the day, a brief review of the International Congress and an urge to participate in the building of the Rush monument.

The editor of THE JOURNAL told his readers that he would have the official minutes in the following week and he begged them to disregard the inaccurate, hasty and imperfect reports of the meeting that had been published by the contemporaries. The personal journalism which was characteristic of that day had invaded the field of medical journalism. Dr. Davis was much annoyed with the telegraphic reports from the convention in Cinncinati to the New York medical periodicals. He did not see the reason for all the hurry. "No one," he said, "can possibly object to an accurate report of the business meeting of the Association, but as the matter now is, it usually takes some months to correct the inaccuracies of one week's issue of some of our electric contemporaries. Inaccuracy is neither condoned nor corrected by telegraph wires, notwithstanding the marvelous therapeutic properties of electricity."

"PATENT" MEDICINE ADVERTISING

At this meeting there came a resolution from the Arkansas State Medical Society condemning the religious press of the nation for its continuous endorsement of "patent" medicines and the fact that the religious press published "serious homilies on prayer and praise side by side with cures for consumption, cancer, Bright's disease and other incurable ailments."

THE RUSH MEMORIAL

The committee on the Rush memorial reported that it knew that every doctor wanted to give a dollar but that the dollars had not been forthcoming and that they had not found out how to get them. The committee, which had started out to get $45,000, had got $392 the first year and $498 the second year but it had now had an expenditure since the last report of $34.73. Some of the state medical societies had made contributions—notably $500 from Pennsylvania—which had paid $100 on account, and $100 had been promised from Michigan but had not yet shown up in the treasury.

TOO MANY SOCIETIES

As the year ended there began to be agitation against the number and variety of medical societies. The difficulty seemed to lie in having too many special societies which were detracting from the national organization. These special societies were apparently not only taking away the harmony from the national organization but also interfering with pronouncements of policy. The *New Orleans Medical and Surgical Journal* of November 1888 said:

> What will be the final effect upon the American Medical Association of the various associations of so-called *specialists*—the American Surgical Association, the Association of American Physicians, the Gynecological Association and all the others? It will be a sad day for the profession of America when the time-honored A. M. A. ceases to be *the* medical institution of the country.

Dr. N. S. Davis charged that those who had taken part in one or more of these specialists' organizations and who had actively promoted the combination of all these in the so-called Congress of American Physicians and Surgeons had been actuated by the desire that the latter should ultimately displace and supersede the American Medical Association. He felt that the leaders in the specialties had never been satisfied with the liberal organization of the American Medical Association. Some of them had tried to restrict the whole business and management of the Association to a council of limited number capable of self perpetuation instead of the representative plan based on the state and local societies. He attacked these specialists for devoting themselves to their special societies rather than giving the major portion of their attention to the sections of the American Medical Association. Too, he was certain that after all the sections of the American Medical Association would triumph because the specialists must depend for much of their patronage on personal contact with the general practitioners, and he concluded:

> Instead of the circle of American associations of specialists, accommodating in the aggregate less than 500 of the 50,000 or 60,000 members of the regular medical profession of the United States, having any serious tendency to supersede the American Medical Association, it will only serve as a convenient and really useful place in which the small but respectable class of exclusionists can work and dine without personal contact with the sunburned and weatherbeaten general practitioners of the healing art.

In THE JOURNAL OF THE AMERICAN MEDICAL ASSOCIATION for Nov. 24, 1888, appears this significant notice:

EDITORIAL CHANGE

Having accomplished all that he had hoped or expected to accomplish when he accepted the editorship of THE JOURNAL OF THE AMERICAN MEDICAL ASSOCIATION in

1883, and feeling the necessity for diminishing his responsibilities and constant work, the Editor of THE JOURNAL tendered his resignation to the Board of Trustees in the latter part of June last, the same to take effect on the 31st day of December, 1888. At a special meeting of the Board of Trustees held in Chicago Nov. 9 and 10, 1888, the resignation was accepted, and John B. Hamilton, M.D., Supervising Surgeon General of the Marine Hospital Service and late Secretary General of the ninth International Medical Congress, was chosen unanimously to fill the place. He will enter upon the discharge of his editorial duties Jan. 1, 1889. We trust he will have a long and prosperous editorial career.

Thus apparently ended the visible leadership of Nathan Smith Davis. But it was only apparent! A study of the minutes of the Association and of the Board of Trustees during the continuing years proved that, as long as there was in him spirit and life, N. S. Davis was wholly devoted to the American Medical Association and its progress.

1889

NEWPORT, R. I.

Prophetic indeed was a little note that appeared in the editorial column of THE JOURNAL OF THE AMERICAN MEDICAL ASSOCIATION for Jan. 12, 1889. It said:

> There are a little more than eighty thousand persons practicing medicine in the United States, of whom more than sixty thousand are regular practitioners. When one third of the regular profession are members of the American Medical Association we can have the strongest organization and the best medical journal in the world.

As the Association faced its hundredth anniversary in 1947, there were about 190,000 physicians in the United States, and of these about 130,000 were members of the American Medical Association. THE JOURNAL had reached more than 130,000 subscribers, a figure representing more circulation than the ten next weekly journals of medicine in the world combined.

In 1889 the British Medical Association was in excellent financial condition. It occurred to the editor of THE JOURNAL to make some comparisons and to point out that a technic like that by which the British Medical Association was organized would be of vital importance to promotion of THE JOURNAL. Yet from various places in the United States came a variety of suggestions, one urging frequent meetings in Washington and the beginning of the first agitation for moving the headquarters of the American Medical Association to that city. The suggestion has never quite died. Again and again it reappears in the various motions and promotions frequently supported by the belief that in some manner the location of the headquarters of the American Medical Association in Washington would result in a sort of influence on the legislative and executive leaders that cannot be secured by any less intimate contact.

THE EDITOR OF THE JOURNAL

It will be remembered that the Board of Trustees of the American Medical Association accepted the resignation of Dr. N. S. Davis at the end of 1888. Dr. John B. Hamilton was elected to succeed him. He served as editor only from January to February of 1889; then he resigned the position for reasons which he stated succinctly in an editorial published in the issue of February 9. At that time the committee on general management, which was the Board of Trustees, took over control of THE JOURNAL.

EDITORIAL NOTICE

When the writer accepted the position of Editor of the Association JOURNAL, although the Marine Hospital Service bill was then pending, as it had been for the past ten years, he had no certainty of its passage, but, on January 4 it passed both houses of Congress and became a law, which by prohibiting any original appointments into the service except to the rank of Assistant Surgeon, has the effect of creating a life tenure in the office of Supervising Surgeon General. He therefore tendered his resignation as Editor to the Board of Trustees and it was kindly accepted by them to take effect on a day named by himself. His editorial connection with THE JOURNAL will therefore cease with the present number, and until further notice the "Committee on General Management" will take charge of the affairs of THE JOURNAL. With the most sincere thanks to those who have sent him kindly letters, his best wishes for the continued success of THE JOURNAL, and the renewed prosperity of the Association, the Editor assumes his life work in the Marine Hospital Service.

JOHN B. HAMILTON.

John B. Hamilton was born in Jersey County, Ill., Dec. 1, 1847, the year in which the American Medical Association was founded. He graduated from Rush Medical College in 1869. Following his graduation he entered the Marine Hospital Service and rose rapidly to the rank of Supervising Surgeon General. His surgical skill won for him a position in Rush Medical College, where he became professor of the principles of surgery and clinical surgery. He obtained special recognition for his operations for hernia and for his skill in surgical diagnosis.

In "American Medical Biographies," edited by Howard A. Kelly and Walter L. Burrage, appears the statement that THE JOURNAL OF THE AMERICAN MEDICAL ASSOCIATION was never more successful than under his four years of editorship. His second term as editor began in 1893. This first period occupied just two months.

In 1889 Dr. Oliver Wendell Holmes gave his private library to the Boston Medical Library. THE JOURNAL OF THE AMERICAN MEDICAL ASSOCIATION recognized the occasion with special editorial notice and suggested to the members of the Association that they might have opportunity to meet the great American author and physician at the next meeting of the Association, which was to take place in Newport, R. I.

PROGRESS IN OBSTETRICS

Significant of the progress of medical science in that year was a lecture given to the Chicago Medical Society by Professor W. W. Jaggard of the Chicago Medical College. Jaggard was one of the greatest teachers of his day. Dr. Joseph B. DeLee derived from him the interest toward improvement in obstetrics which became his life work. The article on "The Prevention of Puerperal Fever" is a demand for thoroughgoing cleanliness which came closely on the demonstrations by Semmelweis and the argument of Oliver Wendell Holmes. Curiously, however, at the conclusion of his article Dr. Jaggard warned physicians to make sure that the woman who was giving birth should not be placed in a room in which there was "communication with' the sewer, since vitiated air is unwholesome under all conditions of human life." He called attention, however, to an aphorism of Kucher, "I would be less frightened by the bursting of a sewer pipe during labor than by the use of a suspicious sponge or an unclean rag on the external genitals." And as a final conclusion, Dr. Jaggard said "These rules are simple and easy of application as well in private as in hospital practice; as well on South Halsted Street as on Calumet Avenue." It would interest Professor Jaggard, should he return today, to discover that South Halsted Street has improved considerably over Calumet Avenue.

Following the resignation of Dr. John B. Hamilton, THE JOURNAL was issued by the Board of Trustees with the advice of N. S. Davis until June 26, when Dr. John H. Hollister of Chicago was elected editor.

PROGRESS OF THE ASSOCIATION

Toward the end of the year THE JOURNAL began a compoign for better control over licensure to practice in the individual states. The editor published a brief review of forty years in the history of the American Medical Association and he listed the following five chief accomplishments of those forty years:

"First. By the early adoption of a Code of Ethics which commends itself to the approval of all medical men, it has clearly defined the rules that should govern, not only among members of the profession, one with another, but also their relations with the people.
Second. It has fostered fraternal fellowship and helped to bring into close and friendly relation the medical men of all parts of this broad Union.
Third. It has always been the earnest advocate of a higher standard of medical education and in every way possible has sought to stimulate original investigation.
Fourth. Its influence has always been helpful to our medical colleges—and it has favored the maintenance of medical societies, both state and local, everywhere.
Fifth. For the purpose of assuring the closest possible relations with the masses of the profession—it even commits its own management to their delegates, as they shall come

fresh from the local societies to express their will, from year to year, rather than to permanent members, who might in time misrepresent their constituencies.

The Association is in accord with the genius of American institutions. It is national in its representation and never sectional in interests. It is in no sense exclusive and yet makes ample provision for those who by reason of talent and culture may best serve the profession as instructors and guides.

In June the editor discovered that some one, taking advantage of the forthcoming annual session of the American Medical Association, began soliciting advertisement for something called "The American Medical Association Annual." It became necessary for the Association to disavow publicly any association with this dubious financial enterprise.

THE SPECIAL ISSUE

THE JOURNAL itself was, however, embarking on a financial enterprise to signalize the occasion that amazed the American medical publishing world. In anticipation of the 1889 convention THE JOURNAL OF THE AMERICAN MEDICAL ASSOCIATION issued an edition of 75,000 copies and mailed one to every physician in the United States. Its purpose was to attract a large number of physicians to the annual meeting in Newport. The other medical periodicals of the country paid compliments to the special issue. One contemporary called attention to the fact that THE JOURNAL was under temporary management and suggested that the Association could scarcely do better than to make the present arrangement permanent.

The final issue of the twelfth volume carried a plea for the sufferers from the Johnstown flood.

The next volume opened with the address of the President of the Association, Dr. W. W. Dawson of Cincinnati. He was concerned with the quality of medical teaching in the United States; with the quality of the young men who were to become medical students; he recognized that there would always be some doctors who were not as good as most of them. The University of Texas had just been liberally endowed. The universities of Virginia, Harvard, Yale, Princeton, Columbia and Cornell and the University of California had made enviable records, but there were now in the United States more than a hundred medical colleges and there was a feeling that medical colleges had increased too rapidly.

President Dawson urged an expansion of THE JOURNAL OF THE AMERICAN MEDICAL ASSOCIATION and a drive for more members. Great praise he poured on the Army Medical Library and Museum and on John Shaw Billings and his development of the *Index Cata-*

logue. "The medical profession," he said, "asks very little of the general government but it does ask that these two institutions shall be made as useful as possible." He saw looming as clouds on the horizon the gradual development of proprietary "patent" medicines which were in every sense of the word nostrums. He saw failure of states to set up systems of licensure as rapidly as they were needed.

THE NEWPORT MEETING

The meeting in Newport was marked by many interesting features. Dr. William Pepper of the University of Pennsylvania gave the address on medicine and devoted it to the life of Benjamin Rush, but the treasurer of the Rush monument committee could only report a total of $1,000, and it was decided to abandon the $1 limit on subscriptions.

The Board of Trustees of the American Medical Association made its report on THE JOURNAL, recognizing that it had now become well established and a credit to the Association. At the beginning of the year the number of pages of THE JOURNAL had been increased from thirty-two to thirty-six weekly.

The American Social Science Association sent in a resolution, which was adopted, urging a more thorough general education antecedent to the study of medicine.

After the reading of the report of the Board of Trustees, the minutes show that Hon. George Bancroft, famous as a historian, entered on the stage and was presented to the members, who arose to receive him.

At that time the resolution was adopted that the American Medical Association should send its representatives to the meeting of the U. S. Pharmacopeial Convention.

BROWN-SÉQUARD AND REJUVENATION

Among the extraordinary manifestations of our civilization is the manner in which a noted scientist who has gained great fame may suddenly hazard all his repute by some sudden aberration as he grows older. This occurred to the great Brown-Séquard, who suddenly claimed that he had discovered the secret of perennial youth and of rejuvenation. THE JOURNAL OF THE AMERICAN MEDICAL ASSOCIATION had recorded his utterances as too absurd to warrant serious consideration, but his ideas began to gain great public interest. THE JOURNAL then announced the report of a citizen who had met sudden death by attempting to rejuvenate himself by the Brown-Séquard technic.

ORGANIZATION

Still experimenting with methods of organization, there was now an attempt to gain strength and support for the American Medical Association by promoting reorganization with branches and societies similar to those of the British Medical Association. It was hoped that the districts and tristate and similar groups could be incorporated into the American Medical Association in some manner so as to assure a great membership with a vast subscription to THE JOURNAL. At the same time the California State Medical Association passed a resolution demanding that the one qualification necessary for membership should be continuous membership in a local medical society. This was the principle which was ultimately to prevail.

CONFUSION AND STRIFE, 1890 TO 1894

NASHVILLE

THE BOUND VOLUME OF THE JOURNAL for the period January to June 1890 contains a list of editorial writers; these no doubt contributed some of the scientific editorials as well as those having to do with the work of the organization.

S. T. Armstrong, U. S. Marine-Hospital Service.
Robert H. Babcock, Chicago.
Henry T. Byford, Chicago.
Archibald Church, Chicago.
J. C. Culbertson, Cincinnati.
Nathan S. Davis, Chicago.
Richard J. Dunglison, Philadelphia.
James M. French, Cincinnati.
Albert I. Gihon, medical director, U. S. Navy.
Junius C. Hoag, Chicago.

John H. Hollister, Chicago.
Bayard Holmes, Chicago.
W. W. Jaggard, Chicago.
Samuel J. Jones, Chicago.
Charles Lodor, Chicago.
Franklin H. Martin, Chicago.
L. L. McArthur, Chicago.
Harold N. Moyer, Chicago.
Wolfred Nelson, New York.
John Shrady, New York.
William L. Worcester, Little Rock, Ark.
Richard M. Wyckoff, Brooklyn.

Here are such distinguished names in the history of the Association as J. C. Culbertson, John H. Hollister and N. S. Davis, all of whom served as editors of THE JOURNAL. They aided with the editorials on the work of the Association.

THE JOURNAL for May 3, 1890, contains a review by James E. Pilcher, assistant surgeon in the United States Army, of "The Annals and Achievements of American Surgery." The review is especially important because it established the place that American surgery was to occupy in the development of surgery throughout the world. Pilcher gives credit to Dr. Philip Syng Physick of Philadelphia for the foundation of American surgery, calling him the father of American surgery. Then came the famous Valentine Mott of New York, whose name is still preserved in the annals of the great metropolis. Indeed, there is a special society dedicated to his memory. Pilcher recorded the great achievements of surgery in the history of American medicine; his review must have taken many hours of research into medical literature. He concludes concerning the American surgeon that "his brilliancy and force as a teacher, his originality and skill as an operator, and his grace and impressiveness as an author have united to secure the high position accorded to him by other nations." The history of the growth of medicine in our modern times reveals the rise of American surgery to great eminence, to leadership throughout the world. But some of the greatest names of those who built American surgery had not yet begun to appear in the Transactions of the American Medical Association!

With May THE JOURNAL OF THE AMERICAN MEDICAL ASSOCIATION issued the special edition which had now become a feature in American medical publishing. This issue, which forecast the program of the convention, was placed in the hands of every regular registered physician in North America. It was made the occasion of still further promotion of THE JOURNAL to the medical profession. The editors took great pride in pointing out that the weight of the paper of the special issue amounted to fifteen and a half tons.

The Rush monument was still not doing well; the collection had just barely gone beyond $1,500, and it seemed that the minimum cost would be not less than $15,000.

PLANS FOR THE CHICAGO WORLD'S FAIR

At this time THE JOURNAL was agreeably surprised to read in the *Cincinnati Lancet Clinic* that a world's fair was to be held in Chicago in 1893 and that it might be a good idea if the American Medical Association, which had always "made Chicago its center," took the leadership in planning an exhibit for demonstration to the public of the great advances that medical science had made during the years. This occasion might serve "to bring into closer relation with us the medical fraternity of Central and South America."

THE NASHVILLE MEETING

The meeting convened in Nashville, Tenn., near the end of May. The President's address, which had been printed in the issue published during the week of the annual session, was a review of the relations of medicine to public health. The President recognized the desirability of representation by the public on state boards of health and he urged strongly a wider extension of public health activities.

There had been much gossip in various portions of the country during the year on the necessity for reorganization of the American Medical Association.

The committee on the Rush monument suggested that failure of the appeal to the general medical profession should probably yield to a specific appeal to a few leading members. If this appeal failed, it would probably be better to determine "whether the memorial shall be the imposing one your committee have in view, or such humbler testimonial as the money they then have in hand shall justify them in obtaining."

The Board of Trustees reported that THE JOURNAL had been under the direction of the committee on management. It now had a weekly circulation of 5,100 copies, with its own printing office. An editor had not been named, but one of the members of the committee on management—apparently Dr. John H. Hollister of Chicago, Trustee—had been filling this function. A resolution came from Ohio for the appointment of a special committee of one from each state to consider THE JOURNAL and to see what could be done to superintend its editorial management and to widen its circulation. This resolution was laid on the table, but it was an indication of underlying dissatisfactions which were to come to a focus later in the year.

There were other political dissatisfactions which became manifest. A resolution was offered to the effect that "at future meetings of this Association, the business of the general sessions shall be conducted from the floor of the house, and no one occupying a seat on the platform shall be recognized by the President, excepting the secretary." This resolution was adopted.

An attempt was made to pass a resolution making every medical society with a membership of more than a hundred a branch of the American Medical Association, but the resolution failed.

THE JOURNAL began to reflect increasingly in its editorials its feeling of unrest. The New York State Medical Society had reorganized under a representative system in which the various divisions of the state society were directly related to the society itself. Now for the first time appeared the suggestion that "our local societies could be represented by delegates in the state societies, and these, in like manner, in the national Association."

CHICAGO OR WASHINGTON

Suddenly in December an announcement appeared in THE JOURNAL to the effect that the Board of Trustees had held a special session in Washington, D. C., to consider whether or not THE JOURNAL should be moved to Washington. Six of the Trustees were present. The first point raised was that Dr. John H. Hollister, while acting as supervising editor, had been receiving $250 a month, a fact which did not appear anywhere in the minutes of the organization. The secretary pointed out that he had no record of any meeting of the board at which such an action was taken. The chairman of the committee on management stated that no meeting of his committee had been held. At the afternoon session Dr. I. N. Love, chairman of the board, recommended removal of THE JOURNAL to Washington. There was much discussion, and it was decided to put the matter before the members of the Association. Finally a group were constituted a committee to prepare a resolution, which read:

Resolved, That the sense of the Committee be that the home of THE JOURNAL of the Association should be permanently at Washington, D. C.

Resolved, That the Trustees incorporate the foregoing resolution in their report to be presented at the next meeting of the Association.

A resolution was then offered by John V. Shoemaker that the Trustees "recommend the members of the Association, or the various state and local medical societies in affiliation with the Association, to contribute or subscribe funds for the erection of a permanent building as a place of meeting as well as a library and office for the American Medical Association."

The Trustees recommended that these resolutions be printed in THE JOURNAL and that members be given opportunity to discuss the subject, with, however, a limitation of individual letters to fifteen lines. Then Dr. Hollister was instructed to make such contracts as might be necessary for the continuation of THE JOURNAL until the next meeting of the Association, and the Board of Trustees went off to pay a visit to the President of the United States.

1891
WASHINGTON, D. C.

Something happened by the time the next volume of THE JOURNAL was published; it bears on its title page the name of J. C. Culbertson as editor and the announcement, a little further along, that J. C. Culbertson is editor and manager.

In the first number for the year the correspondence began with a highly amusing combination of three letters, the first of which, from a doctor in Texas, suggested that THE JOURNAL remain in Chicago; the second, from a doctor in Tennessee, that it be moved to Louisville, and the third, from a doctor in Iowa, who wondered what "occult reason or grounds" demanded removal of THE JOURNAL since the objections to its removal were so strong.

THE JOURNAL began begging for more contributors to this debate, because it was apparently of little interest to the medical profession as a whole. By the middle of January there were seven letters—six for Chicago and one for Washington—and in the next issue nine letters (all for Chicago) and one indicating that apparently a little faction was having a whim in the matter that should not too greatly disturb the majority. The last issue for January turned up with three pages of letters, including among the contributors such distinguished names as William T. Corlett of Cleveland, who simply said "I prefer Chicago," and Henry O. Marcy of Boston, who had about 1,000 words on the subject. Marcy went directly to the point. He felt that the agitation for removal was simply that of one trustee who voted for it because he was pledged to that course of action before his appointment. "Why," said Dr. Marcy, "this agitation for Washington? Is it because Washington is the capital city and the center of the political influences of our country? Some have felt that already the greatest danger to our Association and its journal lies in the fact that a political element has entered into its organization and is seeking control. If there is reason for apprehension in this direction, it would be a strong argument for its removal *from* Washington had it been established there instead of at Chicago."

Dr. Solomon Solis-Cohen of Philadelphia contributed 1,000 words in which he said that THE JOURNAL had not been well edited, that there would be less tendency in Washington to debase THE JOURNAL into a local organ, that America must have a scientific center and that there could only be one center and that was Washington. He argued that any defects in THE JOURNAL were not those of the editors, since they were all first class scientists and that therefore they must be due to the location.

The battle waged through issue after issue, seldom with less than ten letters in each number of THE JOURNAL. Dr. Harold N. Moyer of Chicago made it his special task to answer Dr. Solomon Solis-Cohen. He pointed out that if there was any peculiar miasm around Chicago it probably prevailed equally around Philadelphia, New York, Boston and Baltimore. He congratulated the profession of Washington on being free from this kind of infection. He wrote sarcastically: "As near as we can analyze Dr. Cohen's statement, there seems to be in Washington a great, intangible, psychic entity that has its being as an incorporeal body working in and for the good of the profession but not of it, for they are of the earth, and this is of the spiritual and invisible." Dr. Moyer pointed succinctly out that if there was anything to be done about improving THE JOURNAL it would have to be done through brains and not through transferring the "editing, printing, press-work or binding to either Washington, Oshkosh or Kalamazoo."

The letter of Dr. Solomon Solis-Cohen served to focus the attack on him and to arouse to the defense of Chicago so many that he well nigh defeated the cause by his advocacy of it. On another occasion a similar bitter attack was to gain him overwhelming support. But this time it concerned his attack on proprietary medicine.

By the end of February medical societies were beginning to take action; first was the Chicago Medical Society, which opposed the removal vigorously. A long letter from Charles A. Hough of Ohio began with the statement that Washington had never produced a medical journal, national either in character or in reputation, and that was the very reason "why she is just the place which *can* do it." They then poured satire on the proponents of the removal to Washington and particularly on Dr. Solomon Solis-Cohen. The correspondence is typical of the personal journalism of that period. Dr. Hough feared that there might be infection of the new magazine by the pathogenic germ of the Congressional *Globe*.

A New York physician, Dr. Thomas H. Manley, said that it was for THE JOURNAL to lay plainly on the table the reasons underlying the demand for removal, for " it may as well be generally known that this transference of location cannot be consummated *except through specious, delusive argument, wily manipulating and shrewd diplomacy, with the aid of sharp parliamentary tactics.*"

The letters continued issue after issue, the vast majority of them opposing any removal to Washington and many beginning to inquire more and more into the motives. More societies began introducing resolutions. The presidents of state medical societies began recording themselves in behalf of maintaining the headquarters office in Chicago. Then the suggestion began to be made that the whole question be referred back to the Board of Trustees. Many an important leader in medicine contributed his personal sentiments to the controversy. A leader in American medicine of that day, Dr. Cornelius G. Comegys of Cincinnati, wrote a most enlightening communication of several thousand words in which he made it clear that THE JOURNAL would have to have a full time editor. He pointed out some other objectives, one of them a full time secretary of public health in the President's cabinet. To him the *British Medical Journal* was the ideal that should be followed, but he felt that there was something about Washington that would do more for THE JOURNAL and the Association than seemed apparent. "If its great purpose can be accomplished in Chicago, let it remain; but, I repeat, the consciousness of Chicago is so immensely inferior to that of our political capital that I hope that all of us may see that the great destiny of the Association may more surely be accomplished at Washington."

Nicholas Senn, who was then in Milwaukee, asserted that a vote of the membership would show at least nine out of ten favorable to Chicago. Dr. T. D. Crothers of Hartford, Conn., warned that removal to Washington might destroy the publication and the

Association. A few voices continued to echo the advantages of Washlngton, but by far the majority were now fully committed to remaining in Chicago. Dr. R. Harvey Reed took another hand in the battle in order to reply in extenso to Dr. Comegys; he continued to insist that there were hidden evil forces behind the movement to get THE JOURNAL to Washington. In fact he felt that there was a federal marasmus that is destructive of anything that gets into the nation's capital. He pointed out that the *Index Medicus* was published not in Washington but in Detroit and he announced that private business enterprises which were run on business principles stayed out of the national capital.

The editors of THE JOURNAL in the issue for April 4, 1891, began quoting editorial opinions from other medical periodicals; apparently the great majority of the leading medical publications of the country were convinced that Chicago was the desirable place for the publication.

The Board of Trustees met in the Arlington Hotel in Washington on Saturday, May 2, 1891. A questionnaire had been sent by Dr. R. H. Reed of Mansfield, Ohio, aided by T. D. Crothers, C. D. Beardsley and John F. Fulton of St. Paul. This questionnaire showed an overwhelming majority in favor of retaining the periodical in Chicago, actually a vote of 10 to 1, and E. D. Moffett of Indianapolis shouted in his letter "Remove THE JOURNAL to Washington—No. Remove Washington to THE JOURNAL."

The House of Delegates assembled in Washington, D. C., May 5. Immediately following the president's address the Board of Trustees made a preliminary report on the question of locating THE JOURNAL. They felt that there had been undue excitement, that sectional antagonisms had been engendered and that efforts had been made in stimulating the interest of lukewarm members.

The Board of Trustees on the second day of the session made an additional report. In this they pointed out that the editorial management of THE JOURNAL had continued as before, that the resident members of the Board had acted in the capacity of supervising editor, that they hoped to secure a building for the Association and that in view of increased funds they hoped to raise the professional and literary standards of its editorial department to the equal of any.

A special committee reported on the desirability of a cabinet appointment of a secretary of public health.

A resolution commended Dr. Hollister and the business manager, J. Harrison White, and recommended that they be employed for the ensuing year. It was considered, however, that this would not be mandatory on the Board of Trustees.

A committee was appointed to look into the question of incorporating the American Medical Association and to report in the following year.

Thus the furor over the transfer of THE JOURNAL from Chicago to Washington died without any battle in the House of Delegates. The ventilation of the subject in the columns of THE JOURNAL and the questionnaire to the membership by those opposed to the removal had been sufficient to settle the issue.

MEDICINE IN THE PRESS

Almost as if it might have been written yesterday are the following words from an editorial in THE JOURNAL OF THE AMERICAN MEDICAL ASSOCIATION, July 4, 1891:

> It is apparent to even the careless reader of the daily papers that medical topics are receiving vastly more attention than ever before. It is even hinted that many large daily papers have a medical man on their regular staff; if such is the case they have generally succeeded in concealing the fact by displaying a phenomenal ignorance regarding medical subjects.

This was in connection with an article on the Keeley cure.

ELECTROCUTION

Early in July 1891 there occurred the first four executions by electricity in Sing Sing Prison. They were most satisfactory, at least to the observers, who said that death was instantaneous and painless in each instance. The doctors congratulated the warden and announced that this was unquestionably a method superior to any other yet devised for the purpose.

THE CORONER SYSTEM

In August 1891 appeared the first essay on the coroner system in the United States. Massachusetts was the first state to get rid of the coroner system and to introduce instead the system of medical examiners. The campaign to eliminate the coroner system is still waged in THE JOURNAL, but legislative bodies are loath to make this revolutionary change.

In his address to the Congress of American Physicians and Surgeons, Sept. 18, 1891, Dr. Claudius H. Mastin made it clear that there was no competition between that organization and the American Medical Association. He paid tribute to Samuel David Gross, who had participated greatly in the work of the American Medical Association and who was the founder of the Congress of American Physicians and Surgeons.

In the issue in which he published the proceedings of the American

Congress, the editor of THE JOURNAL congratulated its readers on having such a good magazine.

ANDROLOGY BECOMES UROLOGY

About this time the urologists in the American Congress of Physicians and Surgeons constituted themselves into a section on andrology, which was to be contrasted with gynecology. The editor of THE JOURNAL felt that there was no future for this specialty as long as the general practitioners felt themselves competent to treat these cases.

1892
DETROIT

The periodicals provide the detail of thought and philosophy that prevail in any period. Thus an examination of the pages of THE JOURNAL OF THE AMERICAN MEDICAL ASSOCIATION for the first half of the year 1892 indicates that the publication was being edited by J. C. Culbertson and that he was helped with editorials by Drs. W. S. Christopher, Chicago; T. D. Crothers, New Haven, Conn.; C. A. L. Reed, Cincinnati, and R. M. Wyckoff, Brooklyn.

THE BUSINESS COMMITTEE

Resolutions were proposed several months in advance of the session eliminating the committee on necrology and making the publication of obituary notices the duty of the editor of THE JOURNAL.

Dr. J. C. Culbertson proposed that all business matters of the Association be referred without discussion or comment to an executive committee composed of two members appointed by each state society in affiliation with the Association who should carefully consider and recommend such action as they might deem most advisable. This movement was to culminate in the system of reference committees which has been a feature of modern activities of the House of Delegates of the Association. Through the reference committees any member of the Association has opportunity to appear and express himself before final action is taken on any matter of significance.

POLIOMYELITIS

In 1891 Medin of Stockholm had reported an epidemic in which within five months 44 cases were observed in previously healthy children of a form of paralysis. This was one of the first great outbreaks of infantile paralysis definitely recognized as such; Dr. C. H. Hughes of St. Louis insisted in THE JOURNAL that it must be a form of grip.

THE DEPARTMENT OF HEALTH

Again and again during this year the medical profession was cheered with the belief that legislation would finally pass for the establishment of a department of public health in the cabinet. The measure had been introduced by Senator Sherman. THE JOURNAL OF THE AMERICAN MEDICAL ASSOCIATION had urged all medical societies, individual physicians and others to write to their senators and congressmen and to their special committees urging the passage of this legislation. It was felt that a strong response by the medical profession would ensure passage.

BEHAVIOR PROBLEMS IN THE HOUSE OF DELEGATES

In this period other problems of behavior had to be considered. Dr. Brodie of Detroit offered a resolution permitting the placing of books and other advertising sheets on the seats of members of the American Medical Association when they met in their annual session. This resolution was further amended by Dr. John H. Hollister, who requested that all material be protected by copyright in order to prevent pirating by other professions and other organizations. The first proposals for copyright had been made at the meeting in Nashville in 1890 and now came to fruition.

By this time also THE JOURNAL began urging doctors to bring their wives along to the annual session; the editor pointed out that if a member once did this he would never have another chance to go alone.

FOOD AND DRUG LEGISLATION

In this year also came the first proposals for suitable food and drug legislation to prevent adulteration. THE JOURNAL said that the establishment of a department of health should accompany such a food and drug administration, since under other circumstances it would have to go into the Department of the Treasury. Actually the evolution took just that form. Only in 1947 has a real department been proposed.

THE JOURNAL was having fun editorially with the Ohio legislature, which had rejected an appeal to regulate the practice of medicine in that state principally because it would interfere with itinerant doctors and diminish the advertising receipts of some newspapers. The Ohio legislature, however, before adjournment did appropriate $5,000 to test the Keeley cure and made itself a sort of committee of the whole to investigate. Each member was to be privileged to send 1 patient to take the cure. Here and there the Keeley cure still raises its ugly head. But in 1947 "The Lost Weekend" and "Alcoholics Anonymous" mingled with psychoanalysis bring new aspects to alcoholism.

In May 1892 it was already recognized that registration of hundreds of doctors at the annual session was becoming a problem, and the proposal for registration by mail won great approval. This procedure was ultimately abandoned, only to be restored again in 1947 because so many thousands of physicians indicated they would attend the Centennial Session.

Toward the end of May the Philadelphia County Medical Society on the insistence of Dr. Solomon Solis-Cohen adopted resolutions urging THE JOURNAL OF THE AMERCIAN MEDICAL ASSOCIATION and other leading medical publications to get rid of their proprietary medical advertising. The editor of THE JOURNAL defended the practice and hinted that THE JOURNAL might adopt the rule if the Philadelphia society would make good on the income which would be lost. However, he also defended the advertising of proprietary medicines on the ground that most physicians were prescribing great amounts of these preparations.

At this time American medicine was becoming subject to multiple organizations; the presence of these innumerable bodies was giving great concern to the leaders. In his presidential address Dr. H. O. Marcy of Boston urged that there was a place for all such bodies in American medicine. He emphasized particularly the need for two such groups as the American Congress of Physicians and Surgeons, consisting of organizations of specialists in many fields and of the American Medical Association to represent the great body politic.

THE JOURNAL had now reached a circulation of over 6,000 copies and was beginning to bring some income to the Association. Dr. Marcy traced in detail the development of the movement for a national department of health and expressed the hope that its ultimate establishment was not too far in the future.

DETROIT MEETING

At the 1892 session the movement to bring the New York state societies back into the fold culminated with the establishment of a committee for conference; at the same time a resolution was unanimously adopted directing the appointment of a committee to revise the Code of Ethics and the Constitution and By-Laws of the Association.

There was an extensive report by the committee that had been appointed to urge the establishment of a national department of health which ended with a recommendation that the committee be continued. Resolutions were adopted condemning the giving of testimonials for proprietary medical preparations. The committee on the Rush monument reported that the case was not entirely hopeless. It had received an encouraging donation of $300 from the exhibits at Nashville and the total contributions had now reached over $2,100, but it had only $646.81 left in the treasury. The minutes of the Board of Trustees indicate that Dr. Culbertson had been appointed editor on May 13, 1892. The Trustees had investigated the business of the Association and had made some radical changes. There was much correspondence submitted to the House of Delegates relative to incorporation of the Association, but the committee felt that the incorporation should be delayed until further evidence could be assembled.

It need not be thought that the path which the American Medical Association and THE JOURNAL was treading was entirely without obstructions or difficulties. The *New York Medical Journal*, through its editor, was waging a sort of guerrilla warfare. He ridiculed the quality of material brought before the American Medical Association and praised to the skies the societies of specialists. Nevertheless physicians throughout the country defended the American Medical Association on the ground that it was one organization primarily interested in the work of the general practitioner. The editor of the *New York Medical Journal*, although not a member of the American Medical Association, responded with a statement in which he pointed out that the leaders in American medicine did not attend the meetings of the American Medical Association; indeed, the editor of the *New York Medical Journal* felt that the one essential step toward advancement of the Association would be elimination of the entire Code of Ethics. Here came the old argument that a man would be a gentleman without any Principles of Ethics but forgetfulness of the fact that some men who are not quite gentlemen remain within the borders if they realize that there are no means for detection, trial and elimination.

THE JOURNAL was leaning in its content toward surgery; there were many discussions of proper preparation for specialization. While apparently the editors of THE JOURNAL had authority to omit papers without special interest for their readers, one finds innumerable manuscripts coming from the specialized sections so technical in character that they would be of immediate interest only to the advanced specialists in the fields concerned.

The eminent Dr. Keeley, noted for his "cure for drunkenness," had arrived in London, and he was suing the *Lancet* and the *Press and Circular* for calling him a mischievous quack.

An unusual experiment was an attempt to transplant the skin of a black and tan dog to the head of a woman who had lost a major portion of the integument of her skull.

The desire to advance medical education was still having some troubles because the state board of health in Illinois was allowing a year of credit for study with a preceptor.

THE JOURNAL began to interest itself in the political aspects of the nation and to ask all doctors to find out where candidates stood on the national department of health issue before voting for them.

The committee on ethics submitted the entire code to the medical profession for criticism and with it the Constitution and By-Laws, asking advice as to how best to bring about the necessary revisions.

For the first time there appeared in THE JOURNAL the name of Victor C. Vaughan, the dean of the Medical Department of the University of Michigan, who wrote on "The Kind and Amount of Laboratory Work Which Should Be Required in Our Medical Schools." The discussion on his paper was extensive. But Bayard Holmes, who led the discussion, devoted his part of it mostly to drawings of histologic sections of the nervous system.

1893

MILWAUKEE

A reference to Garrison's "History of Medicine" indicates that the years between 1880 and 1900 were producing many important discoveries throughout the world; those fundamental discoveries are little reflected in the activities of the American Medical Association. True, there were discussions of treatment of diphtheria and of Koch's tuberculin. Lumbar puncture was introduced abroad in 1891, and several years later it had not yet been mentioned in THE JOURNAL OF THE AMERICAN MEDICAL ASSOCIATION. Particularly was THE JOURNAL lagging in its references to fundamental research in the laboratories of the basic sciences; the newer knowledge of bacteriology is little reflected in its pages. Leadership in medicine was still across the Atlantic.

By 1893 fifteen states in the United States had established medical practice acts requiring examination of all persons desiring to practice medicine. This movement had been received with favor; it was anticipated that soon all states would adopt such laws. An extraordinary editorial in January 1893 inclined to the view that Cohnheim was wrong in his theory of the cause of cancer and that it must be parasitic in origin.

An editorial early in 1893 indicates that the only way to improve the quality of THE JOURNAL is to make certain that members prepare and read better papers. Early in 1893 THE JOURNAL felt called on to condemn the House of Representatives for having removed the funds available for the publication of the Surgeon General's Catalogue from the Surgeon General's Library. Unfortunately succeeding congresses have been just as bad or worse. The Library was compelled year after year to move heaven and earth to obtain enough funds to operate the *Index Medicus* efficiently. Eventually the American Medical Association assumed the obligation and since that time has supported this necessary tool to medical research and advancement.

During the early months of 1893 correspondence waged back and forth on the Principles of Ethics. The discussions of the Principles of Ethics were rather onesided with page after page occupied by some one who signed himself "A Conservative Member." It is difficult to determine with any certainty who this might be; the literary style resembles that of Nathan Smith Davis. The discussions were going on in New York pointing toward a meeting of minds on questions of dispute and it seemed likely that the vagrant members would soon be brought into the fold.

ANIMAL EXPERIMENTATION

About this time also THE JOURNAL began its editorials on animal experimentation, being particularly concerned because Lawson Tait in England had decided to side with the antivivisectionists; thus he did harm which many years would not be able to overcome.

PRINCIPLES OF ETHICS

As the year went on, THE JOURNAL published the new proposed Constitution and By-Laws and the new Principles of Ethics, which were to be the major subject of interest in the annual session in Milwaukee. In presenting the revision of the Constitution and By-Laws THE JOURNAL urged acceptance of the concept that every member of a state society would be a member of the national organization and that the organization itself would be conducted by a delegate body.

As correspondence on the Principles of Ethics continued, it became more and more apparent that there was no real reason to depart from Percival's code as it had been adopted by the Association in 1848 except for such minor modifications as needed to be made to meet some changing conditions. Yet some, including Edward Jackson of Philadelphia, felt that the Principles of Ethics were a bar to a real unity of the profession. The publication of the Principles of Ethics had resulted in only twenty letters, most of which dealt with such matters as the patenting of instruments and advertising by members of the profession. THE JOURNAL concluded, therefore, that "as the clamor for a change in the Code has not materialized in any widespread expression, and as the silence of 99 per cent of the 7,000 members of the Association ought to be counted in favor of satisfaction with the present status, further and detailed consideration of the proposed amendments might be omitted."

MILWAUKEE MEETING

Dr. Hunter McGuire, President of the Association, in his address in Milwaukee, June 6, 1893, felt it desirable that both the Constitution and By-Laws and the Principles of Ethics lie over for a year so that the views of the individual states might be ascertained. He concluded his address by urging again the establishment of a national department of health. A feature of the Milwaukee session was the presence of Mr. Ernest Hart, editor of the *British Medical Journal*.

The committee on creating a department of health in the government reported progress, particularly because Grover Cleveland in dedicating the building of the New York Academy of Medicine had made most complimentary remarks about the medical profession.

The Trustees were having a little trouble about publishing THE JOURNAL because the Association had adopted a resolution calling attention to the fact that the Code of Ethics prohibits all commendatory mention or reference to secret preparations. The Trustees neatly passed the buck by instructing the editor that "when the editor is in doubt of the character of an advertisement, he shall refer the same to the committee on advertising, and that an advertisement of a proprietary medicine shall be accepted in the discretion of the committee when the proprietors thereof shall furnish the complete formula."

The main business of the session was the consideration of the Constitution and By-Laws, on which there were majority and minority reports. However, the whole procedure had, in any event, to lie over for a full year. The same man who presented a minority report on the Constitution and By-Laws, Dr. Henry D. Didama of New York City, presented a minority report on the Principles of Ethics. The situation was, however, well under control. Debate was stopped by the presentation of a report by N. S. Davis of the committee to confer with committees of the Medical Society of the State of New York and the Medical Association of the State of New York. This indicated that there had been no conferences because it seemed likely the situation was well in hand in New York State.

Eight hundred and sixty-seven physicians had registered at the meeting in Milwaukee. THE JOURNAL pointed out that the entertainment had been superb and that the new Pfister Hotel was not surpassed for elegance by any hostelry in any city, being only favorably compared with the princely Waldorf in New York City.

Four new Trustees had been elected, and the editor was not a candidate for reelection, so that his official relation with THE JOURNAL ceased with the last issue of June, 1893. The editor called attention to the difficulties in maintaining membership in relationship to subscription to THE JOURNAL and also to the need for a new legislative body which would be truly representative. THE JOURNAL was confronted with an enormous list of delinquents. Apparently one member, Dr. R. Harvey Reed, had circulated a letter to all the Trustees and officers in Milwaukee calling attention to the fact that THE JOURNAL was in debt $10,000. This the editor classifies as a "dastardly falsehood," since THE JOURNAL had never been in debt $1 beyond the cash funds in the hands of the treasurer. In leaving, Dr. Culbertson announced that he planned to resume his connection with the *Cincinnati Lancet Clinic* and that his latch string would be out in Cincinnati for all the members of the American Medical Association. Dr. John B. Hamilton, who resigned immediately as Trustee, succeeded to the editorship of THE JOURNAL following the retirement of Dr. Culbertson, who had a long list of editorial contributors, including such distinguished names in the Chicago area as those of Harry Gradle, Bayard Holmes, G. Frank Lydston, Harold N. Moyer and George W. Webster and from outside the Chicago area such men as Hobart A. Hare, G. Betton Massey and Frank Woodbury.

One finds for the first time the name of J. L. Rosenberger, Esq. He was for many years responsible for the abstracts of medicolegal decisions, which has come to be one of the most important features in the makeup of THE JOURNAL OF THE AMERICAN MEDICAL ASSOCIATION.

THE JOURNAL AND ITS PROBLEMS

Dr. Hamilton had previously been editor of THE JOURNAL for a brief period; the change in editorship did not accomplish all that was necessary toward improving the makeup or quality of the material in the publication.

The preparation of students for entrance into medical schools was still far below the quality needed to ensure culture. Here are a few examples quoted in THE JOURNAL of essays contributed by students immediately following their graduation:

Treatment of eclampsia: "To keep the patient from stricking his head or limbs against and place the patient in a horzontal position to favor respration circulation. Give bromide of potass. to act as a direct sedative or to excite motor susceptibility of the medula oblongata of the nerve centers and keep perfect qeuiet."

"Cholor infantum is due to a tomen symtom comences with Diarrhea first stools partly soft yet Liquid and stains the clothing a green color with a musty Odor vomiting pain and Rise of temperature and rapid prostration. May efect the brain when the patiant Roles heat and sleep with eyes open give Bromide potass for this first give Hyd chlor mit in small doses every hour and epecac at first and then Bismuth and Shlicylyc acid give stimulent to keep up the strenth."

"In false croup the farinx is not involved there is false membrane we dont get the spasms."

"There are 3 Verietys of pnemonia lobor Lobular interstiscial lobor is where we have all the lobes of the lung involved we have 3 stages. The inflamation extends from below upwards the seat of inflamation is in the alveoli or air vescle. Stage of ingorgement last 24 to 70 days red hepatization 5 days."

"The Teory of diebetis is an eretation upon the floor of the 4th ventrecle, may be do to Violence or High liveing."

Significantly Mr. Ernest Hart before departing for Great Britain gave an interview to the editors of THE JOURNAL in which he pointed out that an increase in the membership of the American Medical Association would automatically result in an improvement in THE JOURNAL. He said "Better papers, more condensation and a larger wastebasket would naturally follow an extended membership." Mr. Hart was convinced that the American Medical Association should have the strongest association and the best journal.

Within a few months THE JOURNAL began to make improvements, adopting some black letter side headings which gave it a much more lively appearance. An interesting essay is contributed by Dr. James B. Herrick, published July 22, 1893, with his observations on an experience with nearly 1,000 cases of typhoid. These were all seen in the Chicago area. In 1945 there were only 13 cases of typhoid in the entire area (now with a population of 3,500,000) and there were only two deaths.

In 1893 Grover Cleveland became ill. He was attended by Dr. Joseph O. Bryant, who refused to give a detailed statement of the President's illness to the reporters. At once the press set up a terrific howl against the Principles of Ethics, which, incidentally, had nothing whatever to do with the case. The editor of THE JOURNAL felt that the responsibility was not at all that of Dr. Bryant but of the family to give to the press such information as it cared to give.

About this time THE JOURNAL apologized to Dr. R. Harvey Reed of Mansfield, Ohio, for the editorial that had been published by Culbertson. It turned out that Dr. Reed had limited the circularization of his letter and had sent it only to the business committee.

Interesting in this period was the announcement by Dr. John B.

Murphy of his button for anastomosing the intestine. The button was at that time a medical sensation.

In New York there was a physician named Robert Lincoln Watkins who was convinced that the germ of tuberculosis was not the cause of the disease. He inoculated himself with a pure culture of the organisms, and THE JOURNAL editorial described him as a "crazy physician."

In the meantime Dr. John C. Culbertson and some of his friends were circulating editorials attacking the American Medical Association, and THE JOURNAL was endeavoring to build up the membership by calling attention to the improved quality of the scientific work and of the publication itself. THE JOURNAL did much to promote the great Pan American Medical Congress that was held in that year in Washington. Incidentally it is amazing that more people did not go because the hotels were charging from $4 to $4.50 a day American plan. The addresses given at the Pan American Medical Congress appeared for the most part in THE JOURNAL OF THE AMERICAN MEDICAL ASSOCIATION, and they represented about the best that American medicine could develop. They were of great aid to the quality of THE JOURNAL.

Dr. G. Frank Lydston devoted several pages to "Muscle Building as Illustrated by the Modern Samson, Sandow" in which he concluded that "Sandow is a wonderful man, but his example is pernicious." Lydston was well in advance of his time in recommending play for exercise rather than muscle culture.

In its coverage of the Pan American Medical Congress, THE JOURNAL printed letters describing the trips and the guests on every one of the special trains that went from Boston, Detroit, Cincinnati and Chicago. An amusing item describes the excursion train that left Chicago for Washington, which was wrecked near Indianapolis. The people on the special trains were entertained en route. In Chicago they had a breakfast at the Palmer House which was mixed up with a breakfast at the Auditorium. Dr. Fernando Henrotin welcomed the visitors in French, Dr. E. J. Gardner in Spanish and Dr. John B. Hamilton in English. At 8:30 in the evening they had a party at Kinsley's, where a male quartet sang funny songs and a mandolin orchestra furnished instrumental music. Then they visited the Chicago Medical College and the Cook County Hospital and all of the other medical schools.

In November 1893 the state of New York began to get rid of its coroner system and to follow the examiner system of Massachusetts.

In its last issue for the year, the editor of THE JOURNAL has one of the most amusing editorials published in the entire history of the organization. A special correspondent of the *British Medical Journal* had called the attention of that publication to the fact that America lacked independent medical journals controlled by medical men and that it lacked also a national or unitary organization. The *British Medical Journal* therefore addressed a communication to the prominent members of the United States offering them the *British Medical Journal* for $8 a year. This annoyed the editor of THE JOURNAL, who replied by pointing out that THE JOURNAL OF THE AMERICAN MEDICAL ASSOCIATION, while it took legitimate advertisements, kept them in the columns devoted to that purpose and did not supply reading notices as was customary in the British publication.

1894

SAN FRANCISCO

With the beginning of 1894 the editor of THE JOURNAL began circulating sample copies to men who were not subscribers with a view to increasing the circulation. In the same issue Dr. N. S. Davis remarked bitterly about the manufacturers of Maltine, who used his picture on a calendar which they circulated to the medical profession. He said "As I have never prescribed an ounce of Maltine nor written a line concerning it in my life, I assume the manufacturers have taken this method to inflict punishment. And certainly they could not have devised a more contemptible or meaner method if they had searched the records of meanness for half a century." The old gentleman must certainly have been angry on this occasion.

The editor of the *New York Medical Record* challenged some of the statements that were used by THE JOURNAL in giving an impression as to the amount of reading material that it gave to the readers. By actually counting the words on the pages, the editor of THE JOURNAL proved that THE JOURNAL OF THE AMERICAN MEDICAL ASSOCIATION was the largest medical journal in America. He challenged the *Record* by telling it that THE JOURNAL had only just started; the editorial ended with the words "Just wait."

In a long letter to THE JOURNAL Dr. N. S. Davis supported the changes that were being proposed for the Constitution and By-Laws; he thought that the time had just about come to stop tinkering with the Constitution and By-Laws.

The editor of THE JOURNAL was alert to protect the interests of the publication. In a brief note he told the editors of the *Philadelphia Medical News* and the *Pittsburgh Medical Review* to mind their own business because they ran an editorial objecting to publication in

THE JOURNAL of an article in two parts. Those were the days of competitive journalism in American medicine, and the battle raged continuously. A week later the editor told the editor of the *Pittsburgh Medical Review* that his ill natured commentary on a note published in THE JOURNAL was unwarranted.

A notable feature of THE JOURNAL OF THE AMERICAN MEDICAL ASSOCIATION for March 24, 1894, was the clinical history of the case of President James A. Garfield by his physician, Dr. Robert Reyburn, who gave a complete description of his case—one of the most important historical documents in its field and yet one hardly mentioned in historical or biographic writings in this country.

In THE JOURNAL for March 31, 1894, an article on the psychophysical relations of man considered from the standpoint of a professor of medicine is just about as modern a review of psychosomatic medicine as can be found in periodicals current in 1947.

FRAUDULENT MEDICAL COLLEGES

On March 31, 1894, the Illinois State Board of Health compiled for THE JOURNAL OF THE AMERICAN MEDICAL ASSOCIATION a list of fraudulent medical institutions. This was the first of the important articles which were to do more to raise the standard of medical education and eliminate low grade medicine in the United States than any other factor.

PROPRIETARY MEDICINES

The medical profession was beginning to be increasingly aware of its responsibility in the promotion of proprietary medicines. Dr. Solomon Solis-Cohen of Philadelphia initiated this fight and constituted himself the leader of the crusade. He was attacked in a vicious letter published in THE JOURNAL OF THE AMERICAN MEDICAL ASSOCIATION for March 24, 1894, which indulged in personalities as to his race and religion. The writer, whose communication was anonymous, said that he would just as leave use Listerine and Phenacetin until the Pharmacopeia gave him something to take their place. By March 31 half a dozen writers alined themselves with Dr. Solomon Solis-Cohen in this crusade. The majority of physicians already favored the elimination of "patent" medicines and low grade proprietaries from the advertising columns of THE JOURNAL. Apparently, "Medicus," who wrote the anonymous letter, overplayed his hand. Issue after issue of THE JOURNAL condemned him for conduct that was unethical in his attack on Dr. Solis-Cohen and for being anything but a gentleman. By the virulence of his attack he rallied to the support of Dr. Solis-Cohen many who might otherwise have paid little attention to the controversy.

PIRATING JOURNAL ARTICLES

The editor of THE JOURNAL called the attention of his competitors to the fact that the papers read in the annual session were the property of THE JOURNAL. Already competitors were asking authors for their papers, offering to publish their articles, to put them in type and to give them free reprints if they would only pull their articles out of THE JOURNAL OF THE AMERICAN MEDICAL ASSOCIATION.

Early in May 1894 the Washington correspondent of THE JOURNAL telegraphed that "Coxey's army," 437 men and 30 horses, fatigued and improperly and scantily fed, without shelter, was camping in an enclosure of 60,000 square feet, recently drained, containing five decomposing manure dumps and abutting on James Creek. There were foul smelling, open sewers and many filthy gutters; there was no shade, and the temperature was about 90 at 10 p. m. The health of the "army" and city was threatened. The editor of THE JOURNAL pointed out that some better place should have been found for General Coxey's army and that the animals at Rock Creek Zoo were better cared for.

ATTACKS ON THE PRINCIPLES OF ETHICS

The discussions on the revision of the Principles of Ethics were growing sharp; many of the older leaders of the American Medical Association began to express themselves with such pseudonyms as "Conservative Member" and "Harmony," while Dr. N. S. Davis kept pointing out that the Principles of Ethics were a part of the fundamental law of the Association and that they could be amended only with the same seriousness as the Constitution and By-Laws.

The address of the President, Dr. James F. Hibberd of Richmond, Ind., was concerned wholly with associational affairs and particularly with the desirability of membership in county and state societies as the basis for representation in the American Medical Association. He was glad to report that the Congress had been made to see the importance of the *Index Catalogue* and to continue the appropriation for its publication. Again he urged the establishment of a department of health in the cabinet. It seemed to him that the future of medicine would be along biologic lines and that biology must be more and more the basis for training in medicine.

The San Francisco session had taken many significant actions. The business of the Association had increased to include a budget of more than $35,000, a figure which was to grow with the years, so that the next fifty years saw this $35,000 grow into millions.

The state medical societies had been asked to consider the Principles of Ethics. Twenty-one had reported opposition to any change; two reported in favor of a change, and two recommended that the subject be laid on the table.

THE TREASURER

Dr. R. J. Dunglison had been for seventeen years the faithful and energetic treasurer of the Association without compensation. A resolution was offered by E. E. Montgomery of Philadelphia that he be given an honorarium of $300 and this was referred to the Board of Trustees.

THE LIBRARY

At this meeting the librarian suggested that the library of the American Medical Association be turned over to the Newberry Library in Chicago, to which Nicholas Senn had previously given his complete library.

ADVERTISING IN THE JOURNAL

The Board of Trustees reported that they were receiving cancellations of five subscriptions daily at the time when Dr. John B. Hamilton became editor but that following his assumption of the editorship THE JOURNAL began to increase in size and was thereafter more successful as an advertising medium. The Board of Trustees felt that it was necessary for them to take some action on the quality of advertisements. The Board found itself in a difficult position. It needed the advertising to pay for THE JOURNAL but it had a resolution from the membership that advertisements should not be accepted for any secret proprietary remedies. They therefore took as their standard what other journals were doing.

The new Constitution and By-Laws came up for consideration. Again Dr. H. D. Didama presented a minority report and his minority report, by vote, became the report of the committee. This threw the entire organization into an uproar. Speeches were made by many of the leaders. Apparently no one was quite certain as to just what had happened, because it ended with the By-Laws being allowed to remain over until the following year. When the consideration of the Principles of Ethics was called up, Dr. Didama again presented a minority report and his minority report was adopted. A motion was then made to lay the whole question on the table, and this motion passed.

The committee that was trying to get a secretary of health for the cabinet was given $400 to go down to Washington and urge its cause.

Then came a battle resulting from a resolution introduced by Edward Jackson of Pennsylvania over the admission of advertisements of proprietary remedies to THE JOURNAL.

In the same issue as appear the minutes of the San Francisco session of 1894 is a report on the question of advertising. This report points out that most of the criticism had come from the *Medical News* of Philadelphia, which was printed by a Philadelphia publisher. This Philadelphia publisher had wanted to get THE JOURNAL under his control. The *American Lancet* defended the Trustees in their policy to keep on publishing somewhat doubtful advertisements, but it felt that this would cost THE JOURNAL $8,000 a year and that the sacrifice was hardly warranted.

The Medical College Association at this time expelled two of its constituent colleges for failing to comply with rules governing the graduation of medical students.

SIGNED REVIEWS AND EDITORIALS

Among the editorial contributors added to the staff in 1894 one finds the significant names of W. A. Pusey and John A. Wyeth. At no time in its history has THE JOURNAL published signed editorials or book reviews. The question has been repeatedly agitated in the columns of THE JOURNAL and before meetings of the Board of Trustees. Without doubt the adoption of this policy has resulted in a freedom of expression in editorials and book reviews which has been for the advantage of American medicine.

RAILROAD TROUBLES

The record of the return home of former President Hibberd from San Francisco to Indiana indicates that travel in that day of the great railroad strike partook of the hazards of pioneer overland trails. The trains and their arrivals and departures resembled a great deal the kind of delays that accompany long airplane trips in these times. Dr. Hibberd's travel was complicated; the train moved along in jumps of 25 to 50 miles. Chicago was cut off entirely from railroad travel. Stages carried the party over the crest of the Rockies; it took from five to seven days to go from Helena, Mont., to St. Paul. One hundred and seventy physicians found themselves unable to leave Yellowstone National Park and failed to receive any mail for ten to fifteen days.

Now began an agitation which was to make obstetrics and gynecology specialties in medicine. The general surgeons revolted and argued that a woman's liver and intestines and stomach were just the same as those of a man and that the general surgeon could do everything necessary surgically in the abdomen, male or female.

Dr. Hamilton devoted himself strongly during the latter half of 1894 to building subscriptions to THE JOURNAL. Every issue urged doctors to subscribe. Premiums were offered to medical students who could secure subscriptions.

THE JOURNAL FINDS A NEW PLANT

In September 1894 THE JOURNAL moved from its quarters on Wabash Avenue in Chicago because the new library building cut off the light and air, making it necessary to burn the gas continuously for the last six months. Because of the cramped quarters it had been necessary to have the editorial work done elsewhere. The editor had been authorized by the trustees to secure better accommodations; the new offices were in the *Times* Building at 84-86 Fifth Avenue (now known as Wells Street). THE JOURNAL purchased its own presses (the best and fastest that could be purchased at the time) and the remainder of the machinery was of the latest and best pattern.

Dr. Hamilton was still combative; he ended his editorial with the statement:

> Carping critics have not infrequently amused themselves by predicting the downfall of THE JOURNAL, but, supported by the Association, it has continued to prosper beyond the most sanguine hopes of its best friends.

In another editorial Dr. Hamilton wrote:

> A medical gentleman on whom a JOURNAL representative called said that he did not care to belong to the Association "because," said he, "the organization is simply a mutual admiration society." Exactly so, and if our fugacious friend wishes to be thoroughly admired, he too should join the Association and assist in the noble work of making it the greatest medical organization the world has yet known.

The editor pointed out that the new press would print 2,300 impressions an hour and that another press would print 2,000 an hour. The Board of Trustees of the Association has more recently authorized the expenditure of some $250,000 to purchase one new rotary press capable of printing ninety-six pages at one time and of turning out 6,000 two-color impressions an hour.

On October 7, 1894, Dr. Oliver Wendell Holmes, the genial autocrat of the breakfast table, died at the age of 85. His passing received editorial comment in every medical journal of the nation. The editor of THE JOURNAL called attention to his "famous report of the committee on medical literature." He had participated in the work of the founding and development of the American Medical

Association, and his contributions to medical advancement insured him a prominent place in medicine's hall of fame.

In his message to the Congress in December 1894 President Grover Cleveland recommended the establishment of a national board of health and a national health officer. Alas, the years have passed and this vain hope is not yet realized. It continues to be one of the leading planks in the platform of the American Medical Association.

THE PERMANENT SECRETARY RETIRES AND DR. GEORGE H. SIMMONS SUCCEEDS

1895

BOOK REVIEWS

BOOK REVIEWS HAVE ALWAYS BEEN a source of serious discussion in medical periodicals. When publishers owned most of the medical journals in the United States a definite relationship prevailed between the character of the review, the owner of the periodical and the publisher. This abuse finally reached such proportions that THE JOURNAL found it necessary in its issue of Jan. 12, 1895, to talk about book reviews and to remind its readers that THE JOURNAL OF THE AMERICAN MEDICAL ASSOCIATION, at least, would publish criticisms and not eulogies of new books. Some publishers had already developed the technic of avoiding distribution of books for review to periodicals which would not guarantee them favorable reviews.

Improvements in medical journals were, however, definitely on the march. In THE JOURNAL for Jan. 26, 1895, the editor announced that he would no longer publish anonymous communications, a rule that has been followed almost invariably since that date. Unless a physician cares to give his name in discussing the work of another physician or some activity of the American Medical Association, he should not wish the editor to take the responsibility for views which, in most instances, when they are to be published anonymously are venomous and hypercritical rather than honest.

Certain themes recur at cycles of five or ten years in the history of the Association. In March of 1895 the editor said:

> A certain number find great fault with THE JOURNAL, others are alarmed at what they call the political ring rule, and others think the Association ethics is a most serious rock of offense.... This is the friction that is a part of all organized movements and indicates growth and progress which is always very promising for the future.

THE FIRST FIRE

On March 31, 1895, the day being Sunday, a fire resulted in serious damage to the equipment and a flooding of the offices of THE JOURNAL. Two of the trustees and the editor arrived in an hour to find the fire practically extinguished. THE JOURNAL appeared on time, but it was quite a strain on the staff. As the year went on, the struggle for improved quality in advertising in medical periodicals began to burst more and more into the open. Letters appeared in various publications with the definite trend towards cleaning advertising pages. The committee in charge of the Rush monument was still at work and still not making much progress. A picture of Benjamin Rush was printed in May 1895, and the committee was urged to collect enough money to build this monument.

In his president's address published May 11, 1895, Dr. Donald Maclean of Detroit devoted himself largely to the history of medicine, with special emphasis on Edinburgh, where he had had his own education. He closed his address with another plea for a national department of health.

THE BALTIMORE SESSION

The annual session, held in Baltimore May 7–10, 1895, was to make history of the greatest importance for the future of medicine in the United States. The population of the United States had increased from 35,000,000 in 1866 to 70,000,000 in 1895. The population of Baltimore had increased from 250,000 to 500,000. Dr. William Osler was chairman of the committee on arrangements, and a number of interesting receptions and visits to educational institutions had been provided.

THE DRIVE FOR CLEAN ADVERTISING

The Medical Society of the State of Pennsylvania had taken the leadership in the attempt to improve the quality of advertising in medical periodicals and had brought a case before the Judicial Council against the practice. The Judicial Council discovered that the trustees and the editor had, perhaps inadvertently, published some objectionable advertisements. Dr. Solomon Solis-Cohen, who had assumed leadership in this movement, asked for a special committee to take up the matter with the Board of Trustees at a later hour in the session. Dr. John B. Hamilton, editor of THE JOURNAL, by a parliamentary procedure, endeavored to prevent the discussion, whereupon Dr. Solis-Cohen said:

> I am speaking to the resolution. The object of this committee is to digest the report; to consider the criticisms that have been offered publicly, and to consider further what the Trustees have to say in relation thereto calmly, deliberately, without prejudice, and then report to the Association at a time when it can again be calmly discussed by the Association with all the necessary data before it. It is to prevent hasty judgment, favorable or unfavorable, that this resolution is offered. It is offered as a means of peace,

as a means of carrying out the will of the Association, as a means of elevating THE JOURNAL of the Association to the proud position that it ought to occupy as the leader and not the follower of the medical press of the United States. Therefore we ask that this resolution be adopted.

After much discussion, the resolution proposed by Dr. Solis-Cohen, that a committee of three work with the trustees, was tabled. Then a new resolution introduced by Dr. E. Fletcher Ingals requesting a committee to consult with the Board of Trustees was passed following a second of the motion by Dr. Solis-Cohen. Dr. Cochran took it that the appointment of such a committee was an indictment of the Board of Trustees. A motion was then made to table the discussion and, following a call for a count, the motion was tabled by a vote of 138 to 108. But the fight was not ended! Following an interlude of discussion on improved rank for medical officers of the Navy, Dr. Leartus Connor of Detroit again introduced the subject and demanded a survey as to the proportion of the membership of the American Medical Association who prescribed secret proprietary remedies. This resolution was briskly discussed and again the question was laid on the table.

The Board of Trustees reported that the editor had been instructed to refuse advertisements of proprietary remedies which were not accompanied by a formula:

> Still further to comply with what appears to be the desire of a large number of those interested in the highest success of THE JOURNAL, the editor, with the termination of present contracts, has been instructed to accept no advertisements of medicinal preparations the proprietors of which do not give a formula containing the official or chemical name and quantity of each composing ingredient to be inserted as a part of the advertisement.

When this report was read, Dr. Solis-Cohen congratulated the trustees on the fact that the Association could "at last stand upon an honest platform." He felt that the Association should demand that every other medical journal should make its pages clean from the shame of "patent" medicines.

> On behalf of the Pennsylvania delegation, as commissioned by them officially, and unofficially on behalf of the hundreds of members who came to me, as well as of various medical societies, to express their desire that we go forward to cleanse THE JOURNAL, I move the approval of the report of the Board of Trustees.

There was great applause and the motion was carried.

And still the issue was not dead. After an interlude of discussion on the raising of the dues, Dr. A. Koenig of Pittsburgh moved a vote of confidence for the Board of Trustees. Dr. Hamilton objected to this motion. There was a lot of discussion back and forth, and finally Dr. Solis-Cohen moved that the whole new discussion be tabled and it was tabled.

AMENDMENTS TO THE BY-LAWS

Next considerable discussion arose over amendments to the Constitution and By-Laws, including a proposal to establish a new section on orthopedic surgery. Dr. N. S. Davis contended that there had been too much carelessness in proposing amendments to the Constitution and By-Laws and that there ought to be more formal proposal of such amendments.

THE INDEX MEDICUS

The *Index Medicus* was again in financial difficulties, and Dr. William Osler offered a resolution requesting members of the Association to support the *Index Medicus*.

THE BATTLE OVER THE SECRETARY

This meeting has also become noted in the history of the Association because of the action that was taken regarding the permanent secretary. There was a provision in the Constitution that the permanent secretary should remain in office until either by death, resignation or removal by a two-thirds vote of the Association a change should take place. The committee on nominations brought in the name of Frank Woodbury of Pennsylvania as secretary. Dr. E. D. Ferguson of New York pointed out that the permanent secretary was really permanent and he moved that the portion of the report pertaining to the permanent secretary be not agreed to. Dr. I. N. Quimby said that the present permanent secretary had served thirty-one years and he concluded with the following emotional appeal:

> Let the sentiment of this Association be *fiat justitia*—exact justice and mercy to every one, whether he be high or low, and let this Association sustain the present secretary, at least for the present. Let us not send him home as though he had some affliction, but let us try to make him feel happy.

This motion was about to pass when Dr. William Osler stood on his chair—the better to be heard—and made the famous speech for which he was hissed, saying bluntly:

> *Fiat justitia* for the Association is all right, but let the quality of mercy be not strained. I stand here and say plainly and honestly before Dr. Atkinson what I and many other members have said behind his back, that he is not an efficient secretary of this Association, and that we have not found him so. [Hisses, followed by applause.] You may hiss if you will, but I unhesitatingly say that no more important step in advance will be taken by the Association than when it changes its secretary. [Cries of Question! Question]

President Maclean put the motion that the present incumbent remain in office, and it was carried by a large majority. Then Dr. I. N. Love moved that the Constitution be amended so that in the future the secretary should be elected annually.

After the vote was taken, Osler left his seat, walked up onto the platform and took Dr. Atkinson's hand and whispered to him for several minutes. Exactly what was said was not recorded, but apparently it was pleasant. However, the meeting must have had some repercussions in the Osler home. Mrs. Osler wrote in a letter to a friend on June 14:

> After you left, my mother soon departed, and she was followed by one relation and friend after another and I only had time to catch my breath and be ready for that— (you know) American Med. Asso. Our plans were changed somewhat as Dr. Osler's sister-in-law died very suddenly and we of course did not take part in any of the entertainments—and Dr. Osler recalled his dinner invitations. Dr. Donald Maclean (A. M. A. President for the year) and his wife stayed here, also Dr. and Mrs. McGuire from Richmond. I hesitate to express my opinion about the A. M. A. probably yours is the same. Thank goodness it cannot come here again while we live here. . . . Dr. Osler distinguished himself by maligning old Atkinson the secretary—I was at the meeting and frightened to death when I heard him pronounce the "secretary absolutely incompetent." It was a benefit to the Association I am told, but I fail to see it.

William B. Atkinson, the permanent secretary, was by temperament and experience really entitled to hold the position that he held for so many years, until the tempest raised by William Osler led to his final resignation. He was born in Pennsylvania in 1832 and was a graduate of the Central High School in Philadelphia and then from the Jefferson Medical College in 1853 after three years of preceptorship with Dr. Samuel McClellan. He had been a correspondent of the *New Jersey Medical and Surgical Reporter*, *New York Medical Times*, the *Nashville Medical Journal* and the *New Orleans Medical Journal* and co-editor with Dr. S. W. Butler of the *Medical and Surgical Reporter*. When Dr. S. D. Gross edited the *North American Medico-Chirurgical Review* he became its obstetric editor. Eventually he published a book of biographies of American physicians. He had been editor of the Transactions of the American Medical Association as secretary, and also editor of the Transactions of the State Medical Society of Pennsylvania when secretary of that organization. His book of biographies called "Physicians and Surgeons of the United States," published in 1878, included the lives of 1,873 physicians, and there had been a second edition in 1880. He held many teaching positions and was the author of a book called "Hints in the Obstetric Practice" and of another called "Therapeutics of Gynecology and Obstetrics." Dr. Atkinson died in Philadelphia Nov. 23, 1909.

PROGRESS WITH THE JOURNAL

In Volume 25 for 1895 the name of Dr. Ludvig Hektoen appeared for the first time as an editorial contributor. There was also the name of Dr. John Ridlon. Dr. Hektoen since 1895 has contributed a number of editorials to the columns year after year and has been especially helpful in training young men to take an interest in journalism and in editorial work.

THE JOURNAL was happy in July of 1895 because it included a double page spread in three colors illustrating pathologic appearances in endarteritis. THE JOURNAL was definitely improving in the quality of its illustrations and in the makeup of its pages.

THE BATTLE OF THE MONUMENTS

The battle of the monuments was now definitely on. The American Surgical Association was behind the movement to erect a statue to Professor S. D. Gross. The monument to Benjamin Rush was still having hard sledding. Then came a movement on the part of the homeopathic group to erect a monument to Samuel Christian Friedrich Hahnemann. The Rush monument fund had now reached $3,357.39.

Interesting is a letter which appeared in THE JOURNAL for Sept. 21, 1895, stating that THE JOURNAL was now too advanced for many of its readers and that it ought to print articles of less scientific value in order to reach a doctor-reader audience. This continued to be a perennial reminder that some physicians are not quite up to others and that men in the lower brackets feel that journals ought to be edited to their levels.

Louis Pasteur, among the most famous of all the names in medicine, died of paralysis at his home in Paris Sept. 28, 1895, aged 73. The first steamer built by the United States government for its quarantine service had been named in his honor. Long before the time of his death it had been recognized that his had been among the greatest of all contributions to the advancement of medical science.

The library of the American Medical Association had been transferred to the Newberry Library of Chicago. The librarian at the Newberry Library discovered in 1895 that it did not even contain a full set of THE JOURNAL OF THE AMERICAN MEDICAL ASSOCIATION or, in fact, even one volume. It had, however, begun to accumulate some excellent incunabula and some complete sets of medical periodicals.

PARLIAMENTARY LAW

The debates in the annual sessions of the previous two years had been so stormy that one member, Dr. A. C. Simonton of San Jose, Calif., in the cooling off period of 1895 wrote a long letter about parliamentary law. He referred particularly to the trustees, who apparently kept copies of Roberts' "Rules of Order" in their pockets and had to refer to them frequently in the midst of debates. Dr. Simonton was seriously interested in parliamentary law, and he felt that it was about time that the rulings in the House of Delegates of the American Medical Association be more in accord with established principles.

1896
ATLANTA

On March 14, 1896, Dr. F. E. Stewart of Detroit proposed that the members of the Association have a permanent badge. He had his own ideas for such an emblem and he invited suggestions from others.

The two year lease of the Association on the rooms at 86 Fifth Avenue terminated April 30, 1896, and it became necessary to move. The stay in the Fifth Avenue headquarters had not been happy. There had been no recovery of anything on account of the damage by fire and water. The power was always breaking down, the halls were dirty, and Dr. Hamilton could not make the owner make good on his verbal promises. A lease was therefore made with the owners of the Dental Building at 61 Market Street, so that the Association occupied the third floor in a new fireproof building. The Association purchased an electric motor so that it could run its own presses. Dr. Hamilton felt, however, that the business necessity of a permanent home for THE JOURNAL was becoming more and more urgent every year. "The bad policy of paying rent," he said, "will be apparent." Thus he urged that the Association take the necessary steps to provide a fund for the purchase of property, the payment of interest and the gradual extinguishment of its debt. "The present move," he said "should be the last move in a rented building. Next time we should go into the permanent home of the Association."

SPECIAL TRAIN TROUBLE

Later in the same month the editor of THE JOURNAL was agitated because some of the members were working independently on the railroads and he had in his responsibility the matter of the special train to Atlanta for the 1896 sesssion. One physician in Chicago who could not get a pass to Atlanta for his wife negotiated with another railroad and tried to work out a special deal with that road. A drug firm in another city, which conducted a medical journal in Chicago, tried to get a special train for that group. This interfered somewhat with the ideas of Dr. Hamilton, and he ended his editorial snappily: "Whether THE JOURNAL ever runs another special to any of the meetings depends upon the view the members take of it."

Now comes the story of a special train which must have given

Dr. Hamilton a maximum of annoyance. The train left Chicago on Sunday night, May 3, by the Big Four Road. Everybody was happy and the train pulled into Cincinnati at 9:05 that night exactly on time. The train was now turned over to the Queen and Crescent Railroad. Here Dr. Hamilton discovered that the train occupied by his group would be held in Cincinnati until another train coming from Detroit—operated under the auspices of a magazine called *Detroit Medicine* and in charge of Dr. Harold Moyer of Chicago and Dr. Whitmore of Parke, Davis & Company—could join with his group. The Detroit party had about 33 people, who started out on the Monon route and were delayed somewhere in Indiana, so that Dr. Hamilton's group was held until 11:30 at night without any supper. (It was supper in those days; dinner came in some time later.) At 11:30 at night everybody got restless and so the Queen and Crescent Railroad brought down a man—"the alleged superintendent," Dr. Hamilton calls him—"a certain Mr. Stephens," to interview the passengers. Mr. Stephens, after some argument, told Dr. Hamilton that the cars belong to the railroad and that he would move them out of the depot when he got ready. "Arguments, persuasion and entreaties were of no avail to the all-powerful Mr. Stephens, who finally, becoming tired of the importunities, sent the train across the river to Ludlow, Ky., where they completed the allotted period of the detention and were finally joined by the delayed contingent as aforesaid." The train arrived in Chattanooga at 10:30 a. m. and finally the people got something to eat. In the nature of a vast understatement, Dr. Hamilton writes "The originators of the trouble, including the alleged Stephens, were not extremely popular with any of the members of THE JOURNAL party." He continues "A number of physicians on the train made up their minds that they had learned something in the matter of travel over certain railroads, and that when it came to advising patients going South for the winter what line to take in order to have the most comfort and humane attention, they would know how to advise them. A more unfeeling and heartless treatment of passengers has seldom been witnessed than that received at the hands of Mr. Stephens of the Queen & Crescent." Were Dr. Hamilton alive today, we would tell him about the special which left Chicago for San Francisco in 1946 and arrived fourteen hours late.

CELEBRATION OF THE SEMICENTENNIAL

At the Atlanta session, among the first of the resolutions offered was one proposing a suitable celebration of the semicentennial meeting in Philadelphia in 1897.

THE PERMANENT SECRETARY

The question of the permanent secretary continued to be agitated by Dr. I. N. Love of St. Louis, but apparently the membership were not yet ready to make a change. Dr. Love in his discussion said that the ruling that had been made at the Baltimore convention to the effect that the Constitution precluded any change in the secretaryship "paralyzed everybody, consequently proper consideration was not given to the question. I know it paralyzed me," he continued, "and I do not easily paralyze." (Laughter.) Questions elicited the fact that the Constitution was so written in 1864. There was a good deal of discussion on the matter. There was some criticism of Dr. Maclean for not having put the question at the Baltimore meeting, and he suggested that in the interest of peace he had avoided it. Then there was a call for the reading of the minutes of the Baltimore session because apparently there was some doubt as to just what was done and there was some question as to whether the minutes as printed in THE JOURNAL were actually minutes of the meeting. The question was particularly agitated by Dr. H. Bert Ellis of California. Eventually the situation was cleared by a resolution to the effect that the minutes as published in THE JOURNAL be recorded as official minutes. The secretary then arose to point out that he kept his minutes in a big book, that he wrote them out every evening before he went to sleep and that the editor published them in THE JOURNAL exactly as they were in the book. He offered to have the book available for inspection but he did not think it essential because such a book would be too cumbersome to carry around from place to place. The discussion continued until it was lost in the midst of a lot of confusion and apparently nothing further was done with it at that session.

There was still more discussion as to moving THE JOURNAL from Chicago to some place else, and Dr. Garcelon of Maine introduced a resolution calling attention to the fact that the trustees had been authorized to establish a building fund and requesting a ballot of the members of the Association indicating a place where they wished THE JOURNAL to be located permanently.

The Atlanta convention was especially notable for the quality of the entertainment, which included a Georgia barbecue, and for a beautiful address given by John Temple Graves. Typical of his discourse are these paragraphs:

> Atlanta is proud beyond expression of her brilliant galaxy of physicians. We support 200 doctors in this happy town, maintain them in the most lavish splendor and the most indolent leisure. There is nothing here for them to do. In the elixir of this incomparable air and under the blue of these cloudless skies there is never an ailment that an old woman's nostrums wouldn't cure.

Our doctors here are almost without exception millionaires. They practice only on the stranger within our gates. They live in stately mansions, drive in splendid carriages and spend their time in thumping the soundest of "livers" and in feeling the steadiest pulses that ever beat in unison with the hope and progress of the healthiest and bravest city in the South.

He concluded:

Turn your stethoscopes upon us; level your heartscopes, your brainscopes, try us with the Roentgen rays of all institutions, and you will find that Atlanta, city of conventions, abating no jot or tittle of the sincerity of any past profession, has held in her heart her last and most loving welcome for the doctors of America.

MORE SPECIAL TRAIN TROUBLE

In the same issue in which he reported the minutes of the convention Dr. Hamilton gave a final curtsy to "superintendent Stephens," who had now become Stevens. He opened up with the quotation from Shakespeare:

> But man, proud man,
> Drest in a little brief authority,
> Most ignorant of what he's most assured.
> His glassy essence, like an angry ape,
> Plays such fantastic tricks before high heaven
> As make the angels weep.

Dr. Hamilton repeated the manner in which the physicians had discussed the delay with Mr. Stevens and then he said:

All these things were explained to the great potentate, but he refused all requests and laughed in our faces, although nearly every male passenger made a personal appeal to him. That his phenomenal brutality should hurt the Queen & Crescent railroad is apparent, and if they are sorry for it they have a plain remedy, that is to repudiate Mr. Stevens, and all his works, at the earliest possible date. It is possible that even the Queen & Crescent railroad may discover that it is not good railroad management to treat a hundred physicians and their families as a trainload of immigrants.

A PERMANENT HOME

Now began the agitation over the permanent home. The trustees had set aside $3,000 to be placed at interest as the commencement of a building fund. All members were sent ballots and requested to vote on the place of the permanent home.

The first page of volume 27 of THE JOURNAL, covering the second half of 1896, reveals the addition to the staff correspondents of several names which were eventually to play highly significant parts in the growth and development of the Association. Among them was that of Emily Cushing, who served for many, many years as an abstracter of literature, and also William Whitford, who was the official reporter until age and illness caused him to discontinue this work.

DIPHTHERIA ANTITOXIN INTRODUCED

Diphtheria antitoxin was now exceedingly prominent as the center of interest, and the American Pediatric Society had conducted quite a modern survey as to its usefulness. The evidence was so convincing that a distinguished committee led by L. Emmett Holt gave the remedy their full support and established a routine dosage. "Antitoxin should be administered as early as possible on a clinical diagnosis, not waiting for a bacteriologic culture," they said.

READING NOTICES

By this time a considerable abuse had risen in American medical journalism which again required years for its correction; it was the so-called "reading notice." The manufacturer of proprietary remedies before signing a contract for purchase of space obtained as a concession a number of editorial notices as to the worthiness of his products. The editor of THE JOURNAL protested, but apparently the abuse was quite outside his ability to correct.

A STANDARD NOMENCLATURE

On Aug. 8, 1896, the editors called attention to the desirability of a standard nomenclature of diseases—a movement which was only to find real accomplishment over forty years later.

THE PERMANENT LOCATION

At the same time the editor published the result of the ballot on the permanent location of THE JOURNAL. Chicago led with 2,128 votes; Washington received 810; New York got only 24, and Philadelphia 48; St. Louis 22 and a good many other cities received just a few votes, including such strange locations as Elmira, N. Y., and Sedalia, Mo.

LEADERS FROM MEDICAL JOURNALISM

Medical journalism at this time occupied a strange place in American medical life. Many of the leaders in American affairs were themselves editors of publications, as for example, Dr. I. N. Love, who was a trustee of the American Medical Association, Dr. Leartus Connor of Detroit and Dr. Harold N. Moyer, a prominent delegate. Much highly personal journalism resulted from the competition. The repartee in such house organs as Merck's *American Medico-Surgical Bulletin,* Parke, Davis & Company's *Medicine,* the *New York Medical Record,* the *New York Medical Journal* and the *Philadelphia Medical News* with the editor of the JOURNAL OF THE AMERICAN MEDICAL ASSOCIATION makes amusing and exciting reading.

MORAL HYGIENE

The hygiene of the period was a moral hygiene more than a scientific medical hygiene. Page after page was devoted to the treatment of inebriety; there were long serial articles published by T. D. Crothers, who conducted an institution for the purpose.

The bicycle was invented about that time and became exceedingly popular. Just as soon as it achieved notice, doctors began to wonder about its medical effects. There were some interesting letters pro and con the bicycle as to what it would do as a cause of vesical and prostatic irritation and how it would react on the reproductive instinct and the sexual appetite of the female. Most of the doctors were convinced however that, regardless of what the bicycle would do to health, the bicycle had come to stay.

THE FIRST EDUCATIONAL NUMBER

The month of September 1896 was highly significant because THE JOURNAL OF THE AMERICAN MEDICAL ASSOCIATION on September 19 published the first report on the medical colleges of the United States, with a description of the Association of American Medical Colleges and the Southern Medical College Association and their requirements together with a statement concerning each school, its tuition fees, its hours of study and its officers. This was perhaps the first Educational Number. Eventually repeated publication of the facts came to be the most important single step in raising the standards of medical education in the United States. Shortly thereafter THE JOURNAL began printing descriptions of diploma mills and to print letters regarding quackery which served to open these successful campaigns.

THE RUSH MONUMENT

The Rush monument project was still doing poorly, and the matter was all the more serious because the homeopaths had raised $75,000 and were in process of building their monument in Washington.

1897

THE SEMICENTENNIAL YEAR; PHILADELPHIA

The editorial pages of THE JOURNAL early in 1897 began to reflect other editorial projects of great significance for the advancement of American medicine. One was the defense of animal experimentation, necessary because Senator Gallinger had begun the introduction of a series of appeals which were to follow year after year, designed to prevent the use of animals in the District of Columbia. The Army and Navy medical departments and the U. S. Public Health Service were compelled to oppose such measures in their own interests. The American Medical Association opposed them also because enactment of such legislation in the District might well set a pattern for the rest of the nation.

In 1947 Senator Lemke had succeeded to the Gallinger toga as champion for the antivivisectionists.

HYGIENIC ASPECTS OF SKYSCRAPERS

THE JOURNAL discussed learnedly the medical aspects of the modern skyscraper. Some tall buildings were going up; the editor was worried not only about the sanitation of these buildings but also because the buildings were built with steel cores; it seemed that the steel might rust through and the building fall down. The height seemed to offer serious thoughts also in relationship to conflagrations. "Tall buildings," said the editor, "are an experiment and it is too early to say with assurance whether the predictions of those who condemn them may be fully justified."

OSTEOPATHY APPEARS

The osteopaths began to appear prominently in various states seeking recognition in legislation. The first editorials jeered at their predictions and compared them with Madam Mapp, a famous "bonesetter" or "shape mistress." There had been bonesetters in New England as early as 1696. The editor of the *New York Medical Record* had written an editorial wondering what this new eccentricity of the West meant. To this Dr. Hamilton commented:

The *Medical Record*, however, should not be too severely criticized for its ignorance of "osteopathy" albeit a female "osteopathist" or "bonesetters" in the days of its editor's youth created a great furor in New York City. The *Medical Record's* knowledge of either medical history or medical science is, it must charitably be admitted, an unstable quantity. It revived Alexander II after his encounter with the nihilist by the use of "oxygen sulfate." A medical journal capable of such a chemical extravaganza can hardly be taken seriously on any subject.

By the end of May, however, the editor of THE JOURNAL OF THE AMERICAN MEDICAL ASSOCIATION began to be disturbed about an osteopathy bill in the state of Illinois, where it had passed the senate.

THE SEMICENTENNIAL MEETING

The really big news of 1897 was the celebration of the semicentennial in Philadelphia. The President was Dr. Nicholas Senn of Chicago, who had already achieved worldwide fame as a surgeon. In his address he recalled the history of the organization. Four members present at the time of its foundation were still alive—Drs. N. S. Davis of Chicago, Alfred Stillé of Philadelphia, J. B.

Johnson of St. Louis and D. F. Atwater of Massachusetts. Dr. Senn recalled the progress that had been made in advancing medical education, in the scientific work of the Association, in its improvement of American medical literature and in its development of its own journal. He praised the Code of Ethics and discussed the difficulties which developed when irregular systems of medical practice were introduced in the nation. "The code has fulfilled the purposes for which it was intended, and will remain a *noli me tangere* for generations to come," he said. He continued:

> I am sure that this feeling will prevail at the centennial celebration fifty years from now, and that our successors will be grateful to us for handing it down to them in an unmutilated form.

He spoke at some length concerning subscriptions to the fund for the Rush monument and urged the erection of a suitable home for the Association with a hall in which its delegates could meet, a library, a museum and other features. He closed with "a glimpse of the future," which is worthy of repetition now that fifty additional years have passed:

> *A Glimpse of the Future.*—Fifty years of steady growth has made the American Medical Association strong. It has passed the experimental stage; it has done a great deal in advancing and diffusing medical knowledge and in the prevention, alleviation and cure of disease. It is the recognized final tribunal which directs and controls all other medical societies and medical educational institutions. It is the final Court of Appeals to which the regular practitioners and the public can look with confidence for the enforcement of a pure discipline and needed protection. It is the highest postgraduate medical institution in this country which without tuition provides a course of instruction annually of a scientific and practical character, well adapted for the busy practitioner, from which every one returns with a firm determination to do more and better work. It is the great bond of fraternal union which binds and cements together the physicians and surgeons and devotees to special departments of medicine and surgery. The Association has done much for the profession and the people in the past, it can and will do more in the future. The organization is now completed and in excellent working order. We can devote in the future all of our time to scientific and practical work. The increase in membership during the last two or three years is unparalleled in the history of the Association. An awakening interest in the usefulness and prosperity of the Association is noticeable on all sides. The papers read in the sections and the discussions are becoming better from year to year. The fiftieth birthday of the Association will give a new impetus to the work and growth of the Association. It is difficult to foretell the possibilities of the second half of the first century of the existence of the Association. It is, however, safe to predict that when the first centennial celebration will be held in this city fifty years from now the membership will have increased from 9,000 to 75,000 or 100,000 and our official organ at that time will be recognized the world over as the most enterprising and best medical journal. Few, if any, who, constituting my audience today, will live to see that day to bear testimony of the proceedings, festivities and incidents commemorating the first semicentennial. The President who will then occupy this Chair and who probably at this time is laboring with his lessons in arithmetic, spelling, geography and grammar in some public school will then review the work of the Association for the first century, and may we trust from the records we shall leave behind that he may adjudge us faithful servants in the cause of science and humanity. Taking up the thread of history from

this day he will chronicle inventions and discoveries of which we have now no conception. The literature of today will be as old and useless as that of fifty years ago. We have the satisfaction of having been permitted to live and labor at a time when the science and practice of medicine and surgery were undergoing a complete revolution. We are now laying the cornerstone and are slowly but surely building the foundation for rational medicine and surgery. The work of the next fifty years will no doubt contribute much toward making what has been sought for ages in vain, the rendering of medicine and surgery exact sciences. The American profession will contribute liberally toward accomplishing this object.

In conclusion, let us implore Almighty God to shower the richest blessings upon the American Medical Association and the labors of all and every one of its present and future members. May it please Him who, during His earthyly career, went from place to place as the Great Physician to heal the sick and maimed, through His boundless mercy and tender sympathies for suffering mankind, to so guide our lives and labors as to imitate His inspiring example in relieving suffering and in adding to the happiness of our fellowman.

The meeting in Philadelphia opened auspiciously with an address of welcome by the mayor and by the Hon. Charles Emory Smith, ex-minister to Russia, who represented the governor of the state. Mr. Smith told the convention that the governor was "detained in Harrisburg in the artistic work of amputating gangrene legislation."

There was a magnificent list of lunches and dinners at which the medical publishers of Philadelphia, the officers of various sections and other distinguished medical organizations were hosts.

After the treasurer of the Rush monument committee made his report, a motion was introduced requesting the American Medical Association to set aside $1,000 each year until a sufficient fund could be raised to build the monument. Dr. J. A. Graham of Colorado made an address pledging the state of Colorado for $2,000, whereupon a roll call of states was made and great numbers pledged anywhere from $2,000 for the state to hundreds of dollars individually. At the end of this great rally Dr. Albert L. Gihon of the U. S. Navy, who had for so many years promoted this fund, thanked the delegates and promised the Association that he would live to see the fulfilment of this work.

The treasurer of the Association made a report indicating a total business of around $56,000 for the year, with $5,000 cash on hand.

Again the question was raised as to the permanent secretary, and Dr. I. N. Love announced that he was not pushing the question. His announcement was greeted with applause. The Association had not yet developed a businesslike method for recording its membership or collecting its dues. There was a tremendous discussion over the fact that the railroad gave half rates to political bodies, synods and Christian Endeavor units but that the best the doctors could get was a fare and a third. In the midst of this discussion it was announced that President William McKinley was about to enter the hall. The proceedings state that:

A moment or two later President McKinley came in arm in arm with Dr. Senn, who had returned to the rear of the stage to perform the office of escort, immediately after quieting down the Association. Dr. Hare preceded Dr. Senn and President McKinley; Mayor Warwick and Governor Hastings and Dr. Pepper and the others of the party attending President McKinley came after. The Association rose and cheered heartily for a minute or two. Quiet being restored, Dr. Senn presented President McKinley, who addressed the Association.

President McKinley merely conveyed greetings and stated that he had paused to pay respectful homage to the noble profession which those present so worthily represented.

Then a brilliant and witty address was made by Governor Hastings of Pennsylvania. A few quotations follow:

> We have all seen the ideal physician, whose presence in the sick room is as welcome as the morning sunshine; his voice is a benediction, his touch an inspiration and his presence emblem of security. To him children turn, and the marks of pain are changed into the expression of love and confidence. The aged reveal to him the secrets of their lives and their hopes of the life hereafter; mothers forget their vigils of the night in loving anticipation for the restoration of their revered or dear ones, or perhaps in the contemplation of the inevitable that the pathway to the tomb shall be strewn with roses in the confidence of a Redeemer's love.
>
> The development of medicine from a layman's point of view has been greater than that of any other science during the last hundred years. There was left a hiatus for a long period of time, when medicine appeared to be nothing but an empiric art. It is very, very different now. I was speaking to you a moment ago about the erection of statues or monuments to our great philanthropists, great soldiers, etc., and allow me to say that I think it is absolutely wrong and decidedly un-American that we do not erect monuments and statues to the great masters of medical science in this country. Then too I have been puzzled at the number of new diseases you have discovered. I read in a history of the fourteenth century by Horner something about diseases of the skin, in which he said there were three diseases of the skin. One was a disease which could be cured by the use of sulfur, a second disease of the skin could be cured by the use of mercury, and the other was a disease of the skin which the devil himself could not cure.

AGAIN CLEAN ADVERTISING

The Board of Trustees reported that some attempt to regulate the advertisements had resulted in a loss of nearly $4,000 because the advertisers felt that "the continued publication of a formula gives every druggist opportunity to enter into competition with the manufacturer of such specialties." The board put up to the Association its willingness to make some change in the manner and standard of advertising. There had been an increase in the membership of the Association. The board had invested $3,000 in a first mortgage on real estate in the city of Indianapolis. Because neither the Association nor the Board of Trustees was a chartered or legal corporation, the investment had to be made in the name of one of the board as trustee for the Association. Owing to a bank failure the funds of the Association had been placed in peril. This offered difficulties because the Board of Trustees did authorize that a charter should be secured.

On motion the report was accepted and action of the board in securing corporation was concurred in.

The convention celebrated with jubilee exercises. Dr. N. S. Davis of Chicago, founder of the Association, appeared on the stage escorted by the presidents of the state medical societies and the presidents of the state boards of medical examiners. Dr. John B. Roberts, chairman of the committee on anniversary exercises, presented Dr. Davis, calling attention to the fact that the fifty-two years that had passed since Dr. Davis's first step toward organization of the Association had been followed by the establishment of a higher standard of education and that there were now medical examining boards in nearly every state of the Union as well as state medical societies. President Senn greeted Dr. Davis on behalf of the Association, then Dr. Davis recited again a brief history of the organization, paying tribute to the many distinguished physicians who had participated in its work. Letters were presented from Drs. Atwater of Springfield, Mass., and John B. Johnson of St. Louis, who had been present at the first meeting.

At this session an action was taken offering a gold medal to members for meritorious work, establishing all addresses delivered before the entire Association as orations to distinguish them from the addresses of the chairmen of the sections and establishing an illustrated lecture to be read on the third evening devoted to some medical subject.

THE AUTHORITY OF THE BOARD

As the session ended, a few matters of great importance for the future of the Association were determined. One was a debate with final action on the decision that all actions of the Association requiring appropriation of funds must go to the Board of Trustees. This included even a motion to print 3,000 copies of the articles of incorporation, the Constitution and By-Laws and the Principles of Ethics.

DECISION BY A WITTICISM

Denver was chosen as the place of meeting. It is rather amusing that this decision was made as a result of a witticism. The competing communities were Columbus, Ohio; Tampa, Fla., and Birmingham, Ala. Those who had been urging Columbus prepared a map showing with what ease it could be reached from those centers. The delegate from Denver merely said, "You will not need a map to find Denver."

ANIMAL EXPERIMENTATION

A significant address at this session was the statement by W. W. Keen beginning the campaign in which he was enlisted the rest of his life in behalf of experimentation on animals. The Association voted to send a reprint of that address to every Senator and Congressman. Dr. Keen reviewed the progress that had been made in medicine and surgery over fifty years. He credited this progress to the advance of medical teaching with the building of libraries and medical literature, the development of the allied medical sciences, the introduction of anesthesia, the development of antiseptic surgery, the rise of bacteriology and immunology, animal experimentation, and the use of instruments of precision. At one point in his address he said:

> Bacteriology would not now exist as a science, nor would accurate modern surgery and a large part of modern medicine be possible, had experiments upon animals been prohibited, as some zoophilous men and women who love dogs better than men and women, and even little children, desire.

He concluded his address with these paragraphs:

> We have discovered the actual cause of tetanus, tuberculosis, erysipelas, suppuration and a host of other diseases and conditions, of the cause of which we were wholly ignorant a few years ago. The causes of many other disorders, both medical and surgical, still remain hidden from our view. We know almost nothing of the origin of benign tumors and are groping to discover the origin of cancer, sarcoma and other malignant growths. When we have discovered the cause, we are nearly half way, or at least a long way, on the road to the discovery of the cure, and I think it not unlikely that in 1947, your then orator will be able to point to the time when a definite knowledge of the causes of these diseases was attained, and probably to a time when their cure was first instituted.
>
> That will be a surgical paradise when we can lay aside the knife and by means of suitable toxins or antitoxins, drugs or other methods of treatment control inflammation, arrest suppuration, stay the ravages of tuberculosis and syphilis, abort or disperse tumors, cure cancer and, it may be, so prolong human life that all of his then audience will die either of accident or old age. Would that you and I could be alive in 1947 to join in the glorious surgical Te Deum!

As the semicentennial passed, Leartus Connor wrote from Detroit congratulating the Association on a tremendous occasion and predicting that the sections and section work might one day be the chief function of the American Medical Association. He pointed out that the Association has one immense advantage over the special societies in the inexhaustible source of its membership.

Leartus Connor, particularly prominent in the affairs of the American Medical Association, was born in New York, Jan. 29, 1843. After graduation from Williams College in Massachusetts he taught for two years as an assistant principal in Mexico Academy of Mexico, N. Y. He studied under Dr. George L. Dayton and then during 1867–1868 in the medical department of the University of Michigan. From there he went to the College of Physicians and Surgeons in New York City and graduated in 1870. In 1871 he moved to Detroit to become teacher of chemistry in the Detroit Medical

College, succeeding eventually to the positions of professor of physiology and clinical medicine and then professor of diseases of the eye and ear. At various times he edited a medical journal known as the *Detroit Review of Medicine and Pharmacy*, the *Detroit Medical Journal*, the *Detroit Lancet* and the *American Lancet*. For seven years he was secretary of the Association of American Medical Colleges. He had also been president of the American Academy of Medicine and of the American Medical Editors Association, chairman of the section on ophthalmology of the American Medical Association and vice president in 1882–1883 and a trustee from 1883 to 1889 and again from 1892 to 1894. He was president of the Michigan State Medical Society in 1902–1903 and chairman of its council from 1902 to 1905. He wrote widely in the field of medicine and contributed many biographies to the "Cyclopedia of American Medical Biography." Dr. Connor died on April 16, 1911.

MEDICAL PATENTS

An interesting item in THE JOURNAL OF THE AMERICAN MEDICAL ASSOCIATION for Sept. 18, 1897 was an article entitled "Is It Ethical for Medical Men to Patent Medical Inventions?" It consisted largely of an attack on proprietary or "patent" medicines, and its tone in general was opposed to secrecy and patents in the field of medicine. When it was read many physicians arose to agree with the speaker. One of the most remarkable speeches was that of Dr. Squibb, founder of the house of E. R. Squibb & Sons. Dr. Squibb said:

> I do not myself think that anything should be patented by either physician or pharmacist. I am sure that the patient would not be benefited thereby. I may say in regard to "patent" medicines that the medical journals themselves are largely responsible for the existence of this class of remedies. If the journals would cease to distribute their advertisements, the sales would fall off 75 per cent. If editors of journals would use their influence to discourage the publication of such testimonials, it would be of great advantage.

1898

DENVER; THE SPANISH-AMERICAN WAR

The JOURNAL OF THE AMERICAN MEDICAL ASSOCIATION began 1898 with an increased number of pages, a new press and some new type. The editor proposed particularly an increased amount of space for society proceedings. He called attention to the fact that some of the newest discoveries in medicine appeared in the proceedings of small societies and that it would be for the reader to differentiate between what was important and what was not.

The battle for animal experimentation had begun to enlist many of the great leaders of American medicine. Dr. William H. Welch of

Johns Hopkins University contributed a notable essay citing his objections to the Gallinger bill. THE JOURNAL was urging doctors everywhere to reach their Congressmen and Senators with messages condemning this legislation.

Late in March THE JOURNAL appeared with an editorial on some medical questions of a possible war. It discussed the tremendous advances that had been made in military science and wondered whether or not human beings would be able to stand the high explosives and steel ships. "In case of hostilities, the sanitary problems on the island of Cuba will be many and full of interest," said the editor and, perhaps satirically, "The march through Spain from Cordova to Madrid will furnish much of interest to the medical profession." In April 1898 the coming of war in Cuba was the chief topic of interest. The editor of THE JOURNAL expressed little fear because Surgeon General Sternberg knew all about yellow fever and he gave good advice about boiling the water. "There is no question," he said, "but immunity from yellow fever can be secured by the rigid observation of sanitary regulations and prompt isolation of any infected case among the troops that may arise through carelessness or faulty hygiene." When the call for volunteers came, THE JOURNAL urged doctors to give their services. "As the number called out is small compared with the population of the country," said THE JOURNAL, "only well grown and perfectly sound men should be accepted."

There was great happiness in the profession because the railroads had finally given the doctors the same rates that they gave to members of the Christian Endeavor for their conventions. The trip to Denver would cost only one way fare plus $2.

THE DENVER MEETING

When the Association met in Denver, President Sternberg was unable to be present because his official duties kept him in Washinton. His address was read for him by Colonel Woodhull of the U. S. Army. In the address George M. Sternberg discussed the progress of medical science. He encouraged the proposal for the establishment of an organization of defense of medical research. He spoke learnedly about the importance of evaluating negative evidence as well as that favorable to new discoveries. He urged greater attention to the use of the laboratory and greater study of the basic sciences. And he concluded that what had been said "would show that there is no room for creeds and pathies in medicine, any more than in astronomy, geology or botany."

In the June issues of THE JOURNAL, Lieut. Col. Nicholas Senn of the National Guard and Illinois Volunteers began his War Correspondence, which was to be a significant feature of THE JOURNAL during the Spanish-American War.

Now THE JOURNAL began printing weekly comments to the effect that the secretary of the business committee, Dr. Bulkley, had failed to turn in the minutes. The permanent secretary had to share the responsibility. In fact, the editor of THE JOURNAL said that it was up to the permanent secretary to see to it that the intense desire of the business committee to conduct the affairs of the Association did not lead its manager to suppress the minutes altogether. Probably the minutes arrived late, because a goodly share of them appeared in the same number in which the editorial complaint is printed.

By this time the technical business of the Association had become so complicated that there began to be complaints that the delegates had no opportunity to attend the scientific meetings. An attempt was made to work out an hourly schedule that would satisfy every one.

Some letters were sent to the editor explaining what had happened to the minutes, and the editor reproved Dr. L. D. Bulkley, telling him that the minutes were the property of the Association and that he had no right to carry them away.

Dr. Richard French Stone of Indianapolis reported that he had worked out a badge for the Association and had it patented so that it would be under the control of the Association. It was an interesting design including a circular spear with a pointed cross. Eventually this design was not adopted.

Dr. William Bailey of Louisville, Ky., offered a resolution to the effect that an active secretary, who could devote his whole time to the work, should be appointed at a salary not exceeding $3,000 a year to work under the present business committee and that the present permanent secretary be retained with the title "honorary secretary." The business committee recommended that his resolution lie over for one year and stated that it would propose changes in the Constitution and By-Laws for the next session. The matter was referred to the Board of Trustees. Out of this came the employment of Dr. George H. Simmons, who was to be the most important force for the next two decades in placing the American Medical Association on the road to financial success and leadership of American medicine.

A motion was passed for the preparation of a membership button.

At the fourth general session there was still more debate over the minutes, which Dr. I. N. Love insisted were not correctly presented.

Members insisted that the reporter was incompetent. Dr. Atkinson was bitterly criticized for leaving out portions of the minutes in his reading. Dr. Atkinson became annoyed and said there would be no trouble in keeping the minutes if the doctors would write out their resolutions and turn them in. The end result was an affirmation of the desirability for having a secretary elected annually and for having an accurate report on the minutes day by day.

Another resolution tried to bring about peace with the disaffected medical societies of New York by rescinding all previous actions in relationship to them. Still another resolution proposed to appoint a committee to go over all textbooks in the field of physiology and hygiene in order to make sure of correctness in their statements. Again came the resolution that all officers of the Association be elected for one year. This was laid on the table.

THE BOARD OF TRUSTEES

The report of the Board of Trustees was exceptional in that it was for the first time a complete statement of comparison of the accomplishments of THE JOURNAL with other publications. It was now clear that THE JOURNAL OF THE AMERICAN MEDICAL ASSOCIATION was publishing more material than other medical periodicals in the United States but was not carrying nearly as much advertising as the *Boston Medical and Surgical Journal* or the *New York Medical Journal* and the *New York Medical Record*. It was estimated that the ruling on proprietary medicines was causing THE JOURNAL a loss of from $8,000 to $10,000 annually, but was nevertheless successful. It had accumulated a great deal of property in the way of machinery and office furniture and it put another $10,000 in the investment fund.

Now Dr. Gihon was able to report that the Rush monument fund had tripled and he now had nearly $12,000.

At this time the Board of Trustees had recommended to the Association that any place that wanted to hold the meeting would have to supply the necessary halls free of expense to the Association.

Practically all resolutions had been referred to the business committee, which rejected the proposal to include anything about the textbooks. The committee put back to the Association as a whole the question of bringing back the New York physicians. Dr. Hobart A. Hare, in an important address, explained the difficulties that prevailed. Dr. X. C. Scott of Cleveland in a reply called attention to the effect that the difficulties with New York involved the Code of Ethics. He was supported by Dr. E. D. Ferguson. There was great heat engendered over this debate with shouts of "No! No!"

and "Yes! Yes!" and with cries of "Good! Good!" Dr. W. P. Munn of Denver spoke passionately and concluded "We have all we can do to keep out the dead rot of commercialism and are we going to be trodden down by this derelict, dead, rotten society of New York, which is continually sending" [cries of "No!" mingled with hisses, the final words of the sentence being inaudible]. Dr. Edward Jackson of Philadelphia hoped that the question would be settled once and for all. Then the question was settled by Dr. W. T. Bishop of Harrisburg, Pa., who pointed out that there could be only one state society in any state and there were two in New York and until New York got together there was no chance to settle the question.

DEATH OF DR. JOHN B. HAMILTON

The issue of THE JOURNAL OF THE AMERICAN MEDICAL ASSOCIATION dated Dec. 31, 1898 opened its editorial column with a black border and the words:

It is our painful duty to record the death of the Editor of THE JOURNAL OF THE AMERICAN MEDICAL ASSOCIATION on the evening of Dec. 24, 1898 at his residence at Elgin, Ill. The immediate cause of his decease was hemorrhage from a perforation of the intestine, communicating with a large abscess outside the bowel, which terminated life after an illness of less than one month.

The concluding paragraphs tell the story of the terrific work in which he engaged during his later years:

The leading sanitarian of the country, in all matters of national interest, his advice was sought in every quarter. No medical gathering of national or international importance was complete without his presence. His vigorous form, his genial countenance, radiant with energy and good will, his persuasive voice, were never to be forgotten features in every such assembly. At home his professional duties, his hospital work, his extensive private practice were enough to wear out any ordinary man; but he was ever ready to expend his energies in behalf of any worthy cause that appealed to him for aid. In this way he gave much time and thought to the organization of the new Public Library in Chicago and was most efficient as President of its Board of Trustees. To the surprise of his friends, despite this accumulation of cares, he accepted, in 1896-1897, the position of superintendent of the Northern Illinois Hospital for the Insane, at Elgin, Ill.—an office that heretofore was always considered sufficient to occupy the whole time of an ordinary official incumbent. But the Doctor speedily showed his mettle by a reorganization of the administration that secured improvement in the care of patients, while leaving time for all his other labors—thus illustrating the old observation that among first class administrators the busiest men still have the most leisure.

Now, alas, this career of action has reached its limit. As we look back upon its years we can more fully than ever appreciate its magnitude and its beneficent efficiency. Dr. Hamilton was fortunate in finding full scope for his remarkable power as a founder and organizer of incipient enterprises. He was fortunate also in being permitted to witness the success of his efforts, and he was doubly fortunate in being called to his reward before age or misfortune or any of the ills of life could dim the splendor of his reputation. He has gone, but his works live and will forever exhibit the impress of his constructive power.

1899

COLUMBUS, OHIO

The first volume for the year 1899 contains a title page which indicates that it was edited for the Association under the direction of the Board of Trustees by George H. Simmons, A.M., M.D. This notice was to continue for the next twenty-five years. There are many stories relative to the selection of Dr. George H. Simmons as editor of THE JOURNAL. The report of the Board of Trustees simply says:

> For the last three months of the year the management was greatly embarrassed by the sickness and death of the late editor, Dr. John B. Hamilton. Under his personal supervision THE JOURNAL had increased to nearly three times its original subscription and had gradually obtained a well equipped plant and a large reserve fund but, more than all, a recognized position among the reputable journals of the country.
>
> On Jan. 1, 1899, shortly after the announcement of the death of Dr. Hamilton, a called meeting of the Board of Trustees was held, at which it was resolved to continue the conduct of THE JOURNAL business under the direction of the resident trustee, Dr. Truman W. Miller, who had very generously, at the sacrifice of his own interests, assumed the management, on the demise of the editor. At the direction of the Board he had the accounts of THE JOURNAL office and the treasurer examined by an expert accountant, who pronounced them correct. At the annual meeting of the Board, February 17 last, after a careful canvass of the available editorial material, Dr. George H. Simmons of Lincoln, Neb., was chosen editor for one year, at a salary of $5,000, with the stipulation that he should move to Chicago and devote his whole time to the work of THE JOURNAL. Your Board congratulates itself that the wisdom of its selection as editor has been efficiently demonstrated by the subsequent progress of THE JOURNAL. The changes that have been made render it more valuable to its patrons and justify the hope of the Board that it shall become the representative medical journal of the world. Other progressive features are under contemplation. A better grade of white paper will be used in the next volume, and the Board has authorized the purchase of two Mergenthaler Linotype machines, at an expense of $6,700, which will insure the use of new type for every issue.

Later in this history a chapter will deal with the details of the life and of the work of Dr. George H. Simmons. According to the best available evidence he was chosen from a considerable group of candidates whose names had been suggested from time to time for the position, including such men as Drs. Bayard Holmes, Harold N. Moyer, Ludvig Hektoen, George M. Gould, G. Frank Lydston and P. Maxwell Foshay. Many of them were interviewed personally by the Board of Trustees. It is understood that Dr. Simmons had the special support of Dr. J. T. Priestly of Iowa and Dr. Joseph Eastman of Indianapolis, who had recognized the merit of his work in the Western Surgical Association.

In 1898 a new weekly Philadelphia medical journal was launched with the financial backing of Musser, Keen, Osler and many others, with George M. Gould as editor. In writing to Musser about that time William Osler said "The J. A. M. A. needs him now more than we do and he could put THE JOURNAL on a first class basis which would be a good thing for the rank and file."

The Board of Trustees discussed the action that had been taken relative to the choice of a full time secretary. It appeared that the minutes of previous action were in such confusion that it was impossible for the Board of Trustees to find their way to a definite conclusion. The Board of Trustees recommended, therefore, an amendment to the Constitution to the effect that the editor of THE JOURNAL OF THE AMERICAN MEDICAL ASSOCIATION should be the secretary of the Association and should serve as such without additional compensation. It was felt that this would be an economical and efficient procedure, since the secretary would have charge of the manuscripts, which he could then turn over to himself in the position of editor. When the Board of Trustees presented this report, Dr. W. B. Atkinson took exception to the statement concerning the confusion in the minutes. He was answered by Dr. T. J. Happel of Tennessee, member of the Board of Trustees, who stated that the trustees had made careful study but had been unable to find minutes sufficient to indicate exactly what the Association had done in the matter in question. The motion was put and carried. Thus Dr. Simmons on June 7, 1899 was confirmed by the Association as editor of THE JOURNAL OF THE AMERICAN MEDICAL ASSOCIATION and as its secretary.

In the period between the death of Dr. Hamilton in December and the time of the meeting of the Board of Trustees in February 1899 THE JOURNAL was conducted under the direction of the resident secretary of the Board of Trustees, Dr. Truman W. Miller, Chicago.

Dr. Truman W. Miller died in 1900 at the age of 60. He had received his medical education at the College of Physicians and Surgeons of New York and his degree of M.D. from the Geneva Medical College. He served in the Civil War and in 1873 was appointed Assistant Surgeon in the U. S. Marine-Hospital Service. In 1877 he was promoted to Surgeon and resigned in 1886. He had served on the staffs of many of Chicago's prominent hospitals. Known as a man of action not much given to writing or speaking but known for a pertinacity of purpose and executive ability, he originated the Chicago Polyclinic.

Significantly, with the assumption by Dr. Simmons of the position of secretary-editor the list of editorial contributors, assistants and other members of the staff of the headquarters office of the American Medical Association disappeared from the pages of THE JOURNAL. Dr. Simmons assumed management of the headquarters office on March 1. THE JOURNAL proceeded without missing a page or an issue. It is not possible to observe any significant changes in the publication from the period of Hamilton until the issue of March 18, when the editorial columns began to contain a number of small notations on medical affairs, now published under the title of "Current Comment." The popularity of these minor comments is indicated by their continuance since that date. In March a department of medical news was introduced into THE JOURNAL and also a section of questions and answers. In April the department of current medical literature was established, with a listing of the contents of other medical publications and abstracts of significant articles. These features have been continuously in THE JOURNAL since that time.

Two interesting articles appeared in THE JOURNAL in April 1899 and are an indication of the trend of thought of the period. The leading article for April 1 was entitled "Some of the Minor Immoralities of the Tobacco Habit." The hygiene of the period was becoming even more teetotalitarian. Here is a paragraph from this extraordinary scientific contribution:

> The vulgarity and licentiousness of the press, with its mercenary pandering to vice, corrupting as it does that very fountain of national strength, the home; the lubricity, the demoralizing baseness of the degraded drama, disfigurement of hoardings by the cigaret-soaked indecencies of the variety stage, making it difficult for our children to walk the streets without contamination, the growing fondness for certain social functions with their flimsy vaudeville adornments, the mockery of and attempted obliteration of personal puritanism, the crass things done by tobacco-biased young people, degradation of seats of learning by the introduction of smoking-rooms, those hotbeds of vice and agnosticism, of ballet dancing and brainless burlesque—imbecility and irreverence under the auspices of fashion—defilement of public buildings by foul receptacles provided for a people so base that it is necessary to ask them to please not spit on the floor, the Negro minstrel methods of some of our churches, the effeminacy of religious periodicals with their venal advocacy of successful quackery and fraud, the prevalence of the gambling mania among women, leveling all ranks, wasting energy, dissipating time so much needed in more ennobling ways, medieval grotesqueries, euchre and wine parties for the spiritual and physical benefit of the outcast and sick, made so by gambling and drink! what, unless completely engrossed in other things, could induce thoughtful men to silently submit to these, but that undiscriminating drowsiness of conscience—"denying nothing, doubting everything," so frequently induced by tobacco?

Another article in an April issue was by Charles J. Whalen of Illinois and dealt with the doctor as a politician. It was a plea that physicians enter politics in order to secure needed medical reforms and politics was an avocation for Dr. Whalen until the end of his interesting career in medical affairs.

Under Dr. Simmons' editorship THE JOURNAL began to assume more definite form and departmentalization. The interest of the members is shown in many letters published as correspondence to the editor. The space devoted to society proceedings was greatly elaborated, as was also the space devoted to editorials and comments.

In 1899 the publication of the *Index Medicus* was discontinued because of lack of funds. THE JOURNAL, as well as other publications elsewhere in the world, expressed sorrow but it was not for many years that restoration of this publication to its present high estate was attempted.

In the May 27, 1899 issue, for the first time, appeared a well ordered announcement of the next annual session of the American Medical Association in Columbus, Ohio, with a map of the center of Columbus, full information regarding transportation, hotels and other data necessary to those who would attend the meeting. A feature of the issue of June 3, 1899 was a review of the previous presidents of the American Medical Association with photographs of many of them and a list of the meetings and those who presided. This interesting feature was contributed by Nathan Smith Davis.

A supplement to THE JOURNAL recorded progress in surgery for fifty years by Rudolph W. Matas and progress in medicine by John H. Musser, in gynecology by Charles A. L. Reed, in obstetrics by Frank Stahl, in therapeutics by Hobart A. Hare, in physiology by G. N. Stewart, in anatomy by Frank Baker, in pathology by J. Rilus Eastman, in ophthalmology by Casey A. Wood, in otology by T. Melville Hardie, in laryngology by E. Fletcher Ingals and in neurology and psychiatry by a writer whose name for some reason was not given.

There were biographies of the officers of the Association, including the chairman of the Board of Trustees, Dr. Alonzo Garcelon, a complete list of previous members of the Board of Trustees with a group photograph, a brief history of THE JOURNAL and a review of the existing medical periodicals and medical colleges of the country. All this material was included in a special supplement to THE JOURNAL which made it a souvenir number. An editorial reviewed the great progress that had been made in American medicine.

In his president's address Dr. Joseph M. Mathews of Louisville, Ky., made a plea for the removal of the headquarters of the Association to Washington. He thought that it was a mistake to refuse to publish in THE JOURNAL any article read in the Association and that it was up to the readers to select the good from the bad. Dr. Mathews made the suggestion that there be a field secretary to travel about the country and to increase its membership, at the same time soliciting subscriptions to THE JOURNAL. This was to be the most significant of his recommendations. The action favorably taken ultimately on this recommendation led to the most significant steps in reorganization and improvement of membership.

Notwithstanding the tremendous enthusiasm and the numerous contributions that had been made at the meeting in Philadelphia, the Rush monument fund had reached only $10,082.52. Dr. Albert L. Gihon announced that he was leaving for an indefinite residency abroad and resigned as leader for this fund.

The Association had up to this time reached an annual budget of a little over $83,000, and it had more than $18,000 in the treasury. The Association was urging the employment of women nurses in military hospitals. It urged increased rank for the Surgeon General of the Army, support for the *Index Medicus*, and the creation of a national department of public health with a cabinet minister.

A committee was appointed to revise the Constitution and By-Laws. On recommendation of the executive committee the Association voted not to hold its meetings permanently in Washington and that it avoid too many entertainments. The recommendation for a traveling assistant secretary was referred to the Board of Trustees. Actions were taken to make a special review of tuberculosis and urged the development of sanatoriums and to urge compulsory vaccination against smallpox. A motion had been introduced that there be published a list of members of the Association. This was opposed on the ground that this list would be used by the proprietary drug houses for commercial purposes. Dr. Simmons rose for the first time in the House of Delegates and defended the publication of the list on the grounds that he could sell it for $25 a copy. However, the entire consideration was finally laid on the table.

THE SCIENTIFIC EXHIBIT

Among the most significant and important developments for the advancement of medical science has been the Scientific Exhibit. Today it occupies many thousands of square feet of space and has been characterized as the most valuable effort in behalf of graduate medical education attempted by any organization anywhere in the world. It started with small and simple beginnings. At the meeting of the American Medical Association in 1899 a resolution was introduced by Dr. Charles E. Slocum of Defiance, Ohio, in which he said "that this Association hereby commends the efforts of the Indiana State Medical Society in preserving pathologic specimens and exhibiting the same at this meeting. This exhibit is worthy the attention of every member, being a good example of what careful and persistent attention to pathology may accomplish in a short time when well directed. Such efforts are recommended to all societies as conducive to more careful and methodic diagnosis of treatment." On motion this resolution was adopted.

In THE JOURNAL for Dec. 2, 1899, Dr. Frank B. Wynn of Indianapolis wrote to the editor about the Scientific Exhibit. In 1897 an appeal had been made to members of the Indiana State Medical Society for pathologic specimens, and at each annual meeting since that date such specimens have been exhibited, reaching 800 in 1899. The exhibit had attracted so much attention in Indiana that the state society appropriated $300 to take the exhibit to the Columbus meeting of the American Medical Association. Dr. Wynn urged a similar exhibit for each meeting of the American Medical Association and together with such an exhibit the establishment of a section on pathology. He felt that there should be a similar exhibit every year and, he concluded, "in seeking to inaugurate a pathologic museum, the executive officers of the American Medical Association should receive the enthusiastic support of every member of the organization. Start the movement at once! Have an exhibit at Atlantic City next year, even if it is a small one! Let us have a wholesome direction from the selfish commercial exhibits! In conclusion, let me say that Indiana, as the pioneer in this field, stands ready to meet the requirement put on her by the national body."

THE JOURNAL INDEX

The quality of the index to THE JOURNAL OF THE AMERICAN MEDICAL ASSOCIATION notably improved with the second half of 1899 and has come to be recognized as one of the most important general indexes in the field of medicine. With the complete coverage of medical science represented by THE JOURNAL, this index is for most workers in the field of medical bibliography the first line of attack.

DR. BILLINGS BECOMES ACTIVE

Dr. Frank Billings was chairman of the Section on Medicine in 1899. There were eighty-three papers, and he had succeeded in securing fifty-four abstracts. He made the suggestion that a rule be adopted requiring every member who desires to prepare and present a paper at any future meeting to prepare and send to the officer of the section a short synopsis of the paper to be printed in advance of the meeting. He urged that, if possible, the papers should concern original research, but he recognized the value of full reports of cases when possible supported by thorough postmortem examinations.

NEW PROGRESS THROUGH THE JOURNAL

The differences and disagreements in American medicine were being harmoniously resolved. The quality of THE JOURNAL began to improve. Membership was increasing, as were subscriptions to THE

JOURNAL. Dr. Hamilton had been a competent editor, but the quality of the new leadership was clearly apparent. Following leadership by the Chicago *Tribune*, THE JOURNAL began a campaign against Fourth of July accidents, initiating its campaign with an editorial which was to be followed some years later by a careful survey of deaths and accidents as seen by physicians and hospitals throughout the nation.

The enterprise of THE JOURNAL was indicated by publication of the proceedings of the Canadian Medical Association on the same day on which the meeting occurred and distributing it among the Canadian members. The button for the Association was developed following the design originally worked out by Dr. Richard French Stone. This design was later to be discarded for the one now followed.

During the year an attempt was made in Germany to produce an Index Medicus under the name of "Index Medicus Novus." It proved to be a weak effort and quite incapable of replacing the *Index Medicus* that had been developed by John Shaw Billings and Robert Fletcher.

Gradually new departments such as clinical reports and therapeutic notes were added to THE JOURNAL. And still THE JOURNAL improved, with special headings of news and center headings of London, Philadelphia and New York, with improved pictures sometimes occupying full pages. A department of New Instruments was added. The prominence of the consideration given to new discoveries and new activities indicated a journalistic quality in the editor that was in advance of his time.

THE REORGANIZATION, 1900 TO 1901

ATLANTIC CITY

THE YEAR 1900 marked another turning point in the life of the American Medical Association; now came the transition from adolescence to adulthood. This was the beginning of the reorganization!

THE JOURNAL INDEX

The index published in 1899 attracted general attention, the only unfavorable criticism being that the book was now so bulky that there ought to be three volumes a year instead of two. This suggestion was adopted about forty years later. The editor suggested in reply to his correspondents that it might be well to bind the index separately.

In 1900 there were some articles reflecting the newer researches on malaria and the relationship of the mosquito to malarial infections. Bacteriology and parasitology were finding their place in medical science.

DEFENSE OF RESEARCH

At the meeting in 1898 a resolution had been introduced that a committee of five be appointed by the President at his leisure to cooperate with similar committees from other bodies to consider the desirability of formulating plans for the dissemination of knowledge of the value of experimental research in the progress of the science and art of medicine. The committee was appointed in 1900; it included Drs. H. C. Wood of Philadelphia, chairman; W. J. Mayo, Rochester, Minn.; F. H. Wiggin, New York City; J. F. Fulton, St. Paul, and C. A. Powers, Denver. This committee was to be the beginning of the work in defense of animal experimentation carried on so successfully by the American Medical Association since that date.

COMMITTEE ON SCIENTIFIC EXHIBIT

At the same time the President of the Association appointed a special committee to look after the Scientific Exhibit; this first committee included Drs. Joseph Stokes, Moorestown, N. J., chairman; F. B. Wynn, Indianapolis, secretary; Alfred Stengel, Philadelphia, and W. W. Fox, Atlantic City.

PROPRIETARY MEDICINES

The interest in proprietary medicines had not died; the forthcoming meeting of the Pharmacopeial Convention stirred the editor of THE JOURNAL to a consideration of means by which editors could be guided in excluding from their advertising pages products which did not meet the standards of ethics of the medical and pharmaceutic sciences. "The difficulty," said the editorial, "has always been to know where to draw the line." A literal interpretation of professional ethics applied to the patronage and advertising of medicinal articles would exclude the vast majority of them. The editorial on proprietary medicines aroused correspondence indicating that the medical profession was ready for a movement toward scientific standards in the prescribing of remedies.

The announcement of the annual meeting was a reminder of the variety of representation in the Association. The scientific sections had now reached twelve, including

Practice of Medicine
Surgery and Anatomy
Obstetrics and Diseases of Women
Materia Medica, Pharmacy, Therapeutics
Ophthalmology
Laryngology and Otology
Diseases of Children
Physiology and Dietetics
Neurology and Medical Jurisprudence
Cutaneous Medicine and Surgery
State Medicine
Stomatology

There were many applications for places on the scientific programs. It became apparent that some means of restricting the total amount of material to be presented would have to be developed.

An article by P. Maxwell Foshay, editor of the *Cleveland Journal of Medicine*, was devoted to medical ethics and medical journals. He called attention to the multiplicity of such publications which lived primarily by the support of proprietary medicines. "The greed for advertising patronage," he said, "leads the editor only too often to prostitute his pen or his pages to the advertiser, so long as he can secure the coveted revenue. So our journals are filled with articles and editorials containing covert advertisements of this and that remedy." He indicated that many of the proprietary medical houses would not advertise without a promise of reading notices and original articles in support of their remedies. The medical professions were beginning to divide periodicals into honest and dishonest publications; Dr. Foshay urged physicians to patronize the honest periodicals and to write to the editors of dishonest ones asking them to stop sending such periodicals to physicians.

The campaign was on in earnest. In the issue of THE JOURNAL for April 21, 1900 appeared the first of a series of articles designed to correct the abuses from advertising and patronizing unscientific pharmaceutic preparations. The article appears without indicated authorship; apparently it had the full support of the editor of THE JOURNAL. The series included analyses and criticisms of such products as Castoria and Syrup of Figs. These contributions were fighting articles; they were the first shots in the campaign that would lead eventually to the establishment of the Council on Pharmacy and Chemistry of the American Medical Association and to the development of a real science of pharmacology and therapeutics. The repercussions from this series of articles were acute. Pressure began to be made on the Board of Trustees of the Association by representatives of pharmaceutic industries.

The convention was now so large that difficulties were developing in the House of Delegates because it could never be clear just who was a delegate and who was not. A distinctive badge was given to the delegates and an attempt was made to seat them separately in the convention hall, but it was clear that issues of importance were sometimes being settled by the mob rather than by the delegates.

Dr. G. Frank Lydston began a series of articles on medicine as a business which was full of invective and satire, for which he was later to become famous.

ADDRESS BY W. W. KEEN

In his presidential address Dr. W. W. Keen noted that the Association now had 9,000 members and that there were 100,000 regular physicians in the United States. THE JOURNAL had reached a subscription list of 15,000, exceeded only by the *British Medical Journal* with 21,000. Dr. Keen was high in his praise of the quality of THE JOURNAL. He was disappointed with the Rush monument fund because it had now reached only $11,000: too small to go ahead and too large to go backward. He was anxious to see improvement in the membership of the Association. He stimulated the Scientific Exhibit. He urged that the editor and the Board of Trustees be given authority to publish only the papers from the sections that seemed suitable. Most of his address was devoted to the necessity for endowment of medical schools so that they might more nearly fulfil their educational functions. As a final recommendation in his address he proposed the establishment by the American Medical Association of a fund for scientific grants in aid of research. This proposal bore fruit. By 1946 the American Medical Association had given more than $1,000,000 of its funds for such purposes and had set aside as a permanent fund for research more than $2,000,000 additional.

THE ATLANTIC CITY SESSION

More than 2,000 physicians attended the Atlantic City session. The committee on arrangements recognized the excessive number of papers on the programs of the sections and recommended some type of restriction. Dr. George H. Simmons, secretary of the Association, presented in an orderly manner the various communications which had been received by his office. The proceedings were conducted formally. General Sternberg of the U. S. Army spoke to the idea that there need no longer be an *Index Medicus* because many of the journals were now printing good indexes. There was a motion by Dr. Ludvig Hektoen of Chicago for the formation of a new section on pathology and bacteriology. Dr. Donald Maclean of Detroit moved that reports of the treasurer and all secretaries be printed in advance of the time of the session so that time need not be taken in reading them. The name of the Section on State Medicine was changed to the Section on Hygiene and Sanitary Science. It was pointed out that the responsibility for accepting and rejecting papers was fully covered in the By-Laws.

CLEANING THE ADVERTISEMENTS

Toward the end of the session a resolution was offered by Drs. A. A. Eshner and Solomon Solis-Cohen. It read:

> *Resolved*, That the steps taken by the editor and trustees of THE JOURNAL of the American Medical Association looking toward the fulfilment of the expressed will of the Association, excluding from its columns advertisements of nostrums and secret preparations, be cordially approved, and that the editor and trustees be encouraged to continue in this course until the work is completed.

CENSORING THE SCIENTIFIC PAPERS

At the final session of this meeting a furor arose over an action by Dr. Denslow Lewis of Chicago. He had read a paper in Columbus on a gynecologic consideration of the sexual act. This paper had been refused publication in THE JOURNAL although it was included in the Transactions of the Section on Obstetrics and Diseases of Women. Two members of the publication committee of the section had rejected the manuscript, stating that they did so on legal grounds. Denslow Lewis had secured opinions from five attorneys in Chicago and insisted that his paper be published. There was much discussion, in which parliamentary procedure was cited pro and con. The President finally ruled that the whole discussion was out of order, and the resolution was referred to a committee for further report.

On the next day the Lewis paper was again the subject of a bitter battle. The Denslow Lewis paper had been read by the trustees and by the executive committee and all agreed that it should not be published; then the Association voted not to publish the paper.

Thus with the 1900 session the Scientific Exhibit became fully established. The editor of THE JOURNAL in retrospect feared that there were going to be too many sections. Today the number has grown to twenty. It was recognized that the exhibit should include not only pathologic specimens but also apparatus and other materials. Indeed it was pointed out that the aim should be to unify and correlate the scientific work at the meetings. The editor suggested that perhaps the sessions on pathology could be short so that its members might participate in the work of the other sections.

1901
ST. PAUL

The year 1901 marked a new century and gave opportunity for THE JOURNAL OF THE AMERICAN MEDICAL ASSOCIATION to review the progress of medicine in the United States for a hundred years. This statement from the leading editorial is prophetic:

While assured that American medicine in the twentieth century will take an active part in the advancement of medical sciences, the sociologic relations of medicine in this country offer problems of great importance. There is need above all things for a greater public faith in the teachings and the advice of the medical profession in matters relating to hygiene and to the prevention of disease. Hygiene should dictate to legislators and courts of law and not economic interests alone. "Unfortunately on the human race there still weighs that fate by which both preventable diseases and premature deaths, as well as duration of life itself, essentially depend on economic institutions." There is hope that the twentieth century may witness great improvements as knowledge is disseminated and the mass of the people learn to place confidence in medical teaching.

The medical college in the coming century will have to give more attention to the quality than the quantity of its output, if present signs are not misleading. Human nature will not change; there will still be deceivers and their followers, but this will only accentuate the demand for higher qualifications in our profession. The future of science is not in doubt; the world will not stop in its progress nor lose what it has gained, but the future of the medical profession is in its own hands and can only be assured by its living up to its higher ideals.

The quality of THE JOURNAL improved with almost every issue in the style of its presentation and in the character of its editing. Yet the action that was to unite the vast majority of the American medical profession into a single, closely knit unit based on a truly democratic system of representation, had not yet been taken. The minds of many leaders were concentrated on the project but the 1901 reorganization was to be the mechanism by which medical solidarity would be brought about.

Following the meeting of 1900 a committee on organization, consisting of J. N. McCormack of Bowling Green, Ky., P. Maxwell Foshay of Cleveland and George H. Simmons, Chicago, was asked to report on organization. The committee proposed that a business section should be constituted to be known as the House of Delegates which should proportionately represent the state societies according to their numerical strength and with the direct representation of one delegate from each scientific section. It was suggested that the ratio of representation for the state societies be fixed at one delegate to every 500 members. This proposal when adopted finally made the House of Delegates truly representative of the membership of the American Medical Association. The committee pointed out that by the means of committees this House of Delegates could deal exhaustively with all the large problems of state medicine. It would afford opportunity to every state to be heard in full, and free debate would be permitted. The states near the place of meeting would no longer wield a preponderant influence. The House of Delegates could work without interfering with the scientific work of the Association.

The committee had endeavored to provide every possible safeguard for maintaining this new organization as truly representative of the medical profession. Provision had been made against political campaigns, against perpetuation in office and against self election to office.

The committee requested every member of the Association to read carefully the proposed amendments to the Constitution and By-Laws and it prophesied that if the Association would give sanction to its recommendations the profession throughout the country in five years would be welded into a compact organization whose power to influence medicine would be almost unlimited and whose requests for desirable legislation would everywhere be met with that respect which the politician has for organized votes.

In the extensive report the committee analyzed the previous difficulties of the Association and the necessity for reorganization. It was particularly commendatory of the committee on nominations. The report suggested a common plan of organization for each of the state societies and a technic for securing members in county and state organizations. Indeed it went on to suggest forms for organization of such societies and duties for the state organizer.

THE ST. PAUL MEETING

When the Association assembled in St. Paul, June 4–7, 1901 the President, Dr. Charles A. L. Reed, said that by custom the President's address was restricted to a discussion of the affairs of the Association. He found that they were in excellent condition but he was especially pleased because THE JOURNAL of the Association had increased its circulation to 22,000 copies per week. Much of the business improvement had been brought about by the fact that the

Association was now incorporated. He suggested that the articles of incorporation be confirmed by the Association at the St. Paul meeting. Dr. Reed was disturbed by the fact that THE JOURNAL had a circulation twice the membership of the organization. He felt that attention should be given to the handling of the surplus funds and he mentioned the desirability of securing and properly maintaining research and expanding THE JOURNAL. The final portion of his address was devoted to the reorganization, and he recommended the adoption of the new Constitution and By-Laws in their entirety. He pointed out that the committee on reorganization had wisely avoided any attempt to discuss the Principles of Ethics, but he suggested the establishment of a special committee to give consideration to that problem.

As the session opened, Dr. J. R. Pennington of Chicago presented to the Association a portrait of the founder, Dr. N. S. Davis.

Dr. George H. Simmons, secretary, read a report indicating that the membership was over 10,600, the largest increase in any year in the history of the Association.

The general executive committee had been successful in reducing the total number of papers read from 491 to 391. The highest number had been read in 1898, when there were 615 papers listed for presentation. This vast accumulation of papers to be read by title or presented only by listing in the program finally forced the adoption of essential corrective measures.

The Board of Trustees was able to report continuous improvement in THE JOURNAL and also in its advertising standards. All medicines advertised in the newspapers had been refused space in THE JOURNAL. As a result some products formerly advertised only in the public press were now being advertised only to physicians.

At a previous meeting of the Association the Constitution and By-Laws had been amended to provide for a standing committee known as the Committee on National Legislation to be appointed annually by the President. This committee was able to defeat the obnoxious bill against animal experimentation in the District of Columbia. It had also been able to aid in securing second class postage rates for THE JOURNAL OF THE AMERICAN MEDICAL ASSOCIATION, making a total saving of about $30,000 in postage.

NATIONAL LEGISLATION

Attempts were under way to develop uniform medical legislation on the basis of a uniform medical education. The distinguished committee, which included Drs. H. L. E. Johnson, William H. Welch and William L. Rodman, recommended an annual conference in Washington of representatives of state legislative committees to consider general trends in both state and national legislation relating to the medical profession. Such a conference had been held in Washington in February of 1901 with a good representation from many of the states. They had been principally concerned with the army reorganization bill and with the duties of the Marine Hospital Service. They had also been concerned with perfecting an organization which would enable the national legislative committee to cooperate fully with the state committees.

The Rush monument fund had now reached $11,941.88.

A significant occurrence at this meeting of the Association was the presentation of Miss Susan B. Anthony, who spoke briefly on the subject of regulating vice in Manila, Hawaii and Porto Rico. She was readily seconded by Rev. Anna Shaw.

Following the address of the President, Dr. Charles A. L. Reed, the general executive committee, which acted as a reference committee for the session, urged the appointment of a committee of three to revise the Code of Ethics and with instructions to report at the next annual session of the Association. This was, however, laid on the table; apparently there was in the meeting a group which did not wish to have this question raised.

The Association voted a resolution of profound appreciation of the generous gift of John D. Rockefeller, who had given $200,000 for medical research, under the able chairmanship of William H. Welch.

The facts about the reorganization are so fundamental to the progress of the American Medical Association that I requested Dr. George H. Simmons to write the story. He prepared it in 1933, nine years after he had resigned as editor of THE JOURNAL. The article follows:

COMMITTEE CREATED

The annual meeting of the Association for 1900 was held in Atlantic City, June 6 to 10. At the second General Meeting the following resolutions, no preamble, were introduced by Dr. D. R. Brower, Chicago, a member of the General Executive Committee:

Resolved, That a committee be appointed by the Association on the organization of the profession throughout the United States to cooperate with the Committee on National Legislation; this committee to consist of one member from each state and territory represented in the Association.

Reseolved, That a committee of three be appointed by the President to prepare plans in detail for such committee on organization; to enter into correspondence with officers of the various state societies, and to take such action in the premises as it may think advisable, and that the Trustees be requested to appropriate a sum not exceeding $150 for the necessary expenses of the committee.

According to the usual procedure, the resolutions were referred to the General Executive Committee. The following day they were referred back with recommendations for adoption. By motion, a representative was added to the large committee—referred to hereafter as the States' Committee—from the Medical Department of the Army, of the Navy, of the Marine Hospital Service and from the Bureau of Animal Industry, respectively.

The Committee on National Legislation, mentioned in the first resolution, was a standing committee on national—congressional—legislation and would not be concerned with the subject matter in the slightest degree.

There were two purposes in view in creating the States' Committee. First, to represent the state and territorial associations, each of which would be asked to appoint a member. Any plan of organization to include the whole country would require the approval, and cooperation in carrying it out, of all the state organizations. This cooperation would be absolutely essential to a successful outcome; hence the main reason for the States' Committee.

Second, the States' Committee would make a large and representative group to which the Committee on Reorganization would make its report, in the first instance at least, rather than to a General Meeting. It proved an ideal arrangement.

COMMITTEE APPOINTED

The Committee on Reorganization was appointed by the newly elected President, Dr. C. A. L. Reed, and consisted of Dr. W. W. Keen, Philadelphia, the retiring President; Dr. J. N. McCormack, Bowling Green, executive officer of the Kentucky State Board of Health, and Dr. George H. Simmons, Chicago. Presumably Dr. Keen was appointed because of his great popularity (he was loved by all who knew him); his membership on the committee therefore would add confidence in it and its work. He later resigned (the committee was not yet organized) because his professional work made it impossible for him to give to the committee the time and attention required. Dr. P. Maxwell Foshay, Cleveland, secretary of the Ohio State Medical Association, was appointed in his place. As now constituted, each member of the small committee was, or had been, officially connected with a state medical association.

FIRST MEETING OF THE COMMITTEE ON REORGANIZATION

The first meeting of the committee was held in Chicago in October (1900) and organized by electing Dr. J. N. McCormack chairman and Dr. George H. Simmons secretary. It was in session two days, during which it outlined the whole scheme of organization which it proposed to recommend and left the working out of the details to future meetings and to correspondence.

In addition to two or three meetings in Chicago, the committee, after the plan of reorganization had been pretty thoroughly worked out, held one meeting in Cincinnati, one in St. Louis and one in Chicago; to these meetings local men who might be interested were invited for conference. These conference meetings were helpful in many ways. A brief statement on some of the subjects the committee had to consider may be of interest.

PLAN OF ORGANIZATION

The general plan of organization was, of course, the first matter taken up by the committee. The following is an outline of the plan tentatively adopted at its first meeting:

The unit of the organization to be the local society, preferably the county; membership in the county society to carry with it membership in the state association; the state association to create a legislative body or branch to be composed of delegates elected by the component (county) societies. The American Medical Association likewise would create a legislative body, its members to be elected by the legislative bodies of the state associations and one by each of the sections; also appointed representatives of the government services. There was nothing unique—nothing original—in the general scheme; it was in use in its essentials by national, religious and social organizations, by fraternal and secret societies, and, at that time, by the United States Senate. There was no other plan on which the medical profession of the United States could be organized if it was to represent the profession of the whole country.

The Unit.—What shall constitute the unit of the organization? Naturally, the ideal would be the county. But in thinly populated states there were counties without a sufficient number of physicians to constitute a society. This problem could be solved by providing for component multiple county societies.

The opposite condition would be a county containing a large city, so large, geographically and in population, that one component society would not meet the required conditions. Boston, New York, Philadelphia and Chicago were considered.

Massachusetts has its districts, not counties; Boston included two of such districts, each with its district society.

New York City covered four counties: four component societies would be satisfactory; Philadelphia was geographically small and one component society would probably be satisfactory.

Chicago (Cook County) was a more difficult problem. Cook

County is large geographically and even then was thickly populated. The committee recommended that subdivision of such counties should be made.*

Maximum Number of Members in House of Delegates.—This should be sufficiently large to make proportional representation for the thickly populated states, but no larger. Investigation showed that, based on the proportion of one delegate to each 500 members of a constituent association, plus one representative from each of the sections and from each of the three government services, would make the House consist of about 145 members. This would give proportional representation. One hundred and fifty as a maximum was recommended and adopted.

Presiding Officer for the House of Delegates.—It was the unanimous opinion of the committee that the House of Delegates should have its own chairman, one who would be selected for his ability to preside rather than for his scientific achievements or popularity. The office should be more or less permanent; the one selected would be more likely to master parliamentary rules than would be the case if one had to preside for one year only. Then there are certain lines of business that are more or less continuous, and the presiding officer should have knowledge of such matters.

However, while the committee had not changed its views, it concluded that the question was a delicate one and might well be left to the members of the House to decide for themselves.

While acting on the rule it had adopted, that is, to make only such modifications of the By-Laws as were absolutely necessary for working out the essentials of the plan, it is probable that the committee carried this policy too far in some matters, possibly in this.†

---

*After reorganization a special committee recommended that the Chicago (Cook County) Medical Society should be a Councilor District; that each branch should be a component unit of the state association. This plan was successfully carried out, with this important exception: as component societies, each branch would be entitled to send representatives to the House of Delegates of the state society. This right the branches do not have. The delegates of the state body are elected by the Council (the business body) of the Chicago Medical Society. This arrangement is perfect for the latter but not for the state society.

†In a few years a feeling had developed that a permanent presiding officer was desirable. Dr. Happel, then chairman of the Board of Trustees, introduced an amendment to the By-Laws to provide for a chairman for the House of Delegates. It caused resentment, and the chairman of the Board of Trustees was hissed; the proposal was regarded as an insult to the President of the Association, then presiding. It was not until 1916 that a By-Law was passed creating the office of chairman of the House of Delegates. Dr. Hubert Work was elected to the office. In 1918 the word "chairman" was changed to "speaker." Dr. Work resigned in 1920 and became President. He was succeeded by Dr. Dwight Murray, New York, who presided one year (1921) and was reelected but died the following October. Dr. Frederick C. Warnshuis was elected speaker in 1922 and has been reelected each year since.

For instance, the paragraph in the old constitution on "Permanent Members" was retained although it had no meaning in the new. The articles on "Funds" was left intact, one clause of which read "an equal assessment of not more than ten dollars annually on each of the permanent members." The "ten dollars" caused vigorous objections in the States' Committee Conference until it was explained that it had been in the old constitution for as long as the records ran. Even "four vice presidents" were still provided for; it so remained until 1920, when the By-Law was changed to provide for one vice president. The By-Laws also contained incongruities because of the decision to make only such changes as were absolutely essential. As was expected, these incongruities were eliminated as the years passed.

THE REPORTS

The preparation of the preliminary report was allotted to Drs. J. N. McCormack and G. H. Simmons; to Dr. Foshay was assigned the task of suggesting the necessary modifications that should be made in the By-Laws. This separate work was done between meetings, but all matters were later thoroughly discussed by the committee in session. There were two reports: (1) the preliminary report and (2) the official report.

The former was the more important and consisted of two parts, an explanatory preface or introduction, and the "argument."

The preface fully outlined the changes proposed and specifically detailed the more important ones. It was a summary such as would give one a clear idea of what changes were proposed and the results expected, if and when this proposed reorganization became a fact.

The "argument" was an exhaustive review of the conditions in the Association, past and present, that made reorganization necessary; it outlined the benefits that would result from such a reorganization as recommended.

The preliminary report in pamphlet form occupied forty-eight pages, six of which were required by the introductory preface.

The official report was submitted first to the States' Committee Conference and later presented to the General Meeting of the Association; with it was submitted the revised Constitution and By-Laws.

PRELIMINARY REPORT DISTRIBUTED

The Preliminary Report was complete and in form for distribution in April 1901. A copy was sent to each member of the States' Committee, with a special typewritten letter asking for criticisms and suggestions. Included in the letter was a call for the conference to be held in St. Paul, June 3. Also with a similar letter copies were sent to the president of each state and territorial association, to the members of the General Executive Committee, to officers of the Association and to about 400 physicians located in various parts of the country, selected as far as possible from physicians known to be interested in the welfare of the Association. In all letters a request was made for criticisms and comments. A stamped return addressed envelop was an enclosure; also an invitation to attend the States' Committee Conference. Altogether, approximately, 500 letters were sent.

The number of replies received indicated a decided interest in the subject; as I recall, approximately 80 per cent acknowledged receipt of the preliminary report. Before me is a bundle of about 100 of these letters. A few are little more than an acknowledgment of receipt of the preliminary report; some are long: one written in long hand takes ten large letter-size sheets; the longest, however, consists of seven such sheets, typewritten, single space and small type face—a size common at that time.

The general tone of each of these and of a few other letters is a fear of what would happen if the plan proposed was adopted. Practically all contain constructive criticisms and suggestions, many of which were adopted. A comparison of the recommendations in the preliminary report with the Constitution and By-Laws as submitted and finally adopted will show this. The number of letters that may be regarded as absolutely opposed is small and practically without exception are from the older, faithful members—"wheelhorses," using the term in its best sense—of the Association.

One letter I quote—not that it indicates definite opposition, but because it is from the "Father of the Association," a man who did more than any other to improve conditions and to bring about reforms.

Chicago, Ill., May 8, 1901
65 Randolph Street

To George H. Simmons, M.D.

Dear Doctor:—On referring to the report that I made as chairman of a committee on revision of the Constitution of the American Medical Association in 1887, and the action thereon by the Association at the meetings in 1887-88-89, I find that *all* of the *amendments* both to the Constitution and to the By-Laws that were recommended in my report were fully considered and *adopted*, except that *one* relating to the formation of a general committee of two members from each state, territory, Army-Navy and Marine Hospital Service to take the place of the nominating committee and serve as a permanent general committee, which was finally fully discussed and *rejected* at the meeting at Newport, 1889. And I still think if such a *council* or *standing general committee* as proposed in that report of 1887 was adopted to take the place of both the *present business committee* and the nominating committee, it would be more simple and efficient than the scheme outlined in the report you sent to me.

Yours truly,
N. S. Davis.

The report Dr. Davis mentions is the one to which reference was made to the effect that had it been adopted it would have made unnecessary the radical reorganization proposed.

The preliminary report was given its greatest publicity when it was published in THE JOURNAL OF THE AMERICAN MEDICAL ASSOCIATION, May 25, 1901.

THE STATES' COMMITTEE CONFERENCE

The States' Committee met at St. Paul, June 3, 1901, to act on the recommendations of the Committee on Reorganization, and on the revised Constitution and By-Laws. The conference was a large and representative gathering. Two sessions, morning and afternoon, were held.

The conference was called to order by Dr. J. N. McCormack, chairman of the Committee on Reorganization. Dr. H. O. Walker, Michigan, was elected chairman and Dr. George N. Kreider, Illinois, secretary.

As all had received a copy of the preliminary report, they knew the subject to be acted on by the conference. The pamphlet containing the official report and the revised Constitution and By-Laws was distributed. The official report was then read, and the meeting took up, section by section, the revised Constitution and By-Laws. Three or four minor modifications were made, but there was one which could not be regarded as "minor." As has already been stated, the committee recommended that each section should be entitled to one delegate; the conference changed this to two delegates. The idea that the sections still constituted the American Medical Association remained in the minds of the majority. Two years later the By-Laws was changed back to the number recommended by the committee, one delegate from each section.

No organic laws were ever more carefully scrutinized than were the Constitution and By-Laws of the American Medical Association passed on at this conference.*

---

*The official copy of the pamphlet containing the Constitution and By-Laws, in which were written the modifications made during the conference, has written on its title page "Original Copy of Report as handed in by Dr. Walker, Chairman, Joint Committee—Wm. Whitford." (Whitford was for many years official reporter to the American Medical Association.) Attached to this pamphlet is a sheet bearing the signature of members of the States' Committee. It is headed "We the undersigned have examined, and hereby

REPORT PRESENTED TO THE GENERAL MEETING

The next morning the following official report was presented to the General Meeting by Dr. J. N. McCormack:

"*Officers and Members of the American Medical Association:*

"We, your Committee on Reorganization, respectfully submit the following:

"We have keenly felt from the first the magnitude of the task set for us, but in all the months of exacting labor we have been spurred on by the hope that our work would, if wisely performed, and if accepted by you, mark the dawn of a new era in the history of American medicine. After full consideration of the problems before us we early reached the conclusion that it would be useless at this late date to suggest the adoption of either half-way or compromise measures, and, therefore, we have prepared and now submit a completely revised Constitution and By-Laws designed to federate all the state organizations into this Association, to foster scientific medicine and to make the medical profession a power in the social and political life of the republic.

"In a recent issue of THE JOURNAL we submitted for your consideration a full outline of the changes proposed and, in an exhaustive manner, presented the reasons for our recommendations. We earnestly request that every member of the Association, before passing judgment, carefully consider all the facts and arguments presented. Such examination will make it clear that we have been conservative, suggesting only such changes in the organic laws as are essential to the accomplishment of the high purpose for which the Association was organized.

"It will be seen that we have left the Code of Ethics, based on the original resolution of adoption, undisturbed and still in force. We

endorse and approve of the above revised Constitution for the American Medical Association." The following are the signatures:

W. G. Harrison, Alabama	J. W. Aird, Utah
Gould A. Sheldon, Connecticut	George Tully Vaughan, Marine Hospital Service
W. N. Fisher, District of Columbia	H. M. McClanahan, Nebraska
John Palmer, Jr., Delaware	A. Garcelon, Maine
W. W. Grant, Colorado	R. Harvey Reed, Wyoming
A. W. Alvord, Michigan	J. H. Pritchard, Wisconsin
Henry O. Marcy, Massachusetts	J. D. Griffith, Missouri
Henry D. Didama, New York	W. J. Means, Ohio
George Cook, New Hampshire	Charles Richard, U. S. Army
Philip Marvel, New Jersey	Joseph M. Mathews, Kentucky
George N. Kreider, Illinois	J. A. Dibrell, Arkansas
G. W. McCaskey, Indiana	John L. Wills, California
R. E. Conniff, Iowa	J. L. Catterson, Washington
J. A. Crook, Tennessee	John A. Wyeth, New York
A. H. Thayer, West Virginia	G. R. Dean, North Carolina

have carefully preserved the membership of all those now in the Association and have jealously guarded the rights and privileges of each state organization now in affiliation with this body.

"In accordance with your instructions we have also submitted to the larger committee, composed of one member from each state, a detailed scheme for the organization or reorganization of state and county societies, in harmony with, and in completion of the general plan, in which we ask your concurrence.

"The various portions of the scheme of organization proposed are interdependent and should be permitted to stand or fall together. During the time devoted to the preparation of the report, we have considered the various questions in detail and have rejected many propositions that we at first thought worthy of adoption, so that we feel that no amendment can be proposed from the floor which has not already been fully considered. We appreciate the fact that some of the details proposed are to a certain extent experimental, and their true value can only be determined by the test of experience.

"As all the changes outlined, and the reasons for them, have been fully placed before you, no discussion of any part of them will be attempted here, the Constitution and By-Laws clear and distinct in every provision, being submitted as our unanimous report.

"Respectfully,

"J. N. McCormack.
"P. Maxwell Foshay.
"George H. Simmons.

"Committee on Reorganization."

It was at once referred to a joint committee composed of the General Executive Committee and the States' Committee. (This action was following the usual custom although it was referring the matter back to the same group who had acted on it the day before.) The next day this joint committee reported to the General Meeting recommending the adoption of the report of the Committee on Reorganization and the revised Constitution and By-Laws. The report was adopted, with practically no discussion, and the new order went into effect on the adjournment of the St. Paul meeting.

As this was only the first step in the reorganization, the Committee was ordered to continue its work to full completion.

It is interesting to note that this radical change in the organic laws of the American Medical Association was made without being subjected to a discussion—worthy of the name—in a General Meeting. There was no reason, of course, for a discussion; the whole matter had been thoroughly gone over by a group which the General Meeting regarded as competent to advise. Further, those who were in the States' Committee Conference constituted a goodly portion of the members present at the General Meeting, at which the foregoing action was taken.

What happened when the General Meeting—the supreme legislative body of the Association—adopted the Report of the Committee on Reorganization and approved the Constitution and By-Laws suggested by the committee and endorsed by the States' Committee? By this action the General Meeting surrendered its legislative functions to the newly created House of Delegates; also its claim to be the representative body of the medical profession of the United States—in a word, the old organization, in its completeness, went out of existence. As Dr. J. N. McCormack put it, "It will therefore be seen that historically the House of Delegates is the legitimate successor and direct outgrowth of the delegated body known as the American Medical Association."

But the annual meeting of the American Medical Association was held the following year (Saratoga, N. Y., June 10–13, 1902) apparently the same as before; there was the usual Opening General Meeting with the same formalities of welcoming addresses and responses, followed by the usual presidential address; likewise the other General Meetings were held as usual, at which the orations on surgery, medicine and so on were delivered.

Yet there was a difference; there was no business transacted at the General Meetings. That was the only change. This was pleasing to those whose interest was chiefly in scientific medicine. On the other hand, there were some—particularly among the older members—who regretted the innovation.

Exactly as in former years the sections met day by day and carried out their respective programs. The only reminder of a change that the members might notice was that each section was required to elect a representative to the House of Delegates.

There was a change in the registration bureau. No new members were registered as delegates from "Affiliated Societies." Those who became members (Fellows of the Scientific Assembly) that year, and thereafter, did so under the old formula, "Members by Application."

Thus it will be seen that while, as Dr. McCormack said, the House of Delegates succeeded "the delegated body known as 'the American Medical Association,' the Association, as a scientific body, continued to exist and to function essentially as before; it so continues as that branch of the Association known as 'the Scientific Assembly of the American Medical Association. . . .' "

BY LEAPS AND BOUNDS, 1902–1904

WHEN DR. CULBERTSON WAS EDITOR, he had called to assist him a young relative by marriage named Will C. Braun. With the retirement of Dr. Culbertson, Mr. Braun remained as advertising clerk with a salary in 1898 of $1500.00 a year. The value of the services of Mr. Braun, who advanced gradually to the position of Advertising and Circulation Manager and then in 1924 to the position of Business Manager of the American Medical Association, cannot be overestimated. He grew with the Association. At the time of his retirement in 1946 he had seen the annual income from advertising increase from under $10,000 a year in 1898 to $1,750,000 in 1946.

With the incumbency of Dr. George H. Simmons as editor, Will Braun became the editorial right-hand. Many of the most significant steps taken by the Association in the development of the periodicals, the exhibits at the annual sessions, the organization of the printing department and the headquarters office may be credited to his canny intelligence.

When the committee of three, headed by J. N. McCormack and including Drs. P. Maxwell Foshay and George H. Simmons, was assigned the task of reorganizing the American Medical Association, they met frequently in the Old Grand Hotel in Cincinnati with Dr. Charles A. L. Reed, who was then President of the American Medical Association. Cincinnati was chosen because it was one night's run for each of the other members from Chicago, Louisville and Cleveland. The drive of Dr. Simmons was tremendous; he kept the other two members of the committee constantly on their toes. From each of their meetings McCormack and Foshay returned home with a mass of notes, suggestions, emendations and other material over which they would work until the time of the next meeting.

At the meeting in St. Paul in 1901, as has already been mentioned, the general principles and policies outlined in the Constitution and By-Laws were presented and almost immediately adopted. Previous to the meeting the committee had prepared a preliminary report which had been serially published in THE JOURNAL. This preliminary report follows in condensed form; the entire present structure of the American Medical Association is built according to this plan:

THE HOUSE OF DELEGATES

The committee proposed that a business section should be constituted, to be known as the House of Delegates, which should proportionately represent the state societies in accordance with their numerical strength and with the addition as directly representative of the scientific work of the Association of one delegate from each section. It was suggested that the ratio of representation be fixed at one delegate to every 500 members. Later plans were established for reapportionment at regular intervals to meet the tremendous growth in membership and thus to avoid an overwhelming number of delegates in the representative body. The organizational committee indicated that opportunity would be afforded to every state to be heard in full and that there would be free debate. The states near the place of meeting would no longer wield a preponderating influence. The House of Delegates could work without interfering with the scientific work of the Association. The committee attempted to make this body truly representative, to provide against political combinations, against perpetuation in office, and against self election to office.

In order to elaborate a complete and effective scheme for uniting the medical profession, the committee suggested plans for the uniform organization of both state and county medical societies as being directly subsidiary to the plan outlined for the Association itself. The committee was convinced that its plan would weld the profession of the entire country into a compact organism whose power to influence public sentiment would be almost unlimited and "whose requests for desirable legislation [would] everywhere be met with that respect which the politician always has for organized votes."

Many of the fundamental changes incorporated in the original Constitution and By-Laws have remained intact since the day when this enlightened group prepared them. With the presentation, they offered an argument in behalf of the proposals which was so convincing that hardly a voice was raised against it. Nevertheless the committee pointed out that a similar committee had been established at the meeting of the American Medical Association in Chicago in 1887 by Dr. N. S. Davis and that the plan then proposed by Dr. N. S. Davis was just about the same plan that they were now proposing.

The committee clearly intended that the House of Delegates would be to all intents and purposes the legislative body of the Association. It elects all the officers, it has control of the affairs of the Association, it expresses in its resolutions the desires of the profession of the country in regard to business and legislative affairs. It is truly a confederation of the state societies of the country, which, in turn, are confederations of the local societies in the states.

The previous experiences in the representative body of the Association led the committee to the belief that political considerations must, as far as possible, be eliminated from the deliberations of the House of Delegates. It therefore wrote into the By-Laws a decision that "no member of the House of Delegates shall be eligible to any office in the Association." It was believed that by this provision medical politics would be reduced to a minimum.

The committee pointed out that the Board of Trustees would have control of the finances of the Association and would be considered officers of the Association. It was the desire that at least six of the nine trustees could be independent of the existing House of Delegates and be in a position to act independently as a protection should that body in any year recommend some extraordinary expenditure.

With remarkable foresight the committee suggested in those tender days that the secretary could be the editor of the Association and it said "While it is better under present conditions for several reasons that the editor and secretary be one, the time may come in the development of the work of the Association that the duties should be separated, and hence it is thought best to incorporate the matter in the Constitution as above."

The committee recommended also that all officers be ex officio members of the House of Delegates but none of them shall have the right to vote except the President, and he only in case of a tie.

As the years have passed the wisdom of this group becomes increasingly apparent. It planned well. To its planning much of the great growth and power of the organization as it exists today must be accredited.

By 1906 the mechanism was functioning smoothly. By that time the Association had 60,000 members instead of the 11,000 members at the time when the new Constitution and By-Laws were adopted.

A SPEAKER FOR THE HOUSE OF DELEGATES

The committee on reorganization was even convinced unanimously that the House of Delegates should have its own chairman, one who would be selected for his ability to preside rather than for his scientific achievements or his popularity. It was felt that the office should be more or less permanent, since the man selected as speaker of the House of Delegates would be more likely to master parliamentary rules than would be the case if he was to preside for only one year.

Many of the matters that arose in the House of Delegates were considered from year to year. A more or less permanent presiding officer would have knowledge of such matters. When it came to presenting the Constitution and By-Laws to the House of Delegates, however, the committee said that this question was too delicate and that it ought to be left to the members of the House to decide for themselves. Nevertheless one member of the Board of Trustees—Dr. Happel—felt that there should be a chairman or speaker for the House of Delegates and he introduced at a later date an amendment to the By-Laws to provide for this office. The introduction of the amendment caused resentment, and the chairman of the Board of Trustees was hissed. The proposal was regarded as an insult to the President of the Association, who was then presiding. In 1916 a By-Law was passed creating a chairman of the House of Delegates and in 1918 the word "chairman" was changed to "speaker."

The committee also failed to have the courage to eliminate some of the extra vice presidents; the Association continued for a number of years to have four vice presidents. The nomination of these four was always a considerable mental strain on the members of the House of Delegates. Finally in 1920 a new By-Law provided that there be only one vice president.

There were other minor incongruities in the By-Laws, but over the years these were gradually eliminated. In fact, they continue to be eliminated, since a new revision of the By-Laws is contemplated for 1947.

PULLMAN CARS

The state of medical science in 1901 was not amazingly different from the medical science of the last ten years of the previous century. Among other things, Pullman cars had come into use. Dr. J. N. Hurty, then health officer of the state of Indiana, had sent a letter to the American Medical Association for improved sanitation for Pullman cars. He recommended the installation of a little basin and fountain so that people could wash their teeth without using the wash basin for that purpose. He recommended that the blankets be white, so that the users of the bed could have some personal knowledge of their cleanliness.

DEATH OF PRESIDENT McKINLEY

THE JOURNAL had shown great concern because the physicians who had taken care of President McKinley at the time of his assassination had never been paid for their services and had not rendered any bills. The editor felt that Congress should make some sort of appropriation for them.

MEDICAL ABSTRACTS

Some of the Eastern periodicals were criticizing the quality of the abstracts in THE JOURNAL OF THE AMERICAN MEDICAL ASSOCIATION although these were far superior to those published in any other periodical. The editor called attention to the fact that he had not created the department of abstracts but that these had first been created by the *Münchener medizinische Wochenschrift* and that it had been the policy of the editor to make them better and better all the time.

WOMEN PHYSICIANS

Strangely, the editor of THE JOURNAL, harking back to the past, still felt that women could not hold much of a place in medical practice. He said "The whole question of woman's place in medicine hinges on the fact that, when a critical case demands independent action and fearless judgment, man's success depends on his virile courage, which the normal woman does not have nor is expected to have."

THE BOARD OF TRUSTEES

The Board of Trustees of the American Medical Association had been meeting regularly in the Grand Pacific Hotel in Chicago and again at the annual session of the Association. The minutes were kept by the secretary in longhand. The editor and the advertising manager (to which position Mr. Will C. Braun had now been promoted) were being employed year by year. The Association was purchasing linotype machines and a small press. The secretary was authorized to employ stenographers to report the meetings of the Association and to furnish blank forms for the use of officers of the sections.

By 1901 the new editor was beginning to have trouble with some of the advertisements. For instance, the California Fig and Syrup Company objected to being barred from THE JOURNAL; it was finally decided that the advertisements of the California Fig and Syrup Company be accepted provided the proprietor agree to conform with the rules and that the editor was satisfied that the company was not advertising in the lay press.

In the Board of Trustees meetings in the Grand Pacific Hotel apparently not all was salubrious. For instance, observe this statement from the minutes:

> After a general discussion the motion was withdrawn and notwithstanding the persistent [sic] and annoying clammer [sic] and protestations from a subordinate of the hotel for the possession of our present meeting room, for the use of some itinerant dinner party, it was decided to hold the fort, so to speak, and continue the deliberations until the business was finished.

Interesting also is a little note indicating that before the coming of Dr. George H. Simmons the financial affairs of the Association were being somewhat imperfectly administered.

It was stated that no satisfactory report had been received in the matter of old checks, postal notes and money orders, reported some time ago to have been found mislaid about the office, and that recently some new ones had been discovered. Dr. Happel moved, seconded by Dr. Montgomery, that all such checks and postal notes be sent to the Finance Committee, and that all Post Office money orders be sent to Dr. Johnson at Washington, D. C., for collection, and the Editor be, and he is hereby directed, to furnish all information concerning the above to the members named.

NEW MACHINERY

By 1901 Dr. Simmons reported that he had bought a small press and had put individual motors on the folder, two small presses, and the stitcher which relieved the strain on the large motor and facilitated the work. He reported that the circulation was steadily climbing each month and that he could truthfully say that THE JOURNAL had the largest circulation of any medical journal in the world. He was then printing 25,000 copies weekly. It was becoming obvious that THE JOURNAL would have to obtain its own quarters.

RESPONSIBILITY OF THE BOARD

The change in the Constitution and By-Laws raised legal questions as to the responsibilities and authority of the Board of Trustees as compared with the incorporated association. It was felt that it would be necessary to obtain legal advice as to the exact legal status of the organization— a question which was to plague the responsible authorities for a good many years to come.

One action taken by the Board requested the secretary-editor to print a complete list of men who had held offices in the Association either in the House of Delegates or in the sections, so that there might be equitable distribution of honors in the future.

Several members of the Board of Trustees began to be disturbed over their financial responsibilities. It was pointed out that the salary of the editor represented the interest of 6 per cent on $100,000 and that there ought to be a business committee of the board which would take full responsibility for the finances of the Association. This arrangement has been of the greatest possible value to the American Medical Association since that time. To the finance committees of the Board of Trustees must be given much of the credit for the favorable financial position of the Association as the years have passed.

TIGHT FINANCING

The Committee on Reorganization had been voted $400 for its expenses, but the total bills represented $416.89. This gave great concern to the Board of Trustees, which eventually decided to give $400 to the chairman and let him argue it out with the other two members.

In 1902 the Board of Trustees moved its meetings to the Sherman House, presumably because of the "clammer" in the Grand Pacific Hotel. When in that year the Board held its first meeting, the attorney who had been called into consultation to report on the legal status of the incorporation of the Association indicated that there were apparently two organizations in the same concern: the Board of Trustees, with one set of officers, and the American Medical Association and the House of Delegates, with their sets of officers; all of this taken together was not in accord with the corporation laws of the state of Illinois. The legal opinion was profound and the lawyer was willing to suggest a technic whereby an incorporation could be completed with just one corporate body with one president and one secretary. The Board of Trustees directed the attorney to prepare the necessary papers, make the necessary changes and cooperate with the Committee on Organization, to which the By-Laws as adopted had been recommitted with authority to make verbal changes.

MORE ABOUT ADVERTISING

Again there was a considerable discussion over the advertisements of the California Fig Syrup Company, and the representative of that agency agreed to stop advertising it in the lay press. Now came another step in the cleaning of the advertising; a rule was adopted that rules governing advertisement of internal remedies should apply also to the advertisement of external remedies. There were disturbances over the advertisements of Battle & Company's Papine. The editor was authorized by the Board of Trustees to edit the various advertisements with a view to keeping out objectionable expressions regarding the efficiency of the products.

THE FIRST HOME

Dr. E. Fletcher Ingals, as resident trustee, had been looking into the possible purchase of property for the Association. He recommended a space on the northeast corner of Indiana and Dearborn Streets being known as Nos. 95 to 103 on Dearborn Street and measuring approximately 80 by 100 feet. The canny members of the board used part of the buildings on this property and rented the rest, thus receiving enough money out of the rentals to carry a considerable portion of their expenses. Arrangements were made to look further into the purchase of property. Finally a resolution was passed by the Board that the American Medical Association have a flag which should be known as the flag of the American Medical Association and fly over the headquarters whenever the board was meeting. The services of Dr. E. Fletcher Ingals in the development of the first headquarters building and in its equipment have never been suitably recognized by the Association. To him must be given most of the credit for the purchase of the original property and the preparation of the plans for the first building.

1902

SARATOGA SPRINGS, N. Y.

The first meeting of the American Medical Association with its new House of Delegates was held in 1902. The transition, as has been pointed out by Dr. Simmons, was exceedingly smooth. The meeting was held in Saratoga Springs, N. Y., early in June.

Following his resolution to the House of Delegates, Dr. H. L. E. Johnson of Washington, D. C, presented a beautiful banner to the Association. Excellent addresses were made to the House by the speaker of the New York state assembly and by Senator Brackett of New York. The technic for the establishment of reference committees of the House of Delegates was not yet perfected; on the first day of the session a business committee was set up to consist of five members to which would be referred all resolutions after being read.

The President, Dr. Wyeth, suggested an organizer who should act as a national organizer of the profession and who could visit states or territories where as yet medical organizations and society work were practically neglected. This business committee was given the address of the President of the Association and also all the recommendations that he had made.

As secretary of the Association, Dr. George H. Simmons read an extensive report in which he indicated that the same committee that had developed the reorganization had been requested by the President to formulate a Constitution and By-Laws for the state medical societies. This had been done and several state medical societies had already adopted the uniform Constitution and By-Laws. Dr. Simmons urged that all members who were not affiliated with local and state societies be dropped from membership in the Association, that the new Constitution and By-Laws be rigidly enforced. This address was also referred to the business committee.

Then the Board of Trustees reported the great improvement in the affairs of the Association that had resulted from the new methods of organization. They were a little apologetic about the advertising. "To the ordinary JOURNAL reader, it would appear to be an easy matter to lay down an inflexible rule by which the advertising department of any publication should be governed—that this should be like the laws of the Medes and Persians—but when brought face to face with many propositions, it is found to be a very difficult matter to decide what to do in each individual case. The Trustees are endeavoring to eliminate from the pages of THE JOURNAL all advertising that could be considered objectionable from an ethical standpoint."

The trustees were concerned with the overwhelming number of papers for the various sections and the difficulties of providing adequate publication. Finally they reported to the House of Delegates their action in purchasing property for the Association, and their report also was referred to the business committee.

THE PRINCIPLES OF ETHICS

Next came one of the most important actions taken by the Association. It resulted from a resolution introduced by Dr. E. Eliot Harris of New York. He said:

> For more than a year some of the members of the council of the New York State Medical Association have been engaged in a critical examination of the ethical part of the laws of the American Medical Association, resulting in the preparation of a revision of the Code of Medical Ethics. This revision has been approved by the council of the New York State Medical Association, and the delegates have been instructed to present it to the House of Delegates at this session.
>
> *Resolved,* That the President appoint a committee of five to examine and report for final action at the annual session in 1903 the proposed revised code of medical ethics which is herewith submitted in writing;
>
> *Resolved,* That the proposed revised code of medical ethics be published in the Association's JOURNAL three times before the meeting in 1903.

This was accompanied with the complete text of the new Principles of Ethics. These resolutions were referred to a special committee to be appointed by the President. The President appointed Drs. E. Eliot Harris of New York, William H. Welch of Baltimore, T. J. Happel of Tennessee, Nicholas Senn of Chicago and Joseph D. Bryant of New York.

REFERENCE COMMITTEES

Now the business committee on which had been wished the analysis of all the recommendations of the President, the Board and the Secretary and all of the new business, came back with a report that there be appointed instead a series of committees including one on sections and section work, one on revision of the list of members, one on finance, one on the relationship of dentists and pharmacists, one on organization, and one on transportation and place of meeting. This was adopted; it constituted the first step toward the establishment of suitable reference committees for the consideration of the vast business which comes before each meeting of the House of Delegates of the American Medical Association. The committee recommended the apportioning of all the business that had been referred to them to these various committees.

REORGANIZATION

The committee on organization report was presented by Dr. P. Maxwell Foshay, who submitted a copy of the new Constitution and By-Laws as well as the constitutions and by-laws developed for the individual states. This committee also recommended that a national organizer be employed to assist in organizing and developing the medical societies of the country. The report of this committee was adopted; later an organizer was employed.

CONFERENCE ON LEGISLATION

Another important resolution introduced by the committee on legislation called for an annual conference on legislation affecting the medical profession to be held in Washington and to include representatives of the national organization as well as representatives of the individual states.

ORIGINS OF TWO COUNCILS

The business committee in a later report recommended the establishment of two additional standing committees to be appointed by the President of the Association. These were a committee on public health and a committee on medical education. From these groups came eventually the Council on Health and Public Instruction and the Council on Medical Education and Hospitals.

THE NATIONAL EXAMINING BOARD

At this time also came the proposal for a voluntary national examining board, an idea which had apparently originated with Dr. William L. Rodman of Philadelphia. The proposal was opposed by the confederation of Medical Examining and Licensing Boards.

DIVISION OF FEES

On the final day of the session a resolution was adopted against the division of fees, to the effect that any member detected in such misconduct be expelled from his county medical society.

SOLICITATION OF VOTES FOR OFFICE

Another resolution adopted by the House of Delegates of the American Medical Association in 1902 declared that *the solicitation of votes for office is not in keeping with the dignity of the medical profession nor in harmony with the spirit of this Association and that such solicitation shall be considered a disqualification for the election to any office in the gift of the Association.* The resolution then passed has never been repealed. Later the Judicial Council declared that it was also wholly inefficient in preventing the abuse it sought to control.

DR. FRANK BILLINGS BECOMES PRESIDENT

At this session of the American Medical Association, Dr. Frank Billings was elected president. He was from that time on to be one of the most important officers in the building of the Association. Indeed to him must be credited largely the making of peace between the two medical societies in the state of New York, thus giving the Association new strength and more power for the future.

QUERIES AND MINOR NOTES

At the meeting of the Board of Trustees of the American Medical Association held in July 1902, one of the trustees suggested to the editor the desirability of a section of THE JOURNAL to be devoted to questions and answers. This section of THE JOURNAL was carried on for some twenty years with a few answers per week. For the last twenty years it has developed into one of the most significant portions of THE JOURNAL OF THE AMERICAN MEDICAL ASSOCIATION. This department now requires the services of several workers in the headquarters office and represents annually consultations with 400 or 500 experts who supply the replies. The answers are paid for at a space rate, which in no way compensates the author of the answer for the knowledge and investigation required but which represents an expenditure of thousands of dollars each year—indeed often equal to the entire budget of THE JOURNAL for the first few years of the present century.

1903

NEW ORLEANS

The report of the Board of Trustees for 1903 indicates that it had been especially active in straightening out the matter of the incorporation. The editor was being overwhelmed with work and was therefore authorized to secure the services of Dr. J. N. McCormack of Kentucky as a traveling organizer. The board described the manner in which it had purchased the property and the necessary equipment for the headquarters office.

The editor presented the names of half a dozen "patent" medicines which were accepted by other periodicals but the Board of Trustees was firm in its insistence that these not be accepted to the pages of THE JOURNAL OF THE AMERICAN MEDICAL ASSOCIATION. The Board of Trustees presented in toto the complete discussions relative to the articles of incorporation. There had been a considerable movement to cause the Association to incorporate in a national corporation under the laws of the District of Columbia. The attorneys did not recommend such an action.

The traveling organizer, Dr. J. N. McCormack, had visited Wisconsin, Florida, Mississippi, Texas and Arkansas, and Dr. Simmons himself had gone to Missouri. Their travels met everywhere with success; the membership of the Association had increased by three times; it was decided to continue these efforts.

The committee on the Rush monument, through the work of Dr. Frank Billings, had now assembled more than $15,000. It was decided to proceed with the setting up of the monument, and the Board of Trustees appropriated $500 to bear the expenses of the dedication.

FOURTH OF JULY ACCIDENTS

The quality of American medical literature had begun to show definite improvement. The papers in THE JOURNAL OF THE AMERICAN MEDICAL ASSOCIATION were of a distinctly higher order than in the previous decade. About this time the editorials began to call attention to the unnecessary injuries resulting from the celebration of the Fourth of July. Eventually THE JOURNAL developed a campaign which only late in 1940 began to have an appreciable effect. Today most of the states in the United States, as a result of the campaign initiated by THE JOURNAL OF THE AMERICAN MEDICAL ASSOCIATION in 1903, have laws regulating the use of fireworks in celebration of the Fourth of July. While the number of injuries and particularly the number of cases of tetanus have greatly decreased, there are still some states which need to take definite action to diminish these casualties.

CAMPAIGNS

As an example, however, of the manner in which THE JOURNAL had begun to carry on a variety of campaigns, we must take into account the campaign against excessive injuries on the Fourth of July, the campaign for improvement of medical education demonstrated by publication in 1903 of the third annual educational number, and the campaign for better organization of medical societies indicated by the great advancement in county and state organizations. Moreover, the Association began to set aside a small sum of money to be devoted to grants for research. In an issue for 1903 appears the first paper published by a grantee.

NEW ORLEANS MEETING

In 1903 at New Orleans, the House of Delegates was greeted with floods of oratory by the mayor, a representative of the governor and a representative of the local bar association. No one better could have been chosen to respond to these addresses than the first vice president, Dr. J. A. Witherspoon of Nashville, Tenn., who later became President of the Association. His address was punctuated with "applause" and "laughter" in many parenthetical inserts that would have gladdened the hearts of such eminent speakers as Chauncey Depew and Joseph Choate. The concentrated attack on medical educational problems was featured by the address of President Frank Billings on "Medical Education in the United States."

The association was presented with portraits of previous Presidents Drs. T. G. Richardson and Hunter McGuire.

In response to a resolution adopted the previous year, all business introduced was referred to the business committee without debate.

The committee on Scientific Research had selected four grantees who were investigating such subjects as the blastomycotic infections, streptococcic infections, malaria and the secretion of sweat.

More significant than the address by President Frank Billings on medical education was his message to the House of Delegates. By 1903 eighteen states had been completely organized in accordance with the plan of the American Medical Association. Dr. Billings recommended the continued employment of Dr. J. N. McCormack as official organizer. He was able to report that sufficient funds had been collected to construct the Rush monument and to promise its dedication before the end of 1903. A suggestion had been made for the establishment of a national bureau of medicines and foods, and a provisional committee had been established to consider this possibility. Out of these suggestions came the Council on Pharmacy and Chemistry.

The American Medical Association was also urged to prepare a memorial for Major Walter Reed, whose fundamental investigations of yellow fever made his name one of the greatest in the history of American medicine.

The business committee which acted as the sole reference committee for this session was concerned with the question of national incorporation for the American Medical Association. The subject was continued because it did not seem possible to make any definite recommendation.

Dr. Arthur Dean Bevan as chairman of the Committee on Medical Education made an extended report at this session which ended with the recommendation that a committee on education be established with a full time salaried assistant secretary and that they have their headquarters in the office of the American Medical Association. This was the origin of the Council on Medical Education and Hospitals.

An enlarged committee was set up to make a final revision of the Principles of Ethics, with representatives from each state on the committee. The President appointed such a committee.

The move to establish the national bureau of medicines and foods was not successful because the business committee rejected its suggestions. There was much discussion, in which Dr. Philip Mills Jones of California led the movement in favor of such a bureau. Eventually it was referred back to the original committee.

THE REVISED PRINCIPLES OF ETHICS

On the fourth day of the meeting the enlarged committee on a revised Code of Ethics was called for a report. The committee included Dr. E. Eliot Harris, William H. Welch, T. J. Happel and Joseph D. Bryant. Their complete report as it had been worked out with the enlarged committee on the previous evening was read and on motion by E. Eliot Harris, seconded by Charles A. L. Reed of Cincinnati, the revised Principles of Ethics were unanimously adopted. The adoption of these new Principles of Ethics put an end to the controversy in New York, which had been for so many years the basis of contention. Once these new Principles of Ethics were adopted, the President of the Association, Dr. Frank Billings, and the organizer, Dr. J. N. McCormack, through meetings with representative physicians of the two groups in New York, brought about an amalgamation and the ultimate establishment of a single society in that state.

I am indebted to Dr. C. H. Bunting of Hamden, Conn., for this story as to how the revised Principles of Ethics were adopted at the New Orleans session in 1903. The committee of four already mentioned had developed a revision, to which, however, one of the members dissented. That member came to Dr. William H. Welch late in the afternoon before the House of Delegates was to meet and expressed his dissatisfaction with the committee report. Dr. Welch then agreed with him. After the motion to appoint a committee of representatives from the individual states, Dr. Welch retired to his room, took off his coat and laying out the necessary number of long black cigars, went to work and wrote out in longhand the entire code. The committee got the code set in type and printed that night and a copy was on the desk of each delegate in the morning. As the delegates came into the meeting, Dr. Welch stood in back of the hall greeting them and telling them how much better he thought the minority report of the committee was than the original majority report. According to Dr. William Sydney Thayer, it was this lobbying of Dr. Welch for his own handiwork that resulted in the eventual unanimous adoption of the report on the Principles of Ethics.

ANOTHER STEP TOWARD THE COUNCIL ON PHARMACY AND CHEMISTRY

Later in the session Dr. Ellis of California presented a report for the provisional committee on the establishment of a national bureau of medicines and foods. That suggestion had first been made by Dr. F. E. Stewart at the session of the American Medical Association held in 1881. Dr. Ellis proposed that a national organization be formed with representatives of the American Medical Association and of the American Pharmaceutical Association to examine and analyze new remedies and to make certain that labels were truthful and that claims were warranted. The proposal was referred back to the business committee, which now recommended that this committee confer with the American Pharmaceutical Association and with the authorities of the United States and report at the next session.

BIRTH OF "TONICS AND SEDATIVES"

On Aug. 15, 1903, THE JOURNAL OF THE AMERICAN MEDICAL ASSOCIATION published for the first time a column immediately following the editorial section with the heading "Clippings from Lay Exchanges." This was a column of peculiar errors made by the press in discussing medical subjects. It was to appear from time to time in the reading pages and then gradually shifted toward the advertising section of THE JOURNAL. Eventually it was to become the Tonics and Sedatives department, a section of medical humor which has come to be recognized as a unique feature of THE JOURNAL OF THE AMERICAN MEDICAL ASSOCIATION.

Toward the end of the New Orleans session of 1903 the business committee which had been charged with passing on most of the active functions of the Association uttered a word of warning on what it regarded as excessive legislation. "In the past," it said, "when so little could be done, sufficient was accomplished from year to year to keep the Association abreast of the development of the profession. At present we are threatened with just the opposite danger, namely, legislation on a great variety of topics, in which the energy of the Association will be dissipated and very little accomplished. It seems to your committee that the organization of the profession, the strengthening of THE JOURNAL and the welding of the profession into a unit are subjects that will profitably occupy the energies of this House for some years to come."

THE NATIONAL CHARTER

As the year went on there continued to be agitation for the securing of a national charter for the Association, and there were many who still believed that incorporation with a national charter would be desirable. In the meantime the former Committee on Constitution and By-Laws had been changed to a new committee with Dr. M. L. Harris of Chicago as chairman. The report of this new committee was adopted so that the Association had a new Constitution and By-Laws which, with minor modifications, prevails to this time.

VENEREAL DISEASE

The American Medical Association had developed a powerful committee on the prevalence of venereal diseases. This committee presented an extensive report on the prevalence of such diseases. This committee cooperated with other agencies in endeavoring to work up a plan for the suppression of venereal disorders. Until, however, modern scientific medicine developed such aids as the Wassermann test and specific methods of treatment which would control syphilis in a reasonably short time, the outlook for stamping out venereal diseases was not particularly bright.

MORE RESOLUTIONS

Notwithstanding the warning of the business committee, resolutions were introduced to the House of Delegates on a great variety of subjects such as the purification of the mails by the elimination of advertisements for "patent" medicines, on condemning the use of wood alcohol as a dangerous poison, on the control of leprosy, on venereal diseases, on cancer, on the concept of a central committee which would act in an advisory capacity to medical periodicals in purifying their advertising, and on a great number of subjects dealing with the intimate affairs of the Association.

THE DIRECTORY

About this time also a proposal came before the House of Delegates for the publication by the American Medical Association of a directory of the medical profession. A commercial directory was being published in the United States and was supported largely by the sale of advertising space to the same type of proprietary and "patent" medicine advertising that was supporting a considerable number of medical periodicals of the nation. It was the belief of Dr. George H. Simmons and the Board of Trustees of the American Medical Association that it would be desirable to publish a directory which would be free from this unsavory commercial taint and which would be free as well from the promotional blurbs of individual physicians who were not averse to putting their best foot forward in the description of themselves and their activities which they sent to the commercial directory.

The Board of Trustees authorized the editor, Dr. George H. Simmons, to make the necessary investigations and to take the necessary steps toward the development of such a directory. This activity was eventually to bring down on the head of the editor a burst of vilification and personal attack almost unprecedented in the annals of journalism and certainly up to that time unprecedented in medical journalism.

The work of the organizer, Dr. J. N. McCormack, was being continued and insinuations began to be made against him on the charge that he was exploiting the Association. The publishers and editors of medical periodicals which were beginning to see their incomes suffer from the loss of advertising revenue joined in the chorus of attack on the editor. These attacks spread finally to direct assaults on the authority and honesty and the motivations of the members of the Board of Trustees. Moreover, the work which burdened the editor had begun to be insuperable with the growth of the Association, the establishment of a headquarters office and the ownership of a considerable amount of property, both real and mechanical.

One of the charges made against Dr. J. N. McCormack had to do with the fact that he "had been active in the politics of the Association while acting as organizer, and complaints had been presented to the Board of his active work in behalf of special candidates for Association honors."

An attempt had been made on recommendation of Dr. M. L. Harris to get the House of Delegates to select the Northern Trust Company as treasurer for the Association. With this proposal the House of Delegates disagreed and Dr. Frank Billings, a former President of the Association, was then nominated treasurer and elected by the House of Delegates. This was fortunate, because it enabled Dr. Frank Billings as treasurer to sit with the Board of Trustees for many years to come. His influence, his wisdom and his force were to be great assets to the American Medical Association during this period in its development.

1904
DEATHS OF PHYSICIANS

In the issue of THE JOURNAL OF THE AMERICAN MEDICAL ASSOCIATION for Jan. 9, 1904, an editorial was published on the deaths of physicians. This was apparently the first summary of the deaths of physicians—a feature that has come to be an annual feature of THE JOURNAL. It has received frequent notice in the public and medical press throughout the nation and, indeed, throughout the world. It is a natural outgrowth of the directory service and the efforts of the American Medical Association to maintain an adequate accounting of the medical profession of the nation.

ATLANTIC CITY, N. J.

The organizer, Dr. J. N. McCormack, reported that he had already visited Wisconsin, Florida, Louisiana, Mississippi, Texas and Arkansas and that Dr. Simmons had gone to Missouri. The Board of Trustees agreed to retain his services for another year.

A bill was presented to the trustees in favor of the American Printing Company for $16 for printing the Principles of Medical Ethics, which had been given to them by Dr. William H. Welch.

A suitable button was adopted as official for the American Medical Association.

At this time it was apparently the chief function of the Board to concern itself simply with expenditures and not at all with policy. Early in 1904 the Board of Trustees met in Chicago for a regular session. It was first concerned with the income of the Association from the conduct of THE JOURNAL and from other sources. During the year THE JOURNAL had been exceedingly careful in its past selection of advertisements and had rejected advertisements of:

Etna Chemical Company
Duffey Malt Whiskey Company
Mariani & Co.
Oppenheimer Institute
California Fig Syrup Company
Scott & Bowne
Charles Marchand
The Fitchmul Company
Antikamnia Chemical Company
New Animal Therapy Company
Mueller Chemical Company
The Manola Company
Micajah Company

Anasarcin Chemical Company
Osborn-Colwell Company
The Pheno-Bromate Company
New York Pharmaceutical Company
The Ringgold-Reinhart Company
C. W. Edison
Opticulin Company
Gonoseptone Company
Asthma Remedy Company
Bellbrook Sanatorium
Merrill-Hall Company
Carl Reinschild Manufacturing Company
A. S. Valentine Chemical Company

These were rejected because they were considered to be secret proprietaries, but a few others were rejected because they were advertised primarily to the public. The editor pointed out that most of these advertisements had been accepted by other medical journals in the United States.

As a result of the work of organizers and solicitors, more than 5,000 new members had joined the Association. The Association had accumulated much machinery in its own office. The profit of THE JOURNAL now had reached more than $50,000 annually.

Once the Association had begun to buy property, the trustees determined to extend their holdi˙gs; arrangements were made to buy additional houses on Indiana Street, now known as Grand Avenue.

Dr. Charles A. L. Reed as chairman of the Committee on National Legislation (to be discussed later) was given a considerable grant for the expenses of his meetings, but he was told by the board that he could have his stationery printed in the office in Chicago.

There was still much debate as to whether or not the Association ought to have a national incorporation.

PRESIDENT JOHN H. MUSSER SPEAKS

At the meeting in June 1904 in Atlantic City, Dr. John H. Musser devoted his presidential address also to medical education.

THE REFERENCE COMMITTEES

Dr. Frank Billings in an opening address to the House of Delegates presented for the first time a definite plan of organization for reference committees. He pointed out that the business in New Orleans had been greatly delayed by the fact that every proposal had to be submitted to the business committee. He proposed therefore a system of reference committees—eight in number—which prevail to this day, except that the speaker of the House of Delegates is now empowered by the House to appoint additional reference committees if there are special projects to be considered.

THE COUNCIL ON MEDICAL EDUCATION

The committee on medical education now made a definite proposal for the establishment of a Council on Medical Education to consist of five members. The history of that council and its efforts from this time on is covered in the history of the Council on Medical Education and Hospitals, which appears in this volume, written by Dr. Victor Johnson, its present secretary.

THE "PATENT" MEDICINE EVIL

The "patent" medicine evil had developed so seriously that a resolution came in by Dr. H. O. Walker of Michigan, representing the Michigan State Medical Society, requesting the Board of Trustees of the American Medical Association to provide for the analysis of medicinal products of unknown composition and undetermined effects and to publish the results in THE JOURNAL, and requesting also the establishment of a commission which would administer this function. This motion was referred to the provisional committee on establishment of a national bureau of medicines and foods. When this committee reported the results of its conferences with Dr. Harvey Wiley (then chief of the Bureau of Agriculture) and with representatives of the American Pharmaceutical Association, its report was again referred to the committee on legislation.

The report for the establishment of a national bureau failed of adoption after an extended discussion in the House of Delegates sitting as a committee of the whole. As a result, official action was not taken by the House of Delegates, but we shall see that the effects of the pressure brought about by the discussion were sufficient to cause the Board of Trustees to take an action later which resulted in the establishment of the Council on Pharmacy and Chemistry.

THE RUSH MONUMENT COMPLETED

The committee on the Rush monument reported that the monument had now been erected on the grounds of the Naval Museum of Hygiene and Medical School in Washington, D. C., and that plans for the dedication on June 11, 1904, were complete.

DEVELOPMENT OF THE COUNCILS

1905

THE COMMITTEE ON LEGISLATION

FOR SOME TIME THE ASSOCIATION had been served by a committee on medical legislation consisting of Dr. C. A. L. Reed as chairman and Drs. William H. Welch and William L. Rodman. The task of watching medical legislation in Washington and throughout the nation as well was far too great for a committee of this type. The committee had met frequently in Washington; it had established a national auxiliary legislative committee with 2,800 local correspondents. It had established also a national legislative council with representatives of the individual states to agitate whenever action was needed on medical legislation. The legislative counci had not met in 1904 because there had not been questions of medical interest before the Congress. The Committee on National Legislation was, however, disturbed at this time because of an executive order issued by President Theodore Roosevelt concerning activities by public officials in their own behalf. This executive order read:

> All officers and employees of the United States of every description serving in or under any of the Executive Departments, and whether so serving in or out of Washington, are hereby forbidden, either directly or indirectly, individually or through associations, to solicit an increase of pay or to influence or attempt to influence in their own interest any other legislation whatever, either before Congress or its committees, or in any way save through the heads of departments in or under which they serve, on penalty of dismissal from the government service.

The legislative committee felt that there ought to be more doctors in the Congress and in the Senate. The expenses had been considerable. The committee proposed therefore that it be dismissed and that there be established a Bureau of Medical Legislation to be located in the Association building in Chicago. This bureau would act under the secretary of the American Medical Association and under the supervisory direction of a committee on medical legislation. The report of the committee was referred to a reference committee on medical legislation and political action. This committee concurred in the report. Thus the Bureau of Medical Legislation was established in the headquarters office.

MORE ACTION AGAINST THE PROPRIETARY DRUGS

Again the House of Delegates began to receive resolutions relative to the use of nostrums and proprietary remedies; these came from Missouri and California.

Following the introduction of these resolutions the Board of Trustees made its report. The board announced to the House of Delegates that the Council on Pharmacy and Chemistry had been organized at a meeting held in Pittsburgh, February 11, with Dr. George H. Simmons as chairman and C. S. N. Halberg as secretary. This council had been conducting its work much as it is now conducted up to the time of the annual session in June. Already it had exerted a considerable effect on the acceptance of "patent" medicines for advertising by THE JOURNAL OF THE AMERICAN MEDICAL ASSOCIATION.

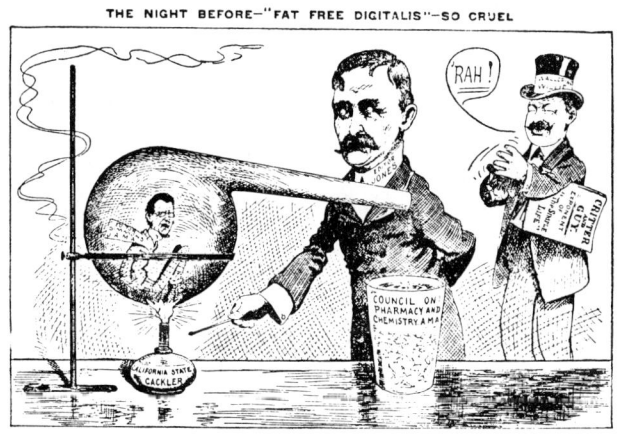

Cartoon from the *American Medical Journalist*, March 1905. Part of the campaign against the formation of the Council on Pharmacy and Chemistry.

The report of the Board of Trustees was referred to a reference committee. The statement of that reference committee, of which Dr. Frank Billings was chairman, is significant. The reference committee said:

> The report of the Board of Trustees on the creation of the Council on Pharmacy and Chemistry is, in the opinion of your committee, the most important and effective measure ever undertaken by this Association to rid the profession of the abuse of the nostrum evil. The personnel of the Council is of such a character as to create a feeling of confidence that the proposed work will be done thoroughly, conscientiously and justly. The publication of the results of the work of the council in book form with annual editions will afford a source of information of inestimable value to the profession.
>
> Therefore we recommend that the House of Delegates indorse the action of the Board of Trustees in the creation of the Council on Pharmacy and Chemistry; that the Trustees be requested to devise a plan through which the council may be made permanent, and that the Trustees request the Secretary of Agriculture of the U. S. government to give

the Council on Pharmacy and Chemistry recognition by authorizing the Bureau of Chemistry to cooperate with the council in its work.

We indorse the work already performed by the Council on Pharmacy and Chemistry in the formulation of rules governing the mode of selection of articles to be investigated and the publication of results already obtained.

We recommend the publication in book form of a list of the preparations not in the Pharmacopeia that are approved by the Council on Pharmacy and Chemistry.

BUDGETS

The minutes of the Board of Trustees for its first meeting in 1905 indicate some of the internecine difficulties. Each time that the editor rejected an advertisement of some proprietary product that had previously been carried there came dire threats of recriminations. The Board of Trustees was, moreover, involved in the purchase of property and with the erection of a new building and with additions to the old building. A separate chapter in this history will be devoted to the story of the gradual development of the headquarters building.

Before the board were the budgets for the councils newly established; these gave much concern to the Board of Trustees in 1905. For instance, the Council on Pharmacy and Chemistry needed $3,000. The sum was granted but with some doubts; today the annual budget of that Council with its various associate councils and laboratory is more than thirty-five times the amount then proposed. The Board of Trustees gave full assent, however, to the rules of the Council relative to the advertising of proprietary products. Then it made the necessary appropriations for a secretary and for an assistant secretary of the Council on Medical Education. The budget of the Council on Medical Education at that time was $750 annually; this has gradually grown to reach more than fifty times the amount required during its first year.

PORTLAND SESSION

At the meeting of the Board of Trustees during the annual session in Portland, difficulties began to develop relative to the employment of the organizer, Dr. J. N. McCormack. The proposal was made to discontinue him as a salaried employee and to reimburse him with an honorarium for each day of service. Dr. McCormack objected to this arrangement and offered either to do the work for nothing or to continue it with the annual honorarium or to discontinue entirely. After reconsideration, the Board of Trustees moved that Dr. J. N. McCormack be reappointed to carry on the work of the Association until the next annual meeting at the same salary as previously.

Now came also for the first time the request to the Association to undertake the publication of a special periodical—the appeal being in this instance from the *Journal of Biological Chemistry*. In proceeding toward the publication of the new directory, the Board of Trustees authorized the purchase of the existing "Standard Medical Directory" for $6,000, and an option had been taken with payment of $750.

THE RUSH MONUMENT

The final and at the same time complete history of the Rush monument appears in the minutes of the House of Delegates for 1905. As has been stated, the turn in its affairs came when the names of Dr. Frank Billings of Chicago, Dr. L. Duncan Bulkley of New York and Dr. William L. Rodman of Philadelphia were added to the committee. They promptly increased its funds to more than $15,000. A site had been obtained for the monument, a bronze statue a little more than life size had been developed and purchased, and the unveiling and dedication took place on Saturday, June 11, 1904 at 5 o'clock. Dr. J. H. Musser, President of the American Medical Association, made a brief address, Dr. J. C. Wilson, chairman of the committee, delivered a eulogy, and the President of the United States accepted the monument as a gift of the medical profession to the nation "in a graceful and interesting address." Music was by the Marine Band.

Much easier had been the collection of funds for a memorial to Dr. Walter Reed. Already more than $18,000 was in the hands of that committee.

THE DIRECTORY

When the Board of Trustees reported to the House of Delegates its action relative to the publication of a directory and its purchase of the "Standard Directory," a complaint arose from the Michigan delegation. At that time the most widely used and commercially profitable directory in existence was published in Detroit.

The report of the Council on Medical Education was well received by the House of Delegates. The members of that first council contained names such as might well command respect and admiration. It included Drs. Arthur Dean Bevan, chairman, William T. Councilman, Victor C. Vaughan, Charles H. Frazier and J. A. Witherspoon.

NATIONAL INCORPORATION

Many pages of the activites of the House of Delegates for this year are concerned with the attempt to incorporate the American Medical Association with a national charter. A bill had been introduced into the Congress for the establishment of such a corporation and had been favorably reported with the change, however, of the right to transact business anywhere in the United States to make it definitely a corporation of the District of Columbia. It was suddenly discovered that the amended bill was a very bad bill. Then Senator McComas of Maryland was induced by Dr. William H. Welch to bring out a bill still further revised. This bill was never reported out in the Senate. There was doubt as to the constitutionality of such a measure. The committee which had the matter in charge says at one place in in its report, "This ends the first lesson in the attempt to secure national incorporation of the American Medical Association by a special act of Congress." In any event the report simply ended by referring the entire matter back to the Committee on National Legislation.

By this time Dr. J. N. McCormack was able to report that the plan of organization promulgated by the American Medical Association had been accepted by practically all the states of the Union except Virginia and Maine.

THE SITUATION IN NEW YORK

As a result of serious efforts by Dr. Frank Billings and Dr. J. N. McCormack, who had met from time to time with various representatives of the two medical societies in the state of New York, the time was approaching when New York would form itself into a single state society and become a constituent of the American Medical Association. Dr. E. Eliot Harris of New York reported to the House of Delegates that before the next annual session of the American Medical Association the medical profession of the state of New York would have united, and he asked that a committee be appointed to apportion a proper number of delegates to that state.

THE "PATENT" MEDICINE EVIL

By this time also many of the great literary publications of the United States, such as the *Ladies Home Journal, Everybody's Magazine* and *Collier's*, had joined with the American Medical Association in the fight on the "patent" medicine evil. The House of Delegates tendered its thanks for their cooperation.

DR. J. N. McCORMACK CONTINUED

As the meeting ended in 1905, a resolution was introduced by Dr. Jones of California asking that the present chairman of the Committee on Organization, Dr. J. N. McCormack, be permitted to continue with his work. Dr. McCormack rose in the House of

Delegates and made a fine address in which he pleaded for unity and in which he said that suspicion of the trustees and the editor was wholly unwarranted; that all were working together with the best interests of the American Medical Association. By a rising vote Dr. McCormack was unanimously recommended for continuation in his work. As evidence of the intensive drive for increase of membership in the American Medical Association, Michigan increased in this

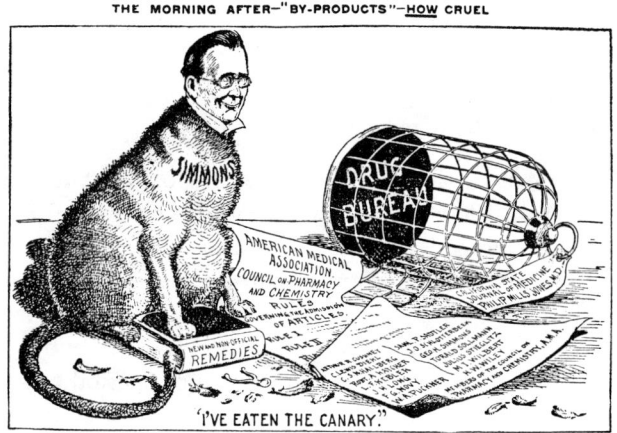

Cartoon from the *American Medical Journalist*, March 1905, refers to the establishment of the Council on Pharmacy and Chemistry instead of the Drug Bureau proposed by Dr. Philip Mills Jones.

year from 452 to 2,100 members, and Texas from 382 to 2,510 members.

At this session of the Association, on nomination by Dr. W. L. Rodman of Philadelphia and E. Eliot Harris of New York, Dr. William J. Mayo was elected unanimously to be president of the Association.

MEMORIAL TO DR. N. S. DAVIS

Through a letter from Dr. Henry O. Marcy of Boston a memorial was recommenced for Dr. N. S. Davis; Dr. Marcy opened the subscription with the first hundred dollars.

A CHAIRMAN FOR THE HOUSE OF DELEGATES

Dr. T. J. Happel offered an amendment to the effect that the House of Delegates should elect a chairman from day to day with the idea of taking this burden from the President. The proposal was hissed. Again it was felt that this would be an implied criticism of the President, and the proposal was rejected.

THE FIRST OPERATION FOR GALLSTONES

At this meeting there was an exhibit of Mrs. Z. Burnsworth of McCordsville, Ind., who was the first person ever operated on for the removal of gallstones. The operation had been done by Dr. John S. Bobbs of Indianapolis.

1906

BOSTON

In 1906 the Council on Pharmacy and Chemistry came to the Board of Trustees with a proposal that it be supplied with a laboratory in the headquarters office.

THE CRIES OF THE WOUNDED

The meeting of the Board of Trustees in Boston at the time of the annual session in 1906 was an indication of the difficulties that are likely to besiege crusaders at all times and in every generation. The purveyors of "patent" medicines, the quacks and charlatans who were beginning to be damaged by the exposés published in THE JOURNAL OF THE AMERICAN MEDICAL ASSOCIATION and by the barring of their advertisements from the medical periodicals, the publishers, the editors and those financially interested in periodicals which were profiting by the publication of these advertisements, the owners of medical schools which were beginning to see their investments and their incomes threatened, and the publishers of medical directories who saw for their activities the handwriting on the wall began to seek legal and other means of forcing the Board of Trustees of the American Medical Association and its editor into abandoning their crusading projects. Now came requests from lawyers and from owners of proprietary medical industries and from other agencies for the right to appear personally before the Board to present their cases. Now began to appear also the publication in competing periodicals of articles devoted to vilification, insinuation and prevarication relative to the work of the American Medical Association. The Board of Trustees properly answered these various agencies when they appeared with a legal representative, that their legal representative could deal with that of the Association. Others were simply told that investigations would be continued and that the facts would be published.

A headquarters was created for the Bureau of Medical Legislation. Preparations were made for the Council on Medical Education, for the new laboratory and for the Committee on Scientific Research.

The sum of $5,000 was appropriated to the California fund for the benefit of suffering physicians. It will be remembered that California had had either an earthquake or a fire—or both—at that time.

The Committee on Scientific Research was granted $483.28, as it was still conducting a small exhibit.

THE PRESIDENT'S ADDRESS

In the meantime Dr. Lewis S. McMurtry of Louisville, President of the Association, made an important address to the House of Delegates dealing with the affairs of the Association. By this time a pattern was beginning to be established: the address of the President at the opening General Meeting was for the public and the medical profession and concerned the advancement of medical science. The president made an address to the House of Delegates at its opening meeting dealing with the work of the organization. Dr. McMurtry found it desirable to point out first to the House of Delegates that the Association was not conducted by either the President or the secretary or both but that the great power of the Association was concentrated in the Board of Trustees.

> Under our organization [he said] the Board of Trustees has sole charge of the extensive property and controls all the financial and business affairs of the Association. This Board also has sole control of the disbursement of all funds in carrying on the publications of the Association—to supply funds for standing committees, to direct scientific investigations—and can mold the policy of the Association at will during the interim of the annual sessions. The present prosperous condition of the financial affairs of the Association, the splendid position and high standard of THE JOURNAL and the efficiency with which the work of the several standing committees is being prosecuted all compose a superb tribute to the ability, good judgment and professional devotion of the present Board.

Fortunately for the American Medical Association the tribute presented by Dr. McMurtry to the Board of Trustees at that session could be repeated year after year to the gradually changing membership of the Board of Trustees. From time to time movements have been initiated to wreck the Board of Trustees, to disturb its activities and to bring about revolution in the Association through action on the Board. Perhaps it is a tribute to the good sense and good judgment of American physicians that even revolutionists who were elected to the Board, once they became familiar with its problems and responsibilities, became among the most effective of the workers in its membership.

Dr. McMurtry was disturbed also by the possibility that a trustee might be at the same time a delegate and also with the possibility that a member of the House of Delegates might be elected to the office of President or Vice President. He said:

The Constitution, article 9, section 3, declares "No member of the House of Delegates shall be eligible to the office of President or Vice President. Such a protection of the interests of the Association against undue influence is so just, and the precaution is so necessary, that it needs no comment for proper appreciation. If such doubling of office in one individual is forbidden by the Constitution as to the President and Vice President, how much more essential is it that the same precaution should be prescribed and enforced as to the trustees, whose power and responsibilities are so much greater? I shall have occasion presently to allude to the attacks now being made on the Association's JOURNAL and the Association's management. These attacks, which you will readily recognize as the result of sinister motives and altogether unjustified in fact, are directed toward work entirely within the control and direction of the Board of Trustees. As the strength and influence of the Association grows, and pressing evils are exposed and corrected, such attacks will naturally increase. Under such circumstances the Board of Trustees should command the confidence of the profession at large, all members of the Board should sustain the same relation to this House of Delegates, which selects them, and they should also be on the same footing with each other. Hence I would recommend that the Constitution be so amended that no member of the Board can occupy the double office of trustee and delegate.

Dr. McMurtry then turned his attention to the attacks that were being made on the Board of Trustees and on the editor. In response to these attacks he said:

So long as the meetings of the American Medical Association consisted almost wholly of section work, with a large general session every day for the adoption of resolutions, with no systematic or persistent work along definite lines, the commendation of the medical press was generally and freely bestowed on the organization. But since the reorganization, when this House of Delegates was established and the membership has increased, and the power of a great organization comes to be intelligently directed toward improving the resources of scientific medicine and advancing the welfare of the profession by organization, certain interests have been interfered with, and the natural course of misrepresentation and abuse has been resorted to by the interests involved. First, and most naturally, THE JOURNAL, owned and controlled by the Association and ably edited and published under the direction of the Board of Trustees, was the object of attack and misrepresentation. For years publishing firms have grown rich by the patronage of the medical profession, and these same firms owned medical journals liberally supported by the profession. That the medical profession should own and publish a journal of its own, and that this journal should attain great popularity and influence, has provoked hostile criticism and misrepresentation. That this hostility, abuse and misrepresentation should be directed against the editor of THE JOURNAL is natural, since he is in the direct line of fire, and, from one standpoint, is the chief offender. That you may appreciate the ridiculous character of these charges, I would refer you to the leading editorial in the last issue but one of a New York weekly which has for years enjoyed the liberal patronage of the profession and which is owned by a wealthy publisher of medical books. The editorial is entitled "The American Medical Directory." After stating that the issuance of a medical directory by the American Medical Association is absolutely without excuse, although mentioning that the Medical Society of the State of New York had advantageously issued a directory of that state, the editor says:

"The Editor-Secretary has also gone into the business of publishing medical books — he might as well drag the Association into the making of shoes. We do not know who authorized this venture—perhaps the managers will take us into their confidence at the Boston meeting in June—but, whether authorized or not, if the Association publishes books it should give them without price to its members."* Comment on this is unneces-

---

*I would state that the weekly New York journal quoted here is not the New York Medical Journal, edited by that veteran medical editor and scholar Dr. Frank P. Foster.

sary. The allusion to Dr. Simmons and the feigned ignorance of the fact that the publication of a medical directory was authorized by a vote of this House of Delegates at Portland last year, shows the unfair methods and animus of the editor who wrote the lines quoted.

But there is another interest which has been offended and which is equally unfair and far more abusive in its attacks on THE JOURNAL and the Association. This is the interest of the manufacturers of "patent" and proprietary medicines. This House of Delegates established a Council on Pharmacy and Chemistry, which, with the cooperation of the Board of Trustees, has secured the services of expert chemists and pharmacists to analyze the various nostrums and proprietary medicines in popular use. Many remedies, widely advertised under a plausible name, were found to be composed of cheap and familiar drugs and sold at a ridiculously high price. The Board of Trustees, by direction of this House of Delegates, excluded from the advertising pages of THE JOURNAL all preparations which did not make public with the advertisement the formula showing accurately the composition of the products advertised. Many of these manufacturers of proprietary medicines have grown rich, and they saw here a serious menace to their interests. Their avenue of assault is through the editorial columns of the medical journals they have subsidized, and their press committee has been very active of late. Here, as in the instance I have cited from the medical publishers, the editor of THE JOURNAL is made the special object of abuse and criticism. In the meantime, the editor's unpardonable offense is that he is doing his duty faithfully, as he is appointed to do, and at all times under the direction of this House of Delegates.

The far-reaching labors of the chairman of your committee on organization, Dr. J. N. McCormack, which have done so much to build up this great organization, have likewise brought on that distinguished physician a goodly share of unjust criticism and abuse.

These attacks on the Association, its work and its officers, abound with allusions to "clique" and "ring" in the organization, which "clique" and "ring" is alleged to be surreptitiously and treacherously running the affairs of the Association. I know not to whom these epithets are intended to apply, but this I do know, that there is no officer or board or committee of the Association which is not directly created by this House of Delegates. Hence, if there be a clique or ring entrenched in power anywhere in this great organization, the responsibility for its existence rests on this House of Delegates and the means for its immediate destruction are in your hands. You represent a constituency of more than 60,000 physicians, and it devolves on you to discharge faithfully the trust you have assumed.

MEDICAL EDUCATION

For the first time the Council on Medical Education now recommended a year of college education before entrance into a medical school.

The Committee on Medical Legislation reported that it had dealt with a number of problems for the medical profession, most important of which were the establishment of a national department of health with representation in the cabinet, the army medical reorganization bill, the pure food and drug bill and the attitude of the postoffice toward nostrums. The Association gave its fullest support to the proposed legislation for a pure food and drugs act, which passed the next session of the Congress.

THE DIRECTORY

In making its report, the Board of Trustees devoted a special section to the new directory. The editorial work on this directory had been placed in charge of Dr. Frederick R. Green. On many occasions the Association had voted to establish a directory, but now for the first time that activity was becoming effective.

ORGANIZATION

Dr. J. N. McCormack reported for the committee on organization. Visits had been made to Minnesota, Oregon, California, Texas, Oklahoma, Tennessee, Illinois and Kentucky, with special meetings in North Dakota, Montana, Washington, Idaho and Arkansas. These trips and their results had been chronicled week by week and month by month in THE JOURNAL.

THE SCIENTIFIC EXHIBIT

By now the Association was holding its seventh scientific exhibit, and a loving cup was presented to Dr. Frank Wynn on behalf of the Board of Trustees.

THE REFERENCE COMMITTEE REPORTS ON THE BOARD

Following a highly favorable report of the work of the Board and of the secretary-editor by a reference committee, headed by Dr. Philip Mills Jones of California, there was an extended discussion in the House of Delegates. Then a motion was introduced from Michigan asking that a special committee be appointed to investigate the criticisms of the Board of Trustees and of the editor, that an auditing expert go over all the books and that an independent study be made of the work of the headquarters office. On motion this was laid on the table. Then Dr. Philip Mills Jones moved a reconsideration of the vote and after some preliminary discussion it was ruled that it could not be reconsidered.

MORE NEW PROJECTS

Again came a mass of resolutions on a variety of topics such as the control of ophthalmia neonatorum, resolutions in behalf of contract surgeons, insurance fees, relief for California sufferers, a resolution to send THE JOURNAL free to medical libraries, a resolution on cancer, a resolution for a national department of health, a resolution on the extermination of mosquitoes, for the establishment of a section on tropical medicine, and many similar subjects.

The Section on Ophthalmology had for the first time printed all its papers in advance of the meeting, a procedure which it followed for many years. Papers were not read but merely presented briefly and then discussed. This innovation attracted much attention and there was extensive discussion of the procedure pro and con.

When the delegates left Boston and the editor returned to his headquarters in Chicago, he found himself sitting on the lid of a boiling pot. Chief agitation came from the commercial interests already referred to, which had begun to feel themselves seriously threatened by the trend in the development of controls. The national pure food bill had passed. It was the first step toward protection of the public against nostrums. Time was to show, however, that advertising made futile any attempts to protect the public by listing of composition or claims made on labels. Not until 1938 were there to be laws which would effectively control false claims made in advertising which were responsible for most of the sales of nostrums and "patent" medicines. These new laws would eventually reduce quackery in the United States to an infinitesimal percentage of that which prevailed in the early years of the twentieth century.

THE MEDICAL RECORD ATTACKS

The *New York Medical Record*, which was at that time owned by the publisher, William Wood & Company, constituted itself the spearhead of the attacks on the Board of Trustees and on the secretary-editor. That journal published a series of editorials questioning the financial management of the Association, accusing the editor of exploitation for personal gain and accusing the Board of Trustees of political manipulation and of operation as a hierarchy. From Detroit came a letter signed by Dr. J. H. Carstens reciting some of the charges made in the *Medical Record;* from Detroit also in the person of Dr. Leartus Connor, one of the older wheelhorses in the advancement of the American Medical Association, came a defense of the Board of Trustees and of THE JOURNAL. When THE JOURNAL published the letter by J. H. Carstens, which was dated August 1, the editor submitted the letter to Dr. T. J. Happel, then chairman of the Board of Trustees. Dr. Happel's reply was restrained and quiet. His most effective sentence was "I agree with the Rev. Sam Jones in cases of such complaints, when he says that 'if you throw a brick into a crowd you can tell who has been hit, because he always makes an outcry.' " However, Dr. Happel submitted in detail a complete statement as to the expenditures of the Association, including the salaries of its editor and its business manager. He told why the trustees had refused to publish complete copies of the payroll. He gave the exact details as to the money paid to Dr. J. N. McCormack for his work in organization. He gave the detail of the problems involved in the printing of the Directory and he indicated why the Board of Trustees thought it desirable that there be established a reserve fund for the Association.

By the second issue in September the editor printed an extended statement on the friends and enemies of the American Medical Association. He listed four different enemies:

1. The Proprietary Association of America, which, it will be remembered, circulated most malicious and libelous attacks on the American Medical Association, sending these to the newspapers all over the country, and which in other ways did all it could to create a public sentiment against the Association. This was because the American Medical Association lent its influence and support to the efforts that were being made to enlighten the public regarding the frauds that were being perpetrated on it by the "patent" medicine men.
2. The so-called "ethical" proprietary medicine men whose products or methods would not bear investigation.
3. Those privately owned medical journals which were more or less dependent on the income received from the foregoing.
4. The firm owning and publishing a medical directory.

The editor had not thought it desirable to reply to the attacks that had been made, "but when members of the Association of years' standing, men like Dr. Carstens, whose sincerity, honesty and loyalty to the Association are beyond suspicion, write letters and ask questions which show plainly that they have been misled and have accepted as facts the vague statements and indefinite insinuations made by those who are interested in creating dissatisfaction and suspicion, and when falsehoods and malicious misrepresentations are being circulated by journals hitherto of good repute and standing, then it is evident that the time has come to state some plain truths in order that the members of the profession may know the facts."

In the September 15 issue of THE JOURNAL the leading editorial was entitled "The Medical Record: An Enemy of the American Medical Association." The editorial was a fiery indictment of William Wood & Company, publishers of the *Medical Record*, and of its editor, who in four editorials had attacked the American Medical Association, its officers and its activity. The editor pointed out that the subscriptions to the *Record* had been steadily falling off and the nostrums in its advertising pages steadily increasing. His editorial accused the editor of the *Medical Record* of insinuations and deliberate misstatements of fact. It accused him of malicious misrepresentations. It called attention to the manner in which minor medical journals joined their own shrill cries of graft, fraud and cliques to the statements of the *Medical Record*. The final point in the editorial was a quotation from the *Medical Record* to the effect that "at Boston a strenuous effort was made to get rid of the editor, and that so great has become the dissatisfaction with his administration that this endeavor might have been successful had the general body any voice in the management of the Association." Here in a single paragraph is the editor's reply—and it is good, strong language:

> This statement is unqualifiedly false, as all who attended the Boston session well know. There was an opposition, it is true, and a bitter one, but it was limited to the horde of nostrum venders who have been getting rich by humbugging and deceiving our profession, and to the owners or attaches of those medical journals nourished by the same brood, who allow themselves to be used as the mouthpieces and tools of proprietary interests. The Editor of THE JOURNAL OF THE AMERICAN MEDICAL ASSOCIATION knows full well that he is hated with a most intense hatred by these gentlemen and their allies, and that they would stop at nothing to secure his "dismissal," but he also knows, and knows thoroughly well, that the "management" was fully and completely endorsed by 95 per cent of the physicians at the Boston session and, for that matter, is endorsed by a like proportion of the physicians of the country who know the truth of what is going on.

The battle against the proprietary medicines had assumed strong proportions. Articles in defense of the policy of the Association were contributed by Dr. Frank Billings, Abraham Jacobi, Jabez N. Jackson and George Dock.

In its attack on the most vicious of the proprietaries manufactured by fly-by-night pharmaceutical organizations, THE JOURNAL reached out occasionally to pick off a product of some of the leading manufacturers. The campaign was beginning to be felt from the very bottom to the utmost heights of the medical profession and the associated industries.

In the meantime the quality of THE JOURNAL was continuing to improve steadily. The councils were rendering regular important reports. The attacks on the American Medical Association being made in the public press were rallying physicians to its defense. Many a lukewarm member was becoming interested in the fight and getting ready to lend a hand on the side of righteousness. Surely this was the cleaning of the Augean stables. Nostrums, quacks, "patent" medicines, bogus medical schools, exploiting directories, unprincipled medical periodicals and commercially tainted manufacturers were being seized by the shovel and the pitchfork. The fierce light of publicity was illuminating the cleansing. The people were beginning to appreciate the sincerity of the profession which had as a fundamental motivation the continuous policing of its own house for their benefit.

There were occasional excursions as well into the quality of English medical writing, the dishonesty of multiple publications of the same article in a variety of medical journals and of plagiarism of articles from foreign publications as well as domestic.

As 1906 came to its end, THE JOURNAL stopped to take stock of the fundamental motivations of the Association as they had developed in the previous sixty years. The American Medical Association had been from the beginning a delegated body. However, it had not really accumulated strength and importance until the reorganization. By the end of 1906 it could report 60,000 members of the constituent state associations and a House of Delegates truly representative of these members. By 1947 it was to report more than 130,000 members.

FUNDAMENTAL MOTIVATIONS

The American Medical Association had been organized primarily to raise the standard of medical education. Year after year by means of resolutions and by the efforts on the part of the medical colleges themselves there had been gradual improvement. However, the first really effective measure was the establishment of the Council on Medical Education and the beginning of regular publication year by year of the status of medical schools considered acceptable to the Council and of the extent to which the graduates of the medical schools were able to pass the state licensing boards.

One of the first questions to come before the preliminary convention in 1847 was the regulation of pharmaceuticals. Repeatedly such resolutions had come before the Association, notably in 1850 and in 1879, but the establishment of the Council on Pharmacy and Chemistry in 1905 and the persistent publication in THE JOURNAL of the exact facts regarding the promotion of nostrums was the fundamental step in improving the quality of medical practice and in freeing the public largely from the hazard of "patent" medicines.

There had never been an official register of physicians, although the need of such a register was felt as early as 1847. A directory had been proposed in 1849. Commercial directories designed to exploit both the public and the medical profession had grown in response to the need. With the inspiration of Dr. George H. Simmons, the publication of an honest directory was undertaken by the American Medical Association. This biographic index maintained from day to day in the headquarters office is one of the greatest assets of the American Medical Association. In every war in which our nation has participated, the American Medical Association has been the possessor of the official roster of the medical profession and has been the fundamental agency in providing our armed forces with a high quality of medical service. It has been invariably necessary for the full time officers of our military services to depend on the vast number of volunteers from the civilian profession to provide medical service during war.

The matter of the establishment of THE JOURNAL as the property of the Association was first proposed in 1852, when Dr. J. B. Flint of Kentucky proposed to amend the Constitution to provide for the establishment and maintenance of a quarterly journal. The gradual development of sentiment toward the publication of a weekly periodical, which culminated with the establishment of THE JOURNAL in 1883, has been traced in the preceding chapters of this history. THE JOURNAL has been the life-blood and the heart of the American Medical Association. Its earnings have paid not only its own expenses but those of the Association as well. Its surplus has been devoted to improvement in the quality of the publication, to obtaining a permanent home and printing plant adequate for the needs of the Association. It has been the powerful voice of the medical profession in raising the standards of medical education, investigating the preparations and composition of drugs and pharmaceutical preparations, compiling and publishing an official directory of the profession and supporting one campaign after another for the advancement of medical science and the provision of medical care to all the people.

1907
ATLANTIC CITY

When the Board of Trustees met in Chicago in its new building early in 1907, the first message was one from W. C. Abbott indicating that it was going to be necessary for the Abbott Company to sell bonds to the medical profession. Dr. Abbott wished to be relieved of any promises given to the Board of Trustees on a previous occasion. The Board promptly moved that Dr. Abbott be notified that the Board would hold itself relieved from any agreements made between the Board and Dr. Abbott previously.

Many minor matters were discussed by the Board of Trustees: for instance, whether or not there ought to be an advertisement on the front cover of THE JOURNAL and whether or not discounts should be given to some advertisers, such as the owners of sanatoriums.

ADDRESS OF PRESIDENT WILLIAM J. MAYO

When the Board of Trustees met with the House of Delegates at the meeting in Atlantic City in June they heard Dr. William J. Mayo, then President of the Association, make a few apt remarks on the work of the organization. First he pointed out that it was a wise provision which placed the real responsibility for the conduct of the affairs of the Association on the Board of Trustees. He congratulated the Association on the work of Dr. George H. Simmons and he said "his courage and fighting for the best interests as a whole, often at a personal sacrifice, must commend itself to every right thinking man." Already, he pointed out, THE JOURNAL was being recognized abroad as a periodical of the highest scientific standards. As he ended this portion of his statment he said "and finally I must pay tribute to the Board of Trustees, not in the perfunctory expressions of one who is about to sever slight official connection wth them, but rather as one who wishes to express his real appreciation of their wise control of the affairs of the Association, a control which has enabled the American Medical Association to become the largest and most powerful medical organization in the world." He emphasized the work of the Council on Medical Education and of the Council on Pharmacy and Chemistry. He indicated the battle that was going on between the medical profession and the insurance companies as to the fees being paid physicians for their examinations, and he concluded by recommending that a committee be appointed to consider measures for expediting the business of the House of Delegates.

By this time the Association had cleaned its advertising pages to such an extent that the Board of Trustees was able to announce that from that time on all proprietary medicines would have to be approved by the full Council on Pharmacy and Chemistry before they could be considered acceptable for advertising in THE JOURNAL.

Most extensive was the report on the publication of the Directory, which had been undertaken at a tremendous cost to the American Medical Association. It was recognized that this was a cost well justified by the importance of the Directory to the organization.

As it came to the end of its report the Board of Trustees emphasized that profits made in any one year must be held at least to some extent to meet lean years. The board said "THE JOURNAL has had a number of years of prosperity, but this cannot always continue, and the only safe refuge will be a strong reserve fund. Any talk about reducing the price of THE JOURNAL before you have placed it on a sound footing is folly. Its business interests should always be carefully guarded." The Board of Trustees was able to report, however, that even though more than $25,000 worth of advertisements had been refused, the total gain from advertisements during the year had been $3,000 over the previous year.

MEDICAL EDUCATION

This was the period when the Council on Medical Education was beginning its most fundamental work inspecting medical colleges and rating them. There were 160 medical schools; 82 had been rated above 70, 46 between 50 and 70 and 32 below 50. The Council condemned medical schools conducted solely for profit, night schools, schools designed to prepare students to pass state board examinations, quiz courses and many other abuses.

MEDICAL LEGISLATION

In the years that occupied the first decade of the twentieth century one of the most important committees in the work of the American Medical Association was the Committee on Medical Legislation. This had been under the leadership of Dr. Charles A. L. Reed of Cincinnati, who had a natural aptitude for such work. He had created a national legislative council which met in Washington, as has already been described, and it kept close contact with every measure of importance introduced into the Congress relating to the medical profession. It had established a Bureau of Medical Legislation in the headquarters office and it was seeking expansion of that agency and of its efforts.

COMMITTEE ON HYGIENE AND PUBLIC HEALTH

The Committee on Hygiene and Public Health of the House of Delegates was concerned with education of the public. The committee proposed a board of public education in the American Medical Association. Interviews with such leaders as President Eliot of Harvard, President Stone of the Associated Press and editors of several Philadelphia newspapers on the need for education of the public regarding medicine, disease and health were reported to the House of Delegates. The committee encouraged the delivery of lectures to the public in schools, colleges and forums. President Eliot of Harvard pointed out that Harvard Medical School had already begun a long course of lectures of this sort given to the public in Boston. The committee proposed to develop a series of pamphlets for education of the public to be sold at reasonable prices. This proposal led to the ultimate formation of the Council on Health and Public Instruction of the American Medical Association. Indeed, promptly following this favorable report by a reference committee, Dr. Alexander R. Craig of Pennsylvania introduced an amendment to the By-Laws for the creation of a board of public instruction on medical subjects.

REFERENCE COMMITTEES PROPOSED FOR EARLY STUDY

At this meeting of the House of Delegates a report was adopted to the effect that reference committees be appointed two months in advance of the annual session and that reports be referred to these committees early enough for consideration. The difficulty of handling the vast amount of work presented to the House of Delegates by the Board of Trustees and the various councils and committees is one that has not yet been suitably surmounted. Apparently the delegates in that day were seeking some sort of solution, but obviously that solution has not yet been found. The reference committee on this occasion, under the leadership of Dr. Philip Mills Jones of California, took occasion in its report to commend the Board of Trustees, no doubt as an answer to some of the criticisms that had been made in the previous year. Thus the reference committee said "Any organization or corporation transacting business can only be successful so long as its affairs are conducted in a careful and up to date businesslike manner, and it is with pleasure that we note the essentially thorough and businesslike manner in which the trustees have conducted the affairs of this Association. We believe that the statement of audit is sufficiently definite and comprehensive and to make public further and more intimate business details would be unwise and poor business policy."

When the section of the report dealing with the work of the Board of Trustees was read, an attack on the Board was opened by Dr. H. W. Coe of Oregon. He accused the Board of Trustees of selecting an auditor and said that the auditor ought to be selected by the House of Delegates. He objected to the listing of inventory as an asset. He wanted to know the meaning of the word "agents." Then Dr. J. W. Grosvenor of New York objected to an item called "sundries." He wanted to know what kind of boxes the American Medical Association was selling. He wanted to see a full copy of the payroll. Dr. M. L. Harris, speaking for the trustees, explained the meaning of the statements which had been questioned and apparently became a little annoyed because he ended his first statement with the words "the gentleman has no business ability or he would not ask such simple questions." At this point the President of the American Medical Association warned him, saying "Be careful, Doctor, what you say; be careful; you are reaching a dangerous point." Dr. Harris then proceeded to explain the meaning of the word "sundries" and of "boxes." After some discussion by members of the House of Delegates who were insistent that the report gave every possible amount of information that might be wanted, the report was passed, and Dr. George H. Simmons was called on for a statement. He began as follows:

> During the last two years I have been accused of everything in the category from being a grafter to a swindler and everything else. Dr. Billings has been grouped with me. Members of the Board of Trustees have been grouped with me. There have been insinuations cast that are not pleasant.

He then continued to explain the technic of auditing the business of the Association and stated that all representatives of the Association were bonded. He pointed out:

> There is not an item paid out at the office of THE JOURNAL that is not represented by a receipt, even if it is a nickel for the boy to pay his street car fare.

Incidentally Dr. Simmons became so sensitive on this point that he continued to sign vouchers covering the purchase of even a paper of pins until he retired in 1924.

When Dr. Simmons finished his speech, Dr. L. S. McMurtry of Kentucky moved that the House of Delegates tender a vote of confidence and thanks. This was seconded by Dr. Coe. Dr. Hubert Work of Colorado moved that the motion include the trustees, and the whole motion was unanimously carried.

Much debate in this House of Delegates concerned suggestion to erect a monument in memory of Dr. N. S. Davis; the whole consideration was postponed for a year.

THE ARCHIVES OF INTERNAL MEDICINE

One of the most significant actions taken by the Board of Trustees at the session in 1907 was the decision to establish a magazine in the field of internal medicine. Some of the leading clinicians in the United States felt that it was desirable that a publication be developed in the field of clinical medicine. Here are such names as Frank Billings, Henry A. Christian, David L. Edsall, W. S. Thayer, Richard C. Cabot, George Dock and James B. Herrick. At the suggestion of Dr. William H. Welch, a committee including Drs. Joseph L. Miller, George Dock, William Sidney Thayer and David L. Edsall was established to report to the Board in October on the publication of such a journal. Dr. Welch suggested that these men should constitute the editorial staff in case the journal was agreed on. When the Board met again in October the committee made an extended report on the publication of such a periodical and suggested that Dr. Joseph L. Miller act as editor. The complete history of the ARCHIVES OF INTERNAL MEDICINE appears as a separate chapter in this history.

1908

CHICAGO

Dr. Joseph D. Bryant occupied the chair when the House of Delegates convened in Chicago in June. Dr. Bryant's presidential address to the House of Delegates complained that there was little for the President to do in the organization. He felt that in some manner the President ought to be more closely tied to the work, but he was much more grieved by the many complaints that had arisen in connection with the exposés of secret remedies and "patent" medicines, which had stirred a furor in the land. There were complaints that businesses were being destroyed, and these were falling on the President of the Association as well as on the Board and the editor.

THE SALARIED ORGANIZER

The Board of Trustees in its report to the House of Delegates felt that the time had come when the Association could and should dispense with the expense of a salaried organizer. Some $40,000 altogether had been expended in building the organization. In recommending discontinuance of the work, the Board said "The American Medical Association will ever owe Dr. J. N. McCormack a debt of gratitude for the great work that he has done in this special department." It recommended that he be employed in securing support for pure food legislation and the need of uniform state laws governing the practice of medicine before the legislators of the different states and as an educator of the public in medical matters.

PUBLIC INSTRUCTION

In this year came the first report of the Board of Public Instruction. This board had prepared an extensive outline of subjects on which the public was to be instructed, covering all the basic sciences, medical and preventive medical problems, and the history of medicine. The board proposed that lectures be provided throughout the country and that outlines of the material that was being extended to the public be included with THE JOURNAL.

Arrangements had been made to have the aid of the laboratory of the Public Health and Marine Hospital Service for the work of the Council on Pharmacy and Chemistry.

The House of Delegates approved a vote of thanks to Hon. George B. Cortelyou, Secretary of the Treasury, "for the interest he had manifested and the active part he had taken in issuing a departmental order recognizing officially the American Medical Association and the work of the Council on Pharmacy and Chemistry, and for his efforts in furtherance of pure food and drug legislation."

THE McCORMACK VALEDICTORY

In making the final report for the Committee on Organization, Dr. J. N. McCormack told of the work that he had done during the year. He had met with opposition and attack because he had carried the campaign against "patent" medicines and nostrums into the county and state societies, and his valedictory was as follows:

> It only remains for me to tell you that when I leave this platform my official connection with the Association is ended. For eight years I have been almost a stranger to my home and my family that I might serve you. My constant regret has been that my capacity for service was not greater. I want to urge on you that this work is in its infancy and that it must be continued year by year until the new generation of students, educated as I am pleading they shall be in these matters, have taken our places, if the profession is ever to obtain the full measure of its usefulness to itself and to the people. As a business

proposition, on a very conservative estimate, I am convinced that my work has added indirectly hundreds of thousands of dollars to your revenues, but that is the smallest part of it, as will one day be known. At least two carefully selected men should be put in the field, and others should be added from year to year until the benefactions of this work are felt, not only by every doctor, but at every hearthstone in this great country—that is, until the profession is really organized.

In conclusion I want to urge you to stand by our great file leader, Dr. Simmons, while he is conducting this reform work to its conclusion. After standing by his side for eight years, often when the result was in doubt, I have been able to know him as no other man ever can. He will make mistakes of the head in the future as he has in the past, but no one will ever be so ready to recognize and right them as he will. I know him, and you can trust him. And to each of you, my co-laborers, and the thousands of my friends you represent in cities, towns and country districts, may I now paraphrase the lines of the Scottish bard and say:

> "The Monarch may forget the crown,
> So lately placed upon his brow;
> The bridegroom may forget the bride,
> To whom so late he made his vow;
> The mother may forget the babe,
> So lately fondled on her knee;
> But I remember thee, my friend,
> And all that thou hast done for me."

When the report on the work of Dr. J. N. McCormack came from the reference committee, it refused to accept the section dealing with the discontinuance of Dr. McCormack as an organizer and recommended as a supplement that he be continued in addition to his duty as organizer.

At this meeting the House of Delegates established a council on the defense of medical research, and later in the session Dr. Frank Billings offered a resolution that the House of Delegates fully and heartily endorsed the work of Dr. J. N. McCormack and recommended the Board of Trustees to continue him in the same capacity for another year.

OPHTHALMIA

Significant in the House of Delegates also for some years had been the report of the Committee on Ophthalmia Neonatorum. This committee, under the chairmanship of F. Park Lewis, did a vital work of introducing the use of silver nitrate for the prevention of blindness throughout the nation.

SIGNED PAPERS FOR THE PUBLIC

For some time the House of Delegates debated in great detail the question as to whether or not papers for education of the public should be signed by their authors. The debate waxed so warm that the entire issue was recommitted to the reference committee for further consideration.

MISCELLANEOUS

For the first time appears the name of Dr. Arthur T. McCormack of Kentucky rising in support of the work of the Council on Pharmacy and Chemistry and calling on the state medical journals to support the Council in the advertisements that they published.

The American Medical Association cooperated in setting up an American committee for the sixteenth International Medical Congress. It agreed to cooperate with the American Association for the Advancement of Science. It endorsed the candidacy of Dr. C. A. L. Reed for senator from Ohio and again agreed unanimously that there ought to be a department of health in the United States government with a secretary in the cabinet. The decision as to whether or not articles for the public should be signed was left to the Board of Public Instruction. A resolution was adopted expressing confidence in and appreciation of the work of the editor.

1909
ATLANTIC CITY

When the Board of Trustees opened its considerations in 1909 it was confronted with another request from Dr. W. C. Abbott to explain his case. He appeared and explained for fifteen minutes. His explanation was referred to a committee of three for report in the following June.

At the meeting of the Board of Trustees in Chicago in 1908 Dr. T. J. Happel was succeeded as chairman of the Board of Trustees by Dr. William H. Welch. He remained, however, as a member of the Board. He was taken ill suddenly during the meeting of the Board in February 1909 and died in May of that year. He had been a member of the Board of Trustees for eleven years and its chairman for seven years.

THE ABBOTT PROBLEM

Dr. Abbott had met with the committee, which now reported to the board that he be placed on the same basis as any other reputable firm in regard to advertising in THE JOURNAL. During this period he had conducted a campaign against Dr. George H. Simmons and the work of the Council on Pharmacy and Chemistry which left feelings of ill will that prevailed for many years.

MORE PRESIDENTIAL SUGGESTIONS

President Burrell was unable to attend the Atlantic City session in 1909, but he sent a special message to the House of Delegates with four specific recommendations involving the work of the Association. He recommended first that the President and President

Elect of the Association be invited to attend all meetings of the Board of Trustees and that the policies of councils and committees, such as those on Medical Legislation, Medical Education and Pharmacy and Chemistry, should be submitted to the Board of Trustees and approved before going to the House of Delegates or to the public. He recommended that expenses of travel of all members of committees and councils be paid by the Association. He deprecated the tendency of members of the Association to use political methods in influencing legislation—state and national—and he was opposed particularly to the placing of a representative in Washington. His exact words were:

> The employment of one individual to serve as a lobbyist in Washington or elsewhere is a mistake; it is the adoption of trade union methods and will sooner or later bring the medical profession into discredit.

Next he suggested for consideration by the Board the separation of the offices of editor and general manager and secretary of the Association. He felt that the limelight of public opinion had been turned on this individual and that it was wrong that he should carry that responsibility. This was not in any sense a criticism of his acts. Indeed, he felt that Dr. George H. Simmons was deserving of the highest possible commendation for his remarkable conduct of an extremely trying double office.

STATE MEDICAL JOURNALS

In 1899 not a single state association owned and published its own state journal. By 1909 nineteen states had developed state medical journals.

The Board of Trustees was able to report that the ARCHIVES OF INTERNAL MEDICINE had begun publication in January 1908 and that it had succeeded beyond expectation from the beginning.

Already it had been found that the headquarters building was inadequate to the growing needs of the Association, and the Board of Trustees had promptly contracted for a new structure. The board was proud to call attention to the fact that the previous ten years had been the most remarkable decade in the history of the organization. The circulation of THE JOURNAL had increased 500 per cent. The Association had now enlarged and outgrown one of the largest medical printing plants, and the assets had been increased to hundreds of thousands of dollars.

The Association had made comprehensive studies of medical education and had elevated standards. It had made itself felt in national legislation. It had laid bare innumerable frauds. It had begun education of the masses in general matters pertaining to medicine. It was stimulating scientific investigation by rewards and grants and by scientific exhibits. In concluding its statement the Board of Trustees called attention to the firm defense that it had been compelled to make against the torrent of ridicule and abuse from proprietary medicine interests.

MEDICAL EDUCATION

By this year the Council on Medical Education had held five annual conferences. It had established minimum standards for medical education and for preliminary education. It had begun to concern itself with the quality of the medical curriculum. As a result of its efforts there had been five important mergers of medical colleges by which nine medical schools had been replaced by four stronger ones. It presented a list of fourteen steps toward improvement of medical education and it had been exceedingly active in improving the quality of medical licensure.

The Committee on Ophthalmia Neonatorum made an extensive report indicating how effective had been its drive toward prophylaxis against blindness resulting from gonorrheal infection during childbirth.

There was an extensive report by the Committee on Patents, the Committee on Drug Reform, the Committee on the Memorial to Nathan Smith Davis, and the Committee on Uniform Regulations of Membership.

At this session the name of the Section on Cutaneous Medicine and Surgery was changed to the Section on Dermatology.

The reference committee whch considered the recommendations of the President, Dr. Herbert L. Burrell, concurred in the suggestion that the President and President-Elect meet with the Board of Trustees. At this time occurred the addition to the Constitution and By-Laws of the important provision which gave the Board of Trustees responsibility for supervision of the actions of committees constituted by action of the House of Delegates between sessions of the House. It was felt that the decisions as to the separation of the offices of editor and general manager and of the secretary were under the authority of the Board of Trustees.

COUNCIL ON DEFENSE OF MEDICAL RESEARCH

The Council on Defense of Medical Research, which included such distinguished names as Walter B. Cannon, chairman, Simon Flexner, David L. Edsall, Harvey Cushing, Reid Hunt and J. A. Capps, reported regulations that it had adopted regarding abuse of experimentation and against misconceptions of its conditions and purposes and concerning the dissemination to the public of the tremendous advances that had been made with the use of animal experimentation.

Incidentally, in the establishment of the Section on Dermatology it was made clear that the subject of syphilis belonged to dermatology and not to urology.

THE MEDICAL TRUST AND OLIGARCHY

ST. LOUIS, 1910

AN AUTOMOBILE NUMBER

THE MOTOR CAR HAD BECOME so definitely an important factor in the practice of medicine by 1910 that THE JOURNAL OF THE AMERICAN MEDICAL ASSOCIATION issued its first automobile number. The section of THE JOURNAL devoted to this purpose appeared in the issue for April 9, 1910; it was entitled "The Choice and Care of an Automobile." It is, in the light of thirty-seven years of subsequent progress with this important appurtenance of medical practice, one of the most amazing collections of information in world history. There are many pictures of the vehicles of that day and some fascinating records of personal experiences of physicians with their vehicles. One section is devoted wholly to the motorcycle, with some debate as to whether or not doctors would do better with motorcycles than with automobiles. One article defends the gasoline propelled vehicle running on railroad tracks. The chapter on the business office pictures some of the advertisements.

THE MEDICAL TRUST

During this year of the presidency of Dr. William H. Welch came the first organized attack on the American Medical Association as a medical trust. The proprietary medical interests had been so seriously damaged by the exposés which were being regularly published in THE JOURNAL OF THE AMERICAN MEDICAL ASSOCIATION that they established an agency known as the National League of Medical Freedom. This organization was designed to defeat the Owen bill for the creation of a national department of health but more particularly to discredit and disrupt the American Medical Association. Its attacks centered on the editor of THE JOURNAL, Dr. George H. Simmons. Detectives were employed to search out his past history, to follow him day by day and to muster public opinion against him. Among the leaders in these attacks were such names, now in excellent repute, as those of Dr. Abbott of the Abbott Laboratories and Mr. Post, inventor of the Post products, out of which has come the great corporation known as General Foods.

These attacks were bitter and vicious; full-page advertisements were purchased in newspapers throughout the nation; it became necessary for the editor of THE JOURNAL to answer them personally and publicly. This he did with a systematic analysis of the nature of the attacks and the powers behind them that carried conviction.

THE BOARD OF TRUSTEES

Incidentally for the first time THE JOURNAL published the minutes of an iterim meeting of the Board of Trustees, so that the members of the Association might keep abreast of the increasing activities of this most powerful body in the affairs of the Association. By this time the multiple affairs of the Association had developed so greatly that Dr. M. L. Harris was drafted to prepare a form for presentation of the report of the Board of Trustees annually. This form was adopted and has been followed since that time.

THE AMERICAN JOURNAL OF DISEASES OF CHILDREN

The success of the American Medical Association with the publication of the ARCHIVES OF INTERNAL MEDICINE led to petitions for the publication of a journal devoted to pediatrics, presented by a committee consisting of Drs. Isaac Abt and F. S. Churchill. The Board of Trustees established a committee including such distinguished names as those of Drs. Abraham Jacobi, L. Emmett Holt and J. P. C. Griffith to investigate the need for such a publication.

A PERIODICAL ON PUBLIC HEALTH

From the Section on Preventive Medicine and Public Health and the Bureau of Medical Legislation came a request for publication by the American Medical Association of a periodical devoted to public health, for the establishment of scholarships in the field of preventive medicine and for similar purposes. It was proposed also that there be established a council to deal with problems of health and preventive medicine and to rate the public health work of the individual states. The council was to be called the Council on Legislation, Organization and Publicity. From a number of leading surgeons of the United States came a request to publish a periodical devoted to surgery; a committee was established to look into this subject.

When the President of the Association, Dr. William C. Gorgas, distinguished sanitarian of the Panama Canal, made his retiring address to the House of Delegates he noted that some question had been raised as to the right of the president to fill vacancies in standing committees that occurred in interims between meetings of the House of Delegates. The rapid growth of the American Medical

Association had resulted in the establishment of too many committees and boards, and there was a tendency to take up new work without completing some of the projects already in hand. Dr. Gorgas was forced to take cognizance that the Association had made bitter enemies of the people engaged in the "patent" medicine business and, "as they command large capital, they are at present making a serious organized fight against us. This is the most altruistic part of our activity for the benefit of others or for the members of the Association."

THE SECRETARYSHIP

In presenting his report to the House of Delegates, Dr. George H. Simmons gave a brief account of his work as secretary of the Association. As far back as 1901 he had wanted to relinquish the position of secretary. In 1904 he suggested again that he resign the secretaryship, but the Board of Trustees advised against this. It had recommended the employment of an assistant to the secretary whose duty it would be to look after the details of that work. The position was filled by Dr. Frederick R. Green, who accepted it and who assumed in 1905 the duties of assistant to the general secretary. Dr. Simmons stated also that he had finally decided that he would not care further to be the secretary of the Association and he now definitely requested the election of a new secretary. He said:

> I realize that it is not usual to refuse a thing, especially an elective office, before it is offered. I think it better, however, to make the announcement now, so that there may be ample time for you to consider carefully whom you shall select for the position.

"For eleven consecutive years," he continued, "I have been unanimously elected general secretary, twice at the general meeting, before the reorganization, and nine times by the House of Delegates." The reference committee recommended to the House of Delegates that Dr. Simmons' desire be respected, but it paid testimony to his work in a few well chosen words:

> **Dr. Simmons** needs no assurance as to the temper and position of this body concerning him personally and officially. It always has stood, and stands today, a solid wall behind him and has no words to express fully its high appreciation of his efficient and faithful service.

The committee recommended that his wish be granted in order that his great ability may be exclusively devoted to the duties of editor of THE JOURNAL OF THE AMERICAN MEDICAL ASSOCIATION—the best medical journal in existence.

When the Board of Trustees made its report, the statement was read by Dr. M. L. Harris, chairman, who presented a vast amount of material in an exceedingly concise and direct form. He listed the special projects which concerned the organization and he indicated that all the work had been reflected from time to time in THE JOURNAL. Especially, however, did he commend the work of the Council on Pharmacy and Chemistry.

THE PUBLIC HEALTH EDUCATION COMMITTEE OF WOMEN

The Board of Trustees had been greatly concerned over the appointment under somewhat doubtful auspices of a special committee known as the Public Health Education Committee of Women. Apparently a resolution had been adopted by the House of Delegates on June 10, 1909, offered by Dr. Charles A. L. Reed, requesting the women physicians of the American Medical Association to take the initiative individually in their respective associations, in the organization of educational committees to act through women's clubs, mothers' associations and other similar bodies for the dissemination of accurate information touching these subjects among the people. They were requested to submit to the House of Delegates a yearly report of such work and elect from among their numbers a committee to take charge of it. The Board of Trustees asked the lawyers for the Association to find out whether or not such a resolution would warrant the women physicians of the American Medical Association in appointing such a committee without having it nominated by the President and further whether or not the Board of Trustees would be warranted in paying expenses already incurred by that committee. The attorneys said that there was no provision for any such action in the Constitution and By-Laws and that therefore such a committee had no legal standing as a committee of the Association. Then came a report from the women's committee, which was read by Drs. Rosalie Slaughter Morton and Mary Sutton Macy. These ladies submitted an extensive report indicating how hard they had been working; apparently they requested some funds as reimbursement for some of their activities. Now the chairman of the Board of Trustees called attention to the misunderstanding; he indicated that it was proposed to establish a council for public health education and that the work of this women's committee would probably come under a secretary's bureau for the purpose.

MEDICAL LEGISLATION

At this meeting of the House of Delegates the Committee on Medical Legislation, headed by C. A. L. Reed, made an extensive report on legislation before the Congress and before the individual states. The committee indicated the great importance of a department of publicity to inform the public on legislation affecting the practice of medicine. At this time Dr. C. A. L. Reed tendered his resignation with an extensive valedictory message based on his eight years of experience. A few wise observations in this little known statement merit thought in modern times:

> The time has passed when any organization, however altruistic its purposes, can throw the whole burden of its duties on a single person and expect to pay the obligation by the honor thus conferred.
>
> For any member of the national organization, not a resident of a given state, to appear before the legislature of that state either for or against a given measure, would, under ordinary circumstances, tend to prejudice the cause at issue before the legislators.
>
> It is hardly worth while to work seventeen years for a food and drugs act if its power to protect the people is destroyed by executive interpretation in the short space of seventeen months.

The Board of Public Instruction on Medical Subjects, which was eventually to be merged into the Council on Health and Public Instruction, had published two popular articles during the year—one on the venereal peril and the other on typhoid. The committee on ophthalmia neonatorum was making great progress toward the acceptance of its proposals by the individual states.

DAVIS MEMORIAL

The new committee on the Davis memorial was having just about the same amount of trouble in getting funds for that purpose as had the committee on the Rush memorial in the last quarter century. Only six states had contributed to the fund, and the total on hand was only a little over $700.

DEFENSE OF MEDICAL RESEARCH

The Committee on Defense of Medical Research had developed some excellent papers on animal experimentation, among them contributions by E. L. Trudeau on tuberculosis, James Ewing on cancer, James R. Angell on the ethics of animal experimentation and W. W. Keen on surgery.

Again the Constitution and By-Laws were completely revised and new arrangements made for a Constitution and By-Laws for the individual states.

ANESTHESIA

A committee on anesthesia had been developed to conduct extensive studies in this field. It concluded that ether was the anesthetic of choice for the general practitioner and for all anesthetists not especially skilled.

A NEW BADGE

In 1910 the Association discarded its insignia which included a red cross and adopted the emblem which is still used. In developing the design the committee suggested that it convey a definite meaning both in color and in form. Scarlet and gold had been considered medical colors since ancient times, and the true ancestral symbol of the healing art was the knotty rod and serpent of Aesculapius. One member of the committee wanted an eagle on the emblem, but other members were opposed to the eagle and it was omitted.

NEW SECTIONS

Petitions came for a new section on physical forces in medicine and for a new section on urology and venereal diseases.

The House of Delegates endorsed the statistical and editorial work of THE JOURNAL leading toward control of Fourth of July fatalities and casualties.

COUNCIL ON LEGISLATION

Now came the organization of the Council on Legislation, Health and Publicity, to consist of five members elected by the House of Delegates on nomination by the President.

SECTION ON GENITOURINARY DISEASES

The committee recommended the establishment of a section on genitourinary diseases; the first officers appointed for that section were Drs. W. T. Belfield, Chicago, chairman; James Pederson, New York, vice chairman, and Dr. Hugh Young, Baltimore, secretary. The reference committee did not believe, however, that the time was opportune for the establishment of a section on physical forces in medicine or for a section on hospitals. These came later.

RATING THE MEDICAL COLLEGES

The House of Delegates authorized publicity for the rating of medical colleges in the United States, and the first rating of class A, B and C colleges was published. This publication was to be of vital significance in eliminating the weaker medical schools and in raising the standards of all the medical schools in the United States.

Again there were calls for elimination of the office of coroner.

DEATH OF RICKETTS

In this year, Dr. Howard Taylor Ricketts died while undertaking investigations into typhus in Mexico; the House of Delegates adopted a memorial in recognition of his death, and THE JOURNAL published important editorials on the significance of his work.

The women's committee made an extensive report on its activities. This was referred to the Reference Committee on Hygiene and Public Health.

SIMMONS RE-ELECTED SECRETARY

When the time came for the election of secretary, a movement began to force Dr. George H. Simmons to retain the office. The movement was successful and he was unanimously elected.

NEW SPECIAL PERIODICALS

As the session ended, the Board of Trustees was encouraged by the House of Delegates to proceed with the publication of a journal of pediatrics and of surgery whenever it should think this step desirable.

Some members feared that publication of these special periodicals would involve losses to the Association, although there was unanimous agreement on the desirability of good scientific periodicals for the encouragement of the specialties. In discussion, Dr. George H. Simmons made it clear that the one purpose of these special periodicals was advancement of the specialties concerned. He said "I believe that we can do nothing that will help scientific medicine in this country so much as the publication of high class scientific journals that private publishers cannot publish, even though it may be done at a loss."

THE BATTLE WITH THE PROPRIETARIES

Behing the scenes were rumblings and turmoil that reflected the activities of the "patent" medicine interests which were trying to disrupt the Association. A communication had come from Dr. G. Frank Lydston insisting that the American Medical Association had no right to meet or to elect trustees or officers outside the state of Illinois. He hinted at procedures by the state's attorney unless his demand be followed. The letter from Dr. Lydston was laid on the table.

A resolution had been developed that there be further modification of the Constitution and By-Laws to make members of county and state medical societies members *ipso facto* of the American Medical Association, and the Board of Trustees was requested to draft a suitable amendment for the purpose. The final action taken with regard to the women's educational committee was to refuse to make any grants for the payment of work of that committee. It was also decided that every committee, council, officer or bureau entitled to funds submit a detailed budget before making expenditures.

1911
LOS ANGELES

The payroll of the American Medical Association as 1911 came on the scene included 23 salaried monthly officers and about 100 other employees in the clerical and mechanical departments. The average wages of printers varied from $20 to $30 a week and of the clerical employees about $15 a week.

By this time the Association was becoming a little touchy on the work of Dr. J. N. McCormack, who was receiving a salary of $6,000 a year for his organization and legislative work. Officially he was employed by the Council on Health and Public Instruction and not by the Board of Trustees. Dr. Alexander R. Craig had been employed as assistant to the secretary. A motion was passed that a periodical to be known as the American Archives of Surgery be published beginning with 1911.

ADDRESS BY DR. WELCH

When the Association convened in Los Angeles in 1911 Dr. William H. Welch made an address to the House of Delegates, contrasting the effectiveness of its actions with those of the general meeting in a previous era. Because of the great importance of actions taken by the House of Delegates he emphasized the desirabilty of selecting the most competent possible representatives for membership in this body.

IMPROVEMENT IN ORGANIZATION

In further development of the compact and efficient organization that he sought for the American Medical Association, Dr. George H. Simmons recommended a technic for transfer of membership when a physician changed his location. He suggested also a reorganization of the Judicial Council as a permanent body authorized to hold meetings when necessary to consider such questions as the secret division of fees, contract practice and advertising.

During the year the Association had moved into its new building.

COUNCIL ON HEALTH AND PUBLIC INSTRUCTION

The first report of the Council on Health and Public Instruction was made by its chairman, Dr. Henry B. Favill of Chicago. This distinguished body included, in addition, Drs. Walter B. Cannon, J. N. McCormack, Henry M. Bracken, W. C. Woodward and a full time employee, Dr. Frederick R. Green, as secretary. Special bureaus devoted to legislation, organization, publicity, protection of medical research and public health had been established under the Council.

Under its auspices addresses had been made throughout the nation, publications had been devoted to the defense of research, legislation had been studied in the national Congress and in the states, bulletins had been issued to the press on a great variety of subjects, and pamphlets had been issued through many state boards of health and of licensure. For instance, the special committee on public health education announced that over 2,800 lectures had been given to more than 230,000 people. Subcommittees considered in addition such subjects as visual standards for pilots, the prevention of blindness due to ophthalmia neonatorum, amblyopia from methyl alcohol, and trachoma. There were reports on blindness due to industrial accidents and faulty eye hygiene.

THE JUDICIAL COUNCIL

The reorganization of the Judicial Council was recommended in some amendments to the By-Laws.

Once the Judicial Council was officially established, the President appointed to its membership Dr. Frank Billings, Illinois; James E. Moore, Minnesota; A. B. Cooke, Tennessee; Alexander Lambert, New York, and Hubert Work, Colorado.

MEDICAL EDUCATION

The Council on Medical Education reported a reduction in medical colleges from 166 in 1904 to 129 in 1911. There were still, however, vast fields to conquer.

The House of Delegates urged the Council on Medical Education to inform the public concerning the status of medical education and the quality of medical colleges, utilizing the forces of the Council on Health and Public Instruction for that purpose.

For the first time the Council on Medical Education recommended the desirability of a five year instruction program, one year of which was to be spent as an intern. The Council urged that medical colleges be requested to adopt such an internship as rapidly as possible.

AMENDING THE PURE FOOD LAW

The Association was urging the Congress to amend the Pure Food and Drug Law so as to prevent false statements in regard to the results to be expected from the use of medicinal agents.

SECTION ON HOSPITALS

A proposal came for the establishment of a scientific section on hospitals.

ALBERT ABRAMS EMERGES

While the Board of Trustees was meeting in Los Angeles it received a remarkable letter from Dr. Albert Abrams of San Francisco in regard to a review of a book printed by him on the subject of spondylotherapy. The book had been somewhat unfavorably reviewed in THE JOURNAL, and the editor had refused the advertising pages of THE JOURNAL to the book. Dr. Albert Abrams threatened to bring suit unless the Board of Trustees reversed the action of the editor. The Board of Trustees approved the action of the editor and of the chairman of the board, Dr. M. L. Harris, in refusing space to Dr. Abrams. The subsequent career of Dr. Albert Abrams in the field of electronic medicine, an unusual form of quackery, indicated the wisdom of this early action in recognizing that he was about to depart from honest medicine into the field of fraud and charlatanism.

THE PHARMACOPEIA

Through its representatives to the U. S. Pharmacopeial Convention the Board of Trustees was initiating action to remove from the U. S. Pharmacopeia preparations of doubtful value. To this meeting of the Board of Trustees came a request from the Council on Pharmacy and Chemistry for funds to be devoted to research in therapy; the Board of Trustees gave its full support to this proposal.

ARCHIVES OF SURGERY

A special committee had met in New York to consider the publication of the ARCHIVES OF SURGERY and was proceeding with its plans, but it felt that a far more elaborate publication was needed than was then contemplated.

THE N. S. DAVIS HALL

As a memorial to Dr. Nathan Smith Davis, the Board of Trustees during this year established the library in the Association building as the N. S. Davis Hall and directed that a bronze bust of Davis be placed therein, the expense of this bronze bust to be paid for out of the Davis fund.

DR. CRAIG MADE SECRETARY

Dr. Alexander R. Craig had become secretary of the Association, and the Board of Trustees fixed his salary.

1912

ATLANTIC CITY

The Association had grown so large and the number of its sections so numerous that it now became necessary to restrict the amount of material published. Up to this time every paper read in a section and approved by the executive committee of the section was published in THE JOURNAL. Moreover, the discussions were lengthy and often of little merit. The Board of Trustees now suggested that discussions published in THE JOURNAL be limited to 500 words and that every possible effort be made to get the executive committees of the sections to limit the length of the papers and to withhold their approval from those that did not represent high quality.

ARGUMENT OVER A SURGICAL PUBLICATION

Now came a petition from 100 of the most prominent surgeons of the country requesting the Board of Trustees to proceed with the publication of the journal of surgery. At the same time, however, came another letter signed by Dr. Lewis S. Pilcher, editor of the *Annals of Surgery*, and Dr. Franklin H. Martin, editor of *Surgery, Gynecology and Obstetrics*, earnestly protesting the establishment by the Association of such a journal. They feared the publication of such a periodical, saying it "would practically put us out of business and leave the field of independent surgical journalism of this country to be occupied solely by journals of a less high scientific character." They said further "We believe it more in keeping with the high purpose of the American Medical Association to foster and forward the honest efforts of its members in the line of medical progress rather than to cripple or destroy them by unnecessary competition."

After hearing these two communications, the Board recommended that a surgical journal be developed along lines similar to those established for the ARCHIVES OF INTERNAL MEDICINE and the AMERICAN JOURNAL OF DISEASES OF CHILDREN.

DR. JOHN B. MURPHY MAKES NEW PROPOSALS

The meeting of the House of Delegates in 1912 brought forth a long address to the House by the President, Dr. John B. Murphy, dealing wholly with the work of the organization and making some revolutionary proposals as to its conduct. These included the breaking up of the Council on Health and Public Instruction so that the functions in regard to medical legislation would go to another council. He wished also a council on organization to be concerned with membership of the Association. He recognized the quality of THE JOURNAL but thought it ought to do much more in the way of answering inquiries and giving information to the medical profession. He made a brilliant attack on fee splitting and felt that the Principles of Ethics should be much more definite in its condemnation of this dishonest practice. He urged clinics in connection with the meetings of the

Association. And he desired particularly that the House of Delegates check the actions of the Board of Trustees, councils, committees and officers to make certain that they were carrying out the requests of the House. He wished to have the President, the secretary and the editor made ex officio members of the Board of·Trustees without voting power, and he urged also that provision be made to give to the House of Delegates complete information as to the action taken by the Board. This action was taken by the House of Delegates and has not been subsequently changed.

NEW COMMITTEES

In the meantime a number of committees appointed through actions of the House of Delegates were studying problems of great importance to the advancement of American medical science. For instance there was a committee to represent the American Medical Association at the third National Conservation Congress. There was a committee on nomenclature and classification of diseases which was conducting systematic studies on this subject. Another committee was concerned with standards in the field of anesthesia. Of this committee Dr. Yandell Henderson was chairman, and at this session of the House of Delegates Dr. Thomas S. Cullen, Baltimore, was appointed to the Committee on Anesthesia. Another committee had been established to consider the completion of the Panama Canal.

The Board of Trustees was able to announce the first publication of its book "Nostrums and Quackery," enlightening the public on frauds and quackeries; more than 10,000 copies had been promptly exhausted.

The Judicial Council, under Dr. Frank Billings as chairman, presented an extensive list of rules for its own procedures. It recommended revisions of the Constitution and By-Laws to improve still further ethical standards of the profession. These amendments concerned particularly the patenting of drugs and instruments, the maintenance of membership being made dependent on conduct in accord with the Principles of Ethics. They condemned the secret division of fees and the giving of commissions and urged amendments as well regarding contract practice.

NEW SECTION ON ORTHOPEDIC SURGERY

As evidence of the growth of scientific work in the Association there came a request for the establishment of a section on orthopedic surgery and another for a section on physical therapeutics. There had come previously a request for a section on proctology. The

House of Delegates established the Section on Orthopedic Surgery but rejected sections on both physical therapeutics and proctology.

THE SCIENTIFIC EXHIBIT

The Scientific Exhibit was growing in quality and in the total number of exhibits, but it was feeling itself a stepchild in the assignment of space at the annual session, and the House of Delegates moved that it be given first choice of location in the exhibition hall.

A JOURNAL OF HEALTH AGAIN PROPOSED

The meeting of the Association of 1910 had heard a recommendation from the President of the Association for the publication of a journal of health. This had finally reached the status of a special committee under Dr. William A. Evans, Illinois, to investigate the possibility of publishing a health journal. The committee urged the Board of Trustees to establish a popular priced health journal. The recommendation was referred to the Board of Trustees of the Association by the House of Delegates. The board replied to the House that, if the House wanted the publication, the board would proceed. Not until 1923 was this objective accomplished.

A JOURNAL FOR GENERAL PRACTITIONERS

In his address to the Association Dr. William H. Welch had suggested the desirability of publishing a small medical journal, because THE JOURNAL OF THE AMERICAN MEDICAL ASSOCIATION was too advanced and too technical for many practitioners. There were at that time 278 medical journals published in this country, many disgraceful to the profession that supported them. The report of the special committee to consider this matter was prepared by Dr. J. N. McCormack. He believed that the best method for meeting the objective would be encouragement by the American Medical Association to the state medical journals and aid to all periodicals conducted in accordance with reasonable rules as to plain honesty in their advertising and reading pages. The committee felt also that the American Medical Association might well aid these smaller publications through providing them with abstracts of the more scientific articles that appeared in the technical publications, of which there were so many in the field of medical science. As a result of these considerations THE JOURNAL OF THE AMERICAN MEDICAL ASSOCIATION undertook at that time the publication of a weekly bulletin of abstracts of important medical articles. This bulletin was sent regularly to smaller medical publications. By the use of these abstracts in the smaller medical journals the advancement of medical science was regularly extended to great numbers of physicians who otherwise would never have come in contact with medical progress.

COUNCIL ON HEALTH AND PUBLIC INSTRUCTION

Again one of the most extensive reports was that of the Council on Health and Public Instruction. This body was clearly attempting functions which, in the light of present day practices, would be grouped under the heading of public relations. It conceived its principal commission to be the development of public confidence in the purposes and work of the American Medical Association and of the medical profession. It conducted a press bureau and a speakers' bureau. It compiled a handbook for speakers. It organized and developed a bureau of literature concerned with the publication of great numbers of bulletins and pamphlets. It distributed educational matter on frauds and nostrums and it enlightened the public on medical legislation. It encouraged membership in the American Medical Association, aided the campaign against the antivivisectionists, collected state laws related to health, offered prizes for the best cartoons on public health subjects and distributed a bulletin, published occasionally, to county and state medical societies regarding the work of the American Medical Association and of this council. The number of its committees was great. They included subjects as profound as resuscitation for electric shock. It had a special committee which cooperated with the National Education Association and a committee on medical expert testimony on railroad sanitation, on vital statistics and on similar subjects. It participated with the Council on Medical Education in a joint annual conference on medical education and legislation, and all of its subcommittees, such as those on the prevention of blindness, visual standards for pilots, public health education among women, cooperation with the National Education Association and uniform regulation of membership, made special reports. Unfortunately the evolution of the work of the American Medical Association in succeeding years resulted in the lapsing of the work of this council, so that some years later it was discontinued by the House of Delegates and its various functions distributed among such agencies as HYGEIA. the Bureau of Investigation, the Bureau of Health Education, the Bureau of Medical Legislation and the Bureau of Exhibits. The special functions having to do with education of the public regarding medical legislation by the use of a speakers' bureau and special publications in that field lapsed entirely until the creation of the Council on Medical Service and, most recently, of a Bureau of Public Relations.

By an action of the House of Delegates taken at this session, the courtesy of the floor of the House of Delegates was extended to the members of the various councils and particularly to the secretaries of these councils so that they might advise the House at any time concerning their work.

DR. J. A. WITHERSPOON MADE PRESIDENT

At the elections on the fourth day of the annual session Dr. J. A. Witherspoon of Nashville, Tennessee, was elected President unanimously.

PRESIDENT JACOBI'S ADDRESS

One of the suggestions made by President Jacobi in his annual address dealt with the desirability of reforestation of the United States as a means of preventing floods. This recommendation was referred to a reference committee of which Dr. Hubert Work of Colorado was chairman. That committee recommended that the American Medical Association urge the Congress of the United States and the individual states to take immediate steps in the direction of extensive reforestation of the country and thereby to protect the country in the future gainst the return of similar calamities. This recommendation was adopted. A good many years later Hubert Work became Secretary of the Interior in the cabinet of President Coolidge. But reforestation began to be taken seriously by our government many years later!

Unusual at this session was a valedictory address by Dr. Abraham Jacobi to the House of Delegates. Some of his remarks were received with great appreciation of his wit. For instance, he said:

> I want you to understand that I am not used to presiding over such a body. I have done the best I could under the circumstances and I have just followed my instincts and what I have seen in inferior places. I am not used to it, because this is a queer place. There is no second and third term where people learn to be disagreeable and make people's lives uncomfortable. So you must excuse me perhaps for not having made things more uncomfortable for you.

He urged particularly that the American Medical Association develop great strength in order to secure the establishment of a department of health in the cabinet. He concluded:

> You want to get home. What I wanted to say was this, that our main position in life should be to wake up our neighbors, particularly the general practitioners, that vast number of men all over the country, and see to it that they participate in public affairs.

During the session of the House of Delegates the Board of Trustees again considered the publication of a health journal but decided that this was much too serious a proposition to be undertaken suddenly. Dr. Simmons was requested to look into the matter. He was never especially desirous of undertaking such a publication and it was not actually begun until just previous to the end of his term as editor. The Board of Trustees referred to the Council on Health and Public Instruction the question of publishing a health journal, and that council said it was not yet ready to give any advice on the subject.

MEETING OF STATE SECRETARIES

A motion was made before the Board of Trustees to provide for an annual meeting of state secretaries at the time of the meeting of the Board of Trustees in October.

GUIDES FOR THE SCIENTIFIC EXHIBIT

The Scientific Exhibit had grown so greatly that the board approved the appointment of guides, who were paid $5 a day, to show doctors around the exhibit.

NEW BUTTONS FOR OLD ONES

A decision was finally made that the button carry the letters A. M. A. and not the entire name of the Association. Then it became necessary to trade in the old buttons for the new buttons, and that had to be settled.

The attorneys of the Association rejected the proposal that the President, secretary and editor of the Association should be members of the Board of Trustees without the right to vote as being a violation of the corporation law of Illinois.

1913

MINNEAPOLIS

The year 1913 was to witness some fundamental changes in the conduct of the work of the American Medical Association resulting in part from the loss of personnel and, secondly, from evolutionary progress. The amount of material coming to THE JOURNAL increased so greatly that the Board of Trustees recommended to the House of Delegates that no more sections be created and, second, that no more than thirty papers be read in any one section. Furthermore, a special approval slip, to be used by the executive committees of the individual sections, was developed so that the executive committee could sign its endorsements for publication. It was felt also that the changing of the secretaries year by year was inadvisable and that they ought to have more permanent office. Finally it was suggested that the secretaries of the sections be assembled at least once each year at a conference and that their expenses be paid for such a conference.

BIRTH OF THE COOPERATIVE ADVERTISING BUREAU

Out of the recommendations that came from the J. N. McCormack committee came a motion to create a bureau of advertising to aid the periodicals that wished to conduct themselves in accord with the principles of the councils of the American Medical Association. The editor and general manager, Dr. George H. Simmons, and the advertising manager, Mr. Will C. Braun, were requested to prepare an outline for such a bureau and to report to the Board of Trustees at a later date.

AN OTOLARYNGOLOGIC JOURNAL

Now came also a request for the American Medical Association to undertake the publication of a periodical in the field of otolaryngology. The disputes that arose over the publication of a surgical journal had now completely blocked progress in that direction, and it was moved that a special committee be set up to study the whole question.

At the end of the February meeting of the Board of Trustees the board authorized Dr. George H. Simmons to take a vacation of ten or twelve weeks during the year. He postponed the vacation until the period following the annual session which was held in 1913 in Minneapolis.

MORE ADVICE FROM DR. JACOBI

The President of the Association, Dr. Abraham Jacobi, had devoted his official address to the question of the prevention of infant mortality. To the House of Delegates when it opened its meeting in 1913 he spoke more definitely of the work of the organization. He felt that the sections could do a better job if they had fewer papers and if the papers could be gathered in symposiums which would draw together the opinions of leaders, and he concluded, "We write too much and debate too little." He urged that the secretaries of the sections be prominent scientific men in the profession and that their term of office be lengthened. He felt that the President of the Association did not have enough to do and that aside from sitting with the Board of Trustees he might well sit with other councils and other agencies of the Association. This suggestion met with great approval by the House of Delegates, which adopted an action to the effect that the President of the Association be asked to attend all meetings of the councils, bureaus and similar bodies in the Association. Dr. Jacobi was moved by the fact that those who attended the House of Delegates simply lost touch with the scientific work of the organization, and he felt that something might be gained if the House would meet for three days previous to the time of the annual session. As

President he had received some letters complaining about the "oligarchy of Chicago and the autocracy of the House of Delegates." He said "If my angry correspondents would pray less and watch more, and would interest themselves in their county and state societies and in the election of their various delegates, they would have less reason to complain of what some of them term the oligarchy of Chicago and the autocracy of the House of Delegates." He was particularly annoyed by the fact that he had received some "epistles of rebuke and expostulation" and that he had "to put up with the wiseacres who were members of no societies and even with those who were not yet citizens of the country." And he said finally, "If you had the benefit of an Ellis Island of your own you would have fewer undesirable citizens of the profession, fewer backbiters, fewer calumniators of persons and aims, fewer enemies of the profession and fewer conspirators."

By this time the American Medical Association had reached a membership of 34,283, but THE JOURNAL had become the primary force in securing membership in the Association.

The recommendations of the Board of Trustees relative to the management of the sections met with a fine welcome from the House of Delegates, which supported the board fully in lessening the number of papers, extending the terms of the secretaries and urging more careful consideration by the executive committees of the sections of the papers that came to them.

The board announced that it was setting up a cooperative medical advertising bureau in the Association headquarters and that it had established a conference of state secretaries. All members of the Association had received copies of the Principles of Medical Ethics, and the publications of the Association were doing very well indeed.

FEE SPLITTING

In an endeavor to determine the status of fee splitting, the Judicial Council had sent a questionnaire to prominent members of the profession throughout the nation. It found great variations throughout the country in this practice. The full report on fee splitting is an extraordinarily interesting document. After discussing every possible phase of the subject, the Judicial Council adopted a resolution to the effect that any member of the American Medical Association found guilty of fee splitting— of giving or receiving division of fees —should no longer be a member of the Association. It also recommended definite action toward the elimination of the abuse of so-called lodge practice. As a part of its report to the House of Delegates at this time the Judicial Council also suggested the desirability of change in the procedure of the House of Delegates, by the election of a speaker who would be responsible for conduct of the affairs of the House of Delegates. The chairman of the Judicial Council which brought in this report was Dr. Alexander Lambert. The Judicial Council included in its membership Drs. A. B. Cooke, James E. Moore, Hubert Work, George W. Guthrie and the secretary of the American Medical Association.

The report of the Judicial Council went to the House of Delegates, which decided to consider the question of speaker by the entire house sitting as a committee of the whole. The House considered the matter of the speaker as a committee of the whole, but there is nothing said in the minutes as to what it did. The other recommendations of the Judicial Council relating to fee splitting were adopted.

The Council on Health and Public Instruction presented again an extensive report of its many activities, which had proceeded along the lines laid down in previous years, and announced a similar program for the year to come. It proposed the establishment of a legislative and medicolegal bureau at the headquarters of the American Medical Association. One of the proposals was a conference of the executive officers of public health organizations to discuss mutual cooperation and proper division of the field. The Council had worked out carefully a long list of organizations interested in public health to which an invitation for a conference was sent. That conference had been held at the American Association for Labor Legislation on April 12 and officers representing thirty-nine national organizations were present. As a result of that conference a committee of fifteen was established to consider the entire question of public health acttivities and the ways in which they could be improved and to report its findings with definite recommendations at a subsequent meeting of the conference.

Among the men on this committee was Dr. S. M. Gunn, whose name appeared at the meeting in 1946 as a maker of the Gunn-Platt report in an effort to coordinate philanthropic organizations related to health and to standardize in some way health activities.

Conspicuous in the activities of this council were its contacts with the government. Much of its work during the year had been devoted to a method of bringing about harmonious cooperation between the Council itself and the special committee on national legislation which had been established by the House of Delegates and the committee of 100, which was concerned with public health problems. It is interesting to observe seven points in the program of this group:

First: Appoint a committee to see President Wilson, tomorrow, May 6, at 10:45, and communicate to him the results of our conference and request him to decide on an administration policy concerning public health legislation.

Second: Recommend to President Wilson that he definitely advocate the establishment of a Department of Health.

Third: That he cooperate with Representative Foster in attempting to secure a Committee on Public Health in the House of Representatives during the present special session.

Fourth: That he call a White House conference on Public Health next fall somewhat similar to the Governors' Conference on Conservation called by President Roosevelt. The object of this conference is to promote the success of the President's policies and if necessary to aid in framing these policies.

Fifth: That at the next regular session the President should send a special message favoring public health legislation or else emphasize it in his regular annual message.

Sixth: That the President should select for the first assistant Secretary of the Treasury some one interested in public health.

Seventh: That in the next regular session we should support the President in securing such public health legislation as he decides to recommend.

The extensive reports of this council deserve to be read in detail by every one who is concerned today with the whole problem of public relations for American medicine.

EDUCATION

The Council on Medical Education continued to make its routine reports of progress toward further standardization of medical education.

The American Medical Association was functioning in relationship to the American Red Cross through a liaison committee.

An attempt had been made to arrange a joint meeting between the American Medical Association and the British Medical Association, but some of the members of the committee had died and the matter was still under consideration.

Already the committee which was working on the establishment of a national department of health was having a little trouble by the fact that the U. S. Public Health Service was trying to divert that activity into an expansion of the U. S. Public Health Service. The committee remarked:

> We, the undersigned, cannot see any virtue in pretending to be for a Department of Health directly and then covertly attempting to get it by an expansion of the great Public Health Service.

The committee that signed that communication included Drs. J. B. Murphy, J. N. Hurty, W. C. Woodward and W. A. Evans.

The House of Delegates had at this time to clarify the functions of the Committee on Health and Public Instruction and the national department of health. It did not agree with the committee that the

Association maintain a paid lobbyist in Washington. It did not concur in the idea that the American Medical Association join with other organizations of a purely commercial nature to maintain a lobby in Washington. This report, which was extensive and which was made by a committee consisting of Drs. E. J. Goodwin, chairman. A. R. Mitchell and Thomas S. Cullen, was adopted. There was much debate, during which the House of Delegates went into executive session. The minutes of the executive session are not available, but at the end the House of Delegates adopted a report placing the responsibility in the Council on Health and Public Instruction and recommending the discharge of the special committee on national public health legislation.

Out of the work of the Reference Committee on Amendments to the Constitution and By-Laws came an action which made it mandatory that a member present only one paper at any annual session.

DR. VICTOR VAUGHAN BECOMES PRESIDENT

At this meeting Dr. Victor Vaughan of Ann Arbor, Mich., was elected President of the American Medical Association. The House of Delegates had great pleasure in hearing an address by Mr. Samuel Hopkins Adams, who spoke on medical advertisements in the public press. The House of Delegates authorized the establishment of the Cooperative Medical Advertising Bureau. It created a new Section on Gastroenterology and Proctology and selected as its officers Drs. Joseph M. Mathews, Louisville, Ky., chairman; J. A. McMillan, Detroit, and A. J. Zobel, San Francisco, secretary.

The Board of Trustees at this session voted not to support a periodical on the ear, nose and throat because the time was not opportune.

DEATH OF E. E. HYDE

After the session ended, Dr. George H. Simmons departed for a trip aboard. During his absence Dr. E. E. Hyde, assistant to the editor, died suddenly of myelogenous leukemia. Following his death, Dr. Malcolm L. Harris, chairman of the Board of Trustees, served as editor until Dr. George H. Simmons returned.

At the meeting of the Board of Trustees in November 1913 Dr. A. R. Craig, secretary of the Association, presented a report in which he called attention to the board of the loyalty of every one connected with the Association following the death of Dr. Hyde and during the absence of Dr. George H. Simmons. In the meantime Dr. George H. Simmons had secured the service of Dr. Morris Fishbein to take the place of Dr. Hyde. Dr. Fishbein had been recommended by Dr.

Ludvig Hektoen and Dr. Frank Billings and had begun his work with the American Medical Association on Aug. 27, 1913.

The Board of Trustees now again took up the question of the Cooperative Medical Advertising Bureau and reaffirmed its original action in establishing this committee and making an appropriation for its work.

In creating the Section on Gastroenterology and Proctology, a motion had been made to the effect that the two existing societies in that field would disband. Apparently, however, these societies did not disband, and the secretary of the Association did not feel that he could create the section unless the societies did disband. Dr. Dwight H. Murray of Syracuse appealed to the Board of Trustees, which felt however, that it could not go beyond the action of the House of Delegates.

Dr. G. Frank Lydston had carried to the courts his desire to force the American Medical Association to hold its meetings and elections in Illinois, so that the trustees authorized publication of the Lydston decision in THE JOURNAL under the authority of the Board of Trustees, to be signed by the secretary and chairman of the board.

1914

ATLANTIC CITY

Because the number of papers at the annual session had been reduced, the restriction of four pages to a section paper was modified now to permit six pages.

The headquarters office was permitted to expand into the old building, which it had been renting to outside parties, because the needs of the Association were continually growing.

Now began a battle over the rental and use of radium, which has continued until this date.

COMPULSORY SICKNESS INSURANCE LOOMS LARGE

In 1913 the American Medical Association began to be interested in the question of sickness insurance. The Council on Health and Public Instruction conceived the desirability of sending one of its employees, Dr. I. M. Rubinow, to Europe to study what was being done there in national health legislation. The Board of Trustees did not think the time was ripe to undertake such studies. An American Academy of Medicine had been formed, and the secretary of that group wanted the cooperation of the American Medical Association in studying medical sociology. This action was referred by the Board of Trustees to the Council on Health and Public Instruction.

At the meeting in Atlantic City the President of the Association, Dr. John A. Witherspoon, announced that he would not make any address because he had just got up from the sick bed.

SECTION TROUBLE

The secretary of the Association reported his troubles over the Section on Gastroenterology and Proctology. The majority of the members of the American Proctological Association were opposed to disbanding when interviewed and indicated that they were not in sympathy with the formation of the section. The Reference Committee on Sections and Section Work, chairman Dr. Hugh Cabot, recommended therefore that there be no Section on Gastroenterology and Proctology. It recommended the division of the sections into two groups—general and special—with the understanding that a member might read one paper before each of these two groups. It recommended finally a committee of five be appointed by the President and be charged with the investigation of the whole matter of sections and section work. The committee had been asked to create a section on hydrotherapy, but it did not feel it desirable to add any more sections.

BOARD OF TRUSTEES REPORT

The Board of Trustees began its report by saying that the past year had been distinguished by no unusual events in the Association. All the activities had been prosecuted with maximum interest to the medical profession. There was trouble because Arbuthnot Lane had recommended Russian mineral oil, and the Council on Pharmacy and Chemistry had found no difference between Russian mineral oil and the liquid petrolatum of the United States. A book had been published called Useful Drugs. Quacks were moving the nation into activity, and the national organization had established vigilance committees to work toward the elimination of frauds in medicine. A special department known as the propaganda department had been established in the headquarters of the organization under the leadership of Dr. Arthur J. Cramp.

The Council on Medical Education reported ten years of excellent progress. It was about to investigate proprietary graduate medical schools and it urged reorganization of the clinical departments of medical schools. A complete arrangement had been made for full cooperation with the American Red Cross.

The Council on Health and Public Instruction again defined the scope of its activities. It recommended, however, as a new activity a survey of public health activities of the federal government to determine exactly what the federal government is doing for public health.

The speakers bureau had sent speakers throughout the nation to cover a wide variety of subjects, which were carefully tabulated. The press bulletin and the bureau of literature had been continued. There was a complete survey of national and state legislation. Somewhat in advance of its time was the report on special activities. This report follows:

> The Council conceives one of its most important functions to be the cultivation, as the official representative of the Association, of friendly relations with other professional organizations and influential bodies. The problem before the Association is exactly that which confronts the individual; namely, the necessity of convincing those whom we would influence of our sincerity and good faith. In a word, the Association and the medical profession, like the individual, must acquire and maintain a reputation for breadth of mind and charity of spirit, as well as for ability and authority in its special field. If we have the confidence and cooperation of the public and if they recognize the honesty of our purpose and sincerity of our motives as a body, almost anything which we may propose will meet public approval. If, on the other hand, the public is suspicious of our motives and skeptical as to our disinterestedness, any proposition emanating from the organized medical profession, no matter how clearly for the public good, will be misunderstood and criticized. The existence of a permanent body with a definite policy and a constant attitude of friendliness toward other organizations is therefore of the utmost importance. The Council feels that, during the short period of its existence, gratifying progress has been made in this direction and that the Association and its activities are gradually coming to be understood and appreciated by intelligent and broadminded citizens.

CANCER

The subcommittees had been effective in their work. A new subcommittee was that on cancer, headed by Dr. Thomas S. Cullen as chairman, and it had begun a series of articles for enlightenment of the public on many phases of cancer.

PATENTS

An attempt had been made to secure participation by the American Medical Association in the holding of patents on medical devices, and the Board of Trustees was requested to look into the matter in cooperation with the Judicial Council.

THE AMERICAN COLLEGE OF SURGEONS

At this time also there came before the House of Delegates information regarding the formation of the American College of Surgeons, with a resolution from the state of Illinois deprecating this organization. The resolution was laid on the table, as was another substitute resolution to the same effect.

The House of Delegates encouraged the Council on Health and Public Instruction to correlate existing national health organizations in the manner proposed and to make the necessary surveys of the health activities of the federal government.

TWO NEW IMPORTANT ACTIONS

As the year went on, the Board of Trustees took two actions of great significance. First it decided to publish a series of monographs on anesthesia for the general information of the medical profession and for the advancement of knowledge of this subject. Next it created a reserve fund containing $125,000 as a first instalment which was to grow and grow as the years went on.

THE WAR—1915 TO 1919

1915

SAN FRANCISCO

AS ONE OF ITS MANY EXPOSÉS of "patent" medicines, THE JOURNAL OF THE AMERICAN MEDICAL ASSOCIATION published in 1914 a report on a product manufactured by the Chattanooga Medicine Company of Tennessee called "Wine of Cardui." The article had been prepared as a joint effort of the laboratory of the Association, the Council on Pharmacy and Chemistry, the Division of Propaganda for Reform and the editorial department. The facts stated were so challenging that the owners of the Chattanooga Medicine Company (the Patten family, one of whom was a leader in the Methodist Church) sued for libel. The record of the suit is told in another chapter. The company also sued Dr. Oscar Dowling, who was secretary of the state board of health in Louisiana. The Board of Trustees determined to make a complete defense in the case and the attorneys for the American Medical Association—Loesch, Scofield and Loesch—were instructed to take charge. Because the proprietors of secret nostrums were now attacking the citadel of American medicine, the Board of Trustees appointed a committee to prepare a special report to the medical profession for presentation to the House of Delegates.

PHYSICIANS AND PUBLIC HEALTH

In opening the annual session for 1915, Dr. Victor C. Vaughan emphasized particularly the need for improvement of postgraduate medical education. He felt that the medical profession might be losing its prestige in relationship to the great advances that were being made in preventive medicine. In Michigan, for instance, the campaign against tuberculosis was being led by a group of whom three were not physicians.

The Board of Trustees indicated that the rapid extension of the interests of the association had so affected its financial status that profits were reaching the vanishing point. The entire profit for the year was less than $4,000. While its work was altruistic, the Board warned the Association that the expenses must not increase but should decrease.

HOUSE OF DELEGATES ATTACKS NOSTRUMS

For the first time in the report of its activities to the House of Delegates a special section was introduced on the law suits of the Association. As has already been mentioned, these will be covered in a special chapter of this history. However, in accordance with the action taken by the Board of Trustees at its session in February, a special report had been prepared on the work of the Council on Pharmacy and Chemistry by a committee of the board, including Dr. W. T. Councilman, Dr. W. W. Grant and Dr. M. L. Harris. Following the presentation of this extensive report the Board of Trustees offered a resolution:

> *Resolved*, We, members of the House of Delegates of the American Medical Association, believe that every effort must be made to do away with the evils which result from the exploitation of the sick for the sake of gain. Earnestly believing that the continued toleration of secret, semisecret, unscientific or untruthfully advertised proprietary medicines is an evil that is inimical to medical progress and to the best interest of the public, we declare ourselves in sympathy with, endorse and by our best efforts will further the work which has been and is being done by the Council on Pharmacy and Chemistry of the American Medical Association in the attempt to eliminate this evil.

The House of Delegates not only endorsed fully the activities of the Council on Pharmacy and Chemistry and of the Board of Trustees in furthering its work but also advised all members of the medical profession to withhold their support from periodicals that advertised proprietary remedies not investigated and accepted by the Council.

SOCIAL INSURANCE

The report of the Judicial Council, under the leadership of Dr. Alexander Lambert of New York, was one of the most extensive in the history of the Association. This report was to have a tremendous effect on the future activities of the Association; it covered such serious topics as the disciplining of Fellows of the Association who received commissions from the manufacturers of drugs and instruments and who thus violated the Principles of Ethics. An elaborate report of many pages dealt with workmen's compensation laws, social insurance in Europe, compulsory sickness insurance and other forms of protection against the hazards of disease and injury. Many pages dealt with industrial insurance in the United States. Attention was called to the difficulties of European physicians, particularly those in Germany, in maintaining a high standard of medical care, insuring free choice of physician and similar basic factors. In concluding its report the Judicial Council stated that its whole purpose was education of the medical profession concerning the trend. The Judicial Council said "In whatever country the social equilibrium has been upset by new laws of compensation there have followed in the wake of compensation for accidents other insurances tending toward the complete insurance systems of England and Germany." The Judicial Council called attention to articles by I. M. Rubinow on social insurance and the medical profession which had been published in THE JOURNAL, and it continued "It is evident, therefore, that once the old social and legal equilibrium has been upset, society tends to follow to the logical conclusion until it reaches a new equilibrium under a new social system." The Judicial Council indicated that we had in the United States a disjointed mass of insurance schemes and pension systems and that in several countries abroad these various social elements had been combined into a single form. The report said:

> In several countries abroad the same various social elements have been combined into some form of workable adaptability by which various accident and sickness insurance, invalidism and old age pensions have been brought together to form social forces which have tended to reduce the destitution of large masses of human beings. These forces unquestionably tend to improve the social condition in any given community, and, for the carrying out of any scheme tending to human betterment, the medical profession must necessarily be included, whether it be to judge of sickness or health insurance, whether it be for the prevention of the intensity of injury in the individual from accident or for the prevention of the spread of disease in a community at large. The medical profession will accept its responsibility in these new social conditions as it has always accepted its responsibilities in the past. The Judicial Council therefore presents this abstract of existing social insurance in this country and abroad.

The reference committee which considered this report recommended that the constituent state societies bring it to the attention of their members as a *"vade mecum* on these important social economical problems."

THE COUNCIL ON HEALTH AND PUBLIC INSTRUCTION

Again the Council on Health and Public Instruction had an extensive report on public health conditions in the United States, public education, the vast work of its speakers' bureau, its bureau of literature, its sections on legislation (both state and federal) and on the work of its many subcommittees. The Council felt that the most valuable work it had done was the coordination and harmonizing of the work of different organizations. There were reports of committees on women's and children's welfare, cancer, expert testimony, the National Education Association, the conservation of vision and similar subjects.

REORGANIZATION OF SECTIONS

Significant also at this session was the effort of a committee headed by Dr. Hugh Cabot to reorganize the work of the scientific sections. The Association must provide not only for the highly trained specialists but also for great numbers of general practitioners to whom it represented their one scientific organization. The committee recommended the establishment of a standing committee or council on section work. This recommendation was accepted by the House of Delegates. The result was the establishment of the Council on Scientific Assembly, which has, since that time, been of the utmost significance in advancing the scientific programs of the Association.

INFANT FOODS

Much attention was attracted by a resolution to control the advertising of proprietary infant foods. Several resolutions urged participation by the Association in the work of medical milk commissions with a view to improving the quality of milk supplied to the nation.

THE NATIONAL BOARD OF EXAMINERS

In his address at this session of the Association Dr. William L. Rodman had recommended the establishment of a national board of medical examiners. The committee to which the report was referred recommended that it be submitted to the House of Delegates for approval. A minority report suggested reference instead to the Council on Medical Education. This report was adopted and the American Medical Association took part, through the Council, in the establishment of the National Board of Medical Examiners.

HARRISON ANTINARCOTIC LAW

The antinarcotic law known as the Harrison Law had been passed and approved on Dec. 7, 1914. The Council on Pharmacy and Chemistry recognized the weaknesses of this law in permitting the sale and use of narcotics when contained in proprietary and stock preparations. On recommendation by the Board of Trustees, the House of Delegates took action to bring this matter to the attention of the Congress of the United States, so that the indiscriminate sale of proprietary and other preparations containing narcotics should not be permitted.

GRADUATE INSTRUCTION

In his address to the House of Delegates President Victor C. Vaughan had indicated the great desirability of participation by the American Medical Association in sending teams of clinical teachers to the individual states to bring general practitioners up to date in medical practice. The Board of Trustees was told to take the matter in hand. Out of that suggestion came a procedure still followed in many states for extending graduate education of physicians in rural areas.

1916

DETROIT; SICKNESS INSURANCE

The first subject to come before the meeting of the trustees early in 1916 was national legislation on sickness insurance. Drs. Alexander Lambert and Henry B. Favill appeared before the board to speak on the subject. Bills had already been introduced in Massachusetts and New York. It was recognized that the relation of the medical profession to any plan of sickness insurance was vital. A special committee appointed jointly by the Council on Health and Public Instruction and the Judicial Council was established to have charge of this investigation; the Board of Trustees requested submission of the plan and of a budget.

The agitation for a presiding officer in the House of Delegates was brought before the Board of Trustees; the Board rightly said that the decision would have to be made by the House of Delegates.

The joint committee on sickness insurance presented a statement. It pointed out that the purposes and duties of this committee would be to make a careful compilation of information concerning health and social insurance and the relation of physicians thereto, and to do everything in its power to secure such constructions of the proposed laws as will work the most harmonious adjustment of the new sociologic relations between physicians and laymen which will necessarily result therefrom. The committee was given great power to study and to act, and an adequate budget to meet all of its needs. It was also recommended that full publicity be given to its work.

In the course of the year President Rodman had died; the vice president, Dr. Albert Vander Veer of Albany, then over 80 years old, served thereafter as president.

ADVERTISING BY PHYSICIANS

As an indication of its seriousness in considering infractions of the Principles of Ethics, the Judicial Council reported publicly that it had taken action in two cases involving the charge of grossly advertising in the public press. One of these involved a physician of Wichita, Kan., who was dropped from the Fellowship roll of the American Medical Association. The second case was that of a former President of the Association, Dr. John B. Murphy of Chicago. Charges had been brought before the Judicial Council that the accused had caused or permitted to appear in a publication with which his name was connected photographs and an article which violated the Principles of Medical Ethics in that they were self laudatory and defied the traditions and were contrary to the ideals of the medical profession. The Judicial Committee condemned this publication as being offensive and in bad taste. Because the testimony indicated that the publication complained of was not intended by the accused to be self-exploiting advertising, the Judicial Council accepted his explanation and apology.

MEDICAL PREPAREDNESS

The most important aspects of the address made by Dr. Vander Veer concerned the preparedness of the medical profession in relation to the threat of war. As Acting President of the Association he had cooperated with other organizations in appointing a strong committee of American physicians to consider plans for civilian medical preparedness. Repeated conferences had been held. Already suitable boards and committees had been established to confer with the President of the United States and to offer to him the services of the medical profession. President Wilson had expressed himself as much pleased with the patriotic actions of the medical profession and assured Dr. Vander Veer that the government would avail itself of the services that were tendered. Base hospitals were being formed, and four such units were ready for mobilization.

PROHIBITION

Through the office of the secretary there came to the House of Delegates a plea for cooperation by the medical profession in combating the liquor evil.

THE BOARD OF TRUSTEES

In its report to the House of Delegates the Board of Trustees called attention to the relationship of the profession to the social state. The Board indicated that it had granted a considerable sum of money mainly for acquiring information. The Board of Trustees said:

> We are entering on a period of great changes in social organization; a period which will necessitate a far closer organization of the people in all forms of activity, and this particularly calls for united strength in opposing disease. It is true we have not so strongly felt the necessity for this as have other nations, but the time has come when we can no longer resist the social movement, and it is better that we should initiate the necessary changes than have them forced on us. On such information, laws regulating social medicine, which will be just both to the medical profession and to the public, whom it serves, must be based. All of our councils have worked in perfect harmony with other bodies, often outside of the profession, which have had the common good in mind.

SPEAKER OF THE HOUSE OF DELEGATES

The Judicial Council recognized the desirability if not necessity, of having for the House of Delegates a presiding officer familiar with the transactions and also with the best methods of expediting the work of the House. The Judicial Council, therefore, recommended that the House take up the election of a speaker and proposed the necessary amendments to the Constitution and By-Laws to make this possible. The House of Delegates approved these recommendations.

COUNCIL ON HEALTH AND PUBLIC INSTRUCTION

In furtherance of the obligations placed on it, the Council on Health and Public Instruction had made a survey of state public health activities begun in 1914 by Dr. Charles V. Chapin. This included a rating sheet of the forty-eight state health organizations and exhaustive tabulations of their various activities, appropriations and expenditures. This action marked the beginning of a movement for elevation of the field of public health as did the first report of the Council on Medical Education in education. A request had come for a similar survey of municipal health departments, but the Council had not been able to devise any feasible plan for the purpose. An attempt had been made also to survey voluntary public health organizations. Such a report had been prepared and published and it had been accepted by the American Public Health Association.

The committee was discharged and a new central committee on public health organization was established to continue such studies. The efforts of the Council in the direction of cooperation had borne fruit; many leading organizations were cooperating fully with the medical profession.

Significant was the report of the subcommittee of the Council dealing with social insurance! Understatement indeed was the opinion that this subject would in all probability be one of the most important to occupy the attention of the medical profession in the next few years both from an economic and from a medical point of view.

The Council had secured the services of I. M. Rubinow, Ph.D., who was chief statistician of the Ocean Accident & Guarantee Corporation and president of the Actuarial Society, as an executive secretary; it had opened a bureau for study of social insurance in New York City. The Council presented a statistical study of the medical profession of the United States. It pointed out, however, that there were not available reliable figures concerning the incomes of physicians and other economic facts of interest. It proposed

to educate the American medical profession in the general principles of social insurance, particularly health insurance, the economic and social significance of the movement to obtain such insurance throughout the United States, and the absolutely essential part which the medical profession must play in a successful adaptation of this new legislation to American conditions.

It seems to have been rather taken for granted that such compulsory sickness insurance laws would be passed in the United States. The committee felt that it should work to avoid the conflicts that had arisen in England at the beginning of a similar movement and which had resulted in a large amount of bitterness between the profession and the public that might easily have been prevented by properly handled action.

In its report on social insurance the committee, under the chairmanship of Dr. Alexander Lambert, presented a report more than thirty-five pages long opposing voluntary sickness insurance and agreeing that only compulsory state insurance would reach the group of people who needed help most. It then discussed in detail the compulsory insurance schemes of all foreign countries in which such systems prevailed, with the majority of the emphasis on the comprehensive system in Germany. The major portion of this extensive report had been prepared by Dr. Rubinow. The report concluded with a consideration of conditions prevailing in the United States for protection against the hazards of sickness among trade unions, lodges, fraternal societies, commercial insurance companies and similar agencies. The report was inclined to accept the conclusion of Drs. B. S. Warren and Edgar Sydenstricker that the democratic character of an effective health insurance system is most pronounced in a governmental system. It was agreed that the experience of European nations with health insurance had shown that governmental systems were the only systems which accomplished the purpose desired. Then came the health insurance act developed by the American Association for Labor Legislation. The report concluded with a general comment to the effect that it had made no attempt to bring together the advantages or disadvantages or to argue for or against health insurance. It favored the German system over that in England and it said

However one may criticize the details, the insurance act has unquestionably improved the health of the working classes which have come under the law.

When this extensive report was turned over to the Reference Committee on Legislation and Political Action, under the chairmanship of Dr. E. J. Goodwin of Missouri, the reference committee recognized the exhaustive character of the report. It was proposed that the Council on Health and Public Instruction should continue to study the subject and to educate the profession concerning it. The reference committee approved such study and approved further establishment by each state association of a committee on social insurance to work in conjunction with the Committee on Social Insurance of the American Medical Association.

COUNCIL ON MEDICAL EDUCATION

Again the Council on Medical Education indicated its progress in merging poor medical schools, raising standards of education and eliminating schools of quackery. Here is a striking statement:

> The largest number of these institutions at present is found in Illinois, where conditions are especially favorable. Besides the class C medical schools which continue to exist there are in Illinois colleges of osteopathy, chiropractic, chiropody, naprapathy, somopathy, physcultopathy, refraction, optics and a legion of others, most of which have for their chief inducement elegantly printed diplomas conferring the degree of "doctor" of this, that or the other. The courses offered for such degrees are in some instances so notably a makeshift as to be ridiculous, and an insult to education. Some are offering courses under two or more titles, and others appear to be doing a retail business in dispensing degrees in all the "forms" or "systems" of healing which may have been or ever shall be enumerated.

The report urged the various states of the nation to protect themselves against such low grade institutions.

Pursuant to the recommendation that had been made by Dr. Rodman, the Council on Medical Education reported the organization of the National Board of Medical Examiners with the assistance of the Carnegie Foundation for the Advancement of Teaching.

A special committee to cooperate with the Red Cross had drawn up a complete arrangement for medical service through the Red Cross.

PUBLICITY AND THE ELECTION OF PRESIDENT

Excitement occurred in the House of Delegates at the meeting to elect officers when a Detroit newspaper announced that Dr. Charles H. Mayo would be elected president three or four hours before the election was held. The publicity had been issued without any activity on the part of Dr. Mayo; he was unanimously elected.

FROM THE MOUTH TO THE STOMACH AND RECTUM

As a recognition of changes in medical interest, the Section on Stomatology was discontinued and a new Section on Gastro-Enterology and Proctology was established.

THE WORLD WAR

The war was prominent on the final day of the convention. Physicians were informed that a citizens military training camp had been established at Fort Benjamin Harrison, Indiana, to instruct doctors in field hospital and sanitation work. Citizens who wished to volunteer to attend this school could do so by paying $1 in addition to the cost of the uniform.

QUARTERLY CUMULATIVE INDEX MEDICUS

During 1916 the support of the Carnegie Foundation for the *Index Medicus* had been discontinued; as a result this valuable tool for workers in medical research was discontinued. At this time Dr. George H. Simmons, as a result of many conferences in Washington and elsewhere, proposed that the American Medical Association establish an index medicus to be published quarterly and cumulated. This would be a large responsibility for the Association. Dr. Simmons presented his proposal to the Board of Trustees, which authorized him to proceed with the publication. The full story of the QUARTERLY CUMULATIVE INDEX MEDICUS is told in another chapter.

ADMINISTRATION OF PATENTS

A resolution was passed by the House of Delegates authorizing the American Medical Association to accept and administer patents. Dr. E. C. Kendall of the Mayo Clinic had just discovered thyroxin, the active constituent of the thyroid, and wished to award the patent to the American Medical Association. This patent was accepted. At a later date, however, it was realized that the function was quite outside the scope of a body such as the American Medical Association. The patent was returned, and the Association has not since undertaken such an activity.

Dr. Charles Mayo, now President of the Association, offered the Association $25,000 which had been contributed by Mr. R. T. Crane for the discovery of the cause and best cure of infantile paralysis. The Association tentatively accepted the funds and the obligation.

1917

NEW YORK CITY

By 1917 the Scientific Exhibit had grown so greatly that the recommendation was made to the Board of Trustees that there be established a special committee on scientific exhibit. The story of the Scientific Exhibit is told also in another chapter.

In this year action was adopted that all papers read at the annual session be treated as volunteer contributions and that they be published in full in THE JOURNAL or rejected or published in abstract, as might seem best. This step was fundamental in improving the quality of THE JOURNAL.

Petitions had come for the publication of journals devoted to ophthalmology and otolaryngology; the board took these under advisement.

The Committee on Social Insurance had found itself heavily obligated because of the thousands of studies necessary. It indicated a wish for additional funds and also the necessity for a full time executive secretary.

When the Association convened in New York in the midst of the war the President of the Association, Dr. Rupert Blue, Surgeon General of the U. S. Public Health Service, told of the activities in which he had participated in the prosecution of the war. Committees had been set up in the various states to cooperate with the Red Cross. A committee of three, consisting of Drs. Arthur Dean Bevan, Alexander Lambert and J. W. Kerr, had been constituted to report on the best way of utilizing the records and activities of the American Medical Association. Letters had been addressed to the presidents and secretaries of all component medical societies urging them to secure medical officers for the armed forces.

THE FIRST CHAIRMAN OF THE HOUSE

The first chairman of the House of Delegates, Dr. Hubert Work, presided. In his opening address he announced his concept of the functions of the office. His was a statesmanlike presentation, free from any political connotations. It established the standards for functioning of the speaker of the House of Delegates since that time.

Most of the report of the Board of Trustees was concerned with the problem of publication of the section papers. Their number had become overwhelming; the price of paper had advanced so greatly that it was not possible with financial safety to publish all the papers. The Board of Trustees informed the House of Delegates that it had passed the resolution relative to volunteer contributions. The editor had been authorized to refer highly specialized papers to the special journals. The board also announced its decision to publish a journal of ophthalmology and otolaryngology.

THE LIBEL SUIT

Then came a report on the defense against the libel suit, which had lasted thirteen weeks. The result was satisfactory not only from the moral standard but also in its financial aspects. Nevertheless the cost of the trial was so great that the auditor's report showed for the first time in twenty-five years an operating loss in the finances of the Association. Fortunately the expense was met largely out of current receipts without impairing the reserve funds of the Association. Nevertheless the Board said:

> This trial demonstrated the wisdom of having a large reserve fund on which to fall back, for the existence of this fund gave courage to carry on a vigorous defense to a successful end. This leads us to suggest that the reserve fund should be still further increased. In times of adversity the absence of such a fund might badly cripple us or force us to suspend temporarily all altruistic work. Not all years are "fat" with prosperity; "lean" years are bound to come, against which provision must be made. No one can foretell the end of the critical period upon which this country has entered; but it is easy to foresee the possibility of a diminished income to the Association. It is quite possible that a large number—perhaps several thousand—of our Fellows will be called to the front for an indefinite period, during which time it is more than likely that there will be a considerable falling off in the subscriptions to THE JOURNAL. Hence it behooves us to husband our resources that there may be no interruption in our more desirable and important activities.

In concluding its report the Board of Trustees presented a memorandum on the death of Philip Mills Jones of San Francisco on Nov. 27, 1916. He had attended a meeting of the Board of Trustees on November 3 and was in his usual good health. Then within three weeks he was dead from pneumonia, and his wife died from the same disease within twenty-four hours. Dr. Philip Mills Jones had become one of the most ardent advocates of clean advertising, although previously favoring a national joint council. He had become so interested in the legal aspect of medical problems that he took up the study of law late in life; in the year previous to his death he had been admitted to the California bar.

THE WAR CHECKS ACTIVITY

As temporary chairman of the Council on Health and Public Instruction, Dr. Frank Billings presented the report, which was greatly condensed, occupying now only two pages of THE JOURNAL. Dr. Frederick R. Green, who had been most active as secretary of this body, had volunteered for military service and had been given a leave of absence by the Board of Trustees. The demands of the war had greatly curtailed all the activities of the Council. Nevertheless, the committee on social insurance presented a report occupying thirty-five pages under the auspices of Dr. Alexander Lambert, the chairman. Two state commissions—California and Massachusetts—had investigated health insurance and had reported favorably on it. Health insurance measures had been introduced into the legislatures of fourteen other states. Most of the extensive report dealt with conditions in Germany. It considered not only health insurance but old age protection and unemployment insurance. The pattern in foreign countries had been a beginning with voluntary insurance, which proved inadequate, then voluntary insurance subsidized by the state, which, although more successful, was still inadequate and, finally, full compulsory insurance. Poorly concealed throughout this report is a plea for early adoption of compulsory sickness insurance in the United States. For instance, the report said:

> Regarding social insurance as a whole, this country is still in the stage of investigation, but the rapidity with which, after a few years—less than a decade—protection against industrial accident was taken up and adopted shows clearly that when the idea is once understood and grasped how rapidly it appeals to all nationalities, although a few years ago the accident insurance was condemned as un-American and the same adjective is being used against the other forms of social insurance today as they are discussed. It has been a noticeable feature that all official investigations in this country have led to the approval of at least the basic principle in the movement for social insurance. There is no question that the enormous modern industrial development has increased the hazards of the wage earner and has increased also the dependence of a large part of the population on their own physical well-being and working capacity. This country today still possesses the strongest development of individualism, but so great has been the collective development of industry and so strong the collective development of labor that the collective protection of the individual against a universal hazard has found ready and vigorous support.

In concluding its report the Council condemned the *Boston Medical and Surgical Journal* for suggesting that medicine be eliminated from social insurance laws. It felt that the intense reaction in many states against sickness insurance or further expansion of social insurance laws in this country was due to the unjustness and cold blooded methods of unfairness under the workmen's compensation laws. The report said, in part:

> Blind opposition, indignant repudiation, bitter denunciation of these laws is worse than useless; it leads nowhere and it leaves the profession in a position of helplessness if the rising tide of social development sweeps over them. The profession can, through its influence in the community, prevent for a time these laws being passed and it can, by a refusal to cooperate, still further retard them, but in the end the social forces that demand these laws and demand an improvement in the social existence of the great mass of the people of the nation will indignantly force a recalcitrant profession to accept that which is unjust to it and that which is to its detriment.
>
> The profession today, in certain states, is acting the part that our school boy history showed of old King Canute sitting on the seashore bidding the rising tide to stop, and King Canute only got wet for his trouble.

The report ended with a resolution:

> *Resolved*, That the House of Delegates of the American Medical Association in the interests of both the wage earners and the medical profession authorize its Council on Health and Public Instruction to continue to study and to make reports on the future development of social insurance legislation and to cooperate, when possible, in the molding of these laws that the health of the community may be properly safeguarded and the interests of the medical profession protected; and be it further

Resolved, That the House of Delegates instruct its Council on Health and Public Instruction to insist that such legislation shall provide for freedom of choice of physician by the insured; payment of the physician in proportion to the amount of work done; the separation of the functions of medical official supervision from the function of daily care of the sick, and adequate representation of the medical profession on the appropriate administrative bodies.

The reference committee expressed its appreciation of this report and recommended the adoption of the resolutions, which recommendation the House of Delegates followed.

This was not a rejection of compulsory sickness insurance; it seems to have been a qualified acceptance. It favored the adoption of compulsory sickness insurance subject to acceptance of the principles related to medical practice which were involved. Behind this report was the influence of Dr. Rubinow. Later came complete repudiation.

THE SECTIONS

Attempts were still being made by the first Council on Scientific Assembly, which included in its membership Drs. E. Starr Judd, chairman, Roger S. Morris, George H. Simmons, J. Shelton Horsley and Alexander R. Craig to organize and coordinate the work of the sections and to assign them relative importance in the number of papers permitted in each. An attempt was made, in fact, to adopt the system which prevailed in Great Britain by which some sections would meet twice, others as often as six times during the session. The reference committee of the House of Delegates accepted the report of the Council on Scientific Assembly with the exception of that portion which distributed units to the different sections. Some of the representatives of the various sections insisted that two units were too few; three units were made the minimum. Later in the session the Section on Preventive Medicine and Public Health objected to being limited to three units and asked for six units, which the House promptly gave it.

THE WAR

Now came resolutions on participation by the medical profession in the war, on the care of infants and children during the war, and on provision of insignia for medical students so that they could continue their studies without being called cowards and slackers.

Other resolutions concerned the operation of quarantine during the war and the appointment of a food commission to act in an advisory capacity to the government in controlling food supplies during the war.

ORGANIZATION OF ARMY MEDICAL SERVICE

In a statesmanlike address to the House of Delegates, Dr. Frank Billings urged the establishment of a committee of five to formulate resolutions whereby better protection could be given to guarding the health of our soldiers. The position of the medical officer in relationship to officers in the line was not such as made it possible for him to secure action on recommendations definitely concerned with the prevention of epidemics. The suggestion of Dr. Billings was unanimously adopted. Many years passed following World War I, and the same difficulties that caused so much distress at that time arose in World War II.

The House of Delegates gave complete support to the Board of Trustees in establishing new journals to be devoted to otolaryngology and ophthalmology.

AIDING THE DRAFT

A special meeting of the Board of Trustees was called in October 1917 to consider a proposal submitted by the War Department through the Provost Marshal General requesting the aid of the American Medical Association in organizing medical boards to conduct medical examinations in connection with the draft. The Board of Trustees accepted the invitation to cooperate with the Provost Marshal General as presented in the letter from Lieut. Col. Hugh S. Johnson, Judge Advocate. A committee of three was appointed to cooperate: Drs. Hubert Work, M. L. Harris and E. J. McKnight. The action was submitted by telegram to the members of the House of Delegates. The committee was empowered to call a meeting of the representatives from every state medical association to discuss the selection of suitable men to constitute such advisory boards. The American Medical Association bore the entire cost.

DAVIS MEMORIAL FUND

Dr. William Allen Pusey appeared before the Board and spoke in behalf of combining the funds held to honor the memory of N. S. Davis by the American Medical Association and the Chicago Medical Society, with a view to establishing a lectureship.

THE POLIOMYELITIS PRIZE

Many applicants had applied for the prize of $25,000 offered by Mr. R. T. Crane to any one who would discover the cause and cure of infantile paralysis, but none had presented sufficient evidence to warrant his being given the prize.

WORLD WAR I

On April 7, 1917 THE JOURNAL OF THE AMERICAN MEDICAL ASSOCIATION noted that war was imminent and called on the medical profession for volunteers. It published the reports dealing with the organization of the Council of National Defense and of the Committee of American Physicians for Medical Preparedness. Dr. Franklin H. Martin had, according to the reports, been selected by a committee of distinguished physicians as the medical representative on the advisory commission of the Council of National Defense. Dr. Frank F. Simpson had been selected as chief of the medical section of the Council of National Defense. Dr. Franklin H. Martin, as chairman, had created an advisory committee which included Drs. W. C. Gorgas, W. C. Braisted, Rupert Blue, J. R. Kean, W. H. Welch, W. J. Mayo and Frank F. Simpson. Dr. William J. Mayo had, in turn, become chairman of the American Physicians for Medical Preparedness, which had organized a special committee of nine men in each state and, under this, county committees. Obviously in this setup the headquarters organization of the American Medical Association had been rather definitely ignored. When it came to functioning, however, the committee was dependent on THE JOURNAL OF THE AMERICAN MEDICAL ASSOCIATION as its voice and on the biographic files of the American Medical Association as the one available source for accurate information concerning the physicians of the United States.

In the issue for April 14 THE JOURNAL discussed in many editorials the organization of the medical department of the Army. The advisory commission of the Council of National Defense would have to utilize the county and state medical societies to carry out the mobilization, and THE JOURNAL urged full cooperation. By this time also Dr. Franklin H. Martin had decided to appoint a general medical board to cooperate with him in coordinating civilian medical activities and to advise with regard to fundamental medical problems in relation to the armed forces of the country. This board included a membership of twenty-four, among whom the only representative of the American Medical Association was Dr. George H. Simmons. In the April 14 issue of THE JOURNAL a special department was created entitled "Medical Mobilization and the War." From that time on many pages were given in each issue to military problems.

In the issue for April 21, by which time war had been declared, THE JOURNAL published a form for application for the medical corps of the Army and also for appointment in the officers reserve corps. An editorial called on physicians of the country to meet the needs of the armed forces. There were reports on the work of the general medical board and on the standardization of general medical supplies; again many pages were occupied by information on medical military activities.

By this time THE JOURNAL began a series of articles which were prepared by Colonel McKnight, who had been assigned to the headquarters of the American Medical Association as a liaison officer. The series was entitled "The Medical Officer of the Army." Later the series of articles was collected in book form and widely used in extending knowledge of military activities to the civilian medical profession.

As the weeks went by THE JOURNAL adopted many technics for promoting interest in medical service, appealing with slogans and editorials to the medical profession. There had been an excellent response to the publication of the application blank. Clearly, however, the greatest function of the American Medical Association in mobilization had been the utilization of THE JOURNAL. Its officers had been largely ignored in places of importance in the mobilization for war. Dr. George H. Simmons, the editor, had been assigned a relatively inconspicuous position on the subcommittee which had to do with assignment of personnel.

It would be impossible to overemphasize the tremendous value of THE JOURNAL, with its extensive circulation, as the important medium in maintaining the dissemination of information concerning military activities and in inspiring the medical profession to the utmost fulfilment of its obligation. The names of all physicians who were enrolled and their assignments to camps were promptly recorded. Special articles dealt with almost every phase of military service. The organization of the base hospitals and the enlistment of physicians in their units were constantly recorded. The formation of the medical officers training camps was fully described, and visits were made to these camps for full reporting of their activities. Special articles were published from the officers in charge of the British and French medical departments. THE JOURNAL enlisted in the campaign for conservation of food. One finds, late in 1917, full page photographs of the medical officers training camps and all of the physicians in attendance. Once more began the campaign for adequate rank for physicians. Week by week the news from every medical front was reported. It is doubtful that there could have been any single effort more important in maintaining medical morale than were the many pages assigned by THE JOURNAL to medical military activities. THE JOURNAL published week by week the orders to medical officers. These were carefully systematized according to the individual states from which the officers came. It required an extensive organization in the editorial functions of the Association to carry out these activities. The Army itself developed no mechanism for contact with medical officers, nor did the Navy. THE JOURNAL during World War I published the photograph and biography of every physician who gave his life in the armed forces, and this procedure was followed also in World War II.

In April 1918 the American Medical Association called a war conference of the secretaries of the constituent state associations. By this time the government had realized the necessity of utilizing the American Medical Association more and more in the enrolment of medical officers. The primary purpose of the conference of secretaries was to enlist the necessary physicians to meet the national need.

An extraordinary contribution was publication by THE JOURNAL of June 1, 1918 of a complete list of civilian physicians in military service, with a tabulation of enrolment by counties and states. The Section on Miscellaneous Topics at the annual session in June was devoted wholly to the reconstruction and rehabilitation of disabled soldiers. When the annual session met in Chicago, a special feature was a military meeting held in the Medinah Temple, at that time the largest assembly hall in Chicago. Over this medical military meeting Dr. Arthur Dean Bevan, President of the Association, presided. Addresses were made by Gen. W. C. Gorgas, Sir James Mackenzie, Sir Arbuthnot Lane, Col. Herbert Bruce of the Canadian army, Major Edouard Rist of the French army, Capt. René Sand of the Belgian army, Admiral William C. Braisted, Surgeon General of the Navy, and President Ray Lyman Wilbur of Stanford University. Dr. Wilbur was especially concerned with food. The final address was made by Major Alexander Lambert, who spoke of the work of the Red Cross.

Another meeting, known as the Patriotic Meeting, was held in the Auditorium Theater. Here Dr. Ludvig Hektoen, president of the Chicago Medical Society, presided, and addresses were made on "Science and the War" by Professor John M. Coulter of the University of Chicago, "The Law and the War" by Judge Charles S. Cutting and "American Ideals" by Bishop Charles P. Anderson.

As the war neared its end, THE JOURNAL became more and more concerned with problems of medical education. Fortunately the war ended in November. The brevity of the American participation made unnecessary the serious considerations that disturbed the profession during World War II, when medical education suffered severely. In World War I, 35,000 physicians had participated.

Almost immediately with the end of the war, THE JOURNAL began calling for the formation of a competent medical reserve corps.

1918
CHICAGO

Early in 1918 the Board of Trustees was mostly concerned with its relationships to the Council on National Defense and to the office of the Provost Marshal. Few activities developed in the American Medical Association. As told elsewhere, Dr. Franklin H. Martin had been alert in hastening to Washington; leadership began and remained with him and leaders of the American College of Surgeons.

A SPANISH JOURNAL

Among new projects brought to the attention of the Board was the possible publication of THE JOURNAL OF THE AMERICAN MEDICAL ASSOCIATION in Spanish, to be circulated in South and Central American countries. Through negotiations by Dr. George H. Simmons with the Rockefeller Foundation, this project was undertaken.

NEUROLOGY AND PSYCHIATRY

The Board of Trustees authorized also the publication of a journal of neurology and psychiatry, and an editorial board was selected for that periodical.

STANDARDIZATION OF HOSPITALS

It was suggested that the Council on Medical Education undertake standardization of hospitals.

AN AUTO EMBLEM

The Board authorized the manufacture and distribution of an automobile emblem for physicians.

WAR SERVICE

The editor and general manager or the secretary were authorized to visit Washington whenever necessary to coordinate more closely the activities of the Association with governmental departments. A special report was made by the war committee, and a resolution was introduced approving the creation of a world war medical conference organization.

THE SPANISH JOURNAL

Extensive discussions were given to the establishment of a Spanish periodical, and Mr. A. A. Moll was selected as supervising editor.

THE WAR MEETING

The 1918 war meeting of the Association was held in Chicago in the offices of the American Medical Association. All five members of the Council on Health and Public Instruction and its secretary were in service, and the activities of the council had been limited to routine work. Its report was brief and the entire section on social insurance had disappeared. It is interesting to think what might have happened relating to social insurance if the war had not intervened.

The President, Dr. Charles Mayo, was also in the armed forces. He felt that there was bickering and disturbance in the profession and a lack of harmony, and he urged cooperation in the battle against Germany. The undercurrent of his address referred to the competition between Dr. George H. Simmons and Dr. Franklin H. Martin, although neither was mentioned by name. He pleaded particularly for coordination between the seventeen different government agencies concerned with medicine.

Dr. Hubert Work, chairman of the House of Delegates, spoke briefly on the war situation and announced that he would present later the report of the war committee. He called the selective draft "the colossal achievement of the times," and he paid high tribute to General Enoch H. Crowder for his magnificent conduct of the draft and also to William C. Gorgas, Surgeon General of the Army.

The secretary of the Association, Dr. Alexander R. Craig, reported on the appointment of the war committee and recommended that it be continued so that it might act for the Association in all matters pertaining to placing the Association at the service of the government for the war. He indicated the numerous facilities in the headquarters of the Association which could be useful to the government and how particularly the biographic data had been utilized in finding physicians for the armed forces.

THE PUBLICATIONS

The Board of Trustees referred to the growth of the publications and emphasized the number of law suits which had been filed against the organization and the manner in which they had been handled in the courts. The active work of the Association in codifying and supplying to the profession and the public information concerning quackery, fraudulent medicines and low standard medical colleges had resulted in threats, intimidation and actual suits. There were six libel suits in sums of $100,000 each.

THE LYDSTON CASE

The Board submitted also a complete record of the case that had been filed by Dr. G. Frank Lydston to oust the trustees of the American Medical Association from office because they had been elected outside the state of Illinois. That case had been decided by the Supreme Court of Illinois in favor of the Association.

PATENTS

A fundamental decision reported by the Judicial Council objected to the acceptance of a patent by the American Medical Association. It declared against the patenting of a medical discovery for commercial gain, and it said "The ethics of patenting a medical discovery is not overshadowed or affected by the use to which the returns from the sale of the patented medicine may be put." Indeed, the Judicial Council declared that it was unethical for the University of Minnesota to accept patents on medical discoveries and that it would be unethical for the Mayo brothers on their part to consummate an agreement of this kind if they would be patenting a medical discovery and using the commercial proceeds therefrom to increase a fund given to the university by them.

The House of Delegates rejected the recommendation of the Judicial Council relative to patents, believing that the Mayo brothers had made their offer in good faith and in the spirit of altruism. It was felt that whatever the University of Minnesota did was a problem for the University of Minnesota.

A NURSE SHORTAGE

Already in World War I there began to be a shortage of nurses, and a resolution was submitted requesting the establishment of a committee to consider the whole question of registering and training nurses with a view to standardizing and simplifying the requirements and with a view to establishing a grade of practical nurses who would receive smaller compensation and take care of the sick, thus relieving graduate nurses for war work.

The meeting approved the commissioning of women physicians in the Army. A resolution was adopted, as offered by Dr. John Ridlon, urging universal military training before the right of suffrage was granted.

In 1918 an amendment to the Constitution had provided for changing the name of "chairman" and "vice chairman" of the House of Delegates to "speaker" and "vice speaker."

At the 1918 meeting Dr. Charles H. Mayo, who was at that time the President of the Association, introduced a resolution into the House of Delegates providing for an ad interim committee to deal with emergency problems, this committee to consist of the President, the president-elect, the chairman of the House of Delegates, the secretary of the Association, the last two living retiring presidents and the chairman of the Board of Trustees. He also proposed that the President of the American Medical Association be authorized to appoint members of committees not provided for by the House of Delegates or the Board of Trustees and that their work be passed on by the ad interim committee. The reference committee on amendments to the Constitution and By-Laws approved this amendment with the exception that they put the last two living ex-presidents on the committee and made it possible for committees appointed by the President to have official existence only until the next meeting of the House of Delegates.

In November 1918 a meeting of the war committee convened in Washington and was reconstituted as a meeting of the Board of Trustees. Since the Armistice had been signed, the war committee was instructed to take steps for using the American Medical Association to constitute a real medical reserve corps, and a special committee was developed for that purpose. When World War II came, the reserve corps had some 18,000 members, but unfortunately 9,000 were incapable of giving active service.

The Association planned for a Victory Meeting in 1919 with distinguished guests from abroad. It was suggested that the Department of State issue invitations to the allied nations to send delegates. Requests were made particularly to invite physicians from the South American nations.

1919

ATLANTIC CITY

Dr. Frank Billings reported for the committee which had been appointed to consider standardization of hospitals that it seemed desirable that such standardization be undertaken in cooperation with the American College of Surgeons. It was felt that it would be desirable to employ a full time man to do this work.

SOCIAL INSURANCE

Then came the question of social and health insurance. A special message had come from the president of the Pennsylvania State Medical Association and from Dr. Alexander Lambert indicating that the situation was becoming pressing. The statement by Dr. Lambert attacked particularly Dr. Edward H. Ochsner of Chicago, who had been the leading opponent of compulsory sickness insurance. Dr. Lambert attacked the Insurance Economic Society of America as the principal camouflage organization now conducting a vigorous campaign against social insurance. Dr. Wendell Phillips called attention to an editorial which had appeared in THE JOURNAL for Feb. 1, 1919 entitled "The Failure of Compulsory Health Insurance." He felt that it did not present the entire subject. Dr. Alexander Lambert, now president-elect of the Association, called attention to the eight pamphlets already published and to the four basic points which he felt must be included in any social insurance system which would be approved by the medical profession.

A SURGICAL JOURNAL

Now that the war had passed there came again a call for the publication of a special journal dealing with the philosophy of surgery in contradistinction to surgical technic. Dr. Lambert urged that such a journal would not be in competition with any journal then being published.

Conferences began to be held between representatives of the American Medical Association and the American College of Surgeons on the standardization of hospitals with a view to cooperation and avoidance of duplication.

In 1918 Dr. Frank Billings, who had served in many capacities, including the presidency of the Association, was elected to the Board of Trustees and his place on the Council on Health and Public Instruction was given to Dr. Ludvig Hektoen.

The Spanish journal had been conducted for three months with considerable success.

The Association had distinguished itself in defending a suit brought by Jenner Medical College for $500,000 damages.

It was felt desirable that the Board of Trustees publish regularly a digest of its minutes in THE JOURNAL and that it would have served a good effect on the medical profession if the report of the conference with the American College of Surgeons had been given adequate publicity in THE JOURNAL.

THE VICTORY MEETING

It became clear that little could be expected in the way of having delegates from foreign countries at the Victory Meeting. Response had been poor, and the secretary of the Association was authorized to send cables to various governments requesting attendance of foreign guests at the 1919 meeting.

The speaker of the House of Delegates made a long address in which he discussed the problems created by the war and the return of men from the war. He recognized the growth of groups of physicians in practice and the evolution of the hospital. He predicted that the greatest future concern of the Association might be in its direction and oversight of hospitals. He suggested the possible establishment of a council on hospitals to be concerned with control of such organizations and with a view to possible elimination of the joint survey of hospitals conducted by the American Medical Association and the American College of Surgeons. He recognized the problems created by the increasing length of the curriculum, and he feared that the duration of medical education was becoming too great. He was equally concerned with the difficulty of securing competent nurses at reasonable costs, and he viewed with alarm the tendency toward specialization and the disappearance of the general practitioner. He conceived it to be the duty of the American Medical Association to assure to the public qualified physicians, nurses and standardized hospitals at prices it could afford to pay. He spoke also of problems in the field of physical education, noting that 30 per cent of registrants appearing before local boards were rejected for military service—a situation which was still a matter of concern in 1946. He was especially concerned with the problems of dentistry as they related to the draft, and he thought the time ripe to give serious consideration to provision of medical care in rural areas.

Dr. Arthur Dean Bevan, who was President of the Association, had been chosen no doubt in recognition not only of his eminence in the field of surgery but also for his many years of leadership in the Council on Medical Education. Both Dr. Work and Dr. Bevan called attention to the manner in which physicians had pledged themselves to the nation for service. He indicated, however, that there must be much closer relationship between the national organization and the individual state organizations. Through the Council on Medical Education a national conference on hospital problems had been developed; this had been of great service through the years in clarifying problems in the hospital field. Dr. Bevan recognized the prominence of THE JOURNAL but he urged again particularly a periodical to be devoted to surgery. As will be seen later, this intensified the competition between the Association and the American College of Surgeons. Dr. Bevan felt that the publication of a surgical journal by the American Medical Association would merely tend to improve all other surgical publications in the field.

In his address as president-elect, Dr. Alexander Lambert announced that he had but two recommendations to make. He urged first a journal on surgery and, second, a popular journal in the field of health—thus intensifying the drive toward such a publication, which had been going on for many years. More particularly he then devoted himself wholly to problems of narcotic addiction; he recommended resolutions leading toward a national conference on the control of narcotic drugs.

The secretary of the Association, Dr. Alexander R. Craig, was concerned with the manner in which physicians returning from the war were being received by their communities.

The introduction by the American College of Surgeons of the letters F.A.C.S. to designate its members had raised the question of a similar designation for fellows of the American Medical Association. The secretary of the Association, therefore, proposed a variety of designations to indicate various qualifications of membership in the American Medical Association.

The Board of Trustees indicated great progress, first by the fact that there had been no loss of membership or subscription to THE JOURNAL during the war. The Spanish edition had been established and had reached a circulation of more than 1,400. The QUARTERLY CUMULATIVE INDEX was operating at a small loss. The Association had been successful in all its law suits. The board announced the decision to develop a new building by adding to its quarters.

At this time the Judicial Council proposed amendments which would more definitely define membership and fellowship in the American Medical Association and which would clarify its wording.

COUNCIL ON HEALTH AND PUBLIC INSTRUCTION

Since the Council on Health and Public Instruction had been relatively inactive during the war because its secretary and most of its members had been in the military service, the chairman found it desirable at this time to present a brief history of the work of the Council since its origin. Since that Council was discontinued some years later, when its activities were turned over to a number of bureaus, it is well to read that summary:

The Council on Health and Public Instruction was organized at St. Louis in 1910. During the reorganization period of the Association from 1902 to 1910 many independent committees had been created dealing with closely related subjects but without any coordination or definite division of functions or jurisdiction. At the 1909 session of the Section on Hygiene and Sanitary Science asked the House of Delegates to create a permanent council on these subjects. The reference committee to which this request was referred called attention to the close relation existing between public education, medical and public health legislation and the development of hygiene and sanitation and recommended the appointment of a committee to consider the advisability of combining the functions of legislation, public instruction, organization and public sanitation in a permanent council. This committee was appointed and reported the following year, recommending the establishment of such a permanent council. The Council on Health and Public Instruction was accordingly created and appointed in June 1910 and held its first meeting and organized in July of the same year. In it were merged the old Committees on Medical Legislation, Public Instruction on Medical Subjects, Defense of Medical Research, Organization, Uniform Regulation of Membership, Visual Standards of Pilots, Public Health Education, Prevention of Blindness and Postgraduate Study. In 1911 the work of the Council consisted in the promotion of the work of Dr. J. N. McCormack, at that time engaged in organization work for the Association; in the development of a series of fifteen pamphlets on the Defense of Medical Research, which, in addition to thirteen already published, formed a standard series of twenty-eight monographs on this subject, and in the development of a bureau on medical legislation by which it was hoped some of the problems in this field could be solved and in studying the problem of public education by state boards and other agencies through popular pamphlets.

At the next session, in 1912, the Council reported that a Press Bureau had been organized and conducted during the past year by which regular press bulletins had been sent to approximately 5,000 daily newspapers each week; the Speakers' Bureau had been organized and in the three months of its existence had supplied speakers for forty-four meetings; nine pamphlets on various public health subjects had been prepared, printed and distributed; a Handbook for Speakers on Public Health had been compiled, printed and distributed to the speakers of the Bureau. The Council also reported the organization, through cooperation with the National Electric Light Association and the American Institute of Electrical Engineers, of the Committee on Resuscitation after Electrical Shock; of the appointment, in cooperation with the National Education Association, of a Joint Committee on Medical Expert Testimony, consisting of representatives of the American Medical Association, the American Bar Association and the Commissioners on Uniform Laws; of a Committee on Rural Sanitation consisting of representatives of the American Medical Association, the Association of Railway Surgeons and the Conference of State and Provincial Boards of Health; of a Committee on Vital Statistics Legislation consisting of representatives of the American Medical Association, the American Public Health Association, the American Bar Association, Commissioners on Uniform Laws and the Bureau of the Census. In addition the Council had done much work along legislatve lines and had represented the Association in a campaign for the establishment of a national department of health.

In 1913 the Council reported the continuation of these activities, showing that speakers had been furnished for 213 meetings during the year; that fourteen pamphlets had been prepared and distributed, and that the various subcommittees of the Council had been functioning successfully during the year. A Committee on Resuscitation from Mine Gases, as the successor of the Committee on Resuscitation after Electrical Shock, had been created at the request of the Federal Bureau of Mines. These committees had stadardized the methods of artificial respiration and the treatment of the drowned and those suffering from gas, electric shock, and so on.

In 1914, after four years of existence, the Council presented to the House of Delegates a definite program in which it endeavored to formulate the duties and activities of the organized medical profession in the public health field. In outlining such a program the Council assumed that the primary object of its existence was to place before the profession and the public of the United States the objects, purposes and work of the organized medical profession as represented by the American Medical Association and its constituent state and component county societies, so as to secure public support and endorsement of our efforts for the improvement of public health conditions in the United States. Three general lines of action were accordingly recommended. These were:

1. A thorough investigation of present public health conditions in the United States with the view to securing more accurate information an all phases of the public health problem than is now available.

2. Education of the public by every possible means in order that the people may understand the enormous advances in scientific medical knowledge during the last generation and the possibilities of utilizing such knowledge in the prevention of disease, the reduction of the death rate and the prolongation of human life.

3. The crystallizing of such educated sentiment in necessary public health laws which

will render possible the conservation of human life commensurate with our advancing knowledge and will render such laws effective through the only force available in this country, namely educated and enlightened public opinion.

Under the first head, namely the investigation of the present public health situation, need for additional knowledge was subdivided into four clases: (a) public health activities of the federal government, (b) state public health activities, (c) municipal health organization and (d) voluntary public health organization.

Under the second head, the education of the public, the Council reported the continuation of the Press Bureau, forty-two bulletins having been sent to 4,900 newspapers at a total cost of approximately $2,300. The Speakers Bureau had been maintained during the year, speakers had been furnished for 133 meetings at a total cost of approximately $1,900, and a standard set of public health pamphlets had been prepared and published for the use of state boards. In addition, a series of twenty pamphlets on Conservation of Vision had been prepared and issued by the subcommittee on this subject. This set of pamphlets has remained in use ever since and has been recognized as a standard in this field. A series of six pamphlets on cancer and its prevention had also been prepared and published. The total number of pamphlets issued during the year was 57,250.

In 1915 the Council reported the continuation of its program, particularly the carrying on of a comparative study of state public health activities by Dr. Charles V. Chapin, health commissioner of Providence, R. I., as the special representative of the Council. Dr. Chapin's report was the first effort to collect data on state health activities with a view to the ultimate standardization and classification of state public health work. Regarding voluntary public health activities, the Council endeavored through a conference of representatives of the various voluntary organizations held in New York on March 13, 1915 to coordinate the numerous organizations in this field. Along educational lines, the Council reported that, at the direction of the general manager, the mailing list of the Press Bulletin had been reduced to 2,200. Owing to the limited appropriation, the amount available for the Speakers' Bureau had been limited to $1,000. For this amount speakers had been furnished for 151 meetings, an average expense of $9.80 a meeting. During the year 285,400 pamphlets have been printed and distributed.

In 1916 the Council reported further development of its program, including the publication of Dr. Chapin's Report on State Public Health Work, with a rating sheet of the forty-eight state health organizations showing their comparative standing in different lines of state public health work, their appropriations, expenditures, etc. A preliminary edition of 1,000 copies of this report was distributed to members of state boards of health and officers of the Association for criticism and suggestions, and the Council expressed the hope that at the end of two or three years a second survey might be made for confirmatory and comparative purposes. Owing to reduced appropriations the Press Bulletin had been suspended, and the plan of the Speakers' Bureau had been modified by asking local organizations to pay the expenses of speakers instead of having these expenses borne by the Association. During the year 1,133,500 pamphlets had been printed and distributed. Cooperative work had been carried on through the Elizabeth McCormick Memorial Fund and the dry-goods stores of the country for child welfare.

Viewing the situation after the war, the Council thought it inadvisable to continue its press bureau and its speakers' bureau since those functions had been developed by other agencies. It proposed to continue the publication of useful pamphlets. It felt that the control of voluntary health organizations was a problem not for the Council but more particularly for the American Public Health Association, which had recently organized a council of representatives of fifty-seven different national public health organizations. It proposed, therefore, to limit its work largely to the routine work of the secretary's office, continuation of the section on legal medicine and medical ligislation, and a survey of public health activities of national, state and municipal, governmental and voluntary agencies. The final section of the report, which was issued under Dr. Victor C. Vaughan as chairman, with Dr. Frederick R. Green as secretary, dealt with social insurance. This report reviewed the existing status of legislation in the field and expressed the point of view of the medical profession in positive terms:

> The attitude of the majority of physicians up to date has been one of unqualified and often unreasoning opposition, without any effort to study the question or to consider the arguments put forward in favor of the proposed plan. Unreasoning opposition or sweeping and often erroneous general arguments against the measure will not prevent its adoption nor will it enhance the influence of physicians. It is of the utmost importance to the medical profession at present that we give this question the most careful, painstaking, patient and disinterested study, that we qualify ourselves as authorities instead of allowing this function to be exercised by the active proponents of social insurance. To this end it is particularly necessary that we study this question dispassionately and critically, discriminating between fundamental principles and nonessential details.

The Council recognized four possible solutions for the problem of illness among persons of low income: (1) increasing the income, (2) reducing the amount of sickness, (3) distributing the costs of sickness among the individual, the industry and the state, and (4) doing nothing. These were classed as the economic remedy, the state public health remedy, social insurance and no remedy at all.

It was recognized that extensive studies would be required from an economic point of view to answer many of the questions in the field concerned. The Council recommended that the House of Delegates give most careful study to the report of its subcommittee on social insurance.

The report of the subcommittee on social insurance leaned largely on statistics that were being developed by insurance companies and by the U. S. Public Health Service. It endeavored to assess the responsibility for sickness in its various proportions to the individual, the community and industry. It discussed the relationships between sickness and economic distress, quoting again largely from such writers as the Webbs, Edward T. Devine, Michael Davis and little at all from writers opposed to state controlled methods of medical care.

The final section of the report was an analysis of the relationship of the medical profession to the problems of social insurance.

The committee seemed to believe that a choice was necessarily between state medicine and health insurance. It recognized the evils prevailing in the plans of other countries and recommended that our medical profession learn from the difficulties that prevailed in

England and Germany. It felt that the decision would rest not with the medical profession but with economic groups and forces outside the medical profession. Thus it said:

> Your committee does not deem that it is its duty to bring forward at this time a method thoroughly worked out in all detail of medical practice under any sickness insurance scheme. In its previous reports it has gone fully into the methods of payment of physicians under such acts. It has pointed out the mistakes made in the administration of medical service by the insurance laws abroad. It must further be emphasized that it is not a question for the decision of the medical profession whether or not these laws shall be put in force. That is a question for economic groups and forces outside of the medical profession. It will be decided when labor and industry agree together sufficiently to demand it of the legislative bodies of the various states. It is, however, of the utmost importance for the medical profession to be ready with constructive suggestions, to meet labor and industry halfway and show to them how the profession may give a greatly improved service to the wage earners and receive a just remuneration in return, and the great mass of unremunerative medical charity may cease to exist. It is also for the profession to decide whether or not it wishes to carry on its existence under some form of sickness insurance or under some method of state medicine. That choice must inevitably be made.

The conclusion was, however, simply a recommendation for further study and for appearance by physicians before all state legislatures having these questions before them so that the point of view of medicine could be adequately presented. This report was signed by four names: Drs. Alexander Lambert, M. L. Harris, F. L. Van Sickle and S. S. Goldwater.

MULTIPLE RESOLUTIONS

By this time it was apparent that so many actions were being taken in the organization and development of the Association that some codification was needed. A resolution was introduced requesting the secretary of the Association to collect all resolutions passed in the previous five years, to index them properly and to add new resolutions as they developed. The resolution was passed with simply an amendment that ten years be codified instead of five.

SOCIAL INSURANCE

The report on social insurance was referred to a reference committee which included Dr. Thomas S. Cullen, Maryland, as chairman, and Drs. Clarence Pierson, Louisiana, and Charles E. Humiston, Illinois. The committee recommended that every member of the House read the report in full. It recognized the stupendous character of the problem. It commended the committee on refraining from making any definite recommendations. Especially, however, it recognized the political character of the situation. It concluded its report by recommending a change in the By-Laws which would make the Reference Committee on Legislation and Political Action instead a Reference Committee on Legislation and Public Relations. The committee said:

> This change is deemed advisable at this time, as the term political action has in some quarters been thought to refer to politics. In the words of Confucius, "Avoid the very appearance of evil. Do not stoop to tie your shoes in your neighbor's melon patch."

SPECIALIZATION

At this session of the Association there suddenly arose a definite recognition of the rise of specialization versus general practice; a resolution was introduced that the House of Delegates encourage the designation of the practice of general medicine or family physician as a distinct and dignified specialty and that the Council on Medical Education consider the possibility of establishing a definite curriculum leading to the degree of practice of this specialty which would materially shorten the course. The House of Delegates referred these to the Council on Medical Education.

THE SPEAKER

When the elections came before the House of Delegates on the concluding day of the session, an unusual situation arose in the proposal of nomination of the speaker for the presidency. A number of the parliamentarians had studied the Constitution and By-Laws and voiced their opinions to the effect that the speaker was not a member of the House of Delegates and that he was therefore eligible. A motion was taken to the effect that the speaker be considered eligible and the motion passed. Then Admiral William C. Braisted of the U. S. Navy was nominated for the presidency and Dr. Hubert Work announced that he was not even a tentative candidate. Admiral Braisted was elected unanimously to the presidency of the Association.

FOREIGN GUESTS

A number of foreign guests had come to the meeting which had been declared a Victory Meeting for the Association. These included six from Belgium, eight from England, three from France, two from China, three from Japan, four from Cuba, one from Norway and one from Sweden. All were elected to Honorary Fellowship in the American Medical Association.

DAYLIGHT SAVING TIME

As the session ended, the Congress of the United States was proposing to repeal the Daylight Saving Act. The House of Delegates officially opposed the repeal of the act and expressed its opinion of daylight saving as follows:

The national experience with the Daylight Saving Act during the past two years has shown in the opinion of the committee that the action of this bill has been wholly beneficial; not only has it added to the total of national health by lengthened hours of recreation in the open air, but it is the belief of the committee that notable economic savings have been made in the use of fuel, thereby materially assisting the conservation of national resources, which still is and always will be essential.

BOARD NEEDS MORE MEETINGS

By this time the multiple affairs of the Association had become so great that the Board of Trustees found it impossible to handle them in the amount of time alloted to its meetings. The Board had been accustomed to meet but twice each year—once in February and once at the time of the annual session. Most of the members of the Board were certain that there ought to be more frequent meetings, primarily because too much opposition was focusing itself on the editor and general manager and that it was unfair to put all the responsibility on the manager. It was felt that the Board of Trustees should meet quarterly and that there ought to be an executive committee which would meet regularly in order to take some of the burden from the editor and the general manager. When Dr. George H. Simmons was asked for his opinion, he pointed out that it was at his earnest suggestion that more frequent meetings of the board were being held. He said that a Board of Trustees consisting of nine men in session once every three months would not do much toward relieving the general manager, or rather the editor, of responsibility; that it is not the general manager, but the editor, that is criticized. He stated that we have a journal second to none in the world, a journal that is a power in the field of medicine, and yet if the editor turns down a paper written by some influential man it has its effect; that what the manager—the editor—wants is some one to shoulder a little of the responsibility—of the blame. He mentioned that there is not as much criticism today as there was fifteen years ago but that there is bound to be some—that it may die down for a time but that it will spring up again. He urged the appointment of a committee of three, living within a reasonable distance of Chicago, to meet once a month—not once in three months—which should act on matters of importance that are coming up all the time and assume part of the editor's responsibility. He stated that it is the editor's position that should be more fully supported.

As a result of these actions the board decided on a technic which would involve four meetings of the full board annually and the meetings of the executive committee once each month—a procedure which has been followed since that time.

DERMATOLOGY JOURNAL

Petitions now had come for a journal in the field of dermatology. For some time the *Journal of Cutaneous Diseases* had been printed in the headquarters office of the American Medical Association and it was felt that publication by the Association would solve many of its financial and editorial problems.

EXECUTIVE COMMITTEE

The first Executive Committee of the Board of Trustees included Drs. Frank Billings (chairman), W. T. Sarles and A. R. Mitchell.

Following the annual session in June of 1919 the Executive Committee met and assumed as its first responsibility advice to the editor relative to passing on papers which had been marked for publication in the Transactions only. THE JOURNAL had begun publishing abstracts from German medical periodicals and Dr. George W. Crile, in association with Drs. F. E. Bunts and W. E. Lower in Cleveland, was opposed to giving any recognition to Germans or German literature. There had been an extensive correspondence on the subject. Dr. Crile was adamant in refusing to countenance any relationships whatever with Germans or any recognition of their science. The Executive Committee of the Board of Trustees agreed with the editor that anything of real importance appearing in the German journals should be brought to the attention of the medical profession.

NEW EDITORIAL BOARDS

The Board of Trustees during this year established editorial boards for the ARCHIVES OF DERMATOLOGY AND SYPHILOLOGY and for the ARCHIVES OF SURGERY.

THE STERNBERG BIOGRAPHY

There was also the problem of printing the biography of General Sternberg, which had been written by Mrs. Sternberg, the costs to be offset by Mrs. Sternberg, and it was agreed to undertake this publication with the understanding that if there were any profits they would be divided equally with Mrs. Sternberg.

WAR BOOKS

At that time the American Medical Association endeavored to get distribution to the medical profession of books which had been printed during the war for the use of medical officers.

It was pointed out by Dr. Frank Billings that he had learned that there were no books on hand but that even if there were any they would be government property and could not be distributed. However, as the nation entered World War II some 8,000 copies of the anatomy prepared during World War I were found in a warehouse on Long Island.

The Ad Interim Committee which had been created during the war to consider emergencies arising during the war presented to the Board of Trustees of the Association an extensive letter from the president of the Association, Dr. Alexander Lambert, which he had received from Gen. Merritt W. Ireland concerning the possibility of deriving some lessons from the experience in the war. It was proposed that a circular letter be sent to all men who had been actually in service and some means be provided for continuing the instruction of men in the medical reserve. At that time Dr. Billings explained some of the problems confronting the medical department of the Army, including representation of the medical department on the general staff, control by the medical department of its own personnel, control by the medical department of supplies, building of hospitals and camps, recognition of the importance of sanitation and preventive medicine in the Army, military medical teaching and suitable recognition of qualifications of officers.

As the year went on there came a request from a group of obstetricians to take over the *American Journal of Obstetrics and Diseases of Women and Children*, but it was decided that the Association already had enough periodicals in hand.

CHANGING VIEWS OF SICKNESS INSURANCE

1920

NEW ORLEANS

BY THE END OF 1919 correspondence began to reach THE JOURNAL opposing the reports that had been issued by the Council on Health and Public Instruction and by its subcommittee on social insurance. The writers charged that these reports were unscientific and more in the nature of propaganda for compulsory health insurance than scientific studies. Comparisons had revealed that many of the statements presented in the pamphlets published by the Council could be found in the propaganda issued by the American Association for Labor Legislation. Attack centered particularly on I. M. Rubinow, who had been secretary of the subcommittee on social insurance and who was responsible for most of the pamphlets. Circulation of the pamphlets was promptly discontinued. It was discovered, incidentally, that Dr. I. M. Rubinow was at the same time in the employ of the American Association for Labor Legislation.

HOSPITAL STUDIES

With much travail, early in 1920 a technic was developed for adding the listing of hospitals to the work of the Council on Medical Education. That task having been successfully accomplished, the function has been carried on continuously since that time.

THE BRAISTED ADDRESS

In his presidential address on Tuesday, April 27, at the New Orleans session, Admiral Braisted of the U. S. Navy read a presidential address which lasted a long time—variously estimated from one and a half to two and a half hours. In the minutes of the Board of Trustees appears a resolution that it is the sense of the Board of Trustees that no address at the opening meeting of the Scientific Assembly should exceed thirty minutes in its delivery. Physicians who were present when Admiral Braisted read his address reported that most of the assemblage listened carefully for the first thirty minutes but that members departed in increasing numbers, so that toward the end the hall presented vast areas of unoccupied seats.

The address was titled "The Obligations of Medicine in Relation to General Education."

THE DIRECTORY REPORT SERVICE

At the suggestion of Mr. Will C. Braun and with the hearty cooperation of Dr. George H. Simmons, the American Medical Association in 1920 introduced its directory report service as a supplement to the directory. The reception of this report service by agencies requiring constant correction of mailing lists was so favorable that the report service has been continuous since that time.

PROHIBITION AND MEDICAL TECHNICIANS

Now for the first time also there came to the Board of Trustees two problems which were to be of great import in the ensuing years. The first was prohibition! The second was the fact that increasingly technicians were administering anesthetics and doing roentgen ray work and that laymen were conducting diagnostic laboratories.

Most of the early portion of 1920 was concerned with increasing costs of paper and labor and with the necessity of increasing the income of the Association by a rise in the price of THE JOURNAL.

THE NEW ORLEANS SESSION

The speaker of the House of Delegates, Dr. Hubert Work, had found some difficulties with the functioning of the Ad Interim Committee; he felt that its prescribed emergency duties might be delegated to the Board of Trustees or perhaps to the Executive Committee of the board. He urged compulsory military training. He pointed out that surgery was becoming dissociated from medicine and that it needed to be reoriented within the science of medicine; it seemed to him that the remedy lay with the American College of Surgeons.

The President of the Association, Dr. Alexander Lambert, spoke to the House of Delegates primarily on the growth and development of the hospital. There had been some resentment among the smaller hospitals to standardizing under the Council on Medical Education and Hospitals.

The report of the Board of Trustees called attention to the need of additional funds to carry on the activities of the organization and particularly to take up the new function of standardization of hospitals.

The Judicial Council had submitted a rewording of the Constitution and By-Laws, primarily with a view to clarity. For this most of the credit attaches to Dr. M. L. Harris of Chicago, chairman of the Judicial Council, whose legal mind was a great asset in such affairs.

SOCIAL INSURANCE

The Council on Health and Public Instruction was suffering from criticisms which had begun to appear in state medical journals, which felt that the Council should have taken a positive position against social insurance. The Council stated that it was not the business of the Council to formulate the policies of the Association. The Council felt, however, that its publications had certainly served to arouse the medical profession to an intelligent discussion of the subject.

NARCOTIC DRUGS

The control of narcotic drugs had become such a difficult problem that a special committee had represented the Association in a conference on the subject; its report occupies some ten pages of THE JOURNAL. This report condemned the ambulatory treatment of narcotic addiction, recommended that heroin be eliminated from all medicinal preparations and urged intensive action by the government to control narcotics.

A LAY MEDICAL JOURNAL

At the meeting of the House of Delegates in 1920 a resolution was offered to establish a lay medical journal. The House recommended postponement.

MORE SOCIAL INSURANCE

Several resolutions from New York condemned compulsory health insurance and any system which would provide for medical service to be rendered contributors or others provided, controlled or regulated by the federal or state government. These resolutions were supported by Illinois and Michigan.

ENDOCRINE PRODUCTS

For the first time there came a resolution demanding some sort of control over the sale of endocrine products.

The Ad Interim Committee, at the request of the Surgeon General, had tried to work out a technic for reconsideration of the medical service in World War I and leading toward the development of the Walter Reed Hospital as a medical education center.

SOCIAL SICKNESS INSURANCE CONDEMNED

When the Reference Committee on Hygiene and Public Health, headed by Dr. J. W. Schereschewsky of the U. S. Public Health Service, made its report, it submitted the following resolution, which was adopted:

Resolved, That the American Medical Association declares its opposition to the institution of any plan embodying the system of compulsory contributory insurance against illness, or any other plan of compulsory insurance which provides for medical service to be rendered contributors or their dependents, provided, controlled or regulated by any state or the federal govermnent.

That policy has remained the policy of the American Medical Association since 1920.

Significant of the elections held at the end of the 1920 session were the unanimous choice of Hubert Work, speaker of the House, as President and the election as the second speaker of the House of Dr. Dwight H. Murray of Syracuse, N. Y.; the latter had long been active in the affairs of the Association.

Again the Association adopted a resolution urging a national department of health.

WHISKY QUESTION LAID ON THE TABLE

Toward the end of the 1920 session a resolution came from the Council on Health and Public Instruction to the effect that the House of Delegates reaffirm a resolution adopted in 1917 that whisky is not necessary for the proper scientific treatment of influenza. This received a tremendous debate and ended by being laid on the table.

THE JOURNAL COSTS

In November a special session of the House of Delegates met to consider the problem of increasing costs in publication of THE JOURNAL. Statements were made by the editor and by Dr. Frank Billings as secretary of the Board of Trustees. Dr. C. J. Whalen, Illinois, and Dr. W. B. Small, Iowa, were the only two delegates opposed to raising the price of THE JOURNAL, and the action was carried overwhelmingly.

AND AGAIN THE LAY JOURNAL

Under the leadership of Dr. Wendell C. Phillips of New York a movement was begun to promote the establishment of a journal for the public in order to disseminate knowledge of scientific medicine and also to employ a field secretary who would carry on the extension of organizational work.

1921

THE CULTISTS' MENACE

Early in 1921 the rise of antivivisectionists, chiropractors, osteopaths and other nonmedical cultists began to give concern not only to the American Medical Association but to many of the foundations prominent in the field of public health. Arrangements were made for a dinner in New York City, attended by representatives of all these foundations, for a general consideration of the subject. It was felt inadvisable that there be any concerted action in this regard, although it was felt also that there ought to be some definite steps taken to enlighten the public regarding the menace of these cults.

THE BOSTON MEETING

In his first official address as speaker of the House of Delegates Dr. Dwight H. Murray of Syracuse urged particularly the establishment of a journal in the field of public health. He thought it possible that the Association might cooperate with the U. S. Public Health Service in such a publication. He believed that it might be possible to publish a periodical of this type as a Sunday magazine with the newspapers and to include questions and answers. He urged the appointment of field secretaries and a mechanism for presenting to the state medical societies the activities of the American Medical Association. His views were reenforced by similar statements from Dr. Hubert Work as President of the Association.

The report of the Board of Trustees gave much attention to the rehabilitation of veterans.

The Council on Health and Public Instruction had held a conference dealing with the provision of medical care particularly in rural areas. It recognized the need for more study and greater cooperation and requested authorization from the House of Delegates to call a national conference on the subject.

An extensive report dealt with the attitudes of the medical profession relative to narcotic drugs, and an even more extensive report concerned the building of hospitals for the indigent.

The Council on Medical Education and Hospitals was also much troubled by such problems as the training of specialists in contrast to the training of general practitioners, and the chairman of the Council was especially disturbed by what he called "outside interference with medical education." He said:

I refer to the introduction of a scheme of organization of the faculties of our medical colleges which has been introduced by great educational foundations and by some of the state universities.

And particularly was he concerned with "the plan of all-time clinical instruction." He continued:

> This plan did not originate in the medical profession. It originated outside the medical profession, and unfortunately it has been forced on the situation largely by money. It is a subsidized plan which has been presented to universities with the statement that they would be given one or two millions of dollars or more, provided they would adopt the all-time clinical plan in their scheme of organization. To be sure, the originators of the plan have presented it as an experiment, but it has not been a fair experiment. A scientific experiment necessarily requires a control. There has been no control here. If, on the contrary, the great foundations would take three schools and give each of them two millions or five millions of dollars and put them on the all-time clinical plan, and another three schools of the same caliber and give each of them the same amount of money and allow them to develop under some plan which has been the outcome of the experience of medical educators the world over, the plan that one might refer to as the Trousseau plan, the Billroth plan, the Osler plan, a plan that has developed from the practical experience of medical educators, it would then be a fair experiment. So far the plan has been introduced at Johns Hopkins and Yale, at Washington University in St. Louis, and it has been adopted by the University of Chicago and by Columbia University. I believe also the new university of Rochester contemplates adopting it, and the plan in a somewhat modified may has been adopted by some of the state universities, notably the University of Michigan.

After this preliminary statement, the chairman said that he was opposed to state medicine but he recognized the necessity for organizing the delivery of medical service for wider distribution and lower costs. His report included this conclusion:

> There is special need that the medical profession develop some method by which the great possibilities of modern medicine, in the way of diagnosis, treatment and prevention of diseases, may be brought within the reach of all people. This function, it is believed, should be preformed by the medical profession and not through any form of state medicine.

Under "New Business" came a group of resolutions on state medicine reaffirming the point of view previously adopted on this subject. The question was considered so fundamental to the future of the American Medical Association that it was considered by the entire House of Delegates as a committee of the whole.

The reference committee suggested, as a substitute for all these resolutions:

> *Resolved,* By the House of Delegates of the American Medical Association, that it approves and endorses all activities and policies of states directed to the prevention of disease but opposes the state treatment of disease, except (*a*) in the institutional care of the delinquent, diseased and defective; (*b*) the treatment of those diseases whose treatment is essential to prevention; (*c*) the recognition and securing the correction of common defects of school children.

However, the committee of the whole made the following substitution which was unanimously adopted:

Resolved, By the House of Delegates of the American Medical Association that it approves and endorses all proper activities and policies of state and federal governments directed to the prevention of disease and the preservation of the public health.

A SECTION ON ANESTHESIA

Resolutions were offered requesting a section on anesthesia.

FULL TIME TEACHING

The reference committee on medical education refused to take a stand on the question of full time versus part time clinical teaching but suggested that experimentation should provide just as much funds in support of one as of the other.

THE LAY JOURNAL

A half dozen resolutions supported the proposal for a periodical in the field of public health, and the entire matter was referred to the Board of Trustees. Other proposals urged extension of the work of the field secretary as well as of full time paid secretaries for state medical societies.

STATE MEDICINE

Now for the first time came before the House of Delegates a definition of the term "state medicine." One of these, emanating from Dr. W. S. Rankin of North Carolina, included eight different types of legislation which had to do in any way with the relationship of the physician to the state. Another, exceedingly brief, came from a New York delegate, Dr. E. F. Delphey, which said succinctly:

> *Resolved,* That the term "State Medicine" be defined by this Association as the practice of medicine by the state by physicians on a salary to the exclusion of all other and individual practice of medicine.

Then came another definition by Dr. James F. Rooney of New York:

> *Resolved,* That the American Medical Association defines "State Medicine" to be any method providing for the practice of medicine under the direction, subsidy or control of the state or national government, excepting those functions having to do with preventive medicine and public health which do not involve the treatment of disease except that which is communicable.

The session of the American Medical Association on June 9, 1921 witnessed one of the peculiar personal attacks which has occurred at fairly frequent intervals in the House of Delegates—this time concerning one of the greatest leaders in the history of American medicine. The man involved was Dr. Frank Billings, and the attack on him was apparently led by Dr. E. H. Ochsner of Illinois. Through some means, not clearly defined, a circular quoting a statement alleged to have been made by Dr. Billings and published in the *American Labor Legislation Review* in 1917 was widely circulated in the House of Delegates. In this statement Dr. Billings was reported to have said that he was "unequivocally in favor of compulsory insurance and the protection of maternity." In 1921 Dr. Billings had published a statement recommending the growth of health centers, which were attacked in the circular as being "the shortest route possible to state medicine." Following this attack, Dr. Frank Billings addressed the House of Delegates. He told the circumstances under which the statement alleged was made and pointed out that it might have been an inaccurate report from a conference held in Washington in 1916. Dr. Billings said:

> Since that time I have declared in published articles that compulsory health insurance was not applicable to the United States, and that I am opposed to it, and that state medicine as related to the treatment of disease I look on in the same way.

Dr. Billings recognized that the attack made on him was in effect a charge of duplicity. He continued:

> I am charged before you and before the profession with writing articles and working for the legal enactment of compulsory health insurance and of state medicine in this country while saying to you and to the profession that I am opposed to it.

He referred to his career in the American Medical Association, including membership in the House of Delegates for eight years, the presidency of the Association and membership on the Board of Trustees since 1918. By unanimous vote the House expressed its confidence in Dr. Billings and referred the circular to the Judicial Council.

THE LAY JOURNAL

The Board of Trustees made a supplementary report that facilities to undertake and publish a health journal would be lacking until the completion of a new building, at which time it proposed to publish such a journal.

COMPOSITION OF THE HOUSE OF DELEGATES

An amendment to the Constitution provided for seating of the trustees and ex-presidents of the Association in the House of Delegates as ex officio members, without the right to vote.

SECRETARY OF HEALTH

Numerous resolutions brought in toward the end of the session dealing with general affairs of the Association were referred to the Board of Trustees, including one which insisted that health should not be submerged in a national department of public welfare but that it have a separate secretary in the cabinet.

ALCOHOL

Again the House of Delegates was concerned with alcohol. One resolution proposed that alcohol be considered a beverage detrimental to the human economy and that its use as a food, tonic or stimulant had no scientific basis and that the Association expressed its disapproval of the acceptance by a small minority of the profession of the position of being purveyors of alcoholic beverages. Another resolution condemned the promiscuous prescribing of alcohol.

The Ad Interim Committee of the Association addressed a message to the President of the United States approving his general attitude toward public welfare and his evident desire to coordinate interdepartmental activities and functions. The committee insisted, however, that there be medical direction in all divisions requiring medical knowledge.

1922

ST. LOUIS

So rapid was the growth of the Association that additions to its buildings had to be considered almost every second or third year. The continuously increasing publications demanded constant supervision, and almost every year the Board of Trustees was compelled to consider changes in the editorial boards because of losses by death or other untoward incident. The growth of the councils required also annual consideration as to changes in membership.

DR. OLIN WEST BECOMES FIELD SECRETARY

With 1922 the general manager, Dr. George H. Simmons, announced that the Board of Trustees, in pursuance of its wish to promote medical organization and medical economics, had secured Dr. Olin West of Nashville, Tenn., then secretary of the Tennessee State Medical Association, to serve as field secretary. He would report in April.

THE ALCOHOL REFERENDUM

So serious had become the debate as to the virtues of alcohol in the treatment of disease that the Board of Trustees had conducted a referendum on the value of alcohol. The Board decided to present to the House of Delegates an abstract of the results of this referendum and with it suggestions for modifications of the Volstead Act which would permit the physician who desired to do so to command a pure drug in the form of whisky or other distilled spirits at a price fixed by the government.

The Association had also conducted negotiations with the commissioner of the Bureau of Internal Revenue on the regulations controlling administration of the Harrison Narcotic Act, with a view to making its administration less onerous to the physician.

ADVERTISING OF COMMERCIAL LABORATORIES

The rise of the commercial clinical laboratories and of fly-by-night postgraduate courses was also giving concern to many agencies interested in standardization of medical science on a high level. It became necessary to adopt regulations governing the advertisements of such institutions.

THE POPULAR JOURNAL

At this time also came debates relative to the popular health bulletin or journal to be published by the Association. The members of the Council on Health and Public Instruction had been requested to submit in writing their concept of such a periodical and its editor, the method of distribution and the prices to be charged for an annual subscription. The opinions were as diverse as the membership itself. Three wanted a magazine that would look like the *National Geographic*. One insisted that the editor be a physician, while the next insisted that the editor be a layman, and still another that he be one experienced in welfare work. Indeed, one member inclined very strongly toward the welfare concept and conceived of a publication in which all national welfare organizations would conduct departments.

A LECTURE BUREAU

With the coming of the new field secretary, it was also proposed that there be established a lecture bureau under his charge and it was agreed that all officers and officials of the Association, as well as the members of the House of Delegates, make their services available to this lecture bureau and that the lecture bureau prepare a syllabus to guide speakers in their presentations.

AMERICAN MEDICAL ASSOCIATION BULLETIN

Next came the question of securing more practical cooperation between officers of county and state societies and the headquarters office. With this object in view, the Board requested the reestablishment of the AMERICAN MEDICAL ASSOCIATION BULLETIN, to be issued as often as once a month for nine months in the year under the editorship of the secretary of the Association and to be devoted wholly to questions of organization and economic, social and ethical questions pertaining to the practice of medicine.

In the meantime the Council on Medical Education and Hospitals was investigating group practice, and the opening of the Cornell Pay Clinic had aroused much disturbance in New York City, which in turn was reflected to the Board of Trustees.

ANNUAL REPORT OF THE BOARD OF TRUSTEES

By this time the work carried on by the Board of Trustees had become so profuse that nearly three hours was required at the meeting of the Executive Committee of the Board of Trustees for the presentation and discussion of the report to be sent to the House of Delegates.

DR. GREEN RESIGNS

In April 1922 Dr. Frederick R. Green, who had served with the Association so long and in so many different capacities, resigned to become associated with Dr. John Dill Robertson of Chicago in the publication of a health magazine. This action caused some consternation, since he had been serving as secretary of the Council on Health and Public Instruction in a capacity which gave him intimate knowledge of the plans of the American Medical Association to publish a similar periodical. The periodical jointly produced by Drs. Robertson and Green suffered a short and financially disastrous career. The publication begun by the Association and eventually named HYGEIA had in 1947 reached its twenty-fifth year of existence.

At the meeting of the Board of Trustees previous to the St. Louis session there came a resolution from the Council on Health and Public Instruction which was to create much concern in ensuing years. It dealt with the prevention of conception and proposed that the American Medical Association take action to secure modification of federal laws which interfered with the right of the physician to give advice by mail on this subject. The Board of Trustees decided at that time that the question was one on which it could not take action.

THE TREASURER

At this meeting of the board Dr. William Allen Pusey, who had served with distinction as treasurer, resigned and was succeeded by Dr. Austin A. Hayden.

ST. LOUIS SESSION

When the House of Delegates convened in St. Louis in May the speaker of the House of Delegates, Dr. Frederick C. Warnshuis, made an address devoted to such topics as education of the public regarding scientific medicine, which discussion he concluded with numerous recommendations regarding the work of the Council on Health and Public Instruction. He discussed compulsory health insurance, asserting that it "never will and never can become an American institution." He considered the trained nurse and nursing problems and recommended that "our Association should assert itself in formulating an acceptable status for the trained nurse and the educational fundamentals requisite for her work of service." He proposed a semiannual meeting of the House of Delegates—a suggestion which was adopted in 1946. He concluded his address with a recommendation that all legislative activities of the American Medical Association be placed in the Council on Health and Public Instruction and that a legislative bureau be established in the headquarters office.

ADDRESS OF DR. WORK

The President of the Association, Dr. Hubert Work, followed with an address in which he pointed out the importance of close liaison between the American Medical Association and state societies. He felt that the councils should be increased in number and most of their work placed on the secretaries. Of organization, he said:

> Periodically the Association is criticized by one, or a small group of members, apparently actuated by destructive motives veiled by a demand for reorganization. The charges are usually built around the complaint that the Association is dictated by a few men in their own interests.

"Part of this statement is true," he said, and then he continued:

> This Association, and all others, even the national government, is directed by a few men for the principal reason that there is no other way to do it. That it is run in the interests of these few men is not true unless the expenditure of time, thought and money, with neglect of personal business, may be so construed. It has uniformly happened that those who have tried to break in, by first breaking down, have been members who have done nothing to build up.

On the subject of state medicine he made a few profound observations:

> The public is entitled to know the legitimate limitations of a state's participation in the practice of medicine. . . . Promiscuous medical treatment of disease . . . is not a state's function, and interference with it through any unit of government should not be tolerated by the public or by physicians. . . . The practice of medicine must remain a process of personal contact, invoking the patient's right of selection and the direct moral responsibility of the physician, with a sympathetic reaction between the two.

PRESIDENT-ELECT DE SCHWEINITZ

Dr. George E. de Schweinitz reviewed many of the activities of the agencies of the Association, showing a thorough knowledge of the work of the councils. He was much concerned that the views of individual members have opportunity for presentation to the House of Delegates, and he endorsed particularly the desirability of a semiannual session of the House.

BOARD OF TRUSTEES

In its report to the House of Delegates the Board of Trustees noted particularly the financial difficulties related to loss of income by many other periodicals and pointed out that during the period the financial condition of THE JOURNAL had been stable. The Spanish periodical was operated at a loss and also with a limited circulation. The QUARTERLY CUMULATIVE INDEX had met with instant favor. Most important, however, was the report on the construction of the new property.

The Board of Trustees recognized the existence of pay clinics, diagnostic clinics and group practice. The Council on Health and Public Instruction had recorded the existence of 139 group clinics and was making an attempt to determine the scope of their work.

The Judicial Council at this session also entered the arena with an extensive report on advertising medical institutions. The problem had reached them because of the existence of new institutes devoted wholly to the treatment of venereal diseases which were endeavoring to secure patients by advertisements in the press. The Judicial Council unhesitatingly condemned such institutions as being both unlawful, practicing as corporations, and unethical because of the nature of their practice.

The Council on Medical Education also paid its respects to so-called group practice and defined it as "the practice of medicine by an organization of physicians in which each member contributes to the group his professional service and receives from the group certain benefits in return and in which the members unite in the diagnosis of cases that indicate need for their combined service." The Council on Medical Education pointed out that less than 700 physicians in the United States were engaged in such practice and said "It is notable also that a large number of 'group practices' are rather short lived. At present, therefore, the group practice movement does not seem to warrant any very great concern on the part of the profession."

The Council on Scientific Assembly refused to make any statement on the therapeutic value of alcohol and recommended that the House of Delegates take no action on such a question. As the floor was thrown open to the delegates for the introduction of new business, there came a half dozen resolutions on the prescribing of alcoholic liquors, a new definition of state medicine, and several proposals for changing the Constitution and By-Laws.

There was an attack on the Sheppard-Towner Maternal Welfare Act as a form of federal bureaucratic interference with the sacred rights of the American home. The House of Delegates adopted resolutions condemning the Sheppard-Towner law and also a resolution on the prescribing of alcohol. This resolution indicated that 51 per cent of physicians consider whisky necessary in the practice of medicine and recommended further that provision be made for supplying bonded whisky for medicinal use only at a fixed retail price to be established by the government.

When the reports of the officers were considered, the reference committee approved the establishment of a bulletin as the official journal of the House of Delegates, to be edited by the secretary of the Association, the field secretary and the speaker of the House. It approved a survey of clinics and group practice, approved enlargement of the Council on Health and Public Instruction and a survey of nursing institutions, but it could see no present need of regular semiannual sessions of the House of Delegates.

DEATH OF DR. J. N. McCORMACK

A special committee had been established to draft a resolution on the death of Dr. J. N. McCormack. He had died on May 4, 1922, at the age of 75. Among other credit given to him was recognition of his magnificent efforts for the organization and reorganization of the American Medical Association and for the fine work that he had done in the state of Kentucky.

> For forty years he gave his time and labor by day and by night to protecting the people from disease and promoting the organization and efficiency of the medical profession.

MEDICAL EDUCATION

The House of Delegates recognized the need for more medical schools. It deplored the tendency toward premature or over-rapid specialization. The relationships of the medical school to the university gave them great concern. The House of Delegates believed that it was especially important that teachers in the clinical departments retain their usual relationships to the medical profession.

GROUP MEDICINE

To meet the rising threat of group clinics which would secure their patients by advertising in the public press, the Judicial Council had proposed an amendment to the Principles of Medical Ethics dealing with the solicitation of patients by physicians which has been a guiding principle in maintaining an ethical standard since its adoption. This section of the Principles of Medical Ethics merits repetition:

> Solicitation of patients by physicians as individuals, or collectively in groups by whatsoever name these be called, or by institutions or organizations, whether by circulars or advertisements, or by personal communications, is unprofessional. This does not prohibit ethical institutions from a legitimate advertisement of location, physical surroundings and special class—if any—of patients accommodated. It is equally unprofessional to procure patients by indirection through solicitors or agents of any kind, or by indirect advertisement, or by furnishing or inspiring newspaper or magazine comments concerning cases in which the physician has been or is concerned. All other like self laudations defy the traditions and lower the tone of any profession and so are intolerable. The most worthy and effective advertisement possible, even for a young physician, and specially with his brother physicians, is the establishment of a well merited reputation for professional ability and fidelity. This cannot be forced but must be the outcome of character and conduct. The publication or circulation of ordinary simple business cards, being a matter of personal taste or local custom, and sometimes of convenience, is not per se improper. As implied, it is unprofessional to disregard local customs and offend recognized ideals in publishing or circulating such cards.
>
> It is unprofessional to promote radical cures; to boast of cures and secret methods of treatment or remedies; to exhibit certificates of skill or of success in the treatment of diseases; or to employ any methods to gain the attention of the public for the purpose of obtaining patients.

WOMAN'S AUXILIARY

From Texas at this session of the House of Delegates came a request that the American Medical Association approve a movement to organize a Woman's Auxiliary to the American Medical Association.

> The object of this auxiliary shall be to extend the aims of the medical profession through the wives of doctors to the various women's organizations, which look to the advancement in health and education; also to assist in entertainment at all medical conventions and to promote acquaintanceship among doctors' families that closer professional fellowship may exist.

This came from the Woman's Auxiliary of the State Medical Association of Texas under the presidency of Mrs. S. C. Red. The House of Delegates approved the resolution. The Woman's Auxiliary thus created had grown by 1947 to a total membership of almost 30,000.

The House of Delegates also urged the Board to proceed as rapidly as possible with its publication of a journal for the public.

SECTION ON MISCELLANEOUS TOPICS

So many specialties had by this time begun to request sections in the Association that the Council on Scientific Assembly had evolved the idea of a special Section on Miscellaneous Topics which would be a tryout area for such new sections. Thus they could hold one or two meetings as the Section on Miscellaneous Topics and when sufficient interest was proved take on the full status of a section.

At this time also the name of the Section on Preventive Medicine and Public Health was changed to the Section on Preventive and Industrial Medicine and Public Health, indicating the new interest that was developing in the field of medical care in industry.

DEFINITION OF STATE MEDICINE

A new definition of state medicine was adopted with the following action:

> The American Medical Association hereby declares its opposition to all forms of "state medicine" because of the ultimate harm that would come to the public weal through such form of medical practice.
>
> "State medicine" is hereby defined for the purpose of this resolution to be any form of medical treatment, provided, conducted, controlled or subsidized by the federal or any state government, or municipality, excepting such service as is provided by the Army, Navy or Public Health Service and that which is necessary for the control of communicable diseases, the treatment of mental disease, the treatment of the indigent sick and such other services as may be approved by and administered under the direction of or by a local county medical society and are not disapproved by the state medical society of which it is a component part.

DR. WILLIAM C. WOODWARD ADDED

The Board had agreed to accept as the first director of the Bureau of Legal Medicine and Legislation Dr. William C. Woodward, formerly health commissioner of Boston.

HYGEIA

The birth pangs of HYGEIA, tentatively known as the people's medical magazine, were a matter of greater travail than was the birth of THE JOURNAL OF THE AMERICAN MEDICAL ASSOCIATION itself. There was, first, the question as to whether or not it ought to be published under the control of the Council on Health and Public Instruction or under the control of the Board of Trustees. Next came the question as to whether or not participation by the American Public Health Association should be authorized. Among others considered for the editorship was Dr. George Dock.

All the members of the Council had been queried as to their attitudes. Such eminent authorities as Dr. Edwin E. Slosson were consulted. Almost every physician, writer on science or public health official whose name had loomed large in the public prints was suggested as a possibility for the editorship.

AN OSTEOPATHIC CHALLENGE

About this time George A. Still, president of the American School of Osteopathy, proposed a challenge to the American Medical Association for a wager of $5,000. He suggested that a number of patients with pneumonia be selected whom the doctors would treat according to their methods and whom the osteopaths would treat by their technics. As with a football game, he proposed that any time an osteopath gave a drug of any sort it might count like an offside play or "clipping," and the osteopaths would be penalized, whereas the use of manipulations by the doctors would be counted as a penalty against them. "Packs," he suggested, "either as flannel jackets, antiphlogistine or any other physical pack will be allowable by either contestant." It was proposed that three unprejudiced laymen be the umpires. In reply Dr. Simmons called attention to the fact that he would not recommend trifling with human life in the manner proposed in order to determine a wager, and he noticed that the Associated Press had already received the communication of Dr. Still before it reached the American Medical Association office.

DR. VAUGHAN BECOMES AN EDITOR

By August it became apparent that the Board of Trustees had authorized Dr. Victor Vaughan to proceed with the publication of the popular medical magazine and had begun to solicit articles from a number of writers and to plan definitely for the publication.

THE FIELD SECRETARY

Dr. Olin West had begun as field secretary to visit the states needing help in organizational efforts. He had been preparing most of the material that was appearing in the AMERICAN MEDICAL ASSOCIATION BULLETIN. Because of the resignation of Dr. Frederick R. Green, he had been serving also as acting secretary of the Council on Health and Public Instruction. The states had been queried as to their desires in relation to the work of the field secretary.

HYGEIA

By this time it had been determined to name the popular periodical HYGEIA. Dr. Vaughan was endeavoring to work out a plan whereby Science Service would cooperate in the publication—a plan which incidentally came to naught. He was being greatly aided by Dr. Edwin E. Slosson with suggestions submitted in writing under the title "Fugitive Hints for HYGEIA."

DEATH OF DR. CRAIG

In the period between the August and September meeting of the Board of Trustees Dr. Alexander Craig, secretary of the Association, died rather suddenly. In an attempt to secure a successor the names of many leading physicians in the United States were considered, including the deans of most of the medical schools.

The new Bureau of Legal Medicine and Legislation was having most of its trouble with the laws regulating the prescribing of alcohol and narcotics and new laws dealing with antivivisection.

The travail of HYGEIA continued. Great numbers of prospective editors were considered, including five or six army officers, three or four public health officials, two or three deans, one neuropsychiatrist and a few newspaper men. There were innumerable problems as to whether or not to purchase material, how the magazine could be circulated, whether or not it should be in color and similar questions.

AMERICAN RED CROSS

In the meantime meeting after meeting of the Board of Trustees and of the House of Delegates had been concerned with working out some sort of an arrangement with the American Red Cross which would clearly define the public health and medical functions of that agency. Through the intermediation of Dr. Hubert Work and Dr. George de Schweinitz with Judge Payne, a satisfactory agreement had been reached as to these functions. Recommendations had been made for a medical advisory committee, but at that time nothing serious was done. In fact, medical advisory committees to the American Red Cross were such in name only and without much in the nature of activity until Mr. Basil O'Connor was made national chairman of the Red Cross. He promptly appointed a competent medical advisory committee, which has been associated with him in the medical functions of the Red Cross since his appointment.

Dr. Olin West had been acting as secretary since the death of Dr. Craig, and it was agreed by the Board of Trustees at their last meeting for 1922 that he would be nominated by the board to the position of secretary.

Special consideration was given to the establishment of HYGEIA. By this time Dr. Victor C. Vaughan had determined to act at least temporarily as editor, and he agreed to serve with the understanding that the members of the Council on Health and Public Instruction would be the editorial board but that he should have the co-operation of Drs. Morris Fishbein and Arthur J. Cramp of the headquarters office in the work of editing the publication.

At this time also there came to the Board of Trustees the suggestion that there be a scientific exhibit for the public in connection with each annual session of the American Medical Association. This idea met with scant interest, however.

At the last meeting in 1922 also a proposal was made to provide group insurance for all the employees of the American Medical Association. The proposal went to the Board of Trustees for consideration, but some twenty years passed before this recommendation became effective.

1923
SAN FRANCISCO

With 1923 a reorganization of the Board of Trustees was considered desirable. The three year term and the election of three members annually permitted much instability in the conduct of the affairs of the Association. In the years 1907-1908 five new and inexperienced men were elected to membership on the Board in a period of twelve months. It was therefore recommended that the members of the Board of Trustees be elected to five year terms with a limitation of two terms to any member and that two trustees be elected each year. These recommendations were to be made to the House of Delegates and amendments to the Constitution and By-Laws submitted to make them effective.

At this time Dr. John M. Dodson was selected as secretary of the Council on Health and Public Instruction. Attempts were being made to find a new field secretary to take the place left vacant by the elevation of Dr. Olin West to secretary.

By this time the attempt to secure a secretary of health in the cabinet was again being actively revived. With the aid of Brig. Gen. C. E. Sawyer, who occupied the position of White House physician in the Harding administration, the proposal was being made that there be a single department of education and welfare. It was agreed that the importance of health in the picture be brought to the attention of the Brigadier General.

For some time the Association had been aiding in the reorganization of the Gorgas Memorial Institute in Panama. Now it reached the phase of a request by Dr. Franklin H. Martin to present the plan of reorganization to the House of Delegates.

In 1923 the Veterans Bureau appealed to have its physicians considered in the same relationship to the American Medical Association as were the physicians of the Army and Navy, with a representative in the House of Delegates.

When the Board of Trustees met previously to the annual session of the Association in San Francisco in 1923, several matters of great moment to American medicine came before it. Among the first was a recommendation that the Council on Health and Public Instruction be discontinued and that there be established in its place a bureau on Health and Public Instruction. The Board's attention on was called to the fact that the functions on organization, legislation and medicolegal affairs had been distributed to other departments of the Association and that its health education function would be largely conducted through HYGEIA. It was therefore suggested that the publication of HYGEIA be placed wholly on the Board of Trustees and that the Council be discontinued. The suggestion met with instantaneous approval. The Board of Trustees agreed to formulate the necessary changes in the Constitution and the By-Laws to make this action effective. It was decided to present directly to the House of Delegates the other questions raised in the consideration.

Dr. Ray Lyman Wilbur had been elected President of the Association to succeed Dr. George E. de Schweinitz.

RESIGNATION OF DR. GEORGE H. SIMMONS

In 1923 at the San Francisco session Dr. George H. Simmons submitted his resignation after having served the Association for twenty-five years. He requested that there be no public announcement, so that the Board might have ample time to select a successor.

WARNSHUIS RECOMMENDS

When the House of Delegates met, the speaker of the House, Dr. Frederick C. Warnshuis, called attention to the death of Dr. Alexander Craig on Sept. 2, 1922. He repeated his recommendation for a semiannual session of the House of Delegates. He spoke at great length on the socialization of medicine. He thought it desirable that there be a large committee to consider the question of a national welfare department in the President's cabinet. He paid glowing tribute to the Board of Trustees, and he recommended that the BULLETIN of the Association be discontinued and that sufficient space be alloted in THE JOURNAL for the necessary organizational material previously published in that periodical. He recommended, as had previous leaders of the Association, the appointment of at least some reference committees thirty days in advance of the annual session so that lengthy reports could be given adequate consideration before the session was held.

PRESIDENT DE SCHWEINITZ COMMENTS

Dr. George E. de Schweinitz paid gracious compliments to the editor and general manager, the Board of Trustees, the Council on Medical Education and Hospitals and other agencies of the Association. He urged that the duties of the President and President-Elect should be more strictly defined. He congratulated the Association particularly on its publication of HYGEIA.

DR. WILBUR REMINDS

As President-Elect, Dr. Ray Lyman Wilbur urged the House of Delegates to remember that it was a legislative and not an administrative body. He felt that there should be more long term planning in the Association and that there should be more responsibility placed on the state organizations. Particularly did he urge that the Association participate in the great projects for Russian relief, which at that time were agitating our country.

THE BOARD PAYS TRIBUTE

Without calling to the attention of the House of Delegates the resignation of Dr. George H. Simmons, the Board of Trustees concluded its extensive report on the projects that have already been mentioned with an appreciation. It said:

> For a period of twenty-five years Dr. George H. Simmons has devoted his entire time and energy to service for the Association. The members of the Board are unanimously of the opinion that an expression of appreciation should be made to him at this time. As editor and Manager, he has manifested remarkable literary ability, and it is due chiefly to his editorial management that THE JOURNAL is recognized as the foremost general medical publication of the world, with a circulation at home and abroad of 80,000 copies weekly. He has shown rare and efficient administrative skill, which has won the respect and confidence of all the general officers, the members of the Board of Trustees, the members of the councils and committees, the personnel at headquarters, and the Fellows of the Association who have been fortunate enough to come in close contact with him. He has been honest, individually unselfish, loyal, and his efforts have been productive of the greatest service to the Association.

The Council on Health and Public Instruction, in what was to be its swan song, called attention to the various actions which it had taken during the year. It indicated that Dr. John M. Dodson, who had been appointed acting secretary of the Council, was also serving as editor-in-chief of HYGEIA.

BUREAU OF LEGAL MEDICINE

For the first time there came an extensive report of the Bureau of Legal Medicine and Legislation, read by Dr. William C. Woodward as executive secretary, to the House of Delegates at the request of the Board of Trustees. He concerned himself with the manner in which the Bureau had been created. He then discussed the National Prohibition Act and indicated that success had been secured in persuading the Commissioner of Internal Revenue to withdraw from warehouses spirits bottled in bond for medicinal purposes. He discussed the regulations of the Harrison Narcotic Act and the relationship of the Veterans Bureau to the training of chiropractors. The Sheppard-Towner Maternity Act had been enacted by the Congress, and the Bureau had been aiding the medical profession of the individual states where opposition to the act was being developed. That act was before the Supreme Court of the United States for the determination of its constitutionality. He outlined in detail the attempt of Brig. Gen. C. E. Sawyer to develop a national department of education and welfare with the hope that it would be known as the Department of Education, Health and Welfare. This matter in 1947 is still before the Congress, the latest legislation calling for the establishment of a Department of Health, Education and Security. The remainder of his presentation was concerned with legislation in the individual states and with the difficulty of animal experimentation.

The House of Delegates approved the recommendation for the change in the manner of electing trustees, but since this required an amendment to the Constitution, it had to lie over for another year.

THE GORGAS MEMORIAL

In accordance with previous arrangements, Dr. Franklin H. Martin discussed at length the work of the Gorgas Memorial, and the House of Delegates by a rising vote pledged the American Medical Association to do everything in its power to assist the Committee on Gorgas Memorial to erect the building.

PRESCRIBING LIQUOR

Following the action of the Commissioner of Internal Revenue in relation to providing whisky bottled in bond for prescription purposes, a resolution was introduced commending the Association for the Protection of Constitutional Rights, for its public spirited efforts in securing this action; also a resolution that in the judgment of the House of Delegates of the American Medical Association every state and county medical association should use its best endeavors to discipline physicians who were negligently or wilfully prescribing liquor otherwise than in accordance with the law and to purge the medical profession of physicians who wilfully under the cloak of their profession prescribe liquor for other than medicinal purposes.

There was the usual resolution condemning the Volstead Act for interfering with doctors in their practice.

There was an appeal to establish the Section on Radiology.

There was a spirited election in which Dr. William Allen Pusey was elected President over Dr. William D. Haggard by a vote of 66 to 62.

THE EAGLETON RESOLUTION

On the closing day of the session came a resolution from the State Medical Society of New Jersey, under the leadership of its president, Dr. Wells P. Eagleton, requesting the Board of Trustees to disassociate the editorship and general management of the Association, placing the editorship entirely separate from the general management of the Association. This communication was referred to the Board of Trustees without objection. The story behind this action is interesting; it may now be told since the two chief characters in the drama are no longer among the living. Dr. Wells P. Eagleton had published a book on the subject of brain abscesses and had requested that the advertisement of that book appear on the front cover of THE JOURNAL. Dr. George H. Simmons had called to his attention the fact that the front cover had been sold under contract to another publisher and that it was not possible to invalidate the contract in order to permit the advertisement of Dr. Eagleton's book. Dr. Eagleton took violent exception to this decision, asserting that the rights of a Fellow of the Association should have precedence over any commercial interest whatever. In proposing the action of the State Medical Society of New Jersey before the House of Delegates, he insisted that THE JOURNAL represent solely the scientific and ethical side of the American Medical Association. He said:

> The editor should devote his entire time to the scientific and ethical aspects of the profession, not to its business.

This step initiated by Dr. Eagleton was to have repercussions for years to come. In 1924 the work of the editor was separated from the activities of the general manager.

ARCHIVES OF OTOLARYNGOLOGY

Following the meeting of the House of Delegates came a proposal for the publication of a journal on otolaryngology, and the Board of Trustees agreed to undertake such a publication.

HYGEIA

In the meantime the Board of Trustees continued to search for an editor for HYGEIA. The editors of leading women's magazines were consulted and six additional candidates were proposed. Dr. Simmons was convinced that the matter should not be too hastily acted on. He agreed to interview the candidates to aid in making a decision.

LEGAL PROBLEMS

At this time the Bureau of Legal Medicine was conducting discussions with the Commissioner of Internal Revenue relative to the right of a physician to deduct from his income tax expenses incurred in attending medical society meetings. There was also the question as to the right of the Commissioner of Internal Revenue to search private professional records under the guise of efforts to collect the federal estate tax from the estates of the physician's deceased patients.

THE ADVERTISING COMMITTEE

In order to conduct more formally the decisions on advertising submitted to THE JOURNAL OF THE AMERICAN MEDICAL ASSOCIATION the Board of Trustees had established in the headquarters office an Advertising Committee consisting of Drs. Arthur J. Cramp, Olin West and Morris Fishbein, Professor W. A. Puckner and Mr. C. H. Mohler of the advertising department. Since that time an Advertising Committee of this type has been a regular feature of the conduct of the headquarters office, the purpose being to give scientific consideration to all advertisements that are not directly within the province of the Council on Pharmacy and Chemistry, the Council on Food and Nutrition, the Council on Physical Medicine and the Council on Medical Education and Hospitals. Indeed the Board of Trustees had authorized the Advertising Committee to reject any advertisements on evidence that a firm was not dealing in complete good faith in its actions toward the medical profession. It was emphasized particularly that all the advertising copy of a manufacturer, as well as the advertisements offered to THE JOURNAL, must meet the standards. In accordance with this action it was recommended also by Dr. Simmons that the publications of the American Medical Association support the councils by refusing to publish manuscripts which promoted the use of nonaccepted products. While this action was not made official it has guided the decisions of the editorial boards in many instances and thus has saved the medical profession from exploitation by manufacturers who were launching untested and untried remedies on the medical profession.

The Board of Trustees was continually concerned with many matters of minor importance to the general progress but which nevertheless had tremendous interest for the health of the American people. It was attempting to secure improvement in the medical service rendered to Indians under the charge of the Secretary of the Interior. It was working with manufacturers as well as with legislators in an endeavor to prevent distribution of lye and other caustic substances without adequate warning labels. It was endeavoring to secure standardization of thermometers and other apparatus used in the practice of medicine. It was holding continual conferences with Director Frank T. Hines of the Veterans Bureau in an endeavor to limit the training of charlatans under the auspices of the Veterans Bureau and to improve the quality of medical service rendered to the veteran himself.

An assistant editor had been secured for HYGEIA. Attempts were being made to secure suitable field secretaries and assistant secretaries, workers in the field of organizations and for many other functions. At the same time the property of the Association was gradually assuming form. An assembly hall had been added to the plans; new presses and much new equipment were being purchased.

MIDDLESEX MEDICAL COLLEGE

In November 1923 the Middlesex College of Medicine and Surgery notified the Board of Trustees of the American Medical Association that it would not permit the Council on Medical Education and Hospitals to make further inspection of the institution and threatened suit for damages should any reference be made to it in the classification of medical schools published in THE JOURNAL. The Middlesex College of Medicine and Surgery continued to be an irritant in the attempt to secure a high standard of medical education until it finally ceased existence by action of the courts of Massachusetts in 1945.

President Harding died toward the end of the year. President Ray Lyman Wilbur of the American Medical Association had been among the physicians who were in attendance at the time of his passing. The press of the nation had intimated that the death was not wholly due to natural causes. As the years have passed it has become more and more apparent that President Harding died of coronary thrombosis, related no doubt to the strenuous existence that he had followed in a country recuperating with great difficulty from a great war and from mental and other stresses too numerous to mention.

As a result of innumerable conferences with Director Hines of the Veterans Bureau, the American Medical Association had been requested to develop a committee to review ratings for disabilities. This was one of the most important functions rendered by the American Medical Association in the postwar period.

In the meantime the American Medical Association through THE JOURNAL had aided in exposing diploma mills in St. Louis and Connecticut and rackets operated by eclectic licensing boards in many states. These crusading activities were vastly important in relation to the public attitude toward the American Medical Association.

1924

CHICAGO; DR. SIMMONS RETIRES

When the Executive Committee met early in January in 1924 Dr. Morris Fishbein, assistant to Dr. Simmons, reported a series of interviews with leading editors in New York City as to the prospects for HYGEIA and indicated other measures that had been taken to extend publicity for the American Medical Association in many ways. Articles had been arranged for publication in the *Woman's World*; contact had been made with *Time* magazine, which then had a circulation of 60,000 weekly, relative to the publication of medical news; columns were to be published by the North American Newspaper Alliance, and in other ways publicity for American medicine was to be issued through various channels.

The Bureau of Legal Medicine, through Dr. William C. Woodward, had made contacts with many organizations of the government, and full reports of these were made to the Board of Trustees. They covered such subjects as income taxes, narcotic laws, patents on nostrums, the care of the Indians, animal experimentation, legislation on lye and the standardization of thermometers.

The Board of Trustees was watching carefully the progress of its numerous special periodicals. It recommended expansion of the AMERICAN JOURNAL OF DISEASES OF CHILDREN so that it would contain not only original articles but also abstracts of articles from other periodicals, news and related material.

The Board agreed early in the year that on retirement Dr. Simmons should be known as the emeritus editor of THE JOURNAL.

By this time the functions of the Association in relation to exhibits were assuming increased prominence. It was being recommended that a Bureau of Exhibits be established with a competent director. Much attention was being given to the formulation of outlines for periodic health examinations. The idea of such examinations was being spread throughout the country by propaganda from many agencies.

HYGEIA had reached 18,000 circulation. Many excellent articles were beginning to be selected. HYGEIA was being widely quoted in the press and in other periodicals, having an influence far beyond its circulation. Moreover the material in HYGEIA was becoming available as reprints and pamphlets, which were extending the circulation to a much more extensive audience.

CHICAGO MEETING

Then came the epoch making meeting of the Association in Chicago in June.

Professor Puckner, secretary of the Council on Pharmacy and Chemistry, was beginning to feel his advancing years, and Dr. Paul Nicholas Leech was made director of the laboratory.

The Board agreed to announce to the House of Delegates the resignation of the editor. At this time the Board of Trustees recognized the necessity for taking immediate action for the conduct of the affairs of the Association following the retirement of Dr. Simmons. The names of several applicants were considered. The board eventually agreed that on the retirement of Dr. Simmons, Dr. Olin West should become acting general manager, Dr. Morris Fishbein acting editor of THE JOURNAL and Mr. Will C. Braun acting business manager, with the understanding that final decisions would be made at a later date.

The House of Delegates convened for the first time in the Assembly Hall of the American Medical Association building in Chicago. Dr. Frederick C. Warnshuis devoted the first portion of his address to the working methods of the House of Delegates. He recommended that the privileges of the floor of the House be granted to the secretaries of councils and bureau heads for brief reports on their own work, so that the House of Delegates might be more familiar with the men who were carrying on the activities of the Association.

Dr. William Allen Pusey, as President-elect, discussed particularly the high costs of nurse and medical training and the problem of supplying adequate medical services in rural districts. His address was long and involved essentially a recommendation for abbreviation in the length of the medical and nursing curriculums with the idea of granting the medical degree within four to five years after leaving high school.

The great length of the report of the Board of Trustees made the House of Delegates impatient; it voted to dispense with reading the report and that instead the responsible officials present them an abstract calling attention to the important features. This met with instant approval from the House and has been followed continuously since that time.

The Judicial Council had been asked to define "sectarian practice" and to define also the term "physician." These definitions follow:

A "sectarian," as applied to medicine, is one who in his practice follows a dogma, tenet or principle based on the authority of its promulgator to the exclusion of demonstration and experience.

A physician is one who has acquired a contemporary education in the fundamental and special sciences, comprehended in the general term "medicine" used in its unrestricted sense, and who has received the degree of Doctor of Medicine from a medical school of recognized standing.

Then came a consideration of the relationships of physicians to cultists—a question which has been raised repeatedly and which, it will be remembered, was the fundamental difficulty that arose in New York and caused for a while two medical societies in that state. The report of the Judicial Council on the relationships of physicians and cultists also bears republication:

> Several communications addressed to the Council have raised various questions as to the relationships of physicians with cultists—the attitude that should be assumed by the physician called into a case under treatment by a cult practitioner, whether a pathologist in a hospital under the direction of regular physicians should refuse to examine material submitted by a cultist, and other questions of more or less similar nature. In the opinion of the Judicial Council, these are questions that are not sharply to be defined by words. In his relations with irregular practitioners, the physician should be bound by the Principles of Medical Ethics, chapter II, article I, section 1, while bearing in mind the considerations set forth in sections 6 and 7 of the same chapter and article, and with due consideration for the observations made in the Conclusion on page 23 of the Principles of Medical Ethics of the American Medical Association. In such matters the policy must be governed largely by the circumstances governing the individual case; by the conditions existing in the special community; and by the realization that the first duties of the physician are the care of the sick and, at the same time, the upholding of the dignity and honor of the profession.

At this time also came before the Judicial Council the question of prescribing of eyeglasses with rebates to the ophthalmologist. The Judicial Council referred this to the Section on Ophthalmology for consideration and a request for a recommendation on the subject. Among the most important of the statements made by the Judicial Council also was a supplementary report at this session of the American Medical Association dealing with the vending of the physician's services through an intermediate agency, such as the Public Health Institute in Chicago and the Life Extension Institute, at that time established in New York. So significant was this report that the House of Delegates decided to consider it as a special order of business at a later session.

In its report to the House of Delegates the Council on Medical Education called attention to the diploma mill scandal which had shocked the nation. Several low grade medical schools had sold diplomas and had then shipped their graduates across the country to Connecticut where the Connecticut eclectic licensing board had arranged for licensure. The situation had been called to public attention by the publication in THE JOURNAL OF THE AMERICAN MEDICAL ASSOCIATION of the statistics of state board examinations.

This had caused the authorities in Connecticut to make an investigation, which resulted in revoking the licenses of 56 physicians and shortly thereafter of another 111, so that 167 physicians in all were declared to have been illegally registered by the eclectic board in that state. Subsequently some of these physicians used their Connecticut licensure to obtain licensure in Arkansas and in Kansas—among them the notorious John R. Brinkley, who at a later date sued the American Medical Association for libel. The Council on Medical Education and Hospitals called attention to the fact that the institutions which were declared to have been involved in the sale of diplomas had long since been in the Council's lowest classification. They were of such low grade that their diplomas were not recognized by the licensing boards of over forty states. Even if those who purchased diplomas had actually matriculated in and attended these medical schools for the required four years and had been regularly graduated, they could not have obtained licenses in more than a few states. That is why the diploma mill ring had to send their "graduates" half way across the continent to get them licensed. Slowly but surely the work of the Council on Medical Education was closing and narrowing the area in which an incompetent physician could attempt to serve the public.

By this time so much interest had developed in anesthesia, radiology and physical medicine that the Council on Scientific Assembly had offered special sessions to these specialties so that they might prove their worth before receiving a section in the American Medical Association.

When a call for new business was made in the House of Delegates, resolutions poured in on the control of cosmetics, on publicity for institutions, on prohibition, on standard methods for reporting deaths in the puerperal state, on the use of zinc stearate dusting powder and on the prescribing of liquor. Again Dr. Franklin Martin addressed the House in behalf of the Gorgas Memorial Institute. At this session the new methods of electing trustees were approved and became a part of the Constitution of the Association. Again the Association appealed for better regulation of the prescribing of liquors.

Dr. Ray Lyman Wilbur, who had been detained so that he could not make an address at the opening meeting of the House of Delegates, attended the second session and addressed the House on the subject of the future of the medical profession. He pointed out that one of the greatest advantages in the United States is the fact that we have forty-eight states so that any state can try an experiment, and, if it is a bad one, it alone suffers. He recommended more experimentation by the medical profession in methods of preventive medicine and medical care. He said:

> It seems to me, too, that we must keep individualism in medicine if it is to advance, and we must keep individual relations between patients and physicians if medicine as an art is to go forward. The minute we allow a bureaucracy to step in between the physician and the patient, it seems to me we have taken the one step that will degrade our profession and that will put us so that we cannot render ideal professional services to patients.

He felt that too much standardization was injurious to medical advancement. As to service to patients in rural areas, he said:

> Now, to me the rural practitioner problem is not one that we can solve. It is a great social question, this transfer of people from the farms to the cities; it comes with more machinery, with better roads, with gasoline and all that sort of thing, with the changed attitudes of people, with the desire to get more education for the children, and so on. If you will study the population curves, you will see that people are going into the cities from the country, and right now we are having an overproduction on the part of the farms; that to me can be solved only by a million or more farmers moving into the city and going into industry, because we have overproduction on the farms.

In considering the report of the Judicial Council, the House of Delegates adopted the principle that "under no circumstances should a regular physician engage in consultation with a cultist of any description."

As to the practice of medicine by corporations, the House of Delegates, sitting as a committee of the whole, said that the practice should be condemned as against the best interests of the public and that every agency of the Association should do its utmost to educate the people as to the desirability of periodic physical examinations. The Association decided to prepare a special manual to aid physicians in this work.

Dr. William D. Haggard was elected President of the American Medical Association. When the time came for the election of trustees, there was evidence of the manner in which a witticism can swing a legislative body. A distinguished pathologist was nominated for trustee, and a general practitioner was nominated as the opposing candidate. In speaking in behalf of the general practitioner, one of the speakers said "The American Medical Association is not dead, and it does not need a pathologist." There was a tremendous burst of laughter, with an overwhelming vote for the general practitioner.

NEW APPOINTMENTS

The House of Delegates at this time referred to the Board of Trustees the ultimate decision on the division of the work of the editor and general manager, and on the concluding day of the session the Board of Trustees announced the action that it had already taken relative to the appointment of Dr. Olin West, Dr. Morris Fishbein and Mr. Will C. Braun.

At the meeting in September Dr. Simmons announced that he was about to leave, and he made a report to the Board of Trustees covering the status of several projects which required action.

The Association was in excellent financial condition. All of its publications were doing well. Dr. Simmons called attention to the fact that the American Medical Association was now in process of

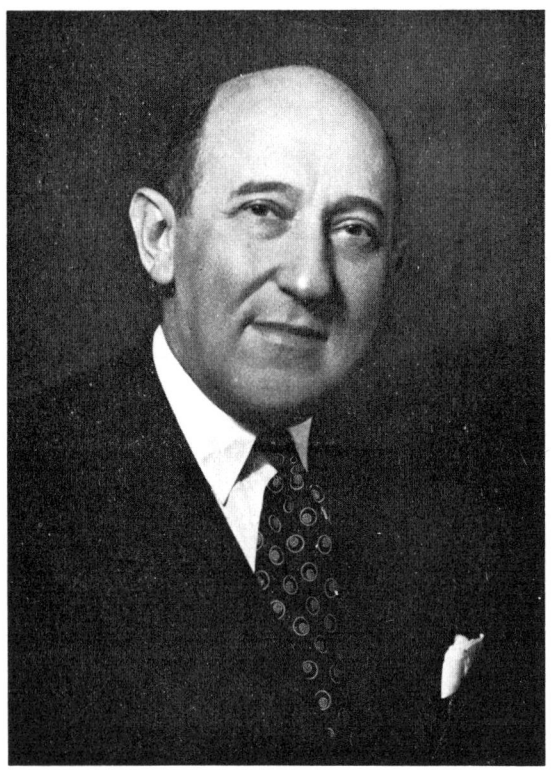

Morris Fishbein, M.D.

developing a package library service, in addition to lending foreign periodicals and furnishing references to literature on various subjects. These services had done much to make available to physicians in remote areas the latest advances in medical science.

At the end of the meeting in September the members of the Board of Trustees appointed a special committee, consisting of Drs. D. Chester Brown, A. R. Mitchell and Charles W. Richardson, to interview candidates for the office of general manager and editor, and the members of the Board were requested to look for available candidates. Dr. Simmons before leaving had prepared an outline of the duties that should be assigned respectively to the general manager, the business manager and the editor.

At this time a considerable disagreement developed between Dr. William Allen Pusey and the Council on Medical Education and Hospitals. Dr. Pusey, as President of the Association, had spoken in behalf of a shortening of the medical curriculum with a view to educating many more physicians and thus supplying the needs of rural areas.

HYGEIA had reached an annual circulation of 25,000.

At the November meeting of the Board of Trustees, after much discussion of many of the pending affairs, the Board met in executive session to consider the appointment of a general manager, an editor and a business manager. The minutes merely record that the board met at 8:30 in the evening and that the discussions were long and arduous. After a session which lasted until dawn, the board adjourned. The minutes state only that the subcommittee appointed to procure names of available men from whom a general manager might be selected presented its report. When the Board reconvened in the morning at 9:30 it was moved that Dr. Olin West be elected general manager. This was seconded and carried. The Board then considered the finances of the Association, after which it was moved by Dr. A. R. Mitchell that Dr. Morris Fishbein be appointed editor of THE JOURNAL, his duties to be those outlined at the time of his election as acting editor. Then it was moved by Dr. Mitchell that Mr. Will C. Braun be made business manager. These officials were called before the Board and notified of their appointments.

DR. GEORGE HENRY SIMMONS—EDITOR

GEORGE H. SIMMONS was born in Moreton, England, January 2, 1852. He came to the United States in 1870 and studied at Tabor College in Iowa in 1870-72 and at the University of Nebraska from 1872 to 1876. While a freshman in the University of Nebraska, he won an important prize for an essay on the sheep industry. He was even at that time interested in writing and editorial work; he acted as editor of the Nebraska Farmer, assistant city editor of the Nebraska State Journal, and field correspondent of the Omaha Republican and the

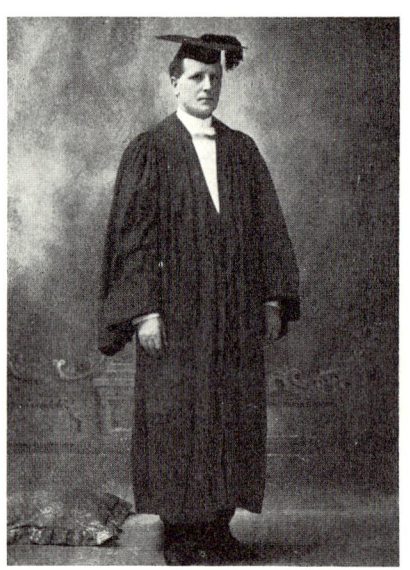

George H. Simmons at graduation from Rush Medical College.

Kansas City Journal while attending college and medical school. With these odd jobs he aided in paying his way. He developed, however, also a taste for the use of printers' ink which followed him throughout his life.

After graduation from the University of Nebraska, he attended the Hahnemann Medical College, Chicago, and received his M.D. degree in 1882. In 1884 he served briefly in the Rotunda Hospital, Dublin, noted for leadership in obstetrics and gynecology. Then in 1884 he returned to Lincoln, Nebraska, and established himself in medical practice. He continued in Lincoln until 1898 but in that intervening period he attended classes in Rush Medical College from time to time and received the M.D. degree from Rush Medical College in 1892.

Early in his life Dr. Simmons became active in medical organizational work; he was secretary of the Nebraska State Medical Society from 1895–99 and also secretary of the Western Surgical and Gynecological Society. In 1896 he established the Western Medical Review and was its editor.

While he was in Lincoln, Nebraska, he became known as a leader in several reform movements. At one time he led an attack to take the government of Nebraska out of the hands of the machine politicians and to restore it to the people. Indeed a resolution adopted by the Chamber of Commerce at a later date admitted the debt of that state to Dr. George H. Simmons for much of its cleanness and financial soundness.

Later in his career when he began to acquire a considerable list of enemies because of his attacks on the advertising of fraudulent nostrums and patent medicines and because of his participation in eliminating proprietary medical schools, Dr. Simmons was made the direct target of innumerable public and private attacks which reflected on his personal integrity and his character. There were, of course, investigations. Some of these attacks were subsidized with considerable sums of money. Fortunately for him and for the American Medical Association, he was able to survive even the most bitter and persistent of these onslaughts on his character.

While in Lincoln, Nebraska, he had briefly conducted an institution which cared for women and in connection with the conduct of this institution, announcements of his work had been published in various medical periodicals. Such announcements were routine in the far western portions of the United States in the days when they were published. Nevertheless, when they were reproduced some twenty-five years after their first publication, they struck amazement and perhaps even horror in the minds of the more conservative physicians of the midwestern and the eastern seaboard areas.

In the course of his life, Dr. Simmons was married at first to a woman physician who later became addicted to the taking of morphine. Apparently she was in some manner drawn into the support of some of the enemies of Dr. George H. Simmons. The charges made by and through this first wife were for him a crown of thorns and a source of continuous suffering. Later he was to marry a second wife with whom he lived a quiet, uneventful, domestic existence until the time of her death. A niece, Miss Annie E. Nicholls, came from England to live with the family and remained to take care of Dr. Simmons following his retirement from his position of editor and general manager of the American Medical Association in 1924 until the time of his death in 1937.

Whenever questions of his personal life were brought to the surface, he refused to be drawn into comment or discussion. He was wont to say that he would never answer a personal attack upon himself but only an attack on the organization for which he worked or on its policies. On one occasion when he was being attacked with exceptional virulence in the course of a campaign to clean up the evils of the proprietary medical industry, he was heard to express the hope that the attacker would refrain from bringing his personal life into the situation.

When he retired from the position of editor and general manager of the American Medical Association in 1924, he destroyed his personal correspondence, memorandums and records. Thus there remain no evidences of his work or his career except such as are embodied in the offical minutes of the Board of Trustees and of the House of Delegates of the American Medical Association. These records indicate the tremendous part that he played in the reorganization of the American Medical Association in 1901, in the establishment of its JOURNAL and headquarters office on a superlative business basis and in creating a firm foundation on which his successors were able to erect the tremendous and efficient organization that exists today.

Mention has been made of the committee on reorganization of which Dr. J. N. McCormack of Kentucky was chairman, Dr. P. Maxwell Foshay a member and Dr. George H. Simmons, secretary. The outline for reorganization which was prepared by this committee was the one presented to the Association with a new Constitution and By-Laws in 1901. In 1901 also Dr. Simmons was made secretary of the Association and later General Manager.

Under his editorship THE JOURNAL began publishing results of the examinations for licensure made by state examining boards. These figures were of vital importance in raising the standards of medical education. He was instrumental in organizing the Council on Medical Education and Hospitals and in initiating the Department of Propaganda for Reform, later to be known as the Bureau of Investigation, which was the spearhead in the attack on frauds and quackery. He participated in the organization of the Council on Pharmacy and Chemistry, becoming its chairman and being closely associated with its work throughout his professional career. While he was General Manager of the American Medical Association he undertook publication of the American Medical Directory which was an outgrowth of the Biographical Department. Several of the special periodicals of the American Medical Association were initiated under his editorship.

When the Army Medical Library and the Carnegie Institution began having difficulties with the continuity of the publication of the Index Medicus he aided in the development of the Quarterly Cumulative Index Medicus so that the discontinuance of the Index Medicus did not leave a gap in medical literature and other medical research. Although he was not personally inclined to the development of a periodical for the public in the field of health education, HYGEIA was initiated when he was General Manager.

To recount in detail the story of his services to the American Medical Association in the period from 1899 to 1924 is, in fact, to tell the history of the American Medical Association in that same period. Until the time when Dr. Simmons became editor of THE JOURNAL, it had been the custom to publish at the end of each volume a list of the medical members of the editorial staff and the names of others who had contributed editorials to the pages of THE JOURNAL. When Dr. George H. Simmons assumed the position of editor and later of general manager, he discontinued any reference to the names of those who were associated with him in his editorial work in any capacity. During the period from 1903 to 1913 he had as an assistant Dr. Edward Everett Hyde. Dr. Hyde was born on Jan. 19, 1875, in Galesburg, Illinois. He graduated with the degree of A.B. from Knox College, Galesburg, in 1896. Then he entered the College of Physicians and Surgeons, Chicago, from which he graduated in 1900. At the same time he was ordained to the Christian ministry and in November 1900 sailed from San Francisco for the Caroline Islands as a medical missionary. On account of the ill health of his wife he returned to the United States in 1902 at which time he became a staff member of THE JOURNAL OF THE AMERICAN MEDICAL ASSOCIATION. His title was Assistant to the Editor. He was accustomed to attend the annual meetings of the Association where he acted as editor of the *Daily Bulletin*. He attended the Minneapolis meeting in 1913 and became ill on his return. Assuming that this illness was only fatigue as a result of a strenuous week, he remained at work. The serious nature of his illness became evident only a few days before his death when it was diagnosed as acute myelogenous leukemia. He died July 4, 1913, aged 38.

During the last three years of this period the name of Dr. Hyde was carried on the stationery of the Association as "Assistant to the Editor." In August 1913, Dr. Morris Fishbein accepted the post of assistant to the editor, with the understanding that the position would be merely temporary until Dr. Simmons should be able to find some other help. Dr. Fishbein has remained in the position as editor of THE JOURNAL since 1924 when he received the appointment.

In 1904 Dr. Arthur J. Cramp became an assistant on the staff of The Journal and was placed in charge of the Department of Propaganda Reform. Practically all of the writing in that department up to the time of Dr. Cramp's retirement on January 30, 1935, was done by Dr. Cramp.

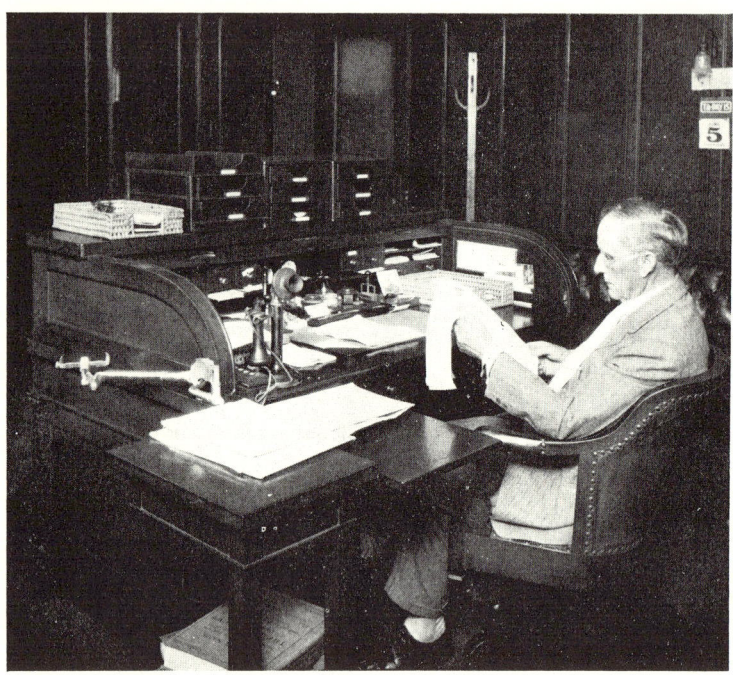

George H. Simmons as editor of THE JOURNAL.

The editorial writers during the period of the incumbency of Dr. Simmons until 1924 included some 40 contributors, of whom, however, just a few did the major portion of the work. During the period from 1913 to 1924 most of the editorials in THE JOURNAL were written by Drs. Lafayette B. Mendel, Ludvig Hektoen and Morris Fishbein. While Dr. Simmons himself seldom wrote an editorial, he would occasionally draft the first statement of an editorial related to the work of the organization. He was not himself a competent writer. He was, however, a meticulous and able editor. Innumerable medical writers could testify to the manner in which he devoted himself personally to the education of younger men in editorial technic. Reference will be made in subsequent chapters of this history to some of the few papers which he published under his own name when they were prepared as addresses before state medical societies or other medical organizations.

In 1908 Dr. Simmons was commissioned a first lieutenant in the Medical Reserve Corps of the U. S. Army. In 1917 when the United States entered the war, he was made major in the Medical Reserve Corps and served diligently in the personnel division. With the onset of the war in 1917 leadership in the organization of the medical profession for services in the war was taken by Dr. Franklin H. Martin, at that time director general of the American College of Surgeons. The story of the continued rivalry for leadership in American medicine between Franklin H. Martin and George H. Simmons is another story not properly included in this history of the American Medical Association. The rivalry was to appear from time to time as a problem for the American Medical Association as will be recorded in the history of the later years. The initiative and drive of Dr. Martin at this time were superior to those of Dr. Simmons. With Martin to think was to act. Thus on the first glimmering of the war clouds on the horizon he was under way to Washington where he became a member of the Advisory Commission of the Council on National Defense. In that position he mobilized various agencies which might be helpful in the prosecution of the war, including the mobile hospitals. When it became necessary to develop personnel to carry on the medical activities of the war, it became necessary also to establish a medical committee for the Council on National Defense. From this committee also the name of Dr. George H. Simmons was eliminated. Later Martin was to create a general medical board with the names of many great American leaders, and we find Dr. George H. Simmons as chairman of the committee on publicity. Still later, however, when it came to securing the necessary personnel, the government found in World War I, as it found also in World War II, that it did not have a roster of physicians in the United States or any means of determining who could be spared or who were competent. Then it was that General Gorgas announced the appointment of an advisory committee on promotions consisting of Drs. William H. Welch, Victor C. Vaughan, John M. T. Finney, William J. and Charles H. Mayo, George H. Simmons, and Franklin H. Martin. This committee met on an average of once each week throughout the war. Its members were recommended by Dr. Gorgas at the end of the war for the Distinguished Service Medal and in 1921, by order of President Harding, Dr. George H. Simmons received this medal in recognition of his work.

For some years Dr. Simmons had been suffering with cataracts and herpes zoster and had been assigning more and more of his editorial responsibilities to his assistant. Finally in 1924 Dr. Simmons resigned as editor and general manager of the American Medical Association and became editor and general manager emeritus. At that time a number of leaders in American medicine arranged for the painting of his portrait which was presented to him at a testimonial banquet in Chicago on June 9, 1924. Hundreds of physicians attended and he received messages of appreciation and congratulation from all over the world.

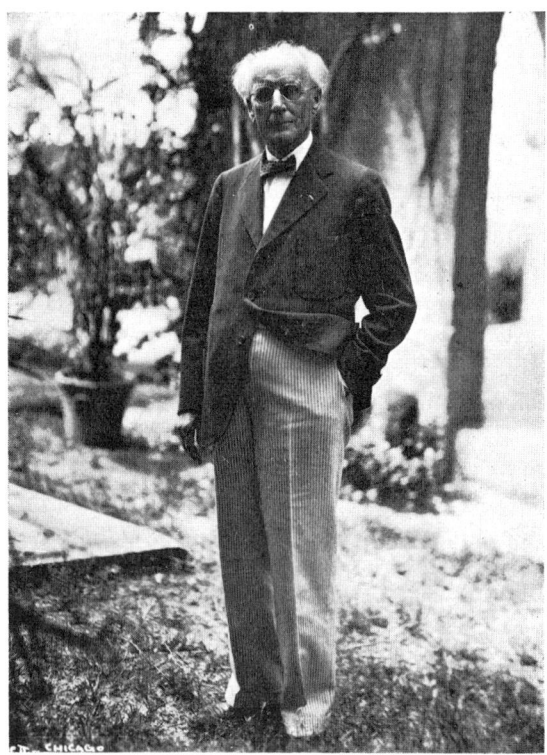

George H. Simmons in Florida.

After his retirement, he traveled extensively for several years, making his residence in Florida but spending some time every other year in Great Britain.

Dr. Simmons died in Chicago September 1, 1937, following an operation for diverticulitis.

This then is briefly the record of Dr. George H. Simmons as an executive and as an administrator. His work for the American Medical Association was characterized by intelligence, unselfishness, and righteousness. He weathered storms of anxieties, criticism and false characterization of his work. He devoted himself completely to the public career which he had chosen. Unquestionably he was the greatest factor in his generation in the development of the American Medical Association. The medical profession of the United States owes him a debt which it could never pay and which he never wished to collect.

THE WAR AGAINST SOCIALIZED MEDICINE—1925-1929

THE FIRST MOTION PICTURE OF THE HEADQUARTERS

INTEREST IN MOTION PICTURES was shown in 1925, when a 16 millimeter film of the various departments in the headquarters office was prepared. This was displayed before state and county medical societies, and did much to inform the medical profession of the growth and multiple functions of the organization.

HYGEIA

Early in 1925 the board, much concerned about the failure of HYGEIA, decided that possibly more could be accomplished toward developing the magazine if the Association's editor were made responsible for the magazine, as he was largely responsible for the special periodicals published by the Association. The House of Delegates gave its full support to the continuance of HYGEIA.

THE DAVIS MEMORIAL

The Nathan Smith Davis memorial fund had now reached more than $4500; the president of the Association, Dr. William Allen Pusey, suggested that the money be used to make a dignified, handsome room of the N. S. Davis library in the headquarters building.

THE FIRST HOUSE ORGAN

At this time also the Association began publication of a house organ, known as "The Little Journal." It also established a library for the employees. By 1925 the publication called "Health" which had been begun by Dr. John Dill Robertson and Dr. Frederick R. Green, had failed.

THREATENED SUITS

Again the Association was threatened with litigation. The manufacturers of a weight reducing bread objected to an exposé which had been published in THE JOURNAL; a Frederick Collins of New Jersey objected to being mentioned in HYGEIA along with other authors in the Macfadden publications. Collins, it appeared, had licenses to practice both osteopathy and chiropractic in New Jersey. He demanded a retraction of a reference to him as not being a physician. The Board of Trustees agreed to make it clear in HYGEIA that Collins was licensed to practice chiropractic and osteopathy.

At this time THE JOURNAL was threatened also with litigation and with an injunction sought by the notorious plastic surgeon charlatan, Henry J. Schireson. These matters were simply referred to the attorneys representing the Association.

THE ATLANTIC CITY SESSION

In his address to the House of Delegates at the Atlantic City session the speaker, Dr. Frederick C. Warnshuis, called attention to the fact that he had published the names of some of the reference committees in The Journal in advance of the session so that more time was available to them for consideration of the material which would be referred to them in the regular order. The speaker also recommended that the secretary of the Association be nominated to the House of Delegates by the Board of Trustees. The House of Delegates introduced the appointment of reference committees thirty days in advance of the annual session but did not support the election of the secretary by the Board of Trustees. The speaker also urged that resolutions be presented, if possible, thirty days in advance of the session and published so that they could come to the attention of the delegates. This also met with the approval of the House of Delegates. He called for much more publicity for medicine in the United States and received the full endorsement of the House of Delegates for such publicity.

ADVANCES IN TECHNIC OF CONDUCT OF AFFAIRS

Dr. William Allen Pusey, the president, called attention to the wisdom of the selection of a president-elect and of the importance that the president-elect should visit as many state societies as possible during his term of office. Both the speaker and the president had recommended that all reports of the councils, officers and standing committees of the Association be made available by publication at least thirty days in advance of the annual session. This, too, met with the approval of the House of Delegates; it has become a routine procedure in the Association, adding greatly to the quality of consideration given to various proposals.

Dr. Pusey was particularly concerned with the policy-making privileges of the councils. He felt it inadvisable that members of the councils meet with the reference committees that discuss their work. He considered it desirable that the councils be enlarged, since the establishment of policies by these councils was of the utmost importance to the future of the Association. With this proposal, the House of Delegates did not agree.

THE PRESIDENT OF THE BRITISH MEDICAL ASSOCIATION

The Association had again the benefit of a visitor from England, Mr. J. Basil Hall, president of the British Medical Association. He included early in his address an interesting anecdote, saying:

"Sir Robert Jones, whom you all probably know as our great orthopedic surgeon, was walking down the Strand the other day, and he suddenly ran into one of the Mayos. 'Hello, Mayo!' he said, 'What are you doing here?'

" 'Oh, Jones, I'm glad to see you. I've been in this place three days and you're the first person that has taken any notice of me.'

"I think you know, gentlemen, that that is a peculiarity of our nation, and you must not take it too seriously."

HEALTH INSURANCE IN GREAT BRITIAN

He then spoke briefly of the passing of national health insurance in Great Britain and of its effects upon the British Medical Association:

"You all know that in 1912 the medical profession in England was suddenly brought face to face with the national health insurance act. Whatever might be said at that time to the contrary, there was no doubt that really it was the shadow or might be the shadow of a state service, a condition of things which we all abhorred. The British Medical Association had been jogging along very comfortably for a great many years. It was poorly organized at that time. I think anybody would admit that. It was suddenly called on to meet this great question. The members of this association disliked the idea of contract service with the government very much indeed. There was a great outcry and we were not going to submit to it. If we had been well organized and if we had been thoroughly united throughout the British Isles, I am sure that that act would have had to be very much modified if not actually withdrawn by Mr. Lloyd George, but our organization was not complete enough and it was too weak to withstand political pressure. Mr. Lloyd George said that if the medical profession as a whole did not come in to work with this act and along the suggested lines, he had up his sleeve sufficient medical men to establish a state se vice and work it on the lines which we wished to avoid of all others.

"Men began to fall away, the organization tumbled to pieces, and finally there was a great panic and every one went into the act. It was rather a pitiful spectacle, not because we went into it, but because we went into it after we said that we wouldn't. The British Medical Association came in for a good deal of abuse; they said we had been weak; they said we had not advised the members wisely, and there was a good deal of mud thrown at us."

That incident had taught the British physicians a lesson. When, at a later date, the Minister of Health had attempted to reduce the capitation fee from 12 shillings 6 pence to 7 shillings and 6 pence, 96 per cent of the physicians resigned. Then the Minister of Health decided to arbitrate. The result of the arbitration was 9 shillings per patient. Mr. Hall ended his address with a plea for unity of the medical profession in the American Medical Association, not only that it might maintain high standards of medical practice in the United States but that its example might be a lesson to all the world.

A MEMORIAL TABLET FOR DR. McCORMACK

The Board of Trustees called attention to the fact that a tablet had been placed in memory of Dr. J. N. McCormack. The inscription read:

TO
J. N. McCORMACK
WHO SERVED AMERICAN MEDICINE
AND THE AMERICAN MEDICAL ASSOCIATION
WITH DISTINGUISHED ABILITY AND FINE FIDELITY
THIS MEMORIAL TABLET
IS ERECTED

Among the resolutions introduced as new business came proposals for eliminating dangerous chemicals from cosmetics, attempts to secure amendments to the Volstead Act, attempts to control the imposition of excess taxes on physicians. An important resolution providing for the establishment of a council on physician therapy.

The president-elect Dr. William D. Haggard, arrived late at the session and in his address dealt with the necessity for adequate medical practice acts, proper defense against malpractice suits, suitable control in the field of workmen's compensation acts, and the whole question of hospitalization of veterans of World War I.

CHANGES IN SECTIONS

At this session of the Association a new section on Radiology was established and the section on stomatology discontinued.

The House of Delegates did not see fit at this time to create a section on physiotherapeutics which had been requested.

NURSES

The address of the president and the report of the Council on Medical Education and Hospitals also had been concerned with the problem of nurse education. The problem of securing an adequate supply of nurses continues to agitate medicine; in 1947 it is still one of the most pressing problems in medical practice. The report of the reference committee contained some interesting comments:

"The present course of nurse education is not providing nurses willing to do the ordinarily accepted duties and accept the ordinarily expected responsibilities of nursing the sick. As in the education of the medical student, science is overshadowing art in a profession which is largely, if not mainly, dependent on art for its successful practice. The plan of a joint committee of nine members from the nursing profession and three members from the medical profession may develop a solution; but, if so, much time will be occupied. It seems possible to your committee that the establishment of numerous small hospitals with their associated training schools for nurses may in a measure, at least in the smaller communities, offer a solution."

As a result of this presentation, the Board of Trustees was urged to give support to a survey of nurse education.

THE SECRETARY OF THE INTERIOR DISCUSSES LOBBYING

At this session also the House of Delegates heard an address by the Hon. Hubert Work, who was now Secretary of the Interior. He paid glowing tribute to the work of Dr. George H. Simmons and Dr. J. N. McCormack. Out of his years of experience in Washington he had a few words to say about lobbying:

"There are many lobbyists in Washington. They all represent a selfish interest. The moment the great American Medical Association, an ethical organization, intended solely for the purpose of eliminating bad tendencies, sends a representative to Washington, he will be that instant known as a lobbyist, and it will be assumed that he is trying to put out things of commercial interest to the medical profession. Commerce and scientific, ethical medicine are not related at all. The study of scientific medicine and the practice of it is a religion; it is a good deal nearer a religion than any other vocation on this earth. It ought to be kept far above the suspicion or the taint of commercialism.

"It would be far better if the congressmen at home were made to feel that the better element of his people want certain things accomplished to protect public health. Make it plain that it is not intended to protect the doctor, and make it plain that we don't care at all who practices medicine or that he practices so long as he is well grounded in anatomy and physiology and knows enough pathology to recognize disease when he sees it. Impress on them that that is our only interest in antagonizing the quack and the upstart and the man who is not qualified. Tell them that it is our purpose to further preventive medicine and explain to them that all medicine in its last analysis is preventive medicine, to prevent death, to prevent invalidism, to prevent deformed cases, and that it is really in the last analysis all preventive.

"If you can make that clear to your representatives in Congress, you don't need any local representative to lobby in Congress for you. In my opinion, it would detract from the dignity of ethical, scientific medicine to do it."

PRESIDENT PHILLIPS' FAMOUS SLIP

At this session of the Association, Dr. Wendell C. Phillips, who had been chairman of the Board of Trustees, was made president elect. In his response to the election, he perpetrated an Irish bull which has become classic in the archives of the Association. He said:

"I am not going to tell you how many years ago, but it was a great many, *I was born barefooted* (Italics ours) on a farm up in the rockribbed valley of the grand old St. Lawrence River, and as a farmer's boy I labored for years. (I am telling you this to show what may sometimes happen to a boy who was born in humble circumstances.)"

COMPENSATION FOR EYE INJURIES

One of the most significant technical reports to come before the Association was the one adopted at this session on compensation for eye injuries. This classic statement still continues to serve in legal and scientific circles whenever the question of compensation for such injuries arises.

ADVERTISING PROPRIETARY INFANT FOODS

For some time the question of the advertising of proprietary infant foods had been debated in the correspondence columns of THE JOURNAL and the question was now brought before the House of Delegates. The House had referred it to the Section on Diseases of Children. At this session the delegate from that section, Dr. Isaac A. Abt of Chicago, made the following report which has since served as a standard:

"A committee, appointed by the Section on Diseases of Children of the American Medical Association, at the annual session of 1924, has made an investigation concerning methods of sale, advertising methods and indications and contraindications for the use of proprietary infant foods.

"1. The committee finds that it is impracticable at the present time to attempt to dispense entirely with all proprietary foods.

"2. It is necessary for the protection of infants to formulate a definite program for the control of the method of advertising in all medical journals and in all periodicals, and especially in those that uphold high ethical standards.

"3. This problem is best attacked at its source, which consists of the education of the medical student in simplified methods of infant feeding. This the committee believes is the fundamental problem.

"4. There should be an increased propaganda among physicians and in lay journals to increase knowledge about breast feeding. Such a propaganda will include the dangers of artificial feeding of infants, particularly when carried on without the supervision of medical men.

"5. There is a disposition on the part of many manufacturers of proprietary foods to cooperate with the medical profession and its medical journals. The committee believes that much good may be accomplished by a better understanding and cooperation between these manufacturers and representatives of the American Medical Association."

The report was signed by Drs. George E. Baxter, Borden Veeder and John G. Foote.

A NEW PERIODICAL FOR PATHOLOGY

A resolution came from the Section on Pathology and Physiology urging the American Medical Association to undertake a publication in the field of pathology. This was referred to the Board of Trustees, which later agreed to establish the Archives of Pathology.

QUALIFIED GRADUATE EDUCATION

The commercial graduate school which gave short courses with fancy diplomas had been attacked by the Council on Medical Education and Hospitals and also by various resolutions introduced into the House of Delegates. The report of the reference committee was strong indeed. It said:

"Your committee is aware that there are still so-called postgraduate schools operated by groups of doctors for the sole purpose of placing in the possession of their 'graduates' documents for exhibition to prospective patients that will inspire unwarranted confidence in the ability of the possessor, such documents being sold at an exorbitant price, but one which it is apparent is satisfactory to the purchaser.

"It is deplorable and disgraceful that there are some prominent members of the profession actively connected with the so-called schools and a larger number willing (for what reason cannot be imagined) to lend the influence of their names as consultants or directors. No professional condemnation can be too strong to apply to those men willing to prostitute the noble, altruistic profession of medicine by assisting for pay the known, grossly incompetent, unscrupulous practitioner to prey upon a trusting public under the disguise of surgery.

"Although condemning without restraint the laboratory or institution which pretends to fit the totally inexperienced in from two to four weeks to practice major surgery and which issues a certificate or diploma to this effect, your committee recognizes that there is a large and legitimate field for the teaching and practicing of surgical technic along special lines, by surgeons competent to give such instruction. As the ability of the growing surgeon increases, there should be some place where he can familiarize himself with the technic of advanced operating which he is desirous of doing. Such laboratory, honestly conducted and with no false pretenses nor documents issued for advertising purposes, should be commended and supported as those previously mentioned should be condemned."

Out of such powerful pronouncements came eventually the certifying boards in the various specialties which now provide our people with specialists whose qualifications have been determined by their peers.

THE COMMISSION ON MEDICAL EDUCATION

At this time new problems in the field of medical education led to the formation of a National Commission on Medical Education; the secretary of the Association, Dr. Olin West, was asked to serve on the commission.

THE COUNCIL ON PHYSICAL THERAPY

At its meeting following the sessions of the House of Delegates the Board of Trustees agreed to establish a Council on Physical Therapy.

COMMITTEE ON COSMETICS

In order to meet the demand for control over dangerous cosmetics, a special committee on cosmetics was established.

INTERNATIONAL ORGANIZATION OF PHYSICIANS

The Board of Trustees was also asked to join an International League of Medical Practitioners which was to constitute in a sense a world medical organization. The Association agreed to take membership in this group, which published reports from time to time until World War II, when its activities were discontinued.

REGULATIONS FOR PROVIDING WHISKY

Much time was spent in discussing the regulations under which physicians could prescribe whisky and other spirituous liquors under the Volstead Act. The Association had been asked to appear as *amicus curiae* in the suit brought by the Association for the Protection of Constitutional Rights.

HYGEIA IMPROVES ITS CIRCULATION

As the year ended, the board heard a report to the effect that HYGEIA, under the new management, had made economies in editorial budget and that there had been an increase in circulation, in advertising and in reader interest, following editorial changes made by Dr. Morris Fishbein, the new editor of the publication.

QUARTERLY INDEX MEDICUS

The Index Medicus in Washington found itself in serious circumstances because of the desire of the Carnegie Institution to withdraw from its support. Conferences had been held by Dr. Charles W. Richardson, a member of the Board of Trustees, with representatives of other agencies concerned, including Dr. Fielding H. Garrison, Dr. L. R. Williams of the New York Academy of Medicine, Dr. William H. Welch of Baltimore, Dr. Victor C. Vaughan, and Dr. J. C. Merriam of the Carnegie Institution. It was considered desirable that there be a combination of the Quarterly Cumulative Index with the Index Medicus. The Board of Trustees appointed a committee consisting of Drs. Richardson, Fishbein and West to deal with the proposed combination.

As 1926 opened, the editor of THE JOURNAL reported that he had been able through conferences with Dr. Fielding H. Garrison and with representatives of the Carnegie Institution to work out a plan for combining the Index Medicus with the Quarterly Cumulative Index into a new publication to be known as the Quarterly Cumulative Index Medicus. The success of the new publication was instantaneous. It has come to be one of the most valuable contributions to medical bibliography in all the world. Its complete story is told in another chapter.

ANOTHER SUIT THREATENED

The Association was again threatened with a suit—this time because of the exposé of certain intravenous solutions. Again the Board of Trustees referred the suit to its attorneys.

NEW ACTIVITIES

The Council on Physical Therapy had organized and the record of its work is likewise told in a special article.

Through its Bureau of Legal Medicine, the Association was still endeavoring to get suitable regulations under the Volstead Act.

At this time Dr. R. C. Dickinson, secretary of the Committee on Maternal Health, appeared before the board to secure assistance in getting changes in the laws regulating contraception. The proposal was laid on the table.

The proposal came that the Association assume leadership in the standardization and control of hospitals.

Some difficulties arose again with the College of Surgeons due to some unfortunate publicity relative to actions taken in the meetings of the American College. The director of the American College of Surgeons, Dr. Franklin H. Martin, expressed his regret but could only say that the report had slipped through the hands of "what we considered an iron-bound committee."

A proposal was made that the Association publish a periodical to be known as the Archives of Medical Economics but the Board of Trustees did not consider this desirable.

A special committee had been appointed to cooperate with the commissioner of internal revenue and the secretary of the Treasury in drafting regulations governing the distribution of medicinal liquor. This committee, after holding three meetings, reported a series of regulations which were then taken by the government officials to the Congress for action.

MORE LIBEL SUITS

Now again the Association had been sued by the Hoxide Cancer Institute and by the Electrophone Corporation. These suits also had been referred to the attorneys for the Association.

1926
THE DALLAS SESSION

The speaker of the House of Delegates opened the session with new emphasis on public education in scientific medicine, a renewed attack on state medicine and contract practice.

Dr. William D. Haggard, president, spoke of the persistent effort to popularize periodic health examinations of the apparently healthy and proposed a plan for securing widespread adoption of this procedure. This plan was heartily endorsed by the House of Delegates.

The president elect, Dr. Wendell C. Phillips, dealt with the great progress of medical science in the United States and called attention to the fact that these great advances had been freely offered to the world and had not been promoted in a nationalistic spirit. He, too, urged renewed emphasis on health education of the public and congratulated the Association on the fine progress being made with HYGEIA.

Attempts to secure favorable action with regard to deductions of traveling expenses and expenses for postgraduate study had been unavailing.

The progress in securing amendments to the Volstead Act had been considerable.

Improvement had been secured in administration of narcotic laws.

The Veterans Bureau had not been in any way inhibited in treating all sorts of injuries not incurred in military service. There had been attempts by the federal government to bring about reorganization of administration without success.

The Sheppard-Towner Act had become widely effective and new bills were in progress to extend its subsidies. Unfortunately the U. S. Department of Labor had designated a chiropractic school as an immigrant school. Osteopaths and chiropractors were trying to force their way into community hospitals.

The action of the Board of Trustees in refusing to accept the proposal from the Gorgas Memorial Institute met with the approval of the House of Delegates.

In order to give the House of Delegates full opportunity to act on the question of a full time representative in Washington, the reference committee suggested that this subject be considered by the House of Delegates as a committee of the whole. By action of the Board of Trustees following the session, it was arranged to provide for representation in Washington through the Bureau of Legal Medicine and Legislation.

An important amendment to the By-Laws at this session made it possible for the Board of Trustees to fill any vacancy of an unexpired term of any of the officers of the Association.

The question of contraception continued to be urged on the Board of Trustees which, however, felt that it was a matter that must be acted on by the House of Delegates.

At a meeting of the Board of Trustees, the editor of THE JOURNAL called attention to the fact that the names of physicians whose licenses to prescribe liquor had been revoked were being printed in THE JOURNAL and that this had caused resentment on the part of some persons. However, the Federal Prohibition Administration had expressed the belief that the publication of the names would be of advantage in enforcing the law. The legal department of the Department of Internal Revenue did not feel that there could be any objection to the issuance of the names for such publication. At the final session of the Board of Trustees during the year, reports were presented from the secretaries of the Chicago Medical Society and the California Medical Society requesting the Board of Trustees to cause the editor to discontinue publishing the names of physicians whose permits to prescribe liquor had been revoked. The editor reported threats against him made in writing and over the telephone because of the publication of names. There was much discussion in in the Board of Trustees of this question. The editor urged that publication be continued for its moral effect. The final action sustained continuation of the publication of the names as long as they should be made available by the federal agencies.

STILL THE MEDICAL TRUST

At this time attention was called to the fact that the periodical called "Physical Culture" was announcing a series of articles "exposing the medical trust."

The Spanish edition had reached a circulation of well over 5000 but was incurring a considerable loss and the support from the Rockefeller Foundation to it was soon to be withdrawn. Under the circumstances the board sought for continuation of the publication for two more years, with the understanding that the periodical would be discontinued at that time if a greater circulation could not be secured. The Rockefeller Foundation agreed to continue.

Early in the year, Dr. R. G. Leland of Toledo was secured as an assistant for the Bureau of Health and Public Instruction.

The study of schools for nursing was well under way.

The Association had called a conference on public health in which some thirty health agencies participated and the board took under advisement a proposal to hold a second such conference.

COOPERATION WITH N. Y. HERALD-TRIBUNE FORUM

The editor of THE JOURNAL was authorized by the board to cooperate with the New York Herald-Tribune in a forum and in the publication of health articles.

1927

THE WASHINGTON, D. C., SESSION

Again the American Medical Association met in Washington. The speaker, Dr. Frederick C. Warnshuis, proposed that a message be sent to the President, Calvin Coolidge, calling his attention to the services of the medical profession to humanity. The speaker was impressed with the progress that was being made in a survey of nursing. He felt that some steps should be taken to standardize surgical procedures. The House of Delegates did not think it desirable that any special committee be appointed for this purpose.

The president, Dr. Wendell C. Phillips, congratulated the Association on the continued progress that had been made since the

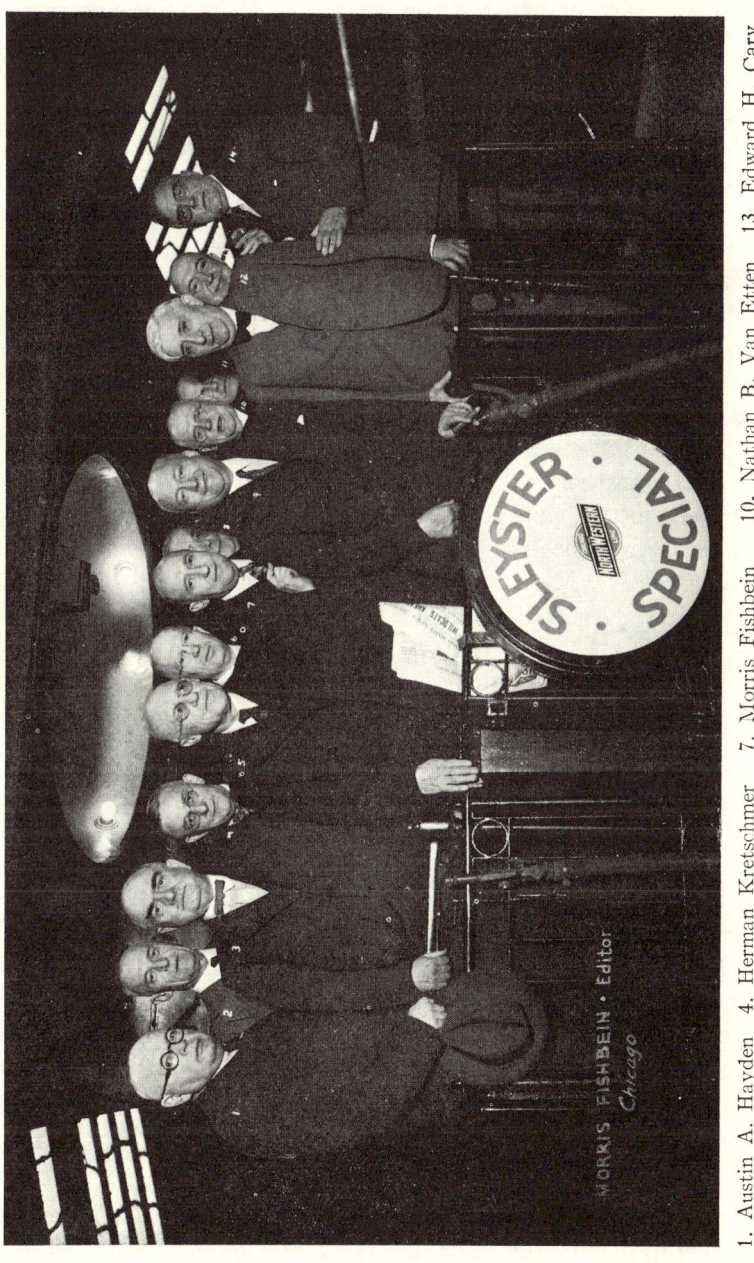

1. Austin A. Hayden
2. Olin West
3. Thomas S. Cullen
4. Herman Kretschmer
5. Will C. Braun
6. Allen H. Bunce
7. Morris Fishbein
8. Roger I. Lee
9. Charles G. Heyd
10. Nathan B. Van Etten
11. Ralph A. Fenton
12. James R. Bloss
13. Edward H. Cary
14. Arthur W. Booth

retirement of Dr. Simmons and he paid a tribute to the officers and staff of the headquarters organization for the quality of their work. He called the attention of the House of Delegates to the public health conference and to the responsibility of the physician in the field of public health. He spoke at length on the attempts that were being made to secure proper regulation of the use of medicinal liquors. He paid tribute to the cooperative work of the Woman's Auxiliary. To all of these tributes the House of Delegates gave its full approval.

The president elect, Dr. Jabez N. Jackson, contrasted the work of the medical profession with other avocations. He urged more frequent publication of the Principles of Ethics and an explanation of these principles to the public so that they might more fully understand the objectives of the medical profession.

The Board of Trustees announced to the House of Delegates that it had assigned a member of the staff of the Bureau of Legal Medicine and Legislation to full time duty at Washington during the sessions of Congress.

Indicative of the new problems which were beginning to concern the medical profession was the report of the Judicial Council under its chairman, Dr. Malcolm L. Harris. It dealt largely with definitions of a clinic and with contract practice.

THE NURSING PROBLEM

Now for the first time came a report of the special committee on nurses and nursing education. It was comprehensive but its only solution to the problem of satisfactory nursing service was the encouragement of visiting nurses service and trial of hourly or part-time nursing. The Committee felt that nursing education should include twenty-eight months, the first four months to be devoted to fundamentals and the succeeding two years to be devoted, as far as possible, to teaching the art of nursing by demonstration, participation and practice. The special reference committee which considered this report told the story of the organization of the committee and recommended that the American Medical Association continue to support the work of the committee for grading of nursing schools.

HOME FOR INDIGENT PHYSICIANS

A special study had been made also of the need for a home for indigent physicians. Dr. George H. Simmons, chairman of the special committee which made this investigation, had studied the matter in every state. Twenty-five states had reported on indigency and in all of the remaining states there were apparently only 41 indigent physicians.

PRESCRIBING OF LIQUOR

Again there were long resolutions on prescribing of spiritous liquors by physicians. Again the House of Delegates resolved that "the American Medical Association declares its adherence to the principle that legislative bodies composed of laymen should not enact restricting laws regulating the administration of any therapeutic agent by physicians legally qualified to practice medicine." This was the basic issue in attempting to secure modification of the Volstead Act.

CONTRACEPTION

The question of contraception again came before the House of Delegates in a resolution recommending alteration of existing laws wherever necessary so that the physician may legally give contraceptive information to his patients in the regular course of practice. The resolution was simply referred to the Board of Trustees, and the Board later simply laid it on the table.

Dr. William S. Thayer was made president elect of the Association.

A PERMANENT EXHIBIT

So successful had become the Scientific Exhibit that there were actions taken to secure the establishment of a permanent Scientific Exhibit. A motion picture theatre had become a function of the annual session but it had gradually lost favor and it was proposed that the money spent on the motion picture theatre might well be spent in improving the quality of the work of the sections.

DEMONSTRATIONS AS MEDICAL PRACTICE

At this time the Board of Trustees agreed to call a second conference on education of the public in health. There had begun to be complaints of so-called health demonstrations on the ground that these tended to take away the practice of medicine from the local medical profession.

COMMITTEE ON THE COSTS OF MEDICAL CARE

This year saw the organization of the Committee on the Costs of Medical Care. Dr. Ray Lyman Wilbur, chairman of that committee, had requested the appointment of the secretary of the Association to membership on the committee. The board authorized the appointment of the secretary to the Committee on the Costs of Medical Care and suggested the employment of a competent economist to aid in these studies.

1928
MINNEAPOLIS

Special problems for the Board of Trustees in the early half of 1928 concerned the resolution on contraception. This had simply been laid on the table but after consideration the Board of Trustees decided to refer it back to the House of Delegates for their consideration.

Trouble seemed to be brewing in relation to the rejection of an advertisement for Spanish ergot which THE JOURNAL had rejected. The suit of the Hoxide cancer cure was not being pressed.

Some of the state medical journals were breaking over the traces and accepting advertisements of products not approved by the Council on Pharmacy and Chemistry and at the same time failing to indicate their desire to depart from the Cooperative Medical Advertising Bureau.

The Board of Trustees was concerned with the selection of an ultimate site for a permanent home for the Association, to be monumental in character.

The program for the second public health conference indicated a new trend in problems for the Association. This program included such subjects as free and part-pay clinics (to be debated pro and con), health demonstrations presented by those who favored them, and a physician who opposed a public health service.

The Association was doing its utmost to secure an economist.

The decision had been made to erect a monumental building on the present property of the Association but the Board of Trustees had wisely secured an additional eighty feet of property on Grand Avenue.

THE ARCHIVES OF OPHTHALMOLOGY

Now came the request for the Association to publish a special periodical in ophthalmology—a request which was granted after conferences between all concerned. The history of each of the publications of the Association is published separately.

BUREAU OF ECONOMICS

Failure to secure a professional economist made it necessary to take Dr. R. G. Leland from the Bureau of Health and Public Instruction and to put him in charge of the Bureau of Medical Economics.

COMMITTEE ON THE COSTS OF MEDICAL CARE

To the Board of Trustees Dr. Olin West reported that protests had been made to the meetings of the Committee on the Costs of Medical Care relative to some of the publications which were being sent broadcast and it was his opinion that many of these publications were pure propaganda. Dr. West stated that the physicians on the committee were doing their utmost to present properly the point of view of the medical profession.

The problem of income tax deduction was still being debated but a final decision had not yet been reached.

SPANISH PUBLICATION DISCONTINUED

After conferences with the Rockefeller Foundation, it was agreed to discontinue publication of the Spanish edition, particularly since surveys indicated that at least one-fourth of the circulation in South America would subscribe for the English edition.

STANDARD NOMENCLATURE OF DISEASE

A communication had come from Dr. George Baehr, chairman of the executive committee of the National Conference on Nomenclature of Diseases, relative to participation by the Association in such a conference. This early step was to lead eventually to taking over by the Association from that conference of the publication of the "Standard Nomenclature of Disease" to which later was added the nomenclature of surgical operations. This standard publication gained wide adoption and is, in 1947, the recognized guide for the governmental services and the accredited hospitals of the United States.

THE MINNEAPOLIS SESSION

The meeting in Minneapolis in 1928 found the speaker of the House of Delegates confessing that he had covered too much territory in his previous addresses. He stated that he had been requested in some instances to make these comments by the president of the Association. He now asked for a ruling by the House of Delegates on the limitations that should be placed on the address of the speaker. He proposed thereafter to confine himself to recommendations dealing solely with parliamentary procedure and business expedients and with the general affairs of the House of Delegates. The House of Delegates agreed with him unanimously.

EDUCATIONAL INSTITUTIONS PRACTICE MEDICINE

The president, Dr. Jabez N. Jackson, reviewed the progress of medical science but condemned particularly the manner in which educational institutions were exploiting the practice of medicine. The House of Delegates agreed with Dr. Jackson that "the time has come (1) when no institution or clinic should permit its attending physicians to be imposed on; and (2) when, whatever the social or other advantage to the physician in the clinic, he should not be permitted to contribute to what is a gross injustice to the profession as a whole."

OVER-ORGANIZATION OF THE PROFESSION

The president elect, Dr. William S. Thayer, dealt with over-organization of the medical profession. Specialism should not be permitted to detract from the work of the national organization. He paid a tribute to two distinguished physicians who had died—Dr. Francis Peabody, professor of medicine at Harvard who was a member of the Council on Pharmacy and Chemistry, and Dr. Hideyo Noguchi who had died while investigating yellow fever in Africa.

The secretary of the Association dealt likewise with a multiplicity of medical organizations.

GOVERNMENT STEPS TOWARD SOCIALIZATION

The attention of the House of Delegates was called by the Bureau of Legal Medicine and Legislation to the manner in which the federal government had begun socialization of medicine through the expansion of the care given to veterans. The Congress had been greatly concerned with legislation affecting medicine and the Bureau of Legal Medicine's reports covered every aspect of such legislation.

From the National Grange at this time came a communication relative to the supply of physicians in rural areas. The Grange had been much impressed by a report made by Lewis Mayers and Leonard V. Harrison dealing with distribution of physicians in the United States. The Grange felt that it might well be a problem for the American Medical Association if possible without lowering medical standards to secure more physicians so that the needs of rural areas could be met.

Again there was much tinkering with the Constitution and By-Laws, largely of a parliamentary character.

TOO MANY HOSPITAL STAFF MEETINGS

The reference committee which considered the multiplicity of medical organizations deprecated especially the multiple scientific meetings of hospital staff organizations. "These," it said, "have tended to limit to small groups the dissemination of medical information and the discussion of medical problems, interfering thereby with the work of organized medical societies." It suggested that the staff meetings of hospitals be devoted preferably to executive discussions of problems relating to hospital economics and records and that members of the American Medical Association make special efforts to stimulate interest in and the development of scientific medicine in the regularly organized county medical societies.

Again there were resolutions on the need for a physicians' home, motion pictures, the teaching of obstetrics, and similar subjects.

At this session Dr. M. L. Harris, who had served the Association in many different capacities, was made president elect.

DISCONTINUANCE OF TRANSACTIONS

Following the discontinuance of the annual proceedings of the American Medical Association, the transactions of the individual sections had been published annually. By 1928 so many of the papers had been found of sufficient quality to warrant publication in THE JOURNAL that the Board of Trustees considered it desirable to discontinue the publication of the annual volumes of transactions. However, the Section on Ophthalmology and the Section on Otolaryngology desired that their annual publications be continued and subscribed for a sufficient number of copies to warrant the exception.

THE PRESIDENT'S MEDAL

The board agreed at this time to prepare a suitable medal to be given to presidents of the Association on completion of their term of office.

A COUNCIL ON FOODS

The rise of our knowledge of vitamins and other constituents of foods had brought increasingly into the advertising pages of THE JOURNAL the announcements of proprietary foods. The subject had become much too unwieldy for the Council on Pharmacy and Chemistry so that there came from the Council the suggestion to the Board of Trustees that food products be removed from the purview of that council. This was the first step toward the ultimate formation of the Council on Foods and Nutrition.

1929

HYGEIA SUCCESSFUL

By this time HYGEIA had begun to yield a small profit over its expense and had achieved a considerable circulation.

Early in January, 1929, the courts dismissed the suit of the Hoxide Institute—a quack cancer cure—against the American Medical Association.

A NEW BOARD FOR ARCHIVES OF INTERNAL MEDICINE

Trouble began to brew with the editor-in-chief of the Archives of Internal Medicine. The difficulties involved concerned the acceptance of articles which did not meet the standards of the publication and failure to cooperate in securing a high standard of literary production from authors of articles.

VETERANS ADMINISTRATION

Meetings were being held regularly with representatives of the Veterans' Administration in an effort to overcome some of the abuses that had developed in that service.

The Board of Trustees was in receipt of a letter from a member of one of the sections, who was also a delegate, who objected to the rejection of his manuscript by the editor of THE JOURNAL.

THE JOURNAL was threatened with a suit for condemning "shotgun" vaccines against influenza. The Board of Trustees told the editor to continue to present the scientific views of the Council on Pharmacy and Chemistry in this matter.

A COMMITTEE ON MOTION PICTURES

The Board of Trustees at this time took up seriously the question of motion picture films. A Committee on Visual and Motion Picture Education had been set up and had conferred with representatives of various organizations interested in the field. It was proposed that certain films be made with the advice of the Association's committee.

THE PORTLAND SESSION

The Portland, Oregon, session heard the speaker, Dr. Frederick C. Warnshuis, limit his address strictly to parliamentary procedures.

The president, Dr. William S. Thayer, again warned against multiplicity of medical organizations. He urged support of the Association for the QUARTERLY CUMULATIVE INDEX MEDICUS and for the Index Catalogue of the Library of the Surgeon General's Office. He closed his address with an appeal for freedom and tolerance in which he said:

"I have been sincerely impressed by the freedom and vigor of the discussions in this House, and at the same time by the fundamental restraint that has marked your actions. These are difficult and anxious days in the world at large, critical days, perhaps, in the history of parliamentary government, of free government by the majority. Here in America we have gone along for upwards of a hundred and fifty years with what we have believed to be a rather happily devised free government, a government by the majority tempered by safeguards allowing a fair measure of local independence. On this model has been formed the constitution of our organization. Government by the majority is wholesome and beneficent so long as it is tolerant and considerate. The strength of our government in the past has been in its elasticity and in that it has allowed much latitude in local self-control, in that it has recognized the right of local communities to settle those questions which relate to their everyday life.

"But there are lengths beyond which a majority may not go. When in a country like ours the national government attempts to legislate for the whole country as to what we may or may not eat or drink, as to how we may dress, as to our religious beliefs or as to what we may or may not read, this is to interfere with rights that are sacred to every English-speaking man. This is no longer republican government; it is tryanny. In the long run we English-speaking people will not endure tyranny. For immediate concentrated mass action such as is necessary in time of war, such government is necessary. We accept it; we *demand* it. But in time of peace we insist on certain local and individual liberties which we regard as rights.

"The Congress of the United States is not made up of men who desire to establish a tyranny. Far from it! But in certain ways, against the warnings of wise and temperate men such as the Chief Justice, they have passed laws which are intemperate, meddlesome and may justly be regarded as tyrannical. As a nation, we have of recent years set a rather sorry example in the passage of inconsiderate, ill considered and intolerant prescriptions and prohibitions, prescriptions and prohibitions some of which may be proper enough in certain localities where they represent the desire of the majority, but which, when applied to the country at large, interfere with the personal liberties of the people. Such laws cannot be enforced; they defeat their own ends. Intolerance is the most fatal enemy of liberty."

DR. M. L. HARRIS ON MEDICAL COSTS

The president elect, Dr. M. L. Harris, was of course impressed by his service with the Committee on the Costs of Medical Care. Dr. Harris said, in part:

"We are all more or less familiar with the question of the cost of medical care or the cost of being sick, which is agitating the public so much at the present time. Articles are appearing almost daily in the popular magazines or the public press, which give expression to the layman's point of view on the subject. In some of these articles, considerable criticism is directed at the medical profession, and the belief is often expressed that it is largely responsible for the present unsatisfactory situation. The national Committee on the Cost of Medical Care is undertaking a thorough study of all the factors that enter into the question, and it is earnestly hoped that the profession will heartily cooperate with the committee in its effort to reach correct conclusions. One of the complaints frequently made against the profession is the lack of suitable provisions for the distribution of high class medical services to the mass of people at a cost within their means. This I hold to be an undisputed obligation of the profession, and I have proposed a plan which I believe will enable it to meet this obligation fully, and which will result in great benefit to the masses as well as to the profession.

"This plan, which has already been published in THE JOURNAL, consists, in brief, in each county medical society incorporating and forming a medical center with a headquarters properly equipped for the diagnosis and treatment of all varieties of ambulatory patients. The organization should be in a sense a pay clinic owned and controlled by the profession. Every person receiving services should pay. Those who are able to pay regular fees should have their own physician, as at present, while those not able to pay regular fees should be treated at the center and should be charged a fee depending on their economic status and the character of the services rendered. Those who are unable to pay anything are charges on the community and should be paid for by the community, at rates to be agreed on by the community and the organization. The center should be managed by a board of directors, which should arrange for the time and service that each is to devote to the work of the center. The income, which will be considerable, after paying the running expenses and upkeep, will go toward paying in an equitable manner those who do the work. Services eventually may be extended to patients of the same class at their homes or in hospitals; in fact, the hospitals, which should be controlled and managed by the profession, should form a part of the general organization. In the large cities, more than one center may be developed, as may be necessary, so as to care for those living in all sections of the city. The whole scheme depends simply on the ability of the profession to organize on a business basis, and to manage its own business of caring for the sick rather than to allow it to pass into the hands of lay organizations or to be controlled by governmental enactment."

These were the opening reverberations of the great battle against compulsory sickness insurance that was to be the outstanding subject for consideration for the next twenty years of the history of the American Medical Association.

The Judicial Council again unreservedly condemned fee splitting.

The Council on Medical Education and Hospitals proposed the essentials of an approved department of radiology or roentgenology.

HISTORY OF THE ASSOCIATION FIRST PROPOSED

When new business was called before the House, it was proposed that there be published a history of the American Medical Association to be available in connection with the dedication of the new building—a project which unfortunately did not at that time come to fruition.

MORE RESOLUTIONS

Resolutions were offered on the care of indigent physicians, on the practice of medicine by corporations, on the dangers of certain gases used in refrigeration, on the teaching of obstetrics, on the policies of the Red Cross. Many of these resolutions were referred by the speaker of the House of Delegates directly to the Board of Trustees—a procedure which was to arouse some difference of opinion at the session of the Association in 1946.

The House of Delegates encouraged the Board of Trustees to proceed with its new building and raised the subscription price of THE JOURNAL $2.00 to aid in financing.

COMMITTEE ON MILITARY AFFAIRS

Perhaps in anticipation of World War II, the Board of Trustees was requested to appoint a special permanent committee to be known as the Committee on Military Affairs in National Defense, to which should be referred all matters of national defense and military preparedness.

There was discussion of expert opinion evidence.

Dr. William Gerry Morgan was made president elect.

PRESCRIPTION LIQUOR PROBLEMS

An investigation made by the general manager of the Association and conveyed to the Board of Trustees following the annual session indicated that there was a sufficient supply of medicinal liquor to last six years and that the time required by law for aging whisky is four years. The prohibition commissioner had thought of securing an opinion from the Association with respect to the advisability of authorizing the manufacture of more medicinal liquor but at the time the communication had not been received. Extended discussion before the Board of Trustees indicated an opinion that the issue was being fought wholly as a political issue between the "wets" and the "drys." Indeed the general manager called attention to the fact that the House of Delegates had provided that all questions dealing with alcohol should be referred to the Council on Scientific Assembly—at least as far as concerned any scientific opinion as to its need in the practice of medicine.

COMMITTEE ON FOODS

The Council on Pharmacy and Chemistry had set up a Committee on Foods, including Drs. H. C. Sherman, New York; L. B. Mendel, New York; W. McKim Marriott, St. Louis; Eugene F. DuBois, New York, and Morris Fishbein of Chicago. This Committee on Foods was to become the progenitor of the Council on Foods and Nutrition.

PATENTS

Toward the end of the year the question of the right of a physician to patent diagnostic apparatus and agents used in the treatment of disease became prominent. The Board of Trustees again felt that it should take under advisement the question of accepting and holding such patents for the public good. However nothing was done other than to consider the subject.

MORE MANUSCRIPT TROUBLE

Again came a protest to the Board of Trustees from a physician relative to the rejection of a manuscript, in this instance involving a paper dealing with anesthesia which was highly controversial. The editor had requested modification of the manuscript, which the author had refused. Again the Board of Trustees sustained the editor in the decision to refuse the manuscript.

A PLASTIC QUACK SUES

At this time a suit for $250,000 was filed by Henry J. Schireson, the Chicago plastic surgeon, against the editor of THE JOURNAL and THE JOURNAL itself. Two or three other suits of a similar character were filed. All were referred to the attorneys of the Association.

STUDY OF CRIME

A request came from the American Bar Association for the appointment of a committee to cooperate with the Bar Association in a study of crime and of expert opinion testimony. Such a committee was appointed.

THOMAS CULLEN BECOMES A TRUSTEE

Due to the sudden death of Dr. Charles Williams Richardson, the Board of Trustees nominated Dr. Thomas S. Cullen to fill the vacancy on the board.

WHITE HOUSE CONFERENCE ON CHILD HEALTH

Toward the end of the year, President Hoover held his White House Conference on Child Health and Protection with Dr. Ray Lyman Wilbur as Chairman, at which time he stated his opinion that public health activities should be carried on, as is education, in individual communities, but that federal subsidies might be necessary for aiding the individual states.

SOCIALIZATION BATTLE INTENSIFIES—1930 TO 1934

THE BOARD OF TRUSTEES early in January, 1930, heard that the medal to be awarded to presidents of the Association was complete; they planned to present such a medal to all ex-presidents at the next annual session. Unfortunately, Dr. W. W. Keen had now reached advanced years and would be unable to be present; he requested that his medal be given to Drs. W. J. Mayo and C. H. Mayo, who would receive it for him.

The Board of Trustees established a Committee on Military Affairs and National Defense, which was far sighted indeed since World War II was still some ten years ahead.

COLOR IN ADVERTISING

At this time the business manager inquired whether or not THE JOURNAL would permit color in its advertising pages. The general manager was opposed to this, feeling that the use of color would arouse the criticism that the Association was emphasizing advertising too much. However, before long colored advertising pages appeared in THE JOURNAL.

DANGEROUS GASES

The coming of the electric refrigerator had introduced into the household the potentiality of poisoning by sulfur dioxide, methyl chloride and other toxic gases. The Association had voted at a previous session to investigate these gases and inform the public concerning them. THE JOURNAL developed a series of articles on the subject, including contributions by Drs. Yandell Henderson and Carey McCord.

COMMITTEE ON FOODS

The Committee on Foods had made a most auspicious beginning. Dr. Morris Fishbein reported that more than 100 food products had already been submitted and that studies were being made of the composition of these foods and of the claims made for them.

NARCOTICS

The problem of narcotic addiction was prominent both before the Congress of the United States and the medical profession. The Hearst newspapers had undertaken a campaign in behalf of the

Porter bills, which would have seriously minimized control. THE JOURNAL OF THE AMERICAN MEDICAL ASSOCIATION had discussed the matter editorially. The president of the Association had given interviews to the press, and the president explained to the Board of Trustees that there had been a misunderstanding of the statements that he had made. Congressman Porter had inserted his letter to the American Medical Association in the Congressional Record before sending it to the Association. As a result of an extended discussion, the Board of Trustees filed a protest against the Porter bills.

PUBLIC HEALTH AND PERIODIC EXAMINATIONS

Plans were being made for a fourth public health conference. The Board of Trustees recognized that many large life insurance companies were offering periodic physcial examinations to all policyholders; this would be most helpful in the campaign for extending this procedure.

As an indication of the many liaisons of the American Medical Association with other organizations, representatives were appointed to attend the Semi-Centennial of the University of Southern California, to go to the American Conference on Hospital Service, the Joint Committee on Health Problems in Education, the Royal Institute of Public Health, the International Trachoma Conference, the British Medical Association and the World Health Sessions of the International Hygiene Congress.

THE CHILDREN'S BUREAU

Already there began to be repercussions from the health activities of the Children's Bureau in the Department of Labor. Following the child health conference held by President Hoover, the Children's Bureau asked for increased appropriations and for an extension of the Sheppard-Towner Act. The American Medical Association urged, as it always had in the past, that there should be only one federal agency for the administration of public health. At the time the United States Public Health Service seemed to be the desirable agency.

The Board of Trustees was still aiding the Committee for the Protection of Medical Research because the perennial legislation had again been introduced into the Congress.

AGAIN THE PORTER BILL

Committees were appointed by the Board of Trustees in March to confer with Congressman Porter relative to his proposed legislation. Following the publication of certain editorials in THE JOURNAL

Congressman Porter had withdrawn his bill and had introduced an entirely new text more in accord with the ideas of the medical profession.

The federal government was still engaged in regulations for the enforcement of the prohibition act.

The Board of Trustees paused in its deliberations to send a telegram of congratulations to Dr. William H. Welch on his eightieth birthday.

DR. JOHN R. BRINKLEY

Early in 1929 THE JOURNAL OF THE AMERICAN MEDICAL ASSOCIATION had published an exposé of Dr. John R. Brinkley of Milford, Kansas. Now Dr. Brinkley had secured a radio station, as had also Norman Baker of Muscatine, Iowa. Baker was promoting a combination of quack cancer cures and announcing regularly that he was out to "bust the medical trust." Letters were pouring into the headquarters office requesting the Association to put a stop to this bogus broadcasting. The Federal Radio Commission had asked that evidence be submitted. The medical societies of Kansas and Iowa had been aroused, and reprints of the exposés made by THE JOURNAL were being widely distributed.

In May the Association was sued by Dr. John R. Brinkley for $600,000 and by Norman Baker for $500,000. These suits eventually came to trial, as will be described in a special chapter of the History.

QUARTERLY CUMULATIVE INDEX

Because of the failure of facilities in Washington in connection with the work of the QUARTERLY CUMULATIVE INDEX MEDICUS, the Board of Trustees approved the taking over of all of the work in the headquarters office of the Association in Chicago. Since that time the work has been done wholly in Chicago.

THE ERGOT CASE

The charges that had been made against the Association for rejecting the advertisements of Howard W. Ambruster, who had cornered the ergot market, had been met by personal testimony given by Dr. Olin West and Dr. Paul Nicholas Leech before a special committee of the United States Senate.

PUBLIC HEALTH CONFERENCES DISCONTINUED

By June it was apparent that there would not be another public health conference, since there was apparently little enthusiasm on the part of public health officials for such a conference.

DIRECTOR OF EXHIBITS

Dr. Thomas G. Hull was employed to take over the responsibility for the Scientific Exhibit of the Association.

THE SHEPPARD-TOWNER ACT

The Board of Trustees proposed to introduce in the House of Delegates a resolution opposing extension of the Sheppard-Towner Maternity and Infancy Act. Other resolutions were adopted against federal aid for complete medical care to veterans regardless of service origin of their disabilities.

DETROIT MEETING

In Detroit the Board of Trustees met on the yacht Mamie O, as guests of Dr. Angus McLean.

When the House of Delegates met, the speaker suggested the possible utilization of a reading clerk so that the messages of the delegates might be better heard by the House of Delegates. The delegates did not approve, although they gave a reader a brief trial.

The president of the Association, Dr. Malcolm L. Harris, indicated that a movement was afoot in Great Britain to create a public medical service under the government. He recognized the drive toward socialization of medicine in Belgium, and he felt that these were trends of which the American Medical Association should be closely observant. "It is unwise," he said, "to put this matter off from year to year while the siege of medicine is drawing its lines tighter and tighter." He reported to the House of Delegates regarding the meetings of the Committee on the Costs of Medical Care and the principles toward which it was tending. He concluded, "There are no more serious and pressing problems confronting the medical profession today than are comprehended under the general term 'medical economics.' Therefore I suggest that this House of Delegates authorize and request the Board of Trustees to establish a Bureau on Medical Economics with a permanent head at the home office whose functions shall be to study all economic matters affecting the profession and that the reports of this bureau be published from time to time in THE JOURNAL so that the profession at all times may be kept enlightened on this most important subject."

President-Elect Dr. William Gerry Morgan urged consideration of a midyear meeting of the House of Delegates in Chicago. He warned against the fact that the hospitals were taking over responsibility for medical care from the medical profession.

The secretary of the Association, Dr. Olin West, was resentful of slurs on the medical profession appearing in periodicals, of the use of the radio by charlatans and faddists, of complex projects developed by well meaning philanthropists, and of the organization of numerous committees, commissions and conferences which were busying themselves with studies and appraisals of the medical profession. He said:

> "Just why this siege has been laid against medicine with its resultant outpouring of proposals of redaction, restriction and degradation of a great humanitarian profession is hard to explain. It may be that in the honest attempt that has been made to educate the public in matters pertaining to medicine we have reached the stage in the program where a certain element of the public feels that it knows enough to make the rules and to dictate the course of procedure. Certainly some of the proposals offered, by individuals and by groups, indicate that a little knowledge is, as it has always been, a dangerous thing. The situation is one that demands that efforts for the information of the public shall be continued and persisted in until the truth shall prevail. This means that compact and efficient organization that will command the undivided loyalty of all reputable physicians must be perfected and maintained, through which information based on scientific fact can be disseminated and misinformation from any source whatever can be combated."

He was disturbed furthermore, as were others, by caucuses and conferences being developed by small sections of the United States. A resolution was presented by Dr. E. C. Thrash, delegate of the Medical Association of Georgia, that the House of Delegates discountenance and disapprove sectional caucuses pertaining to matters that are to be acted on by the House of Delegates.

PRACTICE OF MEDICINE BY CORPORATIONS

The Judicial Council again urged the Fellows of the Association to realize that charges brought before the Judicial Council must be properly prepared. Its most significant statement dealt with the practice of medicine by corporations. On this point the Judicial Council, under the chairmanship of Dr. George Edward Follansbee, said:

> "With regard to the practice of medicine by corporations, it is the opinion of the Judicial Council, based on present evidence, that such practice is detrimental to the best interests of scientific medicine and of the people themselves. When medical service is made impersonal, when the humanities of medicine are removed, when the coldness and automaticity of the machine are substituted for the humane interest inherent in individual service and the professional and scientific independence of the individual physician, the greatest incentive to scientific improvement will be destroyed and the public will be poorly served."

The new chairman of the Council on Medical Education was Dr. Ray Lyman Wilbur. He reviewed the progress of the Council over many years in standardizing medical schools and hospitals. He reviewed as well its action in recognizing clinical laboratories and laboratories of radiology. By this time, of the 162 medical schools which prevailed in 1904, there remained only 75. Medical licensure had been greatly improved, and high standards prevailed generally.

So successful had been the work of the various councils of the Association that there came now a request for a council on medical economics.

ACTIVITIES OF HOUSE OF DELEGATES

The House of Delegates at this time adopted a recommendation from the Board of Trustees that academic green be the official color for all ribbon on emblems used by the American Medical Association.

Again the House of Delegates asserted its view that there should not be a routine midyear meeting but that provision existed for calling such a meeting whenever necessary.

The House of Delegates felt that a campaign should be conducted relative to educating the public and medical profession on the changed relationships of the hospital to the physician.

Because of the necessity for discussing matters in executive session, the House of Delegates at this time adopted a standing rule that the Tuesday afternoon meeting at each annual session be in executive session.

The House approved the creation of a Bureau of Medical Economics. It approved also the statement regarding corporation practice but suggested that the Judicial Council report further on the subject at the next meeting of the House of Delegates. The Association participated in the campaign for physical standards for drivers of motor vehicles by adopting standards of physical fitness. The Committee on Military Affairs urged establishment in each state of similar committees, and the campaign for preparedness went on.

The Federal Radio Commission was urged to give much more care than it seemed to be giving in the granting of licenses to broadcast, and the revocation of licenses of broadcasting stations which seemed to be operating against the public interest was recommended.

MENTAL HYGIENE

Many resolutions dealt with the necessity for better mental hygiene. Already in 1930 resolutions were introduced and adopted urging investigation of all hospitals caring for mental patients.

A special committee was appointed in September to study problems of mental hygiene and mental hospitals.

INDISPENSABLE USES OF NARCOTICS

At the request of the National Research Council, the board had undertaken publication of a series of articles on indispensable uses of narcotics which received wide acclaim and which were widely republished.

THE FRACAS OVER PRESCRIBING WHISKY

Because of a rule that had been adopted by a previous House of Delegates it was impossible for President William Gerry Morgan to read in open meeting a section of his address which dealt with liquor and the use of alcohol in medicine. Unfortunately, before coming to the Detroit session, the president had given out this portion of his address to the Associated Press. When the address was read in executive session, the president of the Association, Dr. William Gerry Morgan, challenged the right of those in charge of publicity for the Association to suppress that portion of his address. Much debate ensued in the executive session of the House of Delegates. The debate was ended by having the House of Delegates refer the ultimate decision to the Board of Trustees. At the September session of the Board of Trustees it was agreed that it would be improper to circulate such materials, since the problems of liquor were so prominent in the public mind that they secured all of the publicity during an annual session. Little attention was paid to either the scientific work or the other fundamental actions of the Association. The final decision was to turn over that portion of the address to the Bureau of Legal Medicine so that it might have the value of the president's opinion in its discussions in Washington.

CERTIFYING BOARDS FOR SPECIALISTS

By this time the specialists in the fields of ophthalmology and otolaryngology had organized certifying boards to determine who were and who were not qualified to practice these specialties. The sections of the American Medical Association had taken a conspicuous part in this movement. Now came a request for the establishment of a similar board utilizing representation from the Section on Obstetrics and Gynecology of the American Medical Association. Sponsorship of the American Medical Association was sought. The Board of Trustees felt, however, that such sponsorship must come from the section and that it was not a function of the Board of Trustees to sponsor formation of a certifying board.

INCOME TAX

The Bureau of Legal Medicine reported that it had a physician, Dr. L. B. Joslyn, of Maywood, Ill., who was desirous of having the American Medical Association support the movement to procure for physicians the right to deduct in the computation of their federal income taxes various expenses incurred in their medical work. The Board of Trustees authorized the Bureau of Legal Medicine to aid Dr. Joslyn in making this appeal.

TOXIC SUBSTANCES

The Board of Trustees gave attention also to proposals for regulating the sale of toxic substances and dangerous appliances used in domestic life and in industry.

COFFEY-HUMBER CANCER TREATMENT

At this time also came a considerable protest to THE JOURNAL OF THE AMERICAN MEDICAL ASSOCIATION against an editorial on the Coffey-Humber treatment of cancer. It was signed by leading physicians of California. However, many physicians in the San Francisco area had disapproved the promotion of the Coffey-Humber treatment and had objected to an editorial endorsing that treatment in the periodical of California known as *California and Western Medicine*. Unfortunately Dr. Ray Lyman Wilbur had aided Coffey in securing a patent. The lawyer for Dr. Coffey was threatening THE JOURNAL with suit for libel in case any reference was made to this letter. The whole procedure was referred to as a scientific scandal. The Board of Trustees supported the editorial and stated that it would watch with interest the results of further investigation of the Coffey-Humber treatment. The years have passed and the method is of little interest now.

SEALS FOR ACCEPTED PRODUCTS

The board heard also that the Council on Pharmacy and Chemistry and the Committee on Foods had created a seal to be used on products accepted by these agencies and sold to the public. The Board approved the use of such seals, which have been of immense service in educating the public regarding the existence of the American Medical Association and the nature of its work.

1931

PHILADELPHIA

The Association had now reached a preeminent position among medical organizations. Independent professional and lay groups throughout the nation appealed to the Association for information. The public began utilizing its services through the various councils, bureaus and departments to an amazing degree. Already it was apparent to the Board of Trustees and to the officers of the Association that the activities in which the Association would engage in the future would be largely extended both in scope and in quantity.

The Association purchased its first rotary press, with a capacity of 96 pages, at a cost exceeding $70,000. Other new machinery was continuously purchased by the trustees in order to keep the physical equipment at optimum functioning efficiency.

The officials in the headquarters office were constantly being called on to address public audiences such as women's clubs, medical groups, student bodies of universities and colleges, and to make many broadcasts. The special journals of the Association were continuing to advance in the quality of their material. The library had grown from a small reference department employing five people concerned chiefly with the preparation of indexes for THE JOURNAL to a staff of almost thirty who were carrying on the QUARTERLY CUMULATIVE INDEX MEDICUS, a periodical lending service, a package library service and many other bibliographic functions. HYGEIA by 1930 had begun to make a small profit and it was being more frequently copied than most other publications. The Committee on Foods had begun to promulgate pronouncements on health questions related to foods, passing on more than 300 foods during the year and issuing general decisions on such questions as the addition of sulfur dioxide to canned foods, the use of the term "sterile," the healthfulness of infant foods of various kinds, and the naming of food products. The Council on Physical Therapy had engaged in many educational activities related to the use of physical devices and had exposed innumerable fraudulent forms of physical apparatus. The Bureau of Health and Public Instruction was promoting education in health over the radio, in meetings and in exhibits by the use of pamphlets, by promoting periodic health examinations and by cooperating with many other agencies, including particularly the National Education Association and the National Congress of Parents and Teachers. Chief among legislative problems continued to be federal subsidies in the health field, narcotic drugs, and veterans legislation.

BUREAU OF MEDICAL ECONOMICS

In accordance with the resolution adopted by the House of Delegates at the Detroit session, a Bureau of Medical Economics had been created. Dr. R. G. Leland was head of the bureau and was undertaking many studies. At the meeting of the previous year, the House of Delegates had provided for the appointment of a Committee on Legislative Activities. The first committee was composed of Drs. D. Chester Brown, E. H. Cary, Thomas S. Cullen, J. H. J. Upham, and C. B. Wright. This committee was cooperating with the Board of Trustees in considering federal legislation.

MENTAL HYGIENE

A Committee on Mental Hygiene had been established to work with the Council on Medical Education and Hospitals in the investigation of mental institutions. This committee included Drs. H. Douglas Singer, F. G. Ebaugh, Walter L. Treadway, J. Allen Jackson and E. J. Emerick.

Other committees were working on such problems as motion pictures, industrial and domestic hazards such as poison gases, care of the veterans, and standardization of clinical thermometers.

THE PHILADELPHIA SESSION

When the Association met in Philadelphia in 1931 the president, Dr. William Gerry Morgan, paid high tribute to Dr. Olin West, the general manager, and urged that he be given an assistant. He spoke also of the great progress of the publications under the editor and of the efficient work of Dr. William C. Woodward in the field of legislation.

Much agitation was again in the air on the question of removal of the location of the headquarters office to Washington. Dr. William Gerry Morgan, as a resident of Washington, advised strongly against moving the headquarters to that city. He felt, however, that the chief office of the director of the Bureau of Legal Medicine and Legislation should be in Washington during the periods when the national Congress was in session. His experience in travelling to various medical societies had convinced Dr. Morgan that it was most desirable that physicians throughout the country be fully informed of the work of the headquarters office and he felt, too, that the work of the president was so arduous that some adequate honorarium should be developed for him during his term of office.

Dr. E. Starr Judd, president elect, emphasized the important place that the American Medical Association had come to occupy in the social and political structure of our country. He urged particularly the development of adequate personnel and of a new building for the headquarters. He reviewed the activities of each of the special councils and bureaus. He felt, however, that not enough Fellows of the Association took advantage of the annual session, and he recommended consideration of county and district clinical meetings as a part of the general functions of the American Medical Association. He felt especially the need of a bureau on the study of problems in connection with cancer, which would affiliate with other agencies and bureaus studying the subject and which would investigate all research on new methods of treatment. It might have charge also of publicity on cancer.

At this session there was a recommendation, made by Dr. Isaac A. Abt, that the name of the Section on Diseases of Children be changed to the Section on Pediatrics; this met with the approval of the House of Delegates.

RISE OF THE HOSPITAL

The Council on Medical Education and Hospitals, under the chairmanship of Dr. Ray Lyman Wilbur, recognized the rise of the hospital to an exceedingly important position in medical practice. It recognized that there was a greater demand for interns than there were graduates available and also the increasing use of resident physicians to carry on the work of the hospital.

REFUGEE PHYSICIANS

Already the rise of totalitarianism in Europe was beginning to bring an increasing number of refugee physicians to the United States. As a result, the Council on Medical Education and Hospitals was requested to draw up a list of foreign medical schools which might be considered acceptable and also to classify foreign medical schools at which great numbers of American physicians were in attendance, so that state boards of licensure might have some guide in admitting the graduates to examination.

MORE THAN 100,000 MEMBERS

In this year the membership of the Association passed the 100,000 mark; the House of Delegates expressed its gratification, and the reference committee highly commended the many expanding activities reported to it by the board.

STILL NO VETERANS' REPRESENTATIVE

At this meeting of the House of Delegates a resolution was introduced to grant to the Veterans Bureau the same type of representation as was given to the Army, Navy and Public Health Service. The reference committee voted three in favor of this procedure and one against. The discussion was profuse and at its end, the entire matter was laid on the table.

LIBRARY OF THE SURGEON GENERAL

Again it was becoming apparent that the structure housing the Library of the Surgeon General in Washington was shabby and a terrible fire hazard. There was a movement either to rebuild the library or to remove it to the Walter Reed Hospital near Washington. Dr. C. B. Wright of Minnesota introduced a resolution urging that the library be built, if possible, on ground adjacent to the Library of Congress. This recommendation was approved by the

House of Delegates. It has recurred at frequent intervals since 1931. By 1947 ground next to the Library of Congress had been secured and plans drawn. It is hoped that a new structure may be forthcoming before 1950.

EXECUTIVE SESSION DISCUSSES LEGISLATION

Now came the first regular executive session of the House of Delegates, established to consider relationships of the medical profession to the federal government and to consider as well problems affecting the operation of the Association itself. The Committee on Legislative Activities made its first report on various measures introduced into the Congress but particularly on the subsidy bills. State medical societies and similar bodies were urged to discuss questions of medical economics and the social relationships of the medical profession. Societies of limited membership were requested to refrain from expressing individual and varying opinions. The medical profession should speak, the delegates believed, as a unit rather than present a divided opinion before legislators and the public.

A number of resolutions dealing with amendments to the Volstead Act were referred to the Board of Trustees for their consideration, through the special committee appointed by the board to deal with these matters.

At this meeting Dr. Edward H. Cary of Dallas, Texas, was made president elect. In his acceptance address to the House of Delegates he expressed his ideals for expansion of the organization. As a trustee he had been particularly concerned with the building of a new home for the Association and he said:

"So let's build a home, some day, as strong as the strength of scientific truth, as lofty as the highest ideals of our art, as broad as the need of man, as beautiful as the hope of service, a tower to inspire all of us to constant and consistent work for the glory of achievement and the lessening of humanity's load of ignorance, pain and disease; an expression of the unified thought of this, our profession, in this our country, in this our century, to stand for us for the ages to come."

1932

NEW ORLEANS

As 1932 came on the scene, the Association was still agitating the amendments to the Volstead Act. The Association was being sued by Norman Baker and John R. Brinkley, and suits had also been filed by one S. Lewis Summers because of what the Association said about a remedy called "Befsal"; by a naturopath named Percival Lemon Clark who had been broadcasting quackery on the radio out of Chicago, and by the Ora-Noid Company which had prepared a powder claimed to be efficient for the control of pyorrhea.

All these charlatans and promoters of nostrums had been issuing literature libeling the Association. Attacks were being made on the headquarters staff with the assertion that their acceptance of remedies and of food products were conditioned by applications for advertising. Most thorough investigations by the Board of Trustees revealed, of course, that these charges were without any basis in fact.

The Committee on Mental Health was preparing to make a survey of mental hospitals in the United States. Some institutions had resented the investigation and were refusing to reply to questionnaires. There were beginning to be rumblings about commercial methods employed in extending corporation and contract practice. The suggestion was made that it might be well for the American Medical Association to make its own study of sickness insurance abroad. The Howard W. Ambruster group was still circulating charges relative to the refusal of the Association to aid a monopoly in Spanish ergot. The Association was cooperating with many other agencies. Dr. John M. Dodson, who had acted as director of the Bureau of Health and Public Instruction, had become ill and Dr. W. W. Bauer who had been secured to act as assistant director, was now made director of the Bureau. Dr. Arthur Dean Bevan, formerly chairman of the Council on Medical Education, was conducting a single-handed campaign against the prescribing of alcoholic liquors but the Association did not feel warranted in supporting him in his campaign. He had nevertheless appeared before Senate hearings on the subject. THE JOURNAL OF THE AMERICAN MEDICAL ASSOCIATION had published an editorial calling attention to some of the strange expressions in these hearings. The Board of Trustees approved the editorial and announced there was no warrant for changing its opinion.

A special committee from the Association had met with the American Legion, and the medical council of the Veterans Administration but it had been found impossible to find a common ground of agreement relative to the care of disabilities that were not of service origin.

CENTRAL SCIENTIFIC EXHIBIT

Following a previous decision by the House of Delegates, an attempt had been made to establish in the headquarters office a Central Scientific Exhibit. The exhibit had been installed but had not apparently attracted many visitors. Hence it was agreed at this time that the exhibit be stored so that it would be available for use in public exhibits but that it would not be desirable to occupy so much of the space in the headquarters office in this way.

PRESCRIBING LIQUOR

Dr. Bevan appeared before the Board of Trustees. He had not made the statement that 90 per cent of the medical profession were writing unethical and illegal prescriptions for alcoholic liquors but he admitted that he did say that 90 per cent of the prescriptions written under the present conditions were used for beverage and not for medicine in the scientific treatment of disease. During the previous year the permits of 977 doctors were revoked for illegal prescribing. THE JOURNAL had been the most active of any publication in the United States in the attempt to control the use of prescribing of liquor by physicians and had pointed out repeatedly that there was a small percentage of doctors who could not be trusted in this respect.

ARCHIVES OF INTERNAL MEDICINE

When the Association met in May in New Orleans, it was confronted with the resignations of the editorial board of the ARCHIVES OF INTERNAL MEDICINE, including Drs. William S. Thayer, J. D. Heard, W. T. Longcope, Richard C. Cabot, J. H. Means, and Walter W. Palmer. By unanimous vote the resignations of this group were accepted and a special committee of the Board of Trustees was established to develop a new editorial board for the ARCHIVES OF INTERNAL MEDICINE. The difficulty with this board had arisen over the failure of the board to renominate for another term the chief editor, Dr. Joseph L. Miller, who had been editor of the publication since its beginning more than twenty-five years previously. Dr. Miller had been having difficulties in the acceptance of material and in the editing of manuscript. He had also attempted to discontinue advertising. The Board of Trustees recognized the necessity of maintaining its own responsibility over the conduct of the publications.

BOOK PUBLICATIONS

The Association was undertaking the publication of several books created largely by various series of articles published in THE JOURNAL, including such subjects as therapy and electrocardiography. The editor had thought that means should be found for gaining wider circulation for these books, perhaps through affiliation with various medical publishers. As the years went on, the problem became increasingly serious. In 1947 the Board of Trustees determined to continue the Association's book publication principally through leading medical publishers.

A plan was prospected for a joint conference of all of the editors of state periodicals with the Board of Trustees during the coming year in order to unify policies and discuss editorial control of these publications.

THE NEW ORLEANS SESSION

The New Orleans session heard the president of the Association discuss at considerable length the preliminary report of the Committee on the Costs of Medical Care. He emphasized the importance of studying contract practice and group practice of medicine. He urged an extension of preventive medicine. He considered the importance of graduate training and of specialization. It was his belief that a method of certification should be devised for each medical specialty.

The president elect, Dr. E. H. Cary, had travelled widely throughout the nation speaking to many medical organizations. He recommended the establishment of a committee to cooperate with the Bureau of Medical Economics and its studies. He urged more extensive development of postgraduate instructional facilities.

For the first time at this meeting there came an extensive report from the new Bureau of Medical Economics. It outlined its purposes, functions and methods of procedure. It had made studies on the care of the indigent sick, of income from medical practice, of capital investment, of collection methods and agencies, and of contract practice.

The Judicial Council had likewise made extended studies of patents and of health and hospital associations.

When new business was called for in the House of Delegates, there were resolutions on the care of veterans, on the appointment of a committee to study birth control, on the hospital and health insurance societies of Cuba.

At this session General R. U. Patterson, surgeon general of the United States Army, made a long and comprehensive plea for support of the Association in securing a new building for the Surgeon General's Library.

The executive session was especially concerned with the report of its Committee on Legislative Activities which discussed in the main legislation related to the care of veterans. It had been concerned with a bill on rural infancy and maternity care.

Then came a resolution on the subject of birth control. It was the opinion of the reference committee that this was a controversial subject and that it would not be advisable to inject this subject before the profession. They, therefore, opposed the resolutions that had been introduced for consideration of this subject.

Toward the end of the session it became apparent that a minor controversy was incubating. Apparently the reference committee on reports of the board of trustees and officers had been given access to the report well in advance of the session and appeared at the annual session with its complete report prepared in mimeographed form. This report it distributed to the House of Delegates immediately. The Board of Trustees at once gave consideration to some of the criticisms that had arisen in the reference committee, drew up a reply to the mimeographed report and, in turn, prepared its own mimeographed reply for distribution to the House of Delegates on the afternoon session of the same day. The reply of the board was comprehensive. The reference committee had expressed its opinion that the need of a new building was not urgent. The Board of Trustees pointed out that this was ultimately a responsibility of the board, which also had full responsibility for the funds of the Association. The charge had been made by the reference committee that some of the activities which the Association was carrying on were inadequately financed. The Board of Trustees pointed out again that it was the responsibility of the board to conserve the funds of the Association and to spend in accordance with a wise budget. The reference committee had suggested that the Committee on Legislative Activities be given authority over the Bureau of Legal Medicine and Legislation. To this came the reply "The Board of Trustees cannot delegate its responsibilities to the legislative committee." The reference committee had suggested that the members of the legislative committee be paid for their work with a generous budget which would be used by the chairman of that committee as he might deem wise and necessary. To this the board replied, "In the past this Association has been served by many idealistic and loyal physicians including members of the House who have given of their services on councils and on committees for the good of the organization and for the benefit of scientific medicine without thought of personal compensation. Such devoted service has been far more effective than any service undertaken for a small fee which the Association might pay possibly could be." And this section of the report concluded:

"It has been the aim of your Board of Trustees to maintain unblemished the great repute of this organization for scientific integrity, for honesty, for dignity, and for devotion to the best interests of the people of this country. In that endeavor it has never descended to any means in legislative activity, or to any means in political manipulation, that it might not report openly and unashamed to this House of Delegates."

Item by item the Board of Trustees answered every one of the criticisms of the reference committee. The House of Delegates fully supported the Board of Trustees and deleted from the report of the reference committee all of the unwarranted criticisms that had been made. The House did recommend that the funds for the Bureau of Medical Economics be increased.

The committee on medicinal alcohol made a special report and received the appreciation of the House of Delegates.

ARCHIVES OF INTERNAL MEDICINE

When the Board of Trustees met following the annual session, it chose a new editorial board for the Archives of Internal Medicine, including Drs. Arthur Bloomfield, San Francisco; Reginald Fitz, Boston; N. C. Gilbert, Chicago; J. H. Musser, New Orleans; and Russell W. Wilder, Rochester, Minn.

The Association had agreed to prepare an exhibit at the Century of Progress exposition which would be held in 1933 in Chicago.

GROUP MEDICINE AND OTHER PROBLEMS

The growth of contract practice and corporation practice of medicine suggested to the Board of Trustees the desirability of a joint conference of all of the official agencies of the Association interested in the subject to consider various means for providing medical and hospital service to the public. Appeals were coming from the conference in charge of developing a standard nomenclature of disease for financial assistance from the Association. There was not, however, any indication that the Association's aid or participation in the work would be especially sought beyond its financial contribution. The Board of Trustees did not feel justified in making such a contribution. Eventually the National Conference on Nomenclature of Diseases requested the American Medical Association to take over the publication of the work, as will be recorded later. Since that time this has been a function of the American Medical Association.

Among other projects for which the Association's aid was sought were the standardization of catgut, overcoming accidents in anesthesia, publications of the Joint Committee on Health Problems in Education of the American Medical Association and the National Education Association, supplying forms for the summer roundup campaign of children. The Milwaukee County Medical Society had formulated a plan providing medical care for persons in the low income group. The special committee appointed to study such plans had studied the Milwaukee program but did not think that the experiment was ripe for national adoption.

As the year went on, the Association was asked to work with the rehabilitation committee of the American Legion, with the Century of Progress, with the International Conference on Goiter. It was asked to survey the publication of the Cleanliness Institute.

The board was asked to consider the exorbitant cost of medical periodicals to libraries, the previews of motion pictures related to medicine. The Committee on Foods was enlarged.

COSTS OF MEDICAL CARE

The editor of THE JOURNAL called the attention of the board to the fact that the final report of the Committee on the Costs of Medical Care would be released for publication on November 29 and asked for instructions as to the attitude which THE JOURNAL should take editorially regarding it. The trustees instructed the editor of THE JOURNAL to take an attitude against any attempt to socialize the practice of medicine. That editorial has since been widely quoted by the proponents of socialized medicine as an indication of the opposition of the Association to any modifications in the nature of medical practice. The report of the Committee on the Costs of Medical Care was an epoch-making document. In order that readers of this history may be fully cognizant of the point of view of the Association the editorial is here quoted in part:

"Both the majority and minority reports recommend continued study of medical economics problems by every type of agency. Certainly the studies already published by the committee indicate the value of such studies and the necessity for having facts on which to base conclusions and recommendations. This would seem to be particularly true in relationship to such studies as are available of various industrial medical services of and of corporate practice. The minority report is paricularly resentful that the majority made recommendations on the basis of inadequate studies in this field. Thus it says:

" 'It is the belief of the minority group that the majority report has presented this question in a distorted manner. The evils of contract practice are widespread and pernicious. The studies published by the Committee show only the favorable aspects. They were selected because they were considered the most favorable examples of this type of practice in the United States. For each of these plans a score of the opposite kind can be found. The evils are inherent in the system although they may be minimized when a high grade personnel is found either among employees or medical group, or both.'

"Specifically, the recommendation of the minority report reads:

" 'The minority recommends that the corporate practice of medicine, financed through intermediary agencies, be vigorously and persistently opposed as being economically wasteful, inimical to a continued and sustained quality of medical care, or unfair exploitation of the medical profession.'

"These two reports represent, therefore, the difference between incitement to revolution and a desire for gradual evolution based on analysis and study. The majority report urges reorganization of medical practice, the development of centers, insurance; if necessary taxation to provide funds; expansion of public health services. The minority is willing to test any plan that may be offered if it conforms to the medical conception of what is known to be good medical practice. Indeed, the minority recommends 'that methods be given careful trial which can rightly be fitted into our present institutions and agencies without interfering with the fundamentals of medical practice.' One seems to hear that famous medical aphorism that has come down through the centuries: 'Prove all things; hold fast to that which is good.' "

1933
MILWAUKEE

By action of officials in Washington, the Army had abandoned its training of reserves in the medical, dental and veterinary corps. The Committee on Military Affairs of the American Medical Association was urging preparedness for war. The Board of Trustees voted to support the Surgeon General of the Army in his efforts to maintain an adequate reserve corps.

The legislative committee had appeared before the Congress and had gone on record as opposing the erection of any additional hospitals for the care of veterans, the provision of free service to veterans whose disabilities were not service connected, and the policy of transporting patients from great distances for examination and service. The legislative committee of the American Medical Association had proposed, moreover, that if the government intended to continue to provide service to veterans, those receiving such service should be permitted to select their own hospitals and their own physicians. When World War II was over, some of these objectives were achieved.

The Board of Trustees determined at this time to obtain a closer insight into the work of the various councils and bureaus of the headquarters office; the chairman of each of these councils was invited to appear before the board and to present the principal problems that concerned him. The Bureau of Medical Economics presented a plan for securing information concerning health insurance systems abroad.

In accordance with a request from motion picture producers, the Association appointed a committee, including representatives in Los Angeles and New York City, to preview motion pictures.

The president of the Association, Dr. Dean Lewis, reported that he had had a conversation with the physician of President-Elect Roosevelt and had gained the impression that Mr. Roosevelt desired to adopt a program of curtailment in veterans' affairs and that he would consider it a definite service if the American Medical Association would appoint a committee to discuss veterans' legislation with him. The Association had also been requested to cooperate with the General Federation of Women's Clubs by appointing a representative and to send a delegate to the fourth international congress of radiology in Zurich. There now came the proposal to provide a medal for the speaker of the House and for members of the Board of Trustees. This the Board of Trustees laid on the table.

The libel suits filed by S. L. Summers, approximating $4,000,000, had been thrown out of court, and the Brinkley suit against Dr. Fishbein because of an address given in Kansas City had likewise been dismissed. Another suit by Dr. John R. Brinkley was being pressed.

The depression, which began in 1929, was beginning to make itself felt in the receipts of the American Medical Association and in its disbursements.

At a meeting of the Board of Trustees early in 1933 the question of group hospitalization insurance came prominently before the Board of Trustees in the form of a resolution by the trustees of the American Hospital Association endorsing the general principle of group payment as applied to hospital service. The Board agreed to bring the question to the House of Delegates for consideration at its next session.

At this meeting came protests from American physicians because of persecution of Jewish physicians in Germany. These, too, were recommended for consideration by the House of Delegates.

Again there came a request for the establishment of a permanent representative in Washington.

The entire subject of medical patents was considered at a joint session of the Board of Trustees with the Judicial Council. The editor of THE JOURNAL was instructed to prepare an editorial on the subject which was to be considered by each member of the board before publication. This editorial said:

PROBLEM OF MEDICAL PATENTS

Recently the question of the desirability of patents of products used in the field of medicine has been hotly debated. The Principles of Medical Ethics of the American Medical Association says specifically, "It is unprofessional to receive remuneration from patents for surgical instruments or medicines." It has been the pride of medicine down the centures that it gave freely of its discoveries for the benefit of mankind. Jenner's contribution of vaccination against smallpox, Pasteur's method for the control of hydrophobia, Withering's contribution of digitalis, becme the property of all who cared to use them for the prevention or treatment of disease.

As the science of medicine developed, however, new elements entered into its work and participated in its endeavors. Physicians began less and less to concoct their own remedies and to depend on the manufacturer of pharmaceuticals for the collection of materials and for their preparation and distribution. In an earlier day the physician who developed new devices or appliances manufactured a few with the aid of some neighboring blacksmith or carpenter. The modern physician is likely to delegate the manufacture to an industry capable of turning out thousands of units, in contrast to the ten or fifteen which might be used formerly. Greater dissemination of medical knowledge creates a greater demand for new drugs and new equipment. Moreover, the situation is complicated by the entrance into medical research of specialties associated with medicine yet not necessarily partaking of the ideals of the medical practitioner. Today the development of a new medicament may involve the participation of chemists, physicists, laboratory technicians, physiologists, biochemists and roentgenologic technicians who may not themselves be concerned at all with the traditions of medicine as a profession. Insulin, for example, was developed by biochemists, physiologists and a practicing physician. Whereas an ethical physician might not derive remuneration from a patent, biochemists or physiologists might do so. Certainly the name of the physician Banting is as much associated with the discovery as those of his colleagues, Macleod, Collip and Best. Finally, if the discoverer fails to patent his discovery, any one else may do so and thus steal both the discovery and the profits. The tremendous advantages of being first in the field with a new medical preparation are well recognized in the pharmaceutical industry.

In a recent issue of *Science*, Dr. Allen Gregg* considered particularly the new questions raised by the patenting of products through universities. In order to avoid possible ignominy and recriminations against physicians who might patent medical discoveries, and especially when the work was done under the auspices of and with equipment provided by universities, it has become customary to have such patents taken out in the name of the university, college or research institution and to control and promote the preparations under boards appointed by these universities. Numerous universities now resort to such patenting to obtain money to support further research but also, possibly, with the idea of rewarding suitably the investigators of products used in medicine. Already medical patents are controlled by Harvard, Toronto, Columbia, Cincinnati, Wisconsin, Stanford, St. Louis, and Northwestern universities, by the Mayo Foundation, and by the Scarlet Fever Foundation of the McCormick Institute for Infectious Diseases.

As Dr. Gregg emphasizes, there may be excellent arguments in favor of such patents, yet their operation has already produced innumerable difficulties. Extraordinary jealousies develop between members of the same research staff because of special advantages accruing to those who derive income from patents A tendency develops to promote new products rather than to examine them critically. The acquisitive desire, inherent in many persons, eventually leads to a psychologic frame of mind described as "royalty crazy."

Vast sums must be accumulated for the protection of patents—to prosecute infringement. Extraordinary secrecy must be maintained, interfering with academic freedom in research. The existence of patents inhibits research on similar products or with the same materials by physicians in practice and by investigators in medical schools and universities. The university, once in the field of patents, as a routine attempts to protect every tiny innovation or result, eventually devoting more time and money to protect old discoveries than is spent on new research or on the studies necessary to determine the actual value of discoveries already made.

Sir Henry Dale,† director of the National Institute for Medical Research in London, accepts the medical tradition as embodying the true ideal, since the ultimate aim of medical research is to provide knowledge for the relief, cure or prevention of human suffering. In a recent address he contrasted the work done by physicians in practice and medical investigators in universities with the type of research carried on in the laboratories founded by industry. Sir Henry Dale expressed his conviction that a general use of patents in all parts of the field of therapeutic research would definitely hinder rather than promote progress. He felt that the greatest danger was in connection with a discovery of the biologic type. Particularly was he inclined to regard the medical patent as a peculiarly dangerous weapon when wielded by the good intentions of the academic amateur. The danger in patents in the chemical field did not seem to him so ominous, because only industrial research and vast organizations can make these preparations generally available at low prices. Nevertheless, only clinical trial in the hands of physicians under controlled conditions can ever determine with certainty the real value of any therapeutic product. Hence the development of such products must be a cooperative effort. This fact should not be forgotten by those who administer patents in the medical field.

Our new order of living in the machine age, the development of specialization in medical practice, the incorporation of great industries for the exploitation of laboratory discoveries, and similar factors seem to make necessary some change in the medical

---

* Gregg, Allen: Science 77: 257 (March 10) 1933.

† Dale, H. H.: Academic and Industrial Research in the Field of Therapeutics, address at the opening ceremony of the Research Laboratory of Merck & Company, Rahway, N. J., April 25, 1933.

point of view concerning medical patents. The control of such patents by universities has to some extent assured standardization of products. Usually only reputable firms capable of developing and exploiting products honestly are granted licenses to participate in the manufacture and sale of products controlled by universities, although there are glaring exceptions. However, as has already been mentioned, there is extreme unevenness in the manner of administration of various patents by the groups involved. Conceivably the best interests would be served if some central body might be developed, wholly altrusitic in character, capable of administrating medical patents for the benefit of the public, and assuring a reasonable remuneration to the investigator, the devotion of much of the profit to research, and adequate returns to manufacturers willing to develop quantity production and distribution in an ethical manner. Such a central body might also set up requirements for adequate clinical research in connection with the development of new products, so that premature launching of unestablished products on the medical profession or on the public might be avoided.

In the opinion of the Council on Pharmacy and Chemistry of the American Medical Association, such premature exploitation is exactly what has occurred in relationship to the use of preparations of copper and iron. Leaving aside the question of priority in the discovery and the difficulties involved in preventing physicians from prescribing mixtures of copper and iron should they wish to do so; diregarding the fact that copper occurs as a natural contaminant in practically all iron preparations, and that too in amounts apparently sufficient to bring about the desired therapeutic results, there still remains for debate the question as to whether or not the discovery is of practical value in the field of therapeutics.

The questions here raised must inevitably concern the scientific bodies of the American Medical Association as well as the Judicial Council, the House of Delegates and the Board of Trustees. Perhaps some suitable means will be evolved whereby the American Medical Association may lend its authority and influence to the establishment of a technic for the control of medical patents in the best interest of the public welfare and for the advancement of scientific medicine.

THE MILWAUKEE SESSION

At the Milwaukee session, the president, Dr. Edward H. Cary, reported that during his term of office he had traveled 99,190 miles on official business and that he had been kept away from his home 340 days—almost an entire year—in keeping eighty engagements in which he was the official representative of the Association. Dr. Cary told of activities maintaining freedom for the physician and his right to prescribe what would be best for the patient. He opposed control of the practice of medicine by a bureaucracy in Washington. He recognized the international character of the narcotic problem. He detailed what had been accomplished in relationship to legislation regarding veterans and the effect of the activities of the President in securing dismissal from veterans hospitals of 15,000 domicilary cases. The economic status of the country had demanded economies in government.

Dr. Cary discussed the report of the Committee on the Costs of Medical Care, pointing out that the minority report had been supported by the Board of Trustees of the Association. He then discussed the relationship of the private physician to health departments and reviewed all of the activities of the headquarters office of the Association.

During the year, Dr. Frank Billings died, also a trustee, Dr. A. R. Mitchell, and the vice speaker of the House, Dr. Albert E. Bulson.

The president elect, Dr. Dean Lewis, also discussed the problems of hospitalization of veterans. He called attention to the fact that more than thirty schemes had been proposed to provide for the periodic prepayment purchase of hospital care. Many of these were proposed by propagandists and promoters who were looking for a profit. He noted that the promoters of various schemes were urging the inevitable failure of voluntary plans and demanding that compulsory sickness insurance be instituted immediately. The medical profession during the two years of depression, he believed, had shown more ability to take care of its own business than any other profession. Of the depression, he said:

"In some ways the depression has rendered a great service, as it has been demonstrated that many of the mechanical aids to practice are not necessary and that the cost of medical service may be greatly reduced and the quality maintained. Sir James Mackenzie stated the case well when he said 'It would be ridiculous to put a man with a cut finger through such a process (a thorough examination) and expect him to pay for it, as it would be to expect an automobile owner to have the entire machine overhauled each time he has a puncture.' Simplification of medical practice should be the aim of this organization. Such simplification will mean a limitation of specialism and the reduction of specialists."

From the state of Pennsylvania came a resolution requesting our national medical organizations to declare their opinions of proposed changes in medical practice through approved channels. This was an effort to secure some unity in expressions of opinion of the medical profession before the Congress. Unfortunately little pressure groups began to form, such as the Committee of Physicians. Statements were also issued by some of the specialistic societies in relationship to the reports of the Committee on the Costs of Medical Care.

The Committee on Legislative Activities, through its chairman Dr. Charles B. Wright, was devoted almost wholly to legislation affecting veterans. The Committee on Mental Health rendered an extensive report concerning psychiatric services and the administration of institutions for mental health.

Now came resolutions urging that the Directory of the American Medical Association indicate specialists who had been certified by the certifying boards.

The abuses of radio broadcasting were condemned.

A resolution was introduced by Dr. G. Henry Mundt of Illinois, which was to have terrific repercussions when the Association would be sued at a later date under the Sherman Act. The Mundt resolution, which was adopted, read:

> "Resolved, That it is the opinion of the House of Delegates of the American Medical Association that physicians on the staffs of hospitals approved for intern training by the Council on Medical Education and Hospitals should be limited to members in good standing of their local county medical societies and that the House of Delegates request the Council on Medical Education and Hospitals to take this under advisement."

From Dr. Henry C. Macatee, delegate from the District of Columbia, came a resolution endorsing the minority report of the Committee on the Costs of Medical Care as expressing in principle the collective opinion of the medical profession. This was also adopted by the House of Delegates.

A resolution for the creation of a committee for the study of birth control was approved by the reference committee on hygiene and public health but the report of the reference committee was laid on the table.

From Indiana came a resolution urging that the curriculums of medical schools include time devoted to training of students in basic business procedures necessary to the conduct of medical practice.

Several resolutions supported the view that there should be unity of opinion in the expression of the medical profession on general social legislative and economic relationships of medical practice. These were adopted.

Again the Board of Trustees reported to the House of Delegates its feeling that a permanent office in Washington was not necessary and the House of Delegates supported this opinion. A special reference committee on medical economics recommended continued discussion of group hospitalization and group medical practice. It urged further teaching of medical economics in medical schools. A complete report on the distribution of hospitals for the mentally disturbed and of physicians associated with such institutions was made available. This was the first complete summary of such studies made by any organization in this country.

In the executive session, the first measure was the adoption of a resolution to the effect that the American Medical Association condemns the persecution of any individual on account of race or religion by any state or under any flag.

In the elections, Dr. Walter L. Bierring was made president elect.

Following the annual session, the Congress of the United States created the agency that was known as the N. R. A. with a blue eagle as its symbol. This was the National Recovery Act. Practically every organization in the country had been asked to draw up a form to conduct its business under the Act. However since the American

Bar Association did not feel that it came under this Act, the Board of Trustees reported that physicians also would be free from its stipulations and that it would be impossible to formulate a code for the activities of the medical profession under this Act.

In an endeavor to secure the cooperation of the Council on Pharmacy and Chemistry in the investigation of new drugs, the editor proposed a plan to be conducted under the auspices of the council whereby commercial companies could submit their products to the council for aid in securing study of these products in hospitals. The Council on Pharmacy and Chemistry was asked by the Board of Trustees to present a plan for further consideration. Eventually following World War II the Council on Pharmacy and Chemistry created its Therapeutic Trials Committee for coordinated and intensified research in the development of new drugs.

At this time the Board of Trustees, after careful consideration of the extent to which cigarettes were used by physicians in practice, voted to accept the advertising of cigarettes.

The editor of THE JOURNAL presented to the Board of Trustees a proposal for the compilation of a history of the American Medical Association.

Toward the end of the year the Board of Trustees began to be interested in the new Food, Drugs and Cosmetics bill. This legislation would, for the first time, control adulteration and misbranding of foods, drugs and cosmetics and with the Wheeler-Lea bill prevent false advertisements of foods, drugs and cosmetics. The passing of this legislation was a tremendous step forward in commercial control of these foods.

Now again came a proposal that there be held an exhibit for the public in connection with the annual session of the American Medical Association. Time did not permit the preparation of such an exhibit for the next annual session but the project was considered a suitable one.

1934
CLEVELAND

The unrest in the medical profession continued to mount apace with 1934. The Bureau of Medical Economics prepared a special report on health insurance, but the nation was still greatly disturbed trying to recover from its economic debacle. Some were urging special sessions of the House of Delegates to consider the problems of the day. The Board of Trustees reaffirmed its faith in the following conclusion:

"It is the sense of the Board that the American Medical Association is now, as it has always been, against the panel system or against state medicine, but feels that in this time of stringency it should not do anything that might interfere with the federal administration in its attempt to work out a recovery program."

The Milbank Fund, under the leadership of John Kingsbury, and the Rosenwald Foundation, under the leadership of Michael Davis, had published misstatements relative to the attitude of the American Medical Association and had made false accusations against its officials. By direction of the board, these were answered in THE JOURNAL.

The Association arranged, with the aid of Dr. Austin A. Hayden, to prepare a motion picture film of the activities of the headquarters office.

The Bureau of Medical Economics prepared an extensive statement on health insurance abroad.

A VISIT FROM THE BRITISH

The British Medical Association was to hold its meeting in Australia in 1935 and arrangements were made to meet the delegation in New York City and to entertain the British visitors suitably in Chicago during their trip. The general manager was instructed to determine the desires of the one hundred or more British physicians who would be in this party.

One of the results of the Century of Progress Exposition in Chicago had been an epidemic of amebiasis resulting from contamination of the water in the Auditorium and Congress Hotels. When the editor of The Journal had received word of this, he had requested immediate submission of a manuscript from the Health Department of Chicago covering the situation. This had been promptly published in THE JOURNAL, notwithstanding threats from attorneys for the corporations against the Association. This was the first water-borne epidemic of amebiasis ever to be recorded.

Arrangements had been made to hold a joint session of the American Medical Association and the Canadian Medical Association in Atlantic City in June of 1935.

The Michigan State Medical Society had sent Drs. Nathan Sinai and Henry Luce to Great Britain to study sickness insurance and they had brought back a report which was, in a way, condemnatory of the attitude of the American Medical Association.

Dr. Harry Benjamin of New York had brought suit against the editor of THE JOURNAL on account of the unfavorable review of Dr. Benjamin's book.

The director of the Bureau of Medical Economics was invited to Cuba to study the Cuban method of sickness insurance.

To the Board of Trustees came requests for liaison and cooperation with many national medical organizations dealing with the health, safety, and welfare of the American people. The Federal Emergency Relief agency had been established with provisions for the care of the sick, and the medical societies of the country were seeking leadership from the American Medical Association in the development of a suitable program.

THE CLEVELAND SESSION

At the Cleveland session in 1934 the president, Dr. Dean Lewis, reported on his visits to many medical societies. He said:

> "We should be concerned today with the quality of medical care. Cheap medicine is often the most expensive, and what is called expensive is often the cheapest, for through the quality are attained the objects of medical practice—decrease in mortality, lessening of morbidity and shortening of the period of disability."

He expressed his belief that the quality of medicine is largely determined during the four years of the medical course but must be maintained by wise planning afterward. He urged that more physicians attend medical meetings.

Dr. Walter L. Bierring, president elect, called attention to the many proposals that were coming forward with a view to changing the nature of medical practice. He said:

> "Well meaning nonmedical advisers have brought you a variety of artificial remedial plans that are supposed to solve every phase of the problem. We well know that no single 'rule of thumb' proposal or method will provide the remedy. The rendering of efficient and complete medical service is still largely governed by the individualistic relation of physician to patient. Furthermore, the practice of medicine is a profession and not a business or a trade."

The Bureau of Medical Economics had made reports on many phases of medical practice and the Bureau of Legal Medicine and Legislation gave many pages of its annual report to the many bills that had been introduced into the Congress affecting the medical profession.

The Board of Trustees recognizing the tremendous extent to which members of the headquarters staff had spoken to medical and lay groups throughout the nation, did not consider it advisable at the time to employ a field secretary.

The Judicial Council was concerned with the extent to which the establishment of the Emergency Relief Administration had invaded the practice of medicine. In its report the Judicial Council said:

> "During the past year, some of the basic beliefs and principles of the medical profession have been attacked and invaded more seriously and extensively than at any time before. An organized and financed campaign for a socialized system of furnishing medical care to a large proportion of the population has apparently crystallized its plans and begun its propaganda with the millions of certain foundations backing the effort. Prac-

tice of medicine by government in all the history of medicine in this country never has invaded the field of the private practitioner with his individual families as has the United States government through the Emergency Relief Administration. This is a complete and undisguised example of 'state medicine.' The avidity with which in general the government's offer was received can be explained only on the basis of an acute economic situation in the profession itself. The occurrence must be considered as a temporary expedient only, due to the unparalleled stress of the times, and must be discontinued as rapidly as the stress on the profession is relieved. A number of societies refused to enter into agreements whereby their members would be bound to provide services and accept compensation directly at the hands of the government. In some instances, official committees of state medical associations and county medical societies have strongly recommended to their members that they continue to provide medical service to all in need and refuse to accept compensation from the government for such services. One of the strongest holds of the profession on public approbation and support has been the age-old professional ideal of medical service to all, whether able to pay or not. That ideal is basic in our ethics. The abandonment of that ideal and the adoption of a principle of service only when paid for would be the greatest step toward socialized medicine and shortly state medicine which the medical profession could take. All our arguments as to better service to the people, freedom of choice of doctor, individual service, and maintenance of high grade medical service by highly qualified doctors would be as naught if such service were not available to a vast proportion of the people."

Before the House of Delegates came new resolutions on the exploitation of roentgenologists in hospitals, definitely related to the introduction of hospital insurance plans. Again there were bills for some type of control of the broadcasting of proprietary remedies over the radio. There were new pleas for a new Army Medical Library. The anesthetists were disturbed at the increasing practice of the administration of anesthetics by others than physicians and dentists. The Mundt resolution, which would bar approval of hospitals for intern training when they have on their staffs other than members of the American Medical Association, was again affirmed into the House of Delegates. The Michigan State Medical Society introduced a digest of its report on sickness insurance based on the visit of its representatives to Great Britain, requested consideration of this report by the House of Delegates. The consideration was referred to the executive session.

From the Judicial Council came amendments to the Principles of Ethics dealing with contract practice and the disposal by a physician of his professional attendance and services to any lay body, organization, group or individual by whatever name called or however organized under terms or conditions which permit a direct profit from the fees, salary or compensation received to accrue to the lay body or individual employing him.

Again came the resolution on contraception.

From Illinois came a resolution condemning the apparent attempt of the Board of Regents of the American College of Surgeons to dominate and control medical practice.

When the executive session convened, the Board of Trustees presented a statement which was a review of the attitude of the American Medical Association toward compulsory sickness insurance as evidenced by actions of the House of Delegates, the Board of Trustees requesting the House of Delegates to express an opinion on the subject. The amendments to the By-Laws proposed by the Judicial Council were adopted. The Judicial Council, having considered the complaint against the American College of Surgeons, requested the Board of Trustees of the American Medical Association and the Judicial Council to ask the Board of Regents of the American College of Surgeons to explain the reasons for their action and to justify the the attempt by this group to legislate for all of the medical profession of the country. There were requests by the House of Delegates that the Board of Trustees appoint a committee to contact the leaders of organized labor with a view to learning their attitudes on sickness insurance.

Other resolutions requested the Judicial Council to make investigations of the ethical practices of institutions. Committees were to be appointed to investigate the control of patents on medical devices. From the District of Columbia came a complaint against the establishment of clinics in government offices and hospitals for government employees. A certifying board for gastroenterology and proctology was sought. The state of New Jersey was supporting the Ambruster attitude on the sale of ergot. Then came a resolution from the Section on Obstetrics and Gynecology and Abdominal Surgery asking the councils of the Association to investigate the virtues and dangers of materials used in contraception. The state of Maine had approved the practice of birth control and wanted studies made of the materials involved.

In the executive session a special committee, headed by Dr. Nathan B. Van Etten of New York, made a complete review of the report from Michigan on sickness insurance. The Bureau of Medical Economics had prepared a report on sickness insurance problems in the United States which contained ten points as bases for the conduct of any social experiment in changing the nature of medical practice. This first ten point program follows:

"First: All features of medical service in any method of medical practice should be under the control of the medical profession. No other body or individual is legally or educationally equipped to exercise such control.

"Second: No third party must be permitted to come between the patient and his physician in any medical relation. All responsibility for the character of medical service must be borne by the profession.

"Third: Patients must have absolute freedom to choose a legally qualified doctor of medicine who will serve them from among all those qualified to practice and who are willing to give service.

"Fourth: The method of giving the service must retain a permanent, confidential relation between the patient and a 'family physician.' This relation must be the fundamental and dominating feature of any system.

"Fifth: All medical phases of all institutions involved in the medical service should be under professional control, it being understood that hospital service and medical service should be considered separately. These institutions are but expansions of the equipment of the physician. He is the only one whom the laws of all nations recognize as competent to use them in the delivery of service. The medical profession alone can determine the adequacy and character of such institutions. Their value depends on their operation according to medical standards.

"Sixth: However the cost of medical service may be distributed, the immediate cost should be borne by the patient if able to pay at the time the service is rendered.

"Seventh: Medical service must have no connection with any cash benefits.

"Eighth: Any form of medical service should include within its scope all legally qualified doctors of medicine of the locality covered by its operation who wish to give service under the conditions established.

"Ninth: Systems for the relief of low income classes should be limited strictly to those below the 'comfort level' standard of incomes.

"Tenth: There should be no restrictions on treatment or prescribing not formulated and enforced by the organized medical profession."

Observance of these ten principles would remove many of the disturbing influences from experiments in administering medical care. Commenting on these principles, the committee said:

"Such restrictions will undoubtedly lower the enthusiasm of many of the present advocates of such schemes. They remove the interest of the politician, the commercial promoter and all those who consciously or unconsciously are seeking to achieve other objectives than better medical care for those unable to provide such care for themselves under present conditions. All these principles are directed toward protecting the character of the service to be given and all are directly designed to guard against abuses which experience shows are bound to arise when these principles are neglected. In most communities it will be found that comparatively few changes in the methods of administering medical care will be necessary. That type of medical practice which preserves the personal relationships between physician and patient, that maintains the practice of medicine as a profession, and that has withstood the test of centuries must be preserved for the best interests of both the public and the medical profession."

Dr. James S. McLester of Birmingham was made president elect.

At the Cleveland session, Dr. Arthur J. Cramp suffered an attack of coronary thrombosis which made necessary his retirement from his position as director of the Bureau of Investigation.

The Council on Physical Therapy was beginning to have more and more calls on its services in relationship to the standardization of equipment, the use of radium and other physical devices.

SICKNESS INSURANCE

The actions taken on sickness insurance by the House of Delegates had had some repercussions in Washington where considerations were under way on the Social Security Act. The President of the United States had appointed a committee to consider the problems of unemployment insurance and old age. An editorial had been published in THE JOURNAL for the week of August 21 commenting on an address made by Miss Frances Perkins over the radio during the preceding week. In that address she had intimated that a group of outstanding physicians and surgeons, who would be available for consultation from time to time, were to be appointed to study the need for sickness insurance. In his letter to Miss Frances Perkins, Dr. Fishbein had said that it would seem highly desirable that the medical profession be adequately represented in any studies of the need for sickness insurance that are made in connection with the President's Committee on Economic Security. He said, further, that there is abroad a vast amount of misinformation as to the methods of medical practice in the country, the statistics concerning medical care in various sections of the country, and similar problems, and that it would seem to be highly desirable also that methods of medical practice be considered in relationship to any plans that might be formulated. In reply Dr. Fishbein received a letter from Miss Perkins in which she said:

"Please be assured that the advice of the medical profession will be obtained on all matters affecting it. Moreover, it is our intention to obtain that advice through the appointment of a group of outstanding physicians and surgeons who will be available for consultation from time to time as the study develops. In this connection, you will be interested to know that Mr. Sydenstricker emphasized the desirability of an arrangement of this sort."

The Board of Trustees wrote to Miss Frances Perkins offering to make available to her the advice of the Association and all of the information available in the headquarters office.

In the meantime, a modest turmoil was developing over the pronouncements by the American College of Surgeons which were at variance with some of the principles expressed by the House of Delegates. Arrangements were being made for a conference between the Board of Trustees of the American Medical Association and the Board of Regents.

At this time also the editor of THE JOURNAL announced that the American Medical Association had been granted time for broadcasting by the National Broadcasting Chain and also by the Columbia Broadcasting Chain. Furthermore, the advice of the Association had been sought by the National Association of Broadcasters relative to more use of radio for educational purposes.

The American Dental Association expressed a desire for closer cooperation with the American Medical Association and liaison committees were appointed for this purpose.

This year had seen the sudden growth of what are called "free medical journals" with controlled circulation. Among these were

"Modern Medicine," "Medical Economics" and "Current Medical Digest." The Board of Trustees and the Council on Pharmacy and Chemistry deprecated lending of their names by distinguished physicians to such periodicals in view of the fact that their advertising was largely of materials which could not possibly be accepted by the Council on Pharmacy and Chemistry.

Conferences were being held with representatives of the American Legion and the Committee on Legislative Activities. Mr. Watson B. Miller, chairman for the Legion, had come to Chicago and was most cooperative.

On June 29, 1934, President Franklin Delano Roosevelt issued an executive order for the establishment of a Committee on Economic Security. The committee included Frances Perkins, Secretary of Labor; Henry Morgenthau Jr., Secretary of the Treasury; Homer S. Cummings, Attorney General; Henry A. Wallace, Secretary of Agriculture, and Harry L. Hopkins, Federal Relief Administrator. Professor Edwin E. Witte of Wisconsin was appointed administrative director. The committee was instructed to report back to the President not later than December 1, 1934. It will be remembered that Miss Perkins made an address on the radio and that the publication of an editorial in THE JOURNAL caused her to request the American Medical Association to submit some names for a medical advisory board. In her book on "The Roosevelt I Knew," Miss Perkins writes:

> "Our Committee had not made a competent, clear report on health and was not prepared to recommend any form of health insurance. Therefore no such measure was included. The bill did include, however, a program for appropriations and grants-in-aid to the states for public health services. The President, in talking with people who came to discuss health insurance with him, spoke in terms of utilizing public money to build hospitals all over the country and to staff them with competent physicians and nurses. He had been impressed with the need for hospital service in many parts of the country and saw this as a substitute for health insurance. I doubt that he was aware at the time of the program, which has become general in the Latin-American countries, of building hospitals, traveling clinics and centralized medical services in lieu of benefit payments under social security."

In John Fulton's "Harvey Cushing: A Biography" he points out that Miss Perkins formed a Medical Advisory Committee to the Committee on Economic Security in October and that this committee was asked to study practicable measures for bringing about better distribution of medical care in the lower income groups of the population and more satisfactory compensation of physicians and others who render medical services to individuals in these groups. Rumor has it, but the evidence cannot be documented, that the President himself was given a long list of physicians and himself selected the men who constituted this committee. On the committee the president of the American Medical Association at the time, Dr. Walter L. Bierring, spoke for the point of view of the medical profession. Fortunately for the American physician, Dr. Harvey Cushing, much against his desire, consented to serve as chairman. In replying to Miss Perkins, he said on October 8:

"I am glad the Committee has thought of establishing such an advisory group, particularly since most of the agitation regarding the high cost of medical care has been voiced by public health officials and members of foundations most of whom do not have a medical degree, much less any actual first-hand experience with what the practice of medicine and the relation of doctor to patient means."

It must be remembered also that previously to the appointment of this Medical Advisory Committee there had been a committee consisting largely of economists and welfare workers who had been inclined to recommend the inclusion of medical care in the social security program.

Dr. Cushing recognized that change in the nature of medical practice was inevitable, but in such change he wished to preserve the fundamental factors which physicians know are essential to a high quality of medical care. Thus on December 14 Harvey Cushing wrote to Dr. Morris Fishbein:

"You have it in your hands more than anyone else to make things run smoothly and to get the profession adjusted to the possibility of some sort of sickness legislation. I am sure that if we bury the hatchet about the C. C. M. C. report and take a fresh start we may be able to get somewhere and preserve the things which most of us regard as precious in our age-long profession. Reassurances from you on this matter from time to time will do more good than anything else."

In the course of the discussions in the committee Dr. Cushing saw fit to write directly to President Roosevelt on November 10, 1934, urging the establishment of a department of medicine in the cabinet. He said:

"May I venture to hand on to you a suggestion for what it may be worth? You are probably aware that there is a sharp difference of opinion between the American Medical Association representing the medical practitioners and the representatives of the Millbank Fund who are agitating and financing a movement for national sickness insurance. This being so, before Mr. Witte's Medical Advisory Committee gets deep in this tangled subject, would it not be a good move just at this time to take into consideration the establishment—if not of a governmental department—at least of a super-bureau of public health to coordinate a number of welfare agencies?

"Such a department would naturally include such scattered interests as infant welfare and the Children's Bureau, old age insurance, possibly the matter of the veterans' hospitals and health compensation, vital statistics, the administration of the Food and Drugs Act, and the existent public health and marine hospital service."

In response to this letter President Roosevelt wrote on November 13:

"I am glad that again your mind runs along with mine. I am giving much thought to the general consolidation of health and allied welfare organizations. Perhaps some day it will be a department, but I doubt if the time is wholly ripe. The difficulty is that, in the meantime, shuffling bureaus between existing departments raises much ruction."

The Medical Advisory Committee, of which Dr. Cushing was chairman, continued to consider the subject through the middle of January, and its final report was sent to the President on January 15. Now a storm of protest developed in the American Medical Association.

COMPULSORY INSURANCE AND AN INDICTMENT—1935-1939

EARLY IN JANUARY the Executive Committee of the Board of Trustees considered compulsory sickness insurance. The group included Dr. Rock Sleyster, Austin A. Hayden, Charles B. Wright, and J. H. J. Upham. Sitting with them were Dr. Herman L. Kretschmer, treasurer; Dr. Olin West, secretary; and Dr. Morris Fishbein, editor. They considered the desirability of calling a special session of the House of Delegates of the American Medical Association to discuss the proposals that were to come from President Roosevelt's Medical Advisory Board. When the full board met in February, they were told that the mail vote taken in January was unanimously in favor of calling a special session of the House of Delegates. The House would meet Friday, February 15, to consider compulsory sickness insurance. The Board of Trustees had prepared six specific questions to be put before the House of Delegates for their consideration.

SPECIAL SESSION OF THE HOUSE OF DELEGATES

That meeting of the House of Delegates in special session, was epoch making in the history of the American Medical Association. Dr. J. H. J. Upham, chairman of the Board of Trustees, read an official statement prepared by the board dealing with the history of compulsory sickness insurance. He reported the considerations of the House of Delegates in 1916, 1917 and 1919 and again in 1922. The board recognized the changes that had occurred in the practice of medicine. They called attention to the report of the Committee on the Costs of Medical Care, to the establishment of the Committee on Economic Security and to the subsequent appointment of the Medical Advisory Board. Dr. R. G. Leland and Mr. A. M. Simons of the Bureau of Medical Economics of the American Medical Association had aided the technical advisory staff of the Medical Advisory Board. That technical staff had included also Messrs. Isidore Falk, Michael M. Davis and Nathan Sinai. The President of the United States on January 17, 1935, had sent a message to Congress relative to security. He said, "I am not at this time recommending the adoption of so-called 'health insurance,' although groups representing the medical profession are cooperating with the federal government in the further study of the subject and definite progress is being made." The Committee on Economic Security had recommended to the President a nationwide preventive medicine and public health program and application of the principles of insurance. Senator Wagner of New York had submitted his first bill, known as the Wagner bill for social insurance.

The Board of Trustees' statement concluded with the following six specific questions for determination by the House of Delegates:

1. Shall or shall not the House of Delegates again declare its opposition to all forms of state medicine, including any form of medical treatment provided, conducted, controlled or subsidized by the federal or by any state government, excepting such service as is provided by the Army, Navy or Public Health Service and such as is necessitated by the control of communicable disease or for the treatment of mental disease or of the indigent sick, and excepting also all such other service as may be approved, administered or conducted by local county medical societies and not disapproved by the state medical societies of which they are component parts?
2. What is the attitude of the House of Delegates toward the eleven principles proposed by the Committee on Economic Security as fundamental to any system of sickness insurance to be established by the federal government?
3. Shall or shall not the House of Delegates of the American Medical Association reaffirm its opposition to the principle of federal subsidies to individual states in relationship to the provision of medical service?
4. Will the House of Delegates express its opposition relative to that provision of the Wagner bill which places the control of medical affairs in the Department of Labor under a nonmedical special board?
5. What attitude shall the House of Delegates take relative to the proposed sickness insurance legislation in the individual states as represented by the Epstein bill of the American Association for Social Security?
6. How may the American Medical Association initiate plans for still further improving the quality of medical service and for obtaining better distribution of medical service for all the people?

Many resolutions came from the individual states opposing government sickness insurance and defining the position of the American Medical Association on this subject. Among those proposing such resolutions were Drs. R. B. Anderson of Texas, H. C. Macatee of the District of Columbia, and Charles H. Goodrich of New York, while from New Jersey came a complete program for meeting the need for medical care.

A special reference committee had been appointed by the speaker of the House to report on the questions raised by the Board of Trustees and by the resolutions which had been introduced on the floor of the House. The report of the reference committee reaffirmed the opposition of the American Medical Association to all forms of compulsory sickness insurance. They condemned the Wagner bill and the Epstein bill and asserted that "there is no model plan which is a cure-all for the social ills any more than there is a panacea for the physical ills that affect mankind." They recommended that physicians be guided by the ten fundamental principles that had been adopted by the House of Delegates at the annual session in June 1934.

In April Dr. Olin West, secretary of the Association, reported to the Board of Trustees that the California Medical Association had adopted a resolution approving the principle of compulsory sickness insurance and declaring that the time had come to apply that principle in California. The bill had been drafted, and the secretary of the California Medical Association had sent a copy of it to the director of the Bureau of Legal Medicine and Legislation for analysis.

In the meantime the American Medical Association was cooperating with many agencies. A national conference had been called by the Federal Communications Commission. The Dental Educational Council of America wanted cooperation. The American Library Association was helped with the preparation of a list of books on health and hygiene.

Plans were being made for the entertainment of the British physicians who were going to tour the United States en route to Australia.

The meeting in Atlantic City was to be a joint meeting with the Canadian Medical Association, which was considering many problems similar to those that were confronting the American Medical Association.

By this time the sickness insurance bill that was prepared for California had been side-tracked, and the California legislature had appointed a committee to study the subject and to report in two years.

The Association was greatly concerned by the number of immigrant physicians who were coming to the United States and was preparing a study of the subject for submission to the House of Delegates.

Senator Copeland had introduced a new food, drugs, devices and cosmetic act, which passed the United States Senate on May 13.

Propaganda from the National Medical Committee on Federal and State Contraceptive Legislation was being circulated widely, and the Council on Pharmacy and Chemistry had given study to the possibility of some type of control over such materials and devices.

AMERICAN COLLEGE OF SURGEONS

Discussions were being conducted with the American College of Surgeons over the pronouncements they had made for the medical profession of the country. During the year the director general of the American College of Surgeons, Dr. Franklin H. Martin, had died. Dr. George Crile wrote that it was "the desire of the College to cooperate in every way with any movement that has for its object the welfare of the medical profession and service to the sick." The American College of Surgeons on June 10, 1934, had proposed a prepayment plan for medical care restricted to hospitals approved by the American College of Surgeons, to members of the staffs of such hospitals and to the physicians acceptable to such staffs.

"PAINLESS PARKER"

During the year an advertising dentist named "Painless Parker" had threatened suit against the editor of THE JOURNAL, but through intermediation of a dentist in California he had decided to withdraw his suit.

THE ATLANTIC CITY 1935 SESSION

At this session of the House of Delegates Dr. Frederick C. Warnshuis was unable to be present because of the death of his son. The vice speaker read his address, referring particularly to the presence in Atlantic City of the Canadian Medical Association.

The president, Dr. Walter L. Bierring, had spoken throughout the United States, traveling some 67,000 miles to meet his engagements. He reviewed the progress of medical science and the rise of the campaign in behalf of federal sickness insurance. He said, "Thoughtful men and women are becoming convinced that private practice will continue to promise the best service for all concerned and insure its high quality." And he continued, "In certain social and economic security measures introduced in Congress, all reference to health or sickness insurance was eliminated, and bills proposing plans for compulsory health insurance presented in one or two state legislatures were unsuccessful and did not even come up for passage."

The president-elect of the Association, Dr. James S. McLester, congratulated the organization on the efficiency of its work. He reviewed the activities of the Association but counseled particularly that the headquarters of the national organization should not be conceived as distinct from or far removed from the state organizations. In his address he discussed nutrition, indicating that proper human nutrition was becoming more and more vital to the health of the nation.

The Bureau of Medical Economics had taken on great activity. It reviewed sickness insurance and called attention to its handbook on the subject. It had considered group hospitalization and indicated that there were a wide variety of schemes in process of development. At that time the bureau had a record of 55 group hospitalization plans operating or discontinued and 44 plans proposed but not yet operating. The bureau reviewed its contact with the President's Committee on Economic Security. It discussed the medical care plans that were being developed in various county societies and reported on its study of the care of the indigent sick.

The Bureau of Legal Medicine and Legislation covered a wide variety of federal laws proposed which had required consideration. These included the Wagner-Doughton-Lewis bill for federal health insurance; the Federal Emergency Relief Administration; the food, drug and cosmetic legislation; narcotic legislation; veterans legislation; vivisection and income tax.

FOREIGN PHYSICIANS

A special report was made on the licensing of foreign practitioners. Inquiry at the Bureau of Immigration had shown that the average number of foreign physicians admitted each year from 1929 through 1934 had been about 300, making a total of 1916. The number coming from Germany had increased from 22 in 1929 to 160 in 1934. Seven hundred and fifty-five of these physicians had announced their destination as New York.

NEW PROBLEMS IN THE HOUSE OF DELEGATES

When resolutions were called before the House of Delegates, they covered a variety of subjects. Of major interest, however, were those dealing with radio broadcasting of medical misinformation, the study of contraception, the care of the indigent and experiments in rendering medical service.

SOLICITATION OF VOTES

The Judicial Council had been asked to pass on the standing rule of the House of Delegates, which provided that "the solicitation of votes for office is not in keeping with the dignity of the medical profession nor in harmony with the spirit of this Association and that such solicitation shall be considered a disqualification for election to any office in the gift of the Association." The Judicial Council brought in a rather long but exceedingly wise report. The council concluded:

"The Council is further of the opinion that in practice the rule is unenforceable. It has, however, been a strong and, at times, an effective moral influence. It has been among our laws for thirty-three years and has never been called on to function, although it is well known, at least to the older members of the House, that violations have not been rare. Disqualification under this rule might be punishment for an offense committed not by the candidate but by overenthusiastic friends and even against his wishes and order. It is common law that no one can be punished for an act of which he had no knowledge or to which he was not a party. It is further common law that no one should be punished without an opportunity to defend himself in a fair trial. The element of time would make this procedure impossible in practice.

"For the reasons detailed, the Judicial Council considers the Standing Rule on 'Solicitation of Votes' to be illegal and of no force and effect. This being so, there can be no violation. There being no violation, the supposed person mentioned in the resolution is legally eligible for nomination or election. The Judicial Council believes that, if the House desires to have our laws disqualify for nomination on a basis of reprehensible solicitation, adequate legislation and phraseology can be found."

This report was unanimously adopted by the House of Delegates.

BIRTH CONTROL

The subject of contraception was discussed in executive session, and as a result of the deliberations a special committee was recommended to be appointed by the Board of Trustees to study the problems and to make a preliminary report in the 1936 session.

SICKNESS INSURANCE

The reference committee which considered all of the resolutions related to the care of the sick and to problems of sickness insurance recommended that every physician give greater study to these problems and that the Bureau of Medical Economics circulate its considerations much more widely.

From California came a special report concerning health insurance delivered by Dr. T. Henshaw Kelly. He called attention to the fact that there is a group of medical men in California "who honestly believe . . . that in compulsory health insurance we have the only way to meet the insurance problem successfully; that if medicine endeavors to solve the costs of medical care on any kind of a budgetary or insurance basis it can be done only by compulsion. . . ." He described in detail the difficulties in securing passage of a suitable bill through the California legislature and indicated his belief that "California probably has the most acute problem."

The American Medical Association's Committee on Legislative Activities presented an extensive report also concerned with problems of medical care, and the Bureau of Medical Economics provided a complete analysis of existing plans in the United States and the difficulties of developing a plan suitable to all areas.

So complicated and intricate were the problems before this session of the House of Delegates that it met repeatedly in executive session, endeavoring to work out standards and principles by which medical care could be made widely available to all.

During this session the differences between the leaders of the American Medical Association and the American College of Surgeons were fully discussed in a special meeting. The report came from the conference that the leaders of the American College of Surgeons had agreed with the action of the House of Delegates of the American Medical Association taken in its special session in Chicago in February 1935.

When the call came for the election of a president-elect, Drs. Charles E. Humiston of Chicago, Dr. J. Tate Mason of Seattle, Dr. J. Norman Henry of Philadelphia, and Dr. Harvey Cushing of New Haven, Conn., were nominated and Dr. J. Tate Mason was elected.

BROADCASTING

During this year there had been negotiations initiated by Dr. Morris Fishbein, representing the Association, and carried on by Dr. W. W. Bauer, with representatives of the National Broadcasting Company. As a result, the National Broadcasting Company agreed to provide a half hour once each week to the American Medical Association for a program on health. This program has been conducted continuously since that time.

THE AMERICAN COLLEGE OF SURGEONS OPPOSES COMPULSORY INSURANCE

Following the meeting of the American Medical Association, Dr. George Crile, chairman of the Board of Regents of the American College of Surgeons, wrote a letter to the President of the United States to the effect that the American College of Surgeons did not favor compulsory sickness insurance. The letter concluded,

"We make this statement to the end that the attitude of the College toward health legislation which has been proposed may be correctly defined and thereby freed from misinterpretation."

STANDARD NOMENCLATURE OF DISEASE

For some time there had been negotiations by the headquarters office of the Association with the National Conference on Nomenclature of Disease, leading to the assumption of this important work by the American Medical Association. The Board of Trustees approved this activity. As a result, the Association at that time undertook the preparation of a new edition of the *Standard Nomenclature of Disease*, which has since been amended by the addition of a *Nomenclature of Operations*. This continues to be one of the most important publications of the Association in standardizing the keeping of case records and the proper use of scientific terms.

THE BRITISH TOURISTS

The British physicians who had come to the United States had enjoyed a pleasant tour across the country. They were met in New York and taken in buses to see the sights of the city and to visit the Grasslands Hospital. In Chicago they were shown the stockyards (at their own special request), but they tired promptly of the stockyards. After being entertained at luncheon by Mr. Swift they were shown through the city in automobiles, given tea at the Edgewater Beach Hotel and a dinner at the Tavern Club. Separate entertainment had been provided later for Lord Horder. It was arranged to invite him as a guest to the Kansas City session in 1936

WORK OF THE BOARD OF TRUSTEES

As a result of action taken in the executive session in Atlantic City, the Board of Trustees constituted a special committee to study contraceptive practices as a joint committee under the Council on Pharmacy and Chemistry and the Council on Physical Therapy. This committee has made great progress since that time.

The Board of Trustees in September received a communication from Dr. Frederick Warnshuis expressing his belief that some form of socilization of medicine was coming and that the subject should be discussed at the session of the state secretaries.

There were requests for cooperation in surveys of chronic diseases by the United States Public Health Service.

Much discussion as to improvement in the buildings of the American Medical Association, caused the board to vote to remodel the building, including refacing and new windows. The completion of this procedure is apparent in the monumental structure which is now the headquarters office of the American Medical Association.

From the Georgia Warm Springs Foundation came a request for cooperation by the American Medical Association. The Board of Trustees constituted an advisory committee to investigate and act in this capacity.

From the Children's Bureau came requests for liaison, and Dr. W. W. Bauer has served since that time as liaison to the Children's Bureau.

California was having some trouble with the practice of radiology in relation to the United States Employees' Compensation Commission and was requesting the American Medical Association to advise with legal counsel on this subject.

The Council on Medical Education and Hospitals had endeavored to inspect osteopathic schools; it was found impossible to secure such inspection through any existing agency.

INCOME AND SOCIAL SECURITY TAXES

The attorneys reported that the American Medical Association was exempt from federal income taxes as a corporation organized and operated exclusively for scientific purposes. It was their opinion that the Association was not liable for taxes either under the Federal Income Tax Law or under the Social Security Act. Subsequently it was determined by an action taken by the state of Illinois that the Association would be liable under the Social Security Act.

1936

As 1936 came upon the scene, into the melee over compulsory sickness insurance came the American Foundation Studies in Government under Miss Esther E. Lape, an intimate friend of Mrs. Franklin D. Roosevelt. Miss Lape had requested the president of the Association, Dr. James S. McLester, and some other officers of the Association to become members of an advisory committee.

There again were some requests for a special session of the House of Delegates, but it was not considered expedient, since the time was close for the annual session in Kansas City.

From New Jersey was coming agitation against some of the decisions of the Council on Pharmacy and Chemistry.

From California came the beginnings of activity against the editor of THE JOURNAL, apparently related in the light of later years to the fact that Dr. F. C. Warnshuis, who was now secretary of the California Association, had been defeated for the speaker's position in the House of Delegates at the Atlantic City session. However, dissatisfaction was expressed by Californians with the syndication of health articles in the California press. The Board of Trustees had been aware of the syndicated articles and considered them useful for education of the public about health. The Board was convinced that the editor had not been at all related to the defeat of Dr. Warnshuis at the Atlantic City session.

With the coming of the Kansas City session an extensive program of addresses on both the Columbia and National broadcasting networks had been developed. The Association was moving more and more into the field of education of the public regarding the work of the medical profession.

As the time approached for the Kansas City session, Dr. J. Tate Mason became seriously ill; it was reported that he might not live to be inaugurated as president. When the Association met in Kansas City, Dr. J. Tate Mason was unable to attend. It became necessary for a substitute to read his presidential address.

This year saw the retirement of Dr. Arthur J. Cramp as director of the Bureau of Investigation and of Mr. E. C. Shelly as cashier. Both had been with the Association more than 30 years.

Among the distinguished foreign guests at Kansas City were Lord Horder and Dr. Leon Asher of Bern, Switzerland.

The name of the Committee on Foods was changed to Council on Foods, since it had by its work achieved full Council status.

THOMAS PARRAN BECOMES SURGEON GENERAL

Dr. Thomas Parran had become surgeon general of the United States Public Health Service. In view of the cooperation required in the survey of chronic illnesses, Dr. Parran was invited to attend a meeting of the Board of Trustees to discuss cooperative efforts. Dr. Parran discussed the health survey being made by the United States Public Health Service. He stated that he had frequently been misquoted in the press on such subjects as medical relief and care of the indigent. He expressed the hope that the physicians of the country would give him their sympathetic interest and work with him in complete agreement as to anything which the federal government might undertake in the broad field of medical care.

Now came difficulties over the Shadid Clinic in Oklahoma City and the Ross-Loos Clinic in California, all of which involved special studies by the Bureau of Medical Economics.

KANSAS CITY MEETING

At the meeting of the House of Delegates in Kansas City in May, the new speaker, Dr. Nathan B. Van Etten, urged the House of Delegates to participate fully in the discussions and in the activities. The president, Dr. James S. McLester, noted the unsettled conditions in the field of medical care and the unsolved problems that lay before many of the councils and bureaus of the Association. From the president-elect, Dr. J. Tate Mason, came a message urging physicians to become more familiar with the activities of the American Medical Association and with the work of its headquarters office. He urged opposition to compulsory sickness insurance:

"The history of other countries clearly shows that voluntary prepayment and insurance schemes, in the hands of the profession at the outset, drift inevitably, as do all plans initiated by private groups, into bureaucratically administered compulsory insurance under government control. . . .

"The medical profession may rest assured that its future depends on the defeat of the present trend toward general socialization and the maintenance in America of at least a moderate individualism. The socialization of medicine is only one phase of the movement toward general socialization and the ultimate abandonment of the American individualistic system. . . ."

At the meeting in Kansas City the candidate for president of the

United States on the Republican ticket, Mr. Alfred Landon, spoke to the American Medical Association and stated his opposition to federally controlled medicine.

The Judicial Council was more elaborate than usual in its reports. It found the need of working jointly with the Council on Medical Education and Hospitals in relation to studies of osteopathy and osteopathic hospitals. The question of medical patents had again reared its ugly head. The trials for unethical conduct against practitioners associated with commercialized clinics and corporations practicing medicine were giving the Judicial Council much concern. They felt that the hospitals were invading the practice of medicine and that there was a tendency "to make the doctor of medicine the servant of the hospital," which "should be stopped." They were especially concerned regarding association of physicians with cultists. On this subject they said, "Such degrading consultation would cheat the patient out of that which he might expect and the subsequent failure of results bring discredit on the science of medicine." And they concluded, "A physical and professional separation as complete as is possible should be established and maintained."

HOSPITALS PRACTICING MEDICINE

Under the heading of new business came the first attacks on the hospitals for undertaking the practice of radiology from several states. There were calls for studies of asphyxia and air conditioning and a number of resolutions on contraception.

Lord Horder spoke before several of the scientific sessions, before women's clubs and with the editor of THE JOURNAL in a joint radio appearance, in which they discussed heart disease.

When the House was in executive session, it gave special consideration to the proposed elimination of legitimacy and illegitimacy from reports of birth. The reports from the Committee on Contraceptive Practices were accepted.

THE DISTINGUISHED SERVICE MEDAL

At this session Dr. Harrison H. Shoulders submitted a resolution providing for the award each year of a Distingushed Service Medal to a Fellow of the American Medical Association who had made noteworthy contributions to the science and art of medicine. The proposal was adopted. Each year since that time a distingished scientist has been honored. The list and the biographies appear elsewhere.

The executive session concerned itself further with the legal activities related to the Harrison Narcotic Act.

The Judicial Council was asked to make a ruling on the question of the installation of Dr. J. Tate Mason. It ruled that the president, Dr. James S. McLester, should formally and officially declare President-Elect J. Tate Mason duly installed in absentia as President and designated a committee to convey to him and the members of his family the action taken.

At this session the chairman of the Reference Committee on Legislation and Public Relations was Dr. R. L. Sensenich. That committee had been concerned with the rendering of medical care in rural districts. It analyzed contract practice and other plans that were being developed to provide medical care to people of low income.

A committee was appointed to study the problem of motor vehicle accidents.

Dr. J. H. J. Upham, who had been for many years chairman of the Board of Trustees, was selected president-elect, and Dr. Charles Gordon Heyd, vice president. This election was especially important, as Dr. J. Tate Mason died June 20 and Dr. Charles Gordon Heyd succeeded to the presidency.

A significant scientific step at this time was the establishment of a central clearing house for the accumulation and recording of information on industrial skin diseases.

LAW SUITS

THE JOURNAL was making a series of exposés of charlatans and was continually being threatened with law suits, most of which, however, failed to reach even the stage of a hearing in court. Among those threatening suit at this time were one Dr. Emanuel M. Josephson, who threatened to sue because THE JOURNAL refused to publish a communication regarding what he alleged was a cure for cataract and another for glaucoma. A charlatan named William F. Koch, of Detroit, who had developed a "cure" for cancer called glyoxylide, was demanding a retraction, which the board did not give.

Pressure groups were being formed to force the adoption of federalized medicine, and everywhere the subject was being increasingly discussed.

Difficulties developed over defining the relative authority of the Committee on Legislative Activities and the Bureau of Legal Medicine and Legislation.

Requests came for closer cooperation with the National Education Association, the National Congress of Parents and Teachers, the National Health Council, the World's Fair in process in New

York City, the American Standards Association and many other groups.

For some time the Association had been publishing a legislative and economic bulletin; apparently it was not being widely read by the members of the Association who received it. Hence there now came an action to return all discussions of medical economics and organizational problems to the columns of THE JOURNAL OF THE AMERICAN MEDICAL ASSOCIATION.

Many complaints came to the Association relative to the extent to which the United States Public Health Service was undertaking the treatment of syphilis.

The Board of Trustees moved toward the establishment of a new council on industrial medicine.

The suit which had been filed by Dr. Emanuel M. Josephson was withdrawn; also the suit of the Civic Medical Center, a group practice association in Chicago, was withdrawn.

CAMPAIGNS OF THE JOURNAL

Year after year the Association had been encouraging the campaign against typhoid fever, and later against both typhoid fever and diphtheria, by publishing in THE JOURNAL the relative ratings of the large cities of the United States in control of these diseases. These campaigns indicated the importance of continuous publicity with accurate facts in relation to harmful practices of many kinds. By such publication THE JOURNAL waged its war against low grade medical schools and fraudulent proprietary medicines. By this technic it conducted the campaign against Fourth of July injuries, against unnecessary deaths from typhoid fever and diphtheria. The campaigns against typhoid fever and diphtheria were first conducted under the leadership of Professor E. O. Jordan of the University of Chicago and more recently by Dr. Henry F. Vaughan of Ann Arbor, Mich.

1937

As 1937 dawned, the Association found itself in the midst of many controversies, most important of which was the question of compulsory sickness insurance legislation. Wisconsin had been selected as one of the battlefields on which this campaign was to be fought; from that state came an appeal for aid from the headquarters office.

The American Medical Association joined with the United States Public Health Service in the preparation of a motion picture film on syphilis and aided in many ways the campaign against that disease.

Again the movement to reorganize governmental activities and to consolidate them into a single agency was being rejuvenated. Miss Esther Lape was about to publish her American Foundation Studies and was anxious to work out some sort of liaison between the American Medical Association and the federal government.

The suit filed by the plastic surgeon Jean Paul Fernel against the editor had been dismissed, and other suits were being threatened for other exposés in THE JOURNAL.

The Department of Commerce had decided to make studies of physicians' incomes.

The Metropolitan Life Insurance Company was undertaking a special attack on pneumonia and developing motion pictures to enlighten the medical profession on the typing of the pneumococcus and the specific serums available against it. Eventually the coming of the sulfonamide drugs and penicillin would make typing obsolete.

Many new activities were under way, including formation of a council on industrial medicine, the studies being made by the committee on contraceptives, and increased activity in the American Society for the Control of Cancer.

THE ATLANTIC CITY 1937 SESSION

When the Association met in Atlantic City in June, it was requested to hear a message from Senator J. Hamilton Lewis of Illinois, who had requested an invitation to the session for the delivery of what he said would be an important message.

The speaker of the House of Delegates, Dr. Nathan B. Van Etten, devoted himself wholly to the work of the house. The president, Dr. Charles Gordon Heyd, analyzed the state of society in relation to medical care. He felt that the chief problem before the medical profession was medical care for the indigent and some type of aid in catastrophic illness.

The president-elect, Dr. J. H. J. Upham, had traveled widely and had become inpressed with "the feeling of unrest in medical circles, manifested in the frequent discussions of the socialization of medical practice, the resentment against the charges of the prevailing inadequacy of medical practice, and medical responsibility for alleged excessive costs of medical care." One step in the solution, he suggested, would be improvement in the quality of medical education and better education of the public regarding the accomplishments of medical science.

At this session a special committee reported on a technic for establishing the Distinguished Service Awards. There were reports on contraceptive practice, motor vehicle accidents and medicolegal blood grouping tests. Then came a series of resolutions, practically all concerned with a national health program, the socialization of medicine, the development of a council on medical ethics and economics, many resolutions dealing with motion picture films, and some proposed changes in the Principles of Medical Ethics dealing with contract practice. From Michigan came a proposal to set up in the headquarters office a department of public relations. New Jersey was annoyed with HYGEIA because it feared that it was giving more health information than it ought to; the reference committee did not agree.

There were extended discussions on the cultists, the use of barbituric acid derivatives, the control of syphilis and prospective legislation. The American Farm Bureau Federation had initiated some conferences on rural medical service.

More consideration was given to the proper relationships of the medical profession in the use of contraceptives. Attempts had been made to discharge the committee. The end result was the establishment of a definite control through the Council on Pharmacy and Chemistry and the Council on Physical Therapy.

SENATOR J. HAMILTON LEWIS BRINGS A THREAT

On the morning of June 10 Senator J. Hamilton Lewis addressed the House of Delegates. He said that he had helped to write, prepare and, as whip and parliamentarian of the Senate, pass the Social Security law. His address, while a little confused, recognized the resentment of the medical profession against federal domination of medical practice. He pointed out, however, that there had been during the previous 45 years a gradual accumulation of government controls of one kind or another in the field of health. He predicted that there would be shortly a system of examination by the federal government of every doctor of America to prove his right to be admitted to practice under federal law. He urged physicians to take into their hands a system by which medical care and hospitalization could be provided for all. In one portion of his address he said:

"I am pleased to tell you that as I left I called the President and told him I was on my way to have a conversation with you gentlemen. I would like to deliver from the President of the United States a message coming direct with his authority. He said that I was authorized to say to you he knew something of your meeting, he had been for some time observing the courses of the doctor, that he was not far removed from constantly keeping up with the features of the profession, and he wished you success as to your undertaking. If I use his exact words, he hoped that you would find a way to cooperate with him in such method as you would jointly find would be to the service of the helpless and the afflicted within such province as you felt government should undertake."

Following the address by Senator J. Hamilton Lewis, the Board of Trustees sent a message to the President of the United States respectfully proffering every cooperation in developing suitable methods for medical care of the indigent, afflicted and sick.

On Thursday the House of Delegates heard an address by the eminent British orthopedic surgeon, Dr. R. Watson Jones. Dr. Irvin Abell was made president-elect of the American Medical Association; a committee was appointed to develop the Distinguished Service Award.

Dr. George Baehr of New York appeared before the Board of Trustees in behalf of having the American Medical Association finally take over the *Standard Nomenclature of Disease*.

THE HOME OWNERS' LOAN COOPERATIVE

At the September session of the Board of Trustees the director of the Bureau of Legal Medicine and Legislation, Dr. William C. Woodward, reported that employees of the Home Owners' Loan Corporation, which had about 2,000 employees in Washington, had organized a cooperative medical service association in Washington called the Group Health Association, Inc., financed in part at least by the Home Owners' Loan Corporation. He suggested that if this corporation should be successful, other similar ones would be formed. This was simply taken under advisement.

The Board of Trustees appointed a committee on resuscitation. An invitation had come from the British Medical Association for delegates from the American Medical Association. The Board of Trustees requested that Dr. Fishbein head the delegation to represent the American Medical Association and that at the same time he visit Sweden, Norway and Denmark to investigate medical practice and medical education in those places.

Attempts were being made to cause the Association to send a questionnaire to every physician in the United States in order to determine his point of view regarding the socialization of medicine.

THE FEDERAL HEALTH PROGRAM

In the meantime Dr. Samuel J. Kopetzky of New York had made some contacts with Miss Esther Lape of the American Foundation Studies in Government, and arrangements had been made for a luncheon of certain physicians at the White House with Mrs. Roosevelt. Drs. Gordon Heyd and Morris Fishbein had sent regrets since acceptance of the invitation seemed to involve undesirable commitments. From that luncheon had come some proposals that the American Medical Association authorize the formation of a committee to formulate a national health policy for submission to the government and to work out some agreement on a health insurance program.

All sorts of offers of mediation were coming from senators and welfare workers and agencies attempting to work out some technic whereby the cooperation of the American Medical Association would be secured in developing a federal health plan.

The Association joined with the American College of Surgeons in a study of the sterility of catgut.

The resolution introduced by Dr. L. J. Hirschman on behalf of the Michigan State Medical Society for establishment of a department of public relations in the headquarters office was endorsed by the reference committee and referred to the Board of Trustees. At this time, however, action was not taken on that resolution. A similar resolution had been introduced by Dr. Fred Moore of Iowa.

Arrangements had been made for an exhibit by the American Medical Association at the World's Fair in New York.

In Kansas osteopaths had been granted the right to prescribe narcotics, and the medical profession was up in arms. In California the antivivisectionists were again on the rampage, and the American Medical Association was helping in the defense of research.

CONTROL OF NOSTRUMS

The food, drug and cosmetic bill had passed, and the Wheeler-Lea Federal Trade Commission bill was about to pass. These two pieces of legislation were together to constitute one of the greatest advances in the control of nostrums and quackery ever developed in the federal government.

Now came a request from Dr. William C. Woodward of the Bureau of Legal Medicine and Legislation that he be permitted to retire on account of advancing age. And in this year Dr. George H. Simmons, who had done so much to build the weak, undernourished American Medical Association into a powerful agency, died in St. Luke's Hospital in Chicago following a surgical operation.

The American Medical Association was also developing an exhibit for the Exposition in California.

From the Board of Trustees to the editor came specific instructions as to his discussion of the report of the American Foundation Studies in Government. There were conferences on public health and radio broadcasting. The Board of Trustees also provided for a conference on health education for the public in the headquarters office. To this came many representative writers.

Now came a suit for $150,000 filed against the Association by Robert Wadlow, the boy giant. This case was to come to trial, as will be described in a later chapter.

AMERICAN FOUNDATION REPORT

THE JOURNAL OF THE AMERICAN MEDICAL ASSOCIATION on October 16, 1937, published an editorial on the American Foundation proposals for medical care. The nature of the editorial had been discussed by the board, and publication approved by the board. Now from John P. Peters, who had, as a member of the Committee of Physicians, established an evangelistic group in behalf of compulsory sickness insurance, came a protest against the editorial.

The Bureau of Health and Public Instruction was now renamed the Bureau of Public Health.

The Group Health Association had created much controversy in Washington, D. C. The American Medical Association was being besought for aid from the District of Columbia Medical Society in meeting the threat of that organization. The board had published a complete description of the Group Health Association, and plans were made to inform the state secretaries and editors concerning its work.

From Dr. Eugene S. Kilgore in San Francisco messages were being sent approving sickness insurance legislation and trying to inoculate the students in the medical schools with this virus.

The Committee of Physicians, about 430 in number, had come out with some "Principles and Proposals," and Harry Hopkins had made a speech in which he said, "I hail the action of the 430 independent physicians who are anxious to turn over to the government the responsiblity for the care of sickness." Letters had poured into the headquaters of the American Medical Association in opposition to these "Principles and Proposals." The Board of Trustees specifically requested the editor to prepare an editorial in reply to these "Principles and Proposals" and to release it to the press for November 21.

The state of Indiana had sent the chairman of its Committee on Study of Health Insurance to Europe, and he had returned absolutely convinced that the practice of medicine under compulsory sickness insurance was a menace to the quality of medical service.

The House of Delegates had adopted a resolution condemning the promiscuous use of barbituric acid and derivative drugs, and the forces of the Association were used to initiate an attack against such harmful activities.

DEATHS FROM ELIXIR SULFANILAMIDE

As the year came toward its end, the nation was horrified by almost 100 deaths resulting from the taking of an elixir of sulfanilamide made with diethylene glycol instead of propylene glycol or ethanol. That terrible disaster had such a profound effect on the Congress that it resulted in almost immediate action in passing the new pure food and drug legislation and the Wheeler-Lea bill.

SOCIAL PROBLEMS

The conference on health education for the public had attracted 35 writers, including five national writers of syndicated columns, five Pulitzer Prize winners, and representatives of practically every important newspaper syndicate. Some made it apparent that they were out of sympathy with the American Medical Association's attitude toward socialized medicine, whereas others appeared greatly to favor it.

The American Public Health Association was calling a conference on health care for the indigent.

A Health Freedom League had been formed in Colorado, which was an encouragement to cultists and charlatans.

And the end of the year saw the battle against socialized medicine approaching a climax!

With 1938 the American Medical Association found itself in a rather anomalous position. It had fought with its back to the wall to stem the tide in behalf of socialized medicine. That movement really swelled in earnest with the report of the Committee on the Costs of Medical Care and the passing of the Social Security Act. The Board of Trustees knew, however, that a completely negative attitude could never succeed and that it was necessary to assume a positive program in order to gain public confidence. Therefore, early in 1938 at the direction of the Board of Trustees, an editorial was prepared calling on the medical profession to initiate, develop and put into practice a comprehensive system of medical care for all the people according to the American plan of medical practice. This was published in THE JOURNAL early in January. Immediately it received favorable comment from medical societies throughout the nation. In addition, a favorable comment appeared in the official organ of the American Federation of Labor. In conferences held with the board, the editor, Dr. Fishbein, felt that it was necessary for the American Medical Association to have tangible evidence to show that it was actually working on the problem. About this time the Committee of Physicians (sometimes known as the Committee of 400) requested a conference with the Board of Trustees of the Association in order to discuss their point of view. As a part of the propaganda in behalf of socialized medicine one social group was trying to organize the students of the United States into an American Medical Students Association. The suggestion was made that THE JOURNAL OF THE AMERICAN MEDICAL ASSOCIATION include a special section for medical students so that they could be kept informed of the issues in the controversy over medical care. Furthermore, there seemed to be wide misunderstanding as to the significance of the hospitalization insurance program and what it might do to medical practice. Following conferences with representatives of the American Public Health Association and the U. S. Public Health Service, the Bureau of Medical Economics of the American Medical Association agreed to undertake a survey of the needs for better medical care for all the people. The proper approach to the subject would be first to determine the needs and then to plan particularly to meet those needs.

When the Board of Trustees convened in February, a committee representing the Committee of Physicians, including Drs. John P. Peters, New Haven; Luther E. Holt Jr., Baltimore; Hugh Cabot, Rochester, Minn.; Hugh J. Morgan, Nashville; Borden S. Veeder, St. Louis; Robert S. Osgood, Boston, and Thomas B. Cooley, Detroit, came before the board. They asserted that they were not in any way related to the American Foundation Studies in Government, and they requested space in THE JOURNAL for their principles and proposals and attitudes.

Dr. Harrison Shoulders, at that time vice speaker of the House of Delegates, appeared before the board with a plan for the care of the indigent. The Wisconsin State Medical Society had determined to send its secretary, Mr. George Crownhart, to Europe to study sickness insurance abroad. There was agitation in the circles devoted to medical education because Dr. Willard Rappleye of New York had suggested the creation of a National Council on Medical Education, Licensure and Hospitals, made of representatives of the universities, medical schools, hospitals, the practicing profession, specialty boards, the state licensing boards and public health agencies. He felt that the government would soon be giving financial support to medical services, teaching and research and that the profession should have in advance an agency which could guide the spending of the money. Up to 1947 this movement had not proceeded further.

For some years the Board of Trustees had been studying the proposal to establish retirement insurance and hospitalization insurance for the employees, and a special committee of the board had been working on that problem.

From Ohio during the annual convention had come a resolution requesting the House of Delegates to clarify the policy of the American Medical Association on group hospitalization and especially on defining and enumerating the services which should not be included, because they were definitely medical services. This resolution pointed to one of the most serious problems in group hospitalization, namely, the proper place of the roentgenologist and the clinical pathologist in such services. The tendency was for the hospitals to employ these specialists as salaried, full-time employees and to derive a profit from their work.

The feeling was increasing that there should be a publicity department in the headquarters office and resolutions had been offered to that effect in the House of Delegates.

The Bureau of Internal Revenue at this time reclassified the American Medical Association as a business league and insisted that the Association pay social security taxes. Several of the state medical societies had been similarly classified.

The attacks being made in THE JOURNAL on charlatans of one kind or another had now accumulated $3,500,000 in libel suits which the Association was defending.

There was again a demand for a midwinter session of the House of Delegates.

RED CROSS COOPERATION

From the Red Cross came a request for a cooperative arrangement with the American Medical Association relative to the payment of physicians in disaster work; it was agreed that the Association present the proposal to the House of Delegates. Through its secretary, Dr. Kingsley Roberts, the Cooperative League of the United States with its Bureau of Cooperative Medicine was requesting conferences with representatives of the American Medical Association. The difficulties in cooperation seemed to lie in the fact that some of the members of this group had departed from the ethics and standards of the Association in their exploitation.

The Committee on Air Conditioning was making its studies. The Board of Trustees viewed a film called "Medicine," prepared by the March of Time, and gave their approval. A variety of ventures in medical publications were called to the attention of the board. The Association was aiding the physicians of California in combatting the antivivisectionists who were promoting an initiative on the so-called California Humane Pound.

A CONFERENCE ON RURAL MEDICINE

What was perhaps the first conference on rural medicine was being scheduled for Cooperstown, New York, in October; the Board of

Trustees was requested to delegate a representative. Later the Association was to initiate its own series of conferences on rural health and to give this movement great impetus.

CONTRACEPTIVES AND OTHER PROBLEMS

As a part of its study of contraceptives, the legislation relating to that subject was analyzed for the board. There were presentations to the board on private plans for sickness insurance. The National Association of Master Plumbers wished cooperation from the Association in prevention of epidemics from inefficient plumbing.

The Association chose as its delegates to the United States Pharmacopoeial Convention Drs. Paul Nicholas Leech and Morris Fishbein. The American Library Association wished a representative from the Association on indexing.

Miss Josephine Roche, then chairman of the Interdepartmental Committee to Co-Ordinate Health and Welfare Activities of the Federal Government, sent an invitation to a national conference on medical care. Miss Roche was invited to come to San Francisco to appear before the House of Delegates but was unable to attend and requested that Dr. Warren Draper be permitted to read her address for her.

The Committee on Legislative Activities was making contacts with many groups, in particular, however, with the American Farm Bureau and its associated women's organization.

1938 THE SAN FRANCISCO SESSION

When the Association convened in San Francisco, the Committee on the Distinguished Service Award reported that it had considered twenty-two names and had submitted five to the Board of Trustees. From these the Board of Trustees selected three, Dr. Simon Flexner, New York, Dr. Ludvig Hektoen, Chicago, and Dr. Rudolph Matas, New Orleans. The House of Delegates selected Dr. Rudolph Matas as recipient of its first Distinguished Service Medal. Dr. Matas, a native of Louisiana, received his degree in medicine from Tulane University in 1880. He had been professor of surgery at Tulane. He was a member of a great many surgical societies throughout the world and the author of innumerable monographs on surgery, particularly of the blood vessels.

The speaker of the House of Delegates, Dr. Nathan B. Van Etten, urged the House of Delegates to mix more sociology with their medicine. He asked the House of Delegates to remember its responsibilities.

The president, Dr. J. H. J. Upham, had continued to visit many organizations throughout the nation and reported a great awakening of the membership to the obligations of medicine and medical practice. "Social questions were intimately intermingled with medical questions," he said. He urged particularly a battle against syphilis and the problem of the care of those with chronic diseases. The questions of medical care for the indigent and the semi-indigent he thought were of chief concern.

The president elect, Dr. Irvin Abell, spoke of the enthusiasm with which the medical profession had greeted the resolution adopted by the Board of Trustees for developing a medical care program. The medical profession was contributing a million dollars a day in medical service to the indigent sick. He realized the great differences in the problem of the care of the sick in different areas. Dr. Abell found it difficult to understand the attitude of the socialistically minded statesmen who would supply medical care at government expense with the lowering of the efficiency and integrity of the medical profession. He felt that improvement in economic conditions for the poor was a more fundamental problem than the problem of medical care. Then he devoted himself to the need for increasing graduate medical education.

The secretary called attention to the request of the Red Cross for advice in the care of people during catastrophes and disasters.

When the call for new business came, resolutions were offered regarding the sale of sulfonamides over the counter. The state of Wisconsin wanted the Council on Foods to change its standards for butter. From Connecticut came a proposal for the establishment of a council on medical care to consider particularly questions of medical service. Iowa supported Wisconsin in the desire for more information about different standards for butter. A motion picture called "The Birth of a Baby" had been produced and great excitement occasioned in various sections of the country over the fact that it seemed to need some censorship. There was a demand from Georgia that the picture be shown only to adult audiences. The State of California wanted again to revise the Principles of Medical Ethics and they wished support for the campaign in behalf of animal experimentation. There were several resolutions dealing with hospitalization insurance. California also asked the establishment of a department of public relations in the Bureau of Health Education.

ETHICS

The Judicial Council, acting as a reference committee on medical ethics, spoke wisely on the general subject of the ethics of medicine. They said:

"The ethics of medicine is stated as it should be in principles of conduct instead of rules. To define and interpret these principles so as to cover every relation of the medical man would be to set up an endless system of rules, regulations and laws approaching in character a criminal code, with its invitation to violation by sophisticated reasoning or through technicality. A rule, regulation or law may be circumvented, but the principle underlying the law cannot be avoided by such means. As occasion arises, amendments will doubtless be made in the future as they have in the past, but these are strenuous times of rapid and radical change and no one can predict the immediate or remote future. The Judicial Council, as your reference committee, recommends that 'amplification, clarification, codification and revision of the Principles of Medical Ethics' be postponed."

By this time the former Bulletin of the Association had been incorporated into The Journal as a supplement and had improved the interest in topics related to organization and medical economics.

The Council on Foods was asked to give consideration to suitable standards for butter as well as for oleomargarine and to scrutinize carefully advertising in this field.

There came additional resolutions on chiropody and alcoholic intoxication from Indiana, and a long description of a proposal in Indiana which was offered as a health education program which would be an antidote to state medicine.

THE EDITOR RECEIVES A VOTE OF CONFIDENCE

From New Jersey came a resolution requesting the editor to confine his writings exclusively to the official publications of the American Medical Association. This was brought into the executive session where the subject was discussed at length by many delegates and by the editor of The Journal. When the House of Delegates, which had been sitting as a committee of the whole, arose from the executive session, the report read:

"The committee of the whole recommends that the House of Delegates express its full confidence and respect for the editor of The Journal of the American Medical Association and bid him Godspeed in going forward in the splendid work he is doing."

This was carried by a rising vote which is recorded in the minutes as unanimous.

FURTHER BUSINESS OF 1938 SESSION

From Miss Josephine Roche, chairman of the Interdepartmental Committee to Co-Ordinate Health and Welfare Activities of the Federal Government, came a message which was largely a rephrasing of the report given to her by her technical committee on medical care. It forecast the National Health Conference which had been called in Washington. Miss Roche stated that her program would include more comprehensive public health services and expansion of maternal and child health services. It would discuss the shortage or unequal geographic distribution of medical facilities and medical personnel. It would consider means of providing more adequate medical care to recipients of public assistance, and finally, it would discuss methods of financing the sickness costs of self-supporting persons of limited means.

Then came a report from the Advisory Committee on Supply of Medical Care, presented by its chairman, Dr. William F. Braasch of Rochester, Minn. He described the survey which was in progress to determine the need for medical care and urged the medical profession to support the survey completely.

The question of showing the film "The Birth of a Baby" in various communities was discussed and the House of Delegates properly said that the question was one for each community to determine for itself through consultation with the county medical society.

A reference committee headed by Dr. J. D. Brook of Michigan considered the statement of Miss Josephine Roche. The committee concluded that "No one formula or program can possibly be found adequate to meet the varied needs of medical care." The committee also expressed its satisfaction that representatives of the American Medical Association would be asked to participate in the National Health Conference.

As the session ended, Dr. Rock Sleyster, Wauwatosa, Wis., was made president elect. Dr. Sleyster had served the American Medical Association in many capacities, beginning with the position of county secretary in 1903, becoming a vice speaker of the House of Delegates and a trustee, and finally chairman of the Board of Trustees.

Dr. Ray Lyman Wilbur, chairman of the Council on Medical Education and Hospitals, on the last day of the session indicated the difficulties that were beginning to arise in medical education because of multiple organizations which had come into the field. Among these were the specialty boards, the advisory board on the medical specialties, the American Hospital Association, and the American College of Surgeons.

In his presidential address at this session Dr. Irvin Abell stated succinctly some of the major objectives of the medical profession in the field of medical care. He concluded his address with a brief statement of the aims of the medical profession as they related to the public. He said:

"The aims of the medical profession as they relate to the public may be briefly summarized:

"1. Maintenance of the present high standard of medical education, affording assurance that the graduate is competent to care for the sick.

"2. Adequate provision for graduate education, with specified training for the development of specialists, and continued training for those who are not specialists so that the level of professional efficiency may be raised.

"3. Extension of public health and preventive medicine to cover the field adequately.

"4. Continuation of the practice of ethical scientific medicine on its present high plane.

"5. Protection of the public against medical frauds, falsely labeled foods, drugs and applicances.

"6. The widest possible dissemination of health information to enable the public to act intelligently in the preservation of its health and in the prevention of disease.

"7. The development and consummation of plans for extension of medical service to all groups of the population consonant with our established high standard of quality.'

Mrs. Mabel D. Ahart, then president of the Associated Women of the American Farm Bureau, met with the Board of Trustees on the closing day of the session and stated the objectives of farm women in medical care. This group did not wish a socialized medical program but did feel the need of some organized planning for the provision of medical care.

The representatives of the Connecticut State Medical Association also appeared before the Board of Trustees in behalf of the establishment of a council on medical care. The Board of Trustees pointed out that it had set up an advisory board to the Bureau of Medical Economics which might serve the purpose. Later this movement, begun in Connecticut, was to eventuate in the establishment of the Council on Medical Service of the American Medical Association.

The retirement of Dr. Woodward led to the appointment of Mr. J. W. Holloway as administrator of the Bureau of Legal Medicine and Legislation with the understanding, however, that he would not represent the Association before congressional hearings but that this activity would be carried on by representatives appointed by the trustees in relation to special legislation.

When the Board of Trustees met late in July the representatives who had participated in the National Health Conference—Drs. Olin West, Morris Fishbein and Arthur Booth (chairman of the board)— reported on the meeting and its significance. The editor of THE JOURNAL was authorized to make a full report of the National Health Conference and to give to the medical profession in an editorial the true picture of what took place.

The Association had been investigating vitamins and prepared a special book on the subject.

From Wisconsin came a plea for a national health program developed by the American Medical Association.

Shortly after the National Health Conference, medical societies throughout the nation began indicating their approval of the point of view taken by the American Medical Association in opposition to compulsory insurance. Because of the necessity for definite policies on these controversial questions, a special session of the House of Delegates was called to meet in September.

The Board of Trustees requested its secretary, Dr. Austin A. Hayden, and the editor to secure a suitable press representative who would issue to the public press the attitude of the Association on social and economic matters.

The Board of Trustees considered the five recommendations made by the National Health Conference as reported by Miss Josephine Roche in San Francisco and a plan of the organization of the House of Delegates to hear these five questions was elaborated. From the National Medical Association, representing the Negro physicians of the United States, came a request to participate with the American Medical Association in its considerations. The National Medical Association proposed to stand for the same principles in medical care as did the American Medical Association.

THE INDICTMENT

In the meantime, the Department of Justice had prepared to indict the American Medical Association for its activities in meeting the challenge of government medicine. The newspapers and the radio reported that the Department of Justice of the United States proposed to seek an indictment of the American Medical Association as a monoply unless the Association, through its central organization or its constituent society in the District of Columbia, consented to certain stipulations in regard to medical practice that would be satisfactory to the Department of Justice. The Board of Trustees adopted the principle that the records of the secretary of the Association, of the Board of Trustees, of all of its councils and its various bureaus should be made available to representatives of the Department of Justice on request.

WAR LOOMS AGAIN

In the meantime, the nation had begun to anticipate war. The Selective Service Boards of Missouri, Iowa, Kansas and Nebraska were reorganizing as a part of the program of preparedness.

SPECIAL SESSION OF HOUSE OF DELEGATES

The House of Delegates convened in Chicago, September 16, in special session. The representatives of the National Medical Association—Drs. Roscoe C. Giles, Clarence H. Payne and Carl G. Roberts—were invited to be present and were given opportunity to address the House of Delegates.

In his address to the House Dr. Harrison H. Shoulders, the speaker, told of the platform of American medicine and emphasized to the House of Delegates that they were the policy-making body for the Association.

Dr. Irvin Abell, president, analyzed the problems before the profession and urged continued experimentation with new forms of medical practice, at the same time, however, defending the fundamental principles that the Association had repeatedly declared must guide any form of medical care.

The president elect, Dr. Rock Sleyster, told the special session of the meetings of the National Health Conference and of various attempts that had been made to keep the people informed of the attitude of the American medical profession.

The statement of the Board of Trustees, which was presented by Dr. Arthur W. Booth, its chairman, dealt with the five proposals that had come from the National Health Conference. It suggested that each of them be considered by a special reference committee of the House of Delegates. The House then took under advisement the proposals which had been made by Miss Roche, which were presented to the House in toto.

From several delegates came alternative plans for the distribution of medical care which had been developed in various state medical societies. West Virginia proposed a publicity program against the regimentation of physicians. From Maryland came a recommendation for cooperation in needed improvements in the care of the indigent and from Kansas came a long resolution defining the extent to which the medical profession should participate in a national health program. Dr. Carl F. Vohs of Missouri presented a plan which was in process of development in Missouri, and other recommendations came from Pennsylvania and New Jersey.

The Bureau of Medical Economics indicated the present status of plans for medical care in various portions of the United States.

The medical profession of Minnesota favored extension of medical care but was definitely opposed to any form of tax-supported health insurance. The state of Wisconsin urged the Association to lend its funds and its efforts to experimentation with new methods of providing medical care.

By noon of the second day, each of the reference committees had provided a comprehensive report on some one of the five phases of Miss Roche's health program. In its editorial comment, subsequent to this special meeting of the House of Delegates, THE JOURNAL OF THE AMERICAN MEDICAL ASSOCIATION summarized these considerations:

Briefly, the House of Delegates recommended expansion of public health services, as related to the control of certain infectious diseases, maternal and infant welfare, and similar projects, with the definite understanding that the need be established and that they be efficiently handled and economically controlled. The House of Delegates approve the principle of hospital insurance, again with the understanding that it cover only the facilities of the hospital and that professional standards be maintained. It approved the principle of *cash indemnity insurance* for meeting sickness costs, provided these efforts meet the requirements of state laws and that they have the approval of the county and state medical societies under which they operate. The House of Delegates again recognized the need for complete medical services to the indigent, at the same time emphasizing the desirability of local control. The House recognized that the necessity for state aid might arise in poorer communities and that the federal government might need to provide funds when the state is unable to meet these emergencies. The needs of the medically indigent were considered, and a definition of medical indigence was supplied. Here the House felt that the determination must be made locally as to the group covered by this term, that control of the service should lie with local administration, and that available facilities should be utilized before new facilities were provided. Thus, the House of Delegates felt that there was but little need for the building of new hospitals or the establishment of new diagnostic centers, provided better utilization of hospitals and laboratories already functioning can be devised.

Again the House of Delegates stated its firm opposition to any compulsory sickness plan. Finally, it approved protection against loss of income during illness.

The Board of Trustees presented to the House of Delegates the statement concerning the proposed investigation by the Department of Justice. The statement had been made repeatedly that the American Medical Association was ready for investigation by any authorized agency. It was reliant in the belief that its actions were in accordance with its constitutional organization, that they had been taken in the interest of the public health and welfare, and that it had never violated the established laws of this country. The House of Delegates expressed its firm conviction in the truth of these statements and urged the Board of Trustees to oppose with its utmost power, even to the courts of last resort, this apparent attempt to convict the American Medical Association in the eyes of the people of being a predatory, antisocial monopoly.

In October the government subpoenaed the Association in connection with its suit.

THE CLIP SHEET

The new Bureau of Publicity began publishing a special weekly clip sheet to be sent to newspapers and periodicals throughout the nation.

The secretary stated that the actions of the House of Delegates taken at the special session had been communicated to the President of the United States and to Miss Josephine Roche.

The Surgeons General of the Army, Navy and the President of the United States had been notified in connection with the development of Selective Service that the American Medical Association had made available its records of the physicians of the country in the event that mobilization of physicians for service in the Army and Navy was deemed necessary. The Surgeons General had called in the headquarters office of the Association to take note of the available records. Again this fundamental service of the American

Medical Association was the main reliance of our government in securing physicians in time of war.

As December 1938 closed an exciting year, the so-called Committee of Physicians for the Improvement of Medical Care, Inc., had begun issuing its own analysis of the National Health Conference and its condemnation of the action taken by the House of Delegates of the American Medical Association.

A Grand Jury had met in Washington to indict the American Medical Association under the Sherman Antitrust Act. Physicians everywhere were protesting the activities of the Committee of Physicians. In the midst of this turmoil, THE JOURNAL continued to appear week after week with the news and facts relative to both scientific and socio-economic aspects of medical science. The multiple councils, bureaus and other agencies of the Association were active in carrying on their special activities. The Board of Trustees was watching closely the finances of the Association with a view to meeting the tremendous demands that were foreseen.

1939

What to do with the refugee physicians who were coming from Europe? How to respond to the government in relationship to the indictment of the American Medical Association? Should doctors patent medical discoveries? These were some of the questions which greeted 1939 for the American Medical Association. From all over the country came messages of encouragement to the Association in relationship to the indictment by the government. One Florida physician sent $10.00 as a sign that he was ready to support the American Medical Association in its legal battle. Conferences were planned with the trustees and representatives of associated organizations, like the American College of Physicians, for it was felt that the American medical profession must, if possible, present a united front to meet the situation. Furthermore, it was felt that there was need to develop new technics of medical care for the American people.

The Committee on Legislative Activities was at the same time being primed to present the case for American medicine to the Ways and Means Committee of the Congress. Then came a conference between the Board of Trustees of the American Medical Association and the directors and representatives of the American Hospital Association, the Catholic Hospital Association and the Protestant Hospital Association. There were mutual expressions of confidence and agreement on many problems in the field of medical care.

Many agencies were moving seriously into the health field. A conference on health education had been called by the National Health Council to consider adequate training of personnel for health educators and to prevent wasteful overlapping of functions and destructive competition and to develop a curriculum in schools on health.

There were requests for representatives from the National Council for Mothers and Babies, from the boys' clubs, from the National Congress of Parents and Teachers, from the American Association for the Advancement of Science, from the U. S. Chamber of Commerce, and from many other organizations of public as well as wholly scientific objectives.

The Association had determined to call a nation wide conference on the nomenclature of disease in order to stimulate the development and use of the standard nomenclature. The Association was asked to develop a periodical in the field of industrial health which would be associated with the work of the Council on Industrial Health but it did not seem appropriate at this time to undertake that publication.

In the meantime, the conference of state and provincial health authorities of North America had approved some of the principles of the National Health Program but it stated definitely objection to the creation of a new federal administrative health agency in the Social Security Board. Senator Wagner had begun to push Senate Bill 1620 but by May two state associations—those of Washington and of Missouri—had stated their objections and their determination to oppose.

A conference was held in April with the Board of Regents of the American College of Physicians on the subject of graduate medical education. Arrangements were in process for a similar conference with the Board of Regents of the American College of Surgeons.

Previous to the meeting of the House of Delegates at the St. Louis session in 1939, the Board of Trustees considered many pending problems. There had been one request that the American Medical Association support citizenship as a prerequisite for licensure. The hospital associations had agreed to oppose the Wagner Bill. The committee on patents had developed a statement which included some of the difficulties involved in granting exclusive patents on medical discoveries. Fee schedules were again up for consideration. The Red Cross had asked approval of its first aid manual. The Council on Physical Therapy was involved in the standardization of technics for artificial respiration.

THE ST. LOUIS SESSION

When the House of Delegates met, Dr. Harrison H. Shoulders, speaker, inspired the House with a eulogy of the principles of ethics and a plea for faith in the ideals of the American Medical Association.

The president, Dr. Irvin Abell, was again concerned with graduate education. He told of the conference with Miss Josephine Roche and her Interdepartmental Committee and of another visit, made by the committee which had been appointed by the speaker of the House of Delegates, to President Franklin Delano Roosevelt. Dr. Abell said:

> "President Roosevelt was most gracious and affable and discussed both his interest in an increase in hospital facilities and a wide distribution of medical care on a basis of need and as well the budgetary difficulties which the program entails."

The president-elect, Dr. Rock Sleyster, urged more attention to the fundamental principles for which the American Medical Association was organized. He was particularly concerned that many specialistic organizations had lost touch with the county medical societies and the national organization. He felt that it was unfortunate that some officers of other national organizations without any due authority to speak for their groups had voiced opinions definitely in opposition to the policies of the American Medical Association.

THE "THROW AWAY" JOURNALS

In this period there suddenly developed in the United States several periodicals having what was called "controlled circulation" paid for entirely by their advertisers and given free to the medical profession. On these publications, Dr. Sleyster said:

> "Thirty years ago there were no medical journals whose advertising pages could be considered a credit to the medical profession. Today not only the greatest medical journal in the world but the state journals and many independent journals show by their clean advertising the imprint of the Council's efforts in furthering rational therapy and enhancing the scientific treatment of the sick.
>
> "In contrast are the pages of certain little magazines sent without subscription charge to all members of the profession—magazines usually referred to as 'throw away' journals. Most of the advertising in these journals is not acceptable to the American Medical Association. This of course is the reason for their existence. They have no doubt been extremely profitable to their private owners for they have furnished to their advertisers a large audience which could not be obtained through the American Medical Association journals. One of them has repeatedly attempted to undermine the councils and committees that have attacked nostrums and made therapy scientific. Some publish the names of an 'advisory board'—names of leading members of this organization. All publish articles or abstracts written by our members. It is hard to believe that members of this organization will lend their names to the promotion of publications of this type."

In response, the House of Delegates voiced their approval of his opinion.

DISTINGUISHED SERVICE MEDAL

At this session of the House of Delegates, the second physician to be honored with the Distinguished Service Award was Dr. James B. Herrick for his work on coronary thrombosis. The other nominees included Dr. Chevalier Jackson of Philadelphia, noted for his work in developing bronchoscopy, and Dr. Edward Jackson of Denver who had made monumental contributions in the field of ophthalmology.

THE GRAND JURY INDICTS

The trustees reported to the House that the American Medical Association, the Medical Society of the District of Columbia, the Harris County Medical Society of Texas, and certain members of the medical societies of the District of Columbia and of the administrative personnel of the American Medical Association had been indicted. The House of Delegates in special session had been informed that the Association had engaged counsel and would exert all possible efforts to make proper defense before the courts.

The Board of Trustees had also appealed a ruling from the Bureau of Internal Revenue to the effect that the American Medical Association was liable for the payment of taxes under the Social Security Act.

Among other subjects the Judicial Council had been asked to give a definition of a diagnostic clinic. It submitted the following report to the House of Delegates:

"1. A diagnostic clinic is an organization of physicians whose sole work in the clinic is to make or supervise diagnostic examinations of patients referred to the clinic by doctors of medicine, or to collaborate in general diagnostic surveys.

"2. The reports of the diagnostic clinic on examinations and tests are made only to the referring physician unless he requests that the case and the recommendations for treatment be discussed with the patient as a part of a professional consultation at which the relationship of the results of the diagnostic studies to the general condition of the patient is open for discussion. In such case, discussion is only by a member of the staff.

"3. The staff of the diagnostic clinic should include representatives from all the specialties that are of recognized diagnostic usefulness. Every clinical examination, laboratory test or x-ray procedure is made by a physician who specializes in that field or under his supervision. The clinic must be equipped to allow the various specialists to exercise fully their abilities.

"4. The control of the clinic must be vested in one or more members of the professional staff. Any profits are to be appointed only to the members of the staff actually engaged in the work of the clinic. There must be no dividends, bonuses or salaries paid any individual except for services rendered.

"5. The clinic must be governed in its activities by the same ethical principles as apply to an individual member of the American Medical Association.

"It is recognized that under this definition only in cities large enough to support the various specialists needed can a diagnostic clinic be established or maintained. Unless the specialists are available it is not a diagnostic clinic worthy of the name."

The House of Delegates adopted that report unanimously.

SPECIALTY BOARDS AND OTHER REPORTS

Constantly advancing in its point of view in relationship to many problems of medical education, the Council on Medical Education and Hospitals now presented, under the leadership of Dr. Ray Lyman Wilbur, a revised list of essentials of a registered hospital, of approved residencies and fellowships, and of approved examining boards in the specialties. The final procedure was one of the most important actions taken by the Council since it brought into the control of these examining boards the point of view of the entire membership of the American Medical Association.

An extensive study had been made by the Council on Medical Education and Hospitals jointly with the Bureau of Medical Economics on the provision of medical care in the state of Mississippi. This report occupied many pages of the annual statement of the Council to the House of Delegates.

Through resolutions offered by individual delegates, the House of Delegates again expressed its opinion of attempts to socialize the medical profession through the Wagner national health bill.

One resolution, offered by Dr. James M. Flynn of New York, called on the Association to take action which would not deny membership to any physician solely on the basis of race, color or creed. The reference committee did not feel that there should be arbitrary action implying that the county medical society should not in effect have the right of selection of its own members, which is a fundamental principle of the American Medical Association.

Especially important was the report of the Committee on Legislative Activities made by its chairman, Dr. Edward H. Cary of Dallas, Texas. This dealt particularly with the Veterans' Administration and medical relief through the Farm Security Administration. The members had appeared before Senate committees in behalf of the secretary of health in the cabinet and the committee had given much consideration to the so-called national health bill.

Up to this time members of the Council on Medical Education and Hospitals had been chosen by the House of Delegates for nomination by the president of the Association. At this session of the House of Delegates, it was proposed that these prospective members be nominated by the Board of Trustees to the House of Delegates—the hope being that this Council might be still further removed from any possible influence through political pressure.

The Committee on Medical Care which was searching for new technics which would aid a better distribution of medical practice made a report through its chairman, Dr. William F. Braasch, calling attention to the survey of medical care that had been made by the American Medical Association and indicating that working alliances were being developed among the various agencies which were particularly concerned with such problems.

The executive session was concerned wholly with the Wagner health bill. The reference committee which reported on the subject had analyzed the bill thoroughly; it presented to the House of Delegates twenty-two distinct arguments against this type of legislation.

On the final day of the session, Dr. Nathan B. Van Etten of New York was made president-elect.

Dr. Rock Sleyster, who had been for many years concerned with the subject of psychiatry and perhaps in anticipation of what was to become the fundamental medical problem of World War II, spoke on "The Mind of Man and His Security," in his presidential address. His peroration was a challenge and a promise. "How great a price," he asked, "are we prepared to pay for what is called security?" And he concluded:

> Today the American people stand before the world as a nation of free men where the processes of individual initiative, freedom of thought, controlled research and independent character have placed us in the very forefront of all the peoples in the world in science, in health, in our scale of living, in recreation and in the ability to enjoy life. It is true, as some of our statesmen have said, that not all the people are possessed of all these advantages, yet taken as a whole the statement is true of the vast majority of our people. By the same forces which have brought us to this high place we should be able to overcome the deficiencies of those who have not yet realized these great advantages and to give to them much of that which is enjoyed by the majority. To this purpose the American medical profession has repeatedly dedicated itself. The solutions of the problems of the nations so far as they concern medical care are the responsibility of the medical profession. That is a responsibility which a free medical profession has never avoided and to which it is at this very time giving its most serious consideration. The responsibility for restoring to this nation an economic status in which more and more independent citizens will be able through their new employment and through the returns coming from that employment to supply themselves with the necessities of life is a responsibility which must rest on the leaders of the nation in industry, in finance and in government. With these leaders also American medicine is ready and willing to cooperate in doing all that can be done to spread more widely the benefits of American life and living.

MULTIPLE PROBLEMS

There were many extraordinary proposals for the Board of Trustees to consider. There were requests to meet with the American Dental Association and a commendation from the Catholic Hospital Association. There was a request for Dr. Dafoe to discuss the quintuplets at the next annual meeting of the Association. The board gave consideration to the program of the Women's Auxiliary. It appointed members to the various councils and bureaus, studied expenditures of government on health, participated in erecting the Museum of Science and Industry in Chicago. It considered the report on spas and health resorts and the proposed Congress on Education for Democracy. The board had under advisement an insurance plan covering the employees of the Association, a bibliography on air condition, several new publications, and a prospective conference with the Board of Regents of the American College of Surgeons.

The Committee to Study Motor Vehicle Accidents had a report. Another committee was standardizing Wassermann tests. There was the problem of compensation of physicians employed in venereal disease clinics under the W. P. A. Several opinion research corporations were requesting the opportunity to conduct surveys for the Association. And again the perennial problem of a national department of health! An American Physicians Art Association had been formed and wished space in the annual exhibit. Every so often there was a fire in the headquarters office. This year it struck the laboratory; the loss was small. Dr. W. C. Woodward was again seeking to retire from the Bureau of Legal Medicine and Legislation. Dr. Arthur J. Cramp had retired from the Bureau of Investigation. The editor reported that the Reader's Digest was cooperating with HYGEIA in the development and publication of articles. Again the advertising committee of the headquarters office had developed rules, which the board approved, governing the acceptance of advertising. These rules had to be constantly revised to meet changing conditions and new discoveries. From one state medical society after another and from many counties came resolutions urging the Association to stand firm in its policies against government medicine. The "Standard Classified Nomenclature of Disease" had been published and a conference was to be called in 1940 to revise it and to add a nomenclature of operations. The Committee of Physicians continued sniping at the American Medical Association and continued to urge cooperation with Senator Wagner. It had enlisted in its support the pen of Michael Davis.

On November 16 the Board of Trustees met with a group of members from the Board of Regents of the American College of Surgeons under the chairmanship of Dr. Irvin Abell. Many plans were discussed in relation to policy and particularly in developing a cooperative plan for the collection of information regarding hospitals. The American College of Surgeons called attention to the work that it had been doing through its Commission on Industrial Medicine and Traumatic Surgery.

From the Bureau of Internal Revenue came a decision that the American Medical Association was liable for social security taxes although exempt from income taxes.

At this time the editor of THE JOURNAL brought to the attention of the board the fact that there had been formed a voluntary body of physicians known as the National Physicians Committee for the Extension of Medical Service, which seemed to be in accord with the objectives of the Association in the development of a health program for the nation. The Board of Trustees authorized a statement in THE JOURNAL regarding the development of the National Physicians' Committee, its officers and its background.

From the Offices of the Surgeons General of the Army and Navy came assurances that they would be glad to have the American Medical Association take the leadership in any efforts that might be made to be helpful if mobilization became necessary. The Association had also offered space in the headquarters office to any personnel of the Army or Navy who might be needed in this work.

On December 8 the Executive Committee of the board met with representatives of the various hospital associations to discuss the implications of the platform of the American Medical Association for the improvement of the national health. This was the first of a series of drafts of the National Health Program which moved gradually toward 1946 when a final ten-point program evolved.

1940—NEW YORK CITY

EARLY IN 1940 the committee which had been appointed by the speaker of the House of Delegates to meet with the President of the United States on a previous occasion met again to consider the question of building hospitals. These preliminary conferences led eventually to the Hill-Burton act for construction of hospitals and health centers.

The National Physicians' Committee was fighting federalized medicine powerfully with discussions in county and state medical societies all over the nation. Word came that the Mexican government was contemplating restriction of two powerful radio stations which had been built on the border by John R. Brinkley and Norman Baker. THE JOURNAL had repeatedly exposed these charlatans; again it called attention to the fraudulent character of their operations.

Early in 1940, also, the editor suggested to the board that the Atlantic City session of the American Medical Association in 1942 be a Pan American meeting. The Department of State was making an effort to establish more cordial relations between the United States and the countries to the south. The Board of Trustees concurred in the proposal and authorized the necessary planning for its accomplishment.

The speaker of the House of Delegates, Dr. H. H. Shoulders, analyzed the reasons for the greatness of the American Medical Association. He conceived that its ethical principles, its fundamental objectives and its spirit of democracy were the factors primarily responsible for its importance.

The president, Dr. Rock Sleyster, introduced a new note in the House of Delegates when he spoke of preparedness. He told how the Association had cooperated with the government in the first World War in securing adequate personnel for the medical departments of the Army and Navy.

"Today our nation is again preparing to defend itself to the utmost against any type of aggression from without. The medical profession, through its House of Delegates, I know, will pledge itself to give, as it has always given in the past, every iota of service that it is capable of rendering."

In response to this challenge, the House of Delegates said:

"Your reference committee would urge on this House of Delegates the absolute necessity of following the advice of the President of our Association in unstinting support of the federal government in the campaign for preparedness in the present chaotic state of a world in which right and reason have been cast to the winds and only brute force is recognized and heeded."

The chairman of the committee that prepared this report was Dr. Walter E. Vest of West Virginia.

In a long statement relative to the public relations of the American Medical Association, Dr. Rock Sleyster told of its many accomplishments. He repeated the platform of the Association in a capsule form!

> The great health movements of this country were initiated, fostered and promoted by the medical profession. We believe, however, that the proper function of government under a democratic system is the protection of its people from hazards to health, the promotion of standards of living which are favorable to health, and leaving to a free people the free choice of medical care when illness comes unless indigence prevents. We believe that the most profitable expenditure of government effort and means in the cause of the sick would be attained, as it has been in the past, through efforts toward the prevention of disease. Let government fight disease at its source as it should; protect the well from the hazards of contact; insure a mode of living which supplies the requirements of proper food and adequate clothing; eliminate the hazards of slum and tenement; provide proper housing; offer wholesome recreation; instruct the masses to avoid the dangers which go with ignorance; educate them to take advantage promptly and intelligently of means now available when threatened with illness, and protect them from the appalling toll of senseless and unnecessary accidents. Let government concentrate its every effort on these sources of mortality and morbidity, and the cause of health, life and happiness will be advanced countless times more than it can be furthered by placing the sick under any form of political control.

The president elect, Dr. Nathan B. Van Etten of New York, spoke of love of country and love of freedom. He explained the need for more hospitals and encouraged the development of the eight point platform. He again pleaded that there be a secretary of health in the cabinet and he stated as his principle:

> "I believe that the medical profession should go along with the government as far as possible for the common good without sacrificing its individual interests in the care of the sick and its collective interests in the prevention of disease."

From the Bureau of Legal Medicine and Legislation came the usual complete analyses of legislation and from the Bureau of Medical Economics a tremendous report of many pages dealing with its publications, experimental medical service plans, group hospitalization, private insurance companies, hospital and medical expense insurance for individuals, professionally controlled credit and collection agencies, medical fee schedules and technics for financing arrangements for medical care.

By this time the Association had incurred a number of libel suits which, as has been said elsewhere, will be accumulated in a single report. In 1940 there were pending libel suits totaling $4,-500,000 brought by plastic surgeons, a giant, a gland quack and a manufacturer of a cosmetic preparation.

In Washington, the legal difficulties had reached the stage of having the Supreme Court deny the petition of the Association for a writ of certiorari so that the Association would have to stand trial in the U. S. District Court. The defendants were instructed to be in Washington on June 14, 1940, to make an appearance before the court, and the Board of Trustees authorized the general manager to enter a plea of "Not Guilty" on behalf of the Association.

The clouds of war loomed ominously. The Board of Trustees introduced a resolution on preparedness for passage by the House of Delegates and for discussion in executive session.

The House of Delegates found it necessary on this occasion to request that all resolutions dealing with such subjects as public relations efforts, legal difficulties, contraception and the relations of the organized medical profession to the federal administration be read by title and that the speaker rule whether or not the resolution should be considered in executive session. Many such resolutions came before the House of Delegates and the executive session was long and arduous.

New sections had been added to the Association so that there were now sixteen specialties and a Section on Miscellaneous Topics. The latest additions were the sections on radiology and on anesthesiology.

In the executive session the House of Delegates authorized the appointment of a Committee on Medical Preparedness. It had heard a report from Colonel George C. Dunham as ' ꞌ the needs of the Army and it urged cooperation in securing medi͏ ꞌersonnel. Resolutions were offered for the protection of the ꞌtices of physicians who might be called to military service.

HOSPITAL CONSTRUCTION

In the absence of the chairman, Dr. Irvin Abell, a report of the committee to confer and consult with the proper federal representatives on hospital construction was submitted. The committee included Drs. E. H. Cary, Walter F. Donaldson, Frederic E. Sondern, Walter E. Vest, Fred W. Rankin and Irvin Abell. Dr. Austin A. Hayden had been appointed to fill a vacancy created by the illness of Dr. Henry A. Luce. There were also in attendance Dr. Olin West, secretary of the Association; Dr. R. G. Leland of the Bureau of Medical Economics, and Dr. W. D. Cutter of the Council on Medical Education and Hospitals. There were also representatives of the U. S. Public Health Service, of the American Catholic and Protestant Hospital Associations and the Surgeon General of the Navy, Ross T. McIntire. Out of this conference came ultimately, as has previously been stated, the Hill-Burton bill. The President of the United States had developed a particular idea as to how hospitals should be built. His proposal included 50 to 100 bed hospitals in communities where such facilities did not exist. The buildings were to be fireproof, and one-story in height. President Franklin D. Roosevelt had estimated that such a hospital could be built for $1500 a bed. Indeed, he had himself drawn sketches of such hospitals, Ultimately, Senators Wagner and George introduced a hospital construction bill seeking to make the President's program effective; that bill, however, failed of enactment.

DISTINGUISHED SERVICE MEDAL

At this meeting of the House of Delegates, Dr. Chevalier Jackson of Philadelphia was elected to receive the Distinguished Service Award. The other candidates were Drs. James Ewing and Ludvig Hektoen.

COMMITTEE ON MEDICAL PREPAREDNESS

As the session ended, the House of Delegates authorized the Board of Trustees to create a committee on medical preparedness to consist of ten members of the House of Delegates, with the president of the Association, the chairman and secretary of the board, the secretary of the Association and the editor as ex officio members.

In the elections, Dr. Frank H. Lahey of Boston became president elect of the American Medical Association.

ADDRESS OF VAN ETTEN

At this session, the president, Dr. Nathan B. Van Etten, discussed "Better Health for America." He considered our facilities in medical personnel and equipment, and he concluded:

"The American Medical Association stands for orderly and continuous progress toward better health for every American citizen. It stands for the elimination of every influence which may be destructive of the public health. It stands for the elimination of every communicable disease. It stands for the elimination of quackery. It stands for better general understanding of personal health problems. It stands for the promotion of research into fundamental causes of disease and curative therapy. It stands for better education of all physicians, not only the undergraduate but the general practitioner who has been long in service. Its platform stands for the coordination of all government health functions in order to promote efficiency and eliminate duplication of effort and wasteful extravagance of the people's money. It stands for the treatment of the sick in their homes by local physicians and welfare agencies—where the real individual troubles are known—and it desires as little interference by the central government as may be consistent with constructive relief of personal suffering. Its program is entirely forward looking and it seeks to carry it on in conformity with the best traditions of an advanced democracy."

During the year, the Board of Trustees lost one of its members, Dr. Charles B. Wright. He had been an exceptional member of the board—one of those who was elected on a platform of reorganization and reconstruction and who became eventually one of the most consistent and stable members of what is essentially a most stable group.

SOCIAL SECURITY TAX

One of the printers of the American Medical Association sought action to cause the Association to undertake social security payments for its employees. This petition was to be carried from court to court in the state of Illinois with ultimate ruling in behalf of the classification by the Commissioner of Internal Revenue that the Association was a business league and would have to pay social security taxes for its employees.

During the year a considerable number of libel suits against the Association were concluded. The John R. Brinkley suit had been settled in behalf of the American Medical Association. Norman Baker had been found guilty of using the U. S. mails to defraud and was sentenced to prison and fined $4000. The suit of the cosmetic manufacturer had been withdrawn. One of the suits of a plastic surgeon had simply passed into innocuous desuetude. However, a new suit for $50,000 had just been filed by a practitioner who was exploited as a "miracle man" in a popular magazine. After a few months the case of the "miracle man" was dismissed by a New York Court.

Following the 1939 annual session of the Association in New York City another member of the Board of Trustees, Dr. Austin A. Hayden, who had been secretary for several years and one of the most efficient workers of the Association died rather suddenly from nephritis and coronary thrombosis.

At this time Dr. Fishbein reported to the Board of Trustees that he had been asked by the National Research Council to be chairman of its Committee on Information in relationship to procedures of research and standardization to be carried on by the National Research Council during the war. The Board of Trustees authorized acceptance of this appointment.

The Committee on Medical Preparedness met and considered the publication of a questionnaire to be sent to every physician in the United States.

Dr. Fishbein presented to the board a request from the National Research Council for the publication of a periodical which would deal with research and military medicine. From this movement came the journal known as *War Medicine*.

In the midst of the activities in behalf of medical preparedness, all of the personnel in the headquarters office who had been indicted found themselves required to spend much of their time in Washington, traveling back and forth to keep wheels moving in Chicago and to be present at the trial.

By this time, medical societies in more than eighteen states had developed medical service plans. Furthermore, a resolution had come from the Michigan State Medical Association urging the American Medical Association to undertake coordination of these plans. This was the beginning of the movement that resulted eventually in the formation of Associated Medical Care Plans, Inc., under the auspices of the Council on Medical Service of the American Medical Association.

Following the death of Dr. Austin A. Hayden, Dr. Ernest E. Irons was elected to fill the unexpired term as secretary of the Board of Trustees.

The Association was taking an active part in the study of hearing aids and audiometers, initiated by Dr. Hayden.

1941
CLEVELAND

Throughout the nation there now arose a call for more attention to the general practitioner, to better education for general medical practice and for the creation of a section on general practice in the American Medical Association. This movement persisted through the end of the hundred year period in 1947. At that time, following the end of World War II the problem of proper recognition for general practitioners came to be one of the most significant problems in American medicine.

On January 14, Dr. Paul Nicholas Leech, secretary of the Council on Pharmacy and Chemistry and Director of the Division of Foods, Drugs and Physical Therapy died suddenly following a cerebral hemorrhage. The appointment of a successor to this young man who had grown up in the work of the American Medical Association and who had proved to be an exceedingly able administrative officer and a competent scientist, gave the Board of Trustees great concern.

Movements began to develop for greater cooperation between medicine and pharmacy and indeed for cooperation of medicine with all of the basic sciences.

The Board of Trustees authorized the editor of THE JOURNAL to begin the publication of a Spanish edition of THE JOURNAL at a suitable time. The board also authorized conferences with Mr. Nelson Rockefeller, Coordinator of Commercial and Cultural Relations between the American Republics, and with other government agencies with a view to working out final details of such a magazine. The editor pointed out the difficulty of attempting such a publication during the trial which was still going on and on in Washington and which will be described in another chapter. The Pan-American Medical Association offered its complete cooperation in this venture.

The first issue of *War Medicine* received commendation from the Army and Navy, from the British and American Research Councils. Its story is told in a separate chapter.

The Council on Industrial Health was considering industrial accidents. Many small matters arose to disturb the Board of Trustees. They were asked their view of a motion picture which would portray the lives of the Mayo brothers. Other projects included cooperation with the food and nutrition division of the National Research Council, special issues of all the special periodicals, but especially the work of the Committee on Medical Preparedness. Next came a request from the Selective Service administration for the appointment of a member of the Board of Trustees on the medical committee of the Selective Service System and another request for representatives on the national rehabilitation committee.

THE END OF THE TRIAL

The trial of the American Medical Association in Washington ended early in April. When the executive committee of the board met in May, Dr. Olin West reported that he and Drs. Fishbein, Cutter and Leland had spent about eight weeks in the District Court of the United States in Washington during the preparations for and the hearings of the trial of the case in which the U. S. brought suit on criminal charges. The verdict was rendered late on the night of April 4. All individual defendants had been found not guilty but the American Medical Association and the Medical Society of the District of Columbia were found guilty. The Board of Trustees had naturally to arrange for presentation of this report to the House of Delegates.

FOOD AND NUTRITION CONFERENCE

The President of the United States, it had been indicated, was about to call a national conference on nutrition and the cooperation of the American Medical Association was sought. The Council on Foods and Nutrition had agreed to cooperate. The Federal Security Administrator had acknowledged the offer of cooperation with a statement that the President of the United States appreciated the letter and that the Association would be asked to cooperate in this conference on May 26.

As the Board of Trustees assembled to meet with the House of Delegates in Cleveland in June, negotiations were still under way for publication of a Spanish medical periodical. A complete program had been drawn up and plans had been made to hold a session with guests from Latin America in 1942.

A conference was arranged with representatives of the pharmaceutical profession on medical-pharmaceutical relationships. From many states came messages commending the work of the administrative officers of the Association and expressing their appreciation of the burden carried by these men in the trial in Washington.

New projects were invitations to cooperate in an American Museum of Health and in the work of the National Noise Abatement Council.

Through the American Red Cross had come a request for physicians to work with the British Army and the British Emergency Medical Service. The American Red Cross had requested the cooperation of Dr. Morris Fishbein in developing a list of physicians for such service and the board authorized this cooperation.

THE CLEVELAND SESSION

In the Cleveland session such a multitude of physicians attended that it was necessary to secure D & C boats to lie on the lake front to accommodate the numerous physicians who were unable to find rooms.

For the Distinguished Service Award, Dr. James Ewing of New York was chosen, with Dr. Ludvig Hektoen of Chicago and Dr. Simon Flexner of New York as the other nominees.

The president of the Association, Dr. Nathan B. Van Etten, told of the growth of the Association in 95 years of progress. He spoke of the platform that had been formulated in 1939 as an evolution of the platform first developed in 1934. Dr. Van Etten called attention to the campaign against the policies of the American Medical Association and indicated to the House of Delegates that if there was any hierarchy in the Association, it lay in the House of Delegates. He felt that every delegate owed it to the Association to enlighten public opinion in his own home as to the democracy that prevails in the organization. In its defense he said:

"I have sat with your Trustees for eight years and I have observed the meticulous and exhausting patience with which they try in every way to carry out the spirit and the letter of the authorized actions of this House. Your Trustees handle your affairs without personal bias. They come from all regions of the country at great personal sacrifice, some of them every month, to concentrate their best intelligence on the execution of your decisions. Only one of them, Dr. Irons, lives in Chicago. Dr. West, Dr. Fishbein and Mr. Braun are executives. I have never heard or seen any of them attempt to originate any policy of the American Medical Association. I have heard these men called a 'Triumvirate of Dictators.' Mr. Braun could double your advertising if you would let him. Ethical advertising could yield to large volumes of uncensored advertising. Dr. Fishbein could travel in far more attractive financial fields than in those in which he is limited by his strict loyalty to the service of American medicine, to which he has dedicated his brilliant talents. Dr. West has been called a 'Pooh-Bah' by some loose thinking space writers, possibly because he has been inflexible in his devotion to the principles that have been evolved in this house. He has frankly and forcibly expressed his convictions on many occasions, but he has never dictated policy.

"Authors whose mental processes seem to have been influenced by Moscow or Berlin have written volumes of destructive criticism concerning the policies of the American Medical Association and the personalities of your executives. If these strictures on these characters who are so vital to the success of your organization have gained any credit in your minds, you should bring your doubts or your questions before the House for appropriate action. If you deny the truth of these allegations, you should at this time express your high appreciation of their unselfish devotion."

The president elect, Dr. Frank H. Lahey, paid great tribute to the American Medical Association. He suggested the desirability of a younger membership for the House of Delegates. He forecast in the conclusion of his address the imminence of the war and called on the American Medical Association for complete dedication to the task of defending our government.

Specialization and the tendency toward more and more specialization disturbed the House of Delegates greatly. Resolutions came asking conferences with the specialty boards; resolutions requesting hospital privileges for general practitioners; resolutions requesting the creation of a section on general practice.

MEDICAL PREPAREDNESS

Most significant in this session was the report of the Committee on Medical Preparedness presented by Dr. Irvin Abell, its chairman. There had been many meetings of the committee and it had cooperated with every government agency requesting aid. THE JOURNAL OF THE AMERICAN MEDICAL ASSOCIATION had established a special section on "Medical Preparedness." Lt. Col. Charles G. Hutter had been assigned to the headquarters office from the Medical Corps of the Army with the Committee on Medical Preparedness. A complete analysis of available medical personnel had been made. Legislation had been considered as it related to the national defense program. There had been complete cooperation with the National Research Council, with the Selective Service System and with the

Army and Navy Medical Departments. The Committee on Medical Preparedness, which served notably throughout the war, included Drs. Irvin Abell, chairman, Stanley H. Osborn, Walter G. Phippen, Harvey B. Stone, James E. Paullin, Fred W. Rankin, Roy W. Fouts, Sam E. Thompson, Charles A. Dukes, John H. O'Shea, and ex officio Nathan B. Van Etten, Arthur W. Booth, Morris Fishbein and Olin West. From this committee came a proposal for the creation of an agency of government to be known as the Procurement and Assignment Agency. The exact words were:

"Resolved, That the United States government be urged to plan and arrange immediately for the establishment of a central authority with representatives of the civilian medical profession to be known as the Procurement and Assignment agency for physicians for the Army, Navy, and Public Health Service and for the Civilian and Industrial needs of the nation."

This resolution was discussed in executive session and received the complete endorsement of the House of Delegates.

The executive session opened with a statement by Mr. E. M. Burke, attorney for the American Medical Association, relative to the indictment and trial. He recapitulated briefly the history of this trial and was directed by the House of Delegates to file an appeal from the judgment.

The Committee on Medical Preparedness had considered resolutions dealing with the medical examination of draftees, uncompensated services, the eligibility of women physicians and surgeons for the medical reserve corps, the services of native American and foreign born physicians, and the continuation of a supply of well trained medical graduates. This was a special appeal that medical students be permitted to continue their medical education during the course of the war so as to meet the need for medical officers in the armed forces.

The Association at this time entertained a representative from the Chilean Medical Association, Dr. Miguel Acuna.

At this session Dr. Fred W. Rankin was made president elect.

After he was installed as president, Dr. Frank H. Lahey spoke of "Current Problems of American Medicine." He began, "Probably few presidents of the American Medical Association have been or will be inducted into the office at more uncertain or more urgent times." Then he turned to military problems and the part that medicine would play should our country be involved in war. He recognized the pending war between capital and labor and he said in conclusion:

"My own opinion, and I believe it is my duty to express it, is that we are already committed to a position, whether we like it or not. I myself like it. We have dared the dictator. It is too late to appease him and the word has no meaning in his language. We should arrive at a conviction concerning isolation. Is it right? It is my conviction that it is not. I prefer destruction if it need be to survival in cowering terror."

His final words were:

"This nation has been gallant in the past and it can be gallant again. I do not believe that there is a safe course. In dangerous times such as these, I would like to make as a closing statement that it is my conviction that a dangerous course has real advantages."

The Board of Trustees was still continuing with its negotiations for a Spanish magazine. An invitation had come from Mexico to attend the national medical and dental congresses, but the board deemed it inadvisable to accept the invitations on account of the critical conditions existing at that time.

Dr. Theodore G. Klumpp had been selected secretary of the Council on Pharmacy and Chemistry and director of the Division of Foods, Drugs and Physical Therapy.

In planning for the Pan American session several foundations had arranged to bring Latin American physicians to attend the meeting. A committee was appointed to study the relationships of medicine and the law, another committee to confer with the specialty boards, and still others to confer with hospital associations. From General George C. Marshall, chief of staff of the United States Army, had come a letter of appreciation of planning by the American Medical Association to develop suitable personnel for the armed forces. Dr. Fishbein reported that President Roosevelt had appointed a committee, known as the Bush Committee, under which had been developed a committee on medical research under the Department of War and that he had been appointed consultant to the Office of Emergency Management of that committee. Plans were being made for the medical care of the wives of men in the service and for the mobilization of physicians and dentists. By this time THE JOURNAL OF THE AMERICAN MEDICAL ASSOCIATION had increased so greatly in its size that protests had come from a book binder in Boston to the effect that the volumes of THE JOURNAL were too thick and that "there are folk who bind the technical part only; that separate paging is not indispensable, but it is an intelligent and orderly arrangement, and in line with modern progress, and provides a means for making four sensible volumes per year." The Board of Trustees instructed the editor to look into this matter; as a result, THE JOURNAL is now bound in three volumes per year.

From Dr. George Baehr, chief medical officer in the Office of Civilian Defense, came an appeal for cooperation of the medical profession in the work of civilian defense. Employees of the headquarters office had been loaned to the office in Washington in order to aid in orderly establishment of this work. The President of the United States had suggested a plan for rehabilitating rejected draftees. Representatives of the American Medical Association, including Drs. Frank Lahey and Morris Fishbein, had been called to sit with the committee of Selective Service which was considering this problem.

PROCUREMENT AND ASSIGNMENT SERVICE

As a result of the action taken by the Committee on Medical Preparedness at the Cleveland session, several preliminary conferences had been held in Washington which resulted eventually in the establishment, through a directive issued by the President of the United States on October 31, of the Procurement and Assignment Service for Physicians, Dentists and Veterinarians. This service was to have an office in Washington and a special office in the headquarters office of the American Medical Association in Chicago. Advisory committees had been established for many agencies. The editor of THE JOURNAL had been selected as chairman of the Committee on Information to work with the general advisory committee.

In December it was reported that Dr. Theodore G. Klumpp had been offered the presidency of a large pharmaceutical manufacturing house. The Board of Trustees elected Dr. Austin E. Smith, who had been associated with Dr. Klumpp in the work of the Council on Pharmacy and Chemistry, to the position of acting secretary of the Council.

More and more personnel were needed in the headquarters office to meet the increasing demands. The Committee on Medical Preparedness had met with the Procurement and Assignment Service. The government desired to create a national roster of scientific personnel and the Board of Trustees authorized the appointment of Drs. West, Fishbein and Leland to aid the National Resources Planning Board in developing a suitably arranged card system.

1942
ATLANTIC CITY

The uncertain economic conditions following the beginning of the war caused the Board of Trustees to take careful account of its financial status as 1942 loomed on the horizon. Military meetings were being held by the American College of Surgeons. The American Medical Association cooperated with its mailing list and other facilities in the promotion of these conferences. Dr. William D. Cutter, secretary of the Council on Medical Education and Hospitals had died; the name of Dr. Herman G. Weiskotten was offered as acting secretary of this Council.

So rapidly had interest in military medicine developed that it became necessary to make the periodical *War Medicine* a monthly magazine. The American Medical Association was being represented in many different capacities before congressional committees dealing with income tax deductions for medical care and similar problems.

EDUCATION IN WAR TIME

Now came a joint session of the executive council of the Association of American Medical Colleges and the members of the Council on Medical Education and Hospitals to develop a suitable program for medical education in the war period. Of principal importance was the consideration of the accelerated curriculum.

At the request of General Lewis B. Hershey, director of the Selective Service System, Dr. R. G. Leland, director of the Bureau of Medical Economics, had become a member of the Health and Medical Committee of that Service. Indeed by this time there were so many requests for liaison representatives of the American Medical Association to other organizations that it became necessary for the full Board of Trustees to authorize the executive committee to make such appointments. Many of these requests demanded immediate action.

Difficulties were developing in the relationships of clinical pathologists to hospitals and of chemists to clinical pathologic laboratories. Nursing education was demanding the cooperation of the medical profession. Since 1938 THE JOURNAL had been publishing a Student Section but now the demands on medical students had become so great and the demands on the Association for the use of its pages had so greatly increased that it was decided to discontinue the Student Section of THE JOURNAL with the end of the year.

The task of the special committee for medical personnel for Britain was ended and thanks had been received from Great Britain and from the National Research Council for the assistance given by the Association.

At this time also there came to the Board of Trustees news of the death of Mrs. Emily Cushing who had made abstracts in THE JOURNAL OF THE AMERICAN MEDICAL ASSOCIATION from 1895 on a part-time basis and from 1907 to 1928 as a full-time employee. She died at the age of 88.

ATLANTIC CITY MEETING

The Distinguished Service Medal for 1942 was given to Dr. Ludvig Hektoen of Chicago. Drs. George Crile and Elliott P. Joslin were the other nominees.

Dr. Frank H. Lahey, the president, paid tribute to the work of the Board of Trustees in their conduct of the affairs of the Association and to the secretary and editor of the Association for the aid and comfort that had been given to him through their years of experience. He told of the work of the Procurement and Assignment Service of which he was chairman, he predicted a long war and warned against optimism. He said:

"We do not suffer from the urgency of the situation that the Japs or the Germans do. They must win or die. There is no urge like that of necessity, and it is my opinion that this country is still not convinced that its situation is one of urgent necessity."

The president elect, Dr. Fred W. Rankin, spoke too of organization for the war in all its aspects and he emphasized the necessity for continuous training of medical students, interns and residents. Finally he suggested the necessity for more clinical conferences and for graduate education of general practitioners.

The program of the Farm Security Administration was presented to the House of Delegates by the Bureau of Medical Economics along with all the work that this Bureau was doing in relationship to military service. An extensive report came from the Committee on Medical Preparedness telling of the participation of the headquarters officials in many agencies of national defense. Thus the report said:

"Dr. Olin West, Secretary and General Manager of the American Medical Association, has acted as secretary of the Committee on Medical Preparedness of the American Medical Association, consultant to officials of the Selective Service System and the Office of Defense Health and Welfare, and member of consultant committee, National Roster of Scientific and Specialized Personnel.

"Dr. Morris Fishbein, editor of THE JOURNAL OF THE AMERICAN MEDICAL ASSOCIATION, has served as chairman of the Committee on Information, Division of Medical Sciences, National Research Council, consultant to the Medical Committee, Office of Scientific Research and Development, consultant to the Selective Service System and Office of Defense, Health and Welfare, chairman of the Committee on Information, Procurement and Assignment Service, editor of War Medicine and vice chairman of the Medical Committee, Civilian Defense, City of Chicago."

The bureaus, councils and other agencies of the headquarters office had been enrolled in many activities related to the winning of the war. Unfortunately the needs of the war had also interfered with several movements in process at the time when the war began. The committee to study the relationship of medicine and the law had had meetings. It had been impossible to create a committee to confer with specialty boards because the war had drawn so many of the important members of such agencies into the service.

The Council on Medical Education and Hospitals had brought out new essentials for an approved internship. Most extensive of all of the reports was that of the Committee on Medical Preparedness. This committee recommended the appointment of a new group to be known as the Committee on Participation of the Medical Profession in the War Effort. Another special committee reported on motor vehicle accidents. Then came resolutions dealing with medical service plans and one on preserving the system of medicine so that men returning from the war would not find themselves in a medical practice that had entirely changed its nature. The roentgenologists were more and more disturbed by the extent by which hospitals were practicing medicine, particularly roentgenology. Other resolutions approved the activities of the National Physicians' Committee for the Extension of Medical Service.

To this session of the House of Delegates came the Surgeon General of the Army to tell of what was being done with medical care in the armed forces. The Hon. Paul V. McNutt, Director of the Office of Defense, Health and Welfare, was particularly concerned with difficulties in the recruitment of doctors. He called for 20,000 more physicians with an average of 3,000 a month for the next six months. In his address to the House of Delegates, he concluded:

"The methods which your officers have recommended and which have been set up in the Procurement and Assignment Service give so much more promise of fairness and equity than any other system which might have been resorted to that I want to see it work! And I give you my pledge, as I gave it to Frank Lahey; I give you my pledge that I will do anything in my power to help make it work.

"Moreover, the success of this program will be reflected in the type of practice which the profession may be expected to resume after the war is over. In boom defense towns such as Radford, Va., Charlestown, Ind., Mobile, Ala., Rantoul, Sparta and other areas, there is little hope that a doctor may count on a long and well established practice. There is money in those towns now, but their economy will certainly sag after the war. We hope it doesn't sag, but if we are frank with ourselves and if we really look at the situation, we think that it will sag. There is need, there is very definite need, for government assistance to provide clinical equipment, facilities for medical care and otherwise to help in bearing the capital costs of servicing these communities. There is a definite responsibility, however, to man those areas with thoroughly competent physicians. I am not talking politics and I am not talking social theory. I am talking only plain, hard facts when I say it will have to be done, on your basis I hope, but, if not, on another basis."

Another resolution, introduced by Dwight L. Wilbur, California, demanded condemnation of rebates by commercial organizations to physicians. The reference committee said:

"It is the opinion of your reference committee that the practice referred to in the resolutions are beneath the dignity of the learned profession, are basically dishonest and are a violation of the Principles of Medical Ethics."

They directed that a copy of this statement be sent to every state medical society.

There were resolutions on safeguarding women in industry, and on the improvement of relations between physicians and insurance companies.

The new War Participation Committee was created with a membership of five members and included the president, president elect, chairman of the Board of Trustees, the secretary and editor as ex officio members.

As this session came to its end, Dr. Emily D. Barringer, New York, received unanimous consent to introduce a new resolution. Her proposal was a demand that more women physicians be allowed to participate in the war and that the editor of THE JOURNAL be requested to write a sympathetic editorial on the subject and that THE JOURNAL print a full and detailed report relative to it from the American Medical Women's Association. After some discussion, the motion was lost.

Dr. James E. Paullin was made president elect.

The president of the Association, Dr. Fred W. Rankin, was concerned with the responsibility of medicine in war time. He discussed every phase of medical care during the war and he concluded:

"Changes, unavoidable and unpleasant, face us in our daily and professional lives; we do not speak of the inevitable essential sacrifices, we speak rather of the glories of service. To serve is our destiny, to serve freely, faithfully and effectively is our wish and ambition. Our duty is plain to see: We shall go forward to our task, and we shall not fail."

From the Coordinator of Information in Washington, D.C., came a request that the editor of THE JOURNAL prepare a news letter every two weeks on the advancement of medical sciences in the United States which was to be sent through the State Department to the Allied Nations with a view to keeping them informed of the progress being made in the United States. The Board of Trustees signified its complete approval of this cooperation. Such a letter was then prepared and has been continued, being circulated in 1947 through the Department of State.

LATIN AMERICAN GUESTS

At the meeting in Atlantic City there had been a fine attendance of Latin American physicians including some of the most distinguished representatives of Chile, Argentina, Brazil, Peru and many of the Central American republics. All had expressed their interest in the medicine of the United States. The movement here initiated was to continue to grow. Unfortunately, however, the Spanish periodical of the American Medical Association has not yet come to fruition because the duration of the war brought about a continuous decrease in the available supply of paper—a situation which still prevailed in 1947. The Association continues to look forward to the possibility of publication of a periodical in Spanish and in Portuguese for distribution to the Latin American nations.

By September of 1942 it became clear that it would not be possible to hold a regular session of the American Medical Association in 1943. The difficulties of transportation and hotel accommodations became increasingly great.

In order that THE JOURNAL might continue to receive the best of material, the editor planned for the development of manuscripts with discussions through the officers of the various sections.

The editor had made an address in Detroit and as a result of reference to osteopathy, suit had been brought by the Wayne County Association of Physicians and Surgeons of Osteopathic Medicine against the editor. After a month or two, that suit was dismissed.

The Association was being asked to set up a special council for testing diagnostic devices. A special committee had been developed for tests of intoxication which was working with the National Research Council. Plans were under way for increased interest of the Association in physical therapy and rehabilitation. The American Association for Health, Physical Education and Recreation was taking up the problem of physical fitness and the Association was engaged in active liaison with this group. This project was to become eventually a national committee on physical fitness under the Federal Security Agency.

There were proposals through the Council on Industrial Health for the safeguarding of women in industry. The War Participation Committee was especially concerned with the medical care of the civilian population and with active work in the field of civilian defense. Meetings continued to be held with the hospital associations dealing particularly with the inclusions of medical surveys as part of services rendered by hospitals and with the inadequacy of available personnel to carry on the work of the hospitals on a high plane. More and more employees were entering military service; the difficulties of carrying on the work of the headquarters office were multiplying. The terrific drive on the medical students through the accelerated program made necessary the development of a special committee on student health.

1943

The war was still engaging most of the interest and attention of the people of the United States. Throughout the nation publishing was becoming more and more difficult because of continuous reduction in the amount of paper available. The periodicals of the Association began to economize by increasing the size of the page, decreasing the size of the type and decreasing the total number of pages. Plans for the meeting of the House of Delegates in lieu of an annual session began to be discussed early in the year.

The State Department was continuously in negotiation with the Board of Trustees on the possibility of cooperation with the American Medical Association in the publication of a Spanish and Portuguese periodical. The entrance of many hundreds of thousands of women into American industry made desirable special action by the Council on Industrial Health. A committee was appointed by the Section on Obstetrics and Gynecology to deal with safeguarding the health of women in industry. Both the Board of Trustees and the Section on Ophthalmology were interested in developing a new program for the conservation of vision. The Council on Medical Education and Hospitals was extending its standardization and survey activities. Among other studies it had completed a survey of ten schools for medical record librarians and had prepared the minimum essentials of an acceptable school.

From Dr. James E. Paullin, president elect, came a plan for the extension of training of physicians both in and out of the armed forces, to be sponsored by the American Medical Association working with the American College of Surgeons and the American College of Physicians. This problem had been first discussed at a meeting of the War Participation Committee of the American Medical Association. As a result of these efforts and with the financial assistance of the American Medical Association graduate education was greatly extended. The young men who were taking the accelerated curriculum in the medical schools were given opportunity in the armed forces to extend their abbreviated courses of training. Dr. Paullin also presented plans for a complete program of postwar medical care not only for the people of the United States but also for its allies and its enemies.

As a part of its contribution to the war effort the Association participated in a National Conference on Planning for War and Postwar Medical Services, which was held in New York City in March 1943. At this conference Thomas T. Mackie presented a paper on "War and the Migration of Tropical Diseases," Thomas Francis, Jr. on "Epidemiology of Influenza," L. T. Coggeshall on "Malaria as a World Menace," John B. Youmans on "Nutritional Diseases as a Postwar Problem," A. R. Dochez on "Trends in Scientific Research." At an afternoon session there were addresses on "Health—A World Problem" by F. P. Keppel, "Work of the Red Cross in Postwar Medical Rehabilitation" by Richard F. Allen, "Inter-American Cooperation" by Nelson A. Rockefeller, and "American Medicine's Contribution to Postwar Medical Service" by Morris Fishbein. This program received nation-wide attention through extension by the press and it had both an inspirational and an educational value.

By this time also it began to be apparent that general practitioners were being gradually shelved because of the rise of the certifying boards in the various medical specialties and the desires of the hospitals to limit their staffs to men who had been thus certified. The problem was presented to the Board of Trustees and was made a special subject of study by the Council on Medical Education and Hospitals.

The problems which concerned the Association were the ever recurring problems of the relationship of medicine to law, the relationship of physician to patient in prepayment hospitalization plans, the problems of hospital corporations which were engaging in the practice of medicine, and relations of physicians to insurance companies.

It was found impossible to continue the publication of the American Medical Directory, which ordinarily would have appeared in 1944, because of the vast number of physicians who were already in the armed forces.

The absence of the annual session of the Association with the hundreds of manuscripts usually presented on such occasions made necessary planning for the preparation of symposiums developed by the editor of THE JOURNAL in cooperation with the officers of the individual sections. By this technic a high quality of medical material was continuously available for publication in THE JOURNAL. Through correspondence, it became possible to publish not only the original contributions but also discussions by selected physicians. It was an annual session *in absentia*.

1943

CHICAGO

When the House of Delegates met in Chicago at the Palmer House, its first task was the election of the recipient for the Distinguished Service Medal. The honor went to Dr. Elliott P. Joslin of Boston, noted for his magnificent contributions to the care of persons with diabetes.

The president, Dr. Fred W. Rankin, who was now brigadier general in charge of surgical services in the Office of the Surgeon

General of the Army, referred particularly to the problems of war but he turned his attention also to the mighty influences that were at work to effect epochal changes in the complexion of medical practice. He recognized that these had long been forming and that the military conflict had hurried their development. "We must face realistically," he said, "these tremendous socioeconomic trends."

The president elect, Dr. James E. Paullin, called attention to the establishment of the Procurement and Assignment Service as a federal agency and to the part played by the American Medical Association in the war services. He was particularly interested in the extension of medical education and in the planning of the wartime medical meetings.

At this meeting Surgeon General Norman T. Kirk spoke of the contribution of the American Medical Association to the war effort.

Mr. George M. Morris, president of the American Bar Association, complimented the American Medical Association on its activities and indicated that the American Bar Association might well be guided by a similar program. Thus he said:

"In connection with the formulation of our procedure and fundamental concepts in the American Bar Association, the experience of the American Medical Association was an invaluable aid. It always seemed an anachronism to me, but nevertheless it was true, that here were the lawyers who would be expected to be the pioneers in a legislative group like this taking their lessons from their brother professionals the medics on how to do the job that the lawyers themselves ought to know how to do. It is a great compliment to the men who have had the management of the American Medical Association under hand for many years that that particular thing should have taken place, and we, therefore, I say on behalf of the American Bar Association, are greatly indebted to you for this example in helping us institute an agency which has meant more to the American Bar Association's successful functioning in its community effort than any single agency that has been brought into that Association in the twenty-one years I have known it."

The genial secretary of the Canadian Medical Association, Dr. T. C. Routley, who for many years visited meetings of the American Medical Association, spoke, too, of the great pleasure he had had in participating in its work and expressed the hope that Canada might well go along with the American Medical Association in achieving its important medical objectives.

No better account could be published of the extent to which the American Medical Association was participating in the war than to quote from the report of the Board of Trustees:

PARTICIPATION IN THE WAR EFFORT

For more than two years the official and administrative personnel of the American Medical Association and of its councils, bureaus and departments have been actively engaged in efforts designed to contribute to the success of the nation's war program.

Members of all the Councils, the members of the Board of Trustees and the administrative personnel in practically every department have served in various capacities on committees or commissions of official standing in Washington or in other ways have been directly concerned with one or another phase of the war effort and in some instances have devoted a large part of their time to such service. Official representatives of the Association have on numerous occasions been called on to participate in official conferences held in Washington and have attempted in that connection and in many other ways to be as helpful as possible to the federal government.

It has been necessary to make certain phases of the work of some departments secondary in order that the greatest possible contribution might be made toward the successful prosecution of the war. The number of male employees of the Association fully eligible for war service has been comparatively small. At the time of the preparation of this report thirty-five employees of the Association including members of its professional staff as well as workers in other capacities have been assigned to active duty with the military forces. Five young women of the Association's personnel have been assigned to duty with the Women's Army Auxiliary Corps, and others are contemplating entering on a similar service.

A suboffice of the Procurement and Assignment Service for Physicians, Dentists and Veterinarians was established some months ago in the headquarters of the Association and is now operating intensively under the direction of Lieut. Col. H. C. Lueth of the Medical Corps of the Army of the United States. Practically all persons engaged in this particular work are Civil Service employees. This suboffice is engaged in compiling material for the use of the Procurement and Assignment Service and for the use of the Army, Navy, Public Health Service and other government agencies that may wish to utilize such data and is otherwise pursuing activities designed to be helpful to the government, to the civilian population and to the medical profession as a whole in its relations to the war program.

Many official releases from various federal offices have been published in THE JOURNAL and several large mailings of informational material have been made from the offices of the Association at the request of responsible officials of government departments.

Thousands of individual communications from physicians and laymen pertaining to medical service with the military forces or to conditions created by the world war have poured in to the Association's offices and, whenever possible and permissible, these communications have received careful attention and replies intended to be helpful to those concerned.

In order that the members of the House of Delegates may be informed as to the specific nature of some of the services that have been performed by officers, members of official bodies and the administrative personnel of the Association in connection with the war program of the federal government, the following information is offered:

The P resident of the American Medical Association, Brig. Gen. Fred W. Rankin, Medical Corps, Army of the United States, has been on active duty assigned to the Office of the Surgeon General in Washington for more than a year. The President-Elect, Dr. James E. Paullin, is a member of the Directing Board of the Procurement and Assignment Service for Physicians, Dentists and Veterinarians and is also a member of one or more committees of the Division of Medical Sciences of the National Research Council. Dr. Harvey B. Stone, a member of the Council on Medical Education and Hospitals, is a member of the Directing Board of the Procurement and Assignment Service. Members of the Council on Pharmacy and Chemistry, the Council on Physical Therapy, the Council on Foods and Nutrition and the Council on Industrial Health are members of important scientific committees working under government auspices in Washington, and some of them are serving in other capacities.

The executive officers of all the councils and the directors of all the bureaus of the Association have attempted whenever opportunity has offered to be helpful to government departments and bureaus in various matters pertaining to war service. Dr. Paul C. Barton, Director of the Bureau of Investigation and assistant to the Secretary, has been on duty in Washington for about four months. In compliance with requests received from several official agencies of the government, the facilities of the Association have been used for the purpose of distributing rather large quantities of informative material.

Under the direction of the Editor of THE JOURNAL, a scientific news letter is prepared every two weeks, which is sent under the auspices of the Committee on Information of the Division of Medical Sciences of the National Research Council to medical officers of the Army, Navy, and Public Health Service. For the Navy, this material is incorporated in a fortnightly letter issued under the title "Bumed," and this letter, in accordance with a special request, is being sent also to the air force of the Canadian army and is issued to the medical officers of that force. The editor of THE JOURNAL also serves as consultant to various offices and committees in Washington and is a member of a committee on drugs and medical supplies of the Division of Medical Sciences of the National Research Council and vice chairman of the Medical Committee of Civilian Defense for the City of Chicago.

The Library of the Association, with the cooperation of the Editorial Department, has assembled material relating to health conditions in various parts of the world for a division of the medical department of the U. S. Army. Through the Current Medical Literature Department bibliographies and abstracts concerned especially with problems of military medicine have been prepared and submitted to federal agencies. From these abstracts collective reports and reviews are prepared which are published subsequently in WAR MEDICINE. A member of the editorial staff has directed the preparation of abstracts issued fortnightly covering progress in medical science for an important government office, and these abstracts are circulated in mimeographed form by that office in a manner that makes the material available in many parts of the world. Some of this material has been republished in periodicals in several countries. The director of the Department of Press Relations is serving as a member of committees or sub committees of official government agencies in Washington and in somewhat similar capacity for the Emergency Medical Services of the Office of Civilian Defense in Chicago.

The Association has attempted to make the greatest possible contribution toward the winning of the war, and the Board of Trustees has authorized the active participation of the Association's administrative personnel in efforts designed to accomplish that end. In extending such cooperation to the government, the Association has received most valuable aid from government officials and desires to express its grateful appreciation of many courtesies graciously extended and for valuable assistance and cordial cooperation offered by those officials.

The House of Delegates heartily commended these activities of the Association which had been so effectively carried out under the leadership of the Board.

Of special significance at this session of the Association was the report of the Bureau of Medical Economics since it not only referred to the vast studies that it had made but also to the many plans for voluntary insurance against the costs of hospitalization and illness which were developing in various states, the dangers to be avoided by such plans, and the vital factors to be recognized and protected. Thus it said:

"A prepayment plan for medical care is complex. It touches closely nearly all emotions, prejudices and customs in our society. It lacks the experience and evolution common to most social institutions. Compulsory sickness insurance systems in every country, and throughout their entire history, have been subject to continuous changes. In spite of their anchorage to legislation and government regulation, none as yet show any signs of approaching equilibrium. It is therefore not surprising that plans of such duration as those of medical societies in the United States are still largely experimental "

HOSPITALS PRACTICING MEDICINE

In a supplementary report by the Board of Trustees was a statement of the many studies that had been made under its direction. Then came a presentation of a most extensive report on the problems of hospital corporations engaging in the practice of medicine. These dealt particularly with the abuses related to the practice of roentgenology and of clinical pathology. During the year the Board of Trustees of the American Medical Association had had a conference with a committee of the American Hospital Association to consider these important questions. The report of that conference was supplemented by studies of plans in various portions of the United States and particularly as they were concerned in these specialties. The report had been largely prepared by Drs. R. L. Sensenich and Ernest E. Irons; its importance cannot be overestimated since it allayed to a considerable extent the unrest that was developing throughout the nation in regard to the manner in which hospital corporations were taking over the practice of these specialties. In 1937 the House of Delegates had approved the following principle: "The subscriber's contract should exclude all medical services; contract provision should be limited exclusively to hospital facilities." Again it was emphasized that this statement is clear and until it is changed by the House of Delegates, must be considered as representing the policies of the American Medical Association.

When the House of Delegates came to the consideration of new proposals, it followed the pattern which had begun to be established by years of experience.

From a number of individual states came resolutions for the establishing of a committee on medical service which would be especially concerned with problems relating to the establishment of prepayment plans for rendering medical care.

At this time also discussions which had been proposed from time to time leading to the establishment of an office of the American Medical Association in Washington began to culminate in resolutions calling on the Board of Trustees to proceed with the establishment of such an office.

As the session went on, there came an address by Brig. Gen. David N. W. Grant, flight surgeon for the Air Force of the Army Medical Department.

Since the activities related to medical service plans, to the federal security law, and to the creation of a council or committee on medical service dealt with matters of intimate importance to the Association, their consideration was brought before the executive session. The reference committee which had the matter for consideration proposed as a solution of the problems of medical service the creation of a council on legal medicine and legislation, to be created at once. The Board of Trustees had met with the reference committee to which this proposal was referred and proposed as an alternative the formation of a Council on Medical Service and Public Relations, stating its composition and defining carefully the duties of this council. An amendment was prepared for the By-Laws to incorporate the council into the formal activities of the Association. The story of this council and its work is told in another chapter.

In the elections, Dr. Herman L. Kretschmer of Chicago was unanimously chosen president elect.

As the war went on, THE JOURNAL's department of "Medicine and the War" continued.

At the annual session of the Association the president, Dr. James E. Paullin, devoted his entire address to the planning of medical service for present needs and future requirements. From the inspiration thus developed by Dr. Paullin came eventually the Committee on Postwar Medical Service which, in turn, was merged into the Joint Committee on Medical Activities.

During the meeting a special war session was held with addresses by representative leaders in the armed forces including the surgeons general of the Army, Navy and the Public Health Service.

THE WAGNER-MURRAY-DINGELL BILL

Just before the meeting of the American Medical Association Senator Wagner of New York for himself and Senator Murray of Montana with the aid of Congressman Dingell of Michigan in the House of Representatives introduced the Wagner-Murray-Dingell social security plan. This was another effort to force compulsory sickness insurance on the people of the United States and it was bitterly opposed by the American Medical Association through all of its agencies.

More and more the activities of the Association turned to problems of the war. The national broadcast of the Association during this year was devoted to "Doctors at War."

The Council on Industrial Health was concerned with absenteeism in industries.

COOPERATIVE ADVERTISING BUREAU

Difficulties began to develop with regard to relaxation of standards of advertising by some of the periodicals which were associated in the Cooperative Medical Advertising Bureau. The Board of Trustees, abiding by the high principles which had animated the creation of this bureau, began to take special interest in its affairs with a view to insisting on the stipulation that all members of this bureau follow the Councils of the American Medical Association in their acceptances of advertising.

The Association was cooperating with the Treasury Department in the sale of War Bonds.

Eighteen thousand copies of THE JOURNAL were being sent to physicians in the armed forces outside the borders of the United States.

DIFFICULTIES IN 1944

Difficulties with labor among the personnel of the headquarters office began to concern the Board of Trustees early in 1944, as they were already beginning to concern every industry in the United States. Constant negotiations were necessary to meet the demands for changes in hours of work and payment.

An Office of Information had been established by the Council on Medical Service in Washington, under Dr. Joseph Lawrence. Its members were meeting frequently with a view to encouraging the development of prepayment medical care plans.

The Association was cooperating with many federal agencies in the war effort. It was aiding in the training of physicians in physical therapy. Its Committee on Postwar Medical Service was meeting regularly to consider particularly the provision of graduate training for physicians as they came from the armed forces. Plans for social security were beginning to agitate many national organizations. The manuals on occupational therapy and physical therapy, prepared by the American Medical Association, were being routinely used by the physicians in the armed forces.

Of particular importance were the relations of officers of the American Medical Association to the Division of Medical Sciences of the National Research Council where they were associated with the development of lists of essential drugs and standards for the control and distribution of food. The problems of the maintenance of an adequate supply of medical students began to concern the Council on Medical Education and Hospitals.

Other members of the personnel of the Association were cooperating with the National Education Association and with the U. S. Office of Education and with the Federal Security Agency in developing a program of physical fitness. The National Advisory Council on Physical Fitness of the Federal Security Agency had asked the Association's cooperation in this program, and Drs. R. L. Sensenich as chairman, Louis A. Buie, Morris Fishbein, George F. Lull and

William D. Stroud were appointed as a committee to fulfil this obligation.

The Board of Trustees also took under advisement the establishment of an office in the headquarters for the dissemination of information on the location and relocation of physicians in the postwar period.

An American Council on Rheumatic Fever had been formed and the Board of Trustees in behalf of the American Medical Association accepted membership on this council and contributed to its formation and delegated representatives to its conferences.

THE CHICAGO SESSION

Again the House of Delegates met in Chicago in a small meeting due to the fact that it was impossible to hold a full session during the war.

The Distinguished Service Medal was awarded to Dr. George Dock of Pasadena, California. The other nominees were Drs. Isaac A. Abt of Chicago and Simon Flexner of New York.

The president, Dr. James E. Paullin, spoke to the House of Delegates on the Wartime Graduate Medical Meetings, postwar planning activities, the supply of medical students and the provision of medical care. The agitation that had developed in the campaign against the Wagner-Murray-Dingell bill had begun to disturb the medical profession and the public. Dr. Paullin ended his address with a plea for unity within the organization.

Dr. Herman L. Kretschmer in his address to the House of Delegates complimented the official staff of the Association, including particularly the editor and the general manager, for their work. He paid special tribute to the vast amount of work being carried on by the Board of Trustees. He emphasized particularly the desirability of better teaching in the prescribing of drugs, and improvement in the scientific medical programs of American medicine.

The Council on Medical Education and Hospitals was now particularly concerned with the prospective shortage of medical students.

The Board of Trustees reported to the House of Delegates the numerous cooperative relationships with such agencies as the Joint Committee on Health Problems in Education of the National Education Association and the American Medical Association; the Advisory Committee to the U. S. Children's Bureau, the National Committee for Boys and Girls Club Work, the National Congress of Parents and Teachers, and many other similar organizations.

The Bureau of Legal Medicine was confronted with new laws relating to obstetrics and pediatric care for the wives and infants of servicemen, with new legislation on the reorganization of the medical services in the armed forces, on additional hospital facilities for veterans, medical care for recruited and migrant farm workers, selective service and training act amendments, nutrition, vital statistics, social security, industrial health, a great variety of taxes and, of course, the Wagner-Murray-Dingell bill.

The Bureau of Medical Economics was similarly concerned with a considerable number of plans for extending medical care. There were special reports of the Committee on Wartime Graduate Medical Meetings, the Committee to Study Air Conditioning, the Committee on Motor Vehicle Accidents, the Committee on Conservation of Vision, and other subjects.

The Council on Medical Education and Hospitals had been compelled to work out many adjustments in its activities in relationship to the acceleration of the curriculum.

Now came also the first report of the Council on Medical Service and Public Relations dealing with its organization and the methods of its work and an extensive supplementary report with the presentation of a national program for the extension of medical care to the American people.

The War Participation Committee and the Committee on Postwar Medical Service also presented extensive contributions of their considerations of these subjects.

A resolution was introduced to create a certifying board for general practitioners. From California came resolutions to create a national department of public health, for a survey of public opinion relative to American medicine and for the support of the United Public Health League which had been developed in California to mold public opinion. There were other resolutions requesting retirement of the secretary of the American Medical Association and limitation of the duties of the editor.

Again the problems of relationship between hospitals and radiologists, anesthetists and pathologists were considered by the House of Delegates.

To the executive session came a plea for recognition of Negro physicians; the reference committee urged the component societies to extend all aid that is practical to the Negro physicians in their communities. It was still recognized, however, that the decision as to membership in the component county medical societies or on hospital staffs was outside the jurisdiction of the American Medical Association.

The resolutions of the California State Medical Association relative to the secretary and the editor were returned to the House of Delegates by the reference committee with the following statement:

"Never before has American medicine been so needful as now of unity. The desire to extend the high quality of medical service to all the people at a reasonable cost is the objective sought by all of us. Your committee is convinced that this can be attained more certainly if physicians throughout the nation would give their loyalty and support to those selected by this House of Delegates as members of the Board of Trustees and to the representatives selected by the Board itself.

"Your committee commends the loyalty and the efficiency with which these officers have for many years served the Association in carrying out the policies established by the House of Delegates. Your committee would also commend the Board of Trustees of the Association for its judgment and wisdom in the management of the affairs of the Association.

"Therefore the Reference Committee on Executive Session recommend that these resolutions be not approved."

To this session of the House of Delegates came a distinguished lieutenant general of the Chinese Army, Robert Kho-sheng Lim, expressing the appreciation of the Chinese for services rendered to Chinese medicine. Again the surgeons general of the Army, Navy and the Air Force addressed the House of Delegates.

By a special resolution, Dr. Roger I. Lee was requested to resign his position as trustee immediately, thereby removing constitutional bars to his eligibility as candidate for president elect.

At the election Dr. Roger I. Lee was unanimously chosen president-elect.

The president, Dr. Herman L. Kretschmer, in his address dealt with American medicine and the war. He spoke of American medicine for our troops, of national nutrition and of the problems of the aged. He condemned socialized medicine and urged greater support of prepayment plans. He spoke of the armed forces and assured them that the Association was doing everything in its power to safeguard the quality of practice in their absence and to aid them on their return.

As the new Council on Medical Service took form, repeated conferences with the Board of Trustees led to the establishment of specific duties.

The Board of Trustees aided the American Red Cross in establishing its blood donor service.

Continuous studies were carried on with a view to developing postgraduate courses for physicians returning from the war. The Board of Trustees began to take under serious advisement the development of retirement and insurance plans for the employees of the headquarters office. Much thought was given to the difficulties of the prepayment plans and arrangements were established to coordinate information concerning all such plans.

The Board began to give special consideration to problems of public relations which were being widely extended through the Bureau of Health Education and other agencies of the Association.

The publications of the Association were finding greater and greater difficulties in meeting the demands upon them because of the shortage of paper and difficulties in printing. The "Handbook of Nutrition," prepared by the Association, had already been translated into Spanish and permission was given also for translation into Chinese.

As the war neared its end, a request came from the Division of Medical Sciences of the National Research Council relative to the establishment of a Therapeutic Trials Committee by the American Medical Association which would be able to carry on the coordinated and intensified study of new products introduced into medicine. The board gave favorable consideration to this proposal.

THE CENTURY ENDS, 1945-1947

WILL C. BRAUN, who had served for fifty-four years in the Business Department of the Association, wished to retire. He requested retirement before December 31, 1945; in connection with this retirement he proposed a plan for continuing the work of this department.

At the same time Mr. Lawrence C. Salter, who had been employed for some years as director of the Bureau of Public Relations in association with the editor of THE JOURNAL, indicated that he wished to retire and Mr. John L. Bach, a newspaperman, was selected to carry on that work.

The plans of the Council on Medical Service and Public Relations had proceeded to the point where they wished to employ a director of medical prepayment insurance.

The Association was requested by the U. S. Public Health Service to participate in considerations on the disposal of surplus properties to health agencies and medical institutions. Dr. Fishbein was delegated to represent the Association in these conferences.

The Wagner-Murray-Dingell bill began to receive special consideration as did also the Hill-Burton bill for the construction of hospitals in the postwar period.

Difficulties with the Veterans Administration were coming to a focus; these led eventually to the passing of a new act for the Veterans Administration and new methods of operation.

It began to be apparent that the publication in Spanish would not be undertaken unless paper could be provided and there did not seem to be any likelihood that paper supplies would be increased.

As June of 1945 came upon the scene, it was apparent that it would not be possible to hold a meeting of the American Medical Association at the regular time because of a lack of transportation and hotel facilities. The Board of Trustees met in Chicago and worked out a technic for continuation of officers until a meeting could be held.

Of principal concern were the work of the Council on Medical Service and the continuous advancement of various prepayment plans.

FELLOWSHIP FOR VETERANS' PHYSICIANS

The members of the medical staff of the Veterans Administration had been seeking for many years to have the same rights of fellowship in the Association as were granted to officers of the Army, Navy and U. S. Public Health Service. The Judicial Council of the Association did not wish to support such fellowship in view of the lower standards that prevailed in conduct of the hospitals in the Veterans Administration. Later with the reorganization of the Veterans Administration, it became possible to extend fellowship to the permanent officers.

Requests had come from the Associated Women of the American Farm Bureau Federation for a committee to cooperate with them in extending medical care to the rural areas.

The Board of Trustees decided to recognize the increase in interest in medical motion pictures and appointed a special committee to consider this subject.

In September the board discovered that it would be possible to hold a meeting of the House of Delegates in December, thus making it unnecessary to pass a year without electing new officers.

RETIREMENT OF OLIN WEST

Toward the end of the session of the board in June, the secretary and general manager, Dr. Olin West, who had been seriously ill for a considerable period, indicated that he would require some help. Dr. George F. Lull, who had been deputy surgeon general during the war and who was available, had been asked to take the position of assistant to the secretary and general manager.

As the time for the December meeting approached, the editors of the state medical journals were invited to meet with the Board of Trustees. A plan for the Cooperative Bureau, prepared by the editor of THE JOURNAL in consultation with the secretary and Mr. Braun, was submitted to them. The plan involved a reorganization of the Bureau and the establishment of new standards. These met with the instant approval and appreciation of the members of the bureau, thus solving a problem that had been much agitated for several years.

THE CENTENNIAL PROGRAM

At this session also the editor presented a statement containing a complete program for the centennial of the Association to be held in Atlantic City in 1947. The Board of Trustees approved the program and agreed to present it to the House of Delegates at its session. This program also met with the approval of the House of Delegates which appointed a committee consisting of five members

(Drs. E. R. Cunniffe, chairman, Walter F. Donaldson, Thomas P. Murdock, Thomas S. Cullen, and Warren F. Draper) to work with the officers in developing the plans.

THE CHICAGO SESSION

The House of Delegates at its meeting in Chicago in December selected for its Distinguished Service Award Dr. George R. Minot, distinguished as the discoverer of a practical method of treatment for pernicious anemia. The other nominees were Drs. A. J. Carlson and Isaac A. Abt.

The speaker of the House of Delegates, Dr. Harrison H. Shoulders, spoke especially of the soul of medicine in an inspiring address which stirred the House of Delegates. He said in conclusion:

> Sociologists, economists and political scientists have made strenuous attempts to bring medicine under the domination of one or all of these groups through the mechanism of legislative enactment. Their efforts have failed. Their lack of success, in my opinion, is due not so much to the fact that their proposals were untried and unpractical as to their failure to recognize and take into account the soul of medicine.
>
> The responsibility for the continued preservation of the best in American medicine still rests largely in the hands of this House of Delegates. Let us again, now as in the past, concern ourselves, with advancing the science of medicine, with maintaining the standards of medical education and with delivering a higher quality of medical service, ever mindful that science without a soul may be cruel and inhumane, whereas science possessed of a soul is the very highest achievement—the apotheosis of humanity.

The president, Dr. Herman L. Kretschmer, urged greater interest by physicians in general in the problems of the medical profession. He attacked particularly the attempts to regiment the practice of medicine. He hoped also for more careful consideration of the programs of county medical societies; he condemned the unscientific use of hormones. He urged less restriction on animal experimentation. He recognized the problems involved in the advancement of medical students and in the care of chronic illness and he spoke particularly of the great question of providing suitably for the returning medical officers:

> "As I view the years that have passed we have not given an inch of ground to the opposition but have gone steadily forward, advancing medical science, extending medical service and gaining leadership in all the world for American medicine. This is no time for retreat. Let us go forward in the firm belief that we are waging a battle for the right, for the ideals on which medicine must stand or fall, for the advancement of the science of medicine and for the elimination of unnecessary suffering and disease."

At this time Major General Paul R. Hawley, the new surgeon general of the Veterans Administration, was introduced to the House of Delegates.

Then the president elect, Dr. Roger I. Lee, spoke to the House of Delegates and dealt largely with its functions as a legislative body in a medical democracy. He urged a midwinter session of the House. He called attention particularly to the multiplication of councils and bureaus and the many functions of the Association which were not well understood by its members. He gave high praise to the publications of the Association, admittedly the best in their given fields.

The Council on Medical Education and Hospitals was now concerned with postwar problems, such as the supply of premedical and medical students and the supply of physicians. It had to consider deceleration as it had formerly considered acceleration of the curriculum. It had to call attention to the continuance of graduate education courses for practicing physicians and the effects of new legislation regarding hospitals and medical facilities. The council recognized the existence of several new medical schools. It had collaborated with many other agencies in consideration of the problems of medical education and particularly with agencies in the field of nursing.

COUNCIL ON MEDICAL SERVICE

An extensive report by the Council on Medical Service indicated that it was entering more and more into the work of the organization. Perhaps the most significant of its developments was a constructive program for medical care which included fourteen major points. Later by condensation and modification this became the ten-point program for the nation's health of the American Medical Association. Further discussion of this program will appear later in this volume.

This council had employed several new officers to be concerned particularly with the extension of voluntary prepayment medical care plans. A conference had been held on public relations and another dealing with the fourteen point program, still others with legislation and with the government's maternal and infant care programs. All these came before the House for its consideration. There were extensive reports on rural medical services and on postwar medical service.

The new resolutions coming before the House of Delegates dealt with the creation of a Committee on Medical Preparedness, on the problems of the veterans and on medical care.

From California came a resolution designed to limit employees of the Association specifically to the positions for which they were appointed.

Major General Paul R. Hawley won encomiums from the House of Delegates in a statement dealing with plans for the organization of the Veterans Administration.

Other resolutions concerned the national health program of the Association, and many others dealt with problems related to medical care.

From California came a half dozen additional resolutions dealing with the relation of the Association to the public and with the functions of the Council on Medical Service.

There were other resolutions dealing with approval by the American Medical Association of the work of the National Physicians' Committee. This voluntary organization had developed tremendously under the leadership of Dr. Edward H. Cary of Dallas, Texas. The purpose of the National Physicians Committee was to defend medicine against federalization and to develop plans for the widest possible extension of medical service.

The resolutions from California were referred to a special reference committee in the executive session which responded by a vote of confidence in the Board of Trustees as an agency devoted to and capable of developing and maintaining the most efficient organization possible in the solution of the Association's present pressing problems, provided it has the support of the membership.

The resolution which would have made the Council on Medical Service and Public Relations the sole agency for interpreting the American Medical Association to the people was rejected by the House of Delegates.

PRESIDENT TRUMAN'S HEALTH PROGRAM

Most significant at this session of the House of Delegates was a consideration of the message sent by President Harry S. Truman to the Congress of the United States on September 19 submitting a national health program. Subsequent to this, there had been introduced a new version of the Wagner-Murray-Dingell bill. The House of Delegates, through its adoption of the reference committee's report, clearly indicated its approval of those portions of the President's program which dealt with suitable extensions of medical care to those in need, expansion of preventive medicine, federal aid for the construction of hospitals and health centers and compensation for loss of earnings due to sickness. The House of Delegates was, however, unanimous in its opposition to the adoption of the Wagner-Murray-Dingell bill or the creation of a federal system of compulsory sickness insurance. It quoted from an editorial in THE JOURNAL OF THE AMERICAN MEDICAL ASSOCIATION in expressing its views:

> No one will ever convince the physicians of the United States that the Wagner-Murray-Dingell bill is not socialized medicine. By this measure the medical profession and

the sick whom they treat will be directly under political control. By this measure the great system of private hospitals and community hospitals that has grown up in our country will depend for their continued operation on funds paid to them by a federal government agency. By this measure the philanthropic efforts for the care of the sick, which have been the pride of our nation, will be forever deterred. Through this measure competent young men who would enter the medical profession will be forced to seek other fields of action still remaining under our democracy which still permit the exercise of individual initiative and freedom of thought and action. By this measure doctors in America would become clock watchers and slaves of a system. Now, if ever, those who believe in the American democracy must make their belief known to their representatives, so that the attempt to enslave medicine as first among the professions, industries and trades to be socialized will meet the ignominious defeat it deserves.

In addition, the reference committee gave the following summary of its point of view:

1. The Wagner-Murray-Dingell bill is founded on the false assumption that solution of the medical care problem for the American people is the panacea for all of the troubles of the needy.
2. This is the first step in a plan for general socialization not only of the medical profession but all professions, industry, business and labor.
3. Positive proof exists from experience in other countries that inferior medical service results from compulsory health insurance.
4. A program such as outlined is enormously expensive. It will result in greatly increased taxes for the entire population of the United States.
5. Voluntary prepayment medical plans now in operation in many parts of the United States and which are rapidly increasing in number will accomplish all the objects of this bill with far less expense to the people, and under these plans the public will receive the highest type of medical care without regimentation.

This committee included Edwin S. Hamilton, chairman, Lloyd Noland, John J. Masterson, Edward L. Bortz and Raymond L. Zech.

PUBLIC RELATIONS SURVEY

In the executive session the reference committee reported to the House of Delegates that the Board of Trustees had secured a public relations counsel to survey the public relations of the American Medical Association.

The address of Dr. Roger I. Lee, president at this session of the American Medical Association, dealt with the subject of "What Is Adequate Medical Care?" He told of his first studies for the Committee on the Costs of Medical Care and of the shifting concepts that were developing with the advance of medical science. He recognized particularly the drift toward specialization and the change in methods in diagnosis and treatment that had come with the years. He concluded:

I appreciate the changing conditions as medical science advances with its seven league boots. I appreciate too that our social standards change. But these considerations to my mind only make such studies more imperative. There should be constant and continuing evaluations of the changing conditions. We must know what place the general practitioner and the specialist has in adequate medical care. At the moment there are trends toward specialism within specialties, particularly in surgery. Yet insulin, liver therapy, the sulfonamides and penicillin tend to return many patients to the general practitioner. Likewise there are trends in the utilization of hospitals which must be considered in evaluating medical care. Social conditions both in the home and in industry create changes to which adequate medical care is always a goal, but as we move forward we push the goal ahead.

With the coming of the war came a tremendous demand on the American Medical Association for copies of its periodicals that had been published during the war years and particularly for copies of the Quarterly Cumulative Index Medicus. Unfortunately the lack of sufficient paper and other printing supplies had exhausted most of the copies of the various publications.

PROBLEMS IN 1946

The problems that opened 1946 were the supply of medical students, and continued study of the Spanish and Portuguese journals. Already "New and Nonofficial Remedies," "The Handbook of Nutrition," "Glandular Physiology" and many other publications of the Association were being translated into Spanish.

The new principles for the Cooperative Medical Advertising Bureau had been adopted and were functioning most satisfactorily.

A new Committee on Rural Medical Service was being expanded and was arranging for conferences with representatives of rural groups.

The Board of Trustees had employed the R. T. Rich Associates to make a survey of public relations. Several other public relations organizations had been considered but since the Rich Associates were the only available agency which dealt with "not for profit" organizations rather than with commercial industries, this was the group chosen.

A request had come to the House of Delegates for support of the International Congress on Tropical Medicine, and the Board of Trustees had been authorized to give it every practicable support.

There were requests for study of the nursing problem which was becoming exceedingly acute in the postwar period.

Plans were being made for two sessions of the House of Delegates annually.

A special technic had been developed for extending education to the public on animal experimentation. Articles were being published in Hygeia and extended in such periodicals as Collier's and Reader's Digest.

The continued study of the national health program which had been developed as a fourteen-point program by the Council on

Medical Service led to the final joint adoption by the Board of Trustees and the House of Delegates of the ten-point program which stands today as the official health program of the American Medical Association. This program appears in its entirety in the section on the Council on Medical Service.

Through a series of conferences of representatives of the Council on Medical Service with the Board of Trustees and with officers of the Association, standards were adopted by the Council on Medical Service for medical care plans. In connection with these standards there was developed an association of medical care plans which limited its membership to those plans which met the standards of the council. This was a vital step toward the creation of a national medical care plan composed of constituent state and county voluntary prepayment plans. The name is Associated Medical Care Plans, Inc.

THE SAN FRANCISCO SESSION

When the Association met in San Francisco early in July, the Distinguished Service Award was given to Dr. A. J. Carlson, noted American physiologist. The other nominees were Dr. Torald Sollmann of Cleveland and Dr. Francis Carter Wood of New York.

Dr. Harrison H. Shoulders had been made president elect so that the speaker who presided was Dr. Roy W. Fouts, formerly vice speaker of the House of Delegates. He concerned himself with the organization and procedure of the House of Delegates.

The president, Dr. Roger I. Lee, was particularly concerned with such legislation as the Hill-Burton bill and the bill for a National Science Foundation. Of the latter he said:

> Again the United States government is manifesting a great interest in science and there is likelihood of a very large expenditure of governmental funds for science. Your association has teamed up with other scientific organizations in favoring the development of a National Science Foundation. But while the intent of such legislation is wholly benevolent, the administration and execution of such legislation may be of a different order. Science is a coy and jealous mistress, and her enduring charms are often not purchasable for a fixed price and do not always go to the highest bidder. Then, too, the practice of medicine is an applied science. While the art of medicine with a dash of science is very old, medical science is new. Like it or not, there is an aristocracy of science, which on occasion may be a bit intolerant.

While the House of Delegates was in session, a committee of the U. S. Senate was completing hearings on the Wagner-Murray-Dingell bill which had been going on for months. Before these hearings, the American Medical Association had sent as its representatives Dr. R. L. Sensenich, Dr. Lowell S. Goin of California, Dr. Victor Johnson, secretary of the Council on Medical Education and Hospitals, and Dr. Walter L. Kennedy of Indiana.

Dr. Roger I. Lee made a plea to the younger members of the medical profession to take an active part in the affairs of the Association because the future would far more greatly concern them than the older members of the Association.

The president elect, Dr. Harrison H. Shoulders, spoke of the problems of reconstruction, of the growth of the voluntary prepayment medical service plans, and he made an earnest plea for statesmanship rather than political interest in the affairs of the Association.

At this session of the American Medical Association the Board of Trustees announced the resignation of Dr. Olin West, after twenty-four years of service, and the appointment of Dr. George F. Lull, associate general manager, to the position of general manager. They announced also the retirement of Mr. Will C. Braun, who came to the American Medical Association in November, 1891.

The Board of Trustees announced the receipt of a portion of the public relations survey that had been made and indicated that this report would be made available to the House of Delegates later in the session.

A resolution was offered by the Board of Trustees providing for a supplemental session of the House of Delegates whenever desirable.

Of special interest to the House of Delegates at this session was a consideration of the National Bituminous Wage agreement which had been established by the United Mine Workers of America and the Coal Mines Administration and the mine owners. This was a mine safety program which incorporated a health and welfare program.

There were other resolutions dealing with medical care plans, the care of veterans and the technic of appointment of reference committees.

Again a series of resolutions from the California delegates dealing with the activities of the councils, the editor of THE JOURNAL and other officers and employees of the Association. These were considered in executive session, to which the Board of Trustees presented its report on the survey of public relations. Following the presentation of the report of the survey by the Board of Trustees and the action that it had taken on the survey, the report was adopted. The California delegation then withdrew its resolutions dealing with the activities of the editor.

As the session ended, Dr. Olin West was unanimously chosen president elect.

The By-Laws of the Association were modified to permit a supplemental session to be held in Chicago in December.

The activities of the headquarters office were being tremendously extended with new agencies.

Requests were coming from all over the world for translation of the publications of the Association into many languages.

A national debate in high schools and colleges was to deal with problems related to medical care and the Council on Medical Service was preparing materials for use by debaters who were opposing federalized medicine.

Following this session the Board of Trustees extended its radio program to include broadcasting on the Mutual Network.

Plans were being developed for the centennial session, for extending considerations of rural medical service, for the establishment of a department of public relations, and for studying the war experience of the medical profession to meet any future needs for the medical profession in an emergency.

When the House of Delegates met in December, 1946, it gave final consideration to the report of the Raymond Rich Associates on the public relations of the Association and to a revision of the Constitution and By-Laws.

The printing problems and the adjustment of difficulties with labor had become so great that it became necessary to begin assignment of some of the numerous publications of the Association to other printing organizations. The increase of subscription to THE JOURNAL and other periodicals had overwhelmed the press capacity of the headquarters office. The councils, bureaus and other agencies had begun expanding their activities so that even the maximum space available in the headquarters office was insufficient to house the many activities in process of development.

In the meantime an election had changed the political aspect of the Congress and Senate; it seemed certain that with this change in membership there would be a change in point of view. The threat of socialization of medicine was less imminent than at any time in the previous thirty years.

The Association had been requested to send representatives to a conference in the State Department and Drs. Roger I. Lee and Morris Fishbein had aided in developing a suitable charter for the World Health Organization of the United Nations.

The Association had been asked to participate in the formation of a World Medical Association consisting of representatives of the national medical organizations of most of the great nations. The Association had accepted this membership and Drs. Louis H. Bauer and E. L. Henderson of the Board of Trustees had been chosen to represent the Association in the first annual meeting of this group.

THE CENTENNIAL YEAR

The problem most prominently in the minds of the medical profession in 1947 was the position that would ultimately be held by general practitioners. Movements were afoot to establish a certifying board for general practitioners and to organize an American college for general practice. The Section on General Practice of the American Medical Association had begun functioning actively. The hospitals were endeavoring in many places to arrange for staff positions for general practitioners and the Council on Medical Education and Hospitals had been requested to study the problem of medical teaching and the internship in relationship to general practice. The Bureau of Information of the American Medical Association was endeavoring to secure general practitioners for rural communities and the Committee on Rural Health had discussed the same problem in several conferences. The Joint Committee on Coordination of Medical Activities had added general practice to its agenda. Out of all these discussions perhaps would come some improvement in the critical situation that prevailed. Young men graduating in medicine had in many instances selected their specialty by the time they had completed the sophomore year and looked forward to following the medical curriculum with an internship devoted exclusively to the specialty and after that an assistant residency and a residency with prompt certification by the board.

The Bureau of Medical Economic Research was constituted anew with Frank Dickinson, Ph.D., and several associates.

So greatly had the circulation of THE JOURNAL increased and also that of HYGEIA that it became necessary to secure an outside printer for the latter publication. The many books published by the Association were also being placed with medical publishers, to permit the presses of the Association to concentrate on THE JOURNAL and the specialized scientific publications.

The American Red Cross had in contemplation the establishment of a five-year plan for making available blood, blood plasma and other blood derivatives to all of the people without cost. The editor of THE JOURNAL had been chairman of the special committee of the Medical Advisory Board of the Red Cross which drew up this program, and the Board of Trustees gave the plan their approval.

The chairman of the board and the general manager were cooperating with educational and welfare agencies in conferences on a proposed bill to establish a department of health, education and security in the cabinet.

The editor and the secretary of the Council on Medical Education and Hospitals had been delegated to confer with representatives of all scientific bodies in conferences on the proposed National Science Foundation bill.

The Council on Industrial Health had interested itself in practically every aspect of industrial medicine and was holding annual conferences on medical education.

A special department of public relations had been opened in the headquarters office with Mr. Charles Swart as executive in charge of this activity. With his associates this department was releasing a weekly bulletin to the press on scientific advances, a letter to the secretaries of county and state medical societies and to the House of Delegates, and general publicity on the work of the Association.

Now the Association had dramatic programs on both the National Broadcasting Chain and the Mutual Broadcasting Chain and was broadcasting health through specially prepared "platters" which were being widely used by individual stations.

The Committee on National Emergency Medical Service, under the chairmanship of Dr. Edward L. Bortz, was making a study of the distribution of medical service during the World War just ended and was working on plans for any future emergencies.

A special committee was established for cooperation with the American Dental Association. A report was received from Drs. Harrison H. Shoulders, Austin Smith and Charles Gordon Heyd who had represented the American Medical Association in the Pan-American Social Congress.

The Centennial meeting was assigned to Atlantic City, June 1947. Distinguished guests featured every one of the scientific programs. Most of the leading nations of the world sent official representatives, including the secretary of the British Medical Association and the editor of the British Medical Journal.

At a dinner given by the Board of Trustees for organizations and interests affiliated with medicine, the program included General Omar Bradley, director of the Veterans Administration, Mr. Basil O'Connor, chairman of the American Red Cross and president of the National Foundation for Infantile Paralysis, and Mr. H. W. Prentis, Jr., president of the Armstrong Cork Company and former president of the National Association of Manufacturers.

The Sunday religious service included as participants Monsignor Fulton J. Sheen, Rabbi Joshua Liebman and Dr. Ralph Cooper Hutchison. Both these programs were broadcast to the nation over national networks.

Advance registration indicated the largest attendance at any medical meeting ever held in the world with approximately 15,000 physicians and thousands of exhibitors and guests.

DOCTOR OLIN WEST

WHEN THE HOUSE OF DELEGATES at the San Francisco session in 1946 tendered to Dr. Olin West, by unanimous choice, the presidency of the Association, it was a highly merited recognition of his devoted service to American medicine.

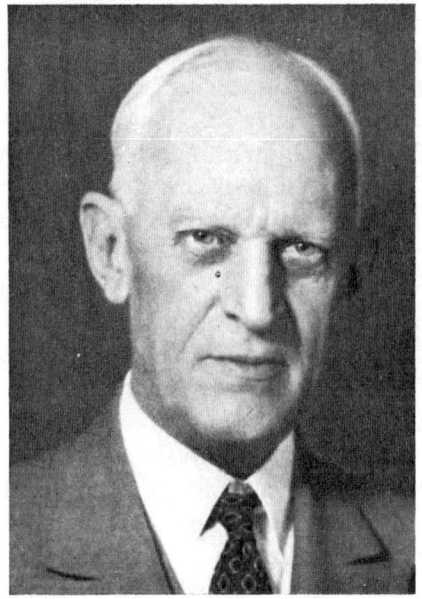

Olin West, M.D.

By an interesting coincidence the first secretary of the American Medical Association, Dr. Alfred Stillé of Philadelphia became president in 1871, and now for the second time in the history of the Association the secretary, Doctor West, after a quarter of a century service, was advanced to the highest honor in the gift of the organized American profession. It was intended that he have the further honor to preside at the Centennial session of the Association at Atlantic City in June 1947.

Dr. Olin West was born July 12, 1874 in Gadsen, Alabama, the son of Rev. Dr. Anson and Sarah Bryant West. He was educated at Howard College in Alabama, and following his graduation he undertook the study of pharmacy in Vanderbilt University, Nashville, Tenn., receiving the Ph. C. degree in 1895, and the degree Doctor of Medicine in 1898. He practiced in Nashville until 1910, during which period he was instructor and associate professor in the medical department of Vanderbilt University. Doctor West served as director of the Rockefeller Sanitary Commission and the International Health Board in Tennessee from 1910 to 1918, and as secretary and executive officer of the Tennessee State Board of Health from 1918 to 1922. He also served as secretary of the Tennessee State Medical Association, and as editor of its journal. Following the death of Dr. Alexander Craig in 1922, Dr. West became secretary of the American Medical Association, and following the retirement of Dr. George H. Simmons, a few years later, he took over the functions of secretary and general manager. His term of service as secretary and general manager of the American Medical Association came to a close on June 30, 1946, when he was succeeded by Dr. George F. Lull, formerly Major General and Deputy Surgeon General, United States Army.

His response as president-elect expressed his strong emotions and gratified appreciation for the high honor that had come to him. He stated that during a quarter century he had watched with pride the growth and expanding opportunities for service of our great association. He was impressed by the constant offensive attitude of the Association during its first hundred years in fighting frauds and fallacies, in providing mediums for the interchange of opinion that would advance the cause of medicine in its efforts to promote the betterment of public health, in defending medicine against the evils of regimentation, and for the establishment and maintenance of high professional and educational standards.

After July 1, 1946, and during his term as president-elect, Dr. Olin West took up his residence in Nashville, Tenn. In March 1947, because of failing health he resigned as President-Elect and was succeeded by Dr. Edward Bortz, Philadelphia.

THE LIBEL SUITS OF THE AMERICAN MEDICAL ASSOCIATION

ONE OF THE HAZARDS OF PUBLISHING is the possibility of being compelled to defend suits for libel or damages by those who have seen their reputations disappear, their profits diminish, their livelihoods destroyed, following exposés. The power of the press should never be minimized. Publication of the facts day after day or even in a single powerful exposé may be sufficient to destroy a false promotional venture in the field of health in a single day.

TWO LOW-GRADE COLLEGES

The campaign of the American Medical Association against unqualified medical schools and against proprietorship in medical education brought two suits against the Association soon after the turn of the century. These suits were filed by medical colleges which found themselves suddenly without students or repute before the state boards of examiners. Evidently those who filed the suits discovered very soon that they had nothing to gain, and the suits were withdrawn. The schools that filed these suits died soon after.

THE "WINE OF CARDUI" SUIT

In 1916 a suit began in the District Court of the United States in the Northern District of Illinois. It was filed by John A. Patten and Zeboim C. Patten, Jr. doing business under the name of the Chattanooga Medicine Company vs. the American Medical Association and George H. Simmons. Two suits were filed, the second by John A. Patten alone against the same defendants.

On April 11 and July 18, 1914, THE JOURNAL OF THE AMERICAN MEDICAL ASSOCIATION published articles dealing with Wine of Cardui, a product manufactured by the Chattanooga Medicine Company. These articles declared, among other things, that the business of the Chattanooga Medicine Company had been built on deceit and that Wine of Cardui was a vicious fraud.

The personal suit of John A. Patten asked $200,000 damages and the company suit asked for $100,000 damages. The cases came to trial on March 21, 1916. In the middle of the trial on April 26 John

A. Patten died and the personal suit automatically ended. The partnership case was continued and the case went to the jury on June 16. The jury brought in a verdict for the plaintiff but assessed the damages at one cent.

This was the first of the important suits defended by the Association. The opening statement for the plaintiff to the jury rehashed the old unwarranted charge that the American Medical Association was a monopoly and a trust, that it was opposed to self-medication and opposed to all sorts of proprietary products. The attorneys for the Association pointed out that neither of the Pattens was a physician, that none of those associated with them was a physician and that their nostrum, sold all over the United States, could not possibly cure the diseases for which it was offered. The attorneys said,

"With full knowledge of the fact that at least one fifth or more than one fifth of every bottle of Wine of Cardui, prior to 1906, that Mr. Patten was putting out on the market, was pure alcohol, he was nevertheless satisfied that the business should continue with the representation to the purchasing public that it was positively non-intoxicating."

The company had put out over 20,000,000 almanacs known as the "Ladies' Birthday Almanac." They had also put out a statement that their "Home Treatment for Women" was a valuable book for the ladies who have any sort of female trouble and their slogan read:

"Lest you may have some serious female trouble that is working on you, buy a bottle of Wine of Cardui today, and be taking it while you are getting this book; price $1.00 a bottle. Or what is better, if you will buy 5 bottles, we will throw in a bottle. All orders cash; nobody trusted."

It had been one of the claims for the Wine of Cardui that it would lift up a fallen womb or uterus.

Mr. John A. Patten was closely connected with the Methodist Church. On this subject Mr. T. J. Scofield commented:

"I do not care whether he is the bishop of the Methodist Church; I do not care whether he is a high layman in the Methodist Church; I do not care whether he is at the head of the book committee of the Methodist Church, when any man tells you that in a case of prolapsed womb, chronically so, with its ligaments stretched until the womb is practically hanging out of the body—that Wine of Cardui, the miserable nostrum that we contend it is, and that we said it was in these articles, and say now, will pull that womb up into its natural position in the human body until it has reached its ascendency and there rests, is a matter of such absurdity that it would seem to me that common intelligence would deny the truth of such representation, and yet that is one of the representations which they (the plaintiffs) make."

I cannot tell here the whole story of the trial or reproduce any considerable amount of the evidence. For the Association appeared some of the leading chemists, toxicologists, gynecologists, obstetricians and other expert witnesses in the entire United States. One finds among them such names as those of Drs. Joseph B. DeLee, Charles A. L. Reed, J. Clarence Webster, Torald Sollmann, Frank Billings, and Hugh McKenna.

The principal ingredient of Wine of Cardui was viburnum prunifolium, a herb remedy, and also another herb known as carduus benedictus. The jury was enlightened on amenorrhea, headaches, puberty and many similar subjects. This case demonstrated, among the earliest of such cases, how difficult it is to make a jury of laymen, uninstructed in any of the medical sciences, understand the problems concerned in the diagnosis and treatment of disease. After Dr. Frank Billings had testified for many hours and just before he left the witness stand, Mr. W. M. Hough, an attorney for the Wine of Cardui company, said to him:

Mr. Hough: Q.—Just before you get off the stand, doctor, will you explain to the jury the difference between puberty and nubility? A.—And what?
Q.—The difference between puberty and nubility? A.—I don't get your last word.
Q.—Nubility. A.—Nubility?
Q.—N-u-b-i-l-i-t-y? A.—Nubility; you've got me.

In preparation for this case the investigators had toured the south and had found great numbers of instances of men who were using this alcoholic nostrum as drink.

Among the amusing evidence was one of the questions placed to Dr. J. Clarence Webster, in his time one of the most distinguished gynecologists in the United States. He was asked particularly as to whether or not it was possible by the taking of any drugs to elevate a uterus which had fallen from its position because of relaxation of the ligaments. He pointed out that it had been impossible in any number of experiments to effect such relaxation by the use of any one of a great number of drugs, including all of those concerned in Wine of Cardui. His cross examination extended for many days since he had actually done experiments with all of the drugs concerned. Apparently the attorneys for the Pattens considered his testimony very damaging. Dr. J. Clarence Webster declared that one could no more raise the uterus by drugs after relaxing of the ligaments than one could put stretch back into a pair of worn out garters by dropping them in alcohol.

In his instructions to the jury, the Hon. Judge George A. Carpenter pointed out that certain statements that had been published in THE JOURNAL for July 18, 1914, had been libelous per se. "Libel," said the court, "is a malicious defamation expressed in writing or by signs or pictures or by epitaphs tending to impeach the honesty, integrity, virtue or reputation of a person and thereby to expose him to public hatred, contempt, ridicule or obloquy and cause him to be shunned or avoided or to injure him in business or reputation." The court continued:

"These statements, I tell you, are libelous per se in that they charge that the plaintiffs were guilty of perpetrating a fraud upon women who purchased Wine of Cardui, in manufacturing and putting the same upon the market as a woman's tonic possessing medicinal value, with full knowledge, actual or constructive, that it was worthless and produced no medicinal effect except from its alcoholic content.

"In order to justify this charge it will be necessary for the defendants to prove: First, that Wine of Cardui is worthless and produces no medicinal effect except from its alcoholic content; and, second, that the plaintiffs had knowledge or should have known of such fact while manufacturing Wine of Cardui and placing it upon the market."

Two defenses had been urged. One was justification and the other qualified privilege or fair comment.

As to the defense of qualified privilege, the Court stated that any person may discuss a matter of private concern provided, first, that he has not been moved by actual malice and, second, that his comment and criticism shall be fair and reasonable. The Court pointed out that the American Medical Association in writing the articles about Wine of Cardui was treating a matter of great public concern. In the discussion of a public matter if any person publishes of another a fair and reasonable comment of his conduct of business and the publisher is not actuated by any element of actual malice, then that publication is privileged, and there may be no recovery whatever because of that publication. Fair and reasonable comment does not include a reckless disregard of the truth or any statement inspired by malice or evil intent. In his charge to the jury, the judge pointed out that if this were the case of John A. Patten, which the court emphasized it was not since John A. Patten had died, complaints might justly have been made that the articles of the defendants did overstep the bounds of fair comment and criticism or qualified privilege. "It was not necessary," said the Court, "in the interest of humanity for the defendants to criticize Mr. Patten in his church relations.". . . "But this suit involves," the Court continued, "purely a business proposition and no consideration may be paid by you to the feelings of the surviving partner, however lacerated they may be, or to the feelings of his family, however keenly his family and relatives may have suffered."

The judge then discussed in considerable detail the question of damages. After being out nearly a week, the jury brought in a verdict for the plaintiff and assessed the damages at one cent.

The Association considered this a notable victory. The public had been enlightened. The worthlessness of the nostrum had been demonstrated. The patent medicine purveyors now realized the Association would not only publish but also fight!

TWO SUITS WITHOUT RECORD

Somewhere in the first ten years of the 1900's two suits were filed by one E. P. Cooke and one Mary A. Duns, but there is no report in any available record of these suits.

HENRY J. SCHIRESON VS. MORRIS FISHBEIN, ET AL.

Shortly after Dr. Morris Fishbein assumed the editorship of THE JOURNAL OF THE AMERICAN MEDICAL ASSOCIATION and undertook an active campaign against quacks, frauds and nostrums of many types, the suits began to multiply. Among the earliest was the suit of Henry Junius Schireson, notorious plastic surgeon with a long record of imposition on the public.

In 1911 Schireson with some other individuals incorporated the "Shirpost Medical Office" in Chicago—a quack concern that advertised in foreign newspapers. At the same time he was connected with the European Medical Institute, also called the People's Medical Dispensary of Cleveland, Ohio. He was also associated with a "medical institute" in Scranton, Pa.

In 1911 he applied to the Illinois State Board of Health for a license to be given to him by reciprocity on the basis of a license issued to him by the Vermont State Board of Medical Registration in February 1909. In his application Schireson stated that he had taken his first and second years in medical college at the Maryland University from October 1902 to May 1904. The actual evidence showed that he had never entered Maryland University until October 1903 when he entered as a freshman but that he failed in all branches, except histology and medical jurisprudence. Further investigation showed that Schireson was not in attendance at the Maryland Medical College for 1904–1905, but that he did attend one course of lectures at the Maryland Medical College in 1905–1906 and was given a diploma from that school in 1906. The Illinois State Board refused to give him a license.

In May, 1912, Schireson was arrested in Detroit because he had obtained a license in Michigan on the basis of forged credentials and his license was cancelled. In Pittsburgh, to which he next moved his headquarters, he ran an advertising office and paid "protection" to two county detectives. He was convicted and sentenced and was pardoned after serving two months because he turned state's evidence. In 1914 he was arrested in New York City for practicing medicine without a license and in 1915 he was sentenced to six months in the penitentiary for violating the penal laws of New York. After leaving the penitentiary, he opened an office in Utica under the name of Dr. Fanning and took in $36,000 in six weeks as a result of "swindling the immigrant population of Oneida County." At the same time he had an office in Schenectady where he took in $14,000. Then he obtained a diploma from a notorious diploma mill in Kansas City, Missouri, and in 1922 got himself a license in Connecticut through the eclectic board of that state. Early in 1924 his Connecticut license was revoked on the ground of fraud and deceit.

In 1921 he had secured a license from the Department of Registration and Education in the State of Illinois in spite of the fact that the state had previously refused him a license. This license was granted during the incumbency of a director of the department, named W. H. H. Miller, who later was convicted of selling licenses and fined $1000.

Now came the heyday of Schireson's career. He set himself up as a specialist in plastic surgery and the straightening of cross-eyes. He hired a press agent who later sued him for $50,000 on a charge that Schireson had never paid him adequately for his press agentry. The press agent charged that he had persuaded Fannie Brice to submit to an operation by Schireson as well as many other notable persons, including Lady Diana Manners. In 1927 Schireson got a lot of publicity in connection with an alleged surgical job on Peaches Browning.

Schireson's biggest mistake came in 1928. A young woman went to him to have a burn on one of her shoulders treated. He suggested to her that he would straighten out her legs. He did the operation at an osteopathic hospital. The legs became gangrenous and both had to be amputated at the knee in order to save her life.

In January of 1930 Schireson was found guilty of fraud, conduct unbecoming a physician and gross malpractice, and his Illinois license was revoked. In 1931 his license was revoked in Ohio following charges of gross immorality, conviction of a felony and grossly unprofessional or dishonest conduct.

His most recent career has been in Philadelphia. The Philadelphia Sunday *Transcript* in 1937 gave a detailed account of Schireson's bankruptcy case; there were so many judgments against him in behalf of former patients who had brought damage suits that he pleaded bankruptcy. In 1939 he was indicted by a Federal Grand Jury in Philadelphia charged with hiding $130,000 from his creditors while filing a petition of bankruptcy in 1937. He was also indicted on a perjury charge as a result of testifying that he was not married and that he did not live in Merchantville, New Jersey. As a result he was sentenced to serve two concurrent terms of eighteen months in the Lewisburg Federal Penitentiary.

This is the charlatan who brought two suits against Dr. Morris Fishbein on the charge that he had been libeled. During his stay in Illinois he brought nuisance suits and tried repeatedly to force the presence of the editor of THE JOURNAL in court, once arranging to have a bailiff serve a subpoena on the editor just after he had boarded the Twentieth Century for an important trip.

As late as June 25, 1946, the Supreme Court of Pennsylvania affirmed the decision of the Court of Common Pleas of Dauphin County upholding the contention of attorneys for the state board of medical education and licensure that the state licensing body had the inherent right to revoke a license obtained by fraud. Schireson had been trying by injunctions to restrain the state board from revoking his license.

The story of Henry Junius Schireson is proof that he is supreme among plastic surgeon quacks.

'None of the suits of Henry J. Schireson against Dr. Morris Fishbein ever came to trial.

HOXIDE CANCER INSTITUTE

Next came a suit of the Hoxide Cancer Institute against the American Medical Association and against Dr. Morris Fishbein. The record of Hoxsey in the field of cancer quackery is one of the longest in the history of American medicine. On January 2, 1926, THE JOURNAL published a three page article dealing with the quack remedy put out by Harry M. Hoxsey. At that time the Hoxide cancer cure was exploited from Taylorville, a town in central Illinois, and was sponsored by the Chamber of Commerce of that town. Hoxsey's father was John C. Hoxsey who had dabbled in veterinary medicine, faith healing and cancer cures. In 1919 John C. Hoxsey died of cancer. In 1924 Harry M. Hoxsey joined with a Dr. Bruce Miller and an insurance man in setting up something called the "National Cancer Research Institute and Clinic." Their treatment was essentially the use of an escharotic or caustic substance with arsenic as its base. The idea of these caustics is that they can eat off a cancer. No such treatment as ever cured a cancer— occasionally the caustic eats off a considerable portion of the skin in additon to the cancer.

After the exposé of the Hoxide cancer cure in 1926 and again in 1929, Hoxsey became associated with Norman Baker of Muscatine, Iowa. Then he headed an alleged cancer clinic in Detroit where he was found guilty May 8, 1931, of practicing medicine without a license and sentenced to serve six months in the Detroit House of Correction.

On July 11, 1941, he was charged in Dallas, Texas, of practicing medicine without a license and fined $25,000 and court costs. He continues at this very time to operate a cancer clinic in Dallas, Texas. No Hoxide libel suit has ever come to trial.

ELECTROPHONE CORPORATION

Next came a suit from the Electrophone Corporation against the American Medical Association. The electrophone was an elaborate device exploited from Chicago. It had been originally called the "De-a-fone." It was put on the market by a concern which was first known as the National Acoustic Laboratories and then as the National Deafone Company and still later as the Electrophone Corporation. The instrument was used in a so-called Audio Institute which advertised, "Hearing restored by the Audio treatment." The electrophone was a bogus hearing device. The suit never came to trial.

PERCIVAL LEMON CLARK

On March 31, 1928, THE JOURNAL OF THE AMERICAN MEDICAL ASSOCIATION published an article about a quack named Percival Lemon Clark who was the promoter of a system of healing called "sanatology." Clark was born in 1866 and had received a diploma in 1889 from the Bennett Medical College, Chicago, which was then an eclectic institution. He conducted a health school and a health home and called himself dean of the world's first university of sanatology. Clark even got some bills introduced before the Illinois legislature to get legal recognition for sanatology. He urged that acidosis and toxicosis are the two basic causes of all disease. He did not believe in the germ theory. He claimed to cure asthma. He also sold a dextrinized health school brand of laxative foods and a "Sanatology Blower," which it was claimed "would dry clean the entire system and rejuvenate."

He exploited a "Sanatology Enema Bag and Attachments" which removed the "toxic poison from the body." This was just a hot water bottle with a hose. The patient would insert the nozzle in the rectum and then sit on the hot water bottle. The weight of the body was supposed to force the water up into the intestines.

He also purveyed "Sanatological Oil," "Laxative Salts," and a book called "How to Live and Eat for Health."

For a while he promoted his health home and his system over the radio station owned by the Chicago Federation of Labor, known as WCFL, a name which it still bears. He used to come on about 7 o'clock at night and utter such slogans as "The whiter the bread, the sooner you're dead." "The more sugar you soak, the quicker you croak."

He filed a suit against the American Medical Association for $3,000,000. Following the discovery by further investigations that he had an unsavory record in Canada where he had on one occasion been involved with the police, the suits that he had filed against the Association were dismissed by the courts in 1933.

ORA-NOID

On March 9, 1929, THE JOURNAL published an exposé of a product called Ora-Noid, said to be synthetic saliva. The suit was filed against Morris Fishbein and the American Medical Association and was for $1,000,000 for libel. The chemists of the American Medical Association had found that Ora-Noid was essentially a mixture of table salt, baking soda, chalk, magnesia, starch and borax. This mixture was being sold as a cure for pyorrhea. In 1933 this case was also dismissed on motion of the plaintiff.

JOHN R. BRINKLEY

John R. Brinkley might well be characterized as the greatest charlatan in medical history. His many suits against Dr. Morris Fishbein and the American Medical Association at different times came to many millions of dollars. His first suit was filed at Junction City, Kansas. Finally a suit came to trial in Del Rio, Texas, on March 22, 1939. That suit was based on an article published in Hygeia entitled "Modern Medical Charlatans."

On May 26, 1942, the Associated Press spread throughout the world the obituary notice of John R. Brinkley, M.D., Ph.D., M.C., LL.D., D.P.H., Sc.D., Lieut. U.S.N.R. Said the A.P.: "Death today closed the turbulent medical, political and radio career of Dr. John Richard Brinkley, 56, rejuvenation surgeon known popularly as 'the goat gland doctor.'" The New York *Times*, perhaps profligate of space, gave him a column and a half with a picture. He was, at the time of his death, one of the most widely known citizens of the United States. He was also by common consent the greatest charlatan the world has ever known.

By his own testimony John Romulus Brinkley, as he later called himself, was born in Beta, Jackson County, in western North Carolina in 1885.

The boy attended the mountain schools of the neighborhood—little one-room shacks with one teacher trying to inform children of many different ages about reading, writing, arithmetic, history, geography, music, drawing and kindred matters and to act simultaneously as school physician, nurse, physical educator and inculcator of etiquette.

When Brinkley was sixteen years old, he obtained a position carrying the mail from the post office in the mountains to the railroad station. Here he became acquainted with the railroad agent, who gave him a chance as assistant to learn telegraphy, railroad bookkeeping and how to run a railroad station.

The next event in the life of Brinkley was no doubt the pivotal point which embarked him on a career of charlatanism. He went from Sylva, North Carolina, to Baltimore to see about getting into Johns Hopkins University; that was the only medical school he had ever heard of at the time. Again I quote:

> "Going up there I found I did not have enough education to enter the school, and I met a man while I was there in Baltimore that had another school there that prepared young men for school entrance requirements, and while I didn't stay there and attend the school with him, yet he furnished me with books to read and outlined a plan of study for me and I went on up to New York City and worked in New York City for quite a while for Western Union. Then I worked for the Central Railroad in New Jersey—Hoboken, New Jersey. During that time I was doing I suppose today what we would call one of these correspondent courses like we have outlined. I would go down to Baltimore occasionally and report how I was getting along and be quizzed and first one thing and another. I left New York in 1906 because my aunt who raised me was in feeble condition. I returned to North Carolina and she died in December of 1906 and was buried, and I married and I went to Chicago and got a job with the Western Union Telegraph Company and found out about Bennett Medical College in Chicago and matriculated in Bennett College in June 1908 and worked for Western Union of a night and went to school of a day. And the first year I was in school there in Bennett Dr. John Dill Robertson, who was president of the school, established a literary department that he called the Jefferson Park College, I believe it was. During our freshman year in Bennett we freshmen that wanted to take literary work outside of our medical work would go over to this Jefferson Park College at three o'clock in the afternoon and spend a couple of hours over there in study until five. I had to leave at five o'clock because I had to be down at the Western Union office at 5:30 to go to work, and that is the way my time was occupied the freshman year."

Brinkley declared under oath that he got his preliminary education at Milton Academy, Baltimore, and was in attendance there from September 1902 to July 1906, when he was given a diploma. Also, when applying for license in California, he did not file any diploma but presented a photograph of a letter written on the letterhead of Milton Academy and purportedly signed by William J. Heaps. Three Baltimore persons deposed that they had attended Milton Academy (day sessions) some time between 1902 and 1906 and did not recall Brinkley. A Doctor Snavely who taught at the school in the same period deposed that he did not remember Brinkley. Also, he said that the alleged signature of Heaps on the photographed letter previously mentioned was a forgery. Heaps was said to have been one of the persons on whom Brinkley claimed to have performed a goat-gland operation. In connection with Milton Academy, there was also what was known as the Milton University, which Brinkley claimed had given him a B. A. degree. The same Mr. Heaps has been quoted as saying that he conferred this on Brinkley as an honorary degree for the work he had done and the reputation that he enjoyed.

Brinkley did not get into the senior year at the Bennett Medical College. He owed a large sum for back tuition. Doctor Robertson was accustomed to permit students to enter short of money, but no one could enter the senior year in debt to the school. It was "pay up or get out," according to Brinkley, so he got out.

Brinkley had entered the Bennett College in 1908, and he remained until the fall of 1910. He missed about six weeks and returned early in November. During those six weeks he was a telegrapher in Montreal and in New York.

The next three years of his life determined his career in quackery. During the summer and fall of 1911 Brinkley practiced medicine in western North Carolina without a license but with a permit of the secretary of the medical board. Brinkley went to Miami for a few weeks in the winter and worked as a telegrapher. Then restlessness seized him. He went back to Whiteville, North Carolina, then to St. Louis, then to Tennessee where he got an undergraduate's license based on three years of the kind of education he had. He was at Danrich, Tennessee, during the first half of 1912, in Knoxville during the last half.

Late in the spring of 1913, John Brinkley was in Chicago. In Lincoln Park a long line of prospective swimmers stood in line to rent bathing suits so they could cool off in Lake Michigan. Among them was Brinkley. The man at the wicket told him the lockers were all rented but that he could, if he wished, share a locker with its occupant. By this adventure, opportunity knocked at Brinkley's door. This was the tide in his affairs which, taken at the flood, led on to fortune. In the locker was James E. Crawford. Brinkley told how he had worked for one Burke, operator of several venereal disease quackeries in Knoxville and in Chattanooga. Crawford and Brinkley decided to return to Burke and set up an establishment under his direction. Together they went to Chattanooga for some graduate study on how to operate a venereal disease quackery; then they opened up in Greenville, South Carolina, with a big sign that read "Greenville Electro Medic Specialists." When they arrived in Greenville, they had ten dollars between them and starvation. They got credit at the drug store for rent and supplies, credit with the press for their advertisements. About this time the American press was informing the world about the advantages of salvarsan and neosalvarsan—"606" and "914"—Ehrlich's magic bullets—for syphilis. The word went out that these itinerant physicians had these remedies, available at twenty-five dollars per injection. Actually according to Crawford, they injected colored water. Crawford it seems had given up mayhem for the more refined career of medical practice. When seen in 1938, he was serving a sentence of eighteen months in the Oklahoma penitentiary for robbery with firearms at the Hotel Mayo in Tulsa. Previously he had a home address in the federal prison at Leavenworth, Kansas, for transporting a stolen motor car. The Council on Medical Education of the American Medical Association has not yet accepted these experiences as prerequisites for medical education and licensure.

Now time plays strange tricks with our memories. Somewhere in the period between 1911 and 1915 Brinkley or a man of the same name was arrested for forgery in Tennessee. He was never able to remember the details. One day he and Crawford departed from Greenville leaving a number of unpaid bills behind them. By the processes of the law they were returned and lodged with the sheriff for forty-eight hours. The sheriff produced a number of rubber checks, the kind that bounce back, signed by the electromedical specialists. Our hero departed for new pastures, greener than Greenville. Somewhere in this period Brinkley was in St. Louis because he turned up with a diploma from the National University of Arts and Science at St. Louis, although even from that nondescript institution one cannot obtain the record showing he was ever a student. His record, full of chicanery and deception, was punctuated with licenses, diplomas, citations, subpoenas, court orders, bad checks, election ballots, bonds and mortgages. In these days of paper shortage, his accumulation would be more valuable as scrap than ever it was for documentary purposes. He had a diploma from the Eclectic College of Medicine or the Eclectic Medical University of Kansas City. When the class graduated, all went, accompanied by a professor, to Arkansas, where they were licensed to practice by the Eclectic Board. In 1921 the Connecticut Eclectic Board gave Brinkley a license. By 1923 it was discovered that many an Eclectic Board was issuing licenses somewhat at random, and Connecticut revoked the one they gave Brinkley. Once he went to California under a temporary license to try his hand at rejuvenating an aging and decrepit publisher. For a few weeks of what turned out to be a useless effort, Brinkley got forty thousand dollars. After he got back to Kansas, where he resided, he was indicted in California, and they sent emissaries to Kansas, but he didn't go back.

In May of 1915 Brinkley was licensed in Arkansas; in June in Tennessee. He tried practice in Memphis without success, moved on to Judsonia, Arkansas, but crops were ruined by a flood; then he went on to Fulton, Kansas, and practiced there, finally arriving in Milford, Kansas—just a wide space in the road—in October 1917. There he remained until 1933. From time to time he visited Chicago and New York. He once visited Shanghai and collected five thousand dollars for a few operations. The Royal University of Pavia, on one of his trips, granted him an honorary diploma which was later annulled. There was also a sort of certificate issued in England, which was also annulled.

On one of the pamphlets issued by Brinkley later in his career appear the letters M. D., C. M., Dr. P. H., Sc.D. following his name. He said the Sc. D. came from the Chicago Law School, the Doctor of Public Health from the Eclectic Medical University of Kansas City. These alphabetic appendages have become the mark of the charlatan. Brinkley also had an LL. D. When asked where he got it, he said, "I will declare I don't know!"

Now how did the famous goat-gland operation originate? Here is his story:

"A very peculiar circumstance happened at Milford, Kansas. I had only been there about two weeks, being a new doctor in town and having a little drug store that I had opened up there, and different country people would drop into the drug store to meet the new doctor and pay me their respects and tell me they were glad I was there and so forth. This one man came in and got to talking with me about sexual weakness. I told him I didn't know anything that would do him any particular good as to sexual weakness. The conversation continued and we got to talking about why couldn't we take some glands out of an animal and put them into a man. I told him it was biologically impossible. He wanted to know why it was impossible. I told him because you couldn't transplant the glands from a higher order of animal kingdom to a lower or vice versa. He wanted to know how I knew you couldn't, and I told him that was what I had been taught and I believed it. To make a long story short, he furnished the animal and I transplanted some glands into him, with good results according to his statements to me. I had advised the man not to have it done and he said, 'You are a surgeon. You can put them in and if they spoil you can take them out.' To me the results were amazing and startling because I expected bad results and disastrous results and instead of that happy results were obtained. The man claimed that he had been sexually dead for sixteen years. His wife verified that statement. A year later I delivered his wife of a fine baby boy, which at least proved that he was fertile, anyhow. Of course the news got around in great fashion, and a cousin of his came to me and asked me to do the same thing on him and I did and he had me to transplant glands into his wife. Then one of their relatives was in the insane hospital in Nebraska. He had been a banker. He was a banker up there, he was a cashier and lost his mind and was placed in an insane institution. They wanted to know from me if I thought glands would do this insane person any good, and I said, 'Lord God no,' and they said, 'We want you to try it' because he had been a masturbator and 'We know it' and they brought him down there, took him out of the institution, and I put those glands into him and that man recovered his mind and today is in charge of one of the biggest banks in Kansas City, Missouri. He came out of the insane asylum in Nebraska and had those glands put in. I published that in an article in a little magazine, and down in Alabama a lady read it. She had a daughter that had been in the insane asylum for ten years in Tuscaloosa, Alabama. She was violently insane at times. When she went to get a permit, she had to get a state permit to get this daughter out of a padded cell, they had to keep her in what is called a padded cell to keep her from doing injury to herself; she was trying all the time to commit suicide. And my wife and I met this lady with her daughter in Memphis, Tennessee, and put her in a drawing room and brought her to Kansas City and over to Milford. I transplanted glands into that young lady. She stayed in my hospital for a month, fully recovered her mental capacity. She didn't want to go home because she felt she was disgraced because of her previous life. She secured a secretarial position in Kansas City, Missouri, and married a physician and today she is healthy and happy and normal."

In the meantime publicity began to come to the scientific sage of Milford. The early 1920's marked the beginnings in the United States of the new profession of public relations council. Publicity hounds of many varieties sniffed their way into the newspapers. The Sunday supplements carried stories of the rejuvenator who preached and who practiced goat-gland science. Brinkley had allied himself closely with the local church. He had given Milford as a gift the Brinkley Methodist Memorial Church bearing a tablet which read, "Erected to God and His Son Jesus in appreciation of the many blessings conferred upon me, By J. R. Brinkley." The Lord takes the blame for many mundane affairs when the responsibility may not always seem clear.

Eventually the fame of the rejuvenator reached California. Here is the story of the beginning of the first Brinkley radio station, KFKB:

"I had been called by Harry Chandler, the owner of the Los Angeles *Times* in Los Angeles, California, who had read a little article I had written or published in some magazine some place and he asked me to come out there; an old employee at the time was sick. Mr. Chandler wanted me to put these glands into him to see if it would do him any good. While I was there, Chandler was having installed KHJ for the *Times*. I think it was the first radio station that was ever put in there in Los Angeles, California. And leaving California and going back to Milford I thought it would be a nice thing to entertain the patients by having a radio station close to the hospital where they could lay in bed and listen in on their earphones, and I bought the station and gave lectures over it, talked about various diseases of the human body and did that up until 1929. I never tried to produce any patients over the radio at all, never even made any effort to. I was using the radio up until 1929 to give musical entertainment and medical lectures and medical advice in a general way. In 1929 I began a series of lectures dealing with the diseases of children. I began to receive an enormous amount of mail from people asking me about this thing and that thing and another thing. I couldn't answer it, and the only way it could be answered was to go on the radio and answer a good bulk of it, and in 1929 from answering those letters over the radio, through the radio, patients began to come to me because of radio advertising."

The right to operate a radio station was easily secured in those early days of commercial radio. Now the growth of the influence of the Federal Radio Commission puts rigid restrictions around broadcasting and station ownership.

Night after night Brinkley mingled with the music from his station announcements concerning the value of goat-gland transplants. His programs were keyed to a listening audience of elderly men likely to be awake attending to various physiological functions between two and four A. M. He had developed the four-phase compound operation, claimed to be "the best thing known for impotency, high blood pressure, large prostate, sterility, neurasthenia, dementia praecox or any disease that is not malignant of the prostate." Patients who came to the hospital on Monday usually left by Friday; next week's patients were not to know how this week's patients were going. The hospital had about fifty beds; the average fee was $750. The glands of a very young species of capricornus might cost $1500. The surgery was crude. A carpenter from New Jersey who had received one of these operations died in St. Louis of tetanus. The Milford technicians had fastened an old rubber heel over his wound to keep the tissues from extruding the goat glands as a foreign substance.

As Brinkley said, people wrote to him in great numbers. He claimed in an interview in 1930 that he was receiving three thousand letters each day. In 1933 he discontinued the goat gland operation.

One of his early cases was Charley Tasine. Let the old doctor tell it:

"The boys in the barber shop were kidding Charley whether he would have an operation or not, and he said he would if he had the money, and I was coming along and I said, 'You don't have to have any money; come up to the hospital and I will give it to you for nothing.' I took him up and the operation was entirely successful. He was a bachelor and he got married right afterwards. He claimed he had become a regular billy goat, twice as good as any other man around Milford. He was one of those boasting fellows, liked to blow off as to his ability." Indeed, the son born to the Tasines was duly named Billy in recognition of his origin.

About 1926 Brinkley organized the Brinkley Pharmaceutical Association. Druggists who joined sold preparations recommended by broadcasts of the Brinkley Medical Question Box. The broadcaster would read the letters received from the sick. He would tell them to get "Women's Tonic No. 50, 67, and 71" or "Men's Prescription No. 60, 87 and also No. 64." The prescriptions were common preparations of ordinary drugs sold under these numbers. The druggist would keep a large portion of the money and send the remainder to Brinkley for advertising the preparation. Thus the doctor prescribed for a patient whom he had never seen, basing his diagnosis on written descriptions of the symptoms. In Doctor Brinkley's broadcast for April 1, 1930, presumably representative of all, he prescribed for forty-four different patients and in all, save ten, he advised the procurement of from one to four of his own prescriptions. Here are two which are typical:

"Here's one from Tillie. She says she had an operation, had some trouble ten years ago. I think the operation was unnecessary, and it isn't very good sense to have an ovary removed with the expectation of motherhood resulting therefrom. My advice to you is to use Women's Tonic No. 50, 67 and 61. This combination will do for you what you desire if any combination will, after three months' persistent use.

"Sunflower State, from Dresden, Kansas. Probably he has gallstones. No, I don't mean that; I mean kidney stones. My advice to you is to put him on Prescription No. 80 and 50 for men, also 64. I think that he will be a whole lot better. Also drink a lot of water."

The preparations prescribed were secret, and the prescriber shared in the profit from the sale. This, from either an ethical or scientific point of view, stinks to high heaven.

The Kansas City *Star* and THE JOURNAL OF THE AMERICAN MEDICAL ASSOCIATION began to tell the truth about the Brinkley broadcasting. Eventually the Federal Radio Commission was moved to action. Brinkley was cited to prove that his programs were in the public interest, convenience and necessity. Off he went to Washington with a trainload of satisfied patients in an attempt to prove to the commission his honesty and scientific ability. He had built his station in 1923; in June 1930 the Federal Radio Commission refused to renew his license. So he sold the station in 1931. He sued the *Star* and THE JOURNAL and their editors for millions and millions of dollars, but these suits never came to trial. He appealed to the Court of Appeals in the District of Columbia, but they sustained the Radio Commission. Then the Kansas Board of Medical Examiners revoked his license to practice. He appealed to the Supreme Court of Kansas. The judges of the Supreme Court spoke with fine diction in announcing their decision. They held that Brinkley was "an empiric without moral sense, and having acted according to the ethical standards of an impostor, the licensee has performed an organized charlatanism until he is capable of preying on human weakness, ignorance and credulity, to an extent quite beyond the invention of the humble mountebank." They spoke of him as one "who was fleecing the defective, the ailing, the gullible and chronic medicine takers who are moved by suggestion, and is scandalizing the medical profession and exposing it to contempt and ridicule."

And now came his candidacy for governor in the state of Kansas. He had lost his radio station, but he toured the state in a truck equipped with a loud speaker, probably the first political candidate to use this technic. He purchased time on other stations. He promised free motor licenses, free textbooks, better roads. Kansas, he pointed out, is a dry state. "If I am elected," he said, "I will build a lake in every county in Kansas. Then the water will be evaporated from these lakes and will pour down as gentle rain on the fertile fields of Kansas." He filed late in his candidacy so that it was necessary to insert his name in writing on the ballots. The election clerks were directed to discard all ballots on which his name was not perfectly spelled, even to dotting the "i." Nevertheless, he polled 183,000 votes, which was some 14,000 less than were polled for the winning candidate. The local politicians have told me that he would have been elected easily if all the ballots had been counted. No doubt they are right, because it is said he received more than 20,000 votes in Oklahoma, and he was not even running in Oklahoma. At a subsequent election he polled 244,000 votes and was almost elected. He then tried to file a third time, but now the people of Kansas had lost interest.

In 1933 Brinkley closed up in Kansas and moved to Del Rio in Texas. I first saw Del Rio myself in 1939. In the hot sunshine lackadaisical Mexicans sleep along the curbstones. The village, for it is that, is typical of all of the towns along the Rio Grande. Along the roadside are signs reading, "This is God's country—don't drive like hell through it." The warning is no doubt necessary, for there is little in Del Rio to hold the casual tourist. In Del Rio Brinkley registered at the hotel and soon began using some of its rooms for his patients. By now he had abandoned the four-phase compound operation which involved the transplantation of the glands of the goat and had undertaken a new procedure based on some of the researches of Steinach, famous Austrian rejuvenator. In this operation Brinkley simply cut the tube leading from the male sex glands and put inside a drop of mercurochrome. A little later the operation was again modified so that the tube was tied with a suture. This he called the Steinach No. 2 operation. Most experts are convinced that the success of the operation in a few cases is due to the power of suggestion.

Shortly after arriving in Del Rio, Brinkley apparently came to terms with the Mexican government and obtained a license for a radio station known as XERA in Villa Acuna, Coahuila, Mexico. This was at its best the most powerful radio station in the North American continent. The Mexicans, who are not wholly a stupid people, built tall steel towers south of his station so that the broadcasts had very little circulation in Mexico. They did, however, have a tremendous reach up into Minnesota, a fact which was particularly annoying to the Mayo brothers. From this station were broadcast not only Brinkley's lectures, read in a strange but compelling monotone, but also all sorts of announcements by patent medicine and similar commercial interests. Special attention was given to garlic tablets for high blood pressure.

The stay of Brinkley in Del Rio was profitable—so profitable indeed that his payroll at the time I visited Del Rio in 1939 had reached $20,000 weekly. During the years from 1933 to 1938 the Brinkley Hospital in Del Rio had taken care of some 15,000 patients, of whom the majority paid $750. This sum the doctor guaranteed by an excellent commercial organization which would accept a mortgage on a farm, an attachment to a bank account, the family jewels or anything that could be made to look like $750. Bear in mind also that $750 was only a minimum. Once the patient was in the hospital a number of interesting devices were developed for promoting what are technically called "extras."

When I saw Brinkley, I observed a little man with a little gray goatee, wearing a gray suit, but the goatee and the suit were the only appurtenances that were not brilliant. On one hand he wore a diamond ring which was said to be fourteen carats, and on the other hand another diamond ring said to be eleven carats. In his tie was a stick pin of a considerable number of carats, and underneath the stick pin was apparently a solid gold tie clasp set with diamonds, the entire device being about two inches long and one-quarter inch wide. From his watch chain there dropped a Masonic emblem with several diamonds also large in carats. Mrs. Brinkley, usually known as Minnie, who in 1921 had also acquired a diploma from the Kansas City college, was likewise somewhat profusely decorated with diamonds. (Remember that diamonds are negotiable everywhere and easily transported when one needs must travel hastily.) In fact, the combination resembled in their brilliance the twin chandeliers of a house of ill fame. The illumination was not limited, however, wholly to the jewelry. Brinkley traveled to and from the court house in a great red sixteen-cylinder Cadillac, on which his name appeared thirteen times—twice on each hub cap, on the front and back, on the trunk and on the sides.

Brinkley would sit quietly in the court room, usually chewing a toothpick and combing his beard with his fingers. In his vest pocket he carried also a combination gold tooth and ear pick, with which he used to explore his teeth, his nose, his ears, and then view the results with a tender, solicitous expression. Usually beside him sat the glamorous Rose Dawn. Mrs. Brinkley did not come in often; when she did, she merely peeked through the door. There sat too beside him on occasion some of the virtuosos of station XERA, including the "Mexican Nightingale" and a sleek Mexican announcer.

Yes, the gland business did well for Brinkley in Texas! He owned three yachts, named John R. Brinkley I, II and III, one of them bought from Joe Schenck of the movies, first used by Douglas Fairbanks. It was a 170-foot job and carried a crew of twenty-one. Brinkley was created an admiral by the governor of Kansas; a picture of Brinkley in his private admiral's uniform hung in the office of the editor of the Del Rio newspaper. Incidentally, Brinkley rented his large yacht to Edward VIII and Wallis Simpson for their honeymoon in the Mediterranean. Brinkley's home and the six acres of ground around it were valued at $200,000. There was a great rose garden artificially irrigated, a swimming pool with colored tile, large greenhouses with orchids, live penguins and tortoises from the Galapagos. On the lawn were great statues of Romulus and Remus with the she-wolf that bred them, purchased by the doctor in Italy after he adopted the name Romulus as a middle name. There was a great marble group of the Three Graces bought in Italy and designed to adorn Mrs. Brinkley's grave at some future date. Two great fountains sparkled in the sun, and at night over each of them an electric sign spelled out the words "Dr. Brinkley." Indeed the repetition of his name on every possible spot in the doctor's vicinity assumed proportions almost pathological. His name was found three times on the swimming pool, once on the pipe organ, twice on the radio station, twice in six inch letters on the house gates, embroidered on the uniform jumpers of the crews of the yachts and painted on all of the yachts in innumerable places. On the great wooden table in his dining room his name was carved where each guest sat; and whose name do you think was on the napkins? J. C. Furnas, who spent some days in Del Rio, is authority for the fact that the name was not carved on the backs of the tortoises.

Brinkley never did quite remember how many motor cars he had, but he estimated that it might be somewhere around thirteen or fourteen.

Eventually the Texas State Board of Medical Examiners began to be annoying, whereupon Brinkley moved his medical establishment to Little Rock, Arkansas. He continued to maintain his home in Del Rio and the radio station in Villa Acuna. Arkansas had long been known for the laxity with which it granted medical licenses. The eclectic board continued to make easy the lives of its licensees. In Little Rock Brinkley bought a country club which he rededicated and called "the most beautiful hospital in the world." It had been built by the Shriners of Little Rock and included a mammoth stone structure fronting on a 100-acre lake, surrounded by 360 acres of golf course. In the town of Little Rock he set up a clinic in an old chain store building which was modernized with glass brick and chrome trim. Here a staff of thirty-five persons handled 2,000 letters daily which came in response to the Brinkley broadcasts. So great had the business become that it was necessary for Brinkley to secure a staff of assistants, most renegade doctors, some of them previously addicted to drugs or alcohol, some of them osteopaths. Closely allied to the clinic was the Romulus Drug Store, with pills for relieving acid stomach at five dollars a hundred and a laxative at three dollars for six ounces.

About this time Brinkley took over a technic that had been developed by a Birmingham doctor named Burr Ferguson. This technique involved the injection of an ampule of what was said to be 1:1000 hydrochloric acid. The patient got five ampules for one hundred dollars, actually worth about twenty-five cents each. The patient was advised to take the ampules to his family doctor on leaving the Brinkley sanatorium, and the family doctor was usually paid well for giving the injections. Unfortunately, the ampules were of a poor quality of glass; when the contents were examined by the chemical laboratory of the American Medical Association, it was discovered that most of the acid had been taken up by the glass of the ampule. What the patient got was essentially a solution slightly blue in appearance, about what he would get if you threw a bottle of bluing into Lake Erie.

Brinkley was accustomed to commute from Little Rock to Del Rio in his own Lockheed monoplane with a pilot and copilot. This was a twelve-passenger ship, for which he paid $58,000 and then added more than $20,000 worth of extras.

In the 1920's Brinkley sued the Kansas City *Star* and the American Medical Association for some millions of dollars, but eventually dropped that suit. In 1938 a description of Brinkley and his work was published in HYGEIA under the title "Modern Medical Charlatans." He then sued the American Medical Association and myself as editor for $250,000, claiming libel. In the testimony given in that suit there came forth many of the facts that have here been told. The suit went to the jury following a remarkable charge by Judge R. J. McMillan which was one of the strongest indictments of charlatanism ever to come from a court. The judge said, at one point, "The words quack and charlatan have substantially the same meaning. Many definitions can be found in the dictionaries or in the reports of the courts. A common definition of the word quack is to make vain and loud pretensions, especially of medical ability; to boast, to vaunt aloud or be a boastful pretender to medical skill or to make extravagant claims for a cure-all; to advertise with fraudulent boasts." Of ethics, the judge said, "Most people know in a general way what you mean by ethics, but few of us think or speak in terms of definitions . . . It has practically always been considered unethical for physicians to advertise, that is to say, to advertise further than to call the attention of the public to the fact that they were ready to practice . . . Advertisements by which prizes are offered to secure patronage or by which claims are made of superior skill or ability are not ethical." And again, "The conduct of the plaintiff Brinkley should not be measured against his own personal ideas with regard to what is proper. It should be measured against the ethics and approved conduct of physicians generally, and to such extent that his conduct as a physician varies from the rules of ethics recognized and observed generally he becomes subject to criticism . . ."

After a short stay in the jury room, the jury found the editor of *Hygeia* to be not guilty of the charge of libel.

On the witness stand in the libel suit Brinkley had testified that his income in 1937 had been more than $1,300,000 and that it had dropped to something like $800,000 in 1938. In an article printed in the *Saturday Evening Post* in April, 1940, J. C. Furnas ventured to predict, "In spite of treaties, medical associations, governments, cold-shouldering civic bodies, hell and high water, it is probably still a bad bet to sell Doctor (Brinkley) short." Brinkley had always been interested in politics. He had done enough for former Vice President Curtis to cause that worthy to go in person to our State Department and to cause them in turn to prevent the Mexicans from interfering with Brinkley's station. His broadcasts during the closing days of station XERA had begun to be devoted to international affairs. He had urged the election of John Garner and had contributed often to the campaign funds of the National Democratic Party. Observe that he aided both Democrats and Republicans. Indeed we find Doctor and Mrs. Brinkley listed among guests at a reception at the White House in 1940. In his politics Brinkley was a hard-shelled isolationist and a chronic Anglophobe. He was opposed to the entrance of the United States into the war. Somewhat later it appeared that he was also a contributor to the funds used by William Dudley Pelley, the anti-Semitic Silver Shirt leader who testified before the Dies Committee that Brinkley had given him $500,000. Yet with all the support that such contributions might have developed, the career of Brinkley, following the libel suit, pursued a course steadily downward. On March 25, 1941, he was confronted in a federal court with claims amounting to more than $1,600,000, and he filed a statement in bankruptcy listing personal property that totaled $46,845.16, 6 head of horses, 90 head of cattle, 1 sow, 6 geese, 2 guineas, 40 ducks, 50 chickens and 20 turkeys, all of which were resident not in Del Rio but in East La Porte, North Carolina. He had sold his last yacht for $110,000 to the United States Navy and his private airplane to the British Purchasing Commission in order to get enough cash to pay some income taxes. The federal government felt that he still owed them more than $113,000 in income taxes. In 1940 he had sold the hospital in Little Rock. His attorneys asserted that the malpractice suits had ruined him, and other judgments against him on such suits were well over $1,000,000. With the loss of his funds came a physical breakdown. He departed for Kansas City and in 1941 opened a school for the teaching of airplane mechanics, which promptly also went into bankruptcy. Then his heart began to disturb him, and a piece of the tissue of the heart breaking away blocked a blood vessel in his leg, that requiring amputation. A few months more and in May 1942 he died.

The conditions that produced John R. Brinkley are not likely to be duplicated again. The licensing boards of the individual states are now, for the most part, above any possibility of such manipulation as was performed when Brinkley was licensed in half a dozen states by the so-called Eclectic Boards. The radio is now controlled by the Federal Radio Commission, and the advertising claims of nostrums and panaceas are subject to the supervision of the Food, Drug and Cosmetic Act of 1937 and the researches of the Federal Trade Commission operating under the Wheeler-Lea bill of the same year. The Post Office Department, through fraud orders, carefully checks on the use of the mails to defraud.

Observe that great charlatans of the Brinkley type are not halted by any increase in public knowledge or by any lessening of human credulity; it requires the social controls exercised by laws with powerful punitive qualities to check a superlative quack.

BEFSAL

On February 21, 1925, THE JOURNAL published an article about a drug called "Befsal," which was exploited by one Dr. S. Lewis Summers of Fort Washington, Pa., and by an agency called Synthetic Organic Products Co., New York City. The product, which was analyzed by the laboratories of the American Medical Association, turned out to be a substance of varying and unreliable composition containing salicylic acid and quinine. It was launched as a special cure for rheumatism. Suit was brought against the American Medical Association and Dr. Morris Fishbein for several millions of dollars for libel but the suit was dismissed when Summers died before it could come to trial He had also filed another suit against Drs. George H. Simmons, Morris Fishbein, W. A. Puckner, Torald Sollmann and others. This suit also failed to come to trial.

NORMAN BAKER VS. THE AMERICAN MEDICAL ASSOCIATION

Norman Baker of Muscatine, Iowa, who headed a number of mercantile enterprises, including the ownership of a radio broadcasting station and an alleged cancer cure, was dealt with, editorially, in THE JOURNAL of April 12 and April 19, 1930, and in *Hygeia* for May, 1930. As a result of these publications, Baker brought suit for libel against the American Medical Association, asking one-half million dollars in damages. This case came to trial in the federal district court in Davenport, Iowa; the trial opened on February 9 and continued until March 3, covering a period of nearly four weeks. Voluminous testimony was offered by the American Medical Association, both through physicians who went on the stand as experts and by scores of depositions that had been gathered by the Association from various parts of the Middle West; much testimony was also put in by Baker. On March 3, the jury returned a verdict for the American Medical Association.

The case was heard before Federal Judge Gunnar H. Nordbye of Minnesota. In this connection, Norman Baker's weekly paper, the *Midwest Free Press*, prior to the trial expressed the editorial opinion that because the case was going to be heard before a judge who was coming from Minnesota, Baker would "not get all that's coming to him." To quote:

"We fear he [Norman Baker] will not get all that's coming to him—Judge Dewey was to hear the case and at the eleventh hour now announces a judge from Minnesota coming to try the case—that may be O. K. but WHY WE ASK, is it necessary to go away out of our district to secure a Federal Judge—we wonder how Dr. Mayo, who is a power in Minnesota would like it if he were in Mr. Baker's place and an Iowa judge from Muscatine section would hear the case—YES WE WONDER—Mr. Baker's formulas have accomplished more than Dr. Mayo ever did for cancer, and Baker will have to fight many years yet to educate the ignorant prejudiced and lazy thinking ones who are dominated by organized medicine." [Capitals as in the original.—ED.]

The implications in this statement are fairly obvious.

The jury before whom the case was heard was a group of substantial farmers or retired farmers and merchants. Counsel for the Association were Messrs. Edward M. Burke and Clement L. Harrell of the law firm of Loesch, Schofield, Loesch and Burke of Chicago, with Mr. C. M. Dutcher of the firm of Dutcher, Walker and Ries of Iowa City, who are the attorneys for the Iowa State Medical Society. Norman Baker was represented by two attorneys, Messrs. Charles P. Hanley of Muscatine and J. C. France of Tipton.

Appearing as medical experts for the Association were Dr. Francis Carter Wood of New York, Dr. Joseph Colt Bloodgood of Baltimore, Dr. Burton T. Simpson of Buffalo, Dr. Max Cutler of Chicago, and Dr. Albert C. Broders of Rochester, Minn. Several other physicians also aided the Association, appearing either as witnesses during the trial or by depositions.

BAKER'S ENTERPRISES

Originally, Baker's enterprises seemed to have been wholly or mainly in the commercial field. He sold radio sets, storage batteries, flour, coffee, canned fruit, silverware, brooms, alarm clocks, overcoats, mattresses, automobile tires, typewriters, paints, and many other things. He advertised his wares not only through printed catalogs and through his magazine, *T N T (The Naked Truth)*, but, more important, over his radio station, KTNT of Muscatine. Baker's first excursion into the medical field seems to have been the use of his radio station to advertise an injection treatment for varicose veins, exploited by a Davenport physician.

Baker had two (and, for a short time, three) alleged treatments for cancer that were being given at Muscatine in the building that was known as the "Baker Hospital." They were (1) a treatment for "external" cancer, an arsenic powder exploited by Harry M. Hoxsey, whose methods* are also dealt with in these pages, and (2) the injection treatment for "internal" cancers of one Charles O. Ozias of Kansas City—who also has received some publicity through THE JOURNAL.† When the American Medical Association, through its Bureau of Investigation, first began warning the profession and the public against the Baker cancer-cure business, Baker made the fantastic claim that the American Medical Association had offered him a million dollars for his "cancer cure," in order that it might be withdrawn from the market, so that sufferers of cancer would be compelled to resort to surgery x-rays, and radium! When Baker himself was on the stand during the first day of the trial, he denied that he had ever made such a statement, but his denial was offset by the presentation of a letter from the files of the Bureau of Investigation, signed "N. Baker" and which Baker had to admit he had dictated. In this letter Baker definitely stated that it was a "fact that the Medical Trust offered one million dollars on January 3rd 1930 to suppress this treatment."

Norman Baker was the first witness to be put on the stand by

---

* The Hoxide Cancer "Cure," J. A. M. A. 86:55 (Jan. 2) 1926. The Hoxide Quackery Again, ibid. 93:400 (Aug. 3) 1929.

† The Ozias Hospital Association, J. A. M. A. 79:1869 (Nov. 25) 1922.

the plaintiff, in order to show that the material published by the American Medical Association had caused him serious financial damage. Baker declared that his monthly receipts from his cancer-cure activities started at $1,380 for October, 1929, climbed to $75,232 for June, 1930, and, following the articles published by the American Medical Association, dwindled until in January, 1932, he took in only $7,008.

BIOGRAPHICAL NOTES ON BAKER

Baker, on cross-examination, admitted that his education went no further than a year and a half of high school work. After leaving school he traveled around the country working in machine shops as a die and tool maker. After two years of this, he went into the vaudeville business, putting on "hypnotism" acts "along psychological lines—mental work." He continued in that field for about eight or ten years, but in 1914 came back to Muscatine, where he started to manufacture calliopes. This work was interrupted for a short time when he went on the road again "putting on an act." In 1920, his factory burned and he then started a mail-order business. His broadcasting station went on the air in November, 1925, at which time he was running the "Tangley Institute," "Tangley Company," "Tangley Correspondence School," and some other things. He had a mail-order "art school," although he admitted that he could not paint a picture for his life. Nevertheless, he advertised to teach "oil painting in ten lessons by mail." Under the name of "Tangley Institute," Baker was broadcasting "to let the world know that varicose veins could be cured without operation." The Tangley Institute went out of existence when the "Baker Hospital" was opened.

From the evidence in the case, it appears that Baker's original intention was to make some financial arrangement with Ozias of Kansas City, whereby the Ozias "injection cure" for "internal" cancer could be used at Muscatine. Such plans, however, never materialized and Ozias testified that he had never sold, loaned or permitted Baker to use the formula. Baker was asked, when on the witness stand, who it was that told him what was in the Ozias mixture; he replied: "I refuse to tell." It was a fact, however, that two persons previously connected with Ozias in the exploitation of the Ozias "cure" were hired by Baker. One of these was a woman, Mary Turner, and the other a chiropractor, Charles Gearing. The Turner woman admitted that she had given thousands of injections of the Ozias "cancer treatment" while in the employ of Ozias; she was employed by Baker to do the same kind of work when she came to Muscatine. Mrs. Turner had no medical training and was not even a registered nurse!

THE FIVE TEST CASES

Baker, on the witness stand, admitted that he broadcast over his radio station that he was going to investigate a cure for cancer (the Ozias "treatment") and that he "wanted five men or women from any part of the United States or Canada who were suffering from cancer to consent to become a test patient for this treatment, that I would pay all of their expenses for them, all doctor bills, nurses' care, medical fee, room and board, and they to pay their own transportation to the hospital (in Kansas City, Mo.) where the treatment would be made." It developed that, as a matter of fact, most of the "test patients" paid their own expenses both in transportation and in fees to Ozias. These "test cases" were dealt with extensively in Baker's *T N T Magazine* and the matter was sent out as a reprint, because, according to Baker, the copies of his magazine containing the material had been sold out. The article was headed in black-faced type, "T N T Magazine Investigation Proves That Cancer Is Curable." The article in question started as follows:

> "Cancer is conquered. The greatest discovery in medical science in years—a positive cure for cancer, that dread disease which has taken toll of millions of lives, caused thousands to commit suicide and driven other thousands to insanity—has been revealed by an investigation conducted by Norman Baker, publisher of T N T magazine and owner of the Norman Baker Enterprises and radio station KTNT, who was assisted by a physician and member of his staff.
>
> "Seeing is believing. Mr. Baker and his fellow investigators have seen with their own eyes enormous and malignant cancers in advanced stages of growth rapidly yield to a new and painless treatment, soften and disappear. They selected the cancer cases themselves for observation after they had determined beyond any doubt that they were authentic cases of cancer. They have watched these true cases of cancer under treatment and have seen the cancers grow smaller and pass away."

Baker then went on to state that "painstaking observation" of the cases that had been selected for the test had "thoroughly convinced Mr. Baker that cancer has been conquered." The article then goes into detail regarding the five test cases, reproducing photographs of the individuals concerned. Here it may be interpolated that all five of the patients are dead and were dead for some time before Baker ceased reprinting his article to prove that "Cancer is Conquered."

THE OPEN-AIR SHOW

One of Baker's advertising stunts was characteristic of a man who had been in the "show business." He broadcast that the Baker Institute would hold an open-air meeting at Muscatine, where it would be demonstrated that both external and internal cancer was curable by the Baker methods. In the June issue of *T N T Magazine*, it was claimed that 32,000 people attended this meeting. In the same issue he purported to describe some of the "wonders" that were shown at that time. One of the more spectacular was thus described:

> "Most amazing and remarkable of all, the entire top portion of the skull of a patient almost in the last stages of cancer was removed and held up for exhibition by the physician before the gasping throng exposing the brains of the entire top of the patient's head."

BAKER'S "EXPERTS"

When the time came for Norman Baker to submit testimony to rebut that which had been put in by the American Medical Association, he called to the stand certain alleged experts. The first of these was E. M. Perdue, M.D., of Kansas City, Mo. Perdue qualified as an "expert" on cancer by stating that he had done special research at Johnson's* Laboratory for Cancer Research at Kansas City, Mo. According to Perdue, the cancer cell differs from the normal cell in that it contains more water, and the way to kill cancer is to remove the water from the cancer tissue! This is done, said Perdue, by applying escharotics or by injecting "certain chemicals which substitute that water and take it out, and the cancer dies."

Perdue testified that he had never done any surgical work for cancer nor had he ever used radium or x-ray, and that he would use none of these methods of treating cancer. He said that he had used escharotics in the treatment of cancer and he submitted as an efficient formula, equal parts of powdered zinc chloride, powdered gum acacia, powdered sanguinaria, powdered galingal and powdered charcoal. According to Perdue, a product of this sort "deaquafies" the cancer, "taking the water out by substituting another chemical for it." Furthermore, according to Perdue's testimony, when escharotics are applied, they do not destroy normal tissue, because the cancerous tissue is selective. Perdue declared that the develop- of cancer was due to an increased alkalinity in the tissues of the person suffering from this disease.

On cross-examination it was brought out that Perdue not only approved of the Koch treatment for cancer, but of the Abrams "electronic" theory; further, that he was using, at various times, what he described as the "Ellis machine," which is apparently one of the many imitations or modifications of the Abrams device.

---

* The Johnson cancer concern is dealt with in the pamphlet "Cancer Cures and Treatments" issued by the Bureau of Investigation of the American Medical Association.

George Starr White* is a personal friend of his, said Perdue, and has taught him "lots of things in diagnosis." Perdue testified that he studied law at the same time that he studied medicine; that he began the study of medicine at the Kansas City Hahnemann Medical College and that he taught histology, anatomy, and dissection at the same time. "I was a good anatomist," he admitted, and when asked where he learned his anatomy, he said that it was part of his course in the Kansas Normal College. He claimed, also, to have gone to the Eclectic Medical University of Kansas City. It was brought out that although Perdue had for years been practicing in the State of Missouri, he held no license from the state board of that state; he claimed that he had a right to practice because he had been in practice twenty years prior to the time that the law went into effect. Perdue also claimed to be a civil engineer and a chemist; to hold the degree of M.D. from two schools—one homeopathic and one eclectic; to have the degrees of Doctor of Public Health from the Eclectic Medical University of Kansas City. He also took "courses" in osteopathy and chiropractic in Kansas City schools now out of existence. He claimed to be an authority on mixing concrete and declared, under oath, that he had "superintended millions of dollars' worth of public work," having laid miles of asphalt paving. He did this civil engineering in the "summertime, between the school sessions."

Another Baker "expert" was J. W. Seip, M.D., of Erie, Pa. Dr. Seip was seventy-two years old, a graduate of Jefferson Medical College, 1883, and licensed to practice in Pennsylvania. Dr. Seip admitted that his practice, up until the time of the world war, had been largely general, but "since then, it has been more psychologic and chronic diseases." He said that he "had never done much of any research work on cancer" but, nevertheless, it was his expert opinion that cancer resulted from the "present devitalized condition of our diet" by which "we rob our blood of its known necessary twelve tissue salts." Dr. Seip further was of the opinion that persons suffering from cancer were nearly all "shallow breathers" and that they were the people who were "living on white bread depriving themselves of the salts of our tissues, which are mainly in bran." He declared: "One reason why cancer is so prevalent today is because people eat white bread, and the whiter the bread, the sooner you are dead." The doctor said that in his own treatment of cancer his "principal reliance is upon the Koch antitoxin." The Bureau of Investigation has in its files advertisements from Erie (Pa.) newspapers of fifteen years ago, reading as follows:

---

* See article: "George Starr White—Quack," THE JOURNAL A. M. A., April 13, 1929.

ERIE'S ONLY
Permanent Office Specialist
For Chronic Diseases

Cures high blood pressure, rheumatism, neuralgia, varicose veins and ulcers, scars and strictures, hemorrhoids, weakness, debility, nervousness, without pain.

Hours: 1 to 4 and 7 to 9 P. M.
DR. SEIP
1031-33 State Street.

A third "expert" called as a witness by Norman Baker was Bruce Miller.* He testified that he was graduated in 1886 by the College of Physcians and Surgeons, Chicago; that he was "out of practice for quite a number of years" but that in 1926, he went to Taylorville, Ill., where he was connected with Harry Hoxsey and his "Hoxside Institute." He practiced for a short period right after graduation and then worked in a factory and as a paper-hanger from 1891 to 1898; that he then "built up quite a large orchestra of ladies, dummies, in connection with a pipe organ" and went to Europe, where he took his "dummy" troupe and exhibited his "automatic orchestra." He was in Europe from 1899 to 1906, when he returned to the United States and entered the real-estate business, in which he continued until about 1918. Dr. Miller testified that the only treatments he administers for cancer are escharotics and that he does not attempt to treat any cases of "internal cancer," although he admitted that cases of that kind were accepted and the patients were given narcotics to make them comfortable.

The fourth "expert" called by Norman Baker was Harry Hoxsey himself. Hoxsey testified that he was thirty years old and that his education had not extended even through the eighth grade; he then worked as a coal miner and, in 1921, he started in the cancer-cure business at Taylorville, Ill. Hoxsey testified that he went to Muscatine with Norman Baker in March, 1930, and stayed at the Baker Institute until September 4, 1930, on a percentage contract basis. He admitted that he treated many patients and even used the hypodermic needle and gave some injections. It was brought out on cross-examination what had been generally known through the newspapers—that Hoxsey and Baker had a disagreement. Hoxsey's explanation of leaving Baker was:

"I told Mr. Baker I refused to be a party any longer to bringing people there to take any other treatment only mine because he had shown no results with any other treatment on external cases and I would truthfully say not one, for I haven't seen one single case of external cancer cured there where the powder was not used."

* Bruce Miller is discussed in the article, "The Hoxide Cancer Cure," already referred to.

He complained that Mr. Bellows, instead of sending the cases that come in for Hoxsey's powder treatment, would "consign them to the needle department where the intramuscular treatment was used." Hoxsey declared that he had sworn: "I have not seen one case of internal cancer leave that institution Baker Institute as cured that did not take my cancer treatment."

Following Norman Baker's "experts," there were put in evidence a number of alleged cases of cancer that were said to have been cured at the Baker Institute. Most of these were of a superficial type and those of the so-called internal type were not satisfactorily diagnosed as cancer. Baker put on the stand some of the individuals who were alleged to have been cured and, at the same time, presented photographs of the "before-and-after" type as confirmatory evidence. Incidentally, during the closing days of the trial, the United States Marshal took a loaded .38 automatic pistol from Norman Baker. Baker's excuse was that he had a permit to carry one, but he was informed that his permit did not extend to the federal courts.

THE CLOSING ARGUMENTS

In the final arguments, Mr. Dutcher, for the American Medical Association, made no attempt to soften the charges that had been made in THE JOURNAL and HYGEIA regarding Baker. "We called Baker a quack and we are not here to apologize for it," Mr. Dutcher declared. He brought out, further, that the State of Iowa had enjoined Baker from practicing medicine without a license and that the Federal Radio Commission had revoked Baker's broadcasting license, because it found that his operation of the station was inimical to the public interests. He reviewed the history of the five "test" patients that Baker had sent to Ozias at Kansas City, Mo., and emphasized the fact that they were all dead at the time that Baker was declaring, either directly or by implication, that they had been cured.

Mr. Dutcher maintained that there was not a single case in the record of the trial in which the Baker Institute could even claim to have cured a case of cancer with its hypodermic injections. Counsel also referred to the fact that Hoxsey and Gearing, neither of whom had any medical training, were known as "Doctors" at the Baker Institute.

Mr. Dutcher also asked why Gearing and Dr. Ozias and numerous other doctors who had been connected with Baker had not been called by Baker to testify in the case. As Mr. Dutcher stated, not a single M.D. who was associated with the "institute" before the date of publication of the alleged libelous articles had been called to testify, except Dr. Statler, who still had a job there. He dwelt on the evidence in the records showing that Statler once cut a woman's breast under the direction of Hoxsey and that in another case, Hoxsey himself cut the breast and the patient died five days later. Mr. Dutcher also dwelt on the case of the young Iowa farmer, who, suffering from what he thought might be cancer, went to the Baker Institute, where Hoxsey started to "treat" him. Not being satisfied that the Baker Institute knew much about his case, the young man went to the State University of Iowa's Dermatologic Clinic, where they found he was suffering from "barber's itch"! This case, as some of our readers may remember, was the subject of a brief article in THE JOURNAL for July 26, 1930.

Baker's attorneys, in their closing speech to the jury, declared that the American Medical Association was malicious in attacking Baker and that it had no right to attempt to interfere with Baker's business or injure his reputation.

The case went to the jury as the court closed on the evening of March 2; the jury was out for a few hours that evening before adjourning for the night. They returned to the jury room at nine o'clock the next morning, and at 10:50, a ballot was taken and the vote was unanimous for the American Medical Association. Their brief formal report to Judge Nordbye was: "We, the jury, find for the defendant."

Subsequently to losing the suit in Iowa, Baker went to Eldorado, Arkansas, where he opened another cure for cancer in an old springs resort. Here he practiced his method, exploiting it with a radio station across the border in Texas for which the call letters were X.T.N.T. Eventually he was tried by the Post Office Department and the government for the promotion of a fraudulent cancer cure and was sentenced to four years in the penitentiary. Shortly after he emerged from the penitentiary, he attempted to launch a fraudulent health institute in Iowa. Once a quack, always a quack!

"PAINLESS" PARKER

Early in 1935 while making an address in California before the Oakland Forum and the California Dental Association, Dr. Morris Fishbein characterized Dr. Painless Parker, a dentist, as a charlatan and a quack. Dr. Parker filed suit for $100,000, which suit was subsequently dropped.

Painless Parker operates a series of dental offices in California. His name had originally been something else but he got it changed to "Painless" Parker so that he could use the word "Painless," which word is contrary to the law in many states.

CHARLES R. WILEY

In June 1935 suit was filed against the American Medical Association by Dr. Charles R. Wiley, practicing medicine in Chicago under the name and style of the Civic Medical Center, asking a large sum of money for damages and for libel. That suit was withdrawn.

JEAN PAUL FERNEL

There have been several suits by Jean Paul Fernel against the American Medical Association and Morris Fishbein requesting at various times damages of $1,000,000 or more for alleged libel.

FERNEL'S PROFESSIONAL RECORD

John Paul Fernel's name originally was Giovanni Furno. He was born in Italy in 1889 and was graduated by the Illinois College of

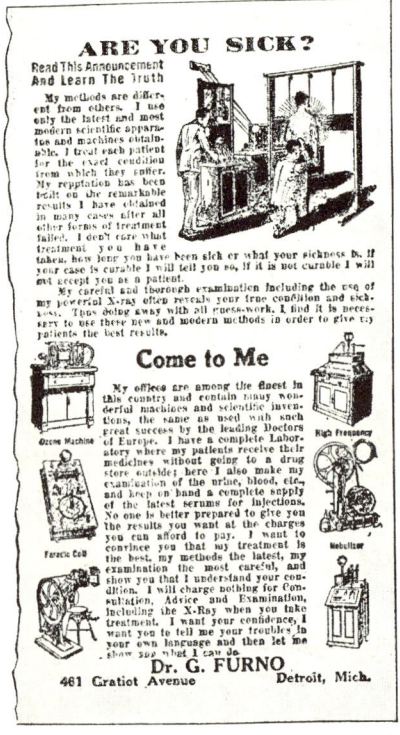

A greatly reduced photographic reproduction of one page of a six page advertising leaflet used by J. P. Fernel when he was in Detroit, Michigan. At that time Fernel had not changed his name from Giovanni Furno to its present form. The other five pages of the leaflet were in as many foreign languages.

Medicine in 1911, receiving an Illinois license the same year and a Michigan license, through reciprocity with Illinois, in 1916. Furno's Illinois license was first revoked in June, 1920, because of dishonor-

[526]

able conduct. Furno's license was restored by the Illinois board in 1922 during the tenure of office of the notorious W. H. H. Miller, who was later convicted of selling licenses, and removed.

For some time prior to 1916, Furno lived in Chicago. About that time he went to Michigan and opened an office in Detroit. In June, 1919, THE JOURNAL received a request from the Detroit authorities for information regarding Furno, who, it was alleged, was at that

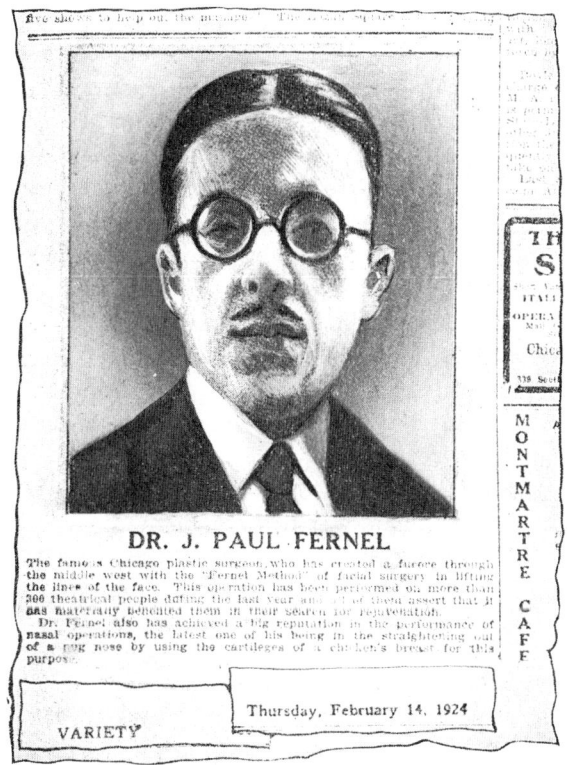

After Giovanni Furno became J. Paul Fernel and moved to Chicago, he went into the "plastic surgery" field, having taken lessons from a Chicago advertiser in the same line of business. Here is reproduced a piece of publicity that appeared in a theatrical publication. The up-to-date seeker of publicity does not purchase advertising space; he hires a press agent, who gets him before the public by means of news stories.

time advertising (as "G. Furno") to treat "nervousness, manly weakness and any other blood disease." Later, according to Detroit officials, Furno was served with a warrant and brought in to the police court, where he pleaded "Not guilty," was bound over to a higher court under $500 bail and, before the case was called to the higher court, "jumped his bail" and left the state. The Detroit officials reported that Furno's method was to get foreigners as patients and compel them to disrobe and enter an adjoining room for physical examination, and while this was going on a confederate (Furno's alleged wife) went through the pockets of the victim to determine the amount of the fee it was possible to obtain. As the result of these methods, the Detroit papers recorded in July, 1919, that nine of Furno's patients started suit against him.

Another part of Furno's scheme, according to the Michigan authorities, was that of collecting additional money from those of his victims who had about reached the limit of their donations, by purporting to have a blood examination made. The Michigan authorities sent the American Medical Association some of the "analytical reports" said to have been used by Furno in furthering this scheme. These bore the legend "International Medical Laboratory, Columbus Building, 32 North State Street, Chicago, Ill." There was no such concern as the "International Medical Laboratory," nor any Columbus Building at 32 North State Street. There is a "Columbus Memorial Building" at 31 North State Street, but there was not and never had been such an institution as the "International Medical Laboratory" in this building.

From Detroit Furno came back to Chicago, and, in October, 1919, is said to have entered into an agreement with a Chicago "plastic surgeon" (of the advertising type) to be taught the gentle art of removing sagging cheeks, baggy eyelids, hump noses, wrinkles, etc. While his preceptor was on a trip out of the state, Furno is said to have seized the opportunity to copy a list of the "plastic surgeon's" patients. On the return of the man from whom he was taking lessons, Furno discontinued his instruction and opened up a competing office in the city of Chicago. This, too, in spite of the alleged fact that he had entered into a contract not to practice "plastic surgery" in Chicago.

In the latter part of 1923, Furno, under his new name Fernel, corresponded with the Michigan authorities, seeking information regarding another Chicago physician who was apparently his most active competitor in the plastic surgery field. This other individual, like Fernel, had previously been in trouble in Michigan, and, also like Fernel, had "jumped his bail" and left the state. Also he obtained his Illinois license during the Miller régimé. The fight between these two "plastic surgeons" was a spirited one, but Fernel's competitor, while having a professional record far worse than Fernel's, seems to have kept the upper hand—so far.

On another occasion he promoted a fraudulent bust developer called "Landa" and on still another occasion a vitamin fraud and a device called the "sleeping brassiere" which contained small, rubber sponges to be worn over the breast and which were soaked with a mixture of various salts and chemicals which were said to be useful in making smaller an oversized bust.

Fernel was in trouble in 1942 when the Circuit Court upheld the action of the State Department of Education and Registration which revoked his license to practice medicine in Illinois. He was in trouble in 1943 for violation of the Federal Food, Drug and Cosmetics Act and he was sentenced at that time to one year in the County Jail and ordered to pay a fine of $500. In 1944 he was again in trouble for violating the Federal Food, Drug and Cosmetic Act and the Circuits Court of Appeals in 1944 affirmed the sentence given by the lower court. Then on December 29, 1944, he was sentenced to prison for three years following his conviction by a jury on twenty-one charges of violating the Food and Drug Act, carrying on a mail order medical business from his home at 1543 N. Wells Street, Chicago.

HERBERT EDWIN SOULE

A suit for some millons of dollars was filed by one Herbert Edwin Soule in 1936 against the American Medical Association claiming libel. Soule was reported to be president of the high-sounding National Health Foundation of Minneapolis. He was widely known for his antivivisection and antimedical propaganda. During the war he gave considerable trouble to the armed forces by his campaigns against inoculations such as were used by the Army to prevent disease among the troops. His suit never was pressed.

ROBERT WADLOW

In 1937 and 1938 came suits by Robert Wadlow, a giant, who claimed that he had been libeled by an article published in THE JOURNAL OF THE AMERICAN MEDICAL ASSOCIATION. The case came to trial in 1939 in St. Joseph, Missouri. Robert Wadlow claimed that he had been libeled in an article published in THE JOURNAL OF THE AMERICAN MEDICAL ASSOCIATION which referred to him as a freak. THE JOURNAL produced several other giants on the witness stand who claimed that they knew they were freaks and made a living at it. A newspaper said, "The parade of giants through this city's federal courtroom, streets and hotel lobbies was climaxed last night when a jury decided against 8-foot, 8-inch Robert Wadlow in a $100,000 libel suit."

Robert Wadlow died in July 1940 when he had an infection in his foot and did not know about it for several days due to the fact that he had lost sensation in his legs, apparently associated with his rapid growth. The boy had weighed $8\frac{1}{2}$ pounds at birth. At the time of his death he was 8 feet, 9½ inches tall and weighed 491 pounds and was definitely credited with being the world's tallest man.

EDNA PURDY FERNEL

In 1938 Edna Purdy Fernel sued the American Medical Association for $100,000. Her case is described in the story of Jean Paul Fernel mentioned previously.

ASA BRUNSON

In 1938 came a trial of the case of Asa Brunson vs. Morris Fishbein for $300,000 libel. This case was tried in the courts at El Paso, Texas, and dismissed by the judge on the fifth day with a fine statement praising the American Medical Association for its attempts to expose quackery. Brunson claimed to be able to cure tuberculosis with a mixture that contained petroleum. A leading periodical was about to publish an article exploiting him when it withdrew the article following a statement by the American Medical Association. Brunson claimed he had been damaged to the extent of $300,000 by failure to publish this article.

HIRESTRA LABORATORIES, INC.

In 1938 (April) also the American Medical Association was sued by the Hirestra Laboratories of New York for $1,000,000 because of an editorial in THE JOURNAL which characterized its product "Endocreme" as "a cosmetic with a menace." Endocreme claimed to contain 0.625 mg. of estradiol per ounce. THE JOURNAL editorial had pointed out the possibility of harm from such a preparation. Such preparations if they contain a sufficient amount of female sex hormone to have an effect are potentially dangerous; if they do not contain enough to have an effect they are fraudulent.

Later came another case by the Hirestra Laboratories for $3,000,000 for conspiracy and libel and then still another suit for $3,000,000 on the theory of conspiracy and libel.

All these suits were withdrawn.

WILLIAM E. BALSINGER

A plastic surgeon named William E. Balsinger sued the American Medical Association in September 1938 seeking $100,000 for libel. Balsinger, who is a plastic surgeon, claimed that he had been restricted in his freedom of practice. Incidentally both Balsinger and Henry J. Schireson claimed that they were the ones who straightened Jack Dempsey's nose. At various times Balsinger had been sued for malpractice by patients upon whom he had operated. The records of all of these cases are available in the files of the American Medical Association. The Balsinger cases have never come to trial.

JEAN FERRELL, INC.

Jean Ferrell, Inc., had tried by a threatened libel suit to prevent the American Medical Association from giving the public the facts relative to its "Concentra Food" which was a mixture of rhubarb, soy bean meal, Irish sea moss, gravel root and dehydrated cranberries. Jean Ferrell was also a cosmetic concern and maufactured another food known as "Bio-vita." The Federal Food and Drugs Administration had obtained judgments against the organization as had also the Federal Trade Commission. In fact, the Food and Drug Administration reported that "Concentra Food" was adulterated, misbranded and falsely and fraudulently represented. The company was fined $2,000.

J. THOMPSON STEVENS

In 1940 damages of $600,000 was sought for libel from Morris Fishbein and the American Medical Association by one J. Thompson Stevens who had been described in the Cosmopolitan Magazine in an article by Rex Beach as a "miracle man." THE JOURNAL OF THE AMERICAN MEDICAL ASSOCIATION published an editorial against unwarranted exploitation of J. Thompson Stevens and his methods. He also filed another suit for $350,000 for libel. These cases never came to trial.

JEAN PAUL FERNEL

In 1941 came another attempt by Jean Paul Fernel to collect $3,000,000 for libel. Nothing came of this!

WAYNE COUNTY ASSOCIATION OF PHYSICIANS AND SURGEONS OF OSTEOPATHIC MEDICINE, INC.

In 1942 the Wayne County Association of Physicians and Surgeons of Osteopathic Medicine, Inc., sued Dr. Morris Fishbein because he had made the statement in a lecture given in Detroit that osteopaths were not acceptable as physicians in the United States Army Medical Department. This case was withdrawn.

DINSHAH P. GHADIALI

The Association was also drawn into a considerable number of suits filed by the United States of America against one Dinshah P. Ghadiali who had repeatedly threatened suits against the American Medical Association because of articles published in the columns of its JOURNAL relative to his promotions of bogus apparatus for treating disease by a system called "Spectro-Chrome Therapy." Ghadiali was also founder of the Spectro-Chrome Institute. He holds the degrees of doctor of chiropractic, doctor of philosophy and doctor of legal law. He is a fellow and ex-vice president of the Allied Medical Association of North America, member and ex-vice president of the National Association of Drugless Practitioners, president of the All Cults Medical Association, president of the American Association of Spectro-Chrome Therapists, president of the American Anti-Vivisection Society, member of the Anti-Vaccination League of London, and member of the American Association of Orificial Surgeons.

Colonel Ghadiali (for he claims to be a Colonel) has a most interesting history. In May, 1925, he was arrested after a pistol battle in Portland, Oregon, charged by the federal authorities with having transported a nineteen year old Portland girl from that city to Malaga, New Jersey, and back for immoral purposes. He was indicted on six counts and found guilty of them all. At the time of his trial it was reported that the girl was engaged as secretary to Ghadiali while he was delivering lectures in Portland on "spectro-chrome therapy."

On December 4, 1925, Ghadiali was sentenced to five years imprisonment in the Atlanta penitentiary. While he was in the penitentiary, there was an outbreak among the prisoners. Because of his services at that time he was released March 1, 1929. He immediately went back to the spectro-chrome quackery and claimed in his advertising that he was pardoned by the President.

In 1931, Ghadiali was arrested in Cleveland, Ohio, and probably since that time he has been arrested and tried in a good many places. He was found guilty in a suit tried in Brooklyn in 1946 and again recently in New Jersey. The federal court at Camden, N. J., found him guilty on all twelve counts after a trial of 42 days. On January 7, 1947, the court fined him $1,000 on each count, making a total of $12,000 fine and also one year imprisonment on each of three counts, the prison terms to run consecutively. At the time of suspending part of the penalty, the judge instructed Dinshah Ghadiali to dissociate himself completely from the Spectro-Chrome Institute and Spectro-Chrome Metry. The court indicated that he must make all records available to the government at all times and that he must turn over all his literature, including some 4,000 copies of an encyclopedia, for destruction. The court then suspended the prison sentence and put him on probation for five years, saying that Dinshah is now an old man, 73 years of age, and because of his age, the judge did not deem it advisable to incarcerate him.

He did not wish to give Dinshah's followers the morbid satisfaction of regarding Dinshah as a martyr. Dinshah filed an appeal based on the theory that the sentence is inhuman and is in violation of the eighth amendment of the Constitution.

SUMMARY

The services rendered by the American Medical Association in its battles against quackery have been widely recognized as one of the most important services in behalf of the people of the United States. The effects of its exposés have been most salutary in preventing quackery and charlatanism which might well have been rampant, at least until the passing of the more recent Pure Food and Drugs Act and the Wheeler-Lea bill.

Week after week down through the years the Association has published its exposés of the charlatans. The evolution of government controls makes it reasonably certain that the future is not likely to see again such charlatans as Albert Abrams, John R. Brinkley and Norman Baker.

UNITED STATES OF AMERICA VS. THE AMERICAN MEDICAL ASSOCIATION ET AL.

ON SUNDAY AFTERNOON, July 31, 1938, delicately timed for Monday morning newspapers, Thurman W. Arnold, then assistant attorney general in the Department of Justice of the United States, released a statement to the press indicating that the Department of Justice proposed to prosecute the American Medical Association under the federal antitrust laws if a grand jury investigation, to be made in the District of Columbia, should result in an indictment of the American Medical Association. He proposed at the same time to indict the affiliated society in Washington and certain leaders of organized medicine. He had previously published two other statements regarding his intentions. In the statement issued on July 31 he offered to the American Medical Association and to the others concerned an opportunity to avoid trial by agreeing to consent to decrees which would assure the cooperation of the American Medical Association in the operation of cooperative clinics. In commenting on this subject, THE JOURNAL OF THE AMERICAN MEDICAL ASSOCIATION said:

> "The statement by the assistant attorney general is in accord with the point of view which he has held for some time in relationship to our government. Apparently it remains to be determined whether or not the federal administration can use the laws and the courts to mold the people of the United States to its beliefs in every phase of life and living."

In the statement by Thurman Arnold he pointed out that Group Health Association, Inc. had been organized in the District of Columbia in 1937 by 2500 government employees to provide prepaid medical care. The group retained its own physicians who were to provide the members with complete medical care. Mr. Arnold charged that the Medical Society of the District of Columbia, the American Medical Association and some of the officers of both organizations were attempting to prevent Group Health Association, Inc., from functioning. This, it was asserted, they did by threatening to expel from the District Medical Society doctors employed by Group Health Association, threatening to expel from the medical society doctors who would consult with the doctors of the Group Health Association staff, and excluding from Washington hospitals the doctors of Group Health Association.

Mr. Arnold claimed that the Group Health Association was being restricted from fulfilling its functions. He said:

> "No combination or conspiracy can be allowed to limit a doctor's freedom to arrange his practice as he chooses, so long as by therapeutic standards his methods are approved and do not violate the law. Organized medicine should not be allowed to extend its necessary and proper control over standards having to do with the science and art of medicine, to include control over methods of payment for services involving the economic freedom and the welfare of consumers and the legal rights of individual doctors."

For the next few weeks syndicated writers of columns and editors of newspapers throughout the nation discussed this impossible indictment pro and con—the titles of their statements indicating largely their point of view. The Indianapolis *Star* called it "New Deal Medical Bluff," the Philadelphia *Record* inquired "Is There a Medical Trust?" the Philadelphia *Inquirer* called this "A New Use for Antitrust Laws" and the Washington *Post* called it "A Very Broad Indictment." Many papers queried the phrase "medical monopoly." The Alton, Illinois, *Evening Telegraph* called it "Regulation Gone Mad" and the conservative New York *Sun* entitled its editorial "Putting the Screws Politely on the Doctors."

THE GRAND JURY

On October 17 the special grand jury in the District of Columbia began its study. The attorneys representing the government included John Henry Lewin, a special assistant selected by the Department of Justice, who had as his principal assistants Allan Hart of Portland, Oregon; Grant W. Kelleher and Douglas B. Maggs.

The District Court Justice James M. Proctor limited the scope of the grand jury investigation by quashing two-thirds of a subpena which the Department of Justice had prepared and which would have brought into the case all sorts of institutions and agencies which had been involved in investigations as far back as 1916. He permitted to stand that portion of the subpena which ordered the American Medical Association to produce all correspondence, memoranda or other documents dating from January 1, 1932, relating to:

> "The Justice Department's investigations of relations of the American Medical Association and the District Medical Society with the Group Health Association Inc. of Washington, D. C.
>
> "Any requirement or proposal of the American Medical Association that hospital staff members belong to local branches of the American Medical Association.
>
> "Instances where approval of hospitals for intern training by the American Medical Association were revoked because of the membership of the staffs of such hospitals."

Later the government presented a revised subpena which the judge permitted to stand.

The special grand jury after conducting its investigation for more than two months returned indictments December 20, charging violation of the Anti-Trust Laws against the American Medical Association, the Medical Society of the District of Columbia, the Harris County (Texas) Medical Society, the Washington (D. C.) Academy of Surgery, and twenty-one individuals. The specific test of applicability of the anti-trust statutes to the medical profession was based on the District of Columbia cooperative, known as Group Health Association, Inc. The indictment charged the defendants with conspiring to "hinder and obstruct Group Health Association, Inc., in obtaining access to hospital facilities for its members." The indictment was signed by Thurman Arnold, Assistant Attorney General of the United States, David A. Pine, United States Attorney for the District of Columbia, and John Henry Lewin, Allan Hart, Douglas B. Maggs and Grant W. Kelleher, special assistants to the Attorney General. According to United Press reports, the indictment charged the defendants with "having combined and conspired together for the purpose of restraining trade in the District of Columbia"; that is to say: "(1) for the purpose of restraining Group Health Association, Inc., in its business of arranging for the provision of medical care and hospitalization to its members and their dependents on a risk-sharing prepayment basis, (2) for the purpose of restraining the members of Group Health Association, Inc. (in Washington), in obtaining, by cooperative efforts, adequate medical care for themselves and their dependents from doctors engaged in group medical practice on a risk-sharing prepayment basis, (3) for the purpose of restraining the doctors serving on the medical staff of said Group Health Association, Inc., in the pursuit of their calling, (4) for the purpose of restraining doctors (not on the medical staff of Group Health Association, Inc.) practicing in the District of Columbia, including the doctors so practicing who are made defendants herein, in the pursuit of their callings, (5) for the purpose of restraining the Washington hospitals in the business of operating such hospitals.

"In so doing, defendants have then and there engaged in an unlawful combination and conspiracy in restraint of trade in and of the District of Columbia, in violation of Section III of the Act of Congress on June 2, 1890, known as the Sherman Anti-Trust Act."

"Plans, understandings and agreements to accomplish the unlawful business herein above described were proposed, discussed and adopted at such meetings" (the indictment apparently refers here to meetings of the Medical Society of the District of Columbia, at which the Group Health Association, Inc., was discussed).

In announcing the decision of the govrenment to press for criminal indictments, Mr. Arnold is reported to have said that such pro-

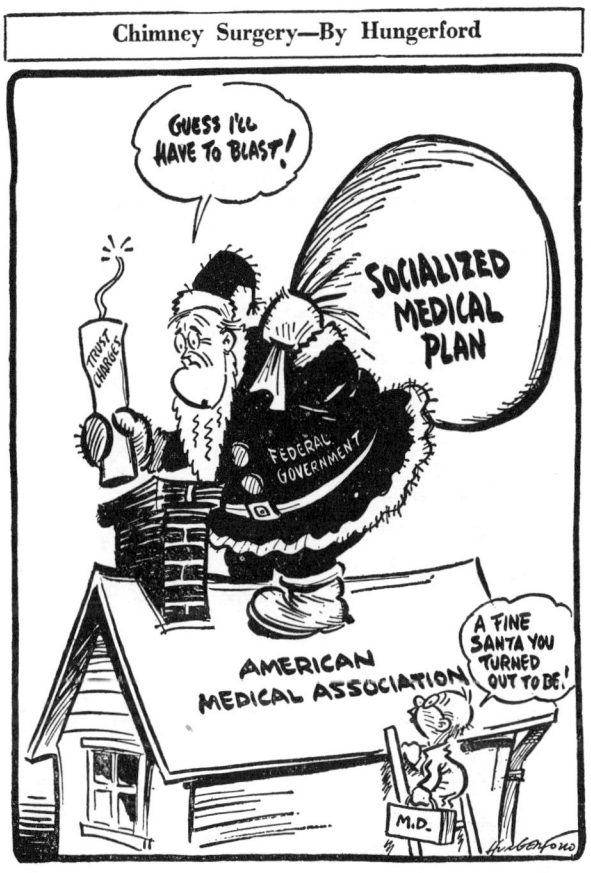

Thurman Arnold, ex-college professor and now trust-busting Assistant Attorney General, has indicted the ruling body of American Medicine on charges of restraining the activities of "group medicine." But if the Medical Association had agreed to "play ball" with Arnold, the indictment would have been shelved. Arnold's system is a brutal combination of the Star Chamber and Nazi bureaucracy. The doctors of America should unite in this fight against a system which jeopardizes the liberties of every citizen.— *New York Daily Mirror.*

cedures seemed the only method to resolve the issues raised in the situation. The individuals indicted include Dr. Olin West, secretary and general manager of the American Medical Association, Dr. Morris Fishbein, editor of THE JOURNAL OF THE AMERICAN MEDICAL ASSOCIATION, Dr. Rosco G. Leland, director of the Bureau of Medical Economics, Dr. William C. Woodward, director of the Bureau of Legal Medicine and Legislation, and Dr. William D. Cutter, secretary of the Council on Medical Education and Hospitals, all from the headquarters of the Association in Chicago. The following remaining individuals named in the indictments are all from the District of Columbia: Drs. Arthur C. Christie, Coursen B. Conklin, James Bayard Gregg Custis, Thomas A. Groover, Robert A. Hope, Leon A. Martel, Thomas E. Mattingly, Francis X. McGovern, Thomas E. Neill, Edward H. Reede, William M. Sprigg, William

The Tyrant

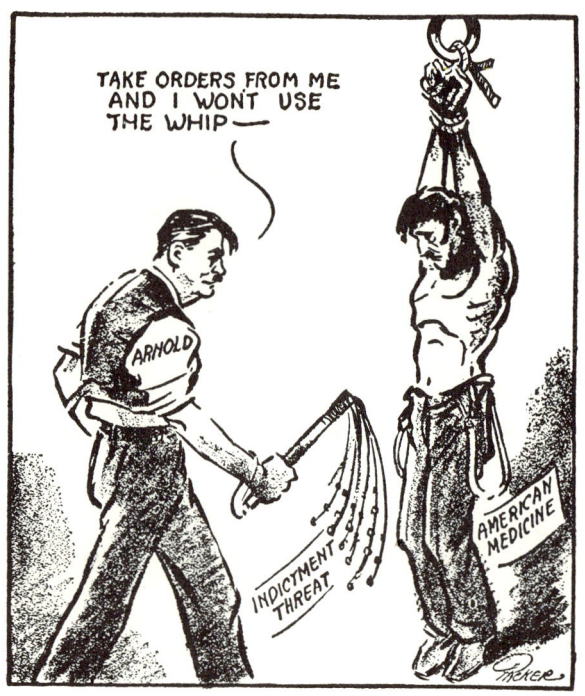

From the Pittsburgh *Post-Gazette*, Dec. 22, 1938.

J. Stanton, John O. Warfield Jr., Prentiss Willson, Wallace M. Yater and Joseph R. Young.

The complete text of the indictment was published in THE JOURNAL OF THE AMERICAN MEDICAL ASSOCIATION December 31, 1938. It was a document of many thousands of words setting forth the specific acts which the government listed as parts of a combination and conspiracy to restrain the activities of the Group Health Association Inc. Then on January 7, 1939, THE JOURNAL OF THE AMERICAN MEDICAL ASSOCIATION published the complete story of the indictment in chronologic order indicating how the Group Health Association had been established through activities of the Twentieth Century Fund, Inc., and all of the relationships of the Group Health Association to the Medical Society of the District of Columbia. There were complete accounts of the various press releases and statements made by the government's attorneys of the difficulties that had arisen in the Congress of the United States concerning some of the expenditures and many other related facts. Again the press of the nation commented widely on the indictment and cartoons throughout the nation referred to the case.

THE DOCTOR AND THE TRAFFIC COP

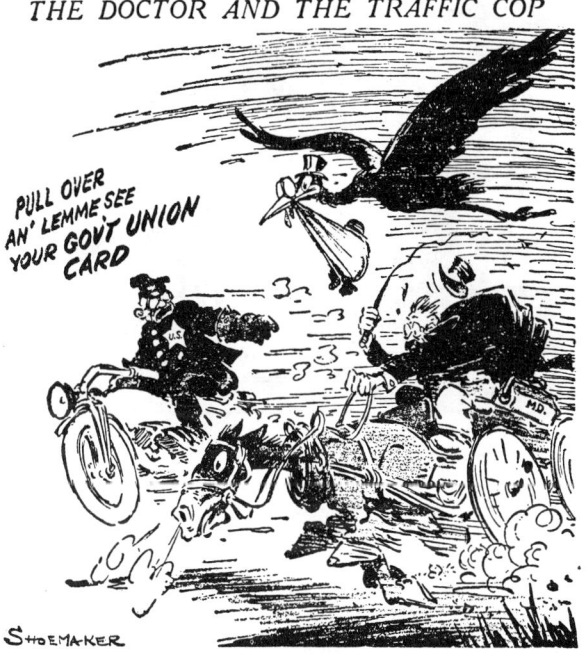

Shoemaker in the Manchester *Union*.

By the slow processes of the law, the next step was a hearing before Justice James M. Proctor who rendered an opinion in the U. S. District Court for the District of Columbia July 26, 1939, on a demurrer to the indictment. It was the opinion of Justice Proctor that medical practice is not a trade within the meaning of section 3 of the Sherman act.

Following this decision, the Department of Justice appeared promptly with another press release and another statement over the radio indicating that it was the intention to appeal from the decision of Justice Proctor. Incidentally Justice Proctor declared that

LOOKING INTO THE PHYSICIANS

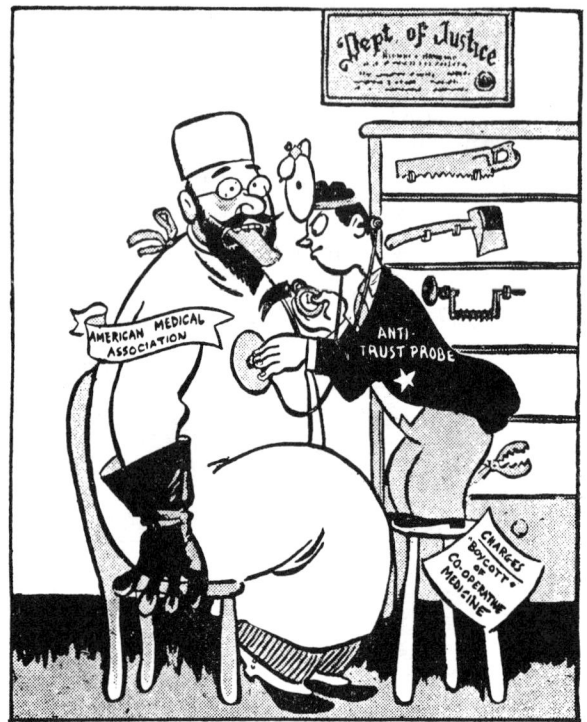

From the New York *Times*.

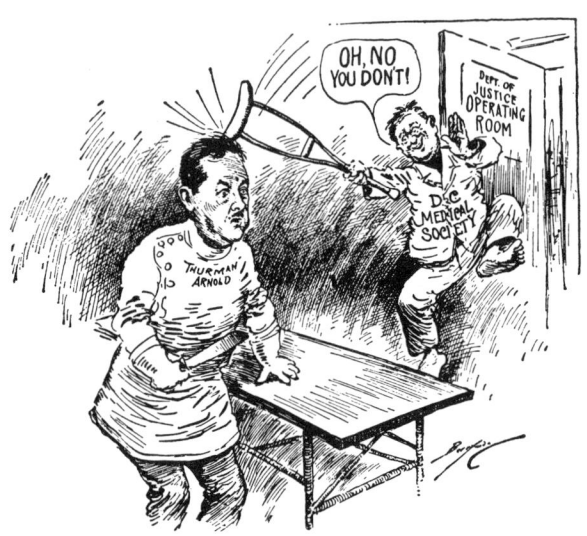

Cartoon in the Washington (D. C.) *Evening Star* July 27, 1939.

"much of the language of the indictment is highly colored, argumentative discourse." THE JOURNAL OF THE AMERICAN MEDICAL ASSOCIATION commented:

"The opinion of Justice Proctor lends encouragement and is an inspiration to continuous effort in behalf of a free profession. The medical profession of this country will not be coerced, threatened, abused or otherwise maltreated, and it will fight to the finish when its high traditions demand a righteous resistance."

Oh, Most Upright Judge!

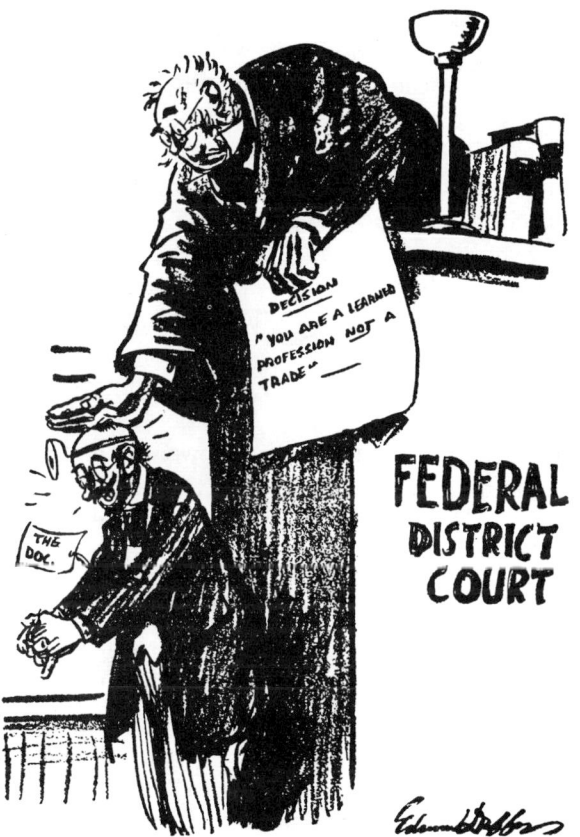

Cartoon in the Baltimore (Md.) *Sun,* July 27, 1939.

The ruling by Justice Proctor again stimulated the editors and the cartoonists to comment. The Dayton, Ohio, *Herald* said, "Our Doctors Go Free;" the Washington, D.C., *Post* called it "A Boomerang Indictment," and the Columbus, Ohio, *Dispatch* called it "A Gratifying Decision."

On October 23 the Supreme Court of the United States indicated that it would not pass on the suit brought by the Department of

Justice since the Department of Justice had appealed directly to the Supreme Court from the decision rendered by Justice Proctor. Next, however, the U. S. Court of Appeals on March 4, 1940, reversed the decision of Justice Proctor that medicine was "a learned profession and, therefore, not within the scope of the Sherman Anti-Trust Act." As part of its decision the Court of Appeals said: "The fact that defendants are physicians and medical organizations is of no significance." At the heart of the litigation was the question whether the law against restraint of trade applies to the medical profession. The court said "We think enough has been said to demonstrate that the common law governing restraint of trade has not been confined, as defendants insist, to the field of commercial activity, ordinarily defined as 'trade,' but embraces as well the field of the medical profession." Again the court said: "It cannot be admitted that the medical profession may through its great medical societies, either by rule or disciplinary proceedings, legally effectuate restraints as far reaching as those now charged." In addition the Court of Appeals held that, while the charge against the American Medical Association may be wholly unwarranted, "For present purposes we must take the charge as though its verity were established; and, in that light, it seems to us clear that the offense is within the condemnation of the statute." The court also said "It certainly cannot be doubted, that Congress intended to exert its full power in the public interest, to set free from unreasonable obstruction the exercise of those rights and privileges which are a part of our constitutional inheritance, and these include immunity from compulsory work at the will of another, the right to choose an occupation, the right to engage in any lawful calling for which one has the requisite capacity, skill, material or capital, and thereafter free enjoyment of the fruits of one's labors." And, it stated, "Congress undoubtedly legislated on the common law principle that every person has individually, and that the public has collectively, a right to require the course of all legitimate occupations in the District of Columbia to be free from unreasonable obstruction, and likewise in recognition of the fact that all trades, businesses and professions which prevent idleness and exercise men in labor and employment for the benefit of themselves and their families and for the increase of their substance are desirable in the public good and any undue restraint upon them is wrong and is immediate and unreasonable and, therefore, within the purview of the Sherman act." Further, the court said, "we are mindful of a generally known fact that under these rules and standards [of the medical profession] there has developed an *esprit de corps* largely as a result of which the members of the profession contribute a con-

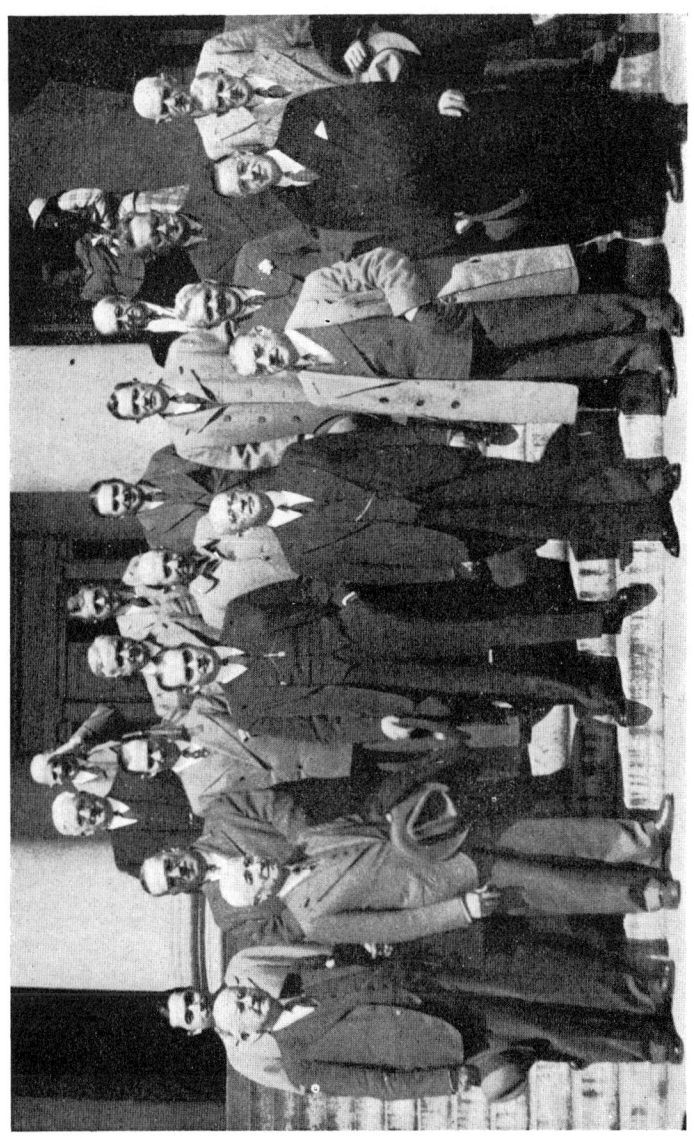

THE DEFENDANTS

From left to right, first row—Drs. W. M. Sprigg, William C. Woodward, Thomas E. Mattingly, William Dick Cutter, R. G. Leland, Daniel L. Boren. Second Row—Drs. J. Rogers Young, Leon A. Martel, Wallace M. Yater, Morris Fishbein, William J. Stanton, J. B. Gregg Custis and F. X. McGovern. Third row—Drs. Thomas E. Neill, Coursen B. Conklin, J. Ogle Warfield, Prentiss Willson, and Olin West. Fourth row—Mr. Theodore Wiprud, Drs. William B. Marbury and E. Hiram Reede. Dr. Borden, Dr. Marbury and Mr. Wiprud were not defendants in fact, but represented organizations which were indicted. Defendants not shown in picture were Drs. A. C. Christie, R. Arthur Hooe, and Thomas A. Groover.

siderable portion of their time to the relief of the unfortunate and the destitute. All of which may well be acknowledged to their credit. Notwithstanding these important considerations, it cannot be admitted that the medical profession may, through its great medical societies, either by rule or disciplinary proceedings, legally effectuate restraints as far reaching as those now charged."

On April 29, 1940, the defendants, including the American Medical Association, filed in the Supreme Court of the United States their petition for a writ of certiorari to review the decision of the Court of Appeals. The Department of Justice opposed this petition and the Supreme Court agreed with them because on June 3 it denied the petition. This was not a decision of the legal issues but merely a refusal to review the decision of the Court of Appeals. This made it necessary to proceed with the trial. At the time when the trial began the attorneys for the prosecution included among others Grant W. Kelleher, John Henry Lewin, Compton Timberlake and Walton Allen. The attorneys for the defense included Charles S. Baker, Edward M. Burke, Adrien Busick, William E. Leahy, Warren Magee, John B. Laskey and Seth W. Richardson.

The first step involved the selection of a jury. As might be expected, a jury chosen by the usual technic involved the assembling of a panel so that the jury when finally chosen comprised twelve persons —two of whom were women—of varying nationalities and occupations. The jury was constituted as follows: Reuben Acton Jr., 33, salesman; Edwin H. Ayers, 46, gas dealer; Jesse Ellis Porter, 45, assistant engineer; Mrs. Madelyn M. McDowell, 44; Mrs. Edna Hayes O'Neil, 51, housewife; Columbus Facchina, 28, secretary-treasurer of the Charles Facchina Tile Company; Joseph F. Taylor Sr., 38, floor manager; Washington W. Horad, 45, mail carrier; Egbert H. Irwin, 39, salesman; Otho T. M. King, 31, salesman; Eugene B. Magruder, 41, foreman; Charles A. Marggraf, 32, salesman.

The opening statement on behalf of the United States was made by John Henry Lewin who did his utmost to emphasize to the court that the issues involved were not medical but business issues. After naming the five employees of the American Medical Association who were defendants, he said: "These five defendants are doctors but they are not generally practicing physicians. The evidence will show that they devote their time and energies as businessmen largely to the policies of this organization, the A.M.A., and to the business side of medical practice." Of the defendant physicians in Washington, he said, "The evidence will show that these defendants induced and coerced the twelve private Washington hospitals to join with the defendants as conspirators to bring about certain of these restraints." He then discussed at great length the American Medical Association and its work, the Group Health Association, classification of hospitals and many other similar subjects. Then his assistant, Mr. Grant Kelleher, traced what he called the background of the case which dealt with the principles of the American Medical Association, its power and its relationship to various forms of clinics throughout the nation.

The opening statement on behalf of the defendants was made by Attorney William E. Leahy who related the history of the organization of the District of Columbia medical society and of the American Medical Association. He told of the House of Delegates, the principles of medical ethics, and then traced, from his point of view, the background and history of the circumstances leading to the trial.

The first witness called by the government was Dr. Hugh Cabot whose examination—direct and cross—occupied many hours on the witness stand.

The trial went on for many weeks and was no doubt the most exhaustive investigation of the evolution of medical practice in the United States ever made. The trial dwindled to its end when the last witness was called on March 31, 1941. Then came the usual "prayer and motions" as the lawyers call them, and following these the argument to the jury. As an example of John H. Lewin's argument to prove conspiracy, note this paragraph:

> Now, what was the A. M. A., the parent body, doing all this time? Just as soon as they heard of it, they condemned it as unethical; they used this horrible word which a normal man might suppose was a charge of immorality. As their past president defined it, the conduct of a gentleman, observing the golden rule, the Ten Commandments. Certainly there was nothing like that involved here, and they sent posthaste from Chicago to Washington their three big men, their full salaried men, their doctor general manager West, their Dr. Cutter, and their doctor lawyer. What to do? Simply to get information? The resolution under which they came showed they were to advise the District Medical Society, and the evidence shows that they did so. And then the Trustees of the American Medical Association, alarmed by this competition, instructs the defendants Fishbein and West, their doctor journalist and doctor general manager, to bring the situation to the attention of the entire medical profession, and an article is to be written, to be published in THE JOURNAL and distributed among their one hundred ten thousand doctors.

As is typical in criminal law cases, he characterized the evidence produced by the defendants as "muckrake, uncorroborative, hearsay on hearsay." He was moved almost to tears by the cases of the patients whom he described and he asked for a verdict in behalf of the government.

Mr. Lewin was followed by Grant W. Kelleher who repeated again the history of the entire case and summarized the evidence.

The argument on behalf of the defendants was made by William E. Leahy. After his opening remarks he said:

You have just heard the oldest profession in the world castigated as though its members were common criminals. You have just heard every motive which has actuated a doctor in the practice of the ideals of his profession dragged down into the common mud and mire of cheap commercialism. You have just listened to a castigation of men who have been drawn into this court room as defendants, the like of whom no jury has ever been called on before to sit face to face with for two months.

You have heard two organizations of professional men which have had for their ideals the protection of your health and mine, the protection of the health and the welfare of the United States, condemned as if they all ought to spend the rest of their lives in disgrace.

There must be some reason for such a thing; there must be some reason why men are thus accused. We are all human, after all. We all have known the medical profession. The medical profession stood by every one of us when we came into this world, and some one of them will be standing beside our deathbed when we leave it. We know that doctors are only human, and we know that sometimes they are actuated by motives which we do not approve of, just as lawyers are, and no one regrets that more than the practitioner because, after all, the profession of medicine has been inspired by the highest ideals under heaven, next to the ideals of those who attend your sick souls.

Why was it, therefore, that this heat was put into the argument in order to arouse you so that you could not review this testimony as jurors with calm deliberation?

I will tell you the reason. It is a reason which every lawyer uses when he cannot talk facts. It is the reason which every lawyer employs when he knows he has not a good case. It is the reason which every advocate employs to try to inflame the jury and get it away from the issues, in order that it may draw you into an unjust and an unfair verdict.

Mr. Leahy then reviewed the entire case from his point of view. Since he spoke as the only attorney for the defense, he had time equal to that occupied by both Mr. Lewin and Mr. Kelleher, and he reviewed the entire case not only as it affected each of the organizations concerned but as it affected each of the individual defendants.

Mr. John H. Lewin made the closing argument on behalf of the United States, after which the court charged the jury.

The jury brought in its verdict at 11 a.m., April 14, 1941. The verdict declared all of the individual defendants to be innocent of the charges, yet found the American Medical Association and the District of Columbia Medical Society guilty. Thereafter the attorneys for the American Medical Association submitted motions to set aside the verdict and to arrest judgment. On May 29 Justice James M. Proctor imposed a fine of $2500 on the American Medical Association and a fine of $1500 on the Medical Society of the District of Columbia. There had been the usual appeals, even to the Supreme Court, which, however, refused to hear the case further and the case was ended when those who had been fined paid their fines.

A few statements from the "charge to the jury" by the court are worthy of quotation in defining to the reader what limitations may be placed on the medical profession in relationship to opposition to various forms of medical practice.

The Sherman Act prohibits combinations unreasonably in restraint of trade. This prohibition extends to undue restraints on the furnishing of medical service to the public. If you find that the defendants conspired together for the purposes charged and employed the means charged, and if you find that the defendants, in seeking to achieve those purposes, intended to prevent Group Health Association from competing with doctors engaged in private practice on a fee-for-service basis in furnishing medical care to members of the public eligible for membership in Group Health Association, then the defendants were engaged in a combination in restraint of trade.

* * * * * *

It is not necessary that all the parties to a conspiracy shall actually meet together at one and the same time and place, or that all discuss its purposes or the means of carrying out its objectives, or whether each party knows all the others. Nor do you need to find that all combined together at the start of the conspiracy. If it is shown that the conspiracy was entered into between two or more of the defendants and that at any later time during its existence new or additional parties, while aware of its existence, united with them for the purpose of aiding in the accomplishment of the scheme, they would then become conspirators too and responsible for the consequences thereof.

In determining whether a conspiracy exists it is not necessary to find there was a written or formal agreement among the defendants or that any participant was bound to another to perform any particular portion thereof. It is sufficient if you find from the evidence that the defendants were voluntarily acting together, however informally, in order to carry out the common objective. Notwithstanding the fact that all the defendants are charged to have participated in the offense, it is not necessary for the Government to prove that all did so, and you are not required to find all guilty. If you find that the offense charged was in fact committed and that some of the defendants on trial were parties to it, you may convict those whom you so find guilty and acquit the others.

* * * * * *

The defendants had the lawful right to combine and form corporations and associations for the improvement of the practice of their profession and to advance their interests. They had the right to make reasonable rules and regulations respecting their profession and to ascertain the qualifications and character of their members. They had the right to discipline members who failed to abide by the regulations or rules adopted by the associations in the formation thereof and to suspend or expel from membership any member who failed to abide by the rules and regulations. The fact that the defendants adopted such rules and regulations and disciplined members does not of itself constitute an unlawful combination in violation of the statute. They must have combined together with the intent to injure, obstruct or restrain trade, or they must have intended to do acts the necessary effect of which would be to injure, obstruct or restrain trade.

The individual defendants as physicians had a right to determine with what other physicians they would consult, and their refusal to consult with any particular physician is not of itself illegal.

Physicians have the right to select the hospital in which they choose to treat and operate on their patients; and the refusal of a physician to do business with any hospital because of the composition of its courtesy staff is not of itself illegal.

The defendants American Medical Association and Medical Society of the District of Columbia have the right to adopt rules for just and fair dealing among their members and the right of enforcement of those rules and regulations by such reasonable penalties as they may provide for violation thereof.

The defendants had the right to reach and attempt to reach their objective of advancing the interests of the medical profession by legitimate persuasion and reasoned argument, and to this end they had the right to tell their side of the story and to persuade others, including the Washington hospitals, other physicians, members of Group Health Association, Inc., and the public to utlilize and use the defendants' method of practicing medicine, and to use peaceful persuasion, publicity, articles in the press, in publications of defendants, including THE JOURNAL OF THE AMERICAN MEDICAL ASSOCIATION, and all lawful propaganda to have their methods of practicing medicine prevail over those of Group Health Association.

The defendants had the right to write letters or other statements among themselves or to other members of the profession or to the public generally, expressing disapproval of or opposition to Group Health Association and the form of medical service offered by it.

* * * * * *

I charge you that the defendants have the lawful right, through action taken in their meetings and conferences, to formulate and adopt rules of medical ethics for the control and government of themselves and the members of their societies in the practice of their profession, and the support and maintenance of such principles of medical ethics by legitimate persuasion and reasoned argument or by enforcement of Society rules, laws, and regulations, without more, would not constitute unreasonable restraints against Group Health Association, its doctors or members.

Any doctor who voluntarily joined the defendant medical societies was required to comply with the constitution, rules and regulations thereof. No doctor would have the right, as against the wishes of the particular society, to retain membership therein regardless of how valuable or advantageous such membership might be to him, and at the same time wilfully violate any provision of its constitution, rules or regulations.

If a doctor desires to retain membership he is bound to obey the constitution, rules and regulations, since membership therein is entirely voluntary; and if, as a result of his nonobservance, he suffers discipline and possible expulsion from the society, any injury, damage or restraint thus suffered by him or by any corporation by which he might have been employed would, without more, not constitute a violation of the statute.

The Washington hospitals are private institutions under private management and control, and the lawful authority to constitute the medical staffs of such hospitals is vested in the governing board thereof. Hospitals have a lawful right to make such reasonable rules and regulations for the operation of the hospitals as to the authorities thereof may seem in their best interests. They are lawfully entitled to require obedience to such rules and regulations by all persons dealing with said hospitals, including doctors permitted by the hospitals to practice their profession therein.

The Washington hospitals had the lawful right, if they so desired, to adopt and enact a rule confining their medical staffs to members of the local medical societies, and any restraint resulting thereby to Group Health Association, its doctors, members or operations, would not in itself be a violation of the Sherman Act.

A member of the medical profession duly authorized by law to practice his profession in the District of Columbia is not by reason thereof entitled to practice in any of the private Washington hospitals. Permission to practice in such a hospital is not a right on the part of an applicant doctor but is only a privilege which can be extended or withheld from him at the will of, or in the discretion of, the particular hospital.

If the Washington hospitals or any of them believed that it was in the best interests of such hospital to adopt and enforce a rule confining appointments to the medical staff to members in good standing of local medical societies any such hospital had a lawful right to adopt and enforce such rule, and any resulting injury or restraint occasioned thereby to a particular doctor or other person would not be a violation of the statute.

The defendant American Medical Association had the lawful right, on request of a hospital, to inspect it for the purpose of approving or disapproving it for intern or resident training, and it had a lawful right to approve or disapprove such hospital based on the inspection so made.

* * * * * *

The Medical Society of the District of Columbia is shown by the evidence to have been a component and constituent society and member of the American Medical Association. As such it was entitled to contact, communicate and advise with the officers and representatives of the American Medical Association with reference to matters affecting or relating to the practice of medicine, and such intercourse between the societies is not a violation of the Sherman Act.

* * * * * *

The defendant Fishbein, the Editor of THE JOURNAL OF THE AMERICAN MEDICAL ASSOCIATION, had a lawful right to publish in THE JOURNAL objections to Group Health Association and its proposed methods of medical practice; and such publication of articles criticizing Group Health and its plan for medical service, even though it may have restrained or injured Group Health Association, its doctors or members, standing alone and without more, would not make Fishbein guilty of a violation of the act.

The American Medical Association and its officers had the lawful right to receive and answer inquiries concerning various so-called contract medicine plans, and the American Medical Association and its officers, in answering such inquiries, were lawfully entitled to state their own conclusions and beliefs with respect thereto, whether favorable or otherwise, and by so doing, without more, the American Medical Association and its officers would not violate the statute.

Evidence has been admitted tending to show the size and scope of the activities of the American Medical Association. Such fact does not raise any inference of wrongdoing or guilty conduct. Whether the American Medical Association is a large corporation or a small corporation does not affect its lawful right under the law; and the evidence is admitted here only for the purpose of showing the possible power, if any, of such corporation to induce and further the alleged illegal conspiracy set forth in the indictment.

* * * * * *

In joining the District Society members assumed the duty of compliance with laws and regulations thereof. The right to practice medicine gave a doctor no right to be a member of the Society. Discipline and control of members of a society, within reasonable bounds, are essential. When applied in good faith, under fair rules, without ulterior purpose to injure the business of a member or others, there is no wrong. However, such rules and regulatory actions cannot be justified where the real purpose, or the natural results, are to interfere with free competition.

The defendant physicians had the individual right to determine with what other physicians they would consult, and refusal to do so with particular physicians is not of itself illegal. Although, if, as alleged, it was done in furtherance of a conspiracy against Group Health and its doctors, it would be illegal. So too a doctor may refuse to treat patients in a particular hospital for any reason at all, but if a group of doctors, pursuant to a concerted scheme, refused so to do to injure the business of the hospital, their acts would be illegal; for in the eyes of the law there is danger to the public interests where many combine and act together to interfere with the free play of competitive forces in business and professions.

There was no duty on the societies, their officers or members, to approve Group Health or its plan of medical care. They could not rightfully oppose in a manner intended to restrain its operations. But they did have the right of legitimate criticism, argument and persuasion, however persistent and severe; either separately or by collective effort; through the medium of speech, letters or print. If their opposition was thus confined and did not take the form of a conspiracy to restrain or was not done in pursuance of such a scheme, there was no violation of the statute.

* * * * * *

The hospitals had the lawful right to prescribe rules and regulations governing the use of their facilities by doctors and patients. In their boards was vested the authority to decide what physicians would be allowed the privileges. A doctor had no right to demand them. To grant or refuse the same rested solely with the hospital. Therefore, if denial of privileges to Dr. Selders, or other members of the Group Health staff, represented the voluntary decision of the boards, no question would arise as to the legality of their acts. However, if refusal was arbitrary and to serve a criminal conspiracy against Group Health or their doctors, it would violate the statute.

* * * * * *

The respective merits of differing methods of medical care are not an issue in this case. Advocates and adherents of each are entitled to their views and may follow their choice. They had the right to support the same by fair competition and to oppose by way of discussion, argument and persuasion. But neither group would be justified in conspiring to restrain the activities of the other.

The legality of Group Health, or its methods of providing medical care, or the quality thereof, or its financial condition, or the grant of money by others to it are not issues in the case.

The defendants, however, had the lawful right to discuss and to argue these matters in opposition to Group Healh Association and its methods of medical care, and to do so would constitute no violation of the statute.

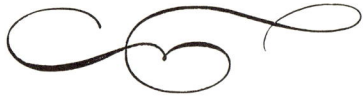

Recipients of the Distinguished Service Medal

BY MORRIS FISHBEIN, M.D.

RECIPIENTS OF THE DISTINGUISHED SERVICE MEDAL

RUDOLPH MATAS

THE FIRST MEDAL FOR distinguished service to scientific medicine to be awarded by the American Medical Association was given to Rudolph Matas, surgeon, of New Orleans, by the House of Delegates in the election held June 13, 1938, at San Francisco.

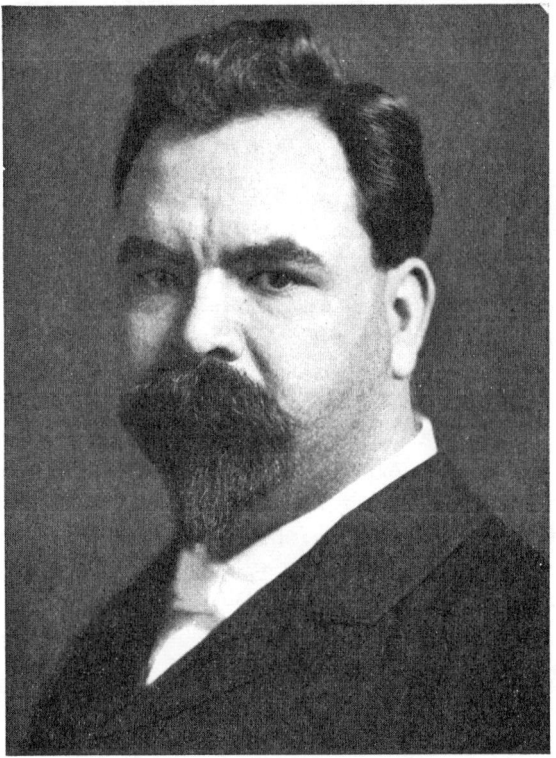

Rudolph Matas, M.D.

Dr. Matas was born in Bonnet Carre, La., Sept. 12, 1860, was educated in Barcelona, Paris, Brownsville (Texas) and New Orleans, and was graduated by the Literary Institute of St. John, Matamoros, Mexico, in 1876. He received his degree in medicine from

Tulane University in 1880 and has had honorary degrees from Washington University, the University of Alabama, Tulane University, the University of Pennsylvania, Princeton and the National University of Guatemala. He began the practice of medicine in New Orleans in 1880 and has specialized in surgery since 1895, when he became professor of surgery in Tulane University.

He has been emeritus professor of surgery at Tulane and consultant at Charity Hospital, New Orleans, since 1928 and honorary chief surgeon of Touro Infirmary since 1935. During the World War he was organizer and director of Base Hospital No. 24. He is a member of innumerable surgical societies throughout the world and at present is president of the Société internationale de chirurgie and honorary president of the International Surgical Congress, which will meet in Vienna next year. He has been decorated by the governments of Venezuela, Spain, France and Cuba. Dr. Matas is recognized as one of the most learned writers on surgery in the world. He is author of many treatises and monographs on surgical subjects, especially in the field of vascular surgery.

JAMES B. HERRICK

The second award of the Distinguished Service Medal and citation by the American Medical Association was tendered during the annual session of 1939 at St. Louis to Dr. James B. Herrick of Chicago.

Dr. James Bryan Herrick was born Aug. 11, 1861, in Oak Park, Ill. He attended Oak Park High School and the Rock River Seminary at Mount Morris, Ill. He then received his A.B. degree from the University of Michigan in 1882. For a time he taught in the Central High School at Peoria, Ill., where he acquired a love of good literature and a facility for expressing himself in the English language. Through an association with Moses Coit Tyler he developed a great interest in Chaucer. Dr. Herrick then took up the study of medicine, receiving the degree of Doctor of Medicine from Rush Medical College in 1888. His internship was served in the Cook County Hospital and in 1889, after completing his internship, he married Miss Zellah P. Davies of Oak Park.

Dr. Herrick has contributed greatly to the periodical literature of medical science, he has taught in his Alma Mater and he is widely known for his contributions particularly to our knowledge of coronary thrombosis. Indeed, it has been said that his articles on coronary thrombosis have done more to force clinical recognition of the condition and to stimulate clinical and experimental study than all other writings on the subject. Probably most significant was the contribution on "Clinical Features of Sudden Obstruction of the Coronary Arteries," published in 1912. In his career as a physician he also has been instructor in medicine at Rush Medical College from 1890 to 1894, adjunct professor from 1894 to 1900, professor from 1900 to 1927, and he is now emeritus. He has been attending physician at the Presbyterian Hospital in Chicago since 1895 and a member of the board of trustees of the Lewis Institute since 1903. He has also been president of the Association of American Physicians, of the Institute of Medicine in Chicago, and of the American Association

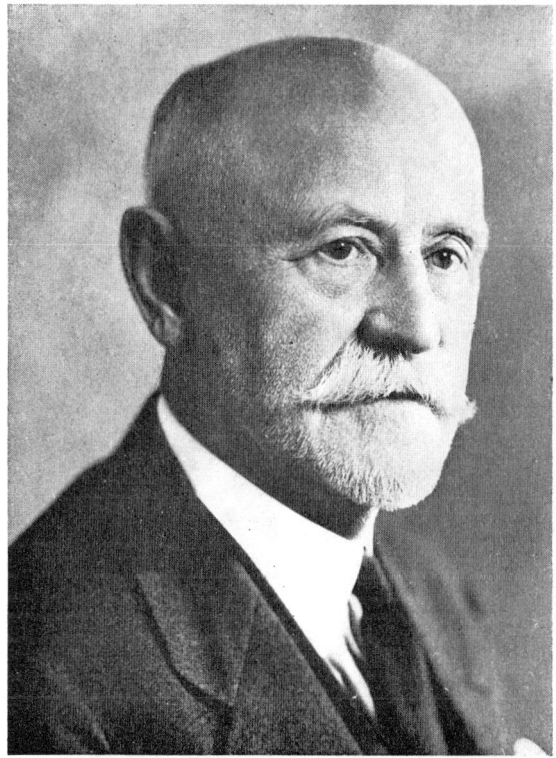

James B. Herrick, M.D.

of the History of Medicine. In 1930 he received the Kober Medal of the Association of American Physicians for Research and Scientific Medicine. In 1931 he gave the sixth Harvey Society Lecture at the New York Academy of Medicine on the Coronary Artery in Health and Disease, and in 1933 he was elected honorary fellow of the New York Academy of Medicine. In 1932 he received the honorary degree of Doctor of Laws from the University of Michigan, and in January 1939, at the 194th convocation of the University of Chicago, the honorary Doctorate of Science was conferred upon him.

Throughout his career he has been of vast assistance to young men and a builder of medical institutions. He was founder and first president of the Chicago Society of Internal Medicine. From 1928 to 1934 he was a member of the Judicial Council of the American Medical Association. By this second award the House of Delegates still further enhanced the significance of its Distinguished Service Medal.

CHEVALIER JACKSON

The 1940 medal was bestowed on Dr. Chevalier Jackson of Philadelphia, known throughout the world as one of the greatest leaders in the field of otolaryngology and especially distinguished for his contributions to bronchoscopy.

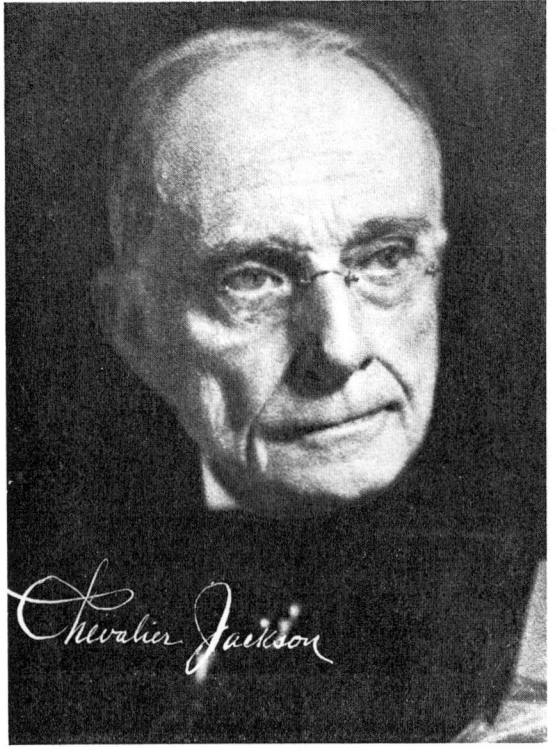

Chevalier Jackson, M.D.

Dr. Jackson received his degree of doctor of medicine from Jefferson Medical College in Philadelphia in 1886. He was professor of laryngology at the University of Pittsburgh from 1912 to 1916 and at Jefferson Medical College, Philadelphia, from 1916 to 1924, when he became professor of bronchoscopy and esophagoscopy at

Jefferson and at the University of Pennsylvania Graduate School of Medicine. He held both positions until 1930. He retired as professor of clinical bronchoscopy at Temple University School of Medicine.

His honors include fellowships in practically every leading organization devoted to his specialty throughout the world. He has been decorated by France, Belgium, Italy and Brazil. His writings include three books devoted to his specialty and innumerable contributions to systems of medicine and to surgery. He also received the Bok award from the city of Philadelphia, given to the resident who in the preceding year has "performed or brought to its culmination an act or contributed a service calculated to advance the best interests of the community."

JAMES EWING

Dr. James Ewing of New York, world famed as a pathologist, was the recipient of the Distinguished Service Award of the American Medical Association for 1941.

Dr. James Ewing was born in Pittsburgh on Christmas Day, 1866. He received his bachelor's degree from Amherst in 1888 and his master of arts degree in 1891. Following his fundamental education, he attended the College of Physicians and Surgeons of New York, now known as Columbia University College of Physicians and Surgeons, and received his degree of doctor of medicine in 1891. He was also honored with honorary degrees of doctor of science by the University of Pittsburgh in 1911, by Amherst in 1923, by the University of Rochester in 1932 and by Union College in 1938 and with the LL.D. degree by Kenyon College in 1931 and by Western Reserve University in the same year. Early in his medical career Dr. James Ewing determined to devote himself to the fundamental sciences. He was a tutor in histology, 1893–1897, and had the Clark fellowship, 1896–1899. He then became instructor in clinical pathology at the Columbia College of Physicians and Surgeons, 1897–1898; he was professor of pathology from 1899–1932, at Cornell University Medical College and from 1932 was professor of oncology. Indeed it was his fundamental work in the field of cancer that has made him most famous. Among other positions which he occupied was the directorship of the Memorial Hospital in New York City. He was a member of such scientific organizations as the National Academy of Sciences, the Association of American Physicians, the American Roentgen Ray Society, the American Association of Pathologists and Bacteriologists, the Society of Experimental Biology and Medicine, the Harvey Society, the

American Association for Cancer Research and the American Medical Museum Society. In 1931, when he was head of the department of pathology at Cornell University Medical College, Dr. Ewing was honored with a dinner and with a testimonial volume including fifty-four articles on cancer written by authorities from all over the world. On that occasion messages were sent by President Hoover, Gov. Franklin Delano Roosevelt and Madame Curie, as well as many others. In 1936 he received the John Scott Award, consisting

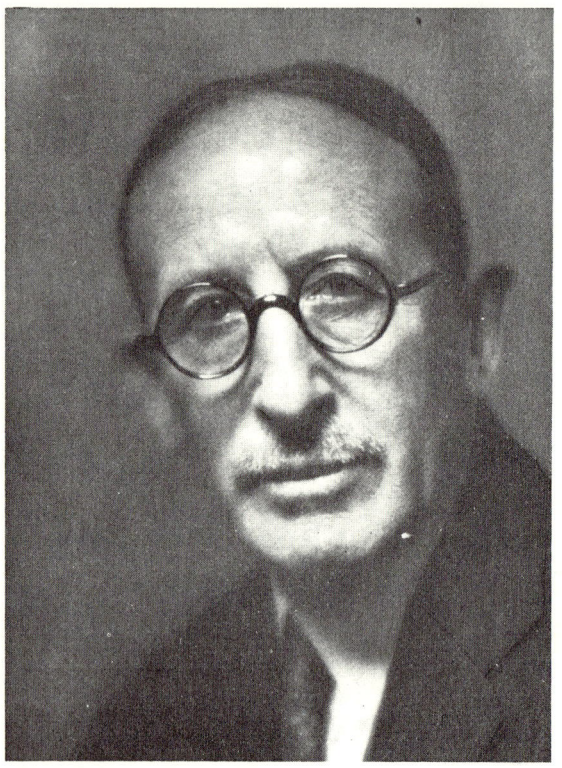

James Ewing, M.D.

of a bronze medal and $1,000, from the Philadelphia Board of City Trusts for his research in classifying tumors. He was appointed in 1937 a member of the National Advisory Cancer Council and he was a member of many other committees in this field. In 1940 he received the Clement Cleveland Medal of the New York City Cancer Committee. Dr. Ewing died May 15, 1943.

His literary contributions include "Clinical Pathology of the Blood," published in 1900; his textbook on legal medicine published in 1910, and his work on "Neoplastic Diseases," first published in 1919. His writings include also innumerable contributions to systems of medicine and to scientific periodicals.

LUDVIG HEKTOEN

The award of the Distinguished Service Medal of the American Medical Association for 1942 was made to Dr. Ludvig Hektoen.

The medical career of Ludvig Hektoen began with a job as druggist in a hospital, which became for him an inspiration to the

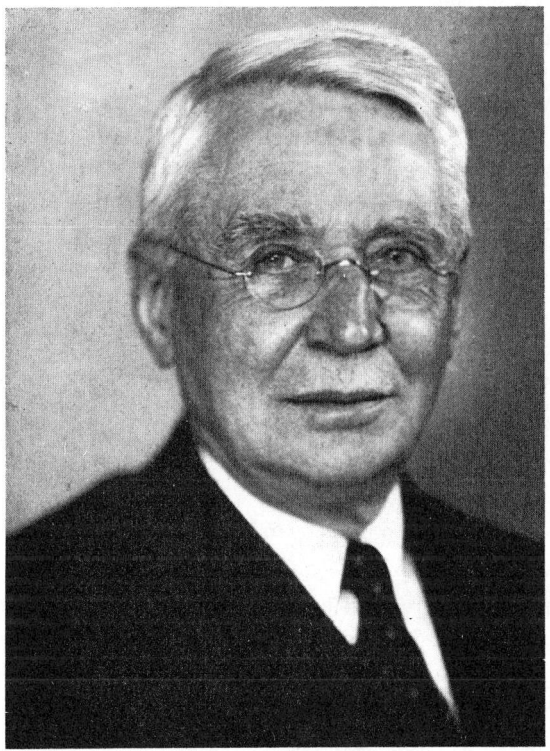

Ludvig Hektoen, M.D.

study of medicine. He graduated in 1887 from the College of Physicians and Surgeons in Chicago, then served as apothecary in the Illinois Eastern Hospital for the Insane and subsequently made first place in the examination for internship at the Cook County Hospital. In this capacity he came under the direct instruction of Christian Fenger and turned naturally to pathology for a career. He was made curator of the museum of Rush Medical College in 1889 and in 1891 he became professor of general pathology in his alma mater. In 1892 he became professor of pathologic anatomy and in 1894 professor of morbid anatomy and director of the laboratory of normal and pathologic histology, bacteriology and hygiene in Rush Medical College. From that time onward his career has been a series of new appointments and new obligations in every field of medical science and public work.

Dr. Hektoen has been pathologist to the Presbyterian Hospital and head of the department in the University of Chicago and of pathology of St. Luke's Hospital. He established in 1902 the John McCormick Institute for Infectious Diseases and became its director. In 1932 he was made a member of the National Advisory Health Council of the U. S. Public Health Service and later became chairman of the Advisory Committee of the National Cancer Institute. In April 1915 he became chairman of the Committee on Scientific Research of the American Medical Association, in which position he has been instrumental in determining grants of funds for research carried on throughout the country. In 1916 Dr. Hektoen gave the Cutter Lecture of the Harvard University Medical School and received the honorary degree of Doctor of Science from the University of Wisconsin. He was president of the American Society for Experimental Pathology. He received in 1920 the honorary degree of Doctor of Laws from the University of Cincinnati. In 1924 he was chairman of the Division of Medical Sciences of the National Research Council and in the same year he was appointed consultant pathologist in the U. S. Public Health Service. In 1926 he served again as chairman of the Division of Medical Sciences of the National Research Council. The Norwegian government gave him its most distinguished recognition, the Order of St. Olaf, in 1929.

Throughout much of his life Dr. Hektoen has been engaged in special work in the field of cancer, serving for many years as a member of the board of directors of the American Society for the Control of Cancer and also as a member of the board of directors and of the advisory board of the Chicago Tumor Institute. In his career, however, he has been interested in every phase of medical science. Essays on pathology have been interspersed with scientific research on bacteriology, parasitology, immunology and cancer. He has maintained a personal and intense interest in medical history and in all problems of social organization which involve medical knowledge. The bibliography of his writings includes many hundreds of references but fails to include innumerable reviews, official documents and miscellaneous writings that give a true picture of the contribution that he has made. He has been editor of the *Journal of Infectious Diseases* since it was first established in 1904 and also editor of the *Archives of Pathology* since its first number in 1925.

He has also been at various times editor of the *Proceedings of the Institute of Medicine of Chicago*, chairman of its board of governors and editor of the *Transactions of the Chicago Pathological Society*. A special issue of the *Archives of Pathology*, dedicated to him at the time of his seventy-fifth birthday, carried the names of more than a hundred physicians who have at one time or another come directly under his preceptorship or inspirational leadership.

As a native of Wisconsin, Dr. Hektoen was awarded the Distinguished Service Award of the State Medical Society of Wisconsin.

ELLIOTT P. JOSLIN

The Distinguished Service Medal and Award of the American Medical Association for 1943 were conferred on Dr. Elliott Proctor Joslin, world famous as a contributor to our knowledge of diabetes and as an educator in that field.

Dr. Joslin was born in Oxford, Mass., June 6, 1869. Following the receipt of the B.A. degree from Yale in 1890 and the Ph.B. from the Sheffield Scientific School in 1891 he was graduated as a doctor of medicine by Harvard in 1895. In 1914 he received the honorary M.A. from Yale and in 1940 the honorary D.Sc. from Harvard. In 1895 he began the practice of medicine in Boston, at the same time serving as an educator in Harvard Medical School, becoming assistant in physiologic chemistry from 1898 to 1900, assistant in theory and practice of physic from 1900 to 1905, instructor from 1905 to 1912, assistant professor of the theory and practice of physic from 1912 to 1921, clinical professor of medicine from 1922 to 1937 and since that time emeritus professor. He has been at the same time consulting physician of the City Hospital and medical director of the George F. Baker Clinic in the New England Deaconess Hospital. During World War I he entered as a major in the medical corps in 1918 and was promoted shortly to lieutenant colonel. He is a member of the Association of American Physicians, the American Academy of Arts and Sciences, the American Physiological Society and other scientific organizations. He was chairman of the Section on Practice of Medicine of the American Medical Association in 1924-25 and president of the Interstate Postgraduate Medical Association in 1936. He is honorary president of the American Diabetes Association. Various important lectures such as the Stephen Walter Ranson Lecture of Northwestern University School of Medicine in 1937, the Harvey Society Lecture in Boston in 1930 and the two Malthe lectures and a clinic in Oslo in 1938 mark his career. From time to time he has traveled throughout the nation extending education about diabetes to the medical profession and to the public. On patients who have survived diabetes for various periods of time he confers bronze, silver or gold medals, recently having conferred such a medal on a woman who had diabetes for more than fifty years. In 1932 Dr. Joslin received the Kober Medal of the Association of American Physicians.

As a part of his contribution to education in his field he published in 1916 the first edition of "The Treatment of Diabetes Mellitus,"

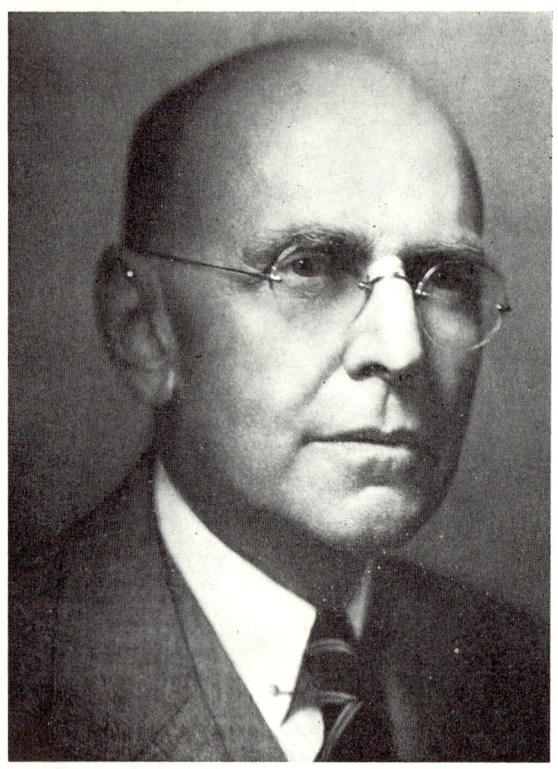

Elliott Proctor Joslin, M.D.

now in its seventh edition; also "A Diabetic Manual" in 1918, which is now in its seventh edition. His publications include more than one hundred smaller contributions to medical literature in his field.

GEORGE DOCK

The Distinguished Service Medal and Award of the American Medical Association for 1944 were conferred on Dr. George Dock, of Pasadena, Calif., famous physician and medical educator.

Dr. Dock was born at Hopewell, Pa., April 1, 1860. He received the M.D. degree from the University of Pennsylvania in 1884, an honorary A.M. from Harvard in 1895, the Sc.D. from the University of Pennsylvania in 1904 and the LL.D. from the University of Southern California in 1936. From 1887 to 1888 Dr. Dock was assistant clinical professor of pathology at the University of Pennsylvania, becoming professor of pathology at the Texas Medical College and Hospital in 1888. He left Texas in 1891 and became professor of the theory and practice of medicine and clinical medicine

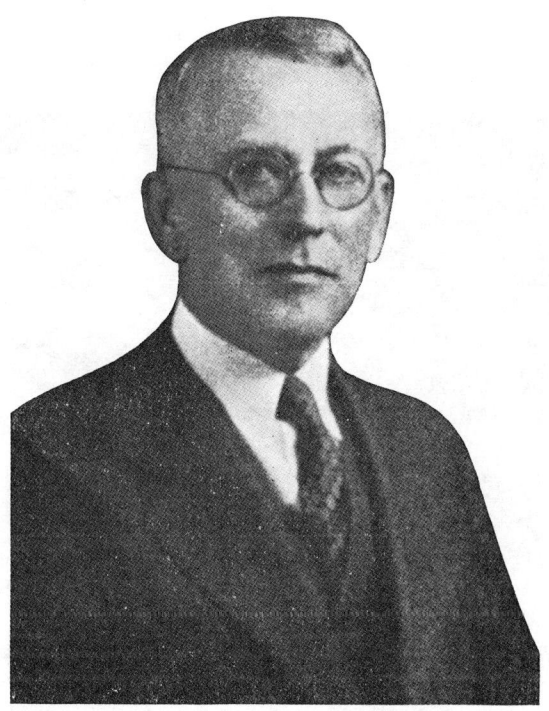

George Dock, M.D.

at the University of Michigan, where he remained until 1908. From the latter year until 1910 he held the same title at Tulane University Medical School. He was professor of medicine at Washington University School of Medicine 1910 to 1922, and dean part of that time. He was instrumental in founding the Archives of Internal Medicine. He is honorary professor of medicine at the University of Southern California and a member of numerous medical societies, including the American Medical Association, American Association for the Advancement of Science and Association of American Physicians, of which he was president in 1916-17.

He is co-author of a book on hookworm disease and of articles and chapters in many textbooks on medicine. A happy conjunction of events led to the celebration of Dr. Dock's eightieth birthday at a dinner at the Los Angeles County Medical Society in April 1940, on which occasion the organization of the Walter Jarvis Barlow Society of the History of Medicine simultaneously held its first public meeting and the birth of the George Dock Lectureship in the History of Medicine also took place, Dr. Dock being the first lecturer.

GEORGE R. MINOT

The House of Delegates at its meeting in 1945 added the name of George Richards Minot to those receiving the Distinguished Service

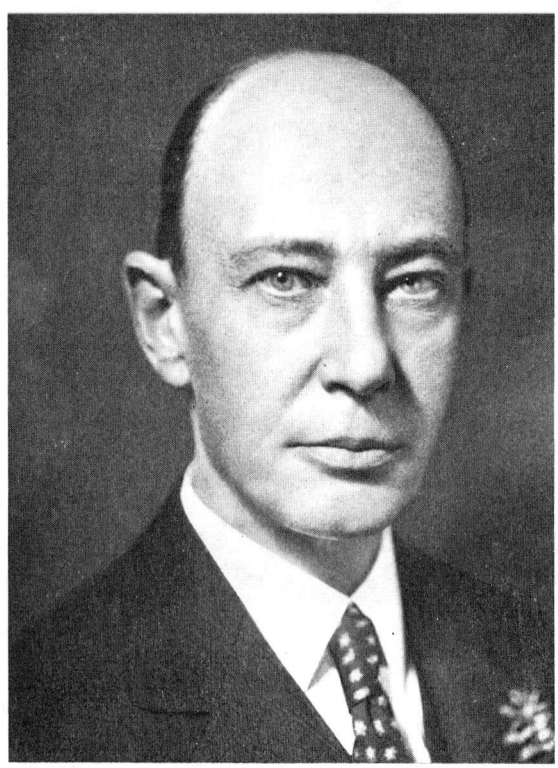

George R. Minot, M.D.

Award. His contribution to our knowledge of the causes and methods of control of pernicious anemia has been recognized throughout the world.

Once every person who developed pernicious anemia died of that disease. Today, by the discovery made by George R. Minot and his associates, those with pernicious anemia are given years of life in which they live to all intents and purposes as normal human beings. This great discovery opened a new pathway into the field of research on blood, along which great numbers of investigators have traveled to build higher and higher the structure of medical science. The significance of Dr. Minot's discovery is perhaps best explained in the following paragraph from his writings:

> Dietary deficiency may arise not only because of an improper intake of one or more substances required by the body but also because established disease may prevent the formation, absorption or utilization, or cause abnormal loss from the body, of necessary substances. The effects of extra demands of organisms are always to be reckoned with. The physiological strain of child bearing requires dietary factors to be often much greater than the standard requirements for women. Moreover, since the material diet in pregnancy and lactation inevitably affects the well being of the infant, the health of the whole population depends to a greater or less extent on the nutrition of the mothers. Fundamental research bearing on nutrition in such fields as chemistry, as well as practical applied studies, offers a basic endeavor for better public health. There are today throughout the world multiple opportunities for the prevention of many sorts of disorders by better nutrition. The partaking of proper food is excellent preventive medicine and upon it depends the integrity of man. Men with different types of training must seek for more information on nutrition and carry forward the work so that the ultimate goal will be nearer for those who follow us.

Dr. Minot has been previously honored with honorary degrees from many universities and medical societies, with the Kober gold medal of the Association of American Physicians, the Cameron prize of the University of Edinburgh, the gold medal of the National Institute of Social Sciences, the gold medal and award of the *Popular Science Monthly*, the Moxon medal of the Royal College of Physicians, London, the John Scott medal of the city of Philadelphia, the gold medal of the Humane Society of Massachusetts and, together with William P. Murphy and George H. Whipple, the Nobel prize in medicine for 1934.

A. J. CARLSON

Dr. Anton Julius Carlson, famous as a leader in physiology, was elected to receive the citation and the Distinguished Service Medal of the American Medical Association in 1946.

Dr. Carlson came to America in 1891 at the age of 16. He received the Bachelor of Science degree from Augustana College in 1898 and the Master of Science in 1899 and the Ph.D. from Stanford University in 1903. After serving as research assistant in physiology at Stanford he became associated with the Carnegie Institution and from 1904 to 1907 worked as instructor in the Woods Hole laboratories. In 1904 he became assistant professor of physiology at the University of Chicago and in 1909 became professor. In 1929 he became Frank P. Hixon Distinguished Service professor and in 1940 retired with the title emeritus.

Dr. Carlson is an Associate Fellow of the American Medical Association and a member of its Committee for the Protection of

Medical Research. He has been president of the American Physiological Society, of the Society for Experimental Biology and Medicine, of the American Biological Society and of the American Association for the Advancement of Science. He has contributed vastly to periodicals in the field of physiology and he has made original studies affecting every possible phase of function in the human body. During World War I he was assigned to the Sanitary Corps as a

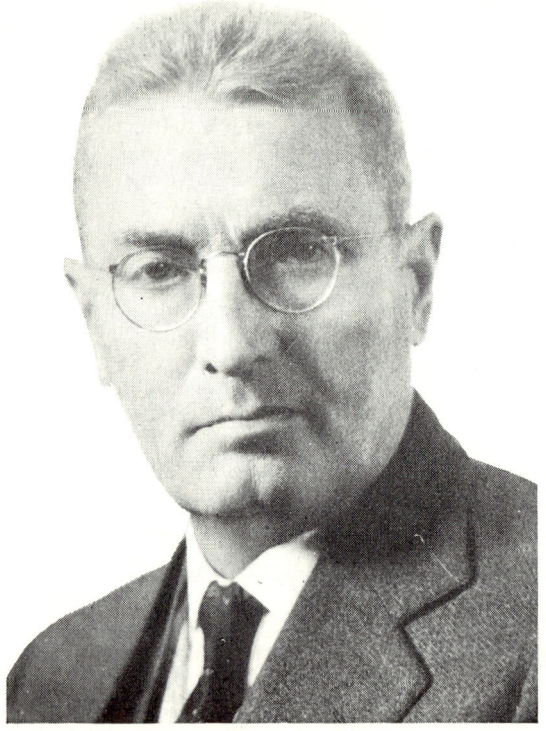

Anton Julius Carlson, M.D.

lieutenant colonel in the U. S. Army and worked with the American Expeditionary Forces in 1919. In addition to his periodical contributions he is the author of a book on "Health in Hunger and Disease" and another on "The Machinery of the Body." His name ranks with that of the great physiologists of all time not only for his scientific studies but also for his leadership as a citizen.

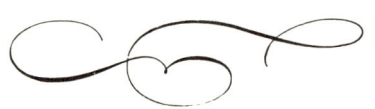

Biographies of the Presidents of the American Medical Association
1847 – 1947

BY WALTER L. BIERRING, M.D.

THE PRESIDENTS OF
THE AMERICAN MEDICAL ASSOCIATION
1847—1947

IN THIS CENTENNIAL YEAR of Association history it is fitting to record in historic perspective the "medical life-story" of the physicians who served as presidents during the first one hundred years.

The selection of each presiding officer was often an index of the trend and leadership in certain fields of medical progress dominant at the time. Again, outstanding service to the Association and advancement of its interests appeared a consideration in the selection. Fourteen of the delegates present at the preliminary convention in New York City in May 1846, and at the organization session in Philadelphia the following year, were later elected to the presidency.*

Three presidents died while in office; the first was Dr. Eli Ives of New Haven, elected in 1860, who died during the interim before the next meeting in Chicago in 1863. No meetings of the Association were held in 1861 and 1862 because of the war between the States. The first vice-president, Dr. Wilson Jewell of Philadelphia (1800–1867) presided during the 1863 session, but was not officially installed.

Dr. William L. Rodman of Philadelphia, presiding at the San Francisco session in 1915, died in March 1916, when he was succeeded by the vice-president, Dr. Albert Vander Veer of Albany, New York, who served until the annual session that year in Detroit.

Dr. James Tate Mason of Seattle, Washington, died within five weeks after his installation as president (in absentia) at the Kansas City session in May 1936, and the vice-president, Dr. Charles Gordon Heyd of New York City, became president.

Twenty-five states and the District of Columbia were represented in the one hundred presidents that served the Association since 1847.

When classified as to special forms of practice it is noted that general surgery predominates, particularly during the earlier years, forty-six being so listed altogether; twenty-two are listed as internists; eight in general practice; six in obstetrics and gynecology; two

---
* Nathaniel Chapman (1847); Alex H. Stevens (1848); James Moultrie (1851); B. R. Wellford (1852); Jonathan Knight (1853); George B. Wood (1855); H. Lindsly (1858); Eli Ives (1860); Alden March (1863); N. S. Davis (1864 and 1865); H. F. Askew (1867); Alfred Stillé (1871); J. L. Atlee (1883); Austin Flint (1884).

in psychiatry (Hubert Work, 1921, and Rock Sleyster, 1939); two in ophthalmology (G. E. deSchweinitz, 1922 and E. H. Cary, 1932), and one each in the following specialties; orthopedics, L. A. Sayre (1880); pathology, W. H. Welch (1910); pediatrics, Abraham Jacobi (1912); biochemistry, V. C. Vaughan (1914); dermatology, W. A. Pusey (1924); otology, W. C. Phillips (1926); gastro-enterology, W. G. Morgan (1930); urology, H. L. Kretschmer (1944), and administrative, Olin West (1947).

The average age of the presidents during their term of office was 59.8 years, the youngest being C. A. Pope (1854) who was thirty-six years old when elected president; the next in the younger group were C. A. L. Reed (1901), and Wm. J. Mayo (1906), each 45 years; N. S. Davis (1864) and D. W. Yandell (1872), 47 years, and J. H. Musser (1904), and Ray Lyman Wilbur (1923), 48 years.

The oldest president in office was J. L. Atlee (1883) who was eighty-four years old; two other presidents were over eighty years old—Eli Ives (1860) and A. Jacobi (1912), each eighty-two years old.

Significant medical developments and many worthy movements are associated with the names of the different presidents. Thirty-five were authors of textbooks in the several special forms of practice; Dr. Nathaniel Chapman (1847) published in 1817 "Elements of Therapeutics and Materia Medica" which passed through seven editions; he was also in 1820 the first editor of the American Journal of Medical Sciences. It was in the surgical clinic of Dr. John C. Warren (1849) at the Massachusetts General Hospital, October 17, 1846, that ether was first used as an anesthetic; following the administration, Dr. Warren made the cryptic statement, "Gentlemen, this is no humbug." George B. Wood (1855) was joint author of the United States Dispensatory in 1845, and published Wood's Practice of Medicine in 1847—the most important work on that subject at the time. Henry Miller (1859) published the first textbook on obstetrics in 1849; Samuel D. Gross (1868) in 1839 published the first American textbook on pathological anatomy, appearing in two volumes. It was largely through the instrumentality of Henry I. Bowditch (1887) that the Massachusetts State Board of Health was established in 1869, the first in the country; the formation of the California State Board of Health the following year was mainly due to the efforts of Thomas M. Logan (1873). The "Elements of Human Anatomy" a volume of 734 pages, published in 1854 by Dr. T. G. Richardson (1878) was the first treatise of its kind published in the Mississippi Valley. Dr. J. Marion Sims (1876) gained international fame by developing a special surgical procedure for the relief of vesico-vaginal fistula. The National Dispensatory, a volume of 1528 pages, was published in 1879 under the joint authorship of Dr. Alfred Stillé (1871) and John A. Maisch, Phar.D. Dr. Austin Flint (1884) originated the binaural stethoscope, and was the first to propose the several diagnostic auscultatory signs that bear his name.

In the development of orthopedic surgery in America, Lewis A. Sayre (1880), will alway be regarded as a pioneer, and Abraham Jacobi (1912) will be accorded the same role in pediatrics.

The following past presidents distinctly enhanced the prestige of American medicine. In surgery, Samuel D. Gross (1868), Donald MacLean (1895), Nicholas Senn (1897), W. W. Keen (1900), John A. Wyeth (1902), W. J. Mayo (1906), Joseph D. Bryant (1907), John B. Murphy (1911), C. H. Mayo (1917), A. D. Bevan (1918), W. D. Haggard (1925), E. S. Judd (1931), Dean Lewis (1933), Chas. Gordon Heyd (1936), Irwin Abell (1938), F. H. Lahey (1941), and Fred W. Rankin (1942); in internal medicine, Frank Billings (1903), J. H. Musser (1904), Alexander Lambert (1919), Wm. S. Thayer (1928), James S. McLester (1935), James E. Paullin (1943), and Roger I. Lee (1945); in ophthalmology, George E. deSchweinitz (1922); in dermatology, Wm. A. Pusey (1924), and in urology H. L. Kretschmer (1944).

William Welch (1900), aside from being the foremost pathologist in America, served as dean of the schools of medicine and of public health, professor of the History of Medicine, and had a medical library named after him at Johns Hopkins University.

Dr. W. L. Rodman (1915) was the founder of the National Board of Medical Examiners. Dr. Ray Lyman Wilbur (1923) is the one university president (Stanford) included in the list. The Association past presidents, Hubert Work (1921) and Ray Lyman Wilbur (1923), were honored with appointments to Cabinet posts by the President of the United States.

All the presidents were graduates of recognized schools of medicine, supplemented in many instances by further study in European medical centers. Many had a prominent part in organizing medical schools, and all but one were at one time or another engaged in medical teaching. The exception was Dr. Henry F. Askew (1867) of Wilmington, Delaware, who was strictly a general practitioner, having at one time the largest practice in Wilmington and the state.

John C. Warren (1849), Reuben D. Mussey (1850) and N. S. Davis (1864–5), were strong advocates of the cause of temperance. H. I. Bowditch (1877) was the friend of Garrison and a militant abolitionist.

The establishment of free public schools in Detroit was one of the principal achievements of Zina Pitcher (1856).

In each of the wars in which the United States has been engaged since the Revolutionary period, Association presidents have taken an honorable part, including the war of 1812, the war with Mexico, 1846; the war of 1861–5; the Spanish American War, 1898–9, and World Wars I and II. In the war between the States, we find them on opposite sides. Hunter McGuire (1893) was Medical Director of the Second Confederate Army Corps; A. Y. P. Garnett (1888) served as Surgeon and Medical Advisor to President Davis and Generals Robert E. Lee and Joseph E. Johnston; D. W. Yandell (1872), T. G. Richardson (1878), and H. F. Campbell (1885) served as Surgeons, and John A. Wyeth (1902) as a private in the Confederate Army. Paul F. Eve (1857) served as a Surgeon in the Mexican War and with the Confederate States Army.

H. I. Bowditch (1877), John T. Hodgen (1881), J. J. Woodward (1882), Wm. Brodie (1886), H. O. Marcy (1892), J. F. Hibberd (1894), Donald MacLean (1895), R. B. Cole (1896), W. W. Keen (1900), and A. Vander Veer (1916) served with the Medical Department of the Northern armies.

In the Spanish-American War Nicholas Senn (1897), W. W. Keen (1900), H. L. Burrell (1908), Victor C. Vaughan (1914), Jabez N. Jackson (1927) served with distinction in the Medical Department of the United States Army. Dr. George M. Sternberg (1898) was Surgeon General of the Army during this war period.

During World War I Rupert Blue (1916) was Surgeon General of the U. S. Public Health Service, Wm. C. Braisted (1920) Surgeon General of the U. S. Navy, and Wm. C. Gorgas (1909) Surgeon General of the U. S. Army.

Some of the outstanding achievements in military medicine in World Wars I and II were largely due to the leadership of former presidents of the Association.

The principal theme in every presidential address throughout the hundred years has been on some phase of medical education. The remarkable evolution in American medical education that has brought it to its present high standards, is in large part due to the constant stimulation of these leaders in the medical profession.

In the last quarter century the economic problems incident to the changing social order, have engaged the thoughtful guidance and judgment of Association officials, to keep the "medical ship" on an even keel.

It may be truly said that the lives and chronicles of a century of presidents exemplify the vigor and accomplishments of the American Medical Association, and thus in large measure form the rich medical heritage that we enjoy today.

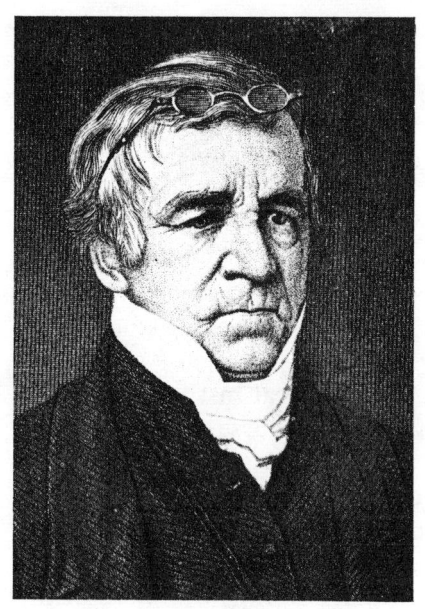

NATHANIEL CHAPMAN, M.D.
Philadelphia, Pa.
1778-1853

First President, A. M. A.
Philadelphia Session
May 5, 6, 7, 1847

AT THE ORGANIZATION session of the American Medical Association, in May 1847, Dr. Jonathan Knight of New Haven was temporary chairman until Dr. Nathaniel Chapman was chosen as the first president, who then presided during the remaining two days of the meeting.

At the time of his election, Dr. Chapman was recognized as the leading physician of Philadelphia. As professor of the Institutes and Practice of Medicine at the University of Pennsylvania, successor to Dr. Benjamin Rush, he had gained a high place among the medical educators and clinicians of his day.

In 1817 first appeared his Elements of Therapeutics and Materia Medica, which passed through seven editions and was widely used as a book of reference.

He became the first editor of the Philadelphia Journal of the Medical and Physical Sciences (later the American Journal of Medical Sciences) in 1820, and by his editorial writings and contributions to the medical literature of his period, he distinctly influenced the standards of the post-colonial practitioners and medical practice in general.

While a native of Virginia, born near Alexandria May 28, 1778, he came to Philadelphia at nineteen years of age and lived the remainder of his life in his adopted city. He became the private and favorite pupil of Dr. Benjamin Rush, graduating from the medical department, University of Pennsylvania, in 1801, which was followed by three years of study abroad—the first year in London as a private pupil of the celebrated Abernathy—then at the University of Edinburgh where he obtained a degree in medicine. Upon his return to Philadelphia in 1804, he began his career as a practitioner and teacher of medicine, first giving a course in obstetrics.

In 1813, at the age of 35, he was elected to the chair of materia medica, and three years later succeeded to the professorship of his distinguished teacher, Benjamin Rush, which he held until 1850 when he retired because of failing health.

In 1817, he founded the Philadelphia Medical Institute, where for twenty-five years he delivered a summer course of lectures. He filled numerous and honorable appointments in medical and learned societies, such as president of the Philadelphia Medical Society, president of the American Philosophical Society, and corresponding member of many learned societies of Europe.

A contemporary colleague writes that "he was not more distinguished for professional attainments than for courtliness and vivacity of manner, with knowledge of the world, and literary tastes." "In the sick chamber, his lively conversation and ever ready joke were often more effective than anodyne or cordial." "As a lecturer he was self-possessed, deliberate, and emphatic and at times became oratorical; he often lectured to 400 students with whom he had an unbounded popularity.

Professor Chapman presided at the opening of the second session of the Association in Baltimore in 1848 and from a brief address is quoted—"This assemblage presents a spectacle of moral grandeur, delightful to contemplate," and added "excited by the generous impulse of the Association's purpose, it comes forward in the majesty of its might to vindicate its rights and redress its wrongs."

Dr. Chapman died at his home in Philadelphia, July 1, 1853 at the age of seventy-five years.

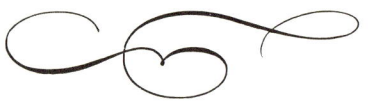

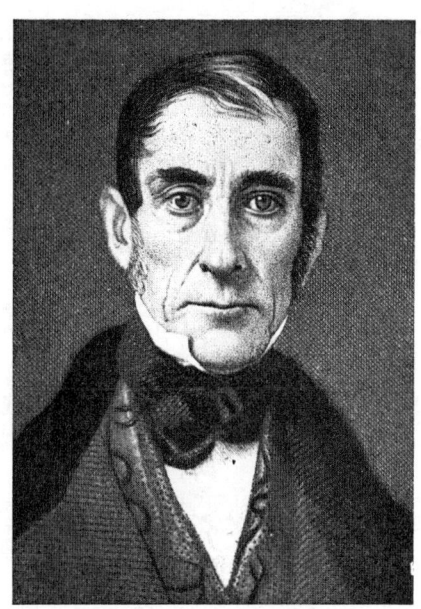

ALEXANDER H. STEVENS, M.D
New York, N.Y.
1789–1869

*Second President, A. M. A.
Baltimore Session
May 2, 3, 4, 5, 1848*

AT THE SECOND meeting in Baltimore, there was a deviation from the custom followed by the Association at its first session and during its early period, of choosing the president from the profession of the city where the annual session was held.

Dr. Alexander H. Stevens, the second president, was a well-known teacher and practitioner of surgery in the City of New York. He was a native of that city, having been born there Sept. 4, 1789; a son of Ebenezer Stevens, one of three who threw tea into the Boston Harbor, and later a Colonel in the Revolutionary War. He was prepared for college by John Adams at Plainfield, Mass., and graduated from Yale College at 18 years of age. His medical studies were carried on at the College of Physicians and Surgeons, New York, for one year, and completed at the University of Pennsylvania from which he received his medical degree in 1811. His graduation thesis on "The Proximate Cause of Inflammation" was highly lauded by Benjamin Rush.

He sailed for Europe in 1811 remaining three years for graduate study under Cooper and Abernathy in London, and Boyer and Larrey in Paris. On the voyage to France in 1811 and returning in 1814, he was captured by a British cruiser and interned as a prisoner each time for a short period at Plymouth, England.

Upon his return to the City of New York he began his career as a teacher of surgery, being appointed surgeon to the New York Hospital in 1818, and in 1825 elected professor of surgery in the College of Physicians and Surgeons.

The records indicate that he gained special distinction more as a teacher of surgery and surgical diagnosis than as an operator. However, his contributions to the surgical literature of his period were not extensive.

In 1841 he was elected president of the College of Physicians and Surgeons of New York, and in 1846 president of the Medical Society of New York. His inaugural or presidential address before the state Society was presented, by request, before both houses of the New York legislature and ordered printed and distributed to "eminent members of the Bar of the State."

In expressing his thanks for the honor conferred as president of the Association, Dr. Stevens spoke as follows: "Our profession, gentlemen, is the link that unites science and philanthropy. It is one of the strongest ligaments that binds together the elements of society. It teaches the rich their dependence and elevates the poor to a sense of the innate dignity of their nature. Its aim is to add to the comforts and length of human life."

Dr. Stevens was a faithful attendant at subsequent meetings of the Association up to the time of his death in New York City March 30, 1869.

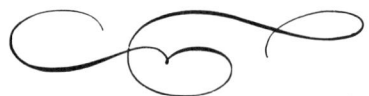

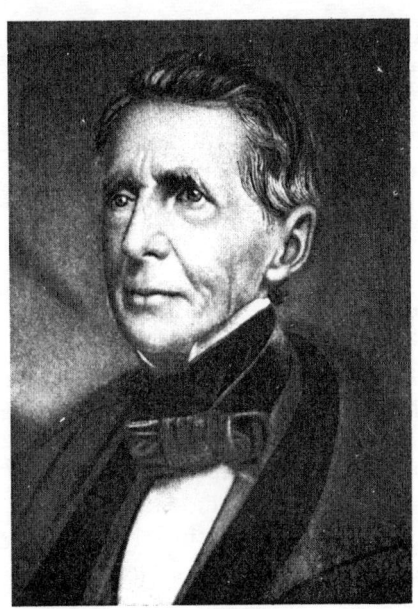

JOHN COLLINS WARREN, M.D.
Boston, Mass.
1778–1856

Third President, A. M. A.
Boston Session
May 1, 2, 3, 4, 1849

DR. JOHN C. WARREN, the third president of the Association, was a natural choice from the profession in the city where the session was held in 1849. Well known as a leading physician and surgeon, he came of a family that were among the earliest inhabitants of Boston and descended from a distinguished lineage of physicians.

His father, Dr. John Warren, was a surgeon in the Revolutionary War and the first teacher of anatomy in New England. An uncle, Dr. Joseph Warren, was killed at the Battle of Bunker Hill.

Dr. John Collins Warren was a native son of Boston, born August 1, 1778, received his preliminary education at the Boston Public Latin School where he was awarded the first Franklin medal for meritorious scholarship and graduated in medicine from Harvard University in 1797. Soon afterwards he visited European medical centers for a period of nearly four years under the tutelage of William Hunter, Sir Astley Cooper and Abernathy in London, the two Monros, Bell and Cullen in Edinburgh, and Bachat, Cuvier and Dubois in Paris, returning to Boston in 1802. Then, only 24 years of age, he began his active career in the full practice of medicine and surgery. He rapidly rose to prominence and in 1806 he became recording secretary of the Massachusetts Medical Society as well as Adjunct Professor of Anatomy, as a colleague of his father. In 1808 with Dr. Jackson he published the Pharmacopoeia of the Massachusetts Medical Society.

In 1810 in conjunction with his father, Dr. John Warren, Dr. Dexter and Dr. Jackson, a request was made of the Government of Harvard University to establish a branch of the medical school in Boston, as it had previously only existed in Cambridge. They also took the first step towards connecting a practical school with the medical institutions by taking charge of the hospital of the Almshouse in Boston.

The first anatomical lectures in Boston were given by Dr. J. C. Warren (1809) over the shop of a chemist, 49 Marlboro Street, and the first public dissecting room was opened in the same place. From this period to about 1820 a series of steps were taken towards the formation of a hospital, and the principal gentlemen of Boston, entering with spirit into the matter, established two hospitals, one for the sick and the other for the insane. The McLean Asylum for the insane was opened at Somerville in 1818, and the Massachusetts General Hospital was opened in September 1821 in Allen Street, Boston. Dr. Jackson was appointed physician, and Dr. John C. Warren surgeon to this institution.

In 1815 upon the death of his father Dr. John Warren, his son Dr. John C. Warren was chosen professor of anatomy and surgery, lecturing at the same time on midwifery and physiology. In the same year, 1815, the Massachusetts Medical College was erected in Boston, a substantial brick edifice belonging to Harvard University, the funds for which were chiefly procured by the appeal of Dr. Warren and Dr. Jackson.

It was in Dr. Warren's surgical service at the Massachusetts General Hospital that the epochal event occurred on October 17, 1846 of the first use of ether as an anesthetic, with Dr. W. T. G. Morton, Dentist, administering the same.

In the same year he resigned as professor of anatomy and surgery, and soon after presented his anatomical museum to Harvard University for the benefit of the medical school, with the sum of five thousand dollars "to keep it in order."

His presidential address before the Association meeting in Cincinnati in 1850 presented a scholarly review of the progress of surgery and the application of ether anesthesia, the importance of clinical teaching with a philosophic discussion of the cause of temperance.

In January 1853 he resigned as surgeon of the Massachusetts General Hospital, whereupon the Trustees presented him a vote of thanks, and placed his bust in their Hall.

Dr. Warren died in Boston May 4, 1856 at seventy-eight years of age.

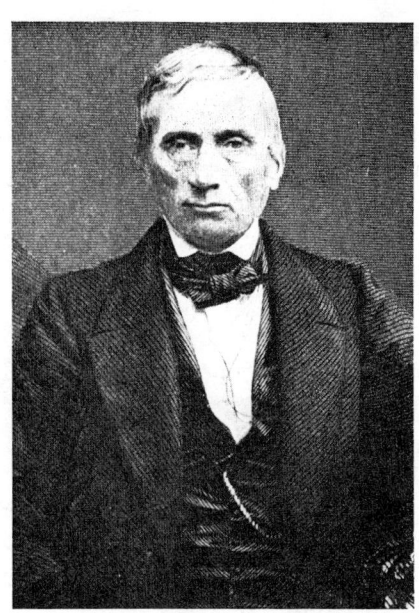

REUBEN DIMOND MUSSEY, M.D.
Cincinnati, Ohio
1780–1866

*Fourth President, A. M. A.
Cincinnati Session
May 7, 8, 9, 10, 1850*

THE ELECTION OF Dr. Reuben Dimond Mussey of Cincinnati as the fourth president of the Association witnessed the first real contest for this position. In following the custom of selecting a president from the profession of the city where the meeting was being held, it evidently was difficult to make a choice as the local profession was divided between two well known physicians in that region west of the Alleghenies—Dr. Daniel Drake and Dr. R. D. Mussey. Both were attending an association meeting for the first time. The choice finally fell to Dr. Mussey, but the record states it was not entirely unanimous. At the time of his election Dr. Mussey was seventy years of age.

His birthplace was Rockingham County, New Hampshire, June 23, 1780, his father Dr. John Mussey being a physician.

Dr. Mussey was an adopted son of Ohio, having come to Cincinnati from New England in 1838 when he was 58 years of age, to become professor of surgery in the Ohio Medical College. That he was called to this important professional post indicated that his high standing in surgery was well established before that time.

He graduated from Dartmouth College in 1803, and received the degree Bachelor of Medicine from the Medical Institute of Dartmouth College in 1805.

After several years of practice at Essex, Massachusetts, he attended further medical lectures at the University of Pennsylvania, obtaining the degree of Doctor of Medicine in 1809. In 1812 Dartmouth College also granted him the same degree.

In 1854, the Dartmouth College conferred upon Dr. Mussey the honorary degree of Doctor of Laws.

After practicing five years in Salem, Pennsylvania, as obstetrician and surgeon, he was named Professor of Theory and Practice of Physic in the medical school of Dartmouth College, and in 1819 he became professor of anatomy and surgery. From 1831 to 1835 he was professor of anatomy and surgery at Bowdoin College and lectured on these subjects in two other medical institutions. For a period of ten years, 1824–1834, he served as President of the New Hampshire Medical Society.

After responding to the call from the Ohio Medical College at Cincinnati in 1838, he continued as professor of surgery in that institution until 1852 when he assumed the same position in the Miami Medical College from which he retired in 1860 at the age of eighty years, moving to Boston where he died June 21, 1866.

Dr. Mussey was a pioneer in several surgical procedures. The first was the successful ligation of both carotid arteries for the removal of aneurismal tumors of the scalp. In 1837 he made the second operation on record in removing a shoulder blade and collar bone because of osteosarcoma. In 1848 he reported 16 operations under chloroform without any "unpleasant symptoms."

Dr. Mussey, like his predecessor Dr. Warren, was an ardent temperance lecturer, and in 1854 a paper of his on "The Effects of Alcoholic Liquors in Health and Disease" was published in the Transactions of the American Medical Association of 1855.

Two of his sons became physicians, one having an active part in the reorganization of Miami Medical College in 1865. A grandson, Robert D. Mussey, is now head of the Department of Obstetrics, Mayo Clinic, Rochester, Minn. Thus four generations have served medicine with distinction.

Dr. Reuben D. Mussey went to live in Boston in 1860 where he died June 21, 1866 at the advanced age of eighty-six years.

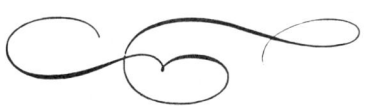

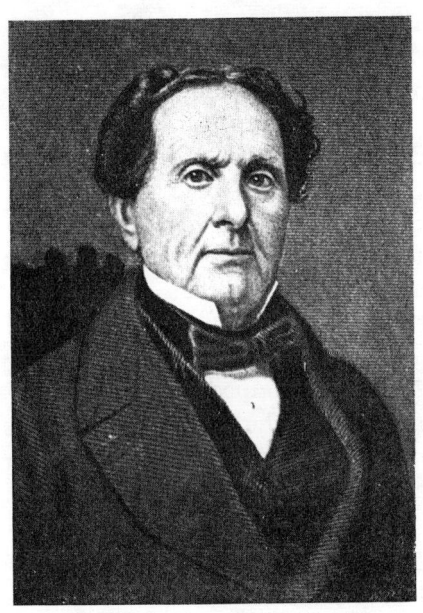

JAMES MOULTRIE, M.D.
Charleston, S. C.
1793–1869

Fifth President, A. M. A.
Charleston Session
May 6, 7, 8, 9, 1851

DR. JAMES MOULTRIE, the fifth president of the Association, was one of the leading medical educators and physicians of his day. A native of Charleston, South Carolina, being born on March 27, 1793, he lived his entire professional life in that city. He was the fourth in four successive generations of physicians, and the names of his ancestry are recorded in the revolutionary as well as the medical history of this country.

He received his early education at home and later in England, which however was interrupted by the encounter of the Chesapeake and the Leopard which later eventuated in the War of 1812.

Soon after his return to Charleston in 1808 he was appointed a Cadet at the West Point Military Academy, but before entering the same became interested in the study of medicine and entered the office of Doctors Barron and Wilson, distinguished practitioners of Charleston; later spent a year in the Marine Hospital, and in 1810 entered the University of Pennsylvania and graduated as Doctor of Medicine in 1812. With the beginning of hostilities with England he was appointed Port physician and surgeon of a battalion of artillery. Soon after returning from Philadelphia he was admitted to the Medical Society of South Carolina, and served successively as Secretary, Treasurer, Vice President, and was elected unanimously as President in 1821 at 28 years of age, serving two years in each position.

While president of the Medical Society of South Carolina he was largely instrumental in establishing the medical college of South Carolina, and became its first professor of physiology. As a lecturer it is stated that "he prepared to sacrifice beauty of diction to the claims of a minute and detailed presentation of the subject." In 1836 he was asked to deliver in the Capitol in Columbia, an essay on the "State of Medical Education in South Carolina," which was a recognition of his leadership in that field of education. His article on the "Uses of the Lymph" published in the first Transactions of the Association was one of his most notable contributions to medical literature of that period.

Through his efforts, in large degree, was formed the Medical Association of the State of South Carolina, and he was named its delegate to the preliminary meeting of the National Medical Convention in New York City in 1846, and also to the organization meeting of the American Medical Association in 1847, where he was elected one of its four vice presidents.

The chair used by Dr. Moultrie after his election as President of the Association in 1851, still remains in Charleston and is used by the President of the State Association whenever it meets in that city. Dr. Moultrie evidently had a profound influence in advancing the standards of medicine, both locally and throughout the country.

He died in his native city May 29, 1869, at seventy-six years of age.

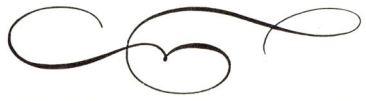

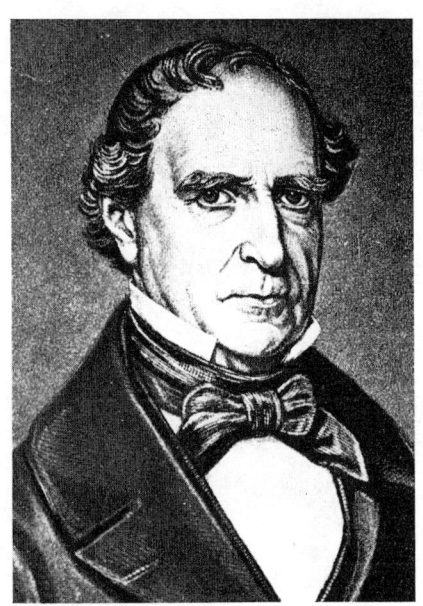

BEVERLY R. WELLFORD, M.D.
Fredericksburg, Va.
1797–1870

*Sixth President, A. M. A.
Richmond Session
May 4, 5, 6, 7, 1852*

DR. B. R. WELLFORD, the sixth president of the Association, was a native of Virginia and was born in Fredericksburg July 29, 1797. He was graduated from the medical department of the University of Maryland in the spring of 1816, and returning to Fredericksburg became immediately associated with his father in the practice of medicine. By devoting himself with enthusiasm and energy to his profession, he soon established himself in the confidence of his colleagues, and by excursions into the kindred fields of science and general literature, enlarged his mind and gained a further liberal education. It is therefore natural that he should sympathize with the movements for medical reform and professional organization by taking an active interest in the Virginia Medical Society which honored him with the presidency in 1851.

He was a delegate to the preliminary convention in New York City in 1846, and to the organization meeting of the American Medical Association in Philadelphia the following year. At the meeting in Richmond in 1852, he was elected president without opposition.

In his presidential address the following year, he reviewed the accomplishments of the Association in the first seven years with special reference to better medical education, proper regulation of the license to practice, and improvement in the registration of vital statistics, closing with the words "In protecting the interests, maintaining honor, advancing knowledge and extending the usefulness of the profession of medicine, you are sustaining the dearest concern of society of your country and of mankind."

In 1854 he was elected to the Chair of Materia Medica and Therapeutics in the Medical College of Virginia, and removed to Richmond where for sixteen years he greatly enhanced his prestige as a teacher and practitioner of medicine.

Death came to him December 27, 1870 while visiting in his native city of Fredericksburg.

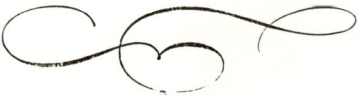

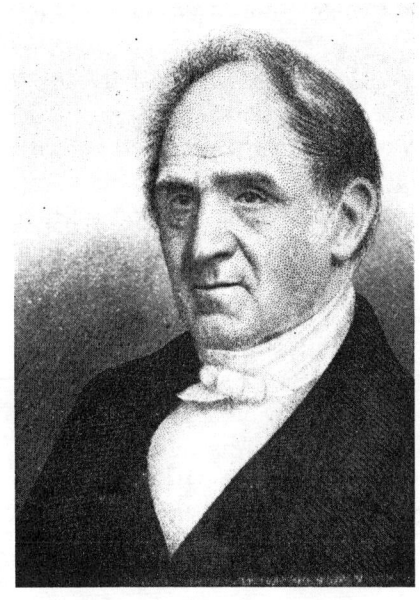

JONATHAN KNIGHT, M.D.
New Haven, Conn.
1789–1864

Seventh President, A. M. A
New York Session
May 3, 4, 5, 1853

DR. JONATHAN KNIGHT, the seventh president, was a familiar name in the annals of the young association. He was president of the preliminary convention to form the American Medical Association, which met in New York City in May 1846, and of the same in Philadelphia May 1847 until the organization was completed. At the time of his election in 1853 he had been a member of the medical faculty of Yale College, New Haven, as professor of anatomy, physiology and surgery for forty years.

At the New York meeting, the nominating committee found the local profession, as at the meeting in Cincinnati, divided, one part advocating the nomination of Dr. Valentine Mott and the other equally zealous for Dr. John W. Francis, both men of the highest standing in the profession. After listening to the arguments on both sides, the member of the Committee from Illinois (N. S. Davis) claimed "that the precedent electing the president from the city in which the meeting was being held was not only tending to beget local partisan faction, but would unjustly restrict the selections to such of the larger cities as could accommodate the annual meetings, while those residing in less populous cities would be excluded however meritorious they might be." During the afternoon session, the nominating committee recommended the election of Dr. Jonathan

Knight of Connecticut, and he was unanimously elected and conducted to the Chair.

Dr. Knight was born in Norwalk, Conn., September 4, 1789, his father and maternal grandfather being physicians. He graduated from Yale College in 1808. After two years of teaching, and one year as tutor in Yale College, he attended two courses of medical lectures, 1811–13, at the University of Pennsylvania. He was licensed to practice by the Connecticut Medical Society in August 1811, and received the honorary degree Doctor of Medicine from Yale College in September 1818. While at Yale College he was a student of the celebrated physicians Dr. Nathan Smith in medicine and Professor Benjamin Silliman in chemistry.

He commenced the practice of medicine in New Haven in 1813, and the same year was appointed Professor of Anatomy and Physiology in the Medical Institution of Yale College. After teaching in these subjects for twenty-five years, he was transferred to the department of Surgery and continued in that Chair until his death August 25, 1864.

When his eulogy was spoken these words appear "There was in him an uncommon correspondence between the outer and the inner man."

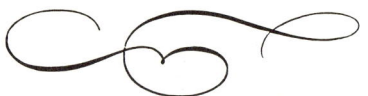

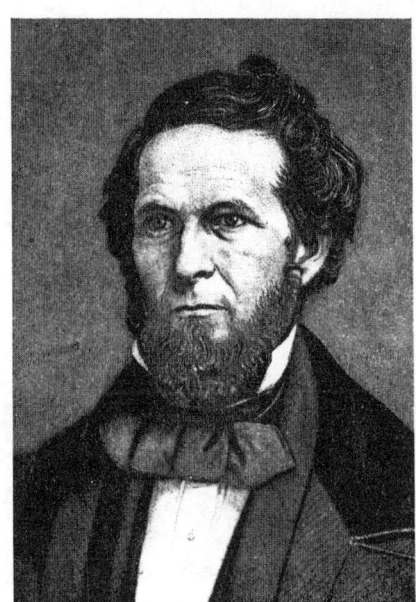

CHARLES ALEXANDER POPE, M.D.
St. Louis, Mo.
1818–1870

Eighth President, A. M. A.
St. Louis Session
May 2, 3, 4, 1854

DR. CHARLES A. POPE, the eighth president of the Association, was only thirty-six years old at the time of his election, and thus the youngest physician to gain that office in the first hundred years of Association history.

Dr. Pope was born in Huntsville, Alabama Territory, March 15, 1818, one year before Alabama was admitted to statehood. He evidently inherited from his parents a liking for both culture and study, receiving his early education in the Green Academy which was chartered in 1812. At fifteen years of age he entered the sophomore class of the University of Alabama, and two years later began his medical studies with Doctors Fearn and Erskine of Huntsville. In later years Dr. Pope often referred to the guidance of the two preceptors in his early professional training. He attended his first organized course of lectures in medicine at the Cincinnati Medical College in 1837–8. Dr. Daniel Drake was then a member of the faculty, and at the height of his fame and popularity as a teacher. He completed his second course of lectures at the University of Pennsylvania, graduating with the degree of Doctor of Medicine in 1839 at twenty-one years of age. His thesis was on "Pathology of the Arteries."

After two years of further study in European medical centers he began the practice of medicine in St. Louis. He soon became interested in establishing a medical school, and in 1842 was one of the founders of the St. Louis Medical College. The father-in-law of Dr. Pope, Colonel John O'Fallon, made the first donation to the medical school, to which Dr. Pope later added a liberal donation.

Evidently his youth prevented his being appointed on the first faculty, but his studious habits, high moral and intellectual attributes soon brought him into popular notice and favor, so that in 1843 when he was 25 years of age he was chosen professor of anatomy and physiology. This appointment was made at the suggestion of Dr. Samuel D. Gross, then professor of surgery at the University of Louisville, who had observed his ability while a student at Cincinnati Medical College. In 1847 he was elected to the Chair of surgery, and two years later became Dean of the Faculty.

The Transactions state that he presided at the Philadelphia session in 1855 "with great dignity and marked familiarity with parliamentary procedure."

In 1856 he was one of ten organizers of the St. Louis Academy of Sciences.

In 1867 when he was under 50 years of age, he retired from the professorship of surgery and moved his residence to Paris. Of this move, Garrison the medical historian, gives the following explanation: "For several years a rivalry had developed between Dr. Pope and Dr. Joseph N. McDowell, the latter a nephew of Ephraim McDowell of ovariotomy fame and brother-in-law of Daniel Drake. He was also the founder of McDowell Medical School of St. Louis. The attitude of McDowell became so acrimonious and vindictive, that it drove the gentle courteous Pope to Paris to die of inanition and desuetude." His death, self inflicted, occurred in Paris July 5, 1870 at fifty-two years of age. His remains are buried in Bellefontaine cemetery, St. Louis.

Dr. Samuel D. Gross in his autobiography pays this tribute to Dr. Pope. "No surgeon of St. Louis ever enjoyed in a higher degree the good opinion of his professional brethren or public at large. He was an innate gentleman, a man of high tone and sterling integrity and well versed in the art and science of medicine."

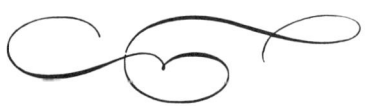

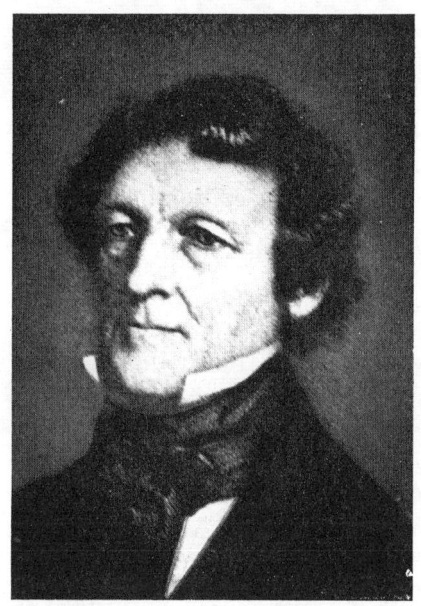

GEORGE BACON WOOD, M.D.
Philadelphia, Pa.
1797–1879

Ninth President, A. M. A.
Philadelphia Session
May 1, 2, 3, 4, 1855

DR. GEORGE B. WOOD, the ninth president, was the second distinguished Philadelphia physician to receive this high recognition from the Association. He was distinctly a medical teacher and while frequently called as a consultant, he never had a large general practice. He disliked obstetrics and never practiced any form of surgery.

Dr. Wood was of English descent and belonged to the Society of Friends, being born in Cumberland County, New Jersey, March 12, 1797. He received his early education at the University of Pennsylvania graduating with "high honors" in 1815, and obtained the degree Doctor of Medicine from the same institution in 1818. There is no record of his following the usual custom of further study in Europe but evidently he soon engaged in teaching, for in 1821 he was elected professor of chemistry in the Philadelphia College of Pharmacy, and ten years later transferred to the chair of materia medica and pharmacy. In 1835 he was called to the professorship of materia medica and therapeutics in the University of Pennsylvania and in 1850 was elected to the chair of theory and practice of medicine upon the retirement of Dr. Nathaniel Chapman.*

In 1847 appeared the first edition of Wood's Practice of Medicine which was the first important text book on that subject published in America. It passed through six editions. His work on Thera-

---

* First President, American Medical Association 1847.

peutics and Pharmacology appeared in three editions from 1856 to 1868. He was perhaps most widely known as the joint author with Dr. Franklin Bache of the United States Dispensatory, a work of vast erudition and research as well as being accurate in every detail. From 1833 to 1870, 13 editions of the Dispensatory were published, the sales amounting to 150,000 copies. The last edition in 1870 was a volume of 1830 pages.

During the greater part of his forty-two years of medical teaching, he was one of the attending physicians to the Pennsylvania Hospital where he conducted medical clinics, which for a time were the only hospital clinics available to medical students in Philadelphia.

A student of that period refers to him "as a fluent speaker with distinct enunciation, expressive and elegant diction, and his descriptions of disease were presented in the choicest language."

In his presidential address in Detroit in 1856, he commended the Medical Code of Ethics and made a protest against calling members of the profession "allopathists."

Dr. Wood held a number of positions of trust and honor in various scientific bodies, such as president of the College of Physicians of Philadelphia (1848–1879), and the American Philosophical Society for a number of years; he was also a manager of the Philadelphia Dispensary and a trustee of the University of Pennyslvania.

His health declined during his later years, and he "suffered much from an enormous accumulation of fat, while his muscular tissues underwent at the same time a fatty degeneration."

He died in Philadelphia March 30, 1879 at eighty-two years of age.

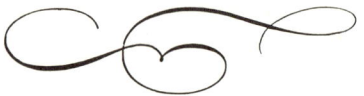

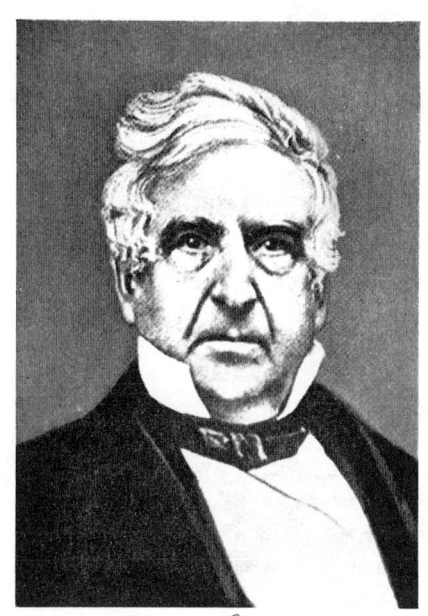

ZINA PITCHER, M.D.
Detroit, Mich.
1797–1872

Tenth President, A. M. A.
Detroit Session
May 6, 7, 8, 9, 1856

DR. ZINA PITCHER, the tenth president of the Association, was one of the pioneer physicians of Detroit and his contributions to the advancement of medical education and practice in the midwest no doubt gained for him the national reputation that led to the presidency.

He was born in Washington County, New York, April 12, 1797, of parents "who endured the many hardships during the struggles by which the Colonies achieved their independence." His father died when he was five years old, leaving a widow with five children. His mother, however, appreciated the value of an education, so that her son Zina received a good academic education, and at the age of twenty-one was able to begin the study of medicine under a private practitioner with whom he spent four years, attending during the time two courses of lectures at the Castleton School of Medicine in Vermont, and in 1822 received the degree of Doctor of Medicine from Middlebury College, Vermont. At the time of his graduation he had not received a single clinical lesson. He soon obtained an appointment as Assistant Surgeon, U. S. Army from President Monroe, and during the administration of President Andrew Jackson he was promoted to the rank of Surgeon. After fifteen years of army service, he became a citizen of Michigan in 1836 and began the practice of medicine in Detroit, and soon took a deep interest in the organization of her educational institutions.

As a Regent of the University from 1837 to 1852 he had a prominent part in the founding of the medical department at Ann Arbor. When the first medical faculty was appointed, his name was listed at his request as Emeritus professor.

One of his principal achievements was the establishment of free public schools in Detroit. He was three times chosen Mayor of that City. Dr. Pitcher was attending physician of St. Mary's Hospital and Surgeon of the U. S. Marine Hospital in Detroit, a member of the City Board of Health, and Associate Editor of the Peninsular Medical Journal. He was a faithful attendant at annual sessions of the Association, and his committee reports on medical education and epidemics were always of a high order.

He was president of the Michigan Territorial Medical Society during fourteen years; president of the Michigan State Medical Society, 1855–56; a founder of the Sydenham Society of Michigan, and a founder and president of the Detroit Medical Society.

Dr. Pitcher was versed in the habits of beasts and birds; his studies on Indian materia medica were classic, for that period. In "Gray and Torrey's Flora of the United States" several new species are named after Dr. Pitcher in acknowledgement of his service to botany.

It can be said of Dr. Zina Pitcher that he represented the finest type of general practitioner and public spirited citizen. Death came to him in Detroit, April 5, 1872, at the age of seventy-five years.

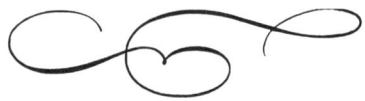

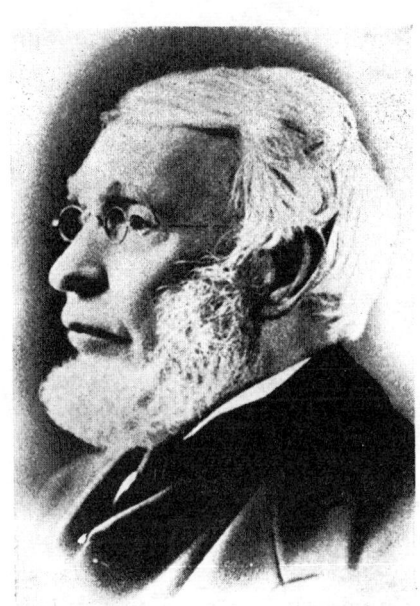

PAUL FITZSIMMONS EVE, M.D.
Nashville, Tenn.
1806–1877

Eleventh President, A. M. A.
Nashville Session
May 5, 6, 7, 8, 1857

AT THE TIME OF HIS election as the eleventh president of the Association, Dr. Paul F. Eve was recognized as one of the leading teachers and practitioners of surgery of his period.

He was often referred to as the "highest type of southern gentleman," with the added glamor of a rich and interesting military experience in three European conflicts and two wars in his native land.

He was born near Augusta, Georgia, June 25, 1806. After completing four years of literary studies in the University of Georgia he began the study of medicine at the University of Pennsylvania, graduating from this institution in 1828. Soon after obtaining his medical degree he left for Europe remaining over three years.

While in London he came under the influence of Sir Astley Cooper, Sir James Paget, Dr. Abernathy and others, and in Paris he followed courses of instruction by Dupuytren, Cruveilhier, Trousseau, Ricord, and Louis. It was during a part of this period that he had some interesting experiences, not directly connected with his graduate medical studies. While in Paris in July 1830 he witnessed the dethronement of Charles X and participated in the short revolution of three days that shook the foundations of France. A year later he volunteered his services to Poland to aid in its struggle for independence from Russia. He came to Warsaw with letters from Lafayette and the Polish Committee in Paris, and was assigned as Surgeon of Ambulances attached to General Turna's division. He was awarded the Golden Cross of honor for his services.

After the capture of Warsaw he was imprisoned for thirty days and upon his release he returned to Paris and soon afterward sailed for the United States. He located in Augusta, Georgia, where his talents were recognized in his appointment as the first professor of surgery in the University of Georgia Medical School in 1832 at twenty-six years of age, remaining in that position for seventeen years.

In the extensive epidemic of yellow fever in Augusta in 1839 he took a courageous and effective part in its control. In 1846 he was appointed the first volunteer surgeon to serve in the war with Mexico. In 1849 he was called to the chair of surgery in the University of Louisville as successor to the distinguished surgeon Dr. Samuel D. Gross. He served in this position only one year when he removed to Nashville, Tenn., as professor of surgery in the Nashville Medical College, later Vanderbilt University, which position he held until within one year of his death in 1876.

After being elected president of the Association May 4, 1857 he returned thanks for the honor conferred on him and closed with the following—"you present again the sublime spectacle of brethren from all sections of this widely extended Union, congregated to devise the best means to relieve suffering humanity and may I add we are here with,

> Our souls by love together knit,
> Cemented, mixed in one:
> One hope, one heart, one mind, one voice."

The year 1859 found Dr. Eve in Italy at the scene of war with Austria, and it is recorded "that the services of Doctor Eve were particularly valuable in the famous battles of Magento and Solferino," the Austrians being defeated in both.

When the flame of battle between the north and south burst forth in 1861, Doctor Eve was appointed Surgeon of Tennessee, later participated in the battle of Shiloh, and subsequently was appointed Chief Surgeon in the Army of General Joseph E. Johnston.

His distinguished career came to a close in Nashville, November 3, 1877 at the bedside of a patient. His remains were buried in Augusta, Georgia, and in that city November 14, 1931 a monument was unveiled to the memory of Dr. Paul Fitzsimmons Eve with impressive ceremonies.

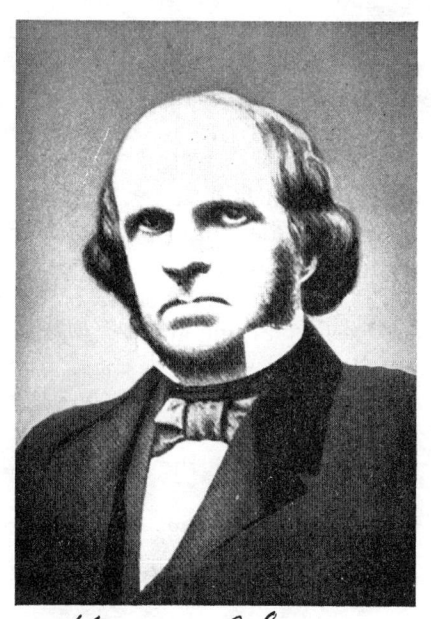

HARVEY LINDSLY, M.D.
Washington, D. C.
1804–1889

Twelfth President, A. M. A.
Washington, D. C. Session
May 4, 5, 6, 1858

AT THE FIRST MEETING of the Association in the Nation's Capital, Dr. Harvey Lindsly of that city was chosen the twelfth president.

In his address of welcome as chairman of arrangements, he expressed "regret that the City was devoid of interest to the medical scientist," but added the prophecy, "the day is not far distant when by the liberality of a great people, our public buildings, our literary and scientific institutions, our national parks and botanic gardens, will be worthy of the grand metropolis of a Nation, which perhaps within the next half Century will be the most populous, powerful and wealthy in Christendom."

He was born in Morris County, New Jersey, January 11, 1804 of English ancestry. After graduating from Princeton University he pursued his medical studies in New York City and Washington, D. C., receiving his degree of Doctor of Medicine from the Columbian Medical College in 1828.

He began the practice of medicine in Washington, D. C. soon after graduation and continued there until his death in 1889.

Dr. Lindsly was one of the founders of the Medical Society of the District of Columbia. From 1839 to 1845 he served as professor of obstetrics and later as professor of the principles and practice of medicine in the Columbian Medical College. For ten years he was president of the Washington Board of Health. He attended the organization meeting of the Association in Philadelphia in 1847, and was a regular attendant in subsequent years. Regarding his presidential address presented at the Washington meeting in 1858 Dr. Nathan S. Davis referred to it forty years later as "one of the best on the records of the Association."

This address expressed real forward thought and leadership referring to the use of the microscope in medical diagnosis, of quinine in intermittent fever, of the stethoscope in auscultation of the chest, of the application of chemistry in medical jurisprudence, of the prevention and control of infectious diseases, urging greater interest in public hygiene, with proper drainage and sewerage of cities, and lastly more careful study of the improvement of the cretin, the idiot and demented, closing with the words, "May our profession keep pace in respectability, progress and usefulness with the unexampled growth of our great country."

Dr. Lindsly died in the city of Washington, April 28, 1889, at the age of eighty-five years.

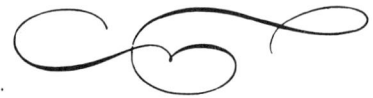

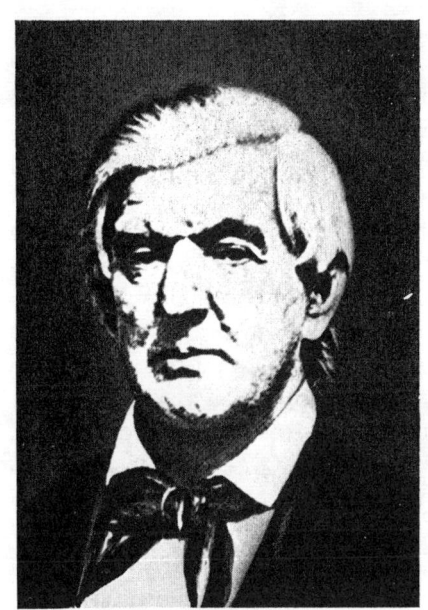

HENRY MILLER, M.D.
Louisville, Ky.
1800–1874

*Thirteenth President, A. M. A
Louisville Session
May 3, 4, 5, 1859*

THE FIRST TIME THAT the Association met in Louisville, Kentucky, Dr. Henry Miller, a prominent physician of that city, was chosen as the thirteenth president. This distinct recognition came to Dr. Miller because of his leadership and pioneer work in the development of scientific obstetrics in the "new West" as it was known in his day. He was born in Glasgow, Kentucky, November 1, 1800, his father being one of the first settlers in the Green River section of Kentucky.

He was denied the advantages of a collegiate training and his education was limited to that afforded by the country schools. At the age of seventeen he began the study of medicine under two local physicians, whose practice extended over a wide area. In the absence of apothecaries, his preceptors were obliged to compound their own medicines, and much of such work was relegated to the apprentice in medicine, including the extraction of teeth and the letting of blood. In this capacity young Miller became the "chief pharmacist, dentist and bleeder for this county." Two years later in 1819, Henry Miller rode on horseback to Lexington to attend the first full course of lectures in the medical department of Transylvania University. At the end of the course, he returned home and was taken into partnership with one of his former preceptors, Dr. Bainbridge. In the fall of 1821 he returned for a second course of lectures, receiving the degree of doctor of medicine in the spring of 1822, he being then twenty-one years of age. After thirteen years of successful private practice in Harrodsburg which at that time was the most popular watering place in the West, he was called in 1835 to Louisville to aid in organizing a medical school there. He was offered the chair of obstetrics and diseases of women and children which he held for a period of twenty-one years.

At the appeal of Dr. Miller, three of the leading teachers of the Transylvania School joined the Medical Institute of Louisville University which added greatly to the prestige of the Louisville school. Later additions to the faculty included Daniel Drake and Samuel D. Gross. In 1858 he resigned in order to devote more attention to his practice, but nine years later he was recalled to assume the professorship of medical and surgical diseases of women and children continuing in this position until his death in 1874.

During his active medical career, he was a frequent contributor to the journals of his day. His first textbook, "A Theoretical and Practical Treatise of Human Parturition," appeared in 1844. In the preface he stated—"To give a full, correct and lurid description of the mechanism of labor is the leading object in writing this book." The classification and nomenclature of foetal presentations and positions which he proposed became largely universal. In 1858 appeared "The Principles and Practice of Obstetrics," in which he championed the specular vaginal examination and the use of anesthetics in labor, both highly controversial subjects at that time.

In his presidential address at the New Haven meeting of the Association in 1860, he referred at length to the existing status of medical education, stating, "The present declension of doctoral standards has contributed to abase the professional office and to multiply the number of schools in the land far beyond all legitimate demands, there being now fifty such schools," and that "their pernicious rivalry is the great obstacle to improvement of medical education."

Samuel D. Gross said of him "he was essentially a strong man, with a well ordered and philosophical mind. Whatever he knew, he knew well." He was evidently a powerful force in advancing the higher medical precepts of his time.

He died in Louisville, February 8, 1874, in his seventy-fifth year.

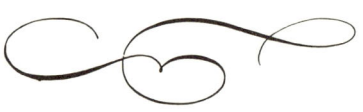

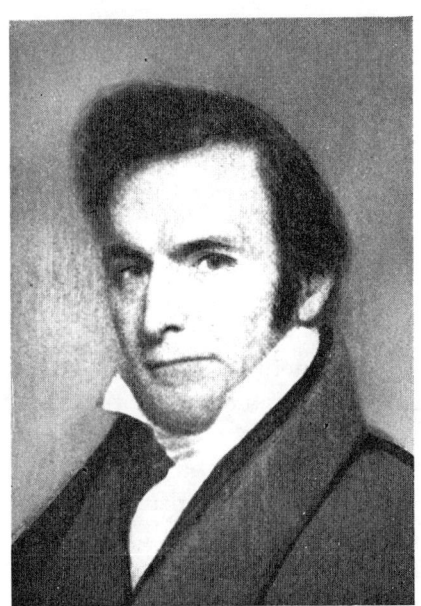

ELI IVES, M.D.
New Haven, Conn.
1779–1861

Fourteenth President, A. M. A
New Haven Session
June 5, 6, 7, 1860

DR. ELI IVES at the time of his election to the presidency of the Association was in his eighty-second year. As he died the following year, his presiding at the New Haven session was probably one of the last official functions of his medical career.

In an address before the Beaumont Medical Club Dec. 16, 1931 Dr. George Blumer* refers to him as "practitioner, teacher and botanist," and states "that the just estimate of the life work and accomplishments of any man can only be made in the light of the professional knowledge and standards of his time," adding, "It happens that the active professional career of Eli Ives is nearly contemporaneous with the first half of the nineteenth Century." He began practice in New Haven in 1802 and became inactive in 1853 when seventy-four years of age.

He was born February 7, 1779 and represented the second in a family which contained five generations of physicians. He received his B. A. degree from Yale College in 1799, being elected to Phi Beta Kappa Society in his senior year.

Eli Ives studied medicine under the tutelage of his father and Dr. Eneas Monson, and early in 1802 began practice with his father. In

---

* Yale J. Biol. and Med. Vol. IV, May, 1932.

this he was evidently successful, because within a few months he established his own office.

He was elected a Fellow of the Connecticut State Medical Society in 1806 and given the honorary degree of M. D. by the same society in 1811.

Dr. Ives was one of the founders of the New Haven Hospital as well as Yale Medical College, in which institution he was professor of materia medica for sixteen years and then transferred to the Chair of practice of medicine serving as a member of the medical faculty from 1815 to 1853. During these 38 years he was a faculty member of the joint Committee of the Connecticut State Medical Society and Yale Medical College which examined candidates for the M.D. degree and license to practice.

His early careful training in botany formed the basis of his continued interest in the purity and standardization of drugs. In 1819 he was named a member of a committee of the County Medical Society "to devise means for establishing an aopothecaries shop" which resulted in the founding of Apothecaries Hall.

Regarding his professional capacity and while he published but little, there seems no doubt that he was thoroughly imbued with the scientific attitude of mind. He was a persistent attendant at medical meetings where he constantly discussed the papers. That he was an excessively modest man is shown by the fact that he did not attach to his name the letters warranted by the various diplomas and honorary degrees bestowed upon him by British and Continental societies. In the words of Dr. Blumer—"One leaves the study of his life with the feeling that here was a man of considerable talent and of great tolerance, who constantly and consistently worked to improve himself and to be of service to his fellow man."

Dr. Eli Ives died in New Haven, October 8, 1861, in his eighty-third year.

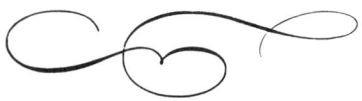

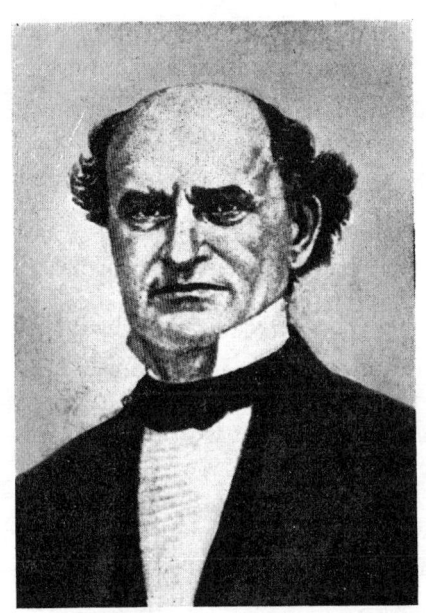

ALDEN MARCH, M.D.
Albany, N. Y.
1795–1869

*Fifteenth President, A. M. A.
Chicago Session
June 2, 3, 4, 1863*

THE ASSOCIATION MET for the first time in Chicago June 2, 3, 4, 1863, no session having been held in 1861 and 1862 because of the war between the States. Dr. Eli Ives the President elected at the New Haven session in 1860 had died in the interim, and the First Vice President, Dr. Wilson Jewell of Philadelphia (1800–1867), presided at the opening of the Chicago session. There is no record of his being advanced to the office of President, but he presented the customary address which was devoted largely to a discussion of Hygiene, and its importance as a branch of study for the practice of medicine.

Of the fourteen presidents previously chosen, all but two had been selected from the profession of the cities in which the meetings were held, and in consequence there was a general expectation that either Dr. Daniel Brainard, prominent surgeon and one of the founders of Rush Medical College, or Dr. Nathan S. Davis, leading physician and Chairman of arrangements, would be elected at the session in Chicago. Dr. Brainard failed to attend the medical meeting and Dr. Davis refused to allow his name to go before the nominating committee because on previous occasions he had opposed the policy of limiting the choice to the place of meeting. The Committee therefore recommended the election of Dr. Alden March of Albany, New York, for President which was unanimously adopted.

Dr. Alden March, the fifteenth president, was one of the charter members of the Association and was nationally known as an operating surgeon and inventor of surgical instruments. He was born in Sutton, Worcester County, Massachusetts, September 20, 1795. His early years were spent on his father's farm. In 1817 it is recorded that he was a teacher of writing and during the vacation periods was quarrying and cutting state stone. He attended his first course of lectures in anatomy and surgery in Boston in 1818 and 1819 and graduated with the degree of M.D. Sept. 6, 1820 from Brown University, Providence, Rhode Island.

After graduation he located in Albany, New York, and soon became known as a teacher and skillful operator in surgery. In 1821 he conducted what is believed to be the first lecture course in anatomy in the State of New York, at Albany, with demonstrations and dissections, having a class of fourteen students.

In 1825 he was appointed professor of anatomy at the Castleton Medical College, Vermont; and two years later was named professor of anatomy in the Albany Medical Seminary. In 1834 he established a practical school of anatomy and surgery in Albany, and five years later in 1839 upon the re-establishment of the Albany Medical School he became the first professor of surgery which position he held for thirty years. It is stated that he was a rapid and dexterous operator and is credited with having performed 7124 surgical operations. In the Transactions of the Association of 1853 he reports a large series of operations for morbus coxarius for which he had devised a special procedure. He performed the first operation in this country for harelip and invented a special forceps for use in this operation.

In his address as retiring president of the Association at the meeting in New York City in 1864, he reviewed the progress of medical education, as well as the procedure of licensing physicians. In conclusion he expressed the hope of an early union between the Northern and Southern states then still in the midst of a Civil War.

Dr. March died in Albany, New York, June 17, 1869, at seventy-four years of age.

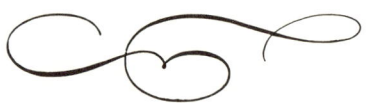

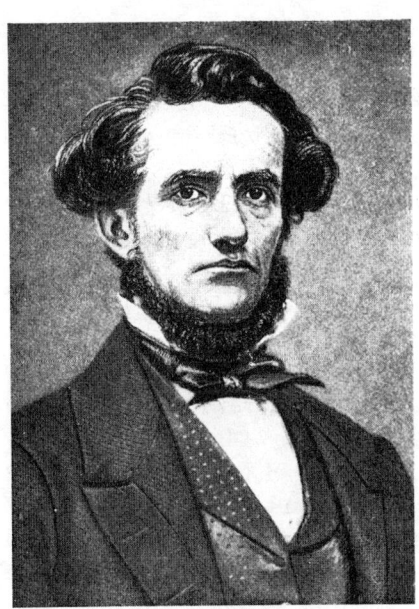

NATHAN SMITH DAVIS, M.D.
Chicago, Ill.
1817–1904

Sixteenth President, A. M. A.
New York Session
June 7, 8, 9, 1864

Seventeenth President, A. M. A.
Boston Session
June 6, 7, 8, 9, 1865

DR. NATHAN S. DAVIS had the unique distinction of serving the Association as president during two years, presiding at the New York Session in 1864 and the Boston meeting in 1865. He was elected president at the beginning of the meeting in New York City June 7, 1864, and presided during the remaining three days of this session. On the last day, the Constitution was so amended that the election of officers should be near the close of each annual meeting and "the president and vice-presidents should assume the functions of their respective offices at the beginning of the annual meeting next succeeding their election, thus giving them one year to prepare for an efficient discharge of their official duties."

Considering that Dr. N. S. Davis is justly styled the Father of the American Medical Association, it seemed eminently fitting that this distinction should come to him.

At the close of the Boston meeting he was given a great ovation for the efficient manner in which he presided at two sessions of the Association. His response voiced the deep appreciation for the honor conferred, and closed with the words: "I feel that the Association as now established can be passed to the next generation and the next, as long as civilization shall last. I hope to come every year, meeting you as long as age shall let me linger with you." This was spoken in 1865; the writer was privileged to meet him at the Columbus, Ohio session in 1899, the last for Dr. Davis, when he still appeared full of life and vigor.

The various publications and exercises connected with commemorating the Association Centennial will bring forth in greater detail the long and active professional career of Dr. Davis, so that this brief sketch will be confined to certain incidents closely related to the origin and growth of the Association to which he devoted his foremost efforts at all times.

He was born in the town of Greene, Chenango County, New York, January 9, 1817, the son of a farmer, spent his boyhood in a log house and until he was sixteen years of age, engaged actively in the varied and laborious pursuits incident to a farmer's life. Endowed by nature with a spare frame, the occupation of his boyhood doubtless contributed much to the acquirement of that physical energy and power of endurance which he enjoyed in his manhood. His early education was limited to such as could be acquired at a backward district school, and by voluntary reading. For pecuniary reasons he could not enjoy those advantages which he so much coveted.

At sixteen years of age he had formed the purpose of preparing himself for the practice of medicine, and with his father's consent he entered Cazenovia Seminary where in a six months course by his earnestness and enthusiasm he added distinctly to his knowledge of English, chemistry, philosophy, algebra and Latin. He then commenced the study of medicine with Dr. Daniel Clark of Smithville Flats. The following year he took his first course of medical lectures in the old "College of Physicians and Surgeons of the Western District of New York." At the close of this course he entered the office of Dr. Thomas Jackson of Binghamton, under whose tuition he remained until the completion of his third term of study when he received the degree Doctor of Medicine in January 1837, being then but a few days over 20 years of age.

He practiced for a short time at Vienna, New York, and then moved to Binghamton where he continued in practice for ten years until his removal to New York City in 1847.

The success that attended Dr. Davis in his new field of labor both professional and social, was all that could be desired. He early showed a talent for writing and was awarded two prize essays—"Diseases of the Spinal Column" and "Physiology of the Nervous System," by the New York State Medical Society. From 1843 to 1847 he was a delegate from the Broome County Society to the State Society. Imbued with the philosophy that "associated action constitutes the main spring and controlling motive power of modern society," it was largely through his instrumentality that a resolution was adopted by the New York State Medical Society, naming a committee to promote a national convention in May 1846 in New York City of delegates from existing medical schools and societies. This preliminary convention led to the permanent organization the following year in Philadelphia of the American Medical Association.

During his two years residence in New York City he served as Demonstrator of Anatomy in the College of Physicians and Surgeons, gave a course in medical jurisprudence, and edited a small semi-monthly medical journal called the "Annalist."

In 1849 he responded to a call from Rush Medical College, located at Chicago, Illinois, as professor of pathology, practice and clinical medicine, and thus began a new chapter in his eventful professional career.

In Danforth's Life of Dr. N. S. Davis* it is stated that as he entered his medical career he had three purposes:

1. Unification of the profession by the creation of the American Medical Association.
2. Founding a medical college with extended graded course of study and a more rational method of teaching, with higher entrance requirements.
3. Publication of a textbook, which would embody his views of the theory and practice of medicine.

The first purpose was accomplished before he left New York State, and the remaining two were realized in his Western medical home.

In 1859 he organized the medical department of Lind University later known as Chicago Medical College, and more recently as the College of Medicine of Northwestern University.

In 1884 appeared his textbook, perhaps his greatest literary effort, entitled "Lectures on the Principles and Practice of Medicine," which passed through several editions.

He prepared the first history of the American Medical Association which was published in 1855. In 1898 he prepared a biography of the 49 ex-presidents of the American Medical Association.

Aside from the above and several textbooks, he published from February 1840 to March 1904, 136 important essays, papers, reports and monographs on medicine and allied subjects. Between the years 1848 and 1890 Dr. Davis was editor of eight different periodicals. He was the first editor of the Journal of the American Medical Association from 1883 to 1888.

The professional life of Dr. Davis is intimately related to the

---

* I. N. Danforth, M.D. Life of Nathan Smith Davis, Cleveland Press, Chicago, 1907.

growth of our Association and the development of its highest ideals during its first half century.

Dr. Nathan S. Davis was the president of the Ninth International Medical Congress in Washington, D. C., in September 1887.

A testimonial banquet was tendered Dr. Davis in Chicago October 5, 1901, attended by three hundred and fifty physicians from all parts of the country. Dr. Davis sat between Dr. Christian Fenger, the toastmaster and Dr. Frank Billings—the one, the highest embodiment of modern surgical pathology, the other, representing all that is progressive and modern in internal medicine.

On Saturday, June 4, 1904, Dr. Davis went to his office at his regular time and appeared in his usual health. On June 16, 1904 his span of earthly life of eighty-seven years, five months and seven days came to a close.

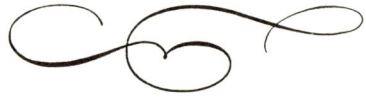

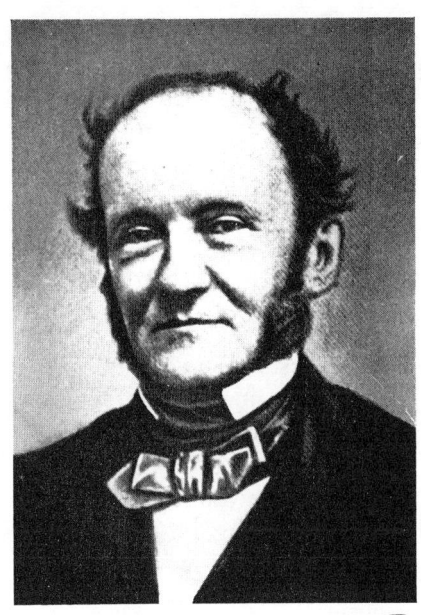

DAVID HUMPHREYS STORER, M.D.
Boston, Mass.
1804–1891

Eighteenth President, A. M. A.
Baltimore Session
May 1, 2, 3, 4, 1866

DR. D. HUMPHREYS STORER, the eighteenth president of the Association, was referred to as one of the most respected and beloved physicians of Boston and particularly well known as an obstetrician and naturalist.

He was born in Portland, Maine, March 26, 1804, and graduated from Bowdoin College in 1822, being granted the degree of Doctor of Medicine by Harvard College in 1825. While in the medical school he was House Student of Dr. John C. Warren. Soon after graduation he began the practice of medicine in Boston with special attention to obstetrics.

He early showed great interest in teaching, and in 1837 in cooperation with Doctors Edward Reynolds, Jacob Bigelow and Oliver Wendell Holmes was most active in the establishment of Fremont Street Medical School as a protest against the formal and insufficent methods of teaching at the Harvard Medical School, where the course of study was limited to one year of four months. As the result of its great success Harvard was forced to take it over bodily and its corps of teachers became highly honored professors of this institution. Dr. Storer was professor of obstetrics and medical jurisprudence (of the Harvard Medical School) from 1854 to 1868, serving as Dean of the school from 1855 to 1864.

A contemporary refers to him "as the best teacher the Harvard Medical School had ever had. While not of the scientific type, he best possessed the secret of being able to communicate his own intense enthusiasm to his students." He served as visiting physician of Massachusetts General Hospital from 1849 to 1858 and as obstetrician of the Boston Lying-In Hospital from 1854 to 1868. Bowdoin College conferred upon him the degree of Doctor of Laws in 1876.

Dr. Storer was to all accounts distinctly a physician of the "old school," wearing his swallow-tail coat and silk hat to the last, yet idolized by his students and held in highest esteem by his medical colleagues. Throughout his professional career he was an ardent and very active naturalist, publishing in 1846 a History of Fishes of North America, and in 1867 a History of Fishes of Massachusetts. His fine collection of shells was presented to Bowdoin College.

He died in Boston September 10, 1891 at the age of eighty-seven years.

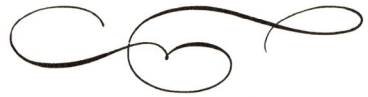

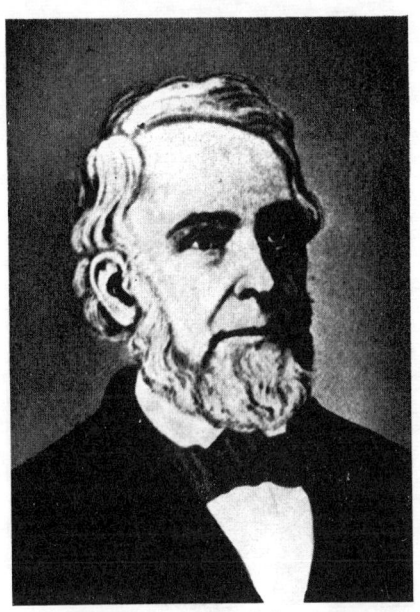

HENRY FORD ASKEW, M.D.
Wilmington, Del.
1805-1876

*Nineteenth President, A. M. A
Cincinnati Session
May 7, 8, 9, 10, 1867*

DR. HENRY FORD ASKEW was the first and only physician elected to the presidency from the State of Delaware. He was a charter member of the Association and distinctly representative of the class of general practitioner, it having been said that at one time he had the largest single practice in Wilmington and the State.

Dr. Askew was born in Wilmington, Delaware, June 24, 1805 of an old Quaker family. He obtained his medical training at the University of Pennsylvania from which institution he graduated in 1826, and soon afterward began the practice of medicine in his native city.

A contemporary biographer has recorded that while he carried on an unusually large general practice, "he was remarkable at all times for his great charm and cheerfulness of manner."

At the meeting in 1868 in a rather lengthy presidential address he reviewed the first twenty years of Association history calling attention to a membership of about three thousand, of which only one-tenth were present at annual meetings. He expressed himself as not in favor of medical specialties except those pertaining to diseases of the eye and ear, and of the skin. He presented a vigorous exposition of his views on medical ethics and other matters pertaining to the welfare of the medical profession.

Dr. Askew died in Wilmington March 5, 1876, at the age of seventy-one years.

SAMUEL DAVID GROSS, M.D.
Philadelphia
1805–1884

Twentieth President, A. M. A.
Washington Session
May 5, 6, 7, 8, 1898

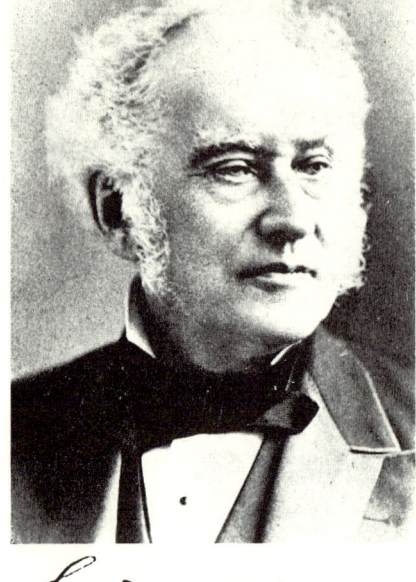

DR. SAMUEL DAVID GROSS was such an outstanding figure in American Medicine that it is difficult to encompass in brief form the proper attributes of this remarkable physician. He was generally regarded as the father of surgical pathology, one of the finest medical writers of the nineteenth century and easily the leading surgical teacher of his day.

He was born near Easton, Pennsylvania, July 8, 1805 of Pennsylvania-Dutch ancestry. His early education was mostly gained at home, and young Gross could hardly speak English until after his fifteenth year. At seventeen he was apprenticed to Dr. Joseph K. Swift of Easton, and launched himself into the study of medicine with an enthusiasm he never lost. Finding that his lack of basic education was a serious handicap, he entered Wilkes-Barre Academy for the purpose of studying English and the classics. After supplementing this with further study at the Lawrenceville, New Jersey, high school he again began the study of medicine at the age of nineteen. His preceptor urged that the formal study of medicine be continued at the University of Pennsylvania, but he chose to cast his lot with the new Jefferson Medical College, graduating from that institution in June 1828 at the age of twenty-three years. The young physician opened an office on Fifth Street and settled down to wait for patients but few found their way to his office. Tiring of inactivity Gross spent the long empty hours in dissection and writing. Within eighteen months after graduation he had translated and published Boyle and Hollard's General Anatomy; Hatin's Obstetrics; Hildebrand on Typhus and Tavernier's Operative Surgery.

The disappointments of practice caused him to close his Philadelphia office and return to Easton an unsuccessful but unbeaten physician. From here in 1830 he published his first original work, Diseases and Injuries of the Bones and Joints. In 1833 fortune smiled on Gross and he received the offer of Demonstrator in Anatomy at Ohio Medical College, which he accepted and thus his career as a teacher had begun.

In 1835 the newly established Cincinnati Medical College included him in its faculty as Professor of Pathological Anatomy. While in Cincinnati he began one of his greatest works, "Elements of Pathological Anatomy," which was subsequently published in two volumes in 1839, being the first book on this subject published in English. The introduction to the first edition contains the following significant statement:

"It is certainly an anomaly in the history of our profession that a science which admits of such extensive application as pathological anatomy and which may be considered as the very foundation of medicine, should still be so neglected as a branch of elementary study in the United States."

So great was the reception of this work that he was elected a member of the Imperial Royal Society of Vienna, and thirty years afterwards, the great Virchow, at a dinner he gave to its then distinguished author, showed this work on pathology as one of the prizes in his library. His reputation thus was made almost overnight. In 1840 he became professor of surgery at the University of Louisville, a post he occupied for sixteen years. He and his colleagues, Daniel Drake and Austin Flint, soon made it the most important medical center in the west, and he was in surgery the "reigning sovereign." In 1851 he published his textbook "Diseases, Injuries and Malformations of the Urinary Organs," to be followed in 1854 by "Foreign Bodies in the Air Passages."

His experiments and monograph on "Wounds of the Intestines" (1843) laid the foundation for the later studies of Parkes, Senn and other American surgeons.

So great had Gross's fame become that he was offered a professorship at the Universities of Louisiana, Virginia and Pennsylvania, all of which he refused. However, in 1856, his Alma Mater called him and he became professor of surgery in Jefferson Medical College.

His work in Philadelphia was considered to be his most outstanding. In 1859 he published his famous System of Surgery, in two volumes containing 936 engravings. In the preface the object is stated "to present a systematic and comprehensive treatise on the science and practice of surgery, considered in its broadest sense." The index was prepared by his son Dr. Samuel W. Gross, a practicing surgeon in Philadelphia. A year later he became the author of an excellent manual on Military Hygiene. In 1861 he gave to the world his monumental work, Lives of Eminent American Physicians and Surgeons of the Nineteenth Century.

As a surgeon he was probably without a peer, and in the course of his 42 years of teaching and practice, he developed many new techniques and was among the first American surgeons to accept Lister's germ theories governing antiseptic surgery.

He established the Pathological Society of Philadelphia, the Philadelphia Academy of Surgery, and the American Surgical Association, of which he was the first president. Foreign honors came to him as to no other physician who was completely educated in America. Cambridge and Edinburgh University each conferred on him the honorary degree of Doctor of Laws.

His address as president of the Association in 1868 exhibits the scholarship and broad scientific viewpoint of this great American physician. It presented the trends of medical thought in distinctly new directions such as higher standards for the education of nurses and establishment of training schools, the education and proper training of veterinary physicians and surgeons, also advocating higher requirements of preliminary education for admission to medical schools and that the faculties of regular medical colleges establish a uniform high grade medical curriculum to be approved by the American Medical Association. He also dwelt at length on the wider recognition of expert medical testimony in medico-legal matters. The address is rich in expressions on the catholic spirit in medicine—"A common heritage and brotherhood recognizing no nationality" using the quotation "Stars need no birthright, no nationality, they belong to all lands and to all nations." He closed with a beautiful tribute to medical leaders in foreign lands, Velpeau, Trousseau, Turck, Faraday, Davy and others, who had recently ended their earthly labors, with these words: "The same God's acre, broad as earth itself, enshrouds their mortal remains as those of their American brethren, the same flowers grow upon their tombs, and the same halo of glory encircles their brows."

He presented a paper at the Detroit session in 1874 of the Association, advocating legislation against the spread of syphilis.

Soon after his death in Philadelphia May 6, 1884 a national monument was erected to him in Washington, D. C.—the first physician so honored.

In the Woodlands Cemetery, Philadelphia, is an urn containing the ashes of Samuel D. Gross with this inscription in part: "A master in surgery. He filled chairs in four medical colleges, in as many states of the union, and added lustre to them all. He recast surgical science as taught in North America, formulated anew its principles, enlarged its domain, added to its art, and imparted fresh impetus to its study."

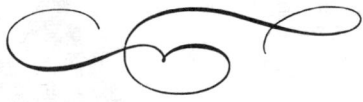

WILLIAM OWEN BALDWIN, M.D.
Montgomery, Ala.
1818–1886

Twenty-first President, A. M. A.
New Orleans Session
May 4, 5, 6, 7, 1869

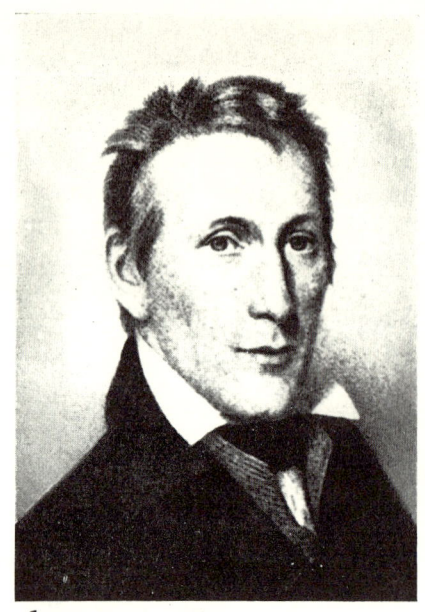

THE SELECTION OF Dr. William O. Baldwin of Montgomery, Alabama, as president, and New Orleans for the annual session was made with the thought of encouraging a larger attendance of members living in the southern states, as well as a renewed interest in the Association. There was the further hope that this meeting, but a few years after the close of the war between the States, would tend to heal the wounded feelings engendered by this great conflict. In the address of welcome by Dr. T. G. Richardson, later president of the Association (1878), were these significant words: "I extend to you a greeting on behalf of a once gay and brilliant metropolis of the South, yet nevertheless can show you in our cultivated gardens a flora unsurpassed in beauty and variety, and exhibit institutions of learning and benevolence of which any city might be proud. And, lastly, we can introduce you to a people whose honest pride has not been broken by defeat, whose recuperative powers are quite equal to the misfortunes they have endured, and whose hearts beat with warmest regard for those whose mission is to heal the bruises and bind up the wounds of our common community."

Doctor Baldwin at the time of his election was just under fifty years of age and comparatively little known by the general profession before the New Orleans meeting. He was born in Montgomery, Ala., August 9, 1818. After receiving a good collegiate education, he began the study of medicine in the office of Dr. McLeod of Montgomery and later attended the medical lectures at Transylvania University at Lexington, Kentucky, graduating with the degree of M.D. from this institution in 1837 at nineteen years of age. He became associated in practice with Dr. Wm. K. Bowling (president A.M.A. 1875) and continued until 1848 when he spent a year in Europe visiting the leading medical centers.

After his return he resumed his practice in Montgomery, and with his studious habits and fine medical preparation he soon attained high rank among the foremost practitioners of his section.

His address as president at the New Orleans meeting expressed his scholarly mind and rare scientific spirit. Evidently deeply conscious of the tragic memories of the moment, one marvels at the tactful phrasing of his opening remarks: "To me, gentlemen, this occasion is one of solemnity and significance; standing here in the great metropolis of the South, I find myself surrounded by men representing nearly every section of a country so lately arrayed in hostile strife. At a time when every other organization has been shaken to its center by the passions of deadliest hate; at a time when the most matured conservatism has been overmastered by the vindictive fury which has swayed the popular mind; you have been drawn hither from homes far distant over highways full of painful historic incidents, through territories watered by the blood and tears of a sorrowing nation and you have assembled here as brothers and friends to unite your offerings to a common science."

The theme of his address was medical education. He deplored the lack of more definite progress in elevating medical education during the twenty-two years of Association history.

He stressed the need of cultural training and better preparation for the study of medicine, expressing it thus: "Natural endowments, individual skill, personal ingenuity, the keen insight of genius all have their value, but a professional man of the present time, much more than ever before, must rely for honorable success on an exact and extended education." He made comparison with the system of European medical education and made a strong appeal to the Association to assume a greater responsibility towards elevating the standards of American medical education.

Following the New Orleans session Dr. Baldwin was a faithful attendant at Association meetings and always had a prominent part in its proceedings.

He had been chosen as one of the Vice-presidents of the Ninth International Medical Congress which was to assemble in Washington, D. C. in 1887, but death came to him at his home in Montgomery, Alabama on May 30, 1886 at the age of sixty-eight years.

GEORGE MENDENHALL, M.D.
Cincinnati
1814–1874

Twenty-second President, A. M. A.
Washington Session
May 3, 4, 5, 6, 1870

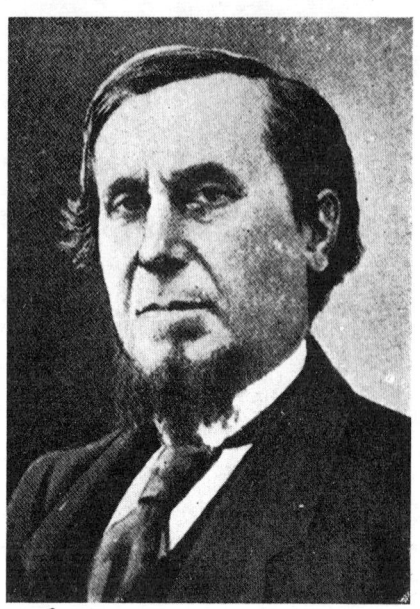

DR. GEORGE MENDENHALL at the time of his election to the presidency of the Association was the leading teacher and practitioner of obstetrics in Cincinnati. He was born in Sharon, Pennsylvania, of Quaker ancestry. In early childhood he was taken with his parents to Columbiana County, Ohio, and received his education there.

He graduated in medicine from the University of Pennsylvania in 1835, as an undergraduate being a special student of Dr. Nathaniel Chapman (first president A.M.A.). Soon after graduation he began practice in Cincinnati with special attention to obstetrics. With the founding of the Miami Medical College in 1852 he became professor of obstetrics and diseases of women and children, remaining until 1857 when he transferred to the Medical College of Ohio, in the same position. When the Miami Medical College was reestablished in 1865, Doctor Mendenhall assumed his original position until 1873 when he became professor emeritus. He also served Miami Medical College as Dean from 1853 to 1857 and again from 1865 to 1874.

His "Students Vade Mecum" published in 1852 passed through eighteen editions.

In his presidential address at the Washington session he referred to the medical profession as "dictators of humanity's guiding star," and "conservators of public health."

Death came to him in Cincinnati June 4, 1874 at the age of sixty.

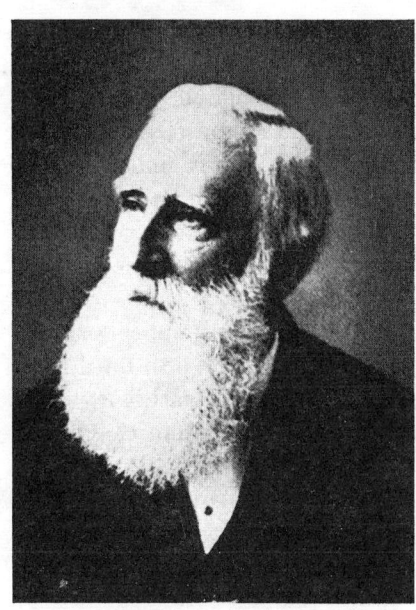

ALFRED STILLÉ, M.D.
Philadelphia
1813–1900

Twenty-third President, A. M. A.
San Francisco Session
May 2, 3, 4, 5, 1871

DR. ALFRED STILLÉ, the twenty-third president of the Association, presided at the San Francisco session in 1871, this being the first meeting on the Pacific Coast. In his address he referred to the meeting of the National Medical Convention in 1846 which he attended as a delegate, when for the first time the medical profession of the whole country had met in common council, adding "while, but a quarter of a century has passed since then, yet today civilization sits by the Golden Gate in a populous and splendid city."

Dr. Stillé was born in Philadelphia October 13, 1813 of Swedish ancestry and lived his entire life in the city of his birth. He received the degree of Bachelor of Arts in 1832 from both Yale College and the University of Pennsylvania, and from the latter institution the degree of Master of Arts in 1835, and Doctor of Medicine in 1836. In 1889 his Alma Mater conferred on him the honorary degree of LL.D.

He came into medicine in an age that ushered in a new pathology and the more exact methods of clinical observation.

As house physician at "Old Blockley" now Philadelphia General Hospital, he was fortunate to come under the tutelage of Dr. W. W. Gerhard, a clinical teacher of the first rank and fresh from the wards of the great Louis in Paris.

Soon after completing his hospital service Dr. Stillé hastened to

Paris to be under the same great teacher and other masters in clinical medicine of the Paris school. After three years of European study he returned to Philadelphia and again became associated with Dr. Gerhard. He had an interesting part in the splendid contribution of Dr. Gerhard—"The differentiation between typhus and typhoid," which was based on an epidemic of typhus in Philadelphia in 1836.

His first teaching experience was as professor of materia medica and therapeutics, and then professor of the practice of medicine in Pennsylvania Medical College.

In 1864 he succeeded to the Chair of Dr. William Pepper (primus) in the University of Pennsylvania, continuing in that post until 1884.

His first important work "Elements of General Pathology" was published in 1848. In 1867 and 1868 appeared two interesting monographs on "Cerebro-spinal Meningitis," and "Cholera and Dysentery." His textbook on "Materia Medica and Therapeutics" was a book of reference for many years. He had an important and fundamental part in the development of that bulky volume of 1628 pages-- the National Dispensatory. Of this work William Osler said "It is a mystery to me how a man with his training and type of mind could have undertaken such a colossal, and one would have thought, uncongenial task."

He was an active participant in the National Medical Conventions of 1846 and 1847, and one of the two first secretaries of the American Medical Association. From his first brief address on medical education in 1846 to his last in 1897 before the Association, he pleaded for better preliminary training and for longer courses of medical study. No one was therefore more rejoiced when the University of Pennsylvania entered upon its new departure of a three year course in 1876.

The Stillé Library at the University of Pennsylvania is a monument to his love of literature and the history of our profession.

Death came to this outstanding figure in American medicine on September 24, 1900 in the city of Philadelphia, at eighty-seven years of age.

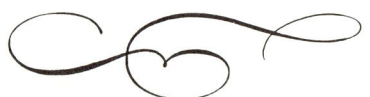

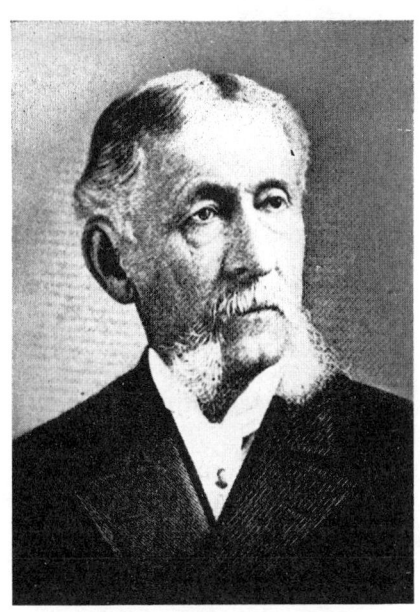

DAVID WENDELL YANDELL, M.D
Louisville, Ky.
1826–1898

Twenty-fourth President, A. M. A.
Philadelphia Session
May 7, 8, 9, 10, 1872

DR. DAVID W. YANDELL, of Louisville, Kentucky, evidently owed his election to the presidency of the Association, at the comparatively young age of forty-six years, to his prominence as a surgeon and teacher as well as his leadership in medical affairs throughout the middle west.

He was born near Murfreesboro, Tennessee, April 4, 1826 and received his collegiate and medical education at the University of Louisville where he was granted the M.D. degree in 1846. After graduation he devoted two years in further study at different European medical centers.

In 1850 he was appointed Demonstrator of Anatomy in the University of Louisville. About this time he established the "Stokes Dispensary," considered one of the first clinical institutions in the West. He was later named Professor of Clinical Medicine serving until the War of 1861–65, when he joined the Confederate Army to become Director of the Medical Division of the Department of the West under General Albert Sidney Johnston.

In 1867 he became Professor of Clinical Surgery in the University of Louisville, which afforded special opportunity for his particular talents as a teacher of clinical surgery.

His operations are described as artistic and carried out with scrupulous cleanliness, and as early as 1870 he prophesied the advent of antiseptic surgery. In 1870 in cooperation with Dr. Theophilus Parvin (president A.M.A. 1879) he established the American Practitioner and was its principal editor for many years. In 1886 he published a classic analysis of 415 cases of tetanus.

Among the many honors that came to him, was the election as president of the American Surgical Association, Honorary Fellow and Corresponding Member of the Medico-Chirurgical Society of Edinburgh, and Fellow of the Royal Medical Society of London. In his address as president at the Philadelphia session of the Association, which was devoted largely to the progress of medical education in the United States, he felt it fitting to recall that as Philadelphia was the cradle of the American Medical Association, it should also be the cradle of American medical education.

His last illness was of five years' duration, due to progressive arteriosclerosis, and he died in Louisville May 3, 1898 at the age of seventy-two years.

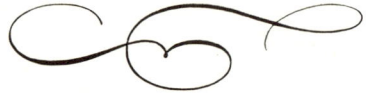

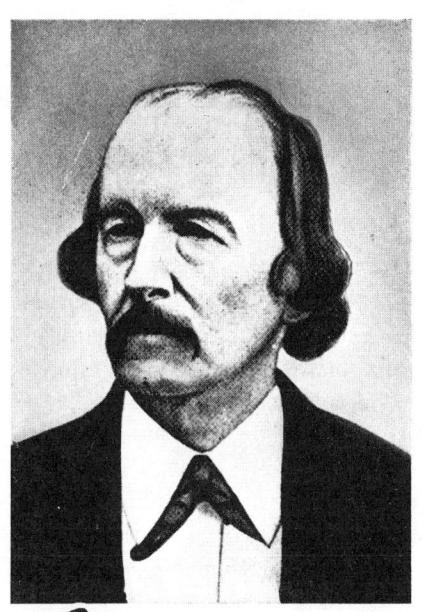

THOMAS MULDROP LOGAN, M.D.
Sacramento, Calif.
1808–1876

Twenty-fifth President, A. M. A.
St. Louis Session
May 6, 7, 8, 9, 1873

DR. THOMAS M. LOGAN of Sacramento was the first California physician to be elected to the presidency of the Association. This recognition came to him largely as the result of his pioneer efforts in medical organization on the Pacific Coast as well as his eminence as a sanitarian and climatologist and founder of the California State Board of Health, the second in the United States.

Dr. Logan was born in Charleston, South Carolina, July 31, 1808, the son and grandson of physicians, and through his mother was of Danish descent. He was educated at Charleston College, and was granted the degree of M.D. in 1828 by the Medical College of South Carolina.

Following his graduation he practiced a number of years in Charleston; then in 1832 he spent nearly a year in further medical study in London and Paris. Upon his return he was appointed lecturer on materia medica and therapeutics at his Alma Mater. A year later he published, with Dr. Thomas L. Ogier, a Compendium on Operative Surgery.

In 1843 he moved to New Orleans where he practiced until 1849 when the discovery of gold attracted him to California, and he came to Sacramento where he practiced the remainder of his life. He became intensely interested in the climatic, social and medical conditions in this new state, and particularly in the status of endemic diseases and in the differentiation between communicable diseases in California and Eastern and Southern states.

In 1870 almost single-handed he put through legislation which brought into being the California State Board of Health. Dr. Logan became the first secretary of the Board, which office he occupied until his death in 1876.

In the meeting of the Association at Philadelphia in May, 1872 he introduced a resolution recommending a National Health Council with a Secretary of Health with Cabinet rank. In the Forty-second Congress December 13, 1872 a bill to establish a Bureau of Sanitary Science in the Department of Education was introduced. While the measure failed to pass, the general awakening throughout the United States in public health resulted in the organization of the American Public Health Association in 1872.

The coming of Dr. E. S. Cooper to California in 1855, and his scientific spirit and interest in medical organization with that of Dr. Logan, led to the organization of the Medical Society of California in 1856—the first meeting being held in Sacramento with one hundred members present. From 1860 to 1870 this Society was rather inactive, but through the efforts of Dr. Logan it was reorganized in 1870 as the California State Medical Society and he was elected to the presidency of the same.

Dr. J. M. Toner, the medical historian of the period, wrote of Dr. Logan, "His name is closely identified with all measures in the direction of public welfare in California for a quarter of a century."

He died of pneumonia in Sacramento February 13, 1876 in his sixty-eighth year.

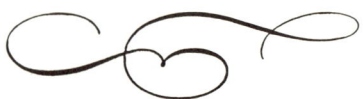

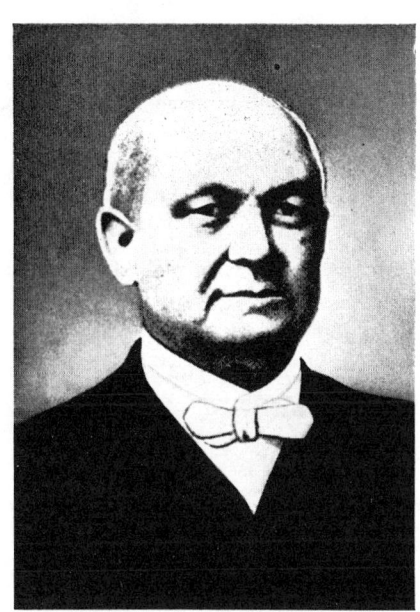

JOSEPH MEREDITH TONER, M.D.
Washington, D. C.
1825–1896

*Twenty-sixth President, A. M. A.
Detroit Session
June 2, 3, 4, 5, 1874*

DR. JOSEPH M. TONER, the second Washington physician to be elected to the presidency of the Association, was the medical historian, bibliophile and librarian of his period.

He was born in Pittsburgh, Pennsylvania, April 30, 1825. He received his collegiate education at Western University of Pennsylvania, graduated in medicine at Vermont Medical College in 1850, and subsequently in 1853 received the degree Doctor of Medicine from Jefferson Medical College, Philadelphia. He located in Washington, D. C. in 1855 and soon acquired a good general practice and became identified with medical societies both local and national.

He developed very high social and literary qualities and became an active and persevering collector of the works of American authors and devised a repository of medical works under the control of the medical profession of the United States. Thus was founded the first library of American medicine deposited in Smithsonian Institution at Washington.

He was the first in this country to attempt the endowment of medical lectureships, founding the Toner Lectures in 1871.

In 1870 he published the necrology of physicians engaged in the War of 1861–5, and the following year a medical register of the United States. As Chairman of the Necrology Committee of the

American Medical Association for 20 years he became the faithful biographer of his medical colleagues.

Some of his important contributions were the History of Smallpox Vaccination 1865, Portability of Cholera 1866, Facts of Vital Statistics in the United States 1872, and Contribution to the Study of Yellow Fever in 1874. In 1895, he published an interesting monograph on "Personal Reminiscences."

In 1882 he presented his entire library consisting of 28,000 books and 18,000 pamphlets to the Congressional Library in Washington. It is said of him "No one ever approached, much less equaled him, in painstaking collection of data, of personal history that might prove of interest and mystery to many, who thus managed to have facts within reach when occasion called for them."

He died while spending a few weeks at Cresson Springs, Penna., July 30, 1896, at seventy-one years of age.

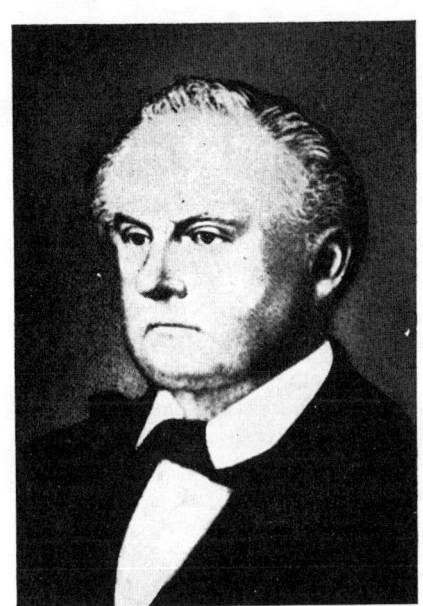

WILLIAM K. BOWLING, M.D.
Nashville, Tenn.
1808–1885

Twenty-seventh President, A. M. A.
Louisville Session
May 4, 5, 6, 7, 1875

DR. WILLIAM K. BOWLING, the second physician of Nashville to be elected to the presidency of the Association, was born June 5, 1808 in Westmoreland County, Virginia, and two years later came to Kentucky. As described by him "like Clay and Drake, I was dropped down in the wilderness of Kentucky and left to fight the battle of life as best I could without education, family influence or patronage."

Most of his early education was obtained from private tutors. After one course of lectures in the Ohio Medical College at Cincinnati he practiced five years and then attended another course at the Medical Department of Cincinnati College receiving the degree Doctor of Medicine in 1836. He then practiced fourteen years in Logan County, Kentucky, which was near the Tennessee line and he soon became widely known in two states. In 1848 he declined the offer of the Chair of Theory and Practice of Medicine in the Memphis Medical Institute, then the pioneer school in Tennessee. Two years later in 1850 he moved to Nashville, Tenn., and established the Nashville Medical School and was elected to the Chair of Theory and Practice of Medicine. Thus a medical school which later became Vanderbilt University School of Medicine and destined to great leadership "was established by the energy of a non-collegebred youth and the wisdom of a backwoods practitioner with the aid of an able corps of teachers in which he became the master spirit."

In 1851 he founded the Nashville Journal of Medicine and Surgery and sustained it with his best efforts for a quarter of a century.

Dr. Bowling at all times was a strong advocate of medical organization, and aside from his eminence as a practitioner and teacher of medicine, he became a leader in all that pertained to the educational social and practical interests of the profession in the Mississippi Valley.

His address as president of the Association in 1875 is described as "a gracious, flowery and eloquent exposition of a cultured gentleman, with a beautiful tribute at the close to the medical pioneers of Kentucky and Tennessee."

He died at his residence on Cumberland Mountain near Nashville, Tennessee, August 6, 1885, at seventy-seven years of age.

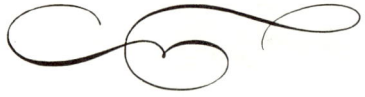

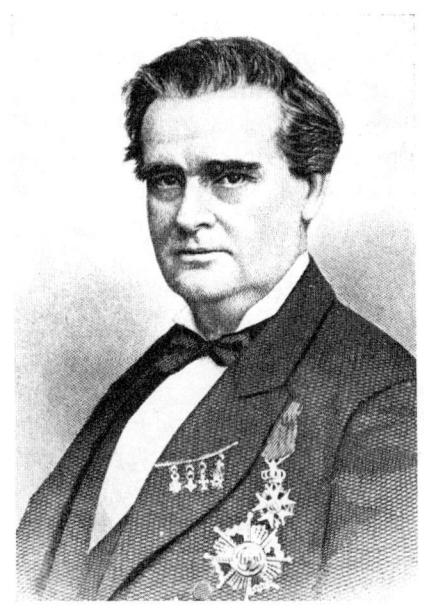

JAMES MARION SIMS, M.D.
New York, N. Y.
1813–1883

*Twenty-eighth President, A. M. A.
Philadelphia Session
June 6, 7, 8, 9, 1876*

THE PHILADELPHIA SESSION of the Association, at which J. Marion Sims presided, was significant also as the Centennial year of the Republic. The spirit of the occasion is reflected in the address of welcome of Dr. William Pepper (secundus), chairman of arrangements and distinguished physician of Philadelphia, in these words—"We are brethren in a great family of the Nation, and fellow citizens of a Republic, which under blessings of Almighty God was established one hundred years ago. May this meeting be inspired with perfect harmony and union which prevades our land today, and with the spirit of purer and higher aspiration which should be the great and lasting good bequeathed by this re-kindling of the fervor of the olden time."

It seemed, therefore, fitting in this city, the birthplace of the Nation and the Association, that the session should be presided over by one of the romantic figures in American medicine, Dr. J. Marion Sims, a son of the southland, then a resident of New York City.

Doctor Sims was born near Lancaster, South Carolina, January 25, 1813, his father serving at this time with the American Army in the War of 1812–14.

After finishing the neighborhood schools, he entered South Carolina College at Columbia, now the University of South Carolina, graduating in 1832. The next year he began the study of medicine at the Charleston Medical College, completing it at Jefferson Medical College and receiving the degree Doctor of Medicine in 1835.

He returned to his home in Lancaster to practice, and thus began a career destined to be one of the foremost in American medicine, yet intermingled with many keen disappointments. His first two patients were infants suffering with "summer complaint" and promptly died, which caused him in despair to take down his "shingle" and throw it in an abandoned well. Thus disgusted with his first experience in medical practice at twenty-two years of age, he turned to Alabama, where he journeyed on horseback for three weeks before reaching Mt. Meigs, twelve miles from Montgomery, remaining one year, when an offer of a partnership took him to Macon County—in a swampy section near Cubahatchee Creek, where several severe attacks of malaria nearly cost him his life.

In 1840 he moved to Montgomery, then a sleepy town of about 4000 people, a third being Negroes. It had recently been chosen as the State capital; there were no paved streets or sidewalks and brawls and public drunkenness punctuated the night life of the town. Tallow candles were the chief means of illumination, and goose quill pens had not been replaced by the steel variety. In therapeutics, quinine and calomel were without rivals, and bleeding was a common treatment. Surgical anesthesia was still unknown. "Malaria poisoning" was supposed to arise from the decomposition of vegetable matter.

In such surroundings Dr. Sims nevertheless developed a good practice and soon became recognized as a surgeon of more than ordinary ability. He was the first surgeon in the South to operate successfully for strabismus and clubfoot, having as early as 1836 operated successfully for abscess of the liver. He helped to rejuvenate the specialty of gynecology, and soon developed the vaginal speculum that bears his name, this being devised from a pewter spoon by bending the handle.

About five years after locating in Montgomery, three Negro slave women were referred to him with vesico-vaginal fistula, all being placed in a little infirmary which he had constructed in his backyard. Other Negro women were added to this list, and for four years he operated many times on these women without success until he began to use silver wire sutures which transformed his former failures into success. Other successful cases followed and the profession was amazed at his accomplishments.

The results were first published in the January 1852 number of the American Journal of Medical Sciences.

At the height of his success, he developed an intractable intestinal disorder, which disabled him for three years and in 1852 he decided to move to New York City. Here an envious profession, although recognizing his talents, kept him from gaining a foothold; his health soon became impaired and he was reduced to poverty, his wife being forced to take boarders.

In spite of all these disappointments he decided to secure a start by establishing a charity hospital for women, where he might demonstrate his ability. With the help of certain wealthy laymen and after two years of hard work and many bitter disappointments, the Woman's Hospital of New York, the first of its kind in the world, opened its doors and from that time Sims prospered and his fame spread throughout the world. On a trip abroad in 1861 he was everywhere given an ovation. He was called upon to operate for vesicovaginal fistulae in Ireland, Scotland, England, France and Belgium. Among his patients were Empress Eugenie, wife of Napoleon III, and the Empress of Austria. His operations were witnessed by such celebrities as Nélaton, Velpeau, Péan and others. He came back to New York City when the war between the states was on in full blast, and as his sympathies were with his people in the South, the conditions were so unpleasant that he returned to Paris. He did not resume his practice in New York City until after the war.

He contributed liberally to the surgical literature of his period and at all times was devoted to the interests of the American Medical Association. In his presidential address at Philadelphia he directed attention to the responsibility of the medical profession in the control of syphilis, the need of establishing State Boards of Health and the prevention of contagious diseases.

As he clasped the hand of his successor in the office of President, Dr. Henry I. Bowditch of Boston, he said "Thank God the day of strife is past forever; once there was bitterness and hate, now there are kindness and affection. What higher proof can there be of this, that at this time Massachusetts and South Carolina can join hands."

The interesting life of J. Marion Sims came to a close in New York City November 13, 1883, at seventy years of age.

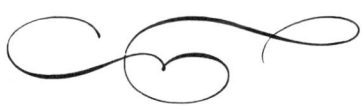

HENRY I. BOWDITCH, M.D.
Boston, Mass.
1808–1892

Twenty-ninth President, A. M. A.
Chicago Session
June 5, 6, 7, 8, 1877

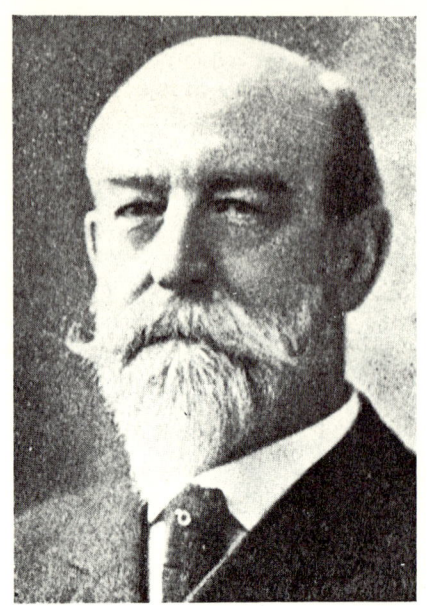

THE ELECTION OF Dr. Henry I. Bowditch of Boston to the presidency was a fitting reward for long and faithful service in the Association and recognition of a distinguished career in several fields of medical endeavor, he being the first Chairman of the Massachusetts State Board of Health, and a pioneer specialist in diseases of the chest.

He was born in Salem, Mass., August 8, 1808, being the third son of the celebrated mathematician, Nathaniel Bowditch. His early life was spent in Salem and in 1823 he moved to Boston. He received his A.M. degree from Harvard College in 1828, and that of Doctor of Medicine from the Harvard Medical School in 1832. While serving as House Officer of Massachusetts General Hospital he came under the tutelage of his revered teacher, Dr. James Jackson. It was upon his advice that he went to Paris in 1832 to become associated with the great clinician Louis for the greater part of two years. As Louis was deeply interested in the teachings of Laënnec, this probably inspired the trend of Bowditch towards the special study of chest diseases and particularly tuberculosis. Upon his return to Boston he became associated with Dr. James Jackson and later succeeded him in 1859 as Professor of Medicine in Harvard Medical School.

In 1835 with Dr. John Ware he founded the Boston Society for Medical Observation, a similar organization to that under the leadership of Louis in Paris. It existed first as a student society, and in 1839 became the Boston Society of Medical Improvement. In the April 1852 issue of the Journal of American Medical Sciences appeared his epoch making article "Aspiration of the Chest in Pleuritic Effusions by Needle and Trocar," introducing the procedure of paracentesis thoracis with which his name will always be associated. This was followed by the publication of his extensive studies on tuberculosis, consumption and phthisis. About this time also appeared the interesting monograph "The Young Stethoscopist."

In 1859 he moved his office and residence to 113 Boylston Street, where he remained until his death in 1892. In this office was held the first meeting of the Boston Medical Library Association December 21, 1874.

As an early student of hygiene he was the natural founder of the Massachusetts State Board of Health in 1869—the first established in this country. He was also one of the founders in 1872 of the American Public Health Association.

His address on State Medicine before the Association in 1874 on "Preventive Medicine and the Physician of the Future" was a review of the grand scope of preventive medicine.

Before the International Medical Congress in Philadelphia in 1876 he presented an address entitled "State Medicine and Public Hygiene in America," which marked an epoch in the history of hygiene and public health in the United States.

In 1877 he presented before the Association a report of an epidemic of diphtheria in New England, of which 85 per cent of the cases occurred in children. He described transmission of the disease from person to person, and recognized that it became more contagious as the epidemic progressed. He noted further that adult carriers could transmit diphtheria to children without having it themselves.

In the light of these facts, he concluded that an epidemic of diphtheria could be controlled as readily as smallpox and scarlet fever.

Dr. Bowditch was deeply religious and a strong advocate of temperance. In his earlier years he was an enthusiastic and militant abolitionist being associated with William Lloyd Garrison in the anti-slavery movement. He had a strong feeling as to the influence of general culture and warned against the danger of "becoming men of one idea." He believed in travel and "consequent humanizing effect of study of men and manners other than our own."

Dr. Bowditch died in Boston January 14, 1892 at the age of eighty-four years.

TOBIAS G. RICHARDSON, M.D.
New Orleans
1827–1892

*Thirtieth President, A. M. A.
Buffalo, N. Y. Session
June 4, 5, 6, 7, 1878*

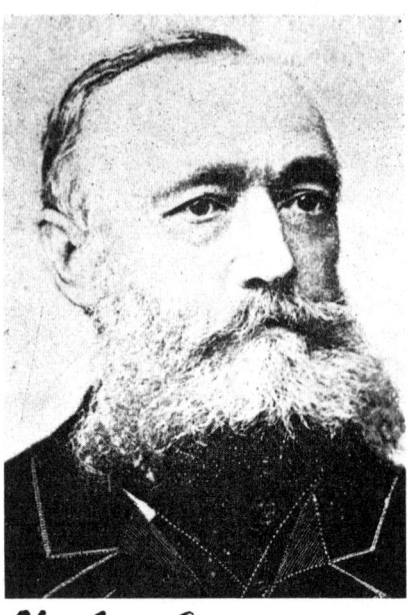

DR. TOBIAS G. RICHARDSON of New Orleans was the first and only president elected from that city. It is stated that his selection to this office was due to his high professional character, and reputation as an anatomist and surgeon, but also in part to the active influence of Dr. Samuel D. Gross, who urged it to more completely obliterate the effects of the previous war between the States.

He was born in Lexington, Kentucky, January 3, 1827, and commenced the study of medicine with Dr. Samuel D. Gross as preceptor, graduating from the Medical Department, University of Louisville in 1848. Soon after graduation he was appointed Demonstrator of Anatomy in the University of Louisville, and while in this teaching position in 1854 he published "Elements of Human Anatomy, General, Descriptive and Practical," an octavo volume of 734 pages with 269 illustrations, the first treatise of its kind published in the Mississippi Valley. In this work he substituted English for Latin terms whenever justifiable.

Aside from his reputation gained as an anatomist he had become favorably known for his surgical ability. As early as 1841 when he was twenty-four years of age it is recorded that he successfully removed the parotid gland and performed a double hip-joint amputation, both without anesthesia.

In 1858 he accepted an appointment as Professor of Anatomy in the Medical Department of Tulane University, and removed his residence to that city. A few years later he became Professor of Surgery and Visiting Surgeon at Charity Hospital. It was in New Orleans that he accomplished his best work both as a teacher and practitioner.

His eloquent and felicitous words of welcome at the New Orleans meeting of the Association in 1869 have been previously referred to. In his presidential address at the Buffalo session he made a plea for more original investigations on the part of the members, and greater attention to public hygiene and sanitation. He referred to the greater number of State Boards of Health that had been formed in the previous ten years; he specially commended the plan adopted in Alabama where the State Medical Society was responsible for the organization of the State Board of Health. He also recommended the incorporation of the Association, and further urged that State laws be enacted requiring licensing examinations of physicians.

Dr. Richardson was a charter member of the American Surgical Association as well as a Fellow of the College of Physicians of Philadelphia.

After his death in New Orleans, May 26, 1892, his widow contributed $170,000 to erect a memorial addition to the Medical School of Tulane University.

THEOPHILUS PARVIN, M.D.
Indianapolis, Ind.
1829–1899

Thirty-first President, A. M. A.
Atlanta, Ga. Session
May 6, 7, 8, 9, 1879

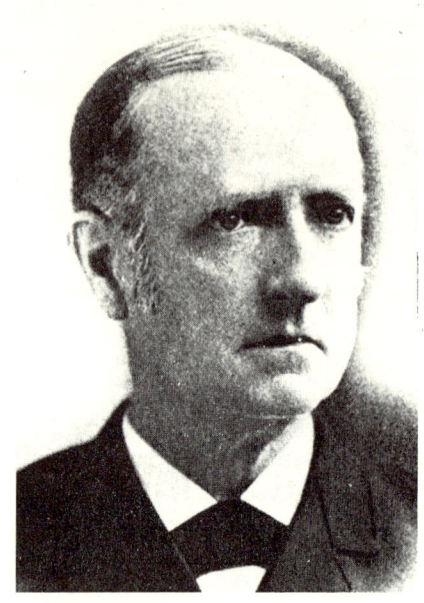

FOR THE FOURTH TIME in the history of the Association a prominent authority in the teaching and practice of obstetrics was chosen for the presidency, those previously selected being Dr. Reuben D. Mussey of Ohio in 1850, Dr. Henry Miller of Kentucky in 1859, and Dr. George Mendenhall of Ohio in 1870.

Dr. Theophilus Parvin was born in Buenos Aires January 9, 1829, while his parents were temporarily residing outside the United States. He received his early education at the University of Indiana and graduated in medicine in 1852 from the University of Pennsylvania. His teaching career began in 1864 when he was appointed Professor of Materia Medica in the Medical College of Ohio at Cincinnati, remaining five years, when he accepted the Chair of Obstetrics and Surgical Diseases of Women, University of Louisville, remaining until 1876 when he became Professor of Obstetrics and Diseases of Women and Children at the College of Physicians and Surgeons in Indianapolis. He was recalled to the University of Louisville in 1882 and in 1883 accepted the Chair of Obstetrics and Diseases of Women and Children at Jefferson Medical College, Philadelphia, where he continued the remainder of his life.

His experience in medical journalism included the editorship of the Cincinnati Journal of Medicine from 1866 to 1867; that of the Western Journal of Medicine, Indianapolis for one year, and co-editor of the American Practitioner, Louisville, from 1869 until his departure for Philadelphia in 1883. His principal publication was his textbook on the Art and Science of Obstetrics, which passed through three editions. Aside from being honored with the presidency of the American Medical Association, he served as president of the Indiana State Medical Society, American Journalists Association, American Academy of Medicine, and Philadelphia Obstetrical Society. He was also Honorary President of the Obstetrical Section of the International Medical Congress in Berlin in 1890 and again in Rome in 1893.

He received the Honorary degree of LL.D. from Lafayette Colledge in 1872, Honorary Fellowship in the Edinburgh Obstetrical Society and Berlin Society of Obstetrics and Gynecology, besides being elected a Fellow of the College of Physicians of Philadelphia and the American Philosophical Society.

He is referred to as an eloquent and earnest lecturer, and in his time conducted in Philadelphia the largest obstetrical clinic in this country.

Dr. Parvin died in Philadelphia January 29, 1899 at seventy years of age.

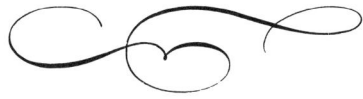

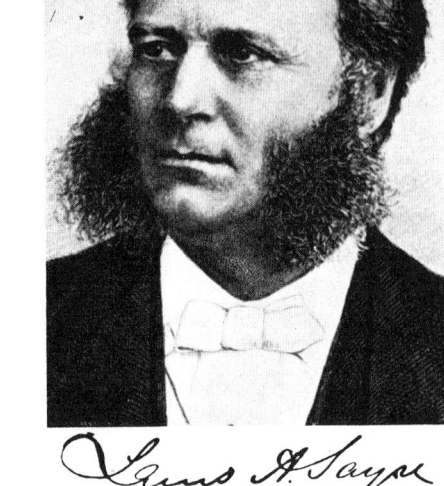

LEWIS ALBERT SAYRE, M.D.
New York City
1820–1900

Thirty-second President, A. M. A.
New York Session
June 1, 2, 3, 4, 1880

DR. LEWIS A. SAYRE has been properly called the father of American Orthopedic Surgery, and also the first and only strictly orthopedic surgeon ever elected to the presidency of the Association.

He was born near Madison, New Jersey, February 29, 1820; his father died when he was 12 years of age and he went to live with an uncle in Lexington, Kentucky, where he received his preliminary education. He returned to New York City in 1839 to enter the College of Physicians and Surgeons, Columbia University, from which he graduated in 1842. He was immediately appointed prosector of surgery under Professor Willard Parker, and carried on this work until 1853, when he was appointed surgeon to Bellevue Hospital. In 1859 he was largely instrumental in founding Bellevue Hospital Medical College, which institution adopted the motto "Clinica Clinice Demonstrada"—"believing that medicine and surgery must be taught by living demonstrations instead of by theoretical disquisitions."

He was elected Professor of Orthopedic Surgery, fractures and dislocations in the new medical school, serving until 1898 when Bellveue Hospital Medical College was amalgamated with New York University, and he was named Emeritus, being succeeded in the chair by his son, Dr. Reginald Hall Sayre. From 1860 to 1866 he was resident physician of New York City (Health Officer) serving under four different Mayors. A contemporary refers to Dr. Sayre's work in this position as being "far ahead of his time in the advocacy of precautions for the preservation of the health of the community. He was a strong proponent of compulsory vaccination; the intelligent disposal of sewage; the sanitary inspection of tenement houses, and quarantine regulations for the control of cholera."

His first paper published October 18, 1842 when he was only 22 years old, showed an originality of thought that characterized all his subsequent writings. This article presented the surgical treatment of abscess of the lung following pneumonia by the removal of four ribs and was the first suggestion of collapse of the lung as a therapeutic measure.

In 1854 he reported the first successful resection of the hip joint in this country. In 1871 he demonstrated this operation at different medical centers in Europe, and before the International Medical Congress in Philadelphia in 1876. The latter was witnessed by Professor Joseph Lister of England, who made the following comment—"I feel that this demonstration would of itself have been sufficient reward for my voyage to America."

His originality was further shown in the treatment of Pott's disease of the spine through rotary lateral curvature which procedure definitely established his fame as the foremost orthopedic surgeon of his time.

His eventful career came to a close in New York City September 21, 1900. From the many obituary notices, the following is quoted from the British Medical Journal. "Few men in this generation accomplished so much for the relief of humanity and his name will go down to posterity with that of J. Marion Sims as amongst the most distinguished benefactors whom the American medical profession has produced for the glory of medicine and the good of mankind during this Century."

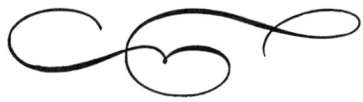

JOHN THOMPSON HODGEN, M.D.
St. Louis, Mo.
1826–1882

Thirty-third President, A. M. A.
Richmond Session
May 3, 4, 5, 6, 1881

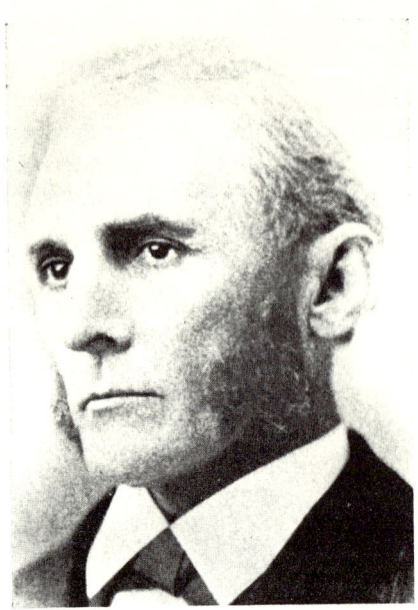

THE THIRTY-THIRD PRESIDENT of the Association, Dr. John T. Hodgen, was a well known surgeon at the time of his election, having attained special recognition at the International Medical Congress in Philadelphia in 1876. His talents as a mechanical genius gave his name to the special wire splint for use in fracture of the thigh, and a forceps dilator for removing foreign bodies from the air passages.

Dr. Hodgen was born in Hodgenville, Kentucky, January 19, 1826, and received his collegiate education at Bethany College, Virginia, and graduated from the medical department of the University of Missouri at St. Louis in 1848. Soon after graduation he located in St. Louis and entered actively into teaching in connection with his practice. Beginning as Demonstrator of Anatomy in the University of Missouri, he became Professor of Anatomy in 1854, and in 1864 was appointed Professor of Anatomy and Physiology in the St. Louis Medical College. In 1875 he became Professor of Surgical Anatomy.

He was recognized as an able teacher, clear and forceful in his expressions and a powerful debater. His presidential address at the Richmond meeting in 1881 emphasized the dangers connected with surgical operations, and included a most comprehensive discussion of tumors and anemia. Less than a year later he developed an acute abdominal condition resulting in peritonitis and his death occurred on April 28, 1882 at fifty-six years of age.

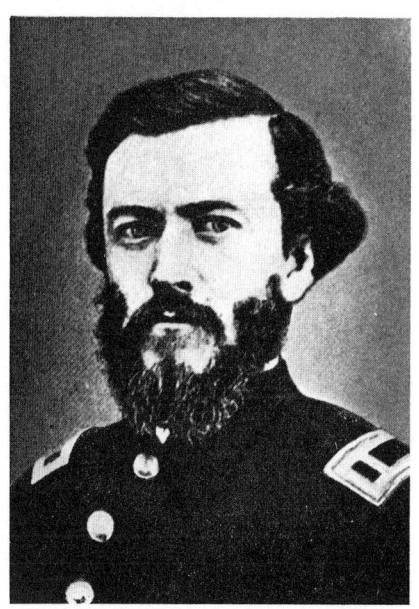

JOSEPH J. WOODWARD, M.D.
Washington, D. C.
1833–1884

Thirty-fourth President, A. M. A.
St. Paul Session
June 6, 7, 8, 9, 1882

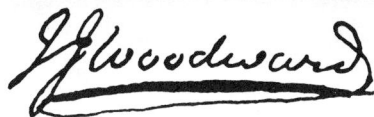

DR. JOSEPH J. WOODWARD, pioneer American medical microscopist, was the first medical officer of the United States Army to be elected to the presidency of the Association. A faithful attendant at annual sessions since 1865, he was prevented by illness from presiding at the St. Paul meeting June 6–9, 1882, and Dr. P. O. Hooper of Arkansas, the first vice president, presided during this entire session.

Dr. Woodward was born in Philadelphia October 30, 1833, and was educated in his native city, receiving the degrees A.B. and A.M. from Central High School, and that of Doctor of Medicine from the University of Pennsylvania in 1853, when he was twenty years of age.

While a student of Professor George B. Wood, he formed a class of instruction in the use of the microscope and the study of pathological histology. He practiced medicine in Philadelphia until 1861 when he was appointed Assistant Surgeon of the Army of the Potomac, later being assigned to duty in the office of the Surgeon General and Army Medical Museum. At the close of the war in 1861–5 he continued with the Medical Corps U. S. Army and remained in this service throughout the remainder of his life. In connection with Colonel George A. Otis he edited the medical and surgical history of the war, the first volume being published in 1870, and the second in 1879. He also prepared the first catalogue of the Surgeon General's Library. His valuable work in microscopy and photo microscopy, in which he was a pioneer, and the publication of the same, won him national and international recognition in this field. He was elected as Honorary Member of the Royal Microscopical Society of London, as well as of the Society of Microscopy of Liverpool and Belgium.

In 1880 his health began to fail and a trip to Europe was advised, without producing any definite improvement. In 1881 he was one of the consultants in the illness of President Garfield.

Dr. Woodward died in Philadelphia, the city of his birth, August 17, 1884, a few months under fifty-one years of age.

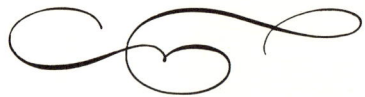

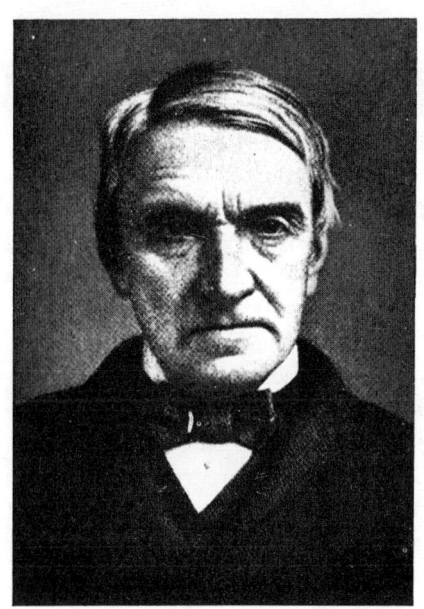

JOHN LIGHT ATLEE, M.D.
Lancaster, Pa.
1799–1885

Thirty-fifth President, A. M. A.
Cleveland Session
June 5, 6, 7, 8, 1883

DR. JOHN L. ATLEE was eighty-three years of age at the time of his election, and the oldest president of the Association to serve in that office. He became a member of the Association at the organization meeting in Philadelphia in 1847, and was a faithful attendant at all subsequent annual sessions. Born in Lancaster, Pennsylvania, November 2, 1799, he lived his entire life in his native city.

His medical studies were carried on at the University of Pennsylvania from which he received the degree Doctor of Medicine in 1820. After graduation he returned to Lancaster, and soon developed a large general practice.

For a number of years he was Professor of Anatomy and Physiology in Franklin and Marshall College at Lancaster. He gained his widest professional recognition in the field of obstetrics. According to the medical historian, Dr. Francis R. Packard, Dr. Atlee revived the operation for ovariotomy in 1843; this operation first performed by the great Ephraim McDowell in 1809 had been regarded with disfavor for some years, as only five cases were reported in the interval.

From 1843 to 1883 Dr. Atlee performed this operation 78 times with 64 recoveries and 14 deaths. During an active practice of sixty-five years, he performed 2125 important operations.

In his presidential address he reviewed the experience of sixty-three years of medical practice, recalling the days as a medical student under Caspar Wistar, the anatomist; Nathaniel Chapman, professor of medicine, successor of Benjamin Rush and first president of the Association; attending also the first courses of lectures in surgery by Philip Syng Physick, pupil of John Hunter. He was a classmate of Isaac Hays, later editor of the American Journal of Medical Sciences, and George B. Wood, for many years Professor of Theory and Practice of Medicine and the ninth president of the Association. He closed with a tribute to the Code of Ethics and its purposes to establish brotherly consideration and kindness—then in retrospect he expressed the conviction after a long life devoted to the study and practice of medicine, understanding its disappointments and uncertainties, that it was still the most satisfying career. "In no other calling could man more fully accomplish his whole duty to God and to his fellow man."

Dr. Atlee died at Lancaster, Pennsylvania, October 1, 1885, within one month of his eighty-sixth year.

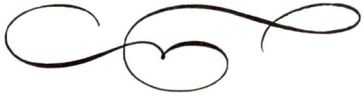

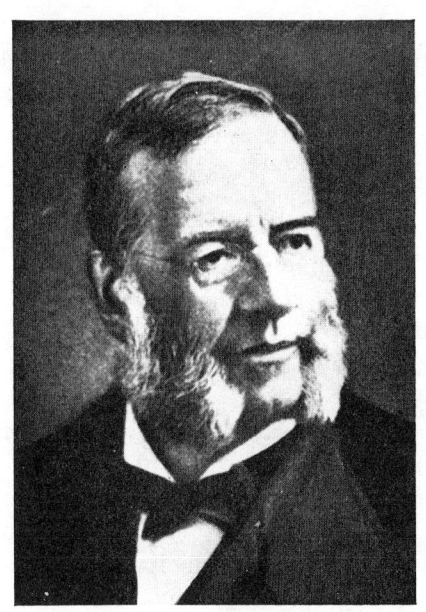

AUSTIN FLINT, M.D.
New York City
1812–1886

Thirty-sixth President, A. M. A.
Washington Session
May 6, 7, 8, 9, 1884

DR. AUSTIN FLINT came of a distinguished medical ancestry being the fourth generation of his line, and was followed by a son Austin Flint, physiologist, and grandson Austin Flint VI, obstetrician, who brought further distinction to American Medicine.

He was a delegate from the University of Buffalo to the New York Convention in 1846 and the Philadelphia meeting in 1847 when the Association was organized, and was the last member of the founders group to be elected to the presidency.

He was born at Petersham, Massachusetts, October 20, 1812, receiving his literary education at Amherst and Cambridge, and graduated in medicine at Harvard College in 1833. He began the practice of medicine in Boston, but within a few years moved to Buffalo, New York, where he began his distinguished career as author, practitioner and medical teacher, that carried him to several medical centers before he finally located in New York City in 1861. In 1836 he became one of the founders of Buffalo Medical College and professor of theory and practice of medicine, continuing to 1852. During this period he was editor of the Buffalo Medical Journal. For one academic year, 1844–5, he served as professor of medicine at Rush Medical College, Chicago.

In 1852 he was called to the chair of theory and practice of medicine at the University of Louisville, where he became associated with

Dr. Samuel D. Gross, who in his autobiography refers to him as "Tall and handsome, with a well modulated voice of great compass, and as a lecturer, at once clear, distinct and inspiring; during his lecture no student ever fell asleep. As a clinical instructor and diagnostician in diseases of the chest, he had few equals, and I know of no one so well entitled to be regarded as the American Laënnec."

During two years 1859–61 he was professor of clinical medicine at the New Orleans School of Medicine. In 1861 he was called to the chair of practice of medicine at Bellevue Hospital Medical School, which he retained until 1886. During seven years 1861–1868 he was also professor of pathology and practice of medicine at Long Island College Hospital.

No American physician was more closely allied to the interests of the American Medical Association than Dr. Austin Flint. An attendant at the preliminary meeting in 1846, at the organization session in Philadelphia in 1847, and at practically every meeting to 1883 when he was honored with the presidency, his principal contributions were first presented at sessions of the Association. In 1852 at the meeting in Richmond he was awarded the prize of the Association for the essay—"on variation of pitch and percussion and respiratory sounds and their application to physical diagnosis"; and in 1858 the prize essay on "clinical study of heart sounds in health and disease."

He was a prolific and forward looking writer, being the first to propose the diagnostic auscultory signs "cavernous respiration"; "broncho-vesicular respiration," and "Austin Flint murmur," and originated the binaural stethoscope. He was one of the earliest advocates in this country of the bacterial origin of certain diseases.

His publications were likewise significant, and added distinction to American medical literature. The compendium on percussion and auscultation in 1865 passed through four editions, diseases of the heart, 1852, four editions, phthisis in 1875; and his well known work —Treatise of Principles and Practice of Medicine, 1866, passed through seven editions.

He served as president of the New York Academy of Medicine and was a member of many learned societies. The Association appointed him general chairman of arrangements for the International Medical Congress to be held in Washington in 1887, and if death had not come to him in 1886, he would no doubt have been the presiding officer of the Congress. He had also been invited to deliver the address in medicine at the next meeting of the British Medical Association.

He died in New York City of apoplexy March 13, 1886. An editorial in the journal of the Association published the following week contained the tribute, "Of many eminent physicians of America, distinguished both as original thinkers and clinicians, none have risen to a higher plane in the esteem and respect of professional men of their country, and indeed of medical men the world over, than Austin Flint."

At the opening of the International Medical Congress the following year, President Nathan S. Davis in his inaugural address referred to Dr. Flint in the following words—"It is my first sad duty to remind you that death has removed from among us one to whom, more than any other, we are indebted for the privilege of having the Ninth International Congress in America. One whose urbanity, erudition, valuable contributions to medical literature and eminence as a teacher, caused him not only to be universally regarded the most influential leader in all the preparatory work, but also the one unanimously designated to preside over your deliberations on this occasion."

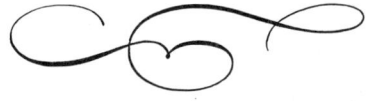

HENRY FRAZER CAMPBELL, M.D.
Augusta, Georgia
1824–1891

Thirty-seventh President, A. M. A.
New Orleans Session
April 28, 29, 30, May 1, 1885

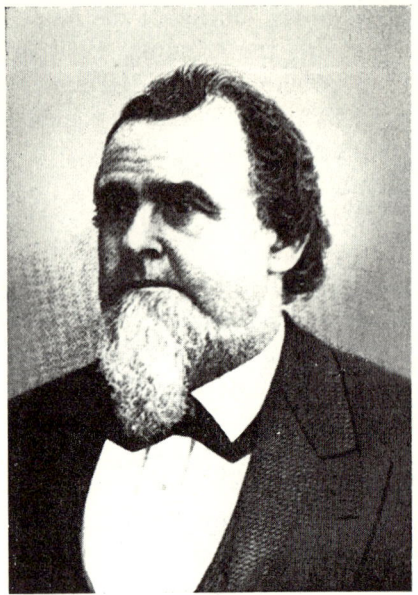

THE ASSOCIATION MET for the second time since the Civil War in New Orleans and again a distinguished southern physician was the presiding officer, one who had gained wide recognition as a physiologist, gynecologist, and an authority on public health.

Dr. Henry F. Campbell was born in Savannah, Georgia, February 10, 1824, his mother Mary R. Eve being the daughter of Mr. Joseph Eve, the inventor of the Brush and Cotton Roller Gin, and a cousin of Dr. Paul F. Eve (Nashville) president of the Association in 1857.

Raised in an environment of culture, he received a very thorough classical education, supplemented by private tutoring, and graduated from the Medical College of Georgia in 1842, at the young age of eighteen years. He always practiced medicine in Augusta, Georgia, except for the period of military service in the Civil War, and the period following when he was professor of anatomy and surgery in the New Orleans School of Medicine.

Soon after graduation he began his career as a medical teacher being appointed Demonstrator of Anatomy in his Alma Mater, serving in that position from 1842 to 1854, when he became Professor of Comparative Surgical and Microscopic Anatomy until 1857, at which time his title was changed to Professor of Anatomy, and he held that chair until 1866.

At the beginning of the War between the States in 1861 he was commissioned a Surgeon in the Confederate Army as well as Consulting Surgeon of the Georgia Military Hospitals in Richmond, Virginia, serving in these two capacities until the close of the war.

After completion of his military service and the period of teaching as Professor of Anatomy and Surgery in the New Orleans Medical College, he returned to Augusta in 1868, having been elected Professor of Operative Surgery in the Medical College, University of Georgia, serving until shortly before his death in 1886.

In 1852 in connection with his brother, Dr. Robert Campbell, he established in Augusta the Jackson Street Hospital—a well equipped institution of fifty beds for chronic and surgical diseases for the colored population.

He always had a large consulting practice which in later years was confined largely to surgery and gynecology. Early in his career he became interested in the physiology of the central nervous system, being credited with the first demonstration of the "excito-secretory" function of the nervous system, published in 1850, and awarded the annual prize essay of the Association in 1859—the title of the thesis being "The Excito-secretory System of Nerves; Its Relation to Physiology and Pathology." This work of Dr. Campbell led to an interesting correspondence with the English physiologist, Dr. Marshall Hall, and the great French scientist, Dr. Claude Bernard of Paris. In 1860 he was elected a corresponding member of the Imperial Academy of Medicine of St. Petersburg, and in 1878 of the Medical Society of Sweden.

He was one of the founders of the American Gynecological Society in 1876. In 1875 he became a member of the Georgia State Board of Health, and at the time of the American Public Health Association meeting in Nashville in 1879, he presented a comprehensive paper on the "Control of Yellow-fever and Dengue," which work entitles him to a place as a pioneer sanitarian.

Dr. Campbell was referred to as a pleasing eloquent speaker and a fine presiding officer. He died in Augusta, December 15, 1891 in his sixty-seventh year.

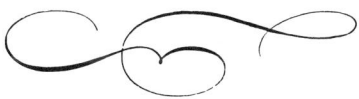

WILLIAM BRODIE, M.D.
Detroit, Mich.
1823–1890

Thirty-eighth President, A. M. A.
St. Louis Session
May 4, 5, 6, 7, 1886

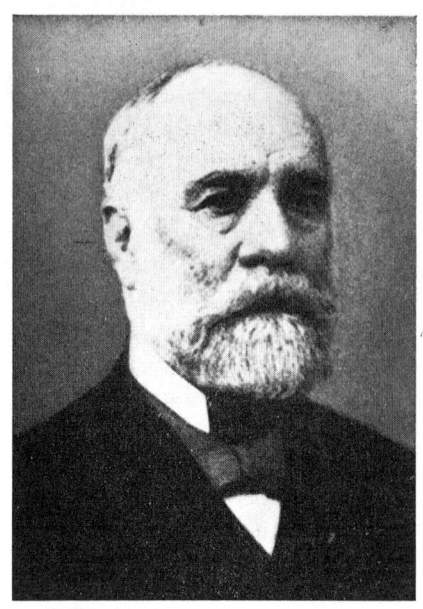

DR. WILLIAM BRODIE of Detroit, the 38th President of the Association and long active in its councils, was a distinguished pioneer physician of the middle-west. He was an Englishman by birth, having been born at Fawley Court July 26, 1823, coming to New York State, near Rochester, in 1832, when he was nine years of age. Here he received his general education and after moving his residence to the new state of Michigan, he became interested in medicine in 1847, as a student of Dr. William Wilson of Pontiac, Michigan. He attended his first course of medical lectures at Berkshire Medical College at Pittsfield, Mass., the second at Vermont Medical College at Woodstock, and completed his medical studies at the College of Physicians and Surgeons, Columbia College, New York City, receiving the degree Doctor of Medicine in 1850.

He began the practice of medicine in Detroit and soon became active in medical society organization. In 1852 he was one of the founders of the Detroit Medical Society, and its President in 1855.

The Michigan State Medical Society elected Dr. Brodie its President in 1876, and the same year he was chosen President of the Wayne County Medical Society, which position he held continuously for twelve years.

Throughout the Civil War he served as Surgeon of the First Regiment of Michigan Volunteers. For a number of years he was Professor of Clinical Medicine in the old Michigan College of Medicine. From 1880 to 1885 he was the editor of the Therapeutic Gazette.

Dr. Brodie attended his first meeting of the Association in 1855, and was a faithful attendant in the following thirty years. In 1857 he served as one of the secretaries, and in 1875 as first vice president of the Association. His presidential address was a comprehensive review of the progress of medical education in America, with special emphasis of the need of uniform and elevated standards of requirements for the degree of Doctor of Medicine.

Dr. Brodie died in Detroit July 30, 1890, at sixty-seven years of age.

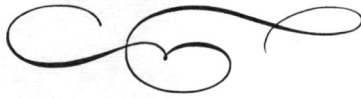

ELISHA HALL GREGORY, M.D.
St. Louis, Mo.
1824–1906

Thirty-ninth President, A. M. A.
Chicago Session
June 7, 8, 9, 10, 1887

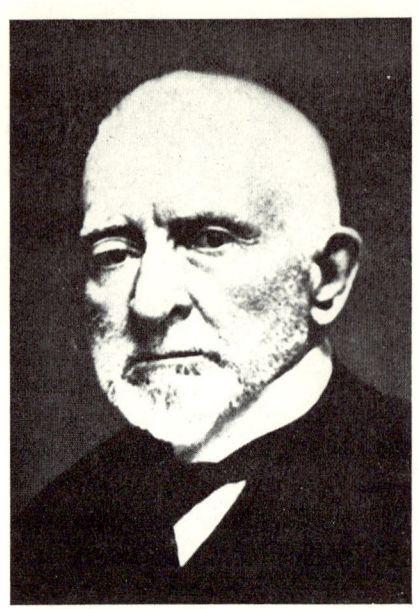

DR. ELISHA H. GREGORY, at the time of his election to the presidency, was a prominent surgeon and medical educator of St. Louis. He was born near Russelville, Kentucky, September 10, 1824, and received his early education in the common schools of Hopkinsville, Ky. and Boonville, Mo. He entered the medical department of St. Louis University from which he graduated in 1849.

In 1851 he joined the teaching staff of his Alma Mater as demonstrator of anatomy, and one year later was appointed professor of anatomy, continuing in that position until 1867 when he was elected professor of surgery. When the Missouri Medical College and St. Louis Medical College were merged in 1899, and became the medical department of Washington University, Dr. Gregory had a large share in bringing about this consolidation. For many years he was surgeon in chief of Mullanply Hospital, St. Louis. He served as president of the St. Louis Medical Society in 1863, and was the first president of the St. Louis Surgical Society. From 1871 to 1875 he was a member of the Board of Health of the City of St. Louis, and after that he served one term as president of the Missouri State Board of Health. His address as president of the Association in 1887 was entitled "Cell Antagonism," containing the interesting statement: "Cell struggle is the gist of modern pathology."

Dr. Gregory was active until his death at Ormond, Florida, from heart disease, February 11, 1906, at eighty-one years of age.

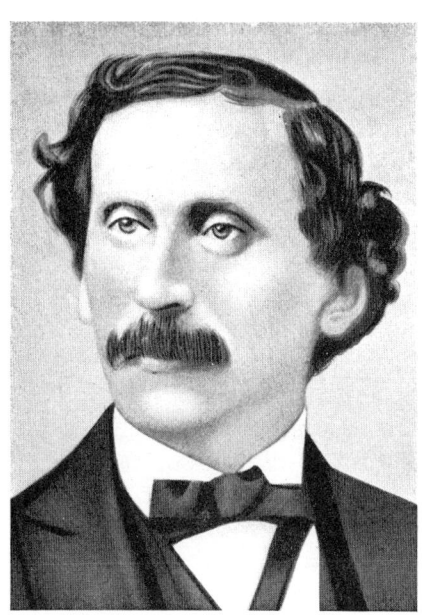

ALEXANDER Y. P. GARNETT, M.D.
Washington, D. C.
1820–1888

*Fortieth President, A. M. A.
Cincinnati Session
May 8, 9, 10, 11, 1888*

DR. ALEXANDER Y. P. GARNETT was one of the most prominent figures in the medical profession of the Nation's capital. He became a member of the Association in 1852 and with the exception of the Civil War years he attended nearly every annual session until his death in 1888; the honor of the presidency came to him during the last year of his life.

Dr. Garnett was born September 19, 1820 in Essex County, Virginia. He received a good liberal education, including private instruction in the classics and the French language, and graduated in medicine from the University of Pennsylvania in 1841. Soon afterwards he joined the United States Navy as Passed Assistant Surgeon serving a period of five years when he resigned and began private practice in the City of Washington. In 1858 he was appointed professor of clinical medicine in the Columbian Medical College. He was known for his ardent sympathies with the South, and when his native State of Virginia seceded from the Union in 1861 he left his lucrative practice and all his earthly possessions north of the Potomac and moved with his family to Richmond. During the war he was the personal physician of President Jefferson Davis, as well as the family physician of Generals Lee and Joseph Johnston, and nearly every member of the Confederate Cabinet and Senate. He was also placed in charge of two Army hospitals. After Lee's surrender he remained with President Davis as a member of his personal staff until after the surrender of General Johnston's army when he returned to Richmond as a paroled prisoner, and resumed practice in that city. All of his property had been confiscated by the United States Government, but upon the inducement of former friends he returned to Washington in the fall of 1865. He soon regained his former high position in professional circles and an extensive practice, particularly among the elite, wealthy and cultured class. The Columbian Medical College promptly re-elected him to the chair of clinical medicine in that institution. In 1874 he was chosen president of the Southern Medical Association.

His writings at all times reflected the scholar and high minded physician. The title of his presidential address at the Cincinnati session was "The Mission of the American Medical Association," and he proposed a radical and thorough reform in medical education, advising an annual conference of medical schools to promote greater uniformity of educational methods. He also recommended a board of medical examiners in each state not connected with medical schools or colleges.

Two months later, his interesting career came to a close at Atlantic City, New Jersey, July 11, 1888, at sixty-eight years of age.

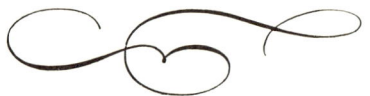

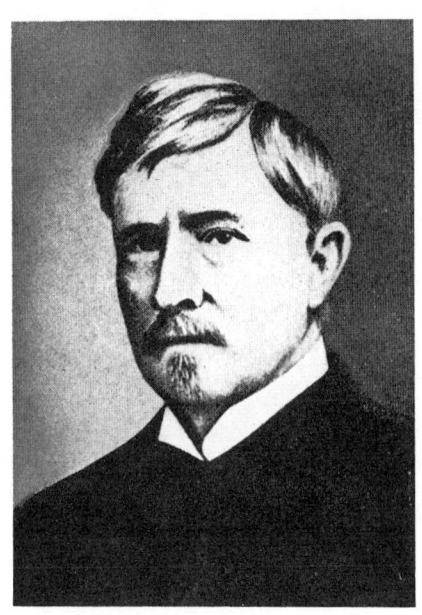

WILLIAM WIRT DAWSON, M.D
Cincinnati, Ohio
1828–1893

Forty-first President, A. M. A.
Newport, Rhode Island Session
June 25, 26, 27, 28, 1889

DR. WILLIAM W. DAWSON came to the presidency of the Association at the height of his career as a skillful operator and well-known teacher in surgery.

He was born December 19, 1828 at Dawson's Mills, Berkeley County, Virginia, and when he was one year of age his family moved to Jamestown, Ohio. He received a good classical education and graduated in medicine in 1850 from the Medical College of Ohio, having taken his first course of medical lectures at the University of Louisville. Soon after locating for practice in Cincinnati, he became interested in teaching and was appointed in 1853 professor of anatomy in the new Cincinnati College of Medicine and Surgery, and in 1860 he was elected to the same post in his Alma Mater—the Medical College of Ohio.

Upon his return from three years of military service in the Civil War in 1864 he was appointed Chief Surgeon of the Cincinnati Hospital, and in 1870 succeeded to the chair of surgery in the Medical College of Ohio. At this time he was recognized as a superior teacher and during the period 1870–1880 he performed many brilliant operations and contributed liberally to the surgical literature of that period. It is recorded that he performed 100 successful lithotomies without a death. He also performed the first recorded successful operation for nephrotomy.

The presidential address of Dr. Dawson at the 1889 session of the Association was of a high order and an able discourse on the future trends of medical education; he referred to the greater number of college graduates entering medicine and the influence of the laboratory in medical training, closing with the strong warning against the too rapid increase of medical schools.

His last years were clouded by a mental illness, and he died in Cincinnati February 16, 1893 at sixty-five years of age.

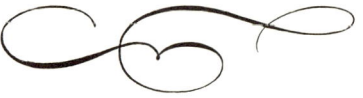

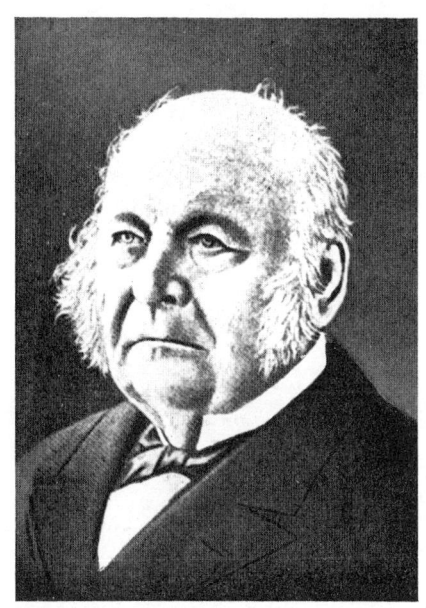

EDWARD MOTT MOORE, M.D.
Rochester, N. Y.
1814–1902

Forty-second President, A. M. A.
Nashville Session
May 20, 21, 22, 23, 1890

DR. EDWARD M. MOORE was a prominent physician of New York State, and at the time of his election had gained a well deserved reputation as a surgeon, teacher and investigator. He was born in Rahway, New Jersey, July 1, 1814, his parents being of the Society of Friends. He received his medical degree at the University of Pennsylvania in 1838. After completing a service as resident physician in "old" Blockley Hospital, Philadelphia, he began practice in Rochester, New York. During these early years he carried on research work with Dr. Pollock of Philadelphia on the mechanism of the heart's action in dogs, which was recognized as a contribution to the knowledge of that subject, as well as his original investigations on blood transfusion. With Dr. W. W. Reid of Philadelphia he worked out the mechanism of reduction of dislocation of the hip joint. His monographs on the fracture and dislocation of the clavicle and the radius were equally notable contributions.

He became professor of surgery in 1842 when he was 28 years of age, at the medical school of Woodstock, Vermont, and soon became recognized as an able teacher of surgery. Later he taught one year, 1853–54 at Berkshire Medical College, and in 1854–55 at Starling Medical College, Cincinnati, and then held the Chair of Surgery at Buffalo Medical College from 1858 to 1883.

He served as President of the Medical Society of the State of New

York, and was one of the founders of the American Surgical Association, serving as President in 1888. In this position he succeeded Dr. Samuel D. Gross.

In 1888–89 he helped frame the constitution and served as the first president of the New York State Board of Health. During nearly fifty years he was Chief of the Staff at St. Mary's Hospital, Rochester, New York. In his presidential address before the Association in 1890 he advocated a National Board of Health based on the United States Marine Hospital Service.

Dr. Moore died in Rochester, New York, March 4, 1902, at eighty-five years of age.

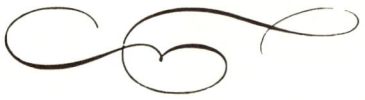

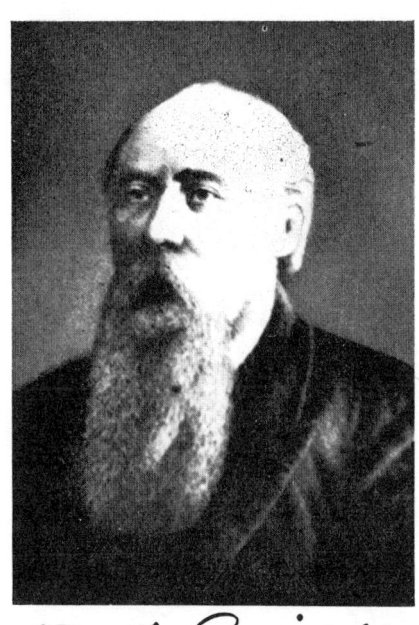

WILLIAM T. BRIGGS, M.D.
Nashville, Tenn.
1829–1894

Forty-third President, A. M. A.
Washington Session
May 5, 6, 7, 8, 1891

DR. WILLIAM T. BRIGGS was another distinguished American surgeon who was honored with the presidency of the Association. He was born in Bowling Green, Kentucky, December 4, 1829, and began the study of medicine at eighteen years of age at the medical department of Transylvania University, graduating from this institution with the degree Doctor of Medicine in 1849, when he was twenty years old. He became demonstrator of anatomy in the medical department of the University of Nashville in 1851, continuing until 1866.

In 1868 he was appointed professor of surgery in the medical department of the University of Nashville, and held the chair until his death in 1894.

Dr. Briggs was one of the founders of the American Surgical Association, and its president in 1885. He was the Chairman of the Section on Surgery of the International Medical Congress in Washington, D. C. in 1887, and one of the vice presidents of the Congress when it assembled in Rome in 1893.

Some of his unusual surgical operations included the removal of both upper jaws in 1863, and ligation of the internal carotid artery in 1871. He also devised a new operative procedure for lithotomy and reported the performing of 254 operations for vesical calculus with only six deaths.

Dr. Briggs died in Nashville June 13, 1894 at sixty-four years of age.

HENRY ORLANDO MARCY, M.D.
Boston, Mass.
1837–1924

*Forty-fourth President, A. M. A.
Detroit Session
June 7, 8, 9, 10, 1892*

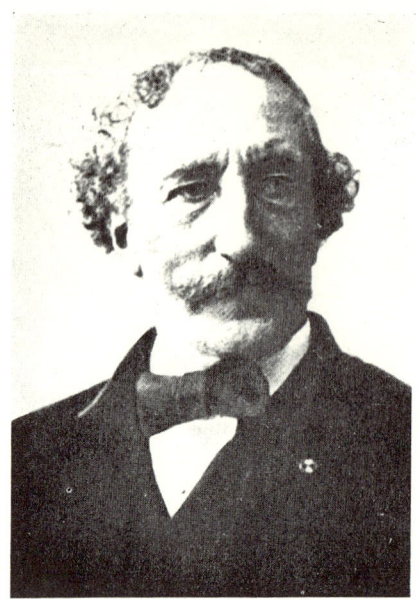

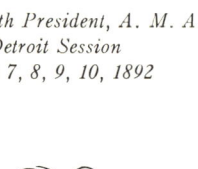

DR. HENRY O. MARCY was a distinguished physician and surgeon of his period; the first American surgeon to introduce antiseptic methods in the treatment of wounds; an extensive writer and promoter of many civic enterprises in his native city of Boston.

He was born in Otis, Massachusetts, June 23, 1837, and received his preliminary and classical education at Wilbraham Academy and Amherst College, graduating from Harvard Medical College in 1863. Soon after graduation he was appointed Assistant Surgeon of the 43rd Regiment of Massachusetts Volunteers, and in November 1863 was commissioned Surgeon of the First Regiment of Colored troops operating in North Carolina; in 1864 he became Medical Director of General Sherman's Carolina Campaign, and in 1864 and 1865 he supervised the sanitary renovation of Charleston, South Carolina. After the close of the Civil War he practiced for four years in Cambridge, Mass., when in 1869 he went to Europe, remaining a year in Berlin as a pupil of Rudolf Virchow, and the following year going to London. He was the first American pupil of Joseph Lister, and upon his return to the United States was the first to introduce antiseptic methods in surgery, devoting nearly ten years to a continuous study of microorganisms in wounds, experimenting with various culture media. Dr. Marcy presented some of the first discussions before the American Medical Association on the "Germ theory of disease"; "relation of micro-organisms to surgical lesions"; and "an experimental study of germicides and their comparative value as antiseptics."

In 1878 he reported an operative procedure for the radical cure of hernia with the antiseptic use of carbolized ligatures. One of his distinct contributions to surgery was the introduction of the buried animal suture.

At the Association meeting in 1884 he strongly advocated a National Board of Health, closing his address with these eloquent words —"Let the profession arise to its just prerogative and power as conservator of the public health,"—"Memorialize Congress to aid in the better solution of the important questions of preventive medicine and have the great wealthy government of the new world rival the old world in a generous emulation in the settlement of questions fundamental to the health, happiness and long life of the citizens."

For many years he conducted the Cambridge Hospital for Women. At the ninth International Medical Congress in Washington, D. C. in 1887, he presided over the Section on Gynecology. His writings on surgery and gynecology form a long list.

His presidential address at the Detroit meeting in 1892 had the title "Evolution of Medicine," and was largely concerned with the evolutionary development of the Association—its relation to the profession, to state societies—the importance of section work and again the need of a national department of health. The entire address was phrased in graceful diction, at times rising to eloquence as in the closing words: "In the ever changing kaleidoscopic pattern, the individual factors of man's personality should intertwine and blend as the colors in perfect symmetry and relationship. To you and me at least it is given to render in no uncertain tone, the fiat of God's own law, unchangeable, repeated from age to age, generation to generation. To us it is given to contribute to the great tripod of human existence, the mental, the moral, and the physical nature of man, upon the harmonic action of which must ever rest the destinies of the human race."

His interest in the affairs of the Association continued until his death in Boston January 1, 1924 at the age of eighty-seven years.

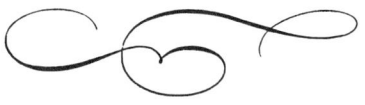

HUNTER HOLMES McGUIRE, M.D.
Richmond, Va.
1835–1900

Forty-fifth President, A. M. A.
Milwaukee Session
June 6, 7, 8, 9, 1893

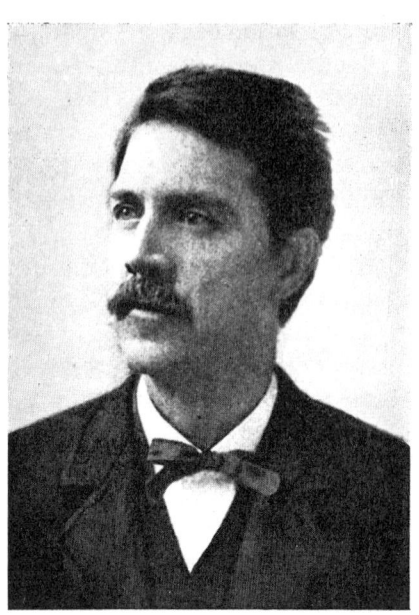

DR. HUNTER H. MCGUIRE of Richmond, Virginia, was one of the last medical officers of the Confederate Army to be chosen president of the Association.* His father Dr. Hugh Holmes McGuire (1801–73) was a charter member of the Association, founder of Winchester, Virginia, Medical College, and also a prominent surgeon of Virginia.

Dr. Hunter H. McGuire was born in Winchester, Virginia, October 11, 1835, in the house which was built by Lord Fairfax when he first came into possession of his Virginia property. When seventeen years of age he matriculated in the Winchester Medical College, which he attended for two years and graduated with the degree Doctor of Medicine in 1855. Soon afterwards he was elected professor of anatomy, teaching two years and practicing with his father. He then decided to go to Philadelphia for further training and entered Jefferson Medical College.

A large proportion of the students of Jefferson Medical College and the University of Pennsylvania were southern men, and sectional feeling flared up when John Brown's body was paraded through Philadelphia in 1859 resulting in frequent riots between students. In December 1859 three hundred medical students led by

---

* Former presidents who served in the Medical Corps of the Confederacy were Paul F. Eve, 1857; W. O. Baldwin, 1869; D. W. Yandell, 1872; W. K. Bowling, 1875; T. G. Richardson, 1878; H. F. Campbell, 1885; A. Y. P. Garnett, 1888, and John A. Wyeth, 1902, who served as a private soldier.

Doctors Luckett and McGuire left Philadelphia in a body and started south. One hundred and forty students matriculated at the Medical College of Virginia, Richmond, fifty-six of whom graduated the following March. Other students went to Atlanta and schools farther south. Doctor McGuire matriculated in the Medical College of Virginia along with the students from Philadelphia and received for the second time the degree Doctor of Medicine at the completion of the session in 1860.

Soon after Virginia seceded he was commissioned in the medical department of the Confederate Army and appointed medical director of the Army of the Shenandoah under General Thomas J. (Stonewall) Jackson. He was Jackson's constant companion in camp and on the march in all his campaigns. When his Chief was mortally wounded at Chancellorsville, Dr. McGuire amputated his right arm and was his constant attendant to the end. Dr. McGuire once said "The noblest heritage I shall hand down to my children is the fact that Stonewall Jackson condescended to hold me and to treat me as his friend." Later Doctor McGuire became Medical Director of the Second Confederate Army Corps, and was with General Robert E. Lee when he surrendered in April 1865. He returned to Richmond and began the practice of medicine. While Doctor McGuire's chief interests and ambitions were along surgical lines, the largest part of his time dur- the first two decades was given to general medical practice, and at one time he had the largest practice in Richmond.

In 1865 he was elected Professor of Surgery in the Medical College of Virginia, continuing in this position until 1878 when he resigned and was named emeritus professor. He however missed the opportunity of contact with medical students, and when in 1892 a new medical school was proposed he readily agreed to take part in the movement.

The following year the University College of Medicine was founded under his leadership. It instituted a three year graded course in medicine, with departments of dentistry and pharmacy. Doctor McGuire was professor of surgery and occupied this position until his death seven years later.

In 1913 the University College of Medicine and the Medical College of Virginia consolidated under the charter of the last named institution, largely through the efforts of Dr. Hunter McGuire's son, Dr. Stuart McGuire, one of the leading surgeons of Richmond.

Dr. Hunter McGuire was one of the first surgeons of his day to accept the germ theory and to adopt the methods of listerism. He was a frequent contributor to surgical literature, particularly in the field of genito-urinary surgery.

In the first American edition of Holmes' "System of Surgery, 1882" he contributed the chapter on gun-shot wounds; to John Ashburst's International Encyclopedia of Surgery 1882, the chapter on contusion, and 1895 the chapter on diseases of the bladder and prostate, and to William Pepper's System of Medicine in 1885, the chapter on intestinal obstruction. He was a charter member of the American Surgical Association, and its president in 1887; president of the Southern Surgical and Gynecological Association in 1889; an associate Fellow of the Philadelphia College of Physicians, honorary fellow of the D. Hayes Agnew Medical Society, and of the Obstetrical Society of Philadelphia. In 1887 the University of North Carolina, and in 1888 the Jefferson Medical College of Philadelphia, each conferred on him the honorary degree of Doctor of Laws.

Death came to Dr. Hunter H. McGuire September 19, 1900 in his sixty-fifth year. Among the honorary pallbearers at the funeral services was Dr. William Osler of Baltimore. An editorial appearing in the Richmond News contained this tribute: "It is difficult to convey by mere description a just picture of Dr. McGuire's remarkable personality. None more striking has been known to this generation of Virginians. Few men have been seen in these parts whose opinions, professional or other, carried as much weight. It may be doubted whether anybody has lived in Virginia since Lee and Jackson died, who was loved by more people."

On January 7, 1904 a bronze statue of Hunter McGuire was unveiled in the historic Capitol Square of Richmond, near the memorial statues of Washington, Lee, Jackson, Henry Clay, and other eminent sons of Virginia, the only physician in the group.

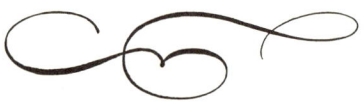

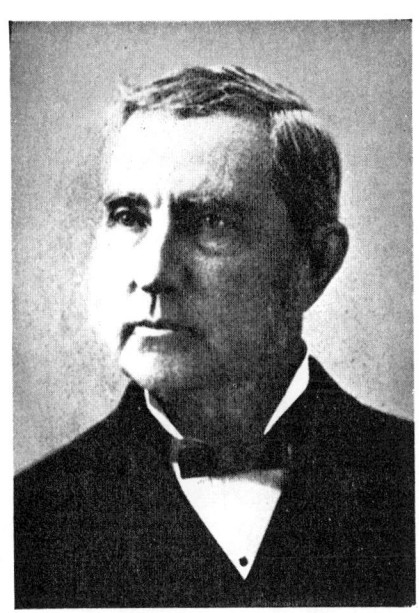

JAMES FARQUHAR HIBBERD, M.D.
Richmond, Indiana.
1816–1903

Forty-sixth President, A. M. A.
San Francisco Session
June 5, 6, 7, 8, 1894

THE HONOR OF THE PRESIDENCY came to Dr. James F. Hibberd towards the close of a long and successful career in the practice of medicine. As one of the original "forty-niners" of California it seemed most fitting that he should preside at the San Francisco meeting of the Association.

Dr. Hibberd was born in Monrovia, Frederick County, Maryland, November 4, 1816 of English-Quaker ancestry. From his tenth to his twentieth year he lived with an uncle in Berkeley County, Virginia, working on a farm and in a woolen mill, yet able to complete a course of study in the Hallowell Classical School at Alexandria, Virginia.

He entered Yale University Medical School in 1838, and after completing two years of study at this institution, he began the practice of medicine in Salem, Ohio, continuing in this location until 1847. Responding to the urge for further medical training he entered the College of Physicians and Surgeons of Columbia University, and graduated with the degree Doctor of Medicine in 1849. Soon afterwards he was appointed surgeon on the S.S.Senator and after a seven and a half months voyage around Cape Horn, he came to California, caught the "gold fever" and was voted a "forty-niner." He practiced in San Francisco until 1855, successively combining with it several commercial enterprises; it being said of him, "that he showed great executive ability and skill not too common among the fraternity." After leaving California in 1855, he returned again to New York City for a short course of graduate study, and then located in Dayton, Ohio, where he remained until June 1856, when he moved to Richmond, Indiana, which became his permanent home. Here he soon acquired a large and lucrative practice. For one year, 1860–61, he was professor of physiology and general pathology at the Ohio Medical College, Cincinnati. In 1862 he published an interesting monograph on "Inflammation as seen by the light of cellular pathology."

Early in his career he was one of the founders of the Ohio State Medical Society and later was one of the chief organizers of Indiana State Medical Society. In 1863 he became a member of the American Medical Association and served as first Vice-President in 1865. He was a member of the American Public Health Association for twenty years after its organization in 1872. During the years 1845–46–47 he was a member of the Ohio legislature.

In 1869 he was absent for one year visiting Europe, Asia Minor, Palestine and Egypt, and also attended, as a delegate, the International Medical Congress in Florence. In 1875 and 1876 he served as Mayor of Richmond, Indiana, and its health officer in 1881. The University of Indiana conferred on him the degree Doctor of Laws in 1885.

Dr. Hibberd was an extensive writer, some of his important publications being "The Anatomy and Surgical Treatment of Hernia"; "The Peritoneum, its Anatomy and Surgical Treatment"; and the "Semi-Centennial of the Introduction of Antiseptic Surgery in America."

His presidential address in 1894 was a mature and scholarly presentation of problems confronting the Association; he made a strong plea for better support by Congress, and a permanent home for the Surgeon General's Library; the establishment of a National Bureau of Public Health; wider application of vaccination for smallpox, and finally a revision of the constitution to provide better representation of constituent State societies.

Dr. Hibberd died at home in Richmond, Indiana, September 8, 1903, at the age of eighty-seven years.

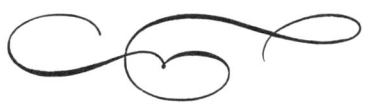

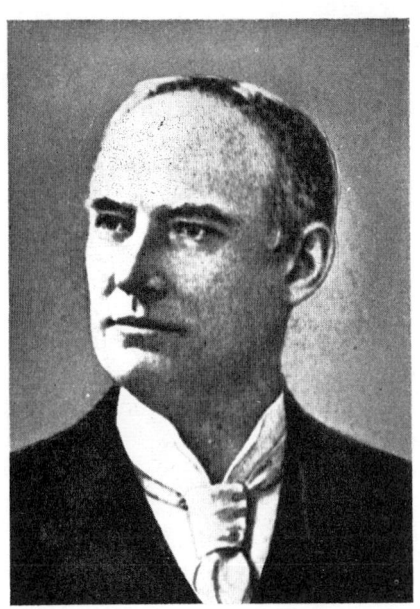

DONALD MacLEAN, M.D.
Detroit, Mich.
1839–1903

*Forty-seventh President, A. M. A.
Baltimore Session
May 7, 8, 9, 10, 1895*

DR. DONALD MACLEAN, the distinguished mid-west surgeon and teacher, was of Canadian birth, having been born in Seymour, Ontario, December 4, 1839. At six years of age he was sent to the famous Oliphant's school for boys in Edinburgh. After six years he returned to Canada and attended schools at Coburg and Belleville, entering at sixteen years the academic department of Queens University, Kingston, Ontario. After obtaining his academic degree he taught for a year in a country district school, and in 1858 he returned to Scotland for the study of medicine at the University of Edinburgh. Here he lived in the old homestead, 21 Albany Street, which had been occupied by the MacLeans for over two hundred years. During his medical course he devoted special attention to pathology and anatomy as a foundation for surgery. In 1862 he graduated from the University of Edinburgh with the degrees M.B., C.M. and Lic. R.C.S. Edin. He was appointed House Surgeon at the famous Royal Infirmary and assistant to Professor James Syme, to whose inspiring influence he attributed much of his later success.

Soon after his return to Canada in 1863, he was appointed Assistant Surgeon of the U. S. Army and served for one year in General

Army hospitals in St. Louis, Louisville and Harrisburg, Pennsylvania.

In 1864 he was appointed professor of clinical surgery at the Royal College of Physicians and Surgeons, Kingston, Ontario. He soon acquired a large practice and while still a young man gained an enviable reputation as a teacher and writer. In 1866 at the request of Professor James Syme, the eminent Scottish surgeon, he edited the American edition of Syme's Surgery.

In 1872 when 33 years of age, he received the appointment of professor of surgery in the College of Medicine, University of Michigan, which opened up special opportunities for his professional talents. He soon gained the highest recognition as a teacher of clinical surgery and a bold and skillful operator.

After seventeen years of teaching at Ann Arbor, he resigned because of differences with the Medical Faculty in advocating the moving of the two clinical years to Detroit. He decided to locate in Detroit, where he soon acquired a large consulting and surgical practice.

He became Surgeon-in-chief of the Michigan Central and Grand Trunk Railway systems. In 1884 he served as President of the Michigan State Medical Society, and in 1887 as President of the Detroit Library Association. He was an honorary F.R.C.S. of England; also an honorary member of the New York and Ohio State Medical societies, as well as the British Medical Association. In 1893, Queens University conferred on him the honorary degree of LL.D.

In his presidential address at Baltimore in 1895, he presented the theme "A few living issues affecting the history of medicine and what came of them" as they concerned matters medical, philosophical and humanitarian. From his own professional cognizance of forty years, he referred to the influence of Syme, Simpson and Playfair—great masters of his student days; he spoke of the far-reaching conception of Darwinism and how it had forcibly and permanently affected every department of medical thought. He referred further to "the striking evolution in the theory and practice of medicine through the abandonment of bloodletting and all concomitant so-called antiphlogistic expedients on which the profession had so confidently and comfortably anchored its faith from time immemorial, and resultant therapeutic reformation."

Through the epoch-making discoveries of Pasteur, Tyndall and Lister on the germ theory of disease and different problems of immunity, eminent authorities in medicine, themselves, were passing through a radical and complete change of belief and practice. He spoke his conviction that the remarkable evolution in medical education was due to the efforts of the Association in that field of activity. In closing he repeated the plea for the establishment of a National Bureau of Health.

Such was the spirit of the true Highlander that graced the office of President, a man of warm friendships and relentless hatred; who opposed everything that savored of charlatanism, quackery, and professional advertising. The human side of Dr. MacLean was strong and he thoroughly enjoyed the social amenities of everyday life; by anecdote and speech he lent charm to the banquet table, rarely equalled. He died in Detroit July 23, 1903, from gastro-enteritis at the age of sixty-three years.

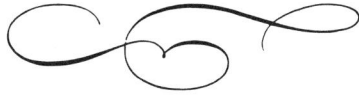

RICHARD BEVERLY COLE, M.D.
San Francisco, Cal.
1829–1901

Forty-eighth President, A. M. A.
Atlanta Session
May 5, 6, 7, 8, 1896

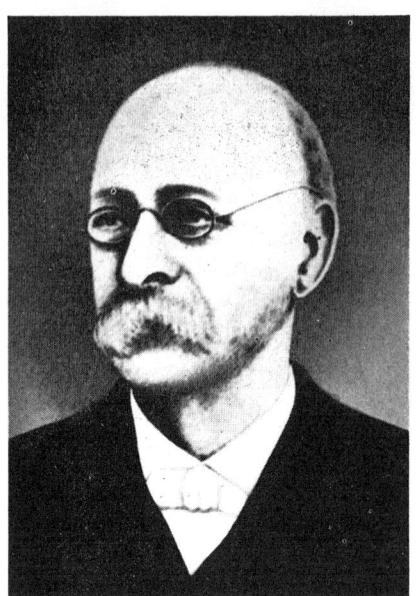

DR. RICHARD B. COLE, one of the pioneers of medical education in California, was born in Manchester, Virginia, August 12, 1829, his parents soon afterwards moving to Philadelphia where he received his literary education. He graduated from Jefferson Medical College in 1849 before his twentieth year, studying later in France, Germany and England.

He was married in Philadelphia and practiced there for one year, when the gold fields of California attracted him westward. He reached San Francisco via Cape Horn in 1851, and immediately opened his office for practice.

He had an adventurous young life, being named Surgeon General of the celebrated Vigilants Committee in 1852, when only 23 years of age. In 1858 he was appointed professor of obstetrics and gynecology in the University of the Pacific, beginning an unbroken career of 43 years of successful medical teaching. In 1866 he assumed the same chair in the Faculty of Toland Medical College which in 1873 became the Medical Department of the University of California, where he continued until his death in 1901.

His practice was limited to surgical gynecology, and he gained his greatest recognition in that field. He was a member of the Royal College of Surgeons of England; Fellow of the Obstetrical Society of London and the British Gynecological Society. He also served as president of the American Association of Obstetricians and Gynecologists.

Dr. Cole was a member of the California State Board of Health and one of the principal promotors of the City and County Hospital of San Francisco.

In his presidential address in 1896 he reviewed the progress of medical education and strongly urged greater uniformity of registration for practice and reciprocal licensure without examination between states, Canada and the United States, as well as between Great Britain, Germany, France and this country.

Death came to this leader of medicine on the Pacific Coast on January 17, 1901 at the age of seventy-two years.

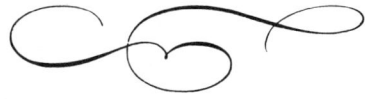

NICHOLAS SENN, M.D.
Chicago
1844-1908

*Forty-ninth President, A. M. A
Philadelphia Session
June 1, 2, 3, 4, 1897*

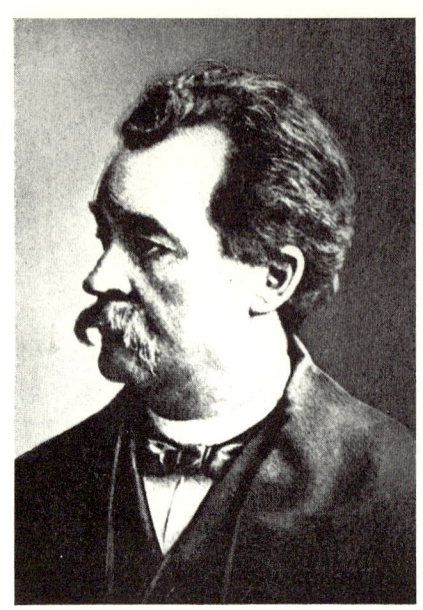

DR. NICHOLAS SENN will always be regarded as an important landmark in American surgery; his work in experimental surgery and surgical pathology distinctly influenced the surgery of his time. In another sense he was a Samuel D. Gross *redivivus*.

He was born in Buchs, Canton St. Gall, Switzerland, October 31, 1844, and emigrated with his parents to the United States in 1852 coming to Fond du Lac, Wisconsin. Here he received a grammar school education and after teaching two years began to read medicine in the office of Dr. Funk, and at the same time studied the local flora of that area. In 1866 he entered Chicago Medical College (later Northwestern University Medical School) graduating with the degree of M.D. in 1868, receiving the first prize for his thesis on "Modus Operandi of Digitalis Purpura."

Following graduation in medicine, he served eighteen months as resident physician in Cook County Hospital, Chicago, and then began the practice of medicine in Ashland, Wisconsin. In 1874 he moved to Milwaukee where he was appointed attending physician of the Milwaukee Hospital.

In 1877 he went to Germany for further study, entering the University of Munich where he became the special student of Professor von Nussbaum, and received the degree Doctor of Medicine, *cum laude*, in 1878. After two more years of special work on surgical pathology and clinical surgery, he returned to the United States in 1880. He was then 36 years of age. Soon after his return to Milwaukee he was appointed professor of surgery at the College of Physicians and Surgeons, Chicago, and in 1884 the title was changed to professor of principles and practice of surgery. During this time he continued his residence in Milwaukee, and two days of each week travelled the 88 miles to Chicago. His lectures were very popular because of their masterly presentation, illuminated by his wide knowledge of surgical history, pathology and surgical principles. He cultivated pathology diligently and brought it into living touch with his surgery. In 1887 he received the degree Doctor of Philosophy from the University of Wisconsin.

In 1888 he was elected professor of surgery and surgical pathology in Rush Medical College, and in 1891 succeeded Dr. Charles T. Parkes as head of the department of surgery. This was regarded at the time as the most important surgical appointment in the midwest.

From the beginning of his professional career he had an unusual and remarkable interest in experimental investigation. This had its beginning in a laboratory constructed under a sidewalk by his Milwaukee home, where night after night he carried on his original investigations. He always maintained that proficiency in abdominal surgery could only be acquired by operating on living tissues.

It was during the decade 1880–1890 that he made his most important contributions to abdominal surgery. He developed the use of hydrogen gas to test intactness of the digestive tract after gunshot wounds of the abdomen. His experiments on the pancreas demonstrated the feasibility of surgical interference in a number of well defined lesions. It became customary during this period to refer to Dr. Senn as the "great master of abdominal surgery."

In 1889 after returning from Europe where he had an opportunity to study bacteriology in its relation to surgery, he published an admirable book on "Surgical bacteriology" which passed through several editions. A year later appeared his textbook on the Principles of Surgery, which was the first work of its kind published in English; previous American surgical books had been devoted largely to the practical side of surgery, neglecting the underlying principles.

The amphitheatre clinics of Dr. Senn became one of the attractions of medical Chicago. He was eminently a teacher of the arena, and was never so happy as when standing in the large upper amphitheatre at Rush Medical College, with a seating capacity of 400, as a rule crowded with students and visitors. Beginning promptly at two o'clock, the first two hours were devoted to showing gross and microscopic specimens from cases in which operations had been done at previous clinics. Great stress was placed on a thorough knowledge of surgical pathology and bacteriology; this would be followed by the presentation of patients in the hospital and dispensary, making a careful examination and diagnosis of each, after which the treatment indicated was discussed. In these clinical conferences he introduced the German custom of calling down students to take part. At four o'clock he would begin operating, usually on a long list of patients, which would continue until six o'clock, and occasionally an hour later, the majority of the students and visitors remaining until the close.

Dr. Senn was very positive in his statements particularly as regards diagnosis and therapy; therein probably was the evidence of his strength as a great surgical teacher—by being definite, clear and emphatic, he was of greatest service to students.

The statement was made by Lord Moynihan, who was probably more familiar than any other British surgeon with surgeons in this country, that "the two greatest teachers of surgery were Nicholas Senn and John B. Murphy."

Dr. Senn was very familiar with medical history and had met personally many of the prominent surgeons of his period. He was probably the most travelled medical man in this or any other country. In 1887 he spent four months visiting important English, Scottish, and European clinics, which he described in an interesting series of letters to his friend and colleague, Dr. Christian Fenger, which were later published under the title "Four Months Among the Surgeons of Europe."

He had an extraordinary capacity for work, and stood sponsor for 23 published books and 316 articles, every word being written by his own hand and with his pen. We quote from the words of a colleague, Dr. Wm. E. Quine—"He was of heroic mold"—"The pomp and formalism of military parade fascinated him," and "the insignia of military rank allured, charmed and enthralled him."

In his presidential address at the Philadelphia session in June 1897 he spoke on the subject "The American Medical Association past, present and future," and gave further evidence of his wide knowledge of its history and development during the first fifty years; he predicted that "our country will become the center of medical education in 25 years." In the same prophetic spirit he added "when the first centennial celebration will be held in this city (Philadelphia) fifty years from now, the membership will have increased from 9000 to 75,000 or 100,000 members, and our official organ will be recognized the world over as the most enterprising and best medical journal. The President who will then occupy the Chair will review the work of the Association for the first century and may we trust, from the records we shall leave behind, he may judge us faithful servants in the cause of science and humanity," "taking up history from this day, he will chronicle inventions and discoveries of which we now have no conception," and "the literature of today will be as old and useless as that of fifty years ago."

As evidence of a noble generosity he left the "Senn Collection" of 40,000 books, and 60,000 pamphlets as a nucleus of a great medical reference library now forming part of the John Crerar scientific library.

He presented Rush Medical College with the Senn Clinical Building, and endowed the Senn Professorship of Surgery, and Senn Fellowship in Surgery, at the same institution.

The city of Chicago remembered him by naming one of the largest high schools the "Nicholas Senn High School."

Death came to him on January 2, 1908. Of the many tributes spoken at the memorial services, perhaps the one by his surgical colleague, John B. Murphy, is most expressive: "He did not found a personal school, but he created a diffuse and general scientific professional sentiment that permeated the western hemisphere."

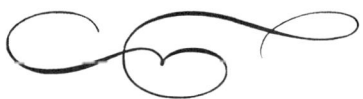

GEORGE MILLER STERNBERG, M.D
Washington, D.C.
1838–1915

*Fiftieth President, A. M. A.
Denver Session
June 7, 8, 9, 10, 1898*

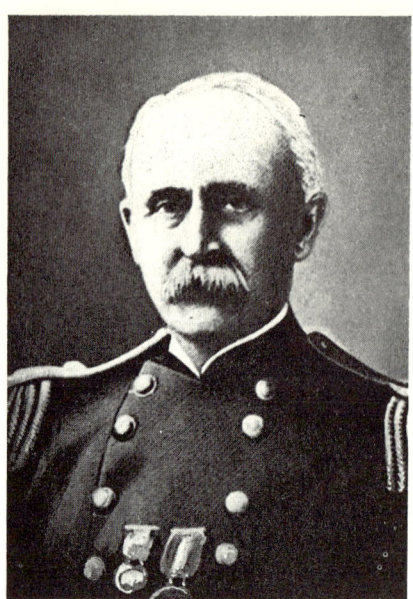

DR. GEORGE M. STERNBERG, America's pioneer bacteriologist and accomplished sanitary expert, was the first Surgeon General of the United States Army to be elected to the presidency of the Association. Because of his duties as Surgeon General and the Spanish-American War, he was unable to attend and preside at the Denver session.

He was born in Hartwick, Otsego County, New York, June 8, 1838, the son of a Lutheran clergyman, and received his preliminary education in Hartwick Seminary. He began teaching at sixteen years, and was able to begin the study of medicine under a local physician, after which he matriculated at the College of Physicians and Surgeons, Columbia University, graduating with the degree Doctor of Medicine in 1860.

He practiced at Elizabeth City, New Jersey, until the outbreak of the Civil War, when he was appointed Assistant Surgeon in the U. S. Army, and continued with the medical corps throughout the remainder of his career. He participated in a number of engagements of the Civil War, being taken prisoner at the first battle of Bull Run and later escaped. He was active in the Indian Campaigns that followed and while stationed at Fort Harken, Kansas, from 1867 to

1871 he had his first experience with a yellow fever epidemic, and later at Barrancas, Florida, where in 1873 he contracted the disease himself. His interest and careful studies led to his being named a member of the Havana Yellow Fever Commission in 1879. While in Cuba, he became intimate with Dr. Carlos Finlay who at that time was fully convinced that yellow fever was propagated by the Stegomyia mosquito. Dr. Sternberg soon began to be recognized for his pioneer work in bacteriology. In 1880, he demonstrated a micrococcus in saliva to which he gave the name Pasteurii, and which when introduced into animals produced a fatal septicemia. Later it was discovered that Sternberg's micrococcus of sputum septicemia was the same as the capsulated micrococcus of rusty sputum in pneumonia discovered by Fraenkel and Weichselbaum.

Later in the same year that Robert Koch discovered the tubercle bacillus, 1882, Dr. Sternberg demonstrated the bacillus with microphotographs for the first time in this country. In April 1884 he was assigned to Baltimore in Newell Martin's laboratory at Johns Hopkins University. Here the culture media and cultures were prepared by his wife, who was his sympathetic co-worker in all his scientific investigations. In 1885 he demonstrated the living motile plasmodium of malaria, discovered by Laveran, five years before. In 1886 he introduced the bacillus of typhoid fever (Eberth) to the profession in a paper before the Association of American Physicians. Also in 1886 he completed his prize work on scientific disinfection, of which it was said—"No one unless familiar with bacteriologic work can have the slightest conception of the magnitude and painstaking labors involved in determining the 'thermal death point' of pathogenic organisms and germicidal value of certain chemical and physical agents." This work was undertaken as chairman of a special committee of the American Public Health Association, and his comprehensive report no doubt led to his election as president of this Association the following year.

In 1890 appeared his work on the etiology and prevention of yellow fever, which was a complete exposition of the knowledge of this disease to that date. His Treatise on Immunity, Protective Inoculation, and Infectious Diseases was published in 1895; the same year appeared the first edition of "Manual of Bacteriology" which became a textbook in 1902, and a valuable guide and work of reference for the early teachers of bacteriology.

While stationed in New York City as consulting bacteriologist in 1893, he received his appointment as Surgeon General of the U. S. Army, marking a new epoch in his distinguished career. During his ten years of service the Army Medical School was founded, and the

Dental Corps and Female Nursing Corps were organized. In the Spanish-American War the entire Medical Corps was under his supervision, the crowning glory of his administration being the organization of the Yellow Fever Commission under the chairmanship of Dr. Walter Reed, in 1900.

The University of Michigan conferred on Dr. Sternberg the degree Doctor of Laws in 1894, and Brown University the same in 1897. In 1905 he was appointed Professor of Preventive Medicine at the George Washington University Medical School. During the International Congress on Tuberculosis in Washington in 1908, Dr. and Mrs. Sternberg were hosts to Professor and Mrs. Robert Koch of Berlin.

Dr. Sternberg was a versatile scholar, acquiring a knowledge of French at forty years, and of the German language at fifty-two years of age. He was a lover of music and a student of botany and archeology.

Death came to him on November 3, 1915 in Washington, D. C. at the age of seventy-seven years.

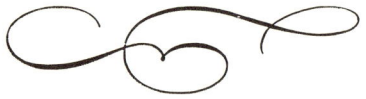

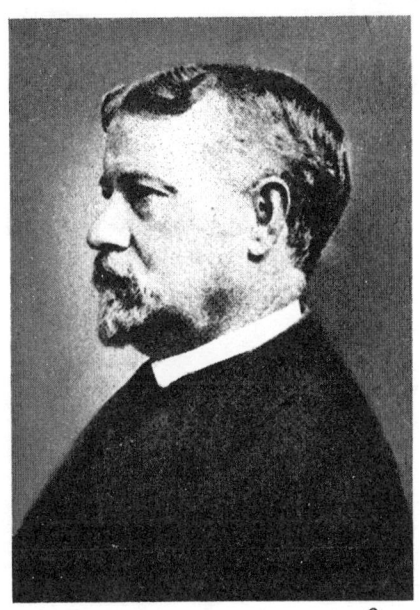

JOSEPH M. MATHEWS, M.D.
Louisville, Ky.
1847–1928

Fifty-first President, A. M. A.
Columbus Session
June 6, 7, 8, 9, 1899

DR. JOSEPH MCDOWELL MATHEWS was a descendant of illustrious ancestry—including Dr. Ephraim McDowell, renowned pioneer abdominal surgeon, and General Joseph McDowell, his great grandfather, a general in the Revolutionary War.

He was born in Henry County, Kentucky, May 29, 1847. His early education was obtained in the public schools of the town of New Castle, and he graduated in medicine at the University of Louisville in 1867 at twenty years of age. After practicing for several years in his native town he returned to Louisville where he continued in general practice until 1877. He then decided to pursue further graduate studies in London where he became interested in the specialty of proctology, which he practiced exclusively in Louisville from 1878 to 1912.

Dr. Mathews was the first physician in this country to limit his practice to the treatment of affections of the terminal bowel. He soon became recognized as an attractive public speaker and excellent teacher and surgeon.

In 1880 he was appointed professor of surgery in the Kentucky School of Medicine, and in 1883 when the Department of Proctology was established, he was chosen as the head of the same. This was the first instance of the kind in this country. In 1887 he delivered the general address in surgery at the annual session of the American

Medical Association. At the session of the Association in 1888 he presented his "Observations on 1000 cases of Hemorrhoids." His "Treatise on Diseases of the Rectum, Anus and Sigmoid Flexure" appeared in 1890 and passed through three editions.

Dr. Mathews organized the American Proctological Society in 1899 and is sometimes referred to as the Father of proctology.

In 1898 he was appointed president of the Kentucky State Board of Health and during a service of ten years initiated many important reforms. He served as president of the Kentucky State Medical Society from 1898 to 1899. For a period of six years he was a member of the Board of Trustees of the American Medical Association.

In 1912 after a trip around the world he retired from practice and moved to Los Angeles, where he continued to reside, except for four years in Seattle, until his death on December 21, 1928, at eighty-one years of age.

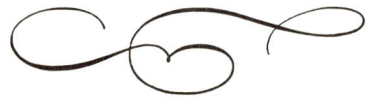

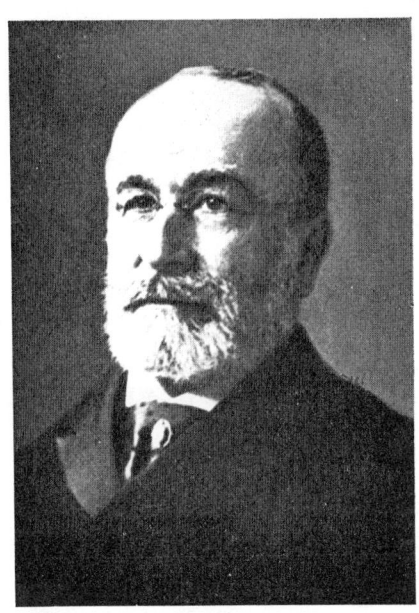

WILLIAM WILSON KEEN, M.D.
Philadelphia
1837–1932

Fifty-second President, A. M. A.
Atlantic City Session
June 5, 6, 7, 8, 1900

DR. WILLIAM W. KEEN was the Dean of American Surgery, of whom any brief record of his accomplishments can only indicate the breadth of his interests and activities during a life span of ninety-five years. Although fragile in frame and diminutive in stature, his intellect coupled with an extraordinary capacity for hard work made him known the world over.

Dr. Keen was born in Philadelphia January 19, 1837. His Swedish ancestor was Joren Kyn (George Keen) who left Sweden 23 years after the Mayflower and settled in New Sweden on the Delaware river. He graduated from Brown University in 1859 and entered Jefferson Medical College in October 1860. It was a time when antisepsis and asepsis were unknown, and bacteriology as Dr. Keen expressed it "was utterly unsuspected." He was fortunate to become a private office student of Drs. Jacob M. DaCosta and John K. Brinton, the former being the ablest clinical teacher of his time; otherwise he would have had no opportunity to percuss or auscult a chest or even look through a microscope.

Dr. Brinton taught him surgery during the first year of medical study and urged him in July 1861 to accept an appointment as Assistant Surgeon of the Fifth Massachusetts Regiment; two weeks later he had his first experience in active warfare in the Battle of Bull Run, and took care of a great many war casualties. He returned to his medical studies in time for the fall term and graduated with

[679]

the degree Doctor of Medicine in March 1862. Soon after graduation he was commissioned Assistant Surgeon U. S. Army, and assigned to duty in U. S. Hospital No. 1 at Frederick, Md., where he assisted his former preceptor Dr. Brinton, in the collection of material for the Surgeon General's Museum, grown since to the finest in the world. In his last year of military service he was stationed at the U. S. Hospital for Nervous Diseases at Turner's Lane, Philadelphia, where he became associated with Dr. S. Weir Mitchell, the leading neurologist at that time. In conjunction with Dr. Mitchell and Dr. George R. Morehouse he published the best known of his earlier works: "Reflex paralysis, Gunshot Wounds, and other Injuries of Nerves," and "Antagonism of Morphia and Atropia." After 1864 he spent two years in Europe rounding out his surgical education. In the laboratory of Professor Rudolf Virchow he received his basic training in pathology which he felt was absolutely essential for rational surgery.

He began practice in Philadelphia in 1866 and soon was appointed to various teaching positions. His first instructorship was in surgical pathology at Jefferson Medical College; at the same time he became the active head of the Philadelphia School of Anatomy, which was a type of extra-mural school giving private instruction to students; he continued this school until 1875 when the buildings were destroyed. During this period Dr. Keen taught nearly 1500 students, five of whom later became professors in medical schools. His practice for a number of years was not burdensome, and he constantly carried on his studies and writing. In 1870 appeared his "Clinical Charts," and "History of Practical Anatomy," and in 1874 the "History of the Philadelphia School of Anatomy" was published. He attended the International Medical Congress in Philadelphia in 1876 and heard Dr. Joseph Lister present his views on wound infection and antiseptic surgery and was fully convinced of their value; he promptly adopted the method at St. Mary's Hospital, and was the first surgeon in Philadelphia to take advantage of Lister's discovery. He was professor of Artistic Anatomy in the Philadelphia Academy of Fine Arts from 1876 to 1889. In 1887 he edited Gray's Anatomy.

As a surgeon he was physiologically minded, and in 1887 he removed the first brain tumor after accurate localization; during his career as an active operating surgeon his contributions to the surgery of the brain, spinal cord and peripheral nerves were recognized as of special merit. In 1893 came the operation on President Grover Cleveland with Dr. Joseph Bryant of New York (carried out with absolute secrecy on board a private yacht in the East River) in which the entire left upper jaw from the first bicuspid to just beyond the last molar was removed, the antrum being filled with a sarcomatous mass; the resulting defect was closed by a cleverly devised rubber plate and the distinguished patient lived for fifteen years thereafter. This story was not known until 1917, when it was published by Dr. Keen.

His monograph published in 1898, "Surgical Complications and Sequelae of Typhoid Fever," attracted wide attention.

In 1905 appeared the first edition of Keen's System of Surgery in 8 volumes, which was repeatedly revised and became an established work of reference for many years.

He served as professor of surgery in the Woman's Medical College from 1884 to 1889, when he was elected professor of surgery in his Alma Mater, Jefferson Medical College, and continued until 1907 when he was named Emeritus professor. He retired also from active practice, being then seventy years of age. He remarked at the time — "No man over 70 has the right to hold human life in his hands."

Even after his retirement from practice and teaching, he continued his historical researches and scientific writings. In 1914 appeared a monograph on Brown University; in 1916 Selected Papers and Addresses, and in 1917 Treatment of War Wounds. The publication in 1914 of his treatise "Animal Experimentation and Medical Progress" was the beginning of his efforts to combat the vicious attacks by anti-vivisectionists; he waged the battle of scientific medicine in this field almost to the hour of his death.

Dr. Keen was honored by numerous organizations in his specialty throughout the world. He was president of the American Surgical Association in 1889; in 1903 he presided at the Congress of Physicians and Surgeons in Washington, and in 1920 at the International Congress of Surgery in Paris. He was elected a corresponding member of the Surgical Societies of France, Belgium and Italy; an Honorary Fellow of the Royal College of Surgeons of England, Edinburgh and Ireland. He was the first surgeon in the United States to accept and have conferred the Honorary Fellowship of the American College of Surgeons.

He was the holder of numerous medals and awards, including Officer, Order of the Crown of Belgium, and Chevalier, Legion of Honor of France. He served as Fellow and Trustee of Brown University from 1873 to 1932. He received honorary degrees from his Alma Mater and the following universities; Northwestern, Toronto, Edinburgh, Yale, St. Andrews, Pennsylvania, Upsala, Harvard and the University of Paris.

Dr. Keen was equally distinguished as a medical officer, physician, teacher, citizen and a socially minded man. He served his country in three wars: Asst. Surgeon U. S. Army 1862–64; Lieutenant M.C.

Spanish-American War 1898-99; and Major M.C., U.S. Army World War I, 1917-18.

His ambition to reach 100 years was thwarted by a failing heart, which made him an invalid the last two years of his life, which he bore with fortitude and maintained his dry humorous attitude throughout.

Dr. Keen appeared the last time before the Association at the Philadelphia session in June 1931, his chair being wheeled on the stage, and he received a great ovation. Death came to him a year later, June 7, 1932, in Philadelphia at the age of ninety-five years.

Many a man who achieves fame and retires from active life at the age of seventy is forgotten until the time when obituaries are transscribed. Invalid though he was, the world continued to talk of Dr. Keen until the moment of his death. His contributions to science and to life are an enduring legacy to medicine and mankind.

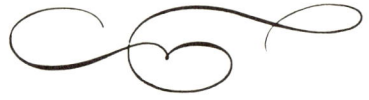

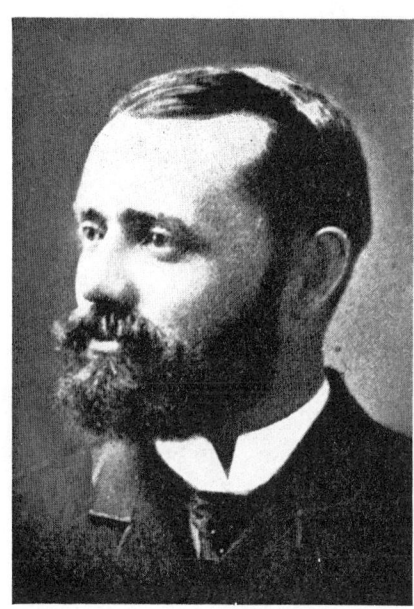

CHARLES ALFRED LEE REED, M.D.
Cincinnati, Ohio
1856–1928

Fifty-third President, A. M. A.
St. Paul Session
June 4, 5, 6, 7, 1901

DR. CHARLES A. L. REED was one of the most interesting and dynamic figures in American medicine. At the time of his election to the presidency he was only forty-four years of age, one of the youngest physicians chosen for that office. He was born in Wolflake, Indiana, July 9, 1856, and received his early education in the public schools of Glendale, and his Arts degree at Miami University, Oxford, Ohio. In 1872 he entered the Cincinnati College of Medicine and Surgery, where his father was professor of materia medica and therapeutics for more than 25 years. He graduated in 1874 with the degree Doctor of Medicine at eighteen years of age. Soon after graduation he began practice in Cincinnati; early in his career he became associated with teaching and organization activities.

He began as a lecturer in pathology and in 1882 was appointed professor of gynecology and abdominal surgery in his Alma Mater. In 1885 he determined to devote his energies to the practice of abdominal and pelvic surgery and with this end in view he became a pupil of the celebrated Lawson Tait of Birmingham, England, remaining about one year. In 1891 he became Director of the University of Cincinnati, when he gave up some of his teaching duties, and devoted all his efforts in merging the then existing medical schools of the city in the College of Medicine, University of Cincinnati. In 1897 he was appointed gynecologist and clinical lecturer on diseases of women of the University Hospital, and in 1902 became professor of clinical gynecology in the medical school, continuing until 1917 when he retired as Emeritus professor.

He early took an active part in the affairs of the American Medical Association, being Chairman of the Section of Obstetrics and Gynecology in 1891, member of the Board of Trustees from 1896 to 1902, and after the House of Delegates was organized in 1901 he served as a member in the sessions of 1902, 1903, 1904 and 1907. As president in 1901 he had a conspicuous part in the reorganization and adoption of the new Constitution and By-Laws of the Association.

The multiplicity of his activities is revealed by his being the founder of the Pan-American Medical Congress of which he was Secretary-General at its first session in Washington, D. C., in 1893, and President at the seventh Congress. He was one of the founders of the American Association of Obstetricians and Gynecologists, and its president in 1898. Because of his thorough knowledge of the French language, he organized the Alliance Francaise of Cincinnati, and was awarded the decoration, Chevalier Legion of Honor of France in 1908. In 1905 he was a member of a special United States Commission to Panama; in connection with this appointment he was a strong supporter of General Gorgas and the Yellow Fever Commission. In 1908 Dr. Reed was a candidate for the U. S. Senate.

His publications covered a wide range of subjects: In 1900 appeared his textbook on Gynecology, and in 1913 his work on Diseases of Women; in the same year he published a monograph on Marriage and Genetics, also a textbook on Diseases of the Stomach and Intestines. In 1919 he published his work on Chronic Convulsive Toxaemias, which reflected his views on epilepsy, which however were not substantiated by other authorities.

In his later years he retired from practice and devoted himself to lecturing and conducting a Health Column in more than a hundred newspapers. He died suddenly from angina pectoris at his summer home in Gloucester, Mass., August 28, 1928 at seventy-two years of age. In his death there passed from the stage one of the most interesting personalities in American medicine.

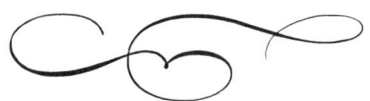

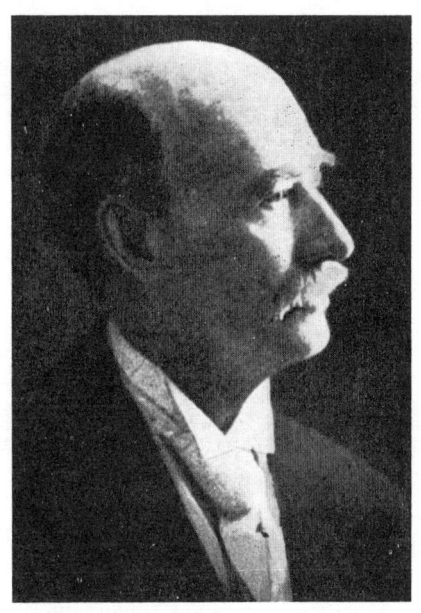

JOHN ALLEN WYETH, M.D.
New York, N. Y.
1845–1922

*Fifty-fourth President, A. M. A.
Saratoga Springs Session
June 10, 11, 12, 13, 1902*

JOHN ALLEN WYETH, distinguished American surgeon, was the last member of the Confederate States Army to be elected to the presidency of the Association.

He was born at Missionary Station, Marshall County, Alabama, May 26, 1845; his early education was obtained in the common schools followed by one year in a military academy. In 1862 at the age of 17 he entered as a private soldier in the 4th Alabama Cavalry, Confederate States Army; fought in each of the engagements at the Battle of Chickamauga, and while following the retreating Federals, was captured and spent fifteen months in the military prison at Camp Morton, Indiana. After peace was declared, he engaged in farming and in 1867 he began the study of medicine under Dr. J. M. Jackson of Gunterville, Ala. He graduated from the University of Louisville Medical School in 1869. He then became a surgeon to a railroad construction company, but after one year gave up the practice of medicine and engaged in various business pursuits from that of pilot on a Mississippi River steamboat to contracting work, and in 1872 erected a public building for the County of Woodruff, Arkansas. He moved to New York in October 1872 and matriculated at Bellevue Hospital Medical College, graduating in March 1873 with the degree Doctor of Medicine—ad eundem. A month later he was appointed assistant demonstrator of anatomy in that institution, and in 1874 prosector to the chair of anatomy, and in 1875 was advanced to instructor. In 1875 he was awarded the Professor James R. Wood $100 prize essay for his work on "the surgical anatomy of the tibia-tarsal articulation with special regard to amputation at the ankle joint"; this was based on consecutive dissections, and published in the American Journal of Medical Sciences April 1876; and he won a prize given by the American Medical Association in 1878 for an essay on "Surgical Anatomy and Surgery of the Great Vessels of the Neck," which was based on 173 dissections of the carotid and subclavian arteries and their branches. Following this initial venture in surgical research, he contributed widely to both lay and medical journals.

Because of ill health he gave up practice and visited Europe from 1876 to 1878. During these two years he studied the plan of postgraduate instruction at the larger medical centers, particularly in Vienna and Berlin, with the thought of establishing a postgraduate school in New York City. In 1880 he became prosector to the chair of anatomy and surgery in Bellevue Hospital Medical College, which position he held until 1897. In 1881 he realized his ambition and organized the first postgraduate medical school in the United States —The New York Polyclinic Medical School and Hospital. Dr. Wyeth became senior professor of surgery and later president of the Faculty. He gathered about him some of the ablest members of the profession, and the school filled a most responsible position in postgraduate training and the development of medical thought under his leadership. William J. Mayo was a postgraduate student here in 1884 and 1885.

In 1886 Dr. Wyeth married Florence Nightingale Sims, daughter of J. Marion Sims, and one of his contributions to medical history was an address on the life and work of his distinguished father-in-law delivered in 1895.

Among his notable papers was an address on medical education in 1890, and at the same time, the description of a method of amputation at hip and shoulder joints. He was the author of Wyeth's textbook on Surgery, the biography of General Forrest—the great cavalry leader of the South—and his own autobiography entitled "With Sabre and Scalpel" published in 1914.

In 1893 he was elected first vice-president of the American Medical Association, and president of the Medical Society of the State of New York in 1900.

The University of Alabama conferred on him the honorary degree of Doctor of Laws in 1900, and in 1908 he received the same honor from the University of Maryland.

During World War I, the postgraduate school was turned over to the Government for hospital purposes, and after the close of the War Dr. Wyeth was especially active in undertaking the reopening of the postgraduate school.

Dr. Wyeth was a man of varied and interesting activities, whose career contains all of the romantic elements, which make up the lives of American medical pioneers. A contemporary wrote of him, "His creed made integrity its cornerstone, and kindness its inspiration."

In his death on May 26, 1922 there passed a conspicuous figure in the development of American medicine.

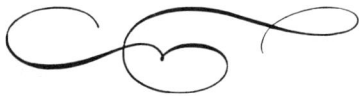

FRANK BILLINGS, M.D.
Chicago, Ill.
1854–1932

Fifty-fifth President, A. M. A.
New Orleans Session
May 5, 6, 7, 8, 1903

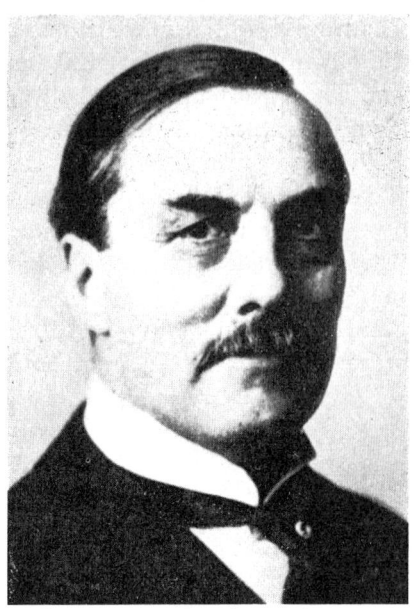

DR. FRANK BILLINGS is best remembered as a leader of medicine in this country during two generations; a builder of medical institutions and organizations and a truly great physician.

He was born on a farm near Highland, Iowa County, Wisconsin, April 2, 1854. His early education was obtained in the public schools and two years attendance at the State Normal School at Plattsville, Wisconsin, after which he taught in the district school and later became the principal of the local high school. In 1878 he matriculated in the Chicago Medical School (later Northwestern University) and graduated with the degree Doctor of Medicine in 1881. In the competitive examinations for the Cook County Hospital internships he was awarded first place. He began the practice of medicine in Chicago, and at once commenced the campaign for better and broader medical education, which he carried on so successfully during his entire life.

From 1882 and in the succeeding twenty years he became associated with Dr. Christian Fenger, and he never failed to acknowledge the influence of this inspiring teacher.

From 1882 to 1885 he served as demonstrator of anatomy in his Alma Mater, and then visited the larger European medical centers for a period of fifteen months. For one of his fine preparation and keen preceptive mind, the opportunities offered for the study of pathology and clinical medicine in these older seats of medical learning must have been most alluring. This period was the so-called "Glanz-periods" of the Vienna school. Upon his return to Chicago late in 1886, he was among the first to demonstrate the special staining technic of the tubercle bacillus before the Chicago Medical Society and the Medical Section of the Association at its meeting in Chicago in June 1887.

From 1886 to 1891 he was professor of physical diagnosis at Northwestern University Medical School, and from 1891 to 1898 professor and head of the department of medicine and dean of the medical school. In 1898 he became associated with Rush Medical College as Professor of Medicine and dean of the school. Soon after this Rush Medical College became affiliated with the University of Chicago, where he served for 25 years as dean and professor of medicine. This medical school affiliation was largely the accomplishment of Dr. Billings through his association with President William Rainey Harper, the builder of this great university of the Middle West. He was further instrumental in the development of Presbyterian Hospital as an educational center, the establishment of the John McCormick Institute for Infectious Diseases, the Durand Hospital, the Otho S. A. Sprague Institute, and later the School for Medical Teaching in the University of Chicago, the Billings Memorial Hospital and the Frank Billings Clinic and Library, as well as the Lasker and Douglas Smith Foundation for Research.

Early in his career he developed an active interest in organized medicine. In 1894 he was elected president of the Chicago Medical Society, then and now the largest county or local medical organization in the world.

At the Columbus meeting of the Association in 1899, Doctor Billings was chosen as Chairman of the Section on the Practice of Medicine; he introduced the abstracts of papers to be presented on the program. In 1902 at the Saratoga Springs (New York session) he delivered the Oration on Medicine. All who were privileged to hear his presidential address on "Medical Education" at the New Orleans session in 1903, recognized that it ushered in a new epoch in American medical education. Dr. Billings advocated a complete reorganization of the four year graded medical curriculum with pre-academic training and one year of approved hospital internship. In proposing these higher standards of medical training he further advocated that the professors in the basic medical sciences be placed on full time, and as soon as possible that the heads of the clinical departments be filled by professors on full time. These recommendations led to the establishment of the Council on Medical Education, which distinctly influenced an evolution in American medical education that was the marvel of the educational world. His term as president was followed by many years of intensive service to the Association. In all this work he closely cooperated with Dr. George H. Simmons, the General Secretary of the Association for a quarter of a century.

In 1903 and 1904 he was a member of the Council on Medical Education; in 1905 he served on the Council on Pharmacy and Chemistry. From 1904 to 1911 he was Treasurer of the Association, and from 1918 to 1924 a member of the Board of Trustees. During this period he served as Secretary of the Board.

In 1927 at the Washington meeting, the Section on Practice of Medicine established a special lectureship, which a year later was named the Frank Billings Lecture in recognition of his eminence in American medicine. The first lecture was presented at the Detroit session in 1930, at which Dr. Billings was present, by Dr. Joseph L. Miller, a former student and assistant.

He was president of the American Association of Physicians in 1906, and in 1907 served as president of the Association for the Study and Prevention of Tuberculosis.

Dr. Billings was instrumental in organizing the Chicago Pathological Society and the Chicago Neurological Society, the Society of Internal Medicine, and the Institutes of Medicine of Chicago. He also established the Ludvig Hektoen and Lewis L. McArthur Lectureships.

He entered World War I as a Major in the Medical Corps of the U. S. Army, having been a First Lieutenant in the Reserve Corps since 1908. In 1917 he served as chairman of a Red Cross Commission to Russia. He was also medical advisor to the Provost Marshal General in establishing the plan of examinations for the draft boards of the United States. At the close of the war he was Chief of the Division of Reconstruction in the Surgeon General's office. He was awarded the Distinguished Service Medal, the Order of Leopold of Belgium and Officer Legion of Honor of France. In 1921 he was advanced to Brigadier General in the National Army of the United States.

Doctor Billings constantly encouraged medical investigation on the part of his pupils and assistants. His studies and clinical observations on spinal cord changes in pernicious anemia, on infectious endocarditis and focal infection, were classic contributions to medical knowledge. Of these the most outstanding is the modern concept of focal infection as related to chronic systemic disease, first presented in 1912.

This constant correlation of experimental investigations with careful clinical observations, advocated by Dr. Billings, distinctly influenced diagnostic procedure for both the medical and the surgical specialist as well as the general practitioner.

He was an inspiration alike to students, interns and young practitioners. At the time of his death in 1932, it was estimated that fully one hundred of the leading medical teachers and clinicians throughout the country bore the stamp of his stimulating personality. During the first World War, six of his former assistants were chief medical officers at the different military cantonments.

The life and service of Frank Billings was perhaps best exemplified by his host of medical disciples sent forth to careers of leadership and the fuller appreciation of those higher professional attributes involved in careful diagnostic conclusions and more complete treatment of patients. He was a big genial sympathetic nature, full of humor and human kindliness, who radiated power in every sphere of human activity.

Death came to him on September 20, 1932, as the result of severe gastric hemorrhage, at seventy-eight years of age.

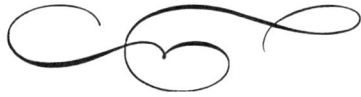

JOHN HERR MUSSER, M.D.
Philadelphia, Pa.
1856–1912

*Fifty-sixth President, A. M. A.
Atlantic City Session
June 7, 8, 9, 10, 1904*

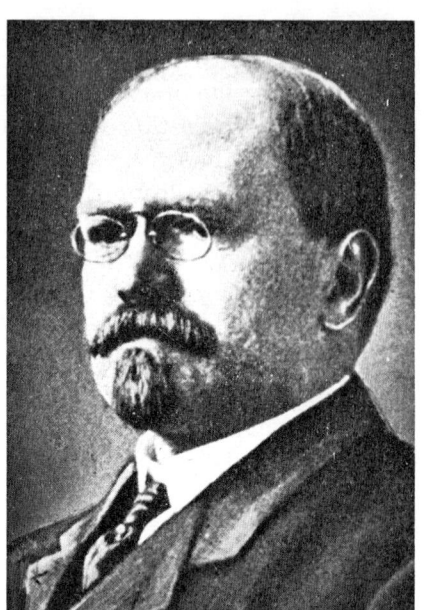

DR. JOHN H. MUSSER of Philadelphia was an eminent internist, a leading consultant in a great metropolis, prominent educator and a pioneer in medical social service. He was born in Strassburg, Penna., June 22, 1856, the son of Dr. Benjamin and Naomi Herr Musser. He came of a line of physicians, his grandfather being Dr. Martin Musser, and great grandfather Dr. Benjamin Musser.

His early education was received at the Strassburg (Pa.) high school and the Millersville State Normal School. He graduated in medicine from the University of Pennsylvania in 1877; after completing an internship at Old Blockley (Philadelphia) Hospital, he began to practice in Philadelphia and soon acquired a very large general practice.

After a few years he became associated with his uncle, Dr. Milton B. Musser, in West Philadelphia, and on his death succeeded to his extensive practice.

The first fifteen years of Dr. Musser's professional life were spent in general practice, after which he devoted his time to internal medicine and consultations.

Dr. Musser was one of a group of able young men that Dr. William Pepper (professor of medicine and provost of the University of Pennsylvania) gathered around him; a group that he taught in his own line of teaching, making them consummate diagnosticians and clinicians of unusual ability.

Doctor Musser early began his medical teaching in his Alma Mater; first as a quiz-master, later as demonstrator and associate professor, and finally as professor of clinical medicine. He was also director of the Department of Research Medicine in the University. He held many pos tions in connection with hospitals, among them those of pathologist of the Presbyterian Hospital; physician to the Philadelphia General, University, and Presbyterian Hospitals; consulting physician to the Jewish Hospital, West Philadelphia, and Mercy Hospital in Springfield, Mass.

In his hospital work, Dr. Musser's studies were chiefly along the line of morbid anatomy and diagnosis. In May 1887 he published an interesting article on two cases of "malignant endocarditis" presenting complete patholog cal and clinical phenomena; the one case having occurred in the practice of his father—Dr. Benjamin Musser, Lancaster, in 1878, and the other at the Philadelphia Hospital, the autopsy findings being reported by Osler, Musser and Dorland. In addition to his many contributions to the medical literature of his period, he was the author of a work on medical diagnosis which passed through six editions; editor of the volume on diseases of the lungs in Nothnagel's Encyclopedia and co-editor with Dr. Aloysius O. J. Kelly of a system of therapeutics. He also was the author of the article on pneumonia in Osler's System of Medicine and of various articles in Hare's System of Therapeutics.

He early became interested in the activities of the Association. At the annual session in Denver in 1898 he gave the Oration on Medicine—the title being "The Essentials of the Art of Medicine."

As president of the Association in 1904 it became his responsibility to appoint the members of the first Council on Medical Education created that year by the House of Delegates, and the successful operation of the Council was largely due to the outstanding leaders in medical education that formed its membership.

It is interesting to note that Dr. Musser's son, Dr. John Herr Musser II, professor of medicine, Tulane University Medical School, has served as a member of this Council since 1934.

Dr. Musser also served as President of the Philadelphia Pathological Society from 1893 to 1897; Philadelphia County Medical Society 1889; American School Hygiene Association 1909; and National Medical Library Association at the time of his death. He was an honorary member of many learned societies in this country and abroad.

The Franklin and Marshall College in 1908 conferred on him the honorary degree Doctor of Laws.

He was a pioneer in social service work in the Hospital of the University of Pennsylvania, and president of the organization in the Presbyterian Hospital.

Dr. Musser died at his home in Philadelphia April 3, 1912, from angina pectoris at fifty-five years of age.

In the Journal of the Association, April 13, 1912, appears this tribute: "In the death of Dr. Musser in the prime of life and at the zenith of his professional career, the medical world has lost an internist and diagnostician of the highest grade; medical education, an enthusiastic, earnest and painstaking instructor; medical literature, a writer of no mean degree; science, a brilliant laborer in its research field, and social service, a pioneer."

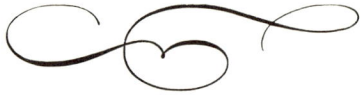

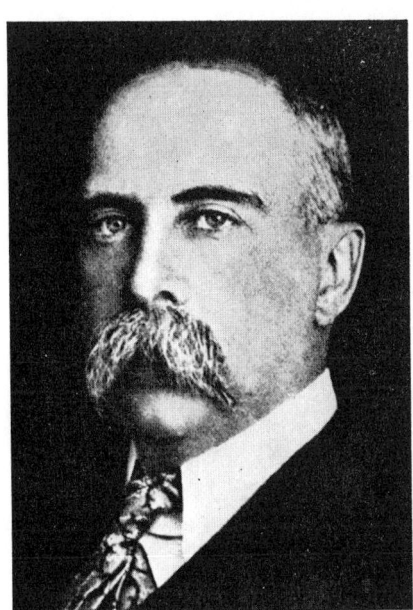

LEWIS SAMUEL McMURTRY, M.D.
Louisville, Ky.
1850–1924

Fifty-seventh President, A. M. A.
Portland, Oregon, Session
July 11, 12, 13, 14, 1905

DR. LEWIS S. McMURTRY, distinguished surgeon of the South, and for many years conspicuous in the Councils of the Association, was born in Harrodsburg, Kentucky, September 14, 1850. He received a liberal education at Center College, Danville, Ky.; a Bachelor of Arts at 19 years, and Master of Arts at 22 years of age. In 1870 he began the study of medicine at Tulane University, and graduated with the degree of Doctor of Medicine after a three year course in 1873. Soon after completing an internship in Charity Hospital, New Orleans, he began practice in Danville, Kentucky, and in 1881 was elected to the chair of anatomy in the Kentucky School of Medicine at Louisville but retained his residence in Danville. In 1883 and 1884, for a period of six months, he carried on special studies in pathological histology and clinical surgery in New York City and Philadelphia. After spending several months in postgraduate study in Europe in 1889, he removed permanently to Louisville and confined his practice to gynecology and abdominal surgery, and became prominently identified with the advancement of this specialty. In 1894 he was elected to the chair of gynecology and abdominal surgery in the Hospital College of Medicine in Louisville, and ten years later assumed the same professorship at the University of Louisville Medical Department. He was elected a member of the first Board of Trustees of the

Association in 1883, serving until 1889 and again from 1893 to 1896. Dr. McMurtry had an important part in founding the Journal in 1882 and selecting Dr. N. S. Davis as the first editor.

He contributed frequently to surgical literature, including several excellent articles on tuberculosis of the peritoneum, the chapter on surgery of the uterus in International Textbook of Surgery, as well as several chapters in Reed's Textbook on Gynecology.

Dr. McMurtry was a member of the American Surgical Association; an honorary member of the Philadelphia Obstetrical Society; an honorary Fellow of the Edinburgh Obstetrical Society and the British Gynecological Society. He was also one of the founders of the International Periodical Congress of Gynecology and Obstetrics.

In 1889 he served as president of the Kentucky State Medical Society; in 1891 of the Southern Surgical and Gynecological Association, and of the American Association of Obstetricians in 1893.

His presidential address in 1905 was largely a tribute to Dr. N. S. Davis, the Father of the Association, who had died that year; he referred also to the new era that had come with the reorganization in 1901, the great increase in membership as a result of the same and expressing a prophecy of 120,000 members in the near future; he referred to the important effect on medical education of establishing the Council on Medical Education the year before, and the first annual educational conference April 20, 1905. He urged the need of cooperation of medical interests and advocated a permanent committee on Legislation, as well as a Council on Pharmacy and Chemistry.

During his later years he served as President of the Kentucky State Board of Health, and maintained his interest and leadership in medicine until his death February 1, 1924, from acute pneumonia, at seventy-four years of age.

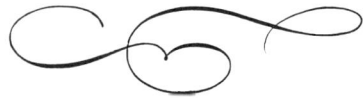

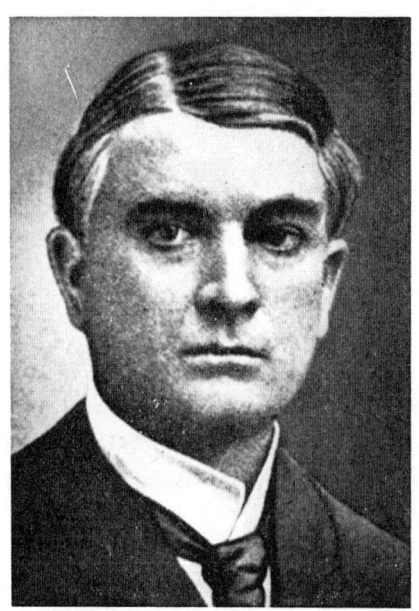

WILLIAM JAMES MAYO, M.D.
Rochester, Minn.
1861–1939

Fifty-eighth President, A. M. A.
Boston Session
June 5, 6, 7, 8, 1906

DR. WILLIAM J. MAYO, the elder of the two famous brothers Mayo, at the time of his election to the presidency had already attained a preeminent place in the councils of the Association, and as one of the leaders in American surgery.

His brother, Charles H. Mayo, followed him in the presidency of the Association eleven years later in 1917. As the two careers were inseparable, what may be said of one can often be spoken of the other, and any biographic record forms the story of the development of the Mayo Clinic and Mayo Foundation. Their passing from life so closely together in 1939 was no doubt as they themselves might have wished it.

The career of Dr. William J. Mayo has been fully recorded in a number of biographies, particularly in "The Doctors Mayo," published by the University of Minnesota Press in 1941, in which many facts are considered that cannot be recorded here.

The father of the two boys, Dr. William Worrall Mayo, was born in Manchester, England, May 31, 1819, and came to the United States in 1845. He studied medicine in Lafayette, Indiana, and received his degree in medicine from the Indiana Medical College at LaPorte in 1850. He received a second degree from the Medical Department of the University of Missouri in 1854, and in 1859 located in LeSueur, Minnesota, and in 1863 moved to Rochester, Minn. He was a competent surgeon, one of the first physicians in the West to use a microscope in his practice, the founder of the Minnesota State Medical Association, and its president in 1873.

The first-born son, William James Mayo, was born June 29, 1861, at LeSueur, Minnesota, the family moving to Rochester when he was slightly over one and a half years old. He attended the public school in Rochester, and the high school, and thereafter spent one year in a private school for languages and sciences, and two years in Nile's Academy.

During their youth, both William and Charles accompanied their father on his rounds and had an opportunity to observe both surgical operations and post-mortem examinations. For a time, both clerked in the drug store. With their father, they learned to use the microscope. In 1880 William J. Mayo went to the University of Michigan at Ann Arbor, completing a three year course which had just been established, and received his degree Doctor of Medicine in 1883 when he was twenty-two years old. During his medical course he had an opportunity to be associated with Ford, the anatomist, Victor C. Vaughan, the biochemist, and Donald MacLean, professor of surgery.

One year later in November 1884 Doctor Will married Miss Hattie M. Damon of Rochester. Through many years the close association of Mrs. Mayo with Dr. William J. Mayo in extending hospitality in the organization of many aspects of the Clinic, and in carrying a great share of the responsibility for his success and happiness, has been widely recognized.

In 1884 Dr. William J. Mayo spent two months in study at the New York Post-Graduate School, and in 1885 he took a course at the New York Polyclinic. For many years he and Dr. Charles alternated in spending week-ends in Chicago with Dr. Christian Fenger. Frequently they travelled abroad to observe surgery as practiced in every nation of the world.

In 1885, Dr. William J. Mayo read his first paper before the Southern Minnesota Medical Association, and his literary contributions to every phase of medical science and art and practice, have been innumerable.

From 1889 until 1905, the Drs. Mayo carried on their work at St. Mary's Hospital in Rochester, an institution which they, with their father, had aided in establishing and one which is now known throughout the world largely because of their work. The records of surgical procedures performed indicate an early tendency toward selection of abdominal surgery by Dr. Will, leaving many of the other fields to Dr. Charles. As Dr. Will himself said, "Charlie soon had driven me to cover by being a better surgeon, and I began to specialize in abdominal work and in operations on the ureters and kidneys." As the repute of their work spread, they soon began to associate with themselves younger men who had shown special predilection for surgical work, the first to be selected being Dr. E. Starr Judd (Pres. A. M. A., 1931), who had charge of the third operating room in 1905. From that time on, the surgical developments in Rochester were so rapid that additional wings continued to be added to the hospital, an annex was opened and additional hospitals were built. As it became apparent that internal medicine and diagnosis, with the work of the laboratory, would be of prime importance, these developments were particularly encouraged. Throughout the record of growth and development of this monumental institution to the proud position which it now occupies, signs of the leadership of Dr. William J. Mayo appear again and again. Early in his career Dr. Will conceived the idea of a permanent endowed institution in Rochester to be connected with a university. He elaborated the concept of the Mayo Foundation and gave freely of himself, of his funds and of his life for its perpetuation.

The honors and recognitions given to him indicate how widely recognized were his achievements for the good of mankind. He was a Fellow of the American Surgical Association, of the Royal Colleges of Surgeons of England and Edinburgh, and of the College of Physicians of Philadelphia. He received the honorary LL.D. from the universities of Toronto, Maryland, Pennsylvania, McGill, Leeds, Pittsburgh, Carleton, Manchester, Temple and Aberdeen. He received the honorary degree of D.Sc. from Michigan, Columbia, Leeds, Harvard, Marquette, and Northwestern Universities. He received the honorary M.D. from Trinity College in Dublin and from the University of Havana. He was also a fellow of the Royal College of Surgeons, Ireland, and of the Royal Academie de Medecine de France. Other recognitions include the gold medal of the National Institute of Social Sciences; the Distinguished Service medal of the United States Army; the Henry Jacob Bigelow gold medal of the Boston Surgical Society; Royal Order of the Commander of the Northern Star, conferred by His Majesty the King of Sweden; the Finlay Congressional Distinguished Service Medal, conferred by Cuba; the cross of the Royal Order of Knight Commander of the Crown of Italy and the citation for distinguished service given by the American Legion with a commemorative plaque, which was presented by the President of the United States in person in 1934.

Dr. William J. Mayo early became associated with medical organizations. He served as president of his County and State medical organizations. In the American Medical Association he was chairman of the Section on Surgery and Anatomy in 1898 and 1899. In 1904 at the Atlantic City session he delivered the Oration on Surgery. He served as president of the Association during the interesting sessions held at the new Harvard Medical School in Boston in 1906. He arranged a dinner for the officers of the Association, including the different scientific sections and distinguished guests, that was a memorable occasion. Among the guests were Professor Trendelenburg, the noted surgeon of Leipzig, and Dr. S. Weir Mitchell of Philadelphia.

In his presidential address, he forecast and considered some of the great problems that concern medical practice in this later day. He attacked abuses of medical care by public service corporations, and the abuse of medical charity by those able to pay. He condemned all attempts by those not trained in the science and art of medicine to dominate its functions. In a note written just a few days before his death, he urged continued work for the advancement and stablization of medical science and the traditions of medical practice.

Dr. William J. Mayo was also president of the Society of Clinical Surgery (1911–1912), the American Surgical Association (1913–1914), of the American College of Surgeons (1917–1919), of the Congress of American Physicians and Surgeons (1925) and of the Interstate Postgraduate Medical Assembly of North America (1932–1933).

During the World War he was commissioned Major in the Medical Reserve Corps on April 9, 1917, and Colonel of the Medical Corps of the National Army on June 15, 1918. He served as chief consultant for all surgical services during the period of the war and was stationed in the office of the Surgeon General in Washington. He was commissioned Brigadier General in the Reserve Corps in 1921 and since then served at various times as consultant in surgery to the War Department.

His memberships in medical organizations, in military organizations and in civic bodies were far too numerous even for listing. Most of the important foreign medical societies of the world had elected him an honorary member.

His contributions to medical literature, previously mentioned, were beyond 600 in number, beginning with a report of an operation for ovarian tumor and covering many phases of medical and surgical science, a wide variety of commencement and honorary addresses, a number of descriptive letters of travel and philosophic contributions to the problems of our day.

In 1915, Drs. William J. and Charles H. Mayo donated $1,500,000 to establish the Mayo Foundation for Medical Education and Research in Rochester in affiliation with the University of Minnesota. In 1919 the brothers formed the Mayo Properties Association to hold all the properties, endowments and funds of the Mayo Clinic to insure the permanence of the institution for public service. Again in 1934 the Mayo Properties Association presented a gift of $500,000 to the University of Minnesota, making a total of $2,000,000 that the brothers had given to the Mayo Foundation. In sending this contribution, Dr. William J. Mayo wrote, in part:

"Our father recognized certain definite social obligations. He believed that any man who had better opportunity than others, greater strength of mind, body or character, owed something to those who had not been so provided; that is, that the important thing in life was not to accomplish for oneself alone, but for each to carry his share of collective responsibility. . . The fund which we had built up and which had grown far beyond our expectations had come from the sick, and we believed that it ought to return to the sick in the form of advanced medical education, which would develop better-trained physicians, and to research to reduce the amount of sickness . . . . The people's money, of which we have been the moral custodians, is being irrevocably returned to from whom it came. The practice of medicine in Rochester is carried on in the same manner as by other members of the regular medical profession throughout the state and nation. All classes of patients, without regard to race or creed, social or financial standing, receive necessary care without discrimination. . . . . ."

These words reflect the great character, the human kindliness, the profound human sympathy that were the part of Dr. William James Mayo. It has been said that opportunity and great occasions make great men. Exception to this rule is present in the lives of Drs. William J. and Charles H. Mayo. They made a small village into one of the most notable medical centers of the world wholly through a genius for surgery and for medical leadership. Throughout their careers they devoted themselves to the advancement of scientific medicine and of the medical profession which they served so nobly, and which gloried so greatly in their achievements.

The Mayo name became a symbol which carried the precepts of American medicine to all parts of the modern world.

When William J. Mayo passed from the stage on July 28, 1939, all the world seemed to pause in the midst of its turmoil and stress, to give him honor and to pay him tribute, so justly his due—a great physician, a superb surgeon, a magnificent leader, a beloved man.

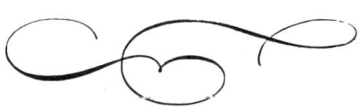

JOSEPH DECATUR BRYANT, M.D.
New York, N. Y.
1845–1914

Fifty-ninth President, A. M. A.
Atlantic City Session
June 3, 4, 5, 6, 7, 1907

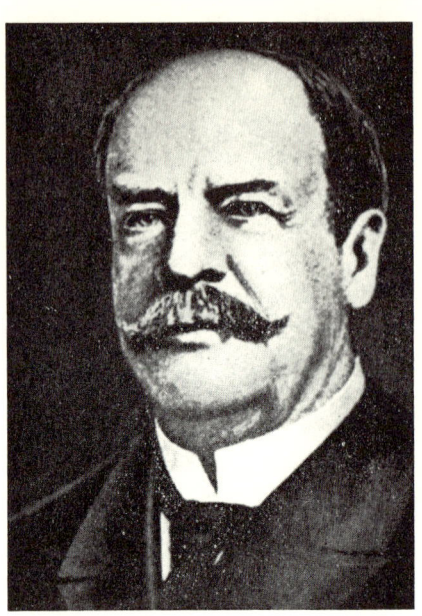

DR. JOSEPH D. BRYANT came to the presidency of the Association with a record of a surgeon of wide renown—thirty-five years as a member of the Faculty of Bellevue Hospital Medical College, formerly Surgeon General of the New York State National Guard, Sanitary Inspector and Health Commissioner of the City of New York, and Commissioner of the New York State Board of Health.

He was born in East Troy, Walworth County, Wisconsin, March 12, 1845. His preparatory collegiate work was done at the Norwich (New York) Academy, after which he entered Bellevue Hospital Medical College, graduating in 1868. After serving an internship in Bellevue Hospital he became assistant to the chair of anatomy in his Alma Mater in 1871, and then passed through the teaching positions of lecturer on surgical anatomy, assistant demonstrator of anatomy, professor of general, descriptive and surgical anatomy, professor of anatomy and clinical surgery and associate professor of orthopedic surgery until 1898, when at the merger of the University of New York and Bellevue Hospital Medical College he became professor of the principles and practice of surgery, operative and clinical surgery, holding this position until his death in 1914.

In addition to his teaching service and extensive surgical practice, he served as sanitary inspector in the Health Department of New

York City for six years followed by a similar period of service as Commissioner of the New York State Board of Health.

In 1873 he was appointed surgeon of the 75th Infantry Regiment, New York State National Guard, and nine years later was made Surgeon General of the State. Due to his special talents for organization, he organized the medical department of the Guard on a basis which placed it in a foremost position among the medical corps of the organized militia of the United States. In 1895 Brigadier General Bryant resigned from the Guard.

He served as president of the New York Academy of Medicine in 1895; president of the New York State Medical Association in 1898, and president of the Medical Society of the State of New York in 1906. He was a Fellow of the American Surgical Association, member of the Association of Military Surgeons, and of many other scientific organizations.

Dr. Bryant was an author of note and his work on operative surgery, which passed through four editions, became one of the textbooks of the period. He was co-author with Buck of the eight volume American System of Surgery, and was also a frequent contributor to surgical literature.

Dr. Bryant was the family physician and warm personal friend of President Grover Cleveland, and was his close associate in his many travel and fishing trips. When the President underwent an operation for malignant tumor of the left upper jaw in 1893, Dr. Bryant was the operator assisted by Drs. W. W. Keen and John F. Erdman. Because of the financial crises at the time, it was necessary to keep it a secret, and it remained so until published by W. W. Keen in 1917.

The President was able to appear before Congress two weeks following the operation, and lived fifteen years afterwards.

Dr. Bryant was a victim of diabetes before the discovery of insulin, but despite his disability was able to keep up his interest in professional and public affairs to the time of his death, which occurred at St. Vincent's Hospital, New York City, April, 7, 1914, at sixty-nine years of age.

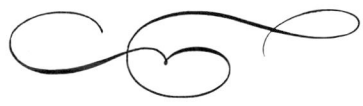

HERBERT LESLIE BURRELL, M.D.
Boston, Mass.
1856–1910

Sixtieth Session, A. M. A.
Chicago Session
June 2, 3, 4, 5, 1908

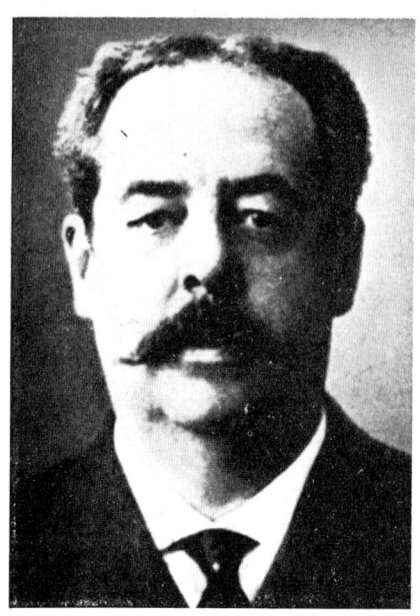

THE SELECTION OF DR. HERBERT L. BURRELL for president of the Association was a fitting recognition of one of the brilliant sons of New England, noted for its sturdy fidelity to the best interests of the profession and its manifold contributions to the science of medicine and surgery. True to heredity and tradition the sons of New England have blazed many a new trail in the field of medicine and in large measure shaped the medical affairs of this nation. Dr. Burrell lived in Boston all his life, being born there April 27, 1856. He received his preliminary education at the English High School in that city and graduated from Harvard Medical School in 1879. After a few years of practice, desiring to take up the teaching of others in the principles and details which he had mastered, he became in 1886 a demonstrator of surgical technic in his Alma Mater. He soon proved that his liking for this field of work was founded on a fitness and thorough preparedness for it. Dr. Burrell gradually advanced in the faculty until he attained the full professorship of clinical surgery in Harvard Medical School. In addition, for many years he gave the systematic course of lectures in surgery. He also served as senior visiting surgeon to the Boston City Hospital; surgeon to the Children's Hospital, as well as consulting surgeon to the Carney Hospital.

One of Dr. Burrell's earliest endeavors was to establish a continued, in place of the short three months, service for attending hospital surgeons. He succeeded early to arrange a continued surgical service at the Boston Children's Hospital and later at the Boston City Hospital. He also brought about a change in the teaching of surgery, formerly consisting of brilliant lectures by surgical leaders, or clinics where the masters of their craft displayed their skill in rare operations to a sensation-loving class, to a system of education comprising the careful study of patients by small groups of students, who under the direction of trained teachers learned thoroughness of observation and skill of hand. Dr. Burrell also worked devotedly to perfect a plan of grouping and arrangement of courses that would give the student some knowledge of everything that was needed for the practitioner, and an opportunity for the more thorough study of that group of subjects which was most important to each individual. He established a system whereby students served as clinical clerks and surgical dressers during the senior year and thereby formed a pattern for similar work in other institutions.

During the early part of his career he was connected with the Massachusetts Volunteer Militia, finally becoming Surgeon General of Massachuetts in 1893. In 1898 Massachusetts sent a hospital ship, the *Bay State*, with her troops to the Spanish-American War, and Dr. Burrell showed himself an efficient surgeon in charge. He directed and commanded three expeditions of relief in returning safely a precious cargo each time of fever-stricken Massachusetts and other soldiers from Cuba and Porto Rico. Among the returning soldiers was Major Victor C. Vaughan of the Medical Corps (president A.M.A. 1914) and he with many others attested that the service and organization was superior to that of the best of hospitals; in fact his relief work in the *"Bay State"* has been called "his most notable achievement."

His society memberships included the American Surgical Association, of which he was secretary for several years; the American Society of Clinical Surgery; American Orthopedic Association; the Boston Society for Medical Improvement; the Boston Society of Medical Science, and the American Association of Pathologists and Bacteriologists. He served as president of the Massachusetts Medical Society, and from 1899 to the time of his death he was president of the Massachusetts branch of the American Red Cross.

Another indication of his power as an organizer was as Chairman of the Committee of Arrangements for the meeting of the Association in Boston in 1906.

All who were privileged to attend this session were impressed with the perfection of the preparations, the success in every detail, the harmony and elaborate preparedness for the meeting; of the many delightful social features, the beautiful afternoon teas served by charming young Boston ladies attired in red and white costumes, on the verandas of the new marble Harvard Medical group of buildings, will be most happily remembered.

As an educator and skillful exponent of American surgery, Doctor Burrell attained a high rank. He was probably the first to make a successful ligation of the innominate artery. Others had re-implanted parts of trephine buttons, but Dr. Burrell was the first to re-implant successfully a whole one. He was among the first to advocate the out-of-door treatment of tuberculosis as equally applicable for surgical as for medical cases. Likewise he was a pioneer in the establishment of an ambulance corps and Massachusetts was the first state to realize this important feature.

He urged a retiring age for the surgeon, and on the other hand often called attention to the danger involved in one's taking up surgery after only a few weeks service in a clinic or postgraduate school. He believed that the public was entitled to good surgery, and constantly labored to make a man's ability to teach the sole criterion by which to judge his value to the institution concerned. Dr. Burrell further urged the education of the public, that it might be fixed in the minds of all that laboratories and research agencies were for the benefit of the people.

Such was the man who honored the office of president of the Association; a man whose life was largely given up to the pursuit of the highest ideals, calculated to uplift the medical profession and to extend its usefulness.

During the last year of his life, Dr. Burrell was an invalid on account of valvular heart disease with kidney complications, and was unable to teach or to practice. At the Atlantic City session of the Associaton in 1909 he was ill and unable to be present and to preside over the House of Delegates and to open the general session. He died at his home in Boston April 27, 1910, at the untimely age of fifty-four years.

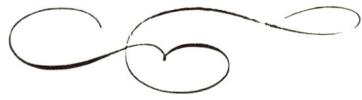

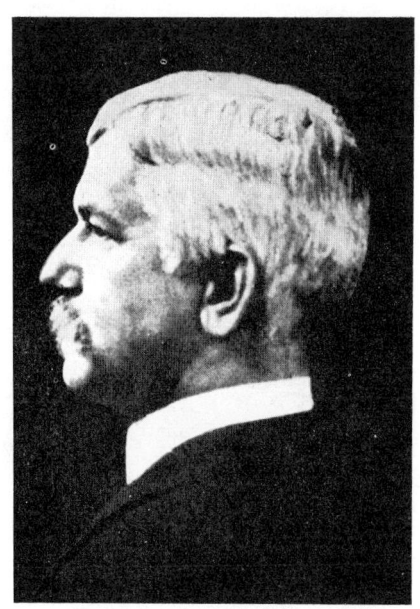

WILLIAM C. GORGAS, M.D.
Washington, D. C.
1854–1921

*Sixty-first President, A. M. A.
Atlantic City Session
June 7, 8, 9, 10, 1909*

THE LIFE AND CAREER OF DR. WILLIAM C. GORGAS forms a chapter in the romance of American medicine: great medical administrator, liberator of the tropics, one who brought to public attention the power of medicine when applied on a large scale and converted the most loathsome spot on the American continent into a place of beauty and a pleasure resort; Surgeon General of the U. S. Army.

Dr. Gorgas was born October 3, 1854 at Toulminville, near Mobile, Alabama, and came of distinguished ancestry; his father was Captain Josiah Gorgas, graduate of West Point Military Academy 1841, a Pennsylvanian, later Major General and Chief Ordnance Officer of the Confederacy; his mother was Amelia Gayle, daughter of John Gayle, Governor of Alabama from 1831 to 1835, a presidential elector in 1840, and later a member of Congress.

It so happened that William Crawford Gorgas spent the most susceptible period of his boyhood amid the exciting atmosphere of Richmond during the war between the States. He was seven years old when the conflict began and eleven when it closed. His father, Brigadier General Gorgas, was stationed there during the war as chief ordnance officer; there the son, William, saw much of the pomp and keenly felt the poverty of war. Holding the hand of his father, in May 1863, he passed the bier of Stonewall Jackson; he often sat on the knee of General Lee, and came in almost daily contact with President Davis and other prominent leaders of the Confederacy.

After Appomatox, the Gorgas family found its way to Baltimore, Maryland; the future medical officer and sanitarian often spoke of this time as—"I first came to Baltimore, a ragged, barefoot little rebel, with empty pockets and an empty stomach."

After the war his father became the president of the University of the South at Sewanee, Tennessee; here the son received his A. B. degree in 1875. He applied for admission to West Point, but failed to secure the appointment, and in the fall of 1876 he enrolled as a student in Bellevue Medical College, New York City, and received the degree Doctor of Medicine in June 1879.

Gorgas made an excellent record as a student. Dr. William H. Welch was then the presiding genius at Bellevue, and the young Alabamian became one of his appreciative pupils. After graduating he served as intern in Bellevue Hospital, and in June 1880 he entered the medical department of the Army. The next eighteen years he spent at Army posts; at one of his early stations, Fort Brown, Texas, in 1882, he had his first contact with yellow fever, where he himself contracted the disease as the result of performing an autopsy. The young lady, Marie C. Daughty, who was later to become his wife, and a niece of the Commanding Officer at Fort Brown, had a severe attack of yellow fever at the same time. Thus early in his career he became immune, and this led to his being afterwards summoned to duty wherever yellow fever appeared. After two years of duty at Fort Randall, North Dakota, he was stationed for thirteen years at Fort Barrancas, Pensacola Bay, Florida, where he had ample opportunity for further study of yellow fever.

During the Spanish-American War, Major Gorgas had charge of the yellow fever camp at Siboney, Cuba, where Dr. Victor C. Vaughan was one of his patients; of this Dr. Vaughan wrote—"It was largely through Dr. Gorgas's skill in the management of yellow fever that the death rate in our army in Cuba was so low. The sight of his kindly face was a stimulant that did much to tone up the muscles exhausted by the exercise imposed upon the body by 'el vomito negro.'"

In 1898 Dr. Gorgas was appointed chief sanitary officer of Havana. One of the first friends Dr. Gorgas made in Havana was Dr. Carlos J. Finlay, who back in 1881 had presented a paper before a sanitary congress in Washington, D. C., asserting that yellow fever was transmitted by the stegomyia mosquito. It was twenty years before this startling theory came to real fruition. This was accomplished by the special commission appointed by Surgeon General Sternberg, headed by Dr. Walter Reed, the other members being James Carroll, Jesse W. Lazear and Aristides Agramonte. Doctor Reed had been trained in bacteriology under the tutelage of Dr. William H. Welch at Johns Hopkins and was splendidly equipped for the work.

After many trials, including the martyrdom of Jesse W. Lazear, Doctor Reed and his associates established the transmissibility of yellow fever by the stegomyia mosquito, following which Dr. Gorgas directed the screening of all yellow fever patients, and destroying the fever bearing mosquitoes by oiling the surface of all pools or collections of water where they were likely to breed. As a result, in three months Havana was freed from yellow fever for the first time in nearly two centuries.

For his work in eliminating the disease from Havana, Dr. Gorgas was made a Colonel and Assistant Surgeon General of the Army by special Act of Congress March 9, 1903.

On March 1, 1904, Dr. Gorgas was appointed Chief Sanitary Officer of the Panama Canal, where he began to fight yellow fever in the jungle in connection with the construction of the Isthmian Canal. Evidently the work of Reed and Gorgas in Cuba had made little impression on the official mind; nevertheless, he succeeded in the face of skeptical criticism when wise men predicted failure.

Because of this official criticism, his recall was recommended to President Theodore Roosevelt, who however depended on the advice of William H. Welch, and particularly his personal friend, Dr. Alexander Lambert of New York, and Doctor Gorgas remained at his post.

Doctor Gorgas carried out the same line of work as in Havana in cleaning up the Isthmus. The death rate from yellow fever was high, and an epidemic was going on when he arrived, and yet in less than a year yellow fever was wiped out and from May 1906 there was not a single case reported.

Doctor Gorgas was made a member of the Isthmian Canal Commission in 1907, and he remained in charge of sanitation until the winter of 1913. When the Canal was about completed Doctor Gorgas and his sanitary engineer, Mr. Joseph L. LePrince, were the first persons to pass through it in a small boat.

In 1908 he was granted an honorary degree, Doctor of Science, from Johns Hopkins University and was honored the same year by degrees from the universities of Pennsylvania, Harvard, Brown, and the University of the South; in the same year the seal of further approval came from the American Medical Association in the election to the presidency.

In 1913 he received an invitation from the Chamber of Mines of

Johannesburg, South Africa, to investigate the high rate from pneumonia among the natives working in the mines of the Rand. While in South Africa, he received a cablegram from President Wilson advising him of his appointment as Surgeon General of the Army January 16, 1914.

Upon his return to England he was specially received by Sir William Osler in Oxford, and there at a convocation on March 23, 1914 he received the honorary degree of Doctor of Science from the University of Oxford. He was complimented by a dinner on March 26, 1914, at which Sir Thomas Barton, President of the Royal College of Physicians of London presided, and attended by the Archbishop of Canterbury, the Lord Chancellor, the American Ambassador Viscount Brice and a distinguished company of physicians and surgeons.

After assuming his duties as Surgeon General, he was raised to the rank of Major General.

In 1916 under the auspices of the International Health Board, Rockefeller Foundation, he spent several months in South America making a preliminary survey of localities still infested with yellow fever.

Doctor Gorgas was awarded the Gold Medal of the Liverpool School of Tropical Medicine in 1907, and that of the American Museum of Safety in 1914.

His society affiliations included membership in the American Medical Association, American Public Health Association, American Society of Tropical Medicine, Association of Military Surgeons and the College of Physicians of Philadelphia.

With the entrance of the United States in World War I in April 1917, Doctor Gorgas entered into the last important work of his life. Fortunately he had begun reorganization of the Medical Corps before the advent of war. He was able to call into the Reserve Corps, as advisors, the leading medical and surgical authorities in this country. It was a record of great credit to the Medical Corps—being marred only by the unusual outbreak of influenza, which prevailed throughout the entire world. He was awarded the Distinguished Service Medal at the close of the first World War.

After his retirement as Surgeon General November 14, 1918, he again became interested with the International Health Board in the investigation of possible breeding grounds of yellow fever in South Africa, from Senegal to the Belgian Congo, and headed a Commission which sailed for London May 8, 1920.

A series of official visits and receptions awaited him on his arrival. He was received by the King and Queen of England, by King Albert and Cardinal Mercier of Belgium. Very soon afterward he was taken suddenly very ill with heart and circulatory failure and died at Queen Alexandria Military Hospital July 4, 1920.

During his illness His Majesty King George of England called at the hospital and conferred on him the insignia of Knight Commander of the Order of St. Michael and St. George.

The funeral service was that of a British Major General in St. Paul's Cathedral. From the lengthy tribute in the London Lancet is quoted: "Thus the ragged, barefoot little rebel who first came to Baltimore in 1865 with empty pockets and stomach—the other day rode up Ludgate Hill sleeping his last on earth, wrapped in the Stars and Stripes," "He passed through the great door through which the sun streams into the nave of St. Paul's, and there he lay with Nelson and Wellington and all that mighty host who came this way and passed into the universe." "They will take him to his own land, but in truth he belongs to us all."

His body lay in state for four days in Washington, and the burial was in Arlington Cemetery.

America can well be proud of having contributed such a man to the field of medicine.

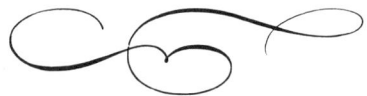

WILLIAM HENRY WELCH, M.D.
Baltimore, Md.
1850–1934

*Sixty-second President, A. M. A.
St. Louis Session
June 6, 7, 8, 9, 1910*

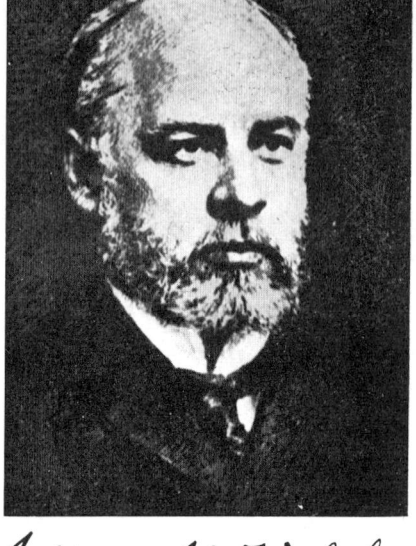

DR. WILLIAM H. WELCH was one of the deans of American medicine, an inspiring leader in three lines of medical endeavor, pathology, public health and medical history, who contributed in large measure towards the evolution of medical education in America during his lifetime, with the introduction of an entirely new attitude towards medicine.

He was born in Norfolk, Connecticut, April 8, 1850, of a remarkable medical lineage for his father, grandfather, and great grandfather were doctors, and he had four medical uncles. The house of his birth, eighty years later, was distinguished by a plaque: "To Dr. William H. Welch, Dean of American Medicine."

If there is something for the race in the great accumulation of energy and of accomplishment, which is possible through the development in successive generations, William H. Welch offers a good example. At sixteen years he entered Yale College, receiving the degree of Bachelor of Arts at twenty. Upon graduation he became a teacher of Latin and Greek, and after a year began his medical studies at the College of Physicians and Surgeons in New York. After attending a few lectures he returned to New Haven for further work in chemistry at the Sheffield Scientific School. After a year of this graduate work he again re-entered the College of Physicians. During his senior year he was appointed an intern at Bellevue Hospital, where he first met

Abraham Jacobi and Francis Delafield, both being an inspiration, and directed his attention toward pathological anatomy. He received the degree Doctor of Medicine in 1875. During the following summer and winter he was asked by Delafield to be curator of the Wood Pathological Museum, and pathologist to the hospital.

On April 19, 1876, he sailed for Europe and remained two years; these were thrilling years and opened up for him a new viewpoint of medicine. The masters he came in contact with determined for him ever afterwards the kind of work and the way of thought that brought him to the high place in American medicine. In Strasbourg he studied under Waldeyer, Hoppe-Seyler and Von Recklinghausen. After this foundation in histology and physiologic chemistry he worked with Ludwig in Leipzig—the great physiologist—and with Cohnheim in Breslau. While in Breslau Dr. Robert Koch came to Cohnheim's laboratory to demonstrate his completed work on the anthrax bacillus. Here he also met Weigert and Ehrlich, as well as Salomonsen, the Danish pathologist and bacteriologist. In Vienna he studied pathology with Chiari, neurology with Meynert, and diseases of the skin with Hebra. He continued his work in Paris and London and returned to the United States in 1878. Soon afterwards he opened a laboratory for micropathology at Bellevue Medical College, which soon became very popular and students attended from all three medical schools. Within a short time a similar laboratory was established at the College of Physicians and Surgeons in charge of Dr. T. Mitchell Prudden. Dr. Welch gained the friendship of Dr. Austin Flint, and in 1880 and 1881 he assisted in revising Flint's Principles and Practice of Medicine—the most consulted medical treatise of its day.

In 1884 came the offer of a full-time professorship in pathology at Johns Hopkins University, Baltimore, and against the advice of his New York colleagues he accepted the appointment. He was allowed a year of further study in Europe in preparation for his new work, particularly in bacteriology and the share taken by microorganisms in the causation of disease. He studied principally with Koch and Flugge bringing back the spirit and impulse that stirred America to enormous efforts and changed the whole aspect of medicine. Since the Johns Hopkins Hospital was not opened until 1889 and the medical school until 1893, a period intervened during which the laboratory of Doctor Welch was the center of medical study in Baltimore. He had much to say in the selection of the clinical professors, William Osler, W. S. Halstead and Howard A. Kelly, who like Welch were all under the age of forty, and later appeared in J. S. Sargent's portrait of "The Four Doctors" (1905), which now adorns the W. H.

Welch Medical Library. Welch became pathologist-in-chief to the hospital and was the first dean of the medical school for five years (1893–8). As a pathologist he had the broadest possible outlook and covered the whole field of this biological science. It was during this period that Dr. Welch made his most significant contributions to the science of medicine, doing research on animal diseases, infections and immunity and gas gangrene; he discovered the Bacillus aerogenes capsulatus in 1892; he worked on hemorrhagic infarction, embolism and thrombosis; experimental work on pulmonary oedema began in 1878, and on glomerulonephritis in 1886. In this period he published "The General Pathology of Fevers" and "Pathology of Bacteria, Infections and Immunity."

It is significant that many of the young men who were associated with him in his early days eventually achieved great fame in the field of medicine. Such names as Councilman, Mall, Nuttall, Abbott, Sternberg, Reed, Flexner, MacCallum, Bolton, were among the first of his students.

With the establishment of the Johns Hopkins University School of Medicine, came a great inspiration for the raising of standards in American medical education. By his leadership Dr. Welch stimulated advancement of research, hospital organization, medical education and public health. His inspiring influence helped to make the pathological laboratory the centre of the modern hospital and the medical school.

By 1894 his repute, although he was but 44 years of age, had already grown, so that honorary degrees were given to him and continued to be awarded to him for many years. He received the honorary M.D. from the University of Pennsylvania in 1894, and LL.D. from Western Reserve University the same year. Yale conferred this degree on him in 1896, Harvard in 1900, Toronto in 1903, Columbia in 1904, Jefferson Medical College in 1907, Princeton in 1910, Washington University in 1915, the University of Chicago in 1916, the University of Southern California, and the University of the State of New York in 1930. He was awarded the Doctorate of the University of Strassbourg in 1923. He also received the degree of Doctor of Sciences from Cambridge in 1923, Western Reserve in 1929, and the University of Pennsylvania in 1930.

His work in pathology and bacteriology was followed by a broader conception of the organization of public health control and the establishment of a new school of hygiene and public health, where he served as director from 1916 to 1926; at seventy-six years of age he became Professor of the History of Medicine and continued until 1931, when he was named emeritus professor. The medical library in the Institute of the History of Medicine at Johns Hopkins University is named in his honor.

Significant in the life of William H. Welch was his immediate contact and guiding influence in many organizations associated with medicine for social, humanitarian or philanthropic purposes. Thus, he was president of the State Board of Health of Maryland from 1898 to 1922, and continued as a member until 1929. He was continuously president of the Rockefeller Institute for Medical Research 1901–1933. He served as a member of the International Health Board and of the China Medical Board of the Rockefeller Foundation and as trustee of the Carnegie Institution.

He was frequently consulted by many foundations having medical interests. His conspicuous achievements were recognized by election to the presidencies of important organizations, including the Congress of American Physicians and Surgeons in 1897, Association of American Physicians in 1901, American Association for the Advancement of Science 1906–1907, the National Tuberculosis Association 1910–1911, The National Academy of Science 1913–1916, the American Social Hygiene Association 1916–1919, the National Committee on Mental Hygiene, and other similar bodies.

His honorary memberships included distinguished medical and sanitary organizations in England, Scotland, Ireland, Austria, Germany, Belgium, France, Italy and Switzerland. Moreover the governments of many foreign countries recognized him by decorations which include those of Japan, Norway, Servia and France, as well as the United States Government.

In the Association, Dr. Welch may be said to have begun with the presentation of the address on State Medicine entitled "Infectious Diseases" at the Newport session in June 1899. As president of the Medical-Chirurgical Faculty of the State of Maryland, he began his official connection. He was a member of the House of Delegates in 1902 and 1903, and served as a trustee of the Association from 1903 to 1909, being chairman of the Board the last year. Doctor Welch was elected unanimously to the presidency in 1909, and in his acceptance he said "that he knew of no nobler work that any member can engage in than to further the interests of the Association." The title of his president's address the following year was "Fields of Usefulness of the American Medical Association," in which he reviewed the achievements accomplished in the decade since the re-organization of the Association; the awakening of interest in a National Department of Health, the progress towards higher standards of medical education, the increasing interest and educational value of the scientific sections and the scientific exhibit—closing with the words: "Our Association has an important part in advancing the happiness and well-being of the country and contributing a beneficent share in the working out of our National destiny."

When the United States entered the World War in 1917 he was commissioned Major in the Medical Reserve Corps, advanced to Lieutenant Colonel in February, and Colonel in July 1918, finally being made Brigadier General in 1921. He served principally as advisor in the Surgeon General's office and in the organization of the special services of pathology and preventive medicine. During his service he visited each of the cantonments and military hospitals in in this country.

In 1920 in commemoration of his seventieth birthday, his published papers and addresses were collected in three memorial volumes and included 411 articles.

The occasion of his eightieth birthday, in 1930, was celebrated by distinguished gatherings not only in Washington, but in many of the capitals of the world. President Herbert Hoover made an address which was broadcast over the radio and celebrations were held in many scientific institutions. The many tributes and addresses were bound in a single volume with the title "Doctor Welch at Eighty."

Doctor Welch died in Johns Hopkins Hospital after a prolonged illness, April 20, 1934, at the age of 84 years. The following is quoted from a tribute published in the Journal of the Association—"The influence of Dr. Welch on American medical education during his career is difficult to overestimate. Certainly he played an important part in the development of the full-time system in the clinical branches, in the development of the medical curriculum on a university basis, in the establishment of schools of public health and hygiene, and in stimulating great financial contributions for the advancement of preventive medicine and public health. No doubt much of his great influence was due to the remarkable geniality of his character. His personality was sparkling, his wit noted, and the twinkle of his eye characteristic. His culture was notable and his familiarity with the literature, music and art in his time was equal to that of many experts in these fields. Such men do not come often in any phase of human life, but when they do appear, the humanistic quality of their greatness brings them universal recognition."

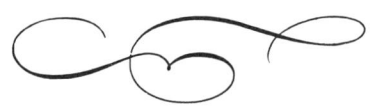

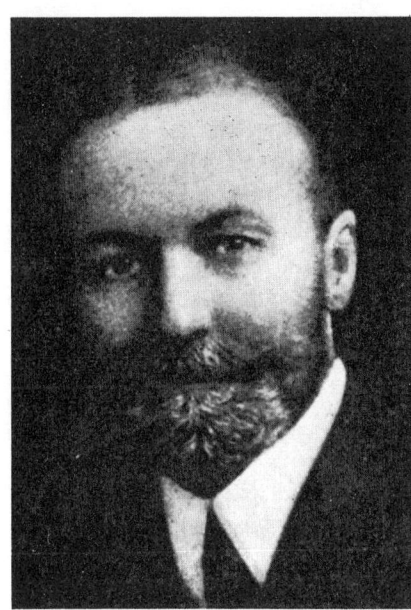

JOHN BENJAMIN MURPHY, M.D.
Chicago, Ill.
1857–1916

*Sixty-third President, A. M. A.
Los Angeles Session
June 27, 28, 29, 30, 1911*

DR. JOHN B. MURPHY, styled by William J. Mayo "the surgical genius of his generation," and by Sir Berkeley Monihan "the foremost surgical teacher of his time," was born of humble parentage, in Appleton, Wisconsin, December 21, 1857, reared on a farm, attended the preliminary schools, graduated from the Appleton High School in 1876, and received the degree Doctor of Medicine from Rush Medical College in 1879. After serving an eighteen months internship at Cook County Hospital, he became associated in practice with Dr. Edward W. Lee, Chicago, until 1882, when he went to Europe where he studied for two years. It was a period when Billroth and Lister were in their prime, when the new science of bacteriology was changing the thought and practice of surgery, and which must have had a stimulating impress on the budding American surgeon.

Soon after his return from Europe in 1884, Dr. Murphy's career as a medical teacher had its beginning when he was appointed lecturer in surgery in Rush Medical College. In 1892 he was made professor of clinical surgery in the College of Physicians and Surgeons, later the University of Illinois Medical School, holding this position until 1901 when he was elected professor of surgery in Northwestern University Medical School and continued in that position until his death in 1916. During an interregnum of three years from 1905 to 1908, he was professor of surgery in the Post Graduate School of Chicago. He was chief of the surgical staff of Mercy Hospital from 1895 to the time of his death. For thirty years he was a member of the attending or consulting staffs of Alexian Brothers Hospital, and for several years attending surgeon to Cook County Hospital, consulting surgeon to St. Joseph's and Columbus Memorial Hospitals, and the Hospital for Crippled Children, Chicago.

In 1892 he startled the surgical world by the introduction of the "Murphy-button" published in his article on "Cholecysto-Intestinal, Gastro-Intestinal, Entero-Intestinal Anastomosis and Approximation without Sutures." He was the first American surgeon to recognize actinomycosis of the lungs; one of the earliest operators for acute appendicitis; made one of the first contributions on echinococcus of the liver. In 1897 appeared the reports of his research and clinical work in suture of arteries and veins, entitled "Resection of arteries and veins injured in continuity; end to end suture; experimental and clinical research."

Doctor Murphy delivered the annual oration on surgery at the Denver meeting of the Association in 1908, his subject being "Surgery of the Lung," in which he advocated the use of nitrogen gas in the production of artificial pneumothorax. His research work in neurologic surgery was published in 1907 under the title of "Surgery of the Spinal Cord." In 1912 was published his most important work on arthroplasty entitled "Contribution to the Surgery of Bones, Joints and Tendons." On February 1, 1912 appeared the first issue of Murphy's Clinics, published monthly, which chronicled his operations and lectures at Mercy Hospital.

Of his rare teaching and surgical talents, the best description is given by Sir Berkeley Monihan, the famous surgeon of Leeds, England, of Doctor Murphy in his clinics: "As he began to speak, one felt a strange sense of disappointment, even of dismay. For while the handsome face and upright figure were things of real beauty, the voice in which he began to speak was quite unpleasant. It was harsh, shrill, apt to wander into other keys ... but as he continued speaking, the voice gradually ceased to distract; it became smoother, quieter, and more evenly pitched, and all thought of it was now lost in rapt attention to the matter. For things were happening—the whole intellectual mechanism underlying a great subject was being shown both in detail and in all the majesty of moving parts. And then Murphy would operate. He was of the true faith; he believed in safe and thorough work rather than in spacious and hazardous brilliance. He was infinitely careful in preparation, and compared with many was inclined to be slow, but every step in every operation which I ever saw him do was completed deliberately, accurately, once for all. It led inevitably to the next step, without pause, without haste; that step completed, another followed. And so when the end came, a review of the operation showed no false move, nor part left incomplete, no chance of disaster; all was honest, sage and simple; it was modest rather than brilliant. During the whole operation, Murphy talked; not wasting time, but expressing and explaining aloud, the quiet, gentle, dextrous movements of his hands and purposeful working of his mind. When the operation was over he would draw his stool near the front row of seats, cross his legs, and talk as only he was able to talk—of surgery in general, of the case in particular, of his own faults and shortcomings, of special experiments made to elucidate, and of doubtful issues. His talk was now quiet, the fervor and passion of the operation gone. Absolute truthfulness was the dominant expression of Murphy's personality—he never looked at truth askance or strangely."

Doctor Murphy served as president of the Chicago Medical Society and the Clinical Congress of Surgeons of North America; he was a member of the Amercan Association of Obstetricians and Gynecologists; a Fellow of the American Surgical Association; a member of the Southern Surgical and Gynecological Association; a life member of the Deutsche Gesellschaft fur Chirurgie; honorary member of the Société de Chirurgie de Paris; an honorary Fellow of the Royal College of Surgeons of England, and a Fellow (Founders Group) of the American College of Surgeons.

In 1902 Notre Dame University conferred on Doctor Murphy the Laetare Medal, in 1905 the degree of LL.D. was given him by the University of Illinois, and the same degree by the Catholic University of America in 1915. The University of Sheffield, England, conferred on him the degree Master of Science in 1908.

Perhaps the most unique recognition that any surgeon has received came to Doctor Murphy in June 1916 from His Holiness, Pope Benedict XV—"the Christian Knighthood and the apostolic blessing"—an honor which was conferred upon him in recognition of his exceptional services to humanity and of his many works of Christian charity.

Those who attended the Los Angeles session of the Association in 1911 were impressed by the scholarly address, handsome appearance and charm of personality. When he received at the President's reception, with his beautiful wife and two charming daughters, it formed a picture to be remembered.

It is distinctly unfortunate that Doctor Murphy did not train a successor, no disciple to carry on his enthusiasm, his glow of life, his fervor and devotion to his work.

His last illness was of several months duration, due to aortitis and severe angina, and the end came while at Mackinac Island, Michigan, August 11, 1916, at the age of fifty-nine years.

After his death friends and Fellows of the American College of Surgeons, established the John B. Murphy Memorial Association which resulted in the building of a John B. Murphy Memorial adjoining the American College of Surgeons at 40 Erie Street, Chicago, and was dedicated with appropriate ceremonies on June 10 and 11, 1926. At the laying of the cornerstone October 23, 1923, William J. Mayo spoke: "This is a fitting monument to the greatest surgeon of his day, John B. Murphy, one of the founders of the College who gave unsparingly of his strength and talents to aid in the establishment of the organization, and whose noble spirit will always sanctify this ground."

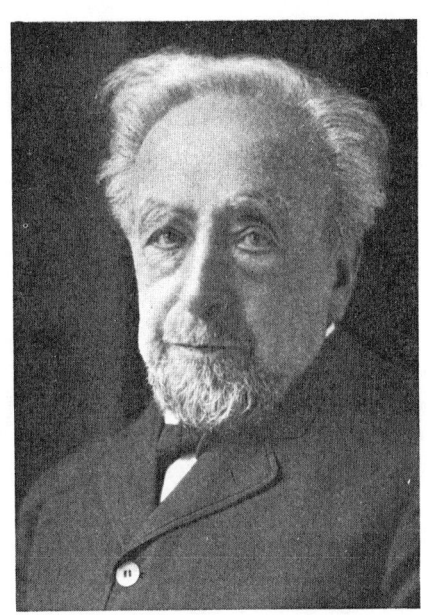

ABRAHAM JACOBI, M.D.
New York, N. Y.
1830–1919

Sixty-fourth President, A. M. A.
Atlantic City Session
June 3, 4, 5, 6, 7, 1912

DR. ABRAHAM JACOBI, the father of Amercan pediatrics, and the only specialist in pediatrics to be elected to the presidency, was for more than sixty years an active member of the Association and one of the most notable figures in American medicine.

He was born at Hartum, Westphalia, Germany, May 6, 1830. He studied at the Universities of Greifswald and Göttingen, graduating in medicine from the University of Bonn in 1851. After receiving his diploma he went to Berlin to take the state examination, and was recognized as having been intimately identified with the German revolutionary movement of 1848; he was promptly arrested and thrown into prison. He spent one and a half years in the fortress at Cologne, later at Minden and Bielefeld. In 1853 he managed to escape to England, and attempted medical practice for a time in Manchester and then migrated to America, settling first in Boston and later moved to New York City.

In 1860 the New York Medical College established the first professorship of infantile pathology and therapeutics, and invited Doctor Jacobi to accept this chair. In 1862 he established a pediatric clinic in the New York Medical College building where it remained for two years. In this way bedside instruction was inaugurated in America, which antedated bedside teaching in internal medicine in the United States. In 1864 Dr. Jacobi accepted a similar position in the University of New York, and in 1870 he became clinical professor of pediatrics in the College of Physicians and Surgeons, Columbia University, holding this position until 1890 when he retired as emeritus professor.

He early became a frequent contributor to medical literature; In 1859 he published a Treatise on Diseases of the Larynx, and Diseases of Women and Children; Dentition in 1862; The Education of Abandoned Children in 1872; Infant Diet, 1872; Diphtheria, 1876; Intestinal Diseases of Infancy and Childhood, 1887; Diseases of the Thymus, 1889; Therapeutics of Infancy and Childhood, 1896-1903; the latter being translated into Italian, Russian and German. History of American Pediatrics, 1902-1913; Cerebro-spinal meningitis, 1905, and History of Pediatrics in New York, 1917.

His most important papers, monographs and addresses were assembled in 1917, in eight volumes, in the Collectanea Jacobi. He was also the founder and first editor of the American Journal of Pediatrics.

During a long career, Doctor Jacobi held practically every honor which the medical profession can give to its members. He was the first president of the American Pediatric Society in 1889, and elected a second time in 1906; the first Chairman of the Section on Diseases of Children of the American Medical Association; President of the New York State Medical Society in 1882; of the New York Academy of Medicine from 1885 to 1889, and President of the Association of American Physicians in 1896. He was a member of many medical societies, both in this and foreign countries. Throughout his life he was associated with many eminent men, and numerous anecdotes are told of conversations with his early friend, Carl Schurz—a German outcast in 1848, of meetings with Austin Flint, Janeway, William H. Welch, William Osler, and may other noted statesmen and physicians. Although a German by birth, Doctor Jacobi was an ardent American. One of the most significant tributes of his life was the urgent invitation extended to him in October 1893, to become professor of pediatrics in the University of Berlin and this position he refused with the historic words—"I was, I am, rooted to the American profession that I have observed to evolve without governmental aid out of its own might to become equal to any on the globe."

In 1873, he married Dr. Mary Putnam, daughter of George P. Putnam (the American publisher). She was the first woman to be graduated from the Ecole de Medicine of Paris, receiving the degree Doctor of Medicine in 1871. As Dr. Mary Putnam-Jacobi she was a noted physician, medical author and teacher.

He was perhaps equally well known as a citizen. Doctor Jacobi was a formidable opponent of prohibition and an ardent advocate of birth control, and in every other matter of public interest he was a conspicuous character.

In his presidential address at the Atlantic City meeting in 1912, he spoke on the theme of infant feeding and particularly the importance of breast feeding. He was then in his 82nd year. The address was interesting, but of some length, and as a few of the audience became a bit restless, he stopped to say—"Gentlemen I have kept you long; if however, you are of the opinion of Cicero, who said that old age makes loquacious, please remember I have waited forty years to tell this story, and I will do so whether you remain or not."

Doctor Jacobi first registered at a meeting of the Association in New Haven in 1860, and was an active participant at annual meetings until the last, in June 1918 at Chicago when he was 88 years of age, and a conspicuous figure at all the meetings. As the years went by, that "leonine" head had become more and more familiar to the physicians of his adopted country.

Doctor Jacobi was in good health up to a day before his death. In September 1918 he had a narrow escape from death when his house at Lake George burned. The next year on his return to Lake George he occupied the residence of his distinguished compatriot, Carl Schurz, and it was in the house of this famous advocate of human freedom that the great and beloved physician died on July 10, 1919.

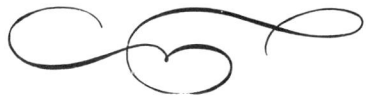

JOHN A. WITHERSPOON, M.D.
Nashville, Tenn.
1864–1929

Sixty-fifth President, A. M. A.
Minneapolis Session
June 16, 17, 18, 19, 20, 1913

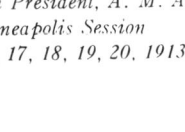

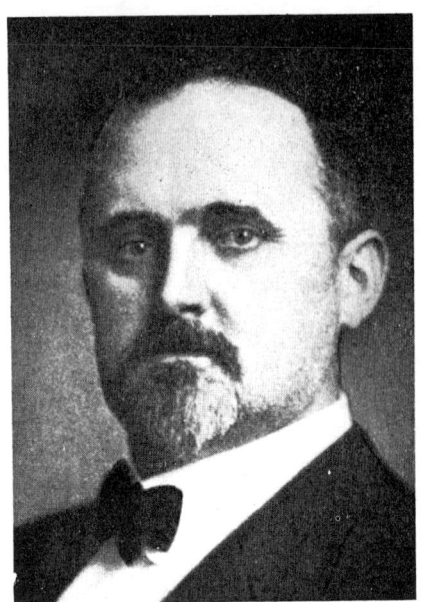

THE SELECTION OF DR. JOHN A. WITHERSPOON for the presidency of the Association was a recognition of his long service as a member of the Council on Medical Education and distinguished record as the leading physician in the South.

He was born in Columbia, Tennessee, September 13, 1864. His preliminary education was received in the local schools, after which he began the study of medicine at the University of Pennsylvania, graduating with the degree Doctor of Medicine in 1887. Soon afterward he began practice in Columbia, Tenn. Evidently his outstanding personality and scholarship won him early recognition and within a short time he was elected professor of medicine at the University of Tennessee College of Medicine at Nashville, but did not move to Nashville until 1895.

At this time efforts were being made to organize a medical school in connection with Vanderbilt University. This engaged the interest of Doctor Witherspoon, and for the remaining thirty-three years of his life he held the position of Professor of Medicine, and had a prominent part in the upbuilding of this medical school.

He furthermore had a substantial influence in gaining aid from various philanthropic agencies toward making this one of the leading medical institutions in the country.

Doctor Witherspoon became a member of the Association in 1890, and the records indicate that he rarely missed a meeting afterwards. In 1902 he was elected to the position of Vice-President, and in 1904 he became a member of the first Council on Medical Education, serving for nine years until 1913 when he assumed the duties of President. His advice and counsel during these formative years distinctly influenced the high standards which this council has maintained from the beginning of its work. He later was a member of the House of Delegates from 1922 to 1928. Doctor Witherspoon for many years was interested in the proceedings of the Association of American Medical Colleges and served as president in 1910–1911.

From 1908 to 1910 he was editor of the Journal of the Southern Medical Association.

His society affiliations included membership and president of the Tennessee State Medical Association; Mississippi Valley Medical Association, and the Southern Medical Association. He was a Fellow of the American College of Physicians.

In 1913 the University of Georgia conferred upon him the degree of Doctor of Laws.

Doctor Witherspoon was a delegate of the Association to the International Medical Congress in Budapest in 1912, where he was chosen the orator at the unveiling of a statue of George Washington erected in that city.

Because of his ability as a pleasing speaker and orator he frequently represented the profession at various ceremonies. Those who heard his eloquent response to the address of welcome at the New Orleans meeting in 1903, or his lecture on "Old Hickory" delivered at The Hermitage, Andrew Jackson's Home, near Nashville and on other occasions will retain the memory of his beautiful phrasing, fine diction and elocution that stamped him as a medical orator of high order.

Doctor Witherspoon likewise attained leadership as a medical educator and practitioner, and at all times lent a dignity and a charm to the profession of medicine.

Death came to him on April 28, 1929, at his home in Nashville at the age of sixty-four years.

VICTOR C. VAUGHAN, M.D.
Ann Arbor, Mich.
1851–1929

Sixty-sixth President, A. M. A.
Atlantic City Session
June 22, 23, 24, 25, 26, 1914

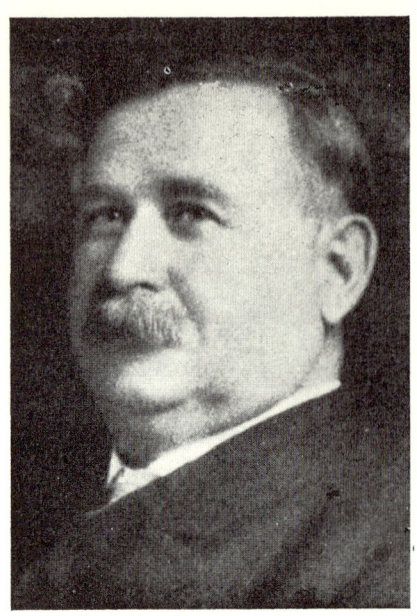

THE LIFE STORY OF DR. VICTOR C. VAUGHAN as physician, administrator, teacher, scientist, epidemiologist and patriot, impressed his personality into so many fields of medicine and thus made him a unique figure in American science and medicine.

No brief chronicle as this can therefore adequately evaluate the effects of his accomplishments on human society.

We learn much of his early life and environment from his delightful autobiography, "A Doctor's Memories," published a few years before his death. His birthplace was Mount Ayr, Randolph County, Missouri, and the date October 27, 1851. He first emerged from the obscurity of youth and adolescence at the age of nineteen as professor of Latin at Mount Pleasant College, Huntsville, Missouri. By accident he acquired a complete outfit for a chemical laboratory, and soon became fascinated with the work so that within a short time he taught chemistry along with his Latin. In 1874 he entered the University of Michigan to pursue his chemical studies, and a year later added the degree of M.S. to that of B.S. obtained in Missouri. In 1876 he received the degree of Doctor of Philosophy, and two years later that of Doctor of Medicine.

As early as 1875 Doctor Vaughan became associated with the medical school of the University of Michigan as instructor in medical chemistry. In 1878 he published a textbook on physiological chemistry which passed through three editions. In 1880 he was made assistant professor, and in 1883 he was promoted to a full professorship with the title of Professor of Physiological and Pathological Chemistry, and Associate Professor of Therapeutics and Materia Medica. He was the first to hold a chair of physiological chemistry in a medical school in this country, and to give chemical instruction from this point of view.

During the first twenty years after graduation, Doctor Vaughan engaged in the active practice of medicine, but his interests were always centered about the laboratory. While evidently a successful practitioner of medicine, and although interested in the individual patient, his heart was in the problems which affected the mass of the people.

His first contribution from the chemical laboratory in 1875 was on the separation of arsenic from other metals. Throughout the succeeding years the study of organic and inorganic poisons held great interest for him. This led to further interest in sanitary measures, the pollution of wells and poisoning from cheese and other milk products. His contributions to these subjects became authoritative, and he was recognized as one of the leading toxicologists in the country, so that his services were in constant demand in cases of medico-legal disputes.

Doctor Vaughan was a pioneer in public health in Michigan and for thirty years was a member of the Michigan State Board of Health. In 1888 he studied in Koch's laboratory in Berlin, visited the laboratories of Pettenkoffer in Munich, and Pasteur and Roux in Paris, who were creating the new science of bacteriology.

In 1889 the new hygienic laboratory was opened at the University of Michigan, and Doctor Vaughan served as director for twenty years. At this time his title was changed to Professor of Hygiene and Physiological Chemistry. As a result of investigation in this laboratory and experience in the field, in 1891 appeared the work with F. G. Novy on ptomaines, leucomaines and bacterial proteins; in 1902 cellular poisons; in 1913 protein split products in relation to immunity and disease; in 1913 infection and immunity, and in 1922 a three volume work on Epidemiology and Public Health with Henry F. Vaughan and George T. Palmer as co-authors.

In 1915 he became the first editor of the Journal of Laboratory and Clinical Medicine. He frequently expressed the view that no physician should practice medicine without laboratory aid, and he lived to see well equipped laboratories as part of every correctly managed hospital.

His service with the University of Michigan Medical School

covered a period of forty-five years as teacher and administrator. From 1891 to 1921, for thirty years, he served as dean of the medical faculty. His ability to gather about him outstanding leaders in the different fields of medicine, made his Alma Mater one of the best known medical schools in America.

During the Spanish-American War he became a victim of yellow fever at Siboney, Cuba, but upon his recovery he was assigned to duty with a Board of Medical Officers consisting of Majors Reed, Vaughan and Shakespeare to investigate the prevalence of typhoid fever in the various military camps. The final report, in two large volumes, was mainly prepared by Major Vaughan, and was a masterpiece of painstaking analysis, as well as an important contribution to knowledge regarding the spread of typhoid fever by flies and direct contact, as well as for typhoid prevention. Later in 1908 he became a member of a board to study anti-typhoid inoculation, which led to compulsory typhoid inoculation in the Army and Navy. This was considered an important factor in the low incidence of the disease during World War I.

During the first World War, Doctor Vaughan was assigned to duty as head of the communicable disease section in the Surgeon General's office. One of the most important services rendered by Colonel Vaughan had to do with numerous sanitary inspections of cantonments and military hospitals. His wide experience and the prestige of his name were of valuable assistance to General Gorgas in the control of the widespread appearance of measles, pneumonia, meningitis and influenza, which prevailed during those troublesome times. He was awarded the Distinguished Service Medal, "for his meritorious and conspicuous service."

In the Journal of the Association April 24, 1920 he published an article "Typhoid Fever in American Expeditionary Forces" being a clinical study of 373 cases, including 270 cases in which patients had received triple typhoid vaccine. The incidence was less than 0.1 per cent as compared with 20 per cent in the Spanish-American War.

All of Dr. Vaughan's five sons were in military service in the first World War. One of the tragedies of war that came to him was the loss of his namesake, Lt. Col. Victor C. Vaughan, Jr., M.C. in France.

His service with the American Medical Association covered a period of a quarter of a century in many capacities. He was a member of the House of Delegates from 1902 to 1906; in 1904 he was chairman of the Reference Committee on Medical Education, which recommended the formation of the Council on Medical Education, and of which he was a member from 1904 to 1913. After serving as president of the Association, he became chairman of the Council on

Health and Public Instruction from 1919 to 1923. During the last year of this period he was in the Association office assisting in the establishing of the new journal Hygiea. He served as chairman of the Division of Medical Sciences of the National Research Council during two years, 1922 and 1925.

Many further honors came to him: In 1897 the University of Western Pennsylvania conferred upon him the degree Doctor of Science and he received the degree Doctor of Laws from the following institutions: University of Michigan, 1900; Central College, Missouri, in 1910; Jefferson Medical College in 1915; and from the University of Missouri in 1923. In 1894 the University of Illinois had conferred upon him the honorary degree of Doctor of Medicine.

He served as president of the American Association of Physicians in 1908 and received the Kober medal in 1928.

His health began to fail in 1927 compelling his withdrawal from all activities, and he died at the home of his son, Dr. Warren T. Vaughan, in Richmond, Virginia, November 21, 1929. In the words of William J. Mayo, a former pupil of Dr. Vaughan: "He not only helped the members of the medical profession to a keener sense of their professional responsibilities, to the individual patient and to sick human beings collectively, but he induced them to live up to a standard of ethics which he himself followed all his life."

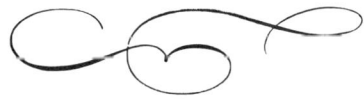

WILLIAM LEWIS RODMAN, M.D.
Philadelphia, Pa.
1858–1916

Sixty-seventh President, A. M. A.
San Francisco Session
June 21, 22, 23, 24, 1915

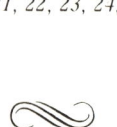

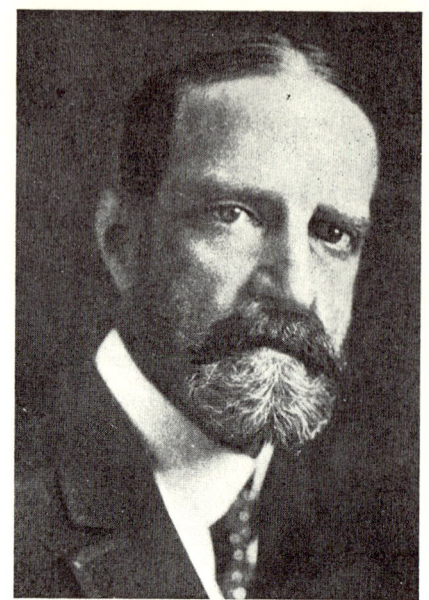

DR. WILLIAM L. RODMAN came to the office of the president after many years of service in the Association, and having gained recognition as a distinguished surgeon, medical educator, and founder of the National Board of Medical Examiners. He was the first president to die in office, and have his term completed by the Vice-President.

Doctor Rodman was born in Frankfurt, Kentucky, September 27, 1858, the son of General John Rodman, for many years Attorney General of Kentucky. His preliminary education was received at the Kentucky Military Institute from which he graduated in 1875 with the degree of Master of Arts. He later received the degree Doctor of Laws from the same institution. He commenced the study of medicine under the preceptorship of his uncle, Dr. James Rodman, and his cousin, Dr. W. B. Rodman, and graduated from Jefferson Medical College in 1879. After a service as interne in Jefferson Hospital, he entered the United States Army as acting Assistant Surgeon and was stationed for two years at Fort Sill, Indian Territory.

In 1882 Doctor Rodman was married to Betty C. Stewart, daughter of Dr. J. Q. A. Stewart, a well known alienist of Kentucky. He then practiced for two years in Abilene, Texas, after which he removed to Louisville and was appointed demonstrator of surgery in the Medical Department of the University of Louisville and clinical assistant to Dr. David W. Yandell (President A.M.A. 1872).

He continued in this position from 1889 to 1893 when he resigned to accept the professorship of surgery in the Kentucky School of Medicine, Louisville. In September 1898 he was elected professor of the Principles of Surgery and Clinical Surgery in the Medico-Chirurgical College of Philadelphia, and moved his residence to that city. From 1900 to 1908 he was also professor of surgery and clinical surgery in the Woman's Medical College of Pennsylvania at Philadelphia.

His first official connection with the Association was as Chairman of the Surgical Section in 1897; at the Denver meeting in 1898 in the absence of the president, Surgeon General Sternberg, he presided during the entire session.

In 1900 he delivered the oration on Surgery at the Atlantic City session on "Gastric Ulcer." He served on the Board of Trustees from 1900 to 1903. He was a member of the House of Delegates from Pennsylvania in 1905 and 1906; he served on the Committee on Legislation for many years, and for seven years was Chairman of the Committee on Reciprocity, until the work of this Committee was taken over in 1904 by the Council on Medical Education.

Doctor Rodman was a surgeon of unusual ability, and was specially interested in the early diagnosis and treatment of cancer. In 1904 he delivered an address on Cancer of the Breast before the British Medical Association. In 1908 he published a monograph on Diseases of the Mammary Gland, and chapters on this subject appeared in the International Textbook of Surgery, Keen's System, and Bryant and Bush System of Surgery.

His society affiliations include membership in the College of Physicians of Philadelphia, the American Surgical Association, International Surgical Association, the Association of Military Surgeons, and a Fellow of the American College of Surgeons (Founders Group).

The crowning achievement of his career was the founding of the National Board of Medical Examiners in 1915, of which he became the first secretary. As President of the Association of American Medical Colleges in 1903 and 1904 he had an opportunity to bring to the attention of medical educators the advantages of a voluntary national examining board maintaining the highest standards, the certificate of which would be accepted by boards of licensing examiners and other qualifying bodies.

In the following years, Doctor Rodman used every occasion to enlist interest in such a board of examiners, presenting it at several annual sessions of the Association, and in his presidential address at the San Francisco session in 1915 he announced the organization of the National Board of Medical Examiners, incorporated in the District of Columbia. The membership comprised representatives from the Council on Medical Education, the Association of American Medical Colleges, the Federation of State Medical Boards, and the three Federal medical services. For support in the early period a grant had been received from the Carnegie Foundation. After being approved by the Council on Medical Education, the Board began operations in 1916. It is fortunate that Doctor Rodman was privileged to see this significant undertaking become definitely established, and it thus will stand as his most enduring movement.

His death was due to an acute pneumonia, and occurred at his home in Philadelphia March 8, 1916, at the age of fifty-seven years.

The By-Laws of the Association provided that in case of the death of the President the vacancy shall be filled by the ranking Vice-President, and therefore Dr. Albert Vander Veer of Albany, New York, became president for the remainder of Doctor Rodman's term.

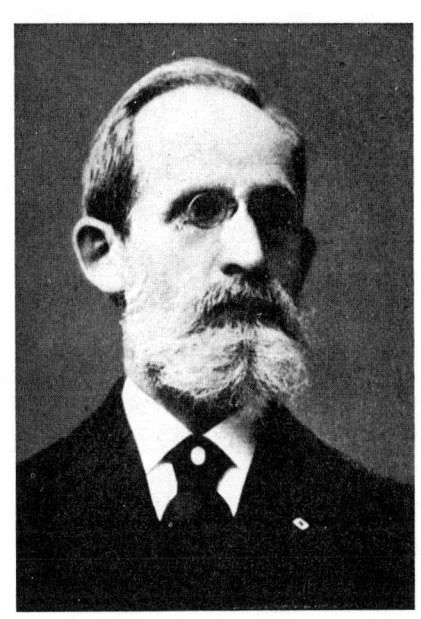

ALBERT VANDER VEER, M.D.
Albany, N. Y.
1841–1929

*Sixty-eighth President, A. M. A.
presiding at opening of
Detroit Session
June 12–16, 1916*

DR. ALBERT VANDER VEER was the first Vice-President of the Association to succeed to the presidency, following the death of President William L. Rodman on March 8, 1916, during his term of office.

He was born in Root, New York, July 10, 1841, and began the study of medicine at the Albany Medical College, but completed the course in the Columbian Medical College (now Medical Department of George Washington University, Washington, D. C.) and was granted the degree Doctor of Medicine in 1862. The Albany Medical College in 1869 conferred upon him the Honory degree of Doctor of Medicine. In 1882 he received a Master of Arts degree from Williams College, and a Doctor of Philosophy from both Union and Hamilton College in 1883. George Washington University conferred upon him the degree Doctor of Laws in 1904.

Soon after graduation in medicine in 1863, he was appointed Surgeon of the 66th New York Volunteers, and thus was the last president of the Association with a record of service in the Civil War.

Following his discharge from the Army he began practice in Albany, New York, and rapidly gained distinction as a teacher and surgeon. In 1869 he was elected Professor of General and Special Anatomy in the Albany Medical College, continuing until 1882, when he became Professor of Clinical and Abdominal Surgery, and in 1902 the title was changed to Professor of Surgery.

From 1896 to 1905 he served as Dean of the Medical Faculty. During most of the period he was Surgeon in Chief of the Albany County Hospital. He was also a Trustee of the Bender Hygienic Laboratory, and Regent of the University of the State of New York from 1895 to 1927, being Vice-Chancellor from 1915 to 1921, and Chancellor from 1921 to 1922.

His society affiliations included—President of the Albany County Medical Society, the Medical Society of the State of New York, the American Surgical Association, and the American Association of Obstetricians and Gynecologists; member of the Southern Surgical and Gynecological Association, International Surgical Association, British Medical Association, and Fellow of the British Gynecological Association, and the American College of Surgeons.

Doctor Vander Veer early in his career became affiliated with the American Medical Association, and was a frequent contributor to its proceedings. At the Nashville session in 1890 he presented an important address on "The Medico-Legal Aspect of Abdominal Section."

President Vander Veer presided at the opening meeting of the Association in Detroit in June 1916, and at the first session of the House of Delegates. In his address he stressed the need of more attention on the part of the profession to Medical Practice Acts, the importance of industrial diseases, and an urgent appeal for military preparedness by the Association and the organization of Base Hospitals by the American Red Cross under the direction of Colonel Jefferson R. Kean of the Army Medical Corps.

Doctor Vander Veer made an impressive record during his short term as president, reflecting a lifetime of leadership in the practice of surgery and civic medicine.

He died at his home in Albany on December 19, 1929, at the age of eighty-eight years.

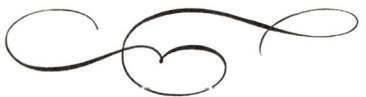

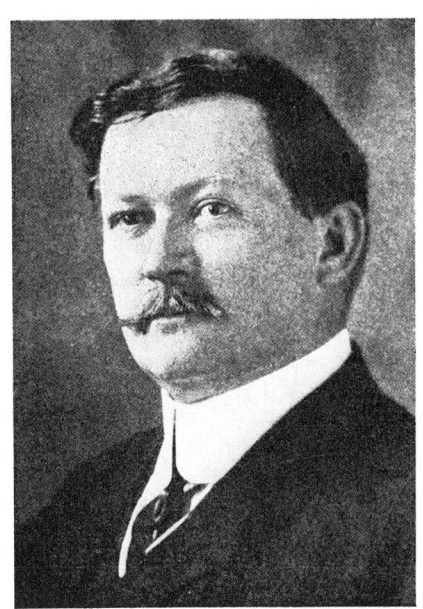

RUPERT BLUE, M.D.
Washington, D. C.
1867–

Sixty-ninth President, A. M. A.
Detroit Session
June 12, 13, 14, 15, 16, 1916

DR. RUPERT BLUE was the first Surgeon General of the United States Public Health Service to be elected for the presidency of the Association, in recognition of the remarkable development of public health work under his direction and particularly for his efficient service in the eradication of bubonic plague in San Francisco in 1903, 1904, 1907 and 1910. Doctor Blue is the oldest ex-president of the Association living in the Centennial year.

He was born in Richmond County, North Carolina, May 30, 1867, his parents moving shortly afterward to Marion, South Carolina. He was educated in the public and private schools, and attended the University of Virginia in 1889 and 1890. Doctor Blue graduated from the University of Maryland with the degree Doctor of Medicine in 1892, and received the degree Doctor of Science from that institution in 1908. Immediately after receiving his medical degree in 1892 he entered the U. S. Public Health Service as intern in a Marine Hospital; became Assistant Surgeon in 1893; Passed Assistant Surgeon in 1897, Surgeon in 1909, and Surgeon General in January 1912. During this time he was stationed at Baltimore, Galveston, Charleston, San Francisco, Portland, Oregon, Milwaukee, New York, Norfolk and New Orleans, having been assigned to hospital, quarantine and other public health duties, which was a fitting preparation for the responsibilities and duties concerned with the office of Surgeon General of this important Government service.

When cholera threatened our shores in 1900 the President of the United States sent Doctor Blue to Italy to study one of the sources of this disease. In 1903 and again in 1907 he was placed in charge of plague eradication measures in California, and handled a difficult situation with the result not only that the disease was controlled, but also that all interests in the State were harmonized. The latter was the most important single work he performed, and during its conduct he advanced and proved the principle that rat proofing is the essential means necessary to prevent plague in urban communities. He demonstrated that the eradication of plague is entirely practicable and, in consequence, that cities may be kept free from the disease.

In 1905 he was second in command of the measures taken in New Orleans and vicinity to eradicate yellow fever.

As Director of Sanitation of the Jamestown Exposition in 1907, Doctor Blue had practical experience in the reduction of mosquito-breeding areas to prevent malaria. After completion of the course in Tropical Diseases at the London School of Tropical Medicine in 1910, he was assigned as adviser to the Governor of Hawaii for the reduction of mosquito-breeding areas in that territory, with the object of guarding against the introduction of yellow fever and malaria after the opening of the Panama Canal. It was from this duty that he was called to become Chief of the Service. In 1910 he was appointed the United States delegate to the International Medical Congress in Buenos Aires, Argentine.

In 1913 he received the honorary degree of Doctor of Science from the University of Wisconsin, and Doctor of Public Health from the University of Michigan.

In his presidential address to the House of Delegates at the New York session in 1917 he urged the appointment of a committee to outline recommendations for the best method of utilizing the facilities of the American Medical Association in preparing for war. This was promptly approved, and a committee appointed comprising Dr. Arthur D. Bevan, Chairman, Dr. Alexander Lambert and Dr. John W. Kerr, which was an important step in mobilizing the medical profession for military service.

After the expiration of his service as Surgeon General in 1919 he was placed in charge of the activities of the United States Public Health Service in Europe, from 1920 to 1923, and represented the Service at the Office Internationale de Hygiene Publique in Paris. During this period he also was the American delegate to the Conference of the League of Nations at Geneva, and served as adviser to the United States Mission at the Lausane Peace Conference in 1922 and 1923.

Doctor Blue is a Fellow of the American Public Health Association, a member of the American Society of Tropical Medicine, and an honorary member of the San Francisco County Medical Society. He was also a member of Phi Beta Kappa Society. In 1925 he received the honor of Chevalier of the Legion of Honor of France.

Since his retirement from the U. S. Public Health Service in 1931, and a career of eminence in every field of public health, he has resided in Washington, D. C.

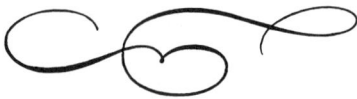

CHARLES HORACE MAYO, M.D.
Rochester, Minn.
1865–1939

*Seventieth President, A. M. A.
New York Session
June 4, 5, 6, 7, 8, 1917*

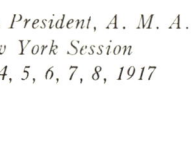

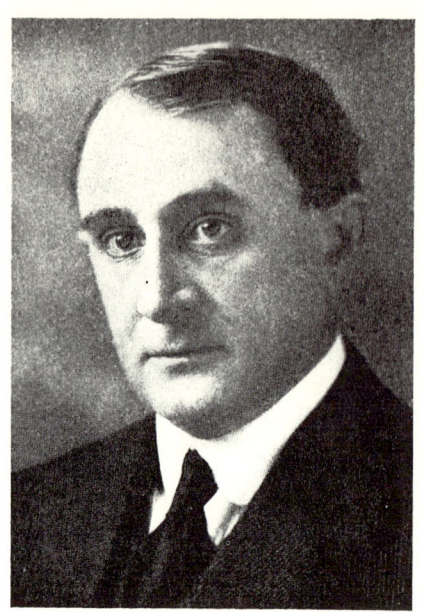

THE HONOR OF THE PRESIDENCY came to Dr. Charles H. Mayo, the younger of the Mayo brothers, in recognition of his great surgical leadership and his constant devotion to the advancement of organized medicine.

He was born in Rochester, Minn., July 19, 1865, the son of Dr. William Worrall Mayo and Louise Wright Mayo. After an education in the Rochester high school and at the Niles Academy, he attended Chicago Medical College, later known as Northwestern University, and received the degree Doctor of Medicine in 1888. He grew up in a medical atmosphere and early became inspired toward medicine as a career. After graduation he returned to Rochester, where his urge toward research and his surgical genius led to innumerable investigations in medicine and surgery. His first published statement was a joint contribution with his brother, Dr. William J. Mayo, entitled "Report of Clinic at St. Mary's Hospital, Rochester, Minn., January 19, 1891" which was published in the Northwest Lancet in November of that year. From that time on hardly a year passed without a contribution by either Dr. Charles H. Mayo alone, or with his brother, or with some of the younger men who soon became attracted to him. These contributions cover every phase of medicine and surgery and in later years embrace as well the fields of philosophy, economics and statesmanship. It has been estimated that Dr. Charles has to his credit 413, and Dr. Will 650, contributions to surgical literature.

In the field of scientific medical organizations Dr. Charles H. Mayo was president of Western Surgical Association in 1904, the Minnesota State Medical Association in 1905, the Society of Clinical Surgery in 1911, the Clinical Congress of Surgeons of North America in 1914, the American Medical Association in 1917, the American College of Surgeons in 1924, the American Surgical Association in 1931, and the Minnesota Public Health Association from 1932 to 1936.

Many of the greatest universities in the world conferred honorary degrees on him. Thus the Master of Arts degree was conferred by Northwestern University in 1904, fellowship in the Royal College of Surgeons in England in 1920 and in the Royal Society of Medicine in 1926, and Master in Chirurgery by Trinity College of Dublin in 1925. He was made Doctor of Public Health by the Detroit College of Medicine and Surgery in 1927 and Doctor of Science by Princeton University in 1917, the University of Pennsylvania in 1925 and the University of Leeds in England in 1909. He also received the honorary degree of LL.D. from the University of Maryland in 1909, Kenyon College in 1916, Northwestern University in 1921, the University of Edinburgh in 1925, Queen's University in Belfast, Ireland, in 1925, University of Manchester in England in 1929, Hamline University in 1930, and Carleton College in 1932.

A number of great nations also honored him with citations for distinguished service, the record including officer de l'Ordre national de la legion d'honneur, France, 1925; officer de l'Instruction publique et des beaux-arts, France, 1925, and Cross of Knight Commander of the Royal Order of the Crown of Italy, 1932, as well as citations from many other countries.

During the first World War he and his brother, Dr. William J. Mayo, alternated between Rochester, where they maintained graduate study for physicians entering the service, and the personnel department in Washington. They served also as consultants in surgery.

Dr. Charles H. Mayo was commissioned Major on April 19, 1917, Colonel June 15, 1918, and Brigadier General Nov. 22, 1921. He received the distinguished service medal of the United States Army on June 7, 1920.

When Dr. Charles H. Mayo gave his inaugural address as president of the Association at the session in New York City in June 1917, he appeared in uniform. The title of his address was "War's Influence on Medicine." It was of historic significance that twenty-five years later when the United States had again become engaged in a World War, the presidential address was given by his son-in-law, Colonel Fred W. Rankin, of the Medical Corps of the U. S. Army.

With Dr. William J. Mayo he received the citation for distinguished service by the National Organization of the American Legion, and was presented with a commemorative plaque, the special ceremony being conducted by President Franklin D. Roosevelt in person August 8, 1934. That the President of the United States should come to Rochester to join in honoring the Mayo brothers seemed to many the culminating triumph of their career. This impressive ceremony was held in the Mayo Park and attended by many of the country's medical and civilian great.

His memberships in distinguished civic and medical organizations, both American and foreign, are far too long to list. He gave freely of himself and of his work to many scientific and general publications. He served as health officer of the City of Rochester from 1922 to 1939 and as a member of the school board of that city.

In 1915 Drs. William J. and Charles H. Mayo established the Mayo Foundation for Medical Education and Research in Rochester, affiliating this organization with the University of Minnesota. Their first contribution was $1,500,000 which was later increased to more than $2,650,000. In order to perpetuate this institution, the Mayo Properties Association was established in 1919 to hold all the property, endowments and funds of the Mayo Clinic, and to insure the permanence of the institution for public service with the understanding that the moneys and property can never inure to the benefit of any individual.

At the time of his death, Dr. Morris Fishbein expressed the following tribute: "Dr. William J. Mayo, Dr. Charles Horace Mayo and their distinguished father made a small village become one of the most notable medical centers of the world. Throughout their careers these distinguished leaders devoted themselves to the advancement of organized medicine. The medical society of the county in which they practiced was founded by Dr. William Worrall Mayo. Dr. Charles H. Mayo was widely known not only as a surgical genius, as a great surgical teacher, as an inspired organizer, as a leader in medical advancement and as a citizen of his city, county, state and of the nation, but also as a warm hearted, genial, faithful, true humanitarian, easily approachable, unostentatious, ready to trade wits and banter, always in the most kindly and sympathetic manner. Such men come but infrequently in any civilization and their places are not easily filled as the world moves on."

Dr. Charles H. Mayo died of acute pneumonia while visiting in Chicago May 26, 1939 at the age of seventy-four years.

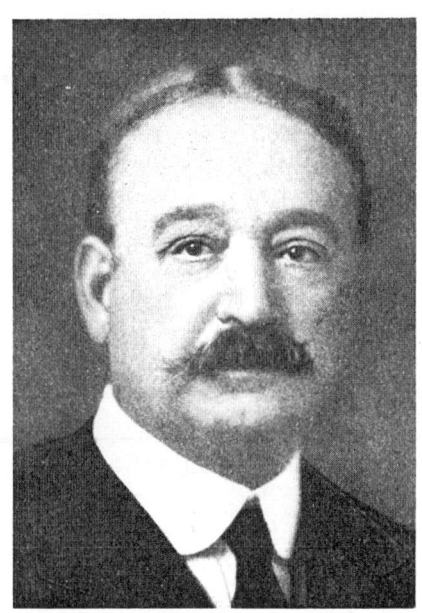

ARTHUR DEAN BEVAN, M.D.
Chicago, Ill.
1861–1943

Seventy-first President, A. M. A.
Chicago Session
June 10, 11, 12, 13, 14, 1918

THE SELECTION OF DR. ARTHUR DEAN BEVAN for the presidency was largely in recognition of his services as the first chairman of the Council on Medical Education, covering then a period of fifteen years and his leadership and eminence in the field of surgery.

He was born in Chicago, August 9, 1861, the son of a physician. His preliminary education was completed at Sheffield Scientific School of Yale University in 1879. After graduating from Rush Medical College in 1883, Doctor Bevan joined the United States Marine Hospital Service, and served until 1888. During this period, for one year, in 1886, he was professor of anatomy at the University of Oregon Medical School, Portland. In 1887 he responded to a call from Rush Medical College to become professor of anatomy, which position he held until 1889 when he was appointed associate professor of surgery, and professor of surgery in 1902. During 1892 and 1893 he visited the surgical clinics of England, Scotland and the principal European medical centers; while in Vienna he formed a friendship with Dr. Anton von Eiselsberg, first assistant of Professor Billroth, which endured through many years. In 1907 he was made head of the department of surgery, and in 1934 the title was changed to Nicholas Senn Professor of Surgery.

His association with Rush Medical College covered a period of forty-seven years, during which he maintained a close affiliation with

Presbyterian Hospital, joining the staff in 1892 as attending surgeon, and serving from 1894 until 1934 as head of the surgical service.

Doctor Bevan was a skillful surgeon, and he evolved many new procedures including the S shaped incision for surgical operations on the liver and bile tracts, and the "hockey stick" incision to expose the gallbladder without cutting through nerves.

It was in Doctor Bevan's service at the Presbyterian Hospital that ethylene-oxygen was first used clinically as an anesthetic. In 1931 he presented a comprehensive paper before the Association entitled "Present Status of the Anesthesia Problem," in which he discussed the method to prevent the possibility of static spark in the operation room.

In 1902 Doctor Wyeth, the president of the Association, appointed Doctor Bevan as Chairman of the Committee on Medical Education, and in 1904 when the Council on Medical Education was created, he was chosen as the first chairman and occupied the position until 1928. The only interruption in his service on the Council was the two years he was president-elect and president of the Association from 1917 to 1919. The only other member who had as long a service on the Council was Dr. Ray Lyman Wilbur (Pres. A.M.A. 1923) who served from 1921 to 1946.

During his long service on the Council on Medical Education Doctor Bevan had an important part in shaping its policies, and in influencing the trend of medical education towards continuing higher standards. It was a period when the Council became the recognized standardizing agency of medical schools. A new classification of schools was inaugurated, resulting in some hundred and fifty medical schools, largely established on a commercial basis, being reduced to half that number, and thus the approved u iversity medical school came into being. It represented an evolution in American medical education that was the marvel of the entire educational world.

Doctor Bevan was a man with a driving personality; a forceful character that gave strength to his leadership for the advancement of medical education. His disdain for personal criticism, and his fearlessness when attacked, did much to promote the great success of the Council on Medical Education in achieving its objectives.

During the first World War, Doctor Bevan served as director of general surgery in the surgical division of the Surgeon General's office in Washington. In recognition of his services as President of the Association, he was made an officer of the Legion of Honor of France.

In 1902 and 1903 Doctor Bevan was a member of the House of

Delegates, and he served as Chairman of the Section on Surgery and Anatomy in 1906 and 1907.

Doctor Bevan had many medical society affiliations; president of the Chicago Medical Society in 1898; membership in the American Association of Anatomists; American Urological Association and Society of Clinical Surgery; he was a founder and member of the first Board of Governors of the American College of Surgeons; president of the Inter-State Post-Graduate Medical Assembly in 1931, and president of the American Surgical Association in 1932. He was also a diplomate of the American Board of Surgery (Founders Group), and at various times was an officer in the American Society for the Control of Cancer.

Aside from Doctor Bevan's numerous contributions to surgical literature, he wrote many articles reflecting his early interest in medical education, the prohibition movement, and other subjects. He was a charter member of the Institute of Medicine of Chicago, and with Dr. Dean Lewis he edited and published "The Lexer-Bevan Surgery."

In 1929 he, with his wife, announced a million dollar gift to Presbyterian Hospital, Chicago, for its expansion program, and principally for the provision of medical services.

After his retirement from the different surgical services in 1934, he was retained as consultant to the time of his death.

He had certain business interests, such as Director of the Diamond Match Company, and others that engaged some of his time in later years.

He remained vigorous and mentally clear, and died at his home in Chicago, June 10, 1943, at the age of eighty-one years, of acute myocardial failure precipitated by an acute respiratory infection.

Of Doctor Bevan it may be said that he played a major role in life and combined well the parts of good citizen, good friend, surgeon and educator.

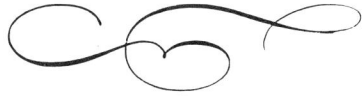

ALEXANDER LAMBERT, M.D.
New York, N. Y.
1861–1939

Seventy-second President, A. M. A.
Atlantic City Session
June 9, 10, 11, 12, 13, 1919

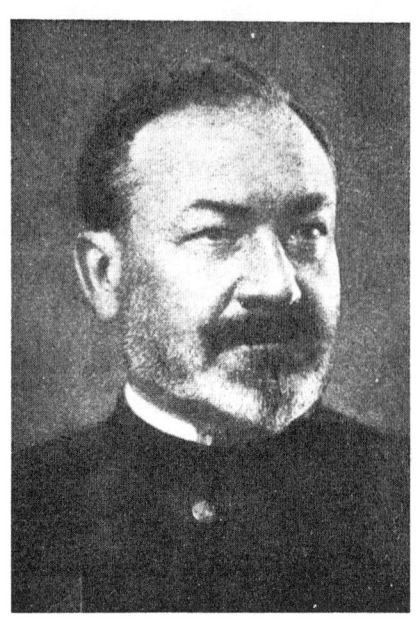

DR. ALEXANDER LAMBERT, distinguished physician of New York City, was honored with the presidency by reason of his outstanding service as Chairman of the Judicial Council, as Director of American Red Cross activities in France and Belgium during World War I, and an earnest worker in the cause of American medicine.

Doctor Lambert was a member of a noted medical family; born in New York City, December 15, 1861, the son of Dr. Edward W. Lambert, for 45 years chief medical advisor of the Equitable Life Assurance Society. His brother Samuel W. Lambert was for many years Dean of the Medical Faculty, College of Physicians and Surgeons of Columbia University, and another brother Dr. Adrian S. Lambert was Professor of Surgery in the same institution.

Doctor Lambert received a very complete literary and professional education. He graduated from Yale University with the degree Bachelor of Arts in 1884, and Bachelor of Philosophy in 1885, the latter degree being awarded for research in metabolism with Professor Russell H. Chittenden. He received the degree Doctor of Medicine from the College of Physicians and Surgeons of Columbia University in 1888.

After graduation in medicine he served one year as intern in Bellevue Hospital, and from 1889 to 1890 as house physician in the Midwifery Dispensary on Broome Street, New York City. He then spent two years in further study in the larger medical centers of Europe. Upon his return in 1892 he became associated with Dr. T. Mitchell Prudden, pathologist, and Dr. William H. Park, bacteriologist, in the investigation of tetanus and diphtheria antitoxin. In 1894 he entered private practice in New York City, and the same year was appointed attending physician at Bellevue Hospital, which service he retained until 1933. In connection with his practice, he was assistant bacteriologist of the New York City Department of Health from 1894 to 1901. He early joined the Faculty of Cornell University Medical College, and for many years until 1931 was Clinical Professor of Medicine.

During his entire medical career Doctor Lambert maintained a keen interest in all matters pertaining to the welfare of physicians and took an active part in medical organization.

In his professional work he was specially interested in the diseases of the heart and the circulation, and in problems concerned with alcoholic and narcotic addiction; for the latter condition he devised a plan of treatment which was usually referred to as the "Lambert Method." He contributed liberally to medical literature dealing with drug addiction and circulatory diseases. In 1927 he served on the Mayor's Committee on Narcotic Addiction, and also as a member of the New York State Commission on the same problem.

Doctor Lambert was an active member of the American Heart Association from the beginning of its organization. His membership in other medical societies included the Association of American Physicians, the Harvey Society, the New York Academy of Medicine, the American Association for the Advancement of Science, the American College of Physicians and the Medical Society of the State of New York, of which he was president in 1917.

His services in the American Medical Association were highly significant and in keeping with his leadership in medical affairs. In 1904 he was Chairman of the Section on the Practice of Medicine; in 1909 he was elected third Vice-President of the Association, and in 1911 served as a member of the House of Delegates. In 1911 he became a member and chairman of the Judicial Council, continuing until his election as President in 1918. In this capacity he served also as Chairman of a Committee on Social Insurance named in 1916 as a subcommittee of the Council on Health and Public Instruction. This report was submitted at the New York session of the House of Delegates in June 1917, and was a most comprehensive analysis of all forms of social and sickness insurance operating at that time in England, Scandinavia, Germany and other European countries. The report covered 34 pages of small type when published in the Journal of the Association June 21, 1917. The final conclusions were significant in the light of thirty years ago; these stated "that the study indicated a world wide movement for social insurance, and had become an important part of industrial legislation in many countries; an evident wide acceptance of the principle that industrial accidents should be compensated, with protection of the worker from the hazards of illness by sickness insurance; that this was of special concern to the medical profession, and therefore recommended that the Council on Health and Public Instruction be authorized to continue the study and make reports on the future developments of social insurance legislation in this country, and urging that such legislation provide for freedom of choice of physician by the insured; that the physician be paid in proportion to the service rendered, and that there be a separation of medical official supervision from the function of daily care of the sick, as well as adequate representation of the medical profession in appropriate administrative bodies."

This report was adopted by the House of Delegates. At this session a further tribute was extended to Dr. Lambert in a resolution prepared by Dr. Arthur T. McCormack of Kentucky, in recognition of his outstanding work on the Judicial Council and his selection as the special representative of the profession with the armed forces over seas.

In 1907 Doctor Lambert became a member of the Medical Reserve Corps, U. S. Army; soon after this country entered the World War in April 1917, Major Lambert was ordered to active duty in France as Chief Medical Adviser of all American Red Cross activities in France and Belgium. He returned to the United States to attend the Association meeting in Chicago in June 1918 to present a further report as Chairman of the Judicial Council. Immediately following the close of the session at which he was chosen president-elect, he returned to his military duties in France. In his address to the House of Delegates in 1919 he spoke of the influence and value of the modern hospital as a teaching institution and advised that a Council on Hospitals be established. This was later incorporated with the Council on Medical Education.

The title of his presidential address at the Atlantic City session in 1919 was "Medicine—A Determining Factor in War." He lauded the remarkable response of the medical profession to the call of duty; the success of preventive medicine in comparison with former wars; the value of lessons learned in determining action for the future, particularly with regard to the educational needs of the medical profession, and finally made a strong plea for the establishment of a National Board of Health.

Doctor Lambert developed a large practice in New York City and numbered many influential citizens among his patients. Early in his career he became closely associated with Theodore Roosevelt, later President of the United States, acting for many years as his personal physician and also accompanying him on hunting and fishing trips.

Doctor Lambert is credited with having been instrumental in influencing President Roosevelt to retain Dr. William C. Gorgas as Director of Sanitary Work during the building of the Panama Canal, after an attack had been made on Doctor Gorgas for his emphasis on mosquito control by some of the lay officials in charge of building the canal; the Secretary of War, William H. Taft, had also advised his recall. President Roosevelt asked Doctor Lambert in regard to the matter and received the terse advice "Keep Gorgas or there will be no canal." After the death of former President Roosevelt in 1919, Doctor Lambert became the Director of the Roosevelt Memorial Association.

Death came to Dr. Alexander Lambert, the distinguished leader in medicine, inspiring organizer and influential physician, on May 9, 1939, at seventy-eight years of age.

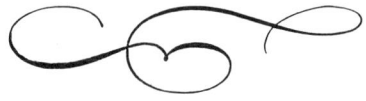

WILLIAM C. BRAISTED, M.D.
Washington, D. C.
1864–1941

Seventy-third President, A. M. A.
New Orleans Session
April 26, 27, 28, 29, 30, 1920

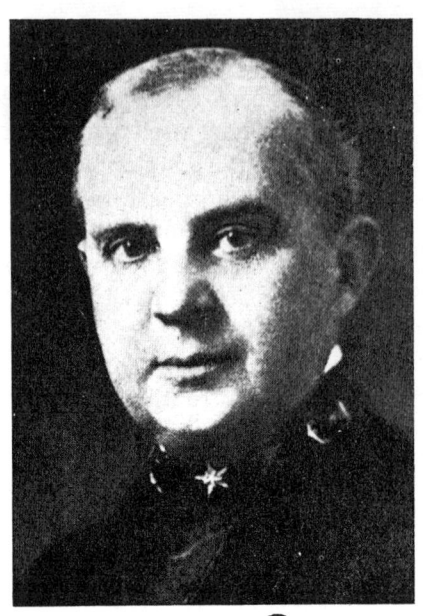

DR. WILLIAM C. BRAISTED, Admiral M.C., U. S. Navy, was the only Surgeon General of the United States Navy elected to the presidency of the Association. His selection was a further recognition of the efficient services rendered by the Medical Corps of the United States Navy during the first World War.

He was born in Toledo, Ohio, October 6, 1864. He received the degree Bachelor of Arts from the University of Michigan, Ann Arbor, in 1883, and the degree Doctor of Medicine from the College of Physicians and Surgeons, Columbia University, in 1886. After the completion of a two year hospital internship at Bellevue Hospital, New York City, he practiced medicine in Detroit from 1888 to 1890, and then entered the Medical Corps of the U. S. Navy as assistant surgeon. He had his full share of sea duty, and served on many naval vessels. His first sea duty was on the celebrated dynamic gunship the "Vesuvius"; it was while serving on this ship that he was decorated by the President of Venezuela for caring for the wounded after a battle at Puerto Cabella during a revolutionary outbreak. In 1904 he fitted out and equipped the Hospital Ship "Relief." During the Russo-Japanese war he was stationed in Japan and represented the medical department of the Navy. His report on the "Naval Medical and Sanitary Features of the Russo-Japanese War" covered 82 pages and was a most accurate and informative narrative and of definite historic value.

In 1906 and 1907, during the administration of President Theodore Roosevelt, he was an attending physician at the White House. From 1906 to 1912 he was assistant chief of the Bureau of Medicine and Surgery, and assisted in its re-organization. Doctor Braisted was fleet surgeon of the Atlantic fleet from 1912 to 1914, when he was appointed by President Wilson, Surgeon General, Chief of the Bureau of Medicine and Surgery with the rank of Rear-Admiral. Thus as Surgeon General he had official responsibilities through the trying times before, during and after the first World War; the personnel of the Navy expanded from 55,000 officers and men to over 600,000; the tasks of the Navy increased in magnitude, including the protection of convoy lanes, the transport of the American Expeditionary forces, and vast quantitites of military material. It required the maintenance of naval patrol in all oceans. All vessels were manned with medical personnel and in addition three hospital ships were fitted out and medical units served with the Marines fighting on the Western front of the Army. For his services as Surgeon General of the Navy he was awarded the Distinguished Service Medal, and he also received a decoration from the Emperor of Japan.

He was elected an honorary Fellow of the Royal College of Surgeons of Edinburgh in 1919. The University of Michigan conferred upon him the degree Doctor of Laws in 1917; Jefferson Medical College, Philadelphia, conferred the same degree in 1918. In the same year he received the Doctor of Science degree from Northwestern University, Chicago. He was a Fellow of the American College of Surgeons (Founders Group). In 1913 he served as president of the Association of Military Surgeons of the United States.

When the National Board of Medical Examiners was organized in 1915, Surgeon General Braisted was chosen as the first president and continued in that position until 1920. While stationed in Washington he served as president of the Board of Directors of Columbia Hospital for Women, and was on the board of visitors of St. Elizabeth Hospital.

The presidential address of Admiral Braisted presented at the New Orleans session in April 1920, while rather lengthy, was a comprehensive exposition of the subject "Obligations of Medicine in Relation to General Education." He emphasized the need of educating the public in matters of health, and the teaching of hygiene in primary and secondary schools; he reviewed the work of the National Board of Medical Examiners of which he was president, for its first five years, and outlined the influence on medical education particularly in stimulating the addition of preventive medicine and public health to the courses of study in medical schools. He also urged the need of a Federal Department of Health.

Doctor Braisted retired from the medical corps of the Navy soon after the end of his term as president of the Association, with the rank of Rear Admiral, and then accepted the offer to become president of the Philadelphia College of Pharmacy and Science, in which position he served until 1926. Several years afterward Admiral Braisted withdrew from all medical and civic activities largely because of impaired health, and died at his home in West Chester, Pennsylvania, January 18, 1941 at the age of seventy-six years.

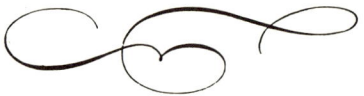

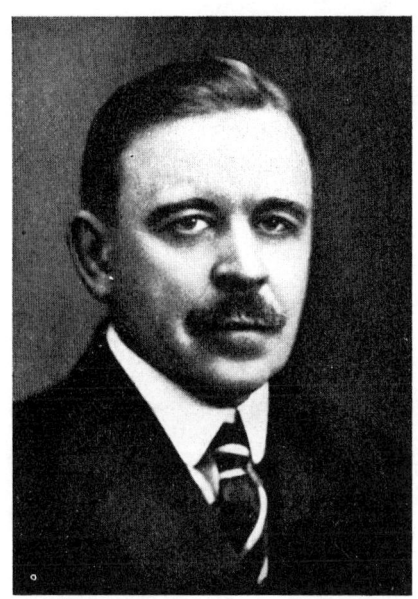

HUBERT WORK, M.D.
Denver, Colo.
1860–1942

Seventy-fourth President, A. M. A.
Boston Session
June 6, 7, 8, 9, 10, 1921

DR. HUBERT WORK was the first speaker of the House of Delegates to be elected to the presidency of the Association. During a service of five years in this position, his special talents as a parliamentarian and presiding officer were recognized, and this coupled with his professional leadership naturally led to his being selected for this high honor.

He was born in Marion Center, Pennsylvania, July 3, 1860. He attended the Indiana State Normal School from 1877 to 1881, and then began the study of medicine at the University of Michigan Medical School, Ann Arbor, but completed his course at the University of Pennsylvania from which he received the degree Doctor of Medicine in 1885. Soon after graduation he began the practice of medicine at Greeley, Colorado. After a number of years he moved to Pueblo, Colorado, to devote his attention mainly to psychiatry, and in 1896 founded the Woodcroft Hospital for nervous and mental diseases, serving for nearly twenty-five years as its physician in charge. He was also superintendent of the Woodcroft School for Feebleminded Children. He rapidly gained recognition as an able clinician and psychiatrist. He was elected a member of the Central Neuropsychiatric Society, and in 1911 Doctor Work served as President of the American Medico-psychological Association which later became the American Psychiatric Association.

He was for many years consulting physician and psychiatrist of the Colorado Fuel and Iron Company Hospital, and the Colorado State Insane Asylum at Pueblo. He also served for a long time as president of the Board of Trustees of the Colorado School for the Deaf and the Blind.

Doctor Work became a Fellow of the American College of Physicians in 1921.

His deep interest in medical developments is further indicated by his service on the Colorado State Board of Medical Examiners from 1889 to 1892, and on the Colorado State Board of Health from 1895 to 1905, serving as president of the Board from 1899–1900. In 1894 he was elected president of the Colorado State Medical Society.

In 1904 he began his first term as a member of the House of Delegates, and from that time served the Association continuously as a member of the House, as a member of the Judicial Council, and then as speaker from 1916 until his election as president in 1920.

It was as Speaker of the House that the members became acquainted with his rare talents as a parliamentarian and his ability to infuse a spirit of progress and cooperation that assured efficient action.

His theme for the address as president of the Association at the Boston meeting in June 1921 was "Some Medical Problems," and reflected a clear concept of the changing order of medical practice; he directed attention to need of more graduate instruction and better service in rural communities. From his experience in public health, he drew the lesson of having better assurance of local health service by the establishment of health centers. He contended that such local health services as well as standardized hospitals were a state and community responsibility.

The increasing extent of group practice was considered another significant trend in medical practice.

During the first World War, Doctor Work rendered meritorious service as medical advisor to the Provost Marshal General. It was in this capacity that his diplomatic qualities were of inestimable service in correlating the work of the medical department of the Army with that of the Provost Marshal General's office. At the conclusion of the War he became a Colonel in the Medical Reserve Corps of the Army.

Important responsibilities took him out of the active practice of his profession, but his faithful attendance at many medical meetings and his loyal devotion to his medical colleagues, attested to his never failing interest in the welfare of the medical profession.

As a citizen he achieved the distinction of candidacy for the United States Senate, being defeated only by a small majority. In

1908 Doctor Work was a delegate at large to the Republican National Convention, and subsequently served as chairman of the Colorado State Central Committee, and member of the Republican National Committee.

In 1921 he was appointed first Assistant Postmaster General by President Harding. A year later he became a member of the Cabinet as Postmaster General, and on March 5, 1923 he was named Secretary of the Department of the Interior, serving in this position until June 24, 1928. The following year he was chairman of the Republican National Committee.

Doctor Work's death in St. Joseph's Hospital, Denver, of coronary thrombosis, December 14, 1942, closed a long and distinguished life. He was a kindly man, endearing himself to everyone by his affability; yet calm and reserved, he inspired cooperation and efficiency and was ever ready for usefulness with kind comment and witty repartee.

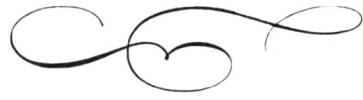

GEORGE E. de SCHWEINITZ, M.D.
Philadelphia, Pa.
1858–1938

Seventy-fifth President, A. M. A.
St. Louis Session
May 22, 23, 24, 25, 26, 1922

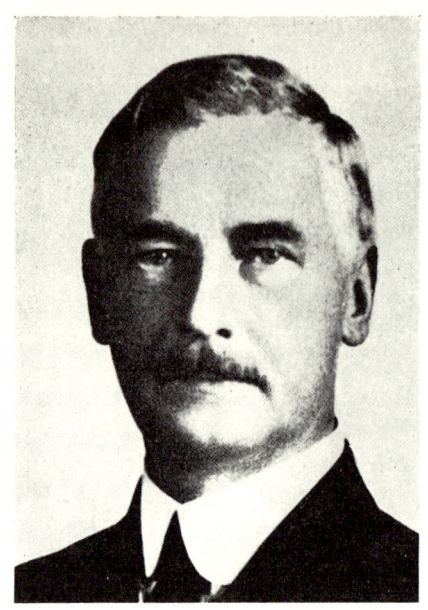

DR. GEORGE E. DE SCHWEINITZ, in the words of a colleague, Casey A. Wood, was the most widely known and the most erudite of American ophthalmologists. His election to the presidency of the Association was a fitting recognition of his specialty, but also of one of the distinguished men in American medicine.

His ancestry goes back to Moravian nobility. He was born on October 26, 1858 in Philadelphia, the son of the Right Reverend Edmund de Schweinitz, Bishop of the Moravian Church. He attended the Moravian Parochial School in Bethlehem, Pennsylvania, and later entered the Moravian College in 1872, receiving the degree Bachelor of Arts in 1876, and in 1878 the degree Master of Arts. Three years later he graduated with honors from the School of Medicine of the University of Pennsylvania, winning the Hodge Gold Medal for "proficiency in anatomy." At the same time he was also awarded the Henry C. Lea prize for his thesis on "Painful Tumors with special reference to Neuromata."

Immediately after leaving medical school, Doctor de Schweinitz was appointed a resident physician in the University of Pennsylvania Hospital, and later to the Children's Hospital, serving these institutions for a period of two years. He began practicing medicine in 1883, and devoted the next four years to general work. During this time under the direction of Dr. William F. Norris he began to devote his attention to diseases of the eye, especially the relation of the eye to general diseases. He developed this important part of ophthalmology in many later contributions. In a very short time he won the respect and confidence of the older men in the profession, who referred many unusual and difficult cases to him for study.

His first experience in teaching medicine began in 1883 as quizmaster on therapeutics. For five years he conducted this most popular and successful quiz in the university, and for three years was prosector to Dr. Joseph Leidy, professor of anatomy and the greatest American student of biology. In 1885 he became ophthalmic surgeon at the Children's Hospital; the following year ophthalmologist to Orthopedic Hospital and Infirmary for Nervous Diseases, where he became associated with Dr. S. Weir Mitchell. In 1887 he was appointed ophthalmologist at the Philadelphia General Hospital (Old Blockley). From 1891 to 1892 he was a lecturer on medical ophthalmoscopy at the University of Pennsylvania, and from 1891 to 1894 was professor of ophthalmology in the Philadelphia Polyclinic and College for graduates in medicine. In 1892 Doctor de Schweinitz was appointed clinical professor of ophthalmology in the Jefferson Medical College, and in 1896 professor of ophthalmology. Then in 1902 he became professor of ophthalmology in the medical school of the University of Pennsylvania, where he served with distinction until 1924, when he became Emeritus Professor.

Because of his unusual ability as administrative officer, he was elected a trustee of the University of Pennsylvania in 1924, and appointed Chairman of its Board of Medical Affairs in 1928.

Early in his career he became closely identified with the work of the profession in many different medical societies, including the Philadelphia County, Pennsylvania State, and American Medical Association; the Philadelphia Pathological and Neurological Societies, and Honorary Fellow of the New York Academy of Medicine; Fellow of the American Academy of Ophthalmology and Otolaryngology, and the American College of Surgeons. He served as president of the College of Physicians of Philadelphia, 1910–1913; of the American Ophthalmological Society in 1916, and the International Congress of Ophthalmology in 1922. He was also a member of the American Philosophical Society, and Vice-President of the Pennsylvania Institute for the Instruction of the Blind.

He was secretary of the Section on Ophthalmology of the American Medical Association in 1891–92, and Chairman 1896–1897. In his election to the presidency in 1921 the Association recognized one of the leading ophthalmologists of the world, and placed at the head of its Scientific Assembly a leader in medical science, who while following a specialty in medicine, had kept in close contact with general medical interests.

His address as president in 1922 was an interesting historical review of American medical achievements, and the activities of the American Medical Association during its first seventy-five years. It was a story of medical progress for that period, remarkable in its accuracy and coverage of the entire field of medicine.

During World War I he was appointed to the Council on National Defense in 1917, and commissioned a Major on April 9, 1917, being advanced to Lieutenant Colonel in May 1918. He was ordered to duty in the Surgeon General's office in September 1917 and went overseas in October, remaining until March 1918. He returned to the office of the Surgeon General as Officer-in-Charge of ophthalmology, and established the School of Ophthalmology in the Medical Officers Training Camp at Fort Oglethorpe. At the end of the war he was appointed consultant in ophthalmology and made a member of the editorial board of the medical history of the war. In April 1919 he was commissioned Colonel, and in 1922 Brigadier General in the Medical Reserve Corps.

During his long and succcessful career, and as a result of the great esteem in which he was held, Doctor de Schweinitz received numerous awards, including several honorary degrees. The University of Pennsylvania conferred upon him the degree Doctor of Laws in 1914; and the Moravian College, the degree Doctor of Letters in Humanity; in 1923 from the University of Michigan, the honorary degree of Doctor of Science, and the same degree from Harvard University.

He was the recipient of the Alvarenga Prize in 1894, awarded by the Philadelphia College of Physicians for his essay on "Toxic Amblyopias"; awarded the bronze plaquette of the Société Française d' ophthalmologie in 1923; the Howe medal in ophthalmology in 1927, and the Huguenot Cross in 1928. He gave the Bowman Lecture before the Ophthalmological Society of the United Kingdom, and was elected an Honorary Member of the society. He was an honorary member of the Ophthalmological Section of the Royal Society of Medicine, London, and of the Hungarian and Egyptian Ophthalmological societies. He gave the Alpha Omega Alpha Lecture in 1931. He was awarded the Leslie Dana Medal for meritorious work among the blind, the medal bearing the inscription "wise, learned, patriotic, teacher and guide." For this award he received the personal congratulations of President Herbert Hoover.

Doctor de Schweinitz was widely known for his contributions to the science of ophthalmology, having devoted his research particularly to toxic amblyopias, the relation of acute intoxication to ocular disorders, pathologic changes of various ocular diseases, relation of cerebral decompression to the cure of choked disk, ocular angiosclerosis, pathogenesis of choked disk, relation of focal infection to ocular diseases, blindness in Guernsey cattle, comparative ophthalmology, ophthalmic surgery and pulsating exophthalmos. For this investigative work he achieved wide recognition.

The greatest literary contribution made by Doctor de Schweinitz was his authoritative "Textbook on Diseases of the Eye," which appeared in 1892 and passed through ten editions. He participated in the editing and publishing of seven additional textbooks in his field, and his original papers numbered hundreds.

He never married, but devoted himself assiduously to his chosen profession. As a consultant, his attitude towards the members of the medical profession was ideal. He was essentially a doctor's consultant. He was in great demand as a public speaker, and his after-dinner speeches were prepared with the same care that he gave his scientific addresses. He was fond of walking, but never participated in any of the popular sports. His principal diversion was reading, and he liked a good detective story.

It will be noted that Doctor de Schweinitz was conspicuous as a recognized leader in every activity in which he took part. He represented the highest type of scholarly gentleman. When he spoke it was with poetic and polished diction and always in behalf of the highest ideals of medical science. His manner was kindly and his presence was the personification of the dignity coupled with the sincerity and humanly characteristics of the truly great physician. His graciousness and nobility was for many years a tradition among physicians.

He died at his home in Philadelphia August 22, 1938, being nearly eighty years of age. Soon after his death the Section on Ophthalmology of the College of Physicians of Philadelphia established a Lectureship in his honor. The first lecture was delivered by Dr. Edward Jackson of Denver on November 17, 1938.

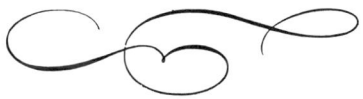

RAY LYMAN WILBUR, M.D.
San Francisco, Calif.
1875–

Seventy-sixth President, A. M. A.
San Francisco Session
June 25, 26, 27, 28, 29, 1923

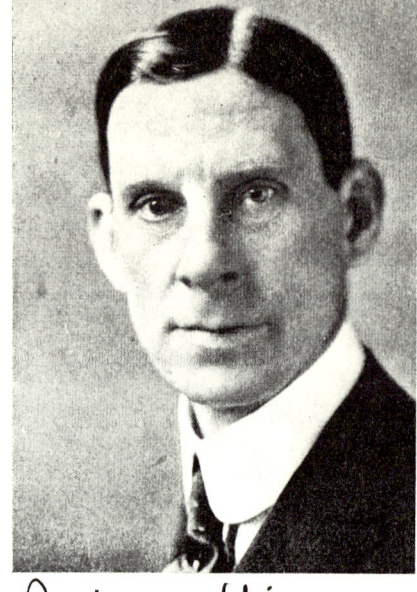

THE SELECTION OF DR. RAY LYMAN WILBUR for president was a fitting recognition of a man typifying the highest ideals in medicine, with a conspicuous talent for administration and leadership. He is the only university president to be elected to the presidency of the American Medical Association.

Doctor Wilbur was born in Boonesboro, adjoining the present city of Boone, Iowa, April 13, 1875, and removed to California when a boy. He graduated from the Riverside High School, and received his A.B. degree from Leland Stanford Junior University in 1896 and the A.M. degree the year following. In 1899 he received the degree Doctor of Medicine from Cooper Medical College of San Francisco, which later became the medical department of Leland Stanford University. He served as instructor in physiology at Stanford University from 1896 to 1897. Soon after his graduation in medicine he was lecturer and demonstrator in physiology at Cooper Medical College from 1899 to 1900, and assistant professor of physiology from 1900 to 1903. At this time he went to Europe studying at Frankfurt and London. Upon his return he began practice in San Francisco, and in 1909 he continued further studies in the University of Munich. In 1909 he was appointed professor of medicine in the Medical School of Stanford University. In 1911 he became Dean of the Medical Faculty. Following the retirement of President David

Starr Jordan of Stanford University in 1913, Professor John Casper Branner, head of the geology department, was made President with the understanding that he was to retire at sixty-five years of age, two years later. At that time, the latter part of 1915, the trustees of Stanford University, in recognition of his extraordinary administrative ability, selected Doctor Wilbur for the position of president. He served in this high office with great distinction until 1942 when he became Chancellor of the University.

With the entrance of the United States into World War I, Doctor Wilbur was called by another Californian, Mr. Herbert Hoover, to assist in one of the fundamental activities necessary to a successful prosecution of the conflict as Chief of the Conservation Division of the United States Food Administration. For this service he earned the gratitude of the entire civilized world.

At the 1920 session of the American Medical Association, Doctor Wilbur was appointed to the Council on Medical Education and Hospitals, and in 1929 upon the retirement of Dr. Arthur Dean Bevan he became Chairman and continued until June 1946, after completing more than a quarter century of service on this Council. In this work he showed a thorough insight and sympathy at all times with the problems of the practicing physician and with the problem of properly coordinating the work of various social agencies with that of the medical profession. In his long period of service on the Council he has had a prominent part in the expansion of its activities as a standardizing agency of medical schools, hospital internships and residencies, and the advisory planning of postgraduate medical education.

His annual reports as Chairman presented to the annual Congress on Medical Education and Licensure were an index of progress during the year in the training of physicians, but likewise gave a clear portent of the problems ahead. Doctor Wilbur has been an outstanding personage in the whole field of medical education in its relation to pedagogy and humanitarian interests.

He served on the California State Board of Medical Examiners in 1902 and 1903; president of the American Academy of Medicine in 1912 and 1913, and president of the California Academy of Medicine in 1917.

In the Association of American Medical Colleges he served as president in 1925, and for many years on the Executive Council. His address as President of that Association at the Boston meeting in 1925 was on the subject "The Future Practitioner" and reflected his clear insight into the problems concerned with medical practice in this country.

As Trustee of the Rockefeller Foundation from 1923 to 1940 and a member of its General Education Board from 1930 to 1940, he was afforded further opportunity for his superior qualifications in education and administration.

When President Herbert Hoover became President of the United States in 1929, he invited Doctor Wilbur to become a member of his Cabinet, as Secretary of the Department of Interior, serving until 1933. This was the second instance of a past president of the American Medical Association being chosen Secretary of the Interior, the first being Dr. Hubert Work in 1923.

From 1927 to 1932 he was Chairman of the Committee on the Cost of Medical Care, which made careful surveys of medical education, public health and the different forms of medical service available to the people of the United States. While the final reports led to considerable controversial discussion, the large amount of fact-finding data collected will be of great value for future reference.

From 1929 to 1931 Doctor Wilbur served as Chairman of the White House Conference on Child Health and Protection, called by President Herbert Hoover, which permitted the assembling of much valuable information from prominent experts concerned with different phases of child health.

He has been a member and enthusiastic worker in the American Social Hygiene Association, and its President since 1936. He received the award of the William F. Snow Medal in 1943. In presenting the citation, Doctor Keyes referred to the recipient of the medal as "experienced and wise in practice, research and teaching of medicine and public health," "Leader in recognizing and adapting new knowledge to social betterment without prejudice or handicap of tradition," and "Wise, farseeing and active in the development and support of sound public policies and effective measures for the welfare of the Nation and its citizens."

Doctor Wilbur has been the recipient of many honorary degrees: Doctor of Laws from the Universities of California and Arizona in 1919, University of Pennyslvania in 1925, of New Mexico in 1928, of Pittsburgh and Chicago in 1929, of Maryland, Duke, Princeton and Rochester in 1930, Puerto Rico, New York and Yale Universities, the University of the State of New York, Southern California and Tusculum College in 1931, and the University of Illinois, Wesleyan and Dartmouth College in 1932. Syracuse University conferred upon him the degree Doctor of Science in 1924, and Western Reserve University in 1931. He received the degree Master of Arts in medicine from Hahnemann Medical College of Philadelphia in 1931.

In 1920 he received the decoration of Commander, Order of

Leopold II, and Chevalier French Legion of Honor, and the Honor Cross of the German Red Cross in 1925.

Doctor Wilbur served as Chairman of the Medical Council of the U. S. Veterans Bureau from 1924 to 1929. In 1928 he was the United States delegate to the sixth Pan-American Conference.

He is a member of Phi Beta Kappa and Sigma Xi societies, and since 1928 has been a director of Alpha Omega Alpha Honor Medical Society. Since 1936 he has been Chairman of the American Institute of Pacific Relations; member of the National Executive Committee, Boys Scouts of America since 1939, President of Motion Pictures Research Council since 1935, and President of California Physicians Service since 1939.

This is by no means a complete list of activities in which this versatile personality is engaged.

Doctor Wilbur is at home at Stanford University, California.

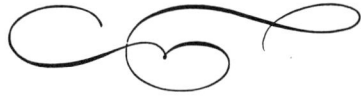

WILLIAM ALLEN PUSEY, M.D.
Chicago, Ill.
1865–1940

Seventy-seventh President, A. M. A.
Chicago Session
June 9, 10, 11, 12, 13, 1924

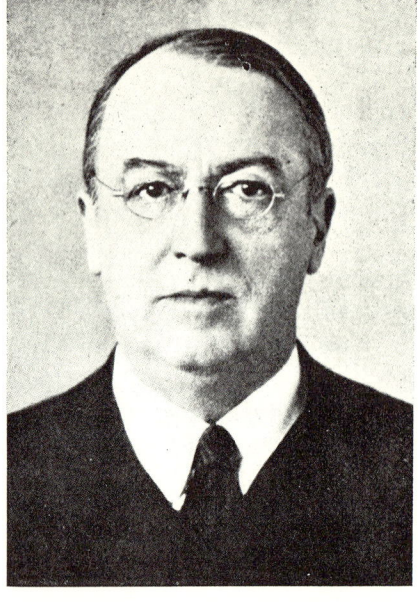

DR. WILLIAM ALLEN PUSEY was a distinguished dermatologist and the only physician practicing that specialty ever to be selected for the presidency of the Association. His election was a further recognition of many years of active service in Association affairs.

Dr. Pusey was born on December 1, 1865 in Elizabethtown, Ky., "in a rural county in the Middle South—a land of red clay hills seamed by fertile valleys." On his mother's side Dr. Pusey was a descendant of the Browns, adventurous Kentucky pioneers who migrated from Virginia in 1782. The Puseys were Quakers, and they were among the pioneers who had come to America with William Penn. At sixteen years of age he entered Vanderbilt University at Nashville, Tenn., from which he received his Bachelor of Arts degree in 1885, and a Master of Arts degree in 1886. In the fall of 1886 he entered the Medical College of New York University graduating in 1888 with the degree Doctor of Medicine. He later published an article on "Medical Education—From the Student's Point of View," in which he forcibly criticized the system of didactic lectures then in vogue and suggested that an effort be made to make of the student an active agent in the exchange of ideas between teachers and students.

After graduation he spent two years working at the Skin and Cancer Hospital in New York, and then planned to continue his studies in Europe. Unfortunately after being in Europe but a few months he was called home because of the death of his father, a physician, to assume his practice and settle the affairs of the estate. After a year of general practice he returned to Europe and remained two years studying under the great teachers in Vienna, Berlin, Paris and London. He settled in Chicago in 1893, the year of the Columbian Exposition, and began the practice of dermatology. He rapidly gained recognition in his specialty, and a year later he became professor of dermatology in the College of Physicians and Surgeons, Chicago. This gave him an opportunity to establish a department and to test his own ideas of medical education. He soon was known as a popular lecturer and an inspiring teacher. He became executive secretary of the medical college, and in that capacity was largely instrumental in effecting the affiliation between the College of Physicians and Surgeons and the University of Illinois, which was a real accomplishment. He occupied the chair of dermatology until 1915, when he resigned because of "other demands upon his time," and he was elected professor emeritus.

Among his important achievements in medicine was his pioneer work with roentgen therapy. From 1900 he reported at intervals on his experiences with roentgen rays in the treatment of a large number of disorders of various types, and in February 1902 Doctor Pusey presented a paper on "Cases Treated by X-rays" before the Chicago Medical Society, which was a clinical demonstration of some forty cases of lupus, carcinoma of the breast and of the head and neck, sarcoma, keloid, leukemia and various kinds of granuloma. This experience was published in book form in 1903, entitled "The Practical Application of the Roentgen Rays in Therapeutics and Diagnosis," which was enthusiastically received and has since been termed as one of the foundations of American reoentgenology.

Doctor Pusey was one of the first (1907) to advocate solid carbon dioxide, "carbon dioxide snow," for use in certain lesions of the skin.

For many years he was dermatologist to Cook County Hospital. He was three times president of the Chicago Dermatological Society, and in 1900 was elected president of the American Dermatological Association.

In 1907 appeared his textbook "Principles and Practice of Dermatology," which passed through four editions. His interest in the activities of the American Medical Association began with his membership in the House of Delegates in 1906. In 1911 he was elected Treasurer of the Association, and continued in that office until 1922.

In 1915 he presented his paper on "Syphilis as a Modern Problem" at the San Francisco session, which was later published as a monograph under the direction of Surgeon General Gorgas. Two years later when the United States became involved in World War I, Doctor Pusey was invited by the Surgeon General of the Army to become his advisor in matters pertaining to venereal diseases. At the suggestion of Major Pusey the work was put in charge of a committee of five members of which he was chairman. An extremely valuable work was written by the Committee entitled "Manual on Treatment of the Venereal Diseases" of which 125,000 copies were distributed by state boards of health all over the country. While he was active in this service he was elected president of the Chicago Medical Society in 1918.

In his inaugural address as president of the Association in 1924, "Some of the Social Problems of Medicine," he pointed out that the social organization was undergoing a revolution, and that medicine was going with it. This was written in 1924—"Medicine is particularly exposed to the dangers of socialization, because the projects of socialism that obtain the first acceptance are those that have to do with health and physical welfare. There is an evident tendency to take the treatment of the sick away from the individual physician's responsibilities and to transfer it to the State; to turn it over to organized movements. If this movement should prevail to its logical limits medicine would cease to be a liberal profession and would degenerate into a guild of dependent employees."

In his address to the House of Delegates he pleaded for a modification of the undergraduate curriculum, so that the medical student could enter the clinical years at an earlier age. His main thesis was the high cost of medical training. The change in the preliminary training to be: "Education in an accredited high school as was required at the time; three years of training in a medical college; internship in a hospital of not less than a year and a half, and lastly, a proper selection of students on the grounds of fitness." According to his plan practitioners were to be turned out in from four to four and a half years after leaving high school. Doctor Pusey would not allow that this program would in any sense lower medical standards. He asserted that rather by proper selection of high grade students and more emphasis and time spent on clinical hospital and bedside work, the end product would be more efficient and would be able to render a higher standard of medical service.

Doctor Pusey suddenly became a public figure, and invitations to address medical and lay audiences came from all over the country, of which he accepted as many as possible, speaking mainly on the topic of medical education and medical economics.

In 1920 he influenced the Trustees of the American Medical Association to publish the "Archives of Dermatology and Syphilology" of which he was the editor in chief for the first sixteen years. A special number, January 1937, was issued in his honor.

Doctor Pusey held honorary membership in a number of state medical societies, and in many foreign societies of dermatology and syphilology. He was a member of Phi Beta Kappa Society and Alpha Omega Alpha Honor Medical Society.

One of his important services in medical education was as a member of the Commission on Medical Education, a body composed of nineteen distinguished educators, lay and medical, headed by President Lowell of Harvard University, which, after five years of study issued its comprehensive report on Medical Education in 1932.

As a member of the Executive Committee, Century of Progress Exposition in Chicago, 1933 and 1934, he accomplished a distinct service for medicine and the allied sciences. Being at the same time a member of the Executive Committee of the National Research Council, he was able to secure the services of about four hundred of the leading scientists of the United States as an advisory group to develop one of the most interesting and informative exhibits of the Century of Progress.

The avocational excursions of Dr. Pusey into the field of history, philosophy and polite literature, revealed him as a man of extensive knowledge of many subjects other than medicine, of refined tastes, cultured and scholarly.

In 1921 appeared his "A Country Doctor of the 1870's and '80's" based largely on the diary of his grandfather, one of Kentucky's medical pioneers. He sketched true to life the noble type of general practitioner, a portrait of the saddle-bag physician of an earlier day.

In his presidential address before the Institutes of Medicine of Chicago in 1907 on the "Importance of being Historically Minded" he takes up the old subject of the science of medicine versus the art of medicine. It forms a sensible discussion of the place and value of research, of bedside practice, of empiricism, and of the true meaning of science. His "History of Dermatology" appeared in 1932, and "History and Epidemiology of Syphilis" in 1933. One of his most interesting efforts was the Prosser-White Oration on "Disease, Gadfly of the Mind," presented in 1934 before the British Association of Dermatology and Syphilology. This reveals a wide knowledge of medicine and the cognate sciences, as well as a mature reflection and historical mindedness of a high order. His last paper of a historical nature was presented before the Institutes of Medicine, January 9, 1940, on "Highlights in the History of Chicago Medicine."

Of Doctor Pusey it may well be said that he met his responsibilities and lived a life of great usefulness. He died in Chicago August 29, 1940, of chronic heart disease at seventy-four years of age.

WILLIAM D. HAGGARD, M.D.
Nashville, Tenn.
1872–1940

Seventy-eighth President, A. M. A.
Atlantic City Session
May 25, 26, 27, 28, 29, 1925

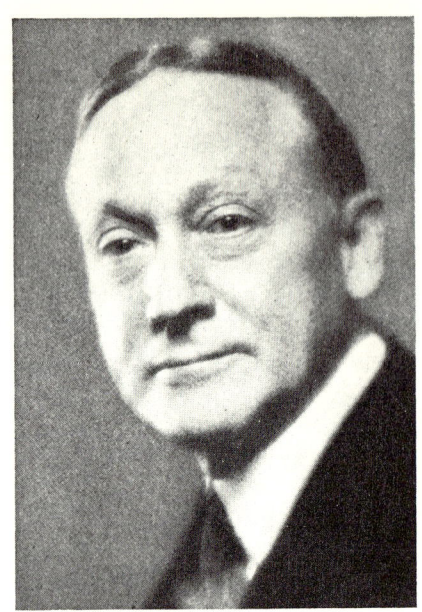

THE SELECTION OF DR. WILLIAM D. HAGGARD for the presidency of the Association was a recognition of his eminence as a surgeon, of the medicine of the South, of his service in the advancement of medical education, and of the qualities of leadership and congeniality which he possessed to a high degree.

He was born in Nashville, September 28, 1872. It is interesting to note that the name of his father, Dr. William David Haggard, appears frequently in the early Transactions of this Association; he was also the first president and one of the founders of the Southern Surgical Association. The son received his preliminary education in the schools of Nashville, and graduated from the University of Tennessee Medical Department with the degree Doctor of Medicine in 1893. Soon afterwards he began practice in Nashville.

In 1896, he was appointed assistant professor of gynecology in his Alma Mater, and in 1900 professor of gynecology and abdominal surgery. He served in the latter capacity until 1912, when he became professor of surgery and clinical surgery at Vanderbilt University Medical School, and served in this position the remainder of his life. He held the position of surgeon and first president of the Staff at St. Thomas Hospital, and that of visiting surgeon at Vanderbilt University Hospital.

After the declaration of war in April 1917, Doctor Haggard was appointed by Surgeon General Gorgas on the Advisory Board of the Division of Surgery and was first on duty in the office of the Surgeon General in Washington. Later he served as Major and Lieutenant Colonel in the Medical Corps of the Army, and acted as surgeon to Evacuation Hospital No. 1 at Toul, France, and later as consultant in surgery at the Mesves Hospital Center.

In the American Medical Association, Doctor Haggard held many positions of importance. In 1898 and 1899 when he was only twenty-six years old, he was chosen secretary of the Section on Surgery; he served again in 1909 and 1910, and as chairman of the Section in 1916-1917. He was a member of the House of Delegates in 1905, 1906, and 1922. In 1912 he became a member of the Council on Medical Education and Hospitals, serving continuously until 1921.

When he was chosen president-elect in 1924, in his brief acceptance speech, he enunciated his great belief in the possibilities of preventive as well as curative medicine, expressing the dictum—"Prevention runs as a thread of gold through the fabric of medicine."

His address as president in 1925 on the "Romance of Medicine" permitted full play for his eloquence and charm of delivery. He originated the activating concept and importance of having a thorough physical examination on one's birthday. Since then the "periodic health examination" has become the accepted educational policy of the medical profession and a slogan of health agencies. This address with other papers was published in book form in 1927.

Through many of his addresses before medical and surgical associations, the theme of preventive medicine was a prominent feature. In his address as president of the Tennessee State Medical Association in 1914 on "Present-day Problems of the Medical Profession" he discussed some new frontiers in the development of public health in this country; the concluding paragraph was significant: "Every physician, no matter how engrossed with the exacting care of those entrusting their lives and health to him, must not fail to interest himself in the larger community interests that relate to the prevention of disease and the wholesome saving of human life."

Doctor Haggard was instrumental in aiding the organization of the American College of Surgery, serving as regent for a number of years, and becoming president in 1933. His address as president entitled "Surgery, Queen of the Arts" with other papers and addresses was published in 1935. His further contributions to medical literature included numerous scientific articles, covering particularly the surgery of appendicitis, goitre and carcinoma.

He was a member of the American Surgical Association, the

Society of Clinical Surgery, and the Southeastern Surgical Congress. Doctor Haggard was further honored with the presidency of the Nashville Academy of Medicine, the Middle Tennessee Medical Association, and vice-president of the Pan-American Medical Congress.

Doctor Haggard was a distinguished gentleman, a masterly surgeon, a facile speaker and raconteur, and widely recognized as a diplomat in medical affairs.

His life's philosophy may be somewhat envisioned by quotations which he gave in beginning and concluding a notable address delivered at the University of Toronto in 1934 on "Seeds of Time"; this was a discussion of the genesis of chronic disease, with a decided philosophical slant. He began by quoting from Macbeth: "If you can look into the seeds of time, and say which grain will grow and which will not, speak then to me," and closed with the quotation, "So live that when thy eternal summons comes, be able and resigned to say: 'Earth you have shown us all; I am ready for the call.' "

Death came to him at Palm Beach, Florida, where he had gone for a brief vacation on January 28, 1940, at the age of sixty-seven years.

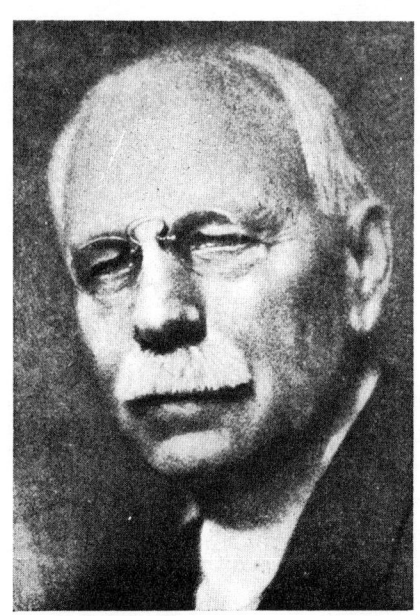

WENDELL C. PHILLIPS, M.D.
New York, N. Y.
1857–1934

Seventy-ninth President, A. M. A.
Dallas, Session
April 19, 20, 21, 22, 23, 1926

THE SELECTION FOR PRESIDENT of Dr. Wendell C. Phillips, distinguished otologist, champion of the cause of hard of hearing, founder of the American federation of organizations for that purpose, was a fitting recognition of his leadership in this field and of many years of service to organized medicine, and of seven years of exceptional service as Trustee of the Association.

He was born in Hammond, St. Lawrence County, New York, June 9, 1857, and received his preliminary education at the Potsdam (New York) Normal School, graduating in 1879; he then began the study of medicine at the University Medical College of New York University, from which he received the degree Doctor of Medicine in 1882. Soon afterward he began the practice of medicine in New York City, continuing for a period of fifty-two years. He promptly devoted himself to diseases of the ear, nose and throat, becoming aural surgeon to the Manhattan Eye and Ear Hospital, of which department he was the head for many years.

For twenty years he was Professor of Otology at the New York Post-Graduate Medical School and Hospital. During these active years he contributed widely to the literature on otology, and was the author of a textbook "Diseases of the Ear, Nose and Throat," which passed through four editions, and was used in a great many medical schools.

In 1914 Doctor Phillips became an officer of the New York League for the Hard of Hearing, serving as a vice-president, as president, and as a director for the last twenty years of his life. Through his connection with this pioneer organization, he became the founder in 1919 of the American Federation of Organizations for the Hard of Hearing, serving as its first president. Under his leadership this federation grew from one member organization in 1919 to nearly one hundred and fifty in all parts of the United States and Canada at the time of his death. Prominent physicians, physicists, educators and social workers, both hard of hearing and normal hearing, were attracted to it and its nationwide program for conservation of hearing, especially in childhood—when, as Doctor Phillips pointed out, impairments of hearing frequently developing later into an economically crippling handicap, actually begin in the majority of cases. The school hearing testing program has been approved by leading medical societies and widely adopted in American municipal educational systems.

He early took an active and conspicuous part in organized medicine, being elected president of the Medical Society of the County of New York in 1909, and of the State of New York in 1912. He was a member of the House of Delegates of the American Medical Association for six years from 1912 to 1917. In 1918 he was elected a member of the Board of Trustees, serving for seven years, the last year as Chairman. He was Chairman of the Section of Laryngology, Otology and Rhinology in 1923 and 1924.

In his address as president presented at the Dallas session in 1926 on "The Physician and the Patient of the Future," is reflected the maturity of his thinking regarding some of the vital problems confronting the medical profession. He recognized the changes in medical practice largely due to rapid progress in medical discoveries, and the more practical employment of sanitation and preventive medicine, effecting a great change in the actual duties of the practicing physician. He urged the preparation of the future physician in the direction of a wide and comprehensive plan of personal and public health education:—"The undergraduate student must learn and recognize the importance of community as well as individual disease, and he must also be trained to treat the body from the standpoint of health as from disease"; he stated further, "The ideal family physician of the future by training, by experience and by expert knowledge of health conservation, will derive a potential power which will qualify him to control and direct the health problems of men." Also, "The maintenance of individual practice in the person of the general practitioner or family physician is of the utmost importance for the survival and continuation of the family home for the foundation of the nation."

His further society affiliations included membership in the New York Academy of Medicine, a Fellow of the American College of Surgeons, and the American Academy of Ophthalmology and Otology. He was a charter member of the American Laryngological, Rhinological and Otological Society, its secretary from 1901 to 1906, and president in 1907.

All those who were privileged to know Dr. Wendell C. Phillips will remember his genial personality, his enthusiastic leadership and unwavering support of organized medicine, and constant devotion to the highest professional ideals.

His death occurred at the Manhattan Eye, Ear and Throat Hospital, November 16, 1934, at the age of seventy-seven years.

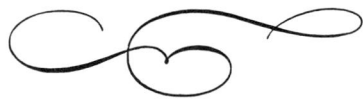

JABEZ NORTH JACKSON, M.D.
Kansas City, Mo.
1868–1935

Eightieth President, A. M. A.
Washington Session
May 16, 17, 18, 19, 20, 1927

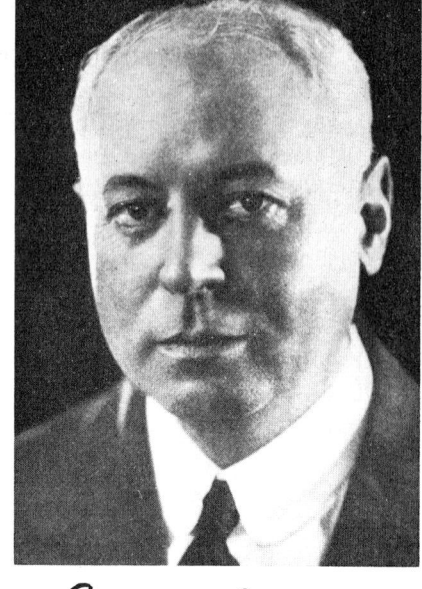

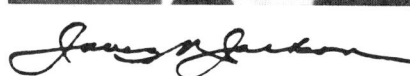

THE ELECTION OF DR. JABEZ N. JACKSON as president of the Association was a recognition of an outstanding surgeon and favorite son of the Southwest and of the high esteem in which he was held by his professional colleagues.

He was born in Labadie, Missouri, October 6, 1868, the son of Dr. John Wesley Jackson, a pioneer physician of Missouri, and a Major of the Union forces in the Civil War. After attending Central College in Fayette, Mo., where he received the Bachelor of Arts degree in 1889, and Master of Arts in 1890, he graduated from the University Medical College of Kansas City with the degree Doctor of Medicine in 1891. This was followed by graduate work at the New York Polyclinic. From 1891 to 1896 he was demonstrator of anatomy at his Alma Mater, then professor of surgical anatomy and adjunct professor of surgery until 1900, when he became professor of principles and practice of surgery from 1900 to 1911. For twenty years from 1891 to 1911 he was a Trustee of the University Medical College of Kansas City, and for several years served as President. From 1893 to 1898 he was assistant surgeon and surgeon in the Third Regiment of the Missouri National Guard, and was a Major and Brigade Surgeon of the United States Volunteer Regiment in charge of the Second Division Hospital of the Second Army Corps during the Spanish-American War.

Doctor Jackson served as a member of the House of Delegates of the American Medical Association in 1903, 1904, 1906, 1919, 1930, 1931, and 1933. As President of the Association he presided at the opening session in Washington, D.C., where President Calvin Coolidge honored the occasion with an address.

Doctor Jackson had a prominent part in organizing the Medical Association of the Southwest, of which he was president in 1898, and was equally active in the establishment of its successor, the Kansas City Southwest Clinical Society. He was president of the Kansas City Academy of Medicine in 1900, of the Missouri State Medical Association in 1904, and the Western Surgical Association in 1913. Among the other medical organizations with which he was affiliated were the American Surgical Association, the Missouri Valley Medical Society, the Pan-American Medical Congress, and the American College of Surgeons (Founders Group). He was surgeon to the Kansas City General Hospital, the Research Hospital, and the Trinity Hospital.

His name is associated with many discoveries in surgical technique and particularly with the elucidation of "Jackson's membrane" in membranous pericolitis, and associated surgical conditions.

In 1926 he was awarded the honorary Doctor of Science degree from Park College, and that of Doctor of Laws from the University of Missouri in 1927.

During the last three years of his life he served most efficiently as the Director of Health of the city of Kansas City, Missouri.

Doctor Jackson died at his home in Kansas City March 18, 1935, at the age of sixty-six years.

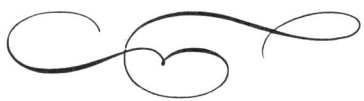

WILLIAM SYDNEY THAYER, M.D.
Baltimore, Md.
1864–1932

Eighty-first President, A. M. A.
Minneapolis Session
June 11, 12, 13, 14, 15, 1928

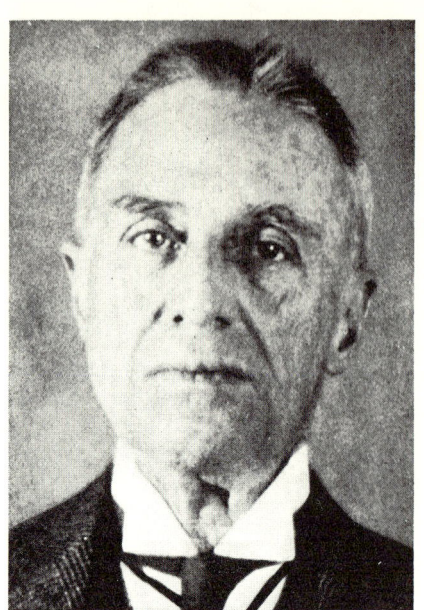

THE ELECTION TO THE PRESIDENCY of the Association of Dr. William Sydney Thayer was a recognition of outstanding achievement in medical science and the conferring of the highest honor on one who had already gained leadership in this country and abroad.

Doctor Thayer was born in Milton, Mass., June 23, 1864. He came from a distinguished family, of which Ralph Waldo Emerson and Oliver Wendell Holmes had been members. His father James Bradley Thayer was professor of law at Harvard, and his brother, Ezra Thayer, became dean of the Harvard Law School. In his physique and character, in his love of scholarship and in his standards and ideals, Doctor Thayer exemplified to a high degree the best that New England blood and training have to give. After an elementary education in a private school in Milton, he attended the Cambridge High School and later Harvard University, where he graduated in Arts in 1885, and received his medical degree from the Harvard Medical School in 1889. Following an internship at the Massachusetts General Hospital, and a period of postgraduate study in Berlin and Vienna, he began as a general practitioner in Boston, but in 1890 was called to Baltimore to join Professor Osler's house-staff in the Johns Hopkins Hospital as a resident physician, which position he held until 1898. He succeeded to the position of attending physician and head of the medical department of the dispensary from 1898 to 1906, at the same time serving as associate professor of medicine and later as professor of clinical medicine. Dr. Thayer did not become the immediate successor of Dr. Osler when he left in 1905 to be the Regius Professor of Physic at the University of Oxford, because at the time Dr. Thayer did not feel able to assume, for financial reasons, a fulltime professorship. However, in 1918, he became professor of medicine in Johns Hopkins University, and physician in chief to the hospitals, resigning in 1921, when he became professor emeritus. He continued to serve as visiting physician to the hospital, and as consulting physician to many other Baltimore institutions.

In later years Dr. Thayer often recalled the fifteen years of intimate association with William Osler—"the Chief" as one of the privileges of his life. Here he made some of his most important investigations, such as his studies of the blood in leukemia (1891), in typhoid (1895), and in malaria (1893–1900). He worked with Lazear in the cultivation of the malaria parasite in Anopheles maculipennis. Here he did his researches upon the third heart sound (1908–9), upon cardiac murmurs (1901–1919), upon the cardiovascular complications and sequels of typhoid fever (1903–4), upon arteriosclerosis (1904), upon chorea (1906), upon heart block (1916), and upon gonococcal endocarditis and endocarditis lenta (subacute bacterial). It was during this period that he attended the International Medical Congress in Moscow in 1897, as a representative of Johns Hopkins University and Hospital. His address was on "The Increase of Eosinophilic Cells in Trichinosis." At that time, he was elected an honorary member of the Therapeutic Society of Moscow.

In the Medical Service of the Army he was one of the 107 charter members of the Reserve Corps who accepted commissions as First Lieutenant on July 5, 1908. He was a member of a medical board with Lieutenants V. C. Vaughan, Wm. T. Councilman, John H. Musser, and Simon Flexner, which in December 1908 recommended vaccination against typhoid fever in the Army and Navy, and that it be compulsory in time of war.

In 1917 he went with Dr. Frank Billings on an American Red Cross mission to Russia; he hesitated at first because of the serious illness of his wife who was in the late stages of cardiac disease, but she urged him to go, both of them fully realizing that this meant their last farewell.

At the beginning of World War I he was commissioned a Major and Chief of the medical service of Base Hospital No. 18, which was organized at Johns Hopkins in 1916, and went to France with it in 1917. In 1918 he was promoted to Colonel and later to Brigadier General, Medical Corps, and Chief Medical Consultant to the American Expeditionary Forces. The Distinguished Service Medal was conferred on him in 1919, and he was awarded the rank of officer in the French Legion of Honor in 1923.

After the war he was Brigadier General of the Medical Section, Officers Reserve Corps, and his title was changed to Brigadier General Auxiliary, U.S.A.

His accomplishments were recognized by election to honorary membership in numerous domestic and foreign medical societies. He was president of the Association of American Physicians, the Interurban Clinical Club, the American Society of Tropical Medicine, and the American Society for Clinical Investigation; also a member of the American Academy of Arts and Sciences, the American Philosophical Society, the American Association for the Advancement of Science, the American Historical Society, and the National Research Council. He was a member of Phi Beta Kappa Society, and Alpha Omega Alpha Honor Medical Society.

He was also an honorary member of the Royal Society of Medicine of London, the Association of Physicians of Great Britain and Ireland, the Royal Medical Society of Budapest, the Academie de Medicine of Paris, the International Tuberculosis Association, and a corresponding member of the Gesellschaft für innere Medicin of Berlin and of Kinderheilkunde in Vienna.

In the American Medical Association Doctor Thayer served as Chairman of the Section on Practice of Medicine in 1902-3. He was a member of the editorial board of the Archives of Internal Medicine from the time this publication first began in 1908 until 1932. He was made a member of the Judicial Council in 1918, and served on that body until his election as President-Elect in 1927.

Great Britain honored Doctor Thayer by asking him to give the Bright Lecture in clinical medicine in 1927. He was for many years a member of the Board of Overseers of Harvard University. He received the LL.D. degree from Washington College in 1907, from the University of Edinburgh in 1927, and from McGill University in 1929. He was appointed by Secretary of Interior Ray Lyman Wilbur to serve as a member of the Education Commission to study the relationship of the national government to education. In 1928 he received the degree of Docteur Honoris Causa from the University of Paris, and during the same year was appointed Gibson Lecturer at the Royal College of Physicians of Edinburgh. He was an honorary Fellow of the Royal Colleges of Physicians of Edinburgh and Ireland.

The University of Chicago in 1907 conferred upon him the honorary Doctor of Science. He gave the Alpha Omega Alpha annual lecture in 1929, and the Frank Billings Lecture in 1932.

In May 1927 a large and representative group of friends and colleagues of Dr. William S. Thayer gathered at the Mayflower Hotel, Washington, D. C., to present to the Johns Hopkins Medical School a lectureship in his honor, to be called "The William Sydney Thayer and Susan Reed Thayer Lectureship in Clinical Medicine."

The contributions of Doctor Thayer were numerous, both to medical and lay literature. He was the author of "The Malaria Fevers of Baltimore" published in 1895, "Lectures on Malaria Fevers," 1897, "Studies of Bacterial Endocarditis," 1925, "America a Poem," 1917, "Other Verse," 1926, and in 1931 appeared that interesting volume "Osler and Other Papers," which contains many of his addresses and his reminiscenses of Osler and frequent affectionate tributes to his "dearest and wisest master." As a writer his style, both in prose and in poetry, was exceptional. His poem on Osler contains the following:

> "A heart whose alchemy transforms the dross
>   of dull suspicion to the gold of love
> A spirit like the fragrance of some flower
> That lingers round the spot that this has graced"

and from the sorrow that came with the loss of his wife came these lines:

> "But ah, how short the day—my light has passed,
> Has vanished as the sun that sets; and now
> Again in darkness and alone. I grope
> Along the sombre way that winds before."

He was a natural linguist, and aside from Latin and Greek he could read and think in French, German and Russian.

He enjoyed the company of congenial persons in dinner clubs and other social groups. To his friends he was known as a lover of books, of people, of sports, and of nature. A rare man of unique personality, high minded, tolerant and lovable, a cultivated man of many talents and of excellent qualities.

Withal he was a great teacher and clinician who left in the minds of many young men an appreciation of the significance of medical service.

He died of heart disease on December 10, 1932, while visiting in Washington, at the age of sixty-eight years. His grave is in Concord, Massachusetts, near that of his New England ancestors.

MALCOM LaSALLE HARRIS, M.D.
Chicago, Ill.
1862–1936

Eighty-second President, A. M. A.
Portland, Oregon, Session
July 8, 9, 10, 11, 12, 1929

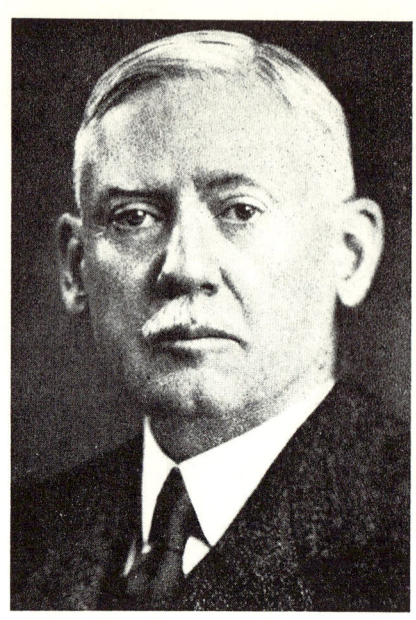

THE HONOR OF THE PRESIDENCY of the Association came to Dr. Malcom LaSalle Harris after a life of service to science and medical organization. He was born in Rock Island, Illinois, June 27, 1862, and received his early education in the public schools of Iowa, and his medical training at Rush Medical College, where he graduated with the degree Doctor of Medicine in 1882; since he was just twenty years of age, he was required to wait one year before taking the examination for licensure. He practiced continuously in Chicago from 1883 until his death.

He early became interested in teaching surgery and principally in connection with postgraduate instruction. This was carried on mostly at Cook County Hospital, and for many years he served as professor of surgery in the Chicago Polyclinic. He served continuously as Secretary of the Board of Trustees of Henrotin Hospital from 1889 until he retired as president emeritus in 1935.

His service with the American Medical Association was unique; following the re-organization of the Association in 1901, he became a member of the House of Delegates, and since that time was in attendance at all sessions, either as a member of the House, of the Board of Trustees, or of the Judicial Council, including his term as President-Elect and President, through 1934. Thus for thirty-five years Doctor Harris was a familiar figure at the annual sessions.

He was a member of the Board of Trustees from 1903 to 1918, most of the time acting as secretary of the Board. He was a member of the Judicial Council from 1918 through 1928, serving also as its chairman. In 1899 at the Columbus Session he served as Secretary of the Section on Surgery and Anatomy with Dr. William J. Mayo as Chairman.

Doctor Harris was credited with what was called a "legal" type of mind, and during his long service as Trustee and Chairman of the Judicial Council, as well as in all his public work, his views regarding form and correct procedure always received the most respectful attention.

His contributions to medical literature included not only the translation and editing of Braun's "Local Anesthesia," and contributions to the Oxford, Keen's and Bryant's Systems of Surgery, but also many periodical contributions in surgery, and in his later years he wrote significant essays in the fields of medical education, medical economics and statesmanship.

As a surgeon he was honored by election to membership in the International Surgical Association, the American Surgical Association, and the Western Surgical Association, of which he was president. He served as president of the Chicago Medical, Chicago Surgical, and Chicago Pathological societies. For a number of years he served as a member of the Illinois State Board of Medical Examiners.

While Doctor Harris seemed naturally diffident and cautious in his intimacies, he gained a wide circle of friends among distinguished political, industrial and medical leaders. He was a clear and forceful speaker, an orderly mind and profound thinker, and evidently shrewd in his estimation of men and their motives. He was highly appreciated by all who knew him well. Early in 1935, while operating at Alexian Brothers Hospital, where he was Chief of Staff, he became suddenly ill from cerebral hemorrhage, and after a prolonged illness died at the Milwaukee Sanitarium, Wauwatosa, Wis., March 22, 1936, at seventy-three years of age.

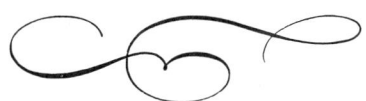

WILLIAM GERRY MORGAN, M.D.
Washington, D. C.
1868–

Eighty-third President, A. M. A.
Detroit Session
June 23, 24, 25, 26, 27, 1930

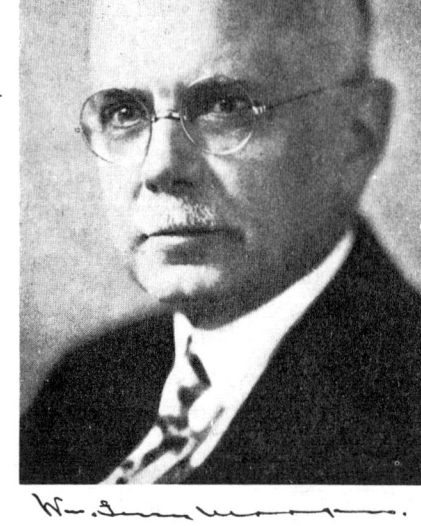

DR. WILLIAM GERRY MORGAN, the well-known gastro-enterologist and leading physician in the nation's capital, came to the presidency of the Association with a wide experience in medical society organization.

He was born in Newport, New Hampshire, May 2, 1868, and received his Bachelor of Arts degree from Dartmouth College in 1890, and that of Doctor of Medicine from the University of Pennsylvania in 1893. After postgraduate work in New York City he began practice in Southport, Connecticut, in 1894, and in 1899 removed to Washington, D.C. where he soon gained a high place in medical circles. He became professor of diseases of the digestive tract in Georgetown University School of Medicine in 1904, and has held that position ever since. From 1931 to 1935 he was Dean of the Medical Faculty. He also served as Regent of the University.

Doctor Morgan has been Associate Editor of Tice's System of Practice of Medicine; and of Lippincott's American System of Medicine and Principles and Practice of Physical Therapy.

During World War I he served as Chairman of the District of Columbia Advisory Draft Board, also as Lieutenant (J.G.) U.S.N. M.R.C. He retired from the Navy Reserve Corps in 1922, and was commissioned a Major in the Medical Reserve Corps U. S. Army, from which he retired in 1932.

In the American Medical Association, Doctor Morgan was a

member of the House of Delegates from 1920 to 1925, serving as president-elect from 1929 to 1930, and president from 1930 to 1931. His inaugural address as president in 1930 was an able presentation of the "paternalistic tendencies of the time as related to the medical profession," and discussed principally the dangers of compulsory health insurance and governmental control of medical practice.

He had a notable record in the American College of Physicians, serving as Regent from 1918 to 1930, member of the Board of Governors from 1930 to 1933, secretary general from 1933 to 1937, and vice-president in 1937, and in 1939 he was specially honored by being elected a Master of the College.

Doctor Morgan has been honored by various special organizations. He was president of the American Congress of Internal Medicine in 1922; president of the American Gastro-Enterological Association in 1933; of the American Therapeutic Association and American Clinico-Pathological Society in 1919; of the District of Columbia Medical Society in 1919; he was vice-president of the Washington Academy of Science in 1919, and Councillor of the Southern Medical Association. He is a member of the Virginia State Medical Society, Washington Historical Society, American Archeological Association, Association of Military Surgeons, and honorary member of the New York Academy of Medicine.

As a member of the International "Gastro-Enterological Society" he attended the Conference in Brussels in 1935 as a representative of the United States.

Doctor Morgan is the author of Functional Diseases of the Alimentary Tract, and the History of the American College of Physicians (1939).

He received the honorary degree of Doctor of Science from Dartmouth College and Georgetown University in 1929, and that of Doctor of Laws from the University of Pennsylvania in 1930.

Doctor Morgan continues his consultation practice in Washington, D. C., and maintains a deep interest in all medical activities.

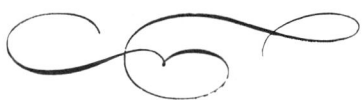

EDWARD STARR JUDD, M.D.
Rochester, Minn.
1878–1935

Eighty-fourth President, A. M. A.
Philadelphia Session
June 8, 9, 10, 11, 12, 1931

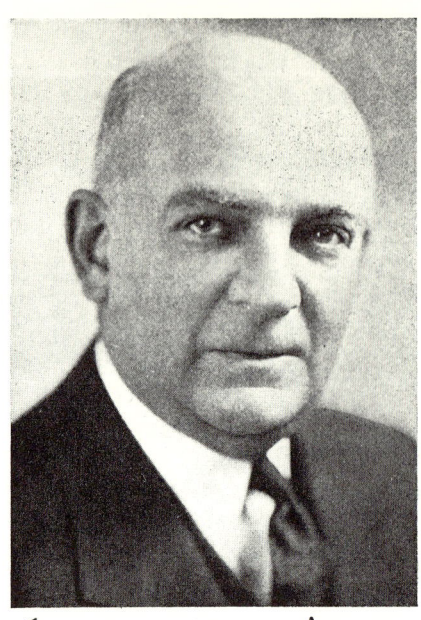

DR. E. STARR JUDD was the third member of the staff of the Mayo Clinic to be chosen for the presidency, and at the time of his election was widely known to the medical profession of America as a competent and practical surgeon; by many regarded as the most dexterous surgeon of his generation.

He was born July 11, 1878 in Rochester, Minn., where he lived and carried on his eventful career. After a preliminary general education in local schools, he entered the University of Minnesota School of Medicine and graduated with the degree of Doctor of Medicine in 1902. He began his professional career at Rochester as intern at St. Mary's Hospital, and in 1903 was appointed first assistant to Dr. Charles H. Mayo. In 1904 at the age of twenty-six years he became head of a section in the Division of Surgery at the Mayo Clinic, and thus gave evidence of becoming Mayo's most distinguished and successful pupil. Later, he was appointed chief of the surgical staff at the Mayo Clinic, as well as professor of surgery in the Graduate School of the University of Minnesota. From 1920 onwards he assumed the main surgical burden of the Clinic. His surgical ability became universally recognized. He was possessed of rare technical ability, an exceptionally keen diagnostic sense, and unusual surgical judgment, which always seemed more like a gift than an acquisition, and thus had the mental equipment as well as the manual dexterity of a master surgeon. Though short of stature he was stockily built, his movements were quick, his decisions decisive, revealing an endless energy. He was capable of maintaining a prodigious surgical output, for many years doing more operations in a single day than any surgeon in the Mayo Clinic. He seemed to have brought the art of economy of movement to perfection. In many ways Doctor Judd had reduced his life to one of machine-like regularity, and it was undoubtedly as a result of this that he accomplished so much.

Another attribute was his quickness to recognize the pathologic condition and to proceed with the operation without needless delay. At all times his chief concern was the patient as an individual, a human being, who had come to him for relief of pain and suffering, an attribute which attracted so many doctors and their relatives to him as patients.

He was greatly in demand at surgical meetings throughout the United States, and as a result his literary output covered a wide field; in all he contributed over two hundred papers to medical literature.

In 1921 Doctor Judd was made a member of the Editorial Board of the Archives of Surgery. He was a member of the Council on Scientific Assembly of the American Medical Association from its beginning in 1915 to 1927. His sound advice was often sought in discussions concerning the arrangement of the scientific program and the policies of this Council.

In the office of president he served with high distinction, ever mindful of the needs of the members of the organization and the objectives which they should hope to obtain if they were to render the highest type of medical service. His presidential address in 1931 "The Obligations of the Medical Profession" was a philosophic discussion of the evident trend of medical education towards scientific medicine and specialization, while not so much time is given to the art of the practice; that the practice of medicine was changing and new methods of medical service were being created, yet he was convinced that this changing character of medical practice had broadened the scope of the usefulness of medical practitioners, who thus became leaders in their communities in public health.

He made a further observation that "the art of caring for a sick person is learned by the student during his service in the hospital, but I fear that too little stress is placed on this form of instruction." "A sick person does not want to be cared for by machine methods, because he feels, and rightly so, that he will not be as well taken care of as though he were having personal attention from his own physician. The practice of medicine, under any scheme must give due consideration to the art of medicine." These were interesting comments from the chief surgeon of a large medical institution.

During World War I he was active as a teacher in the school for developing surgeons, which was established at the Mayo Clinic, and from time to time since the war he took part in work designed to give those continuing in the Medical Corps of the United States Army a more intimate knowledge of diagnostic and operative procedures. He was a Colonel in the Medical Reserve Corps.

Doctor Judd was a member of the American Surgical Association, the American College of Surgeons, the Minnesota Academy of Medicine, the Minnesota Pathological Society, the Western Surgical Association (president 1912), the Southern and Interurban Surgical Associations, the American Society of Clinical Surgery, and the Southern Minnesota Medical Association, and an honorary and corresponding member of several foreign surgical societies.

His untimely death at 57 years on November 29, 1935 was mourned by a host of admiring friends throughout the world.

In 1932 the Edward Starr Judd Lectureship was established at the University of Minnesota by Phi Beta Pi Fraternity. The first lecturer was Dr. Dean D. Lewis, President of the American Medical Association.

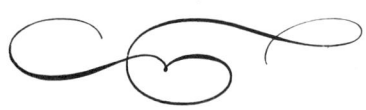

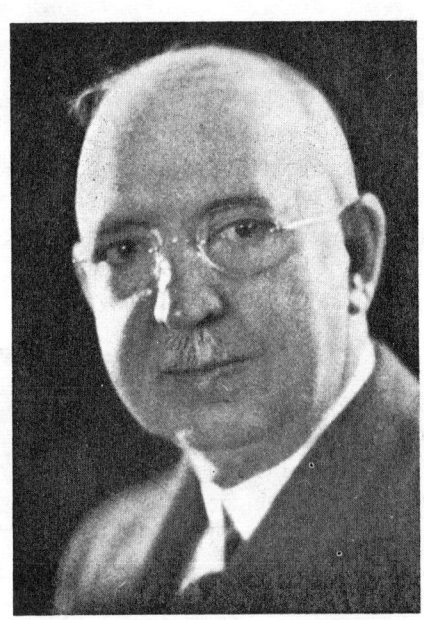

EDWARD HENRY CARY, M.D.
Dallas, Texas.
1872–

Eighty-fifth President, A. M. A.
New Orleans Session
May 9, 10, 11, 12, 13, 1932

THE SELECTION OF DR. EDWARD H. CARY for president of the Association, was in recognition of his accomplishments in the field of medical education, administration and eminence in the specialty of ophthalmology, as a builder of medical institutions, and particularly of his genius for friendship and service.

Doctor Cary was born in Union Springs, Alabama, February 28, 1872. His preparatory education was obtained at Union Springs Academy and high school in New York City, after which he entered Bellevue Hospital Medical College (New York University) receiving the degree Doctor of Medicine in 1898. Following his graduation he served an internship in Bellevue Hospital for one year, and an additional year as house physician at the New York Eye and Ear Infirmary. During the last year he was head of the Ophthalmologic Clinic of the Bellevue Hospital Medical College. He moved to Dallas, Texas, in 1901, and soon afterwards, in 1902, became dean of the Dallas Medical School, and led in the movement to make it a department of Baylor University in 1904. He continued as dean of the Baylor University Medical School until 1929, when he became Dean Emeritus. From 1909 to 1929 he was chairman of the staff of Baylor University Hospital. During all this time, from 1902, Doctor Cary was professor and head of the department of ophthalmology and otolaryngology in both schools. He was instrumental in developing Baylor University Medical School into one of the leading institutions in the Southwest.

In 1942 Baylor University moved its medical school to Houston, Texas, which apparently meant the end of a medical school in Dallas, but such was not to be. Doctor Cary with his characteristic foresight had organized the Southwest Medical Foundation several years before, to be a sponsoring agency for the Baylor University Medical School. With its removal from Dallas, a new medical school was established in connection with the Foundation. A faculty in the different fields was organized, and within a year the school was placed on the approved list of the Council on Medical Education and Hospitals. The new plan included the building of a large teaching hospital, adequate laboratory and other facilities for the equipment of a modern medical school. In all this great undertaking Dr. Cary is the guiding spirit for he is recognized as a builder of institutions of various kinds. He is a director of many corporations, and president of several others; his name being associated particularly with the construction and use of the Medical Arts Building of Dallas—one of the unique office buildings in this country. He is head of the Cary Clinic, and has contributed extensively to the literature of ophthalmology. For many years his annual contribution to the scientific exhibit at Association meetings were of distinct educational value. He was a member of the Board of Trustees for five years preceding his election as president-elect in 1931. During his two years as president-elect and president, he travelled more miles to all parts of the country than any president up to that time.

Since serving as president he has continued his interest and devoted his best efforts to the advancement of Association affairs. He is a member of the House of Delegates, as representative from the Texas State Medical Society, and his mature counsel and experience are welcomed by his associates in the House. As Chairman of the Committee on Legislation, he has distinctly influenced the trend of Federal legislation concerned with medical practice.

His position as Chairman of the Executive Board of the National Physicians Committee has likewise been of great service to the medical profession.

He organized the Baylor Medical Unit which served in France in World War I. In the last World War he was a member of the Appeal Board of Selective Service District No. 7.

The career of Doctor Cary is a record of distinguished service to the profession in different fields of medical endeavor, and recognition has come to him from many societies. He has been president of his County and State medical societies, of the Southern Medical Association, of the American Laryngological, Rhinological and Otological Society, a member of the Council of the American Academy of Ophthalmology and Otolaryngology and a Fellow of the American College of Surgeons. His home is in Dallas, Texas.

Dr. Edward H. Cary of Dallas, Texas, continues a dynamic force in advancing the interests of organized medicine.

DEAN DeWITT LEWIS, M.D.
Baltimore, Md.
1874–1941

Eighty-sixth President, A. M. A.
Milwaukee Session
June 12, 13, 14, 15, 16, 1933

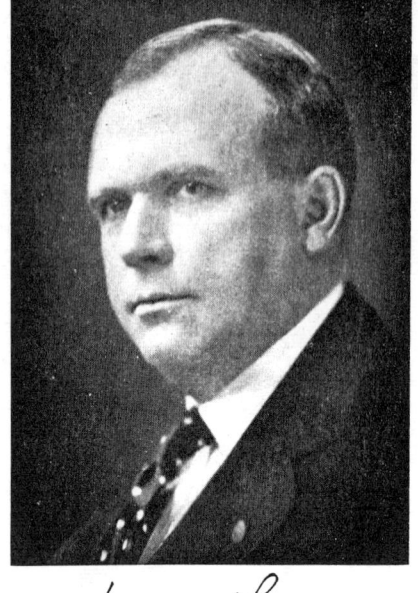

THE SELECTION OF DR. DEAN D. LEWIS to the presidency was a natural recognition of his leadership in medical education, his eminence as a surgeon, and the tribute of a legion of admiring friends everywhere.

Dr. Dean Lewis was born in Kewanee, Illinois, August 11, 1874. He received his Bachelor of Arts degree from Lake Forest University in 1895, and his Doctor of Medicine degree from Rush Medical College in 1899. This was followed by internship at Cook County Hospital, where he served with Doctors Rowan, Kanavel, Besley, Richter, and other well known surgeons of Chicago of that day. Upon completion of this service, he accepted a position as instructor of anatomy at the University of Chicago, and for four years arduously devoted himself to this task. While in this position, he came under the influence of Dr. Bensley, professor of anatomy, and became interested in vital staining of tissues, leading to his report on the "histologic changes and hyperplasia of the chromophile cells in the anterior lobe of the hypophysis, in the case of acromegaly." In this period were included six months of graduate study with Spalteholz the anatomist in Leipzig, Germany, where (by reconstruction models) "the fascia of the kidney" was the subject of study.

From 1903 to 1924 with the exception of the war years, Dr. Dean Lewis taught surgery at Rush Medical College, and carried on an increasing surgical practice at the Presbyterian Hospital. He became professor of surgery in 1920. In the same year he accepted the editorship of the Archives of Surgery, to which he devoted his energies in making it one of the significant surgical journals of his day. He received offers from several medical schools to head their departments of surgery, and in January 1925 he accepted the professorship of surgery at the University of Illinois Medical School. This position he occupied for only six months, as he then accepted the professorship of surgery at Johns Hopkins University, as successor to Dr. William S. Halsted.

A noteworthy event during the period of service at Presbyterian Hospital, Chicago, was the first clinical use of ethylene as an anesthetic by Dr. Lewis, which subsequently was published as "Clinical Experiences with Ethylene Oxygen Anesthesia" by Dr. A. B. Luckhardt, the discoverer of ethylene, and Dr. Dean Lewis in December 1923.

According to one of his biographers, Dr. Vernon C. David of Chicago,—"The first World War played an important role in Dr. Dean Lewis's life, and he often remarked, it was one of its happiest periods. Having a deep regard for his country and for the soldiers of the line, enjoying the society of his fellowmen, resourceful in unexpected situations and having real ability as an organizer and sufficient physical stamina to carry on, made his service a notable one." He was commissioned a Major in the Medical Corps of the U. S. Army in the spring of 1917, and directed to organize Base Hospital No. 13 at the Presbyterian Hospital, Chicago. In December, 1917 he was ordered to active duty with his organization at Fort McPherson, Georgia, and shortly afterward was sent to the University of Michigan to conduct research on regeneration of nerves, with Professor G. Carl Huber. He sailed for France with his unit in May 1918 arriving in June at Limoges, where Base Hospital No. 13 was permanently established. On July 8, 1918 he was assigned to Evacuation Hospital No. 7 at Coulommiers as head of a surgical team; two weeks later he was transferred to Evacuation Hospital No. 6 at Chateau-Thierry, and on August 19 was given command of the surgical service at Evacuation Hospital No. 5, also located at Chateau-Thierry. This hospital was later also stationed at Juvigny to take care of the wounded from the Thirty-second Division during the Verdun offensive, and then moved to Villers-Cotterets to evacuate the wounded from the St. Mihiel sector. Late in September the hospital was moved to LaVeuve, where it took care of the wounded from the Second Division, and from the Thirty-sixth Division during the Champagne offensive. In the final days of the war his hospital was stationed at Staden, Belgium. After the Armistice Major Lewis was returned to Base Hospital No. 13 and was promoted to Lieutenant Colonel of the United States Army. He returned to the United States in December 1918 and was placed in command of U. S. General Hospital No. 28 at Fort Sheridan, Illinois, where a large portion of the service consisted of treatment of nerve injuries and reconstructive surgical procedures. He presented a comprehensive report on the "treatment of peripheral nerve injuries" at the Association meeting in June 1919. He received his honorable discharge from the service in August 1919, and some months later he was accorded the Distinguished Service Medal in recognition of his efficient services.

During his period at Johns Hopkins University and Hospital he contributed largely to the knowledge of the relation of sex hormones to tumor growth. While there he edited the widely used "Practice of Surgery," of twelve volumes, in which appears his own classic work on peripheral nerve injuries and regeneration of nerves.

An expression from one of his colleagues in Baltimore is frequently quoted, "His Friday clinics to the third and fourth year medical students were among the best and most scholarly presentations of surgical discussions ever listened to. In these teaching exercises he displayed a remarkable familiarity with the surgical literature of the whole modern world, and a memory that was astonishing in its accuracy. He was particularly interested in the surgery of peripheral nerves, tendons, joints and bones, and in these fields he showed a mastery of the subject and an operative facility which was remarkable; he always laid great emphasis on the relationship of anatomy to surgery and also on acquaintance with the unusual types of infections such as actinomycosis, sporotrichosis, etc."

In the American Medical Association, aside from the editorship of the Archives of Surgery, he served as a member of the House of Delegates, representing the Section on Surgery—General and Abdominal, in 1915, 1916, and 1917. He was secretary of the Section on Surgery in 1912 and 1913, and Chairman of the same in 1919–1920. In 1931 he became a member of the Council on Medical Education and Hospitals, continuing until he was elected president in 1933.

For many years he had been in demand to speak before medical meetings throughout the country, but during his two years as president-elect and president, he gave liberally of his time and energy to this service, speaking with all the enthusiasm at his command on the teaching function of medical societies, which he regarded as the most valuable postgraduate medical training available to the profession. This theme was further expanded in his presidential address in 1933—"The Place of the Clinic in Medical Practice." In the years following his service as president, he continued his efforts to bring the latest medical knowledge directly to the medical practitioner. In 1926 a testimonial dinner was given for Doctor Lewis in Baltimore, and one of the photographs preserved from this memorable occasion shows him seated between Dr. John M. T. Finney and Dr. Harvey Cushing.

He was affiliated with most of the leading professional associations; a member of the American Surgical Association, the American Association of Anatomists, the American Physiological Society, the Southern Medical Association, the Western Surgical Association. He was an Honorary Fellow of the Royal College of Surgeons of Ireland, the Royal Australian College of Surgeons, the Societa Medico-Chirurgica of Bologna, Italy, and an Ausserordentliches Mitglied der deutschen Gesellschaft für Chirurgie, as well as a foreign member correspondent of the Société des Chirurgiens de Paris. He was made an honorary Doctor of Science by the National University of Ireland at Dublin in 1933.

In 1932 his portrait was presented to Johns Hopkins University, the presentation address being given by Professor John M. T. Finney.

His last illness was prolonged over a period of three years subsequent to cerebral vascular changes; a tragic closing of a life of such vigor and vitality. The end came on December 9, 1941 at his home in Baltimore at the age of sixty-seven years.

One of the many tributes from friends and admirers, a phrase is quoted from a biographic note by Dr. Vernon C. David, a former student of Dr. Lewis: "A host of friends know the greatness of his soul, his loyalty, his matchless spirit, his love of sports, his great ability as a surgeon and his comradeship."

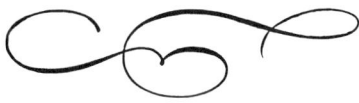

WALTER L. BIERRING, M.D.*
Des Moines, Iowa
1868–

*Eighty-seventh President, A. M. A.
Cleveland Session
June 11, 12, 13, 14, 15, 1934*

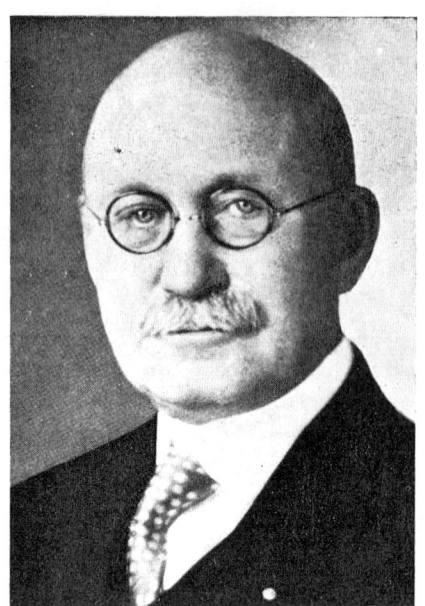

WALTER LAWRENCE BIERRING was born in Davenport, Iowa, July 15, 1868, of Danish parentage. Considering the changes in name, common to many Scandinavian families, from Bering to Bjerring, and to the present Bierring, the same ancestry applies to that of Captain Vitus S. Bering, the discoverer of the sea and northwest passage that bears his name. After preliminary education in the local schools and a short period in the collegiate department of the State University of Iowa at Iowa City, Dr. Bierring began the study of medicine in the medical department in September 1889 and received the degree Doctor of Medicine in March 1892. The medical course was limited to three years of six months each, the instruction being largely didactic with hospital facilities as provided by fifty beds. A few weeks after graduation, he spent twenty months of study mainly in the universities of Heidelberg and Vienna.

About a month after arrival in Vienna in April 1892, he received a letter from the Dean of the Medical Department, University of Iowa, announcing his election to the chair of pathology and bacteriology to begin with the winter term of 1893. His studies at Heidelberg were largely under Professor Arnold in pathology and

---

* The biography of Dr. Bierring was prepared by Morris Fishbein, M.D.

Professor Ernst in bacteriology, the latter being a former assistant of Robert Koch. After a brief winter of teaching and organizing a department of pathology and bacteriology, further study of bacteriology was followed in 1894 at the Pasteur Institute in Paris. Upon return to Iowa City, with the knowledge gained at the Pasteur Institute, diphtheria antitoxin was prepared, and distributed without cost to physicians in the winter of 1894–5, probably the earliest production of anti-diphtheritic serum west of New York City. For a period of seven years a practical (Pasteur) course in bacteriology of one month's duration was conducted each spring, 1895 to 1901, patterned after the work at the Pasteur Institute. The teaching of pathology and bacteriology continued until 1903, during which period two further courses of studies, 1896 and 1902, were pursued in Paris, Prague and Vienna.

In 1903 Dr. Bierring changed to the chair of theory and practice of medicine and clinical medicine. In 1910 an opportunity was offered by Drake University at Des Moines, Iowa, to aid in developing a modern medical school; however, the prospective large endowment did not materialize, and it became advisable to discontinue the medical school at Des Moines and complete a merger with the College of Medicine at the University of Iowa.

This was followed by twenty years of active hospital service and consultation practice in internal medicine until 1933. On July 1, 1933 Dr. Bierring began his service as State Commissioner of Health.

His military experience in the first World War was limited to service as contract surgeon with assignments principally to duty on special boards of diseases of the heart and lungs.

The first meeting of the American Medical Association he attended was the session at Columbus, Ohio, in June 1899, and with the exception of four meetings—Atlantic City, 1900; St. Paul, 1901; Saratoga Springs, 1902, and San Francisco, 1915—he has been a regular attendant.

The first paper he presented before the Association was at the New Orleans meeting in 1903 on "Multiple Chloroma-like Tumors of the Cranial Bones."

In 1905 came the secretaryship, and in 1906 the chairmanship of the Section on Pathology and Physiology; in 1911 vice-chairmanship, and in 1918–19 the chairmanship of the Section on Practice of Medicine.

Membership in the House of Delegates included the years 1904, 1905, and 1906, representing the Iowa State Medical Society; 1910 and 1911, the Section on Pathology and Physiology, and 1922, 1923, 1924 and 1925 as delegate from the Section on Practice of Medicine.

His term of office as president-elect and as president, 1933 to 1935, was strenuous experience. It was not possible to equal the "speeding" record of the preceding president, Dr. Edward H. Cary, yet some 70,000 miles by rail and 5000 miles by air were covered during the two years. His address as president in 1934 was entitled "The Family Doctor and the Changing Order." It was a period when the Social Security Act was under consideration. In October 1934, Secretary Perkins, Chairman of President Roosevelt's Committee on Economic Security, appointed the Medical Advisory Board to advise the committee's technical staff in its study of programs of public health, medical care and health insurance. The membership included the following: Rexwald Brown of California, James D. Bruce of Michigan, George W. Crile of Ohio, Harvey Cushing of Connecticut, Robert B. Greenough of Massachusetts, J. Shelton Horsley of Virginia, James Alexander Miller of New York, Thomas Parran, Jr., of New York, George M. Piersol of Pennsylvania, Stewart R. Roberts of Georgia, and Walter L. Bierring of Iowa; the first meeting was held November 14, 15, 1934 in Washington, and several subsequent meetings during the following winter. To what extent the Medical Advisory Board influenced the final form of the Social Security Act adopted by Congress in August 1935, cannot be detailed; the medical profession is under lasting obligation to Dr. Harvey Cushing for his masterful efforts in having the section or title on compulsory health insurance deferred and omitted in the original Act.

The Commission on Medical Education from 1927 to 1932 included Dr. A. Lawrence Lowell, President Harvard University, Walter L. Bierring, George Blumer, Hugh Cabot, Samuel P. Caper, David L. Edsall, William Darrach, Sir Robert Falconer, Henry G. Gale, M. F. Guyer, Walter A. Jessup, Thos. A. McDavitt, L. B. Mendel, W. A. Pusey, Olin West, Ray Lyman Wilbur, and Hans Zinsser; Dr. W. C. Rappleye, Director.

During the nine years 1931 to 1940, as Regent of the American College of Physicians, he assisted in the organization of the American Board of Internal Medicine in 1936, and served as the first chairman from 1936 to 1939.

With his appointment as president of the Iowa State Board of Health and Medical Examiners in 1913, began an interest in the problems of medical licensure, which resulted in membership in the Federation of State Medical Boards of the United States in 1914; in 1915 began his service as Secretary and Editor of the Federation Bulletin, continuing to the present time. Membership on the National Board of Medical Examiners began in 1916 (as successor to Dr. William L. Rodman, the founder of the Board, who died in March 1916) with continuous service to 1946, except two years in 1930 to 1932.

Early in 1919 a commission of the National Board, consisting of Colonel Louis A. LaGarde, Walter L. Bierring and Colonel Victor C. Vaughan (the latter being prevented from accompanying the commission by reason of the sudden death of his son in France), was appointed to visit England, Scotland and France to study special qualifying examinations for the purpose of promoting some form of reciprocal agreement in matters of medical education. After a return visit of medical representatives from these three countries to the United States in 1920 (Members Sir Humphry Rolleston, Sir Holbert Waring [England], Sir Norman Walker [Scotland], and Professor Gustave Roussy and A. Demarest of Paris), such a reciprocal agreement was accomplished between the National Board and the Conjoint and Triple Qualifying Boards of England and Scotland.

In recognition of these efforts, the Royal College of Physicians of Edinburgh conferred honorary membership on Dr. Bierring in July 1922.

Dr. Bierring has been president of Alpha Omega Alpha Honor Medical Society since 1924. He was appointed Professor Emeritus of the Theory and Practice of Medicine, in the College of Medicine, State University of Iowa in March 1945.

He has served as Trustee at Large for the Frank Billings Lectureship Fund since 1927 and presented the Frank Billings Lecture in 1938 on "Focal Infection: Quarter Century Survey."

Since 1933 he was associated with the State and Territorial Health Officers with the further recognition of the presidency of the Conference of State and Provincial Health Authorities of North America from 1945 to 1947.

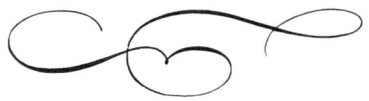

JAMES S. McLESTER, M.D.
Birmingham, Ala.
1877–

Eighty-eighth President, A. M. A.
Atlantic City Session
June 10, 11, 12, 13, 14, 1935

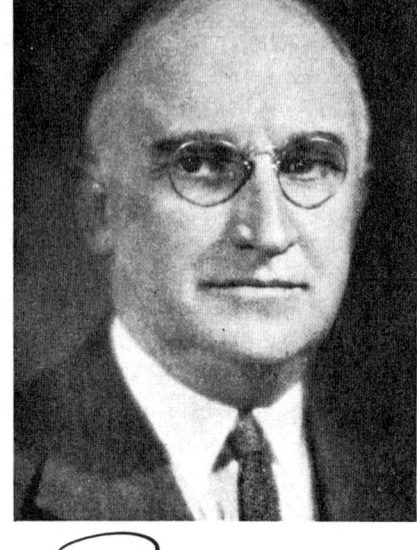

DR. JAMES S. MCLESTER came to the office of president of the Association with a distinguished career of service to organized medicine; furthermore, he had become recognized as an authority on metabolic and nutritional disorders, and attained a high place as a medical educator. Through his election, the great membership of the Association in the South was again honored.

He was born in Tuscaloosa, Alabama, January 25, 1877. His collegiate education was obtained at the University of Alabama where he received his Bachelor of Arts degree in 1896; his degree Doctor of Medicine was granted by the University of Virginia in 1899. This was followed by postgraduate studies at the universities of Göttingen and Freiburg, returning in 1902 to become professor of pathology in the Birmingham Medical College. Within a few years his title was changed to professor of medicine, and he began the practice of internal medicine in Birmingham. In 1907 and 1908 he took further postgraduate work in Berlin and Munich. The Birmingham Medical College was discontinued in 1912, and for a few years Doctor McLester was not actively engaged in teaching.

After the establishment of a School of the Medical Sciences by the University of Alabama, Doctor McLester was appointed professor of medicine in 1919, and has held this position ever since. A few years ago, a four year medical school of the University of Alabama was organized in Birmingham, and the first class was graduated in 1946. In this significant educational development, Doctor McLester has had a prominent part. He early gained recognition for his learning and leadership as he appeared before medical meetings. Dr. Frank Billings, one of the great leaders of American medicine, was a fine judge of men, and back in those early days, said these prophetic words: "You watch that man McLester—he will go far in medicine."

Soon after the beginning of World War I he was commissioned a Major in the medical service in the Base Hospital at Camp Sheridan. Early in 1918 he was promoted to Lieutenant Colonel in the American Expeditionary Forces, becoming Commanding Officer of Evacuation Hospital No. 18. Upon his return from military service in 1919 he resumed his practice in Birmingham, and became professor of medicine in the University of Alabama School of Medical Sciences.

The research and scientific articles of Dr. McLester have dealt chiefly with diseases of nutrition and metabolism. Besides contributing extensively to the literature on these subjects, he has published two books entitled—"Nutrition and Diet in Health and Disease," and "The Diagnosis and Treatment of Disorders of Metabolism." He also contributed the chapter on "Diseases of the Mediastinum," in the Oxford System of Medicine, and the chapter on Syphilis in Cecil's Textbook of Medicine.

Doctor McLester's first official connection with the American Medical Association was as secretary of the Section on Practice of Medicine in 1917 and 1918, and chairman of this section at the annual session in 1920. He served as a member of the House of Delegates from the Section on Practice of Medicine in 1921, and again from 1929 to 1933, inclusive. In 1929 he became a member of the Council on Medical Education and Hospitals, serving until his election as president in 1934.

He has also since 1933 been a member of the Committee on Foods of the Association with the exception of the two years that he was president.

His presidential address in 1935 was a masterly presentation on "Nutrition and the Future of Man," in which he emphasized the importance of an adequate diet in the improvement of racial stock, of undernourished children, of its influence on heredity and environment, and in its implications on certain political and economic factors; adequate nutrition in its last analysis was a problem of education and of Government. Much of this gospel was of significant portent in the great World War then in the offing, when the oft quoted dictum "Food will win the war" came to be realized.

Doctor McLester is associated with many learned societies being a Fellow and Past Regent of the American College of Physicians, a member of the Association of American Physicians, the Society of Clinical Investigation, the American Climatological and Clinical Association, and the Southern Medical Association. He was president of the Alabama State Medical Association in 1920.

It can truly be said that he has at all times added distinction and leadership to American medicine.

Dr. McLester continues his consultation practice and teaching in internal medicine in Birmingham, Alabama.

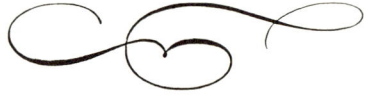

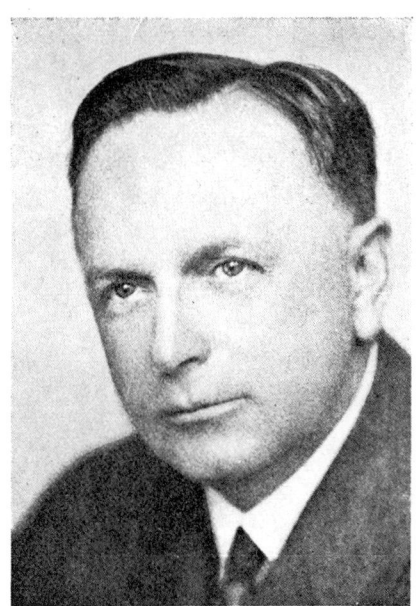

JAMES TATE MASON, M.D.
Seattle, Wash.
1882-1936

Eighty-ninth President, A. M. A.
Kansas City Session
May 11, 12, 13, 14, 15, 1936

THE LIFE STORY OF DR. JAMES "TATE" MASON with its tragic close would cast a dark shadow on this chronicle of Association presidents were it not for the beautiful friendly spirit, the noble attributes of lofty ideals and medical leadership that it exemplified.

He came from a sturdy ancestry in the Old Dominion. His grandfather, Captain Claiborne Rice Mason was a pioneer railroad builder, having constructed the greater part of the Chesapeake and Ohio railroad, served as an engineer with General Stonewall Jackson of the Confederate Army, and the name Mason is still retained in a firm of contractors that built the Coulee Dam in the State of Washington.

Captain Mason's son, Dr. A. S. Mason, "Tate's" father, was a pioneer medical practitioner of Virginia, and also served under General Stonewall Jackson; was wounded and captured, remaining as a prisoner in the North until Appomatox.

James Tate Mason was born May 20, 1882 at Lahore, Orange County, Virginia. At fourteen years of age he entered the Locustdale Military Academy, and began the study of medicine at the University of Virginia Medical School, graduating with the degree Doctor of Medicine in 1905. After two years of postgraduate study at the Philadelphia Polyclinic and Municipal Contagious Hospital, he was appointed ship's surgeon on the S. S. President of the Pacific Coast Steamship Company, and on a voyage around Cape Horn to Seattle he decided to remain in the Northwest. He practiced for two years for the Pacific Coast Coal Company at Franklin and Black Diamond, Washington, after which he located in Seattle, where he practiced from 1909 to the time of his death.

He soon developed an extensive surgical practice, and in 1914 became superintendent and surgeon of the Kings County Hospital, which position he held until 1922. In 1917 he organized the Mason Clinic, and in 1919 he and his associates organized and built the Virginia Mason Hospital, of which he became Chief Surgeon and President.

Doctor Mason was consulting surgeon at the United States Marine Hospital at Seattle for the American Mail Line, the Alaskan Steamship Company, and the Northern Pacific Railroad Company. He served as secretary of the Section on Surgery, General and Abdominal, American Medical Association, from 1923 to 1926, and chairman of this Section in 1927. Doctor Mason was a member of the House of Delegates for six years from 1928 to 1934.

Doctor Mason was a founder and past president of the Pacific Coast Surgical Association, a member and in 1930 vice-president of the American Association for the Study of Goitre, a member of the American Surgical Association, the Southern and Western Surgical Associations, and a Fellow of the American College of Surgeons.

During his year as president-elect he travelled widely across the country on behalf of the Association. These trips were very exhausting and on April 6, 1936 he became suddenly very ill with a severe involvement of his circulatory system, resulting eventually in multiple emboli which occluded blood vessels in the legs and also the brain. Notwithstanding this terrible illness, he sent encouraging messages to the House of Delegates which are recorded in the proceedings, and telegraphed his personal appointments to fill vacancies in the councils of the Association.

His presidential address, delivered by the vice-president, Dr. Kenneth M. Lynch of Charleston, South Carolina, on "Modern Trends in Surgery," was an urgent appeal for the promotion of the highest standards and ideals of American medicine. He was installed as president of the American Medical Association "in absentia," and served a brief period of five and a half weeks—the end coming on June 20, 1936.

This leader of American medicine, chosen for its highest honors, demonstrated by his life and death how well he merited this recognition.

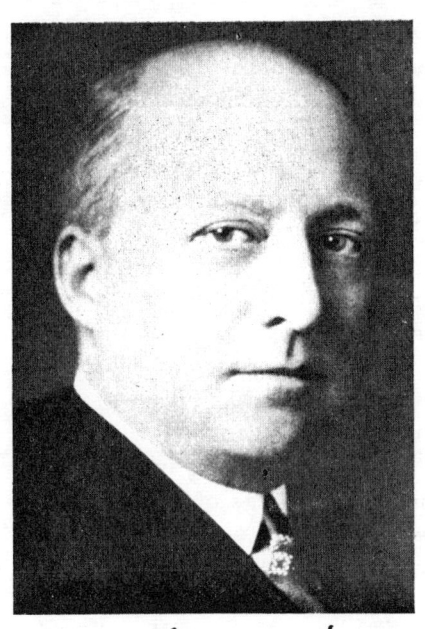

CHARLES GORDON HEYD, M.D
New York, N. Y.
1884—

Ninetieth President, A. M. A.
Atlantic City Session
June 7, 8, 9, 10, 11, 1937

DR. CHARLES GORDON HEYD was the second vice-president to succeed to the presidency in the history of the Association, because of death of the president while in office. In view of the severe character of the illness of President Mason at the time of the Kansas City session, in May 1936, and the certainty that the vice-president, under the By-Laws, would be compelled to officiate in place of the president during most of the term, the House of Delegates recognized its great responsibility, and made a choice for vice-president that was specially significant. Doctor Heyd served as president from June 21, 1936 to June 8, 1937.

He was born in Brantford, Ontario, Canada, August 27, 1884. His preparatory education was received at Brantford Collegiate Institute following which he graduated from the University of Toronto with the degree Bachelor of Arts in 1905. He received the degree Doctor of Medicine from the University of Buffalo in 1909.

Doctor Heyd served as resident house surgeon of the New York Post-Graduate Hospital from 1912 to 1914, when he was appointed adjunct professor of surgery in the New York Post-Graduate Medical School and Hospital, serving until 1920 when he became professor of surgery. At the same time he was appointed professor of surgery in the Postgraduate Medical School of Columbia University.

At the present time he is consulting surgeon to the Woman's

Hospital, New York City, the Dover General Hospital of Dover, New Jersey, and the Norwalk General Hospital in Norwalk, Conn.

In the first World War he was commissioned a Colonel in the Medical Corps, U. S. Army, and was Commanding Officer of Mobile Hospital No. 7 with the American Expeditionary Forces in France.

Doctor Heyd has been a frequent contributor to surgical literature, being co-author of "The Liver and Its Relation to Chronic Abdominal Infection" (with Drs. John A. Killian and Ward J. MacNeal) published in 1924.

He was awarded the Decoration Legion of Honor of France in 1932 and received the honorary degree Doctor of Medical Science from Temple University in 1937. He has served as president of the medical society of the County and of the State of New York. It was at the last session of the State society meeting in New York City that Doctor Heyd, as Chairman in charge of arrangements, revealed an extraordinary executive ability.

He is a Fellow of the American College of Surgeons, serving as vice-president in 1932-33. Doctor Heyd is a member of the American Gastro-Enterological Association, the Southern Surgical Association, and of Alpha Omega Alpha Honor Medical Society.

His address as retiring president in 1937 entitled "Professional Freedom and Social Responsibility" was a further exposition of his scholarly background, clear thinking, accuracy of historic data, and abiding faith in the ideals and future of American medicine. It is fitting to quote briefly from this stimulating address: "In every age and cultural order, the doctor has existed and maintained himself in spite of war, catastrophes and revolution." "From remote times the doctor has enjoyed complete professional freedom and has thereby assumed great social responsibility." "Medicine has the properties of a living organism—it is dynamic and evolves with the spirit of the times—every society throughout history has formulated an ideal of medical service." "One may hopefully anticipate that in this country there shall emerge a progressively advancing type of medical education and medical service which may be called the American system." "The science of medicine and the art of medical practice must retain its freedom and professional liberty."

Following his term as president of the American Medical Association, Doctor Heyd became a member of the Council on Medical Education and Hospitals, in which service his experience in medical education and postgraduate instruction has been specially valuable.

This eloquent and forceful speaker, distinguished educator and genial physician, has before him a life of expanding usefulness to modern medicine and society.

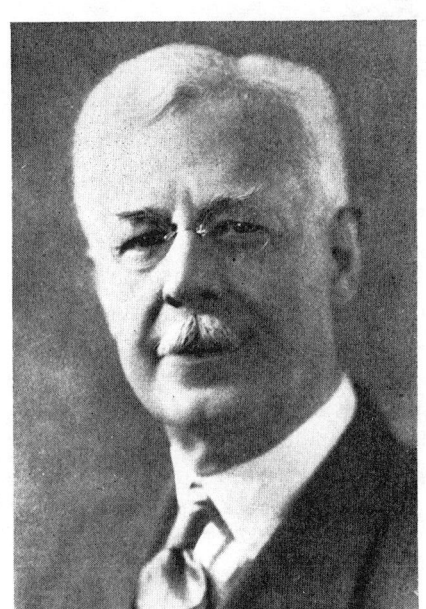

JOHN H. J. UPHAM, M.D.
Columbus, Ohio
1871–

*Ninety-first President, A. M. A.
Atlantic City Session
June 7, 8, 9, 10, 11, 1937*

IN SELECTING DR. JOHN HOWELL JANEWAY UPHAM for president of the Association, the House of Delegates recognized a career of distinguished service in organized medicine, and a notable leadership in the field of medical education and the practice of medicine.

He was born at Trenton, New Jersey, August 12, 1871. After completing his preliminary education he attended the University of Pennsylvania where he received the Certificate of Biology in 1891, and the degree Doctor of Medicine from the same institution in 1894. It was a class that contributed a number of other notable members in high places in the American Medical Association.

Following an internship in Johns Hopkins Hospital in Baltimore from 1894 to 1896, he began the practice of medicine in Columbus, Ohio. In 1897 he entered upon his teaching career as instructor of medicine at Starling Medical College, continuing in that position until 1902. It was during this period that he carried on postgraduate studies in the European medical centers at Prague, Leipzig, and Berlin. From 1902 to 1908 he was associate professor of medicine in the Starling-Ohio Medical College, and then became professor of medicine and clinical medicine. In 1914 he was appointed professor of medicine in Ohio State University College of Medicine. He also served as its Dean for the years 1927 to 1941, when he became Dean Emeritus.

Doctor Upham has contributed in large part to the high place that this medical school has attained in the last twenty years.

Since 1913 he has been a member of the Ohio State Board of Medical Examiners, one of the longest records of service in medical licensure in this country. The advanced standards constantly advocated by the Ohio State Board have likewise been influenced by the stimulating leadership of Doctor Upham. In the Ohio State Medical Association he served as secretary-editor from 1907 to 1913, and president in 1914-15, since which time he has been chairman of the Legislative Committee. He was president of the Columbus Academy of Medicine in 1919.

In the American Medical Association he served on the Judicial Council for a term beginning in 1922; a year later he was elected a member of the Board of Trustees, serving in this important official capacity for twelve years until 1935, the last two years as chairman of the Board.

His address as president on "The Advancement of Medical Education" reflected the experience of forty years of medical practice, and the rapid progress of medicine during that period.

It began under the inspiring influence of that remarkable quartette Kelly, Halsted, Welch and Osler, at Johns Hopkins Hospital, Baltimore; it witnessed the development of the clinical laboratory and of teaching at the bedside with its resultant evolution in medical education; the introduction of special diagnostic measures, knowledge of new diseases and specific therapy; it saw further the organization of the Council on Medical Education and Hospitals, of systematic postgraduate training, and above all the recognized leadership and guidance of the American Medical Association in presenting to the world the highest standards of medical science and medical practice.

He has held positions of trust in many civic organizations. In 1922 he was on the Advisory Committee of the American Red Cross. In 1941 he was honored with the presidency of the Ohio Hospital Association and since 1943 has served as the president and chairman of the Board of Planned Parenthood Federation of America.

Doctor Upham is a member of Alpha Omega Alpha Honor Medical Society, and a Fellow of the American College of Physicians.

The entire medical career of Dr. Upham with its significant accomplishments for the betterment of human welfare has exemplified the highest ideals of the art and science of medicine.

He continues his consultation practice in Columbus, Ohio.

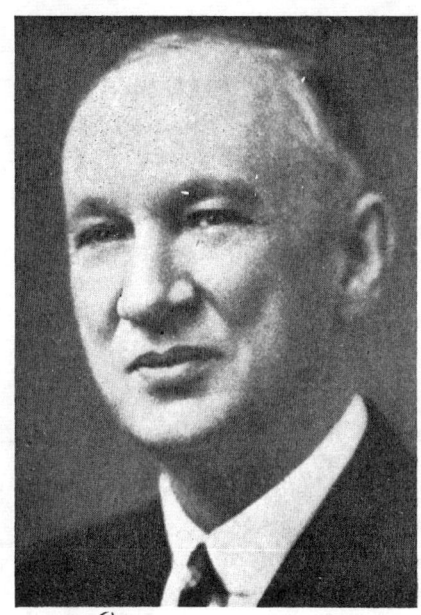

IRVIN ABELL, M.D.
Louisville, Ky.
1876–

Ninety-second President, A. M. A.
San Francisco Session
June 13, 14, 15, 16, 17, 1938

IN THE ELECTION OF DR. IRVIN ABELL for president of the Association, he was unopposed, indicating a remarkable unanimity of action, in keeping with his popularity and long record of service in the medical profession.

Doctor Abell was another son of Kentucky added to the long list of distinguished physicians who had served as president of the American Medical Association.

He was born in Lebanon, Kentucky, September 13, 1876. He received his Master of Arts degree from St. Mary's College, St. Mary, Ky., in 1894, and that of Doctor of Medicine from the Louisville Medical College in 1897, at the age of twenty-one years. He continued his postgraduate studies for a year at the University of Berlin, and in 1900 began to practice in Louisville, Ky.

In 1904 he was appointed Professor of Surgery in the University of Louisville and has served continuously in that position.

Doctor Abell is visiting surgeon of the Louisville Public Hospital and the St. Joseph Infirmary, and consulting surgeon for the Children's Free Hospital and the Kosair Hospital for Crippled Children.

During World War I he was a Lieutenant Colonel, commanding Base Hospital No. 59, then Colonel in the Medical Officers Reserve Corps and Commanding Officer of the U. S. Army Reserve Corps, Hospital No. 59.

His record of service in the American Medical Association has been a notable one. He was a member of the House of Delegates at the annual sessions of 1922, 1924, 1928, 1930 to 1935, and during these years served as member and chairman of many important committees. In 1931 he became a member of the Council on Scientific Assembly, and served as Chairman from 1935 to 1937. During his service as President-elect and President from 1937 to 1939, he was unsparing in his efforts to advance the interests of the Association, appearing at many society meetings throughout the United States, and faithfully fulfilled every obligation that the office required.

His address as president in 1939 on "The Aims of the Medical Profession as they Relate to the Public" reflected his own views and the prevailing thought on the new responsibilities of medical service. He summarized the aims of the medical profession as "(1) maintenance of high standards of medical education, assuring the graduate of competency to care for the sick; (2) adequate provision for graduate education with specified training for the development of specialists; (3) extension of public health and preventive medicine; (4) the widest possible dissemination of health information to enable the public to act intelligently in the preservation of its health and in the prevention of disease; (5) the development and consummation of plans for extension of medical service to all groups of the population, consonant with our established high standard of quality."

As a result of a resolution adopted by the House of Delegates in June 1940, the Board of Trustees created the Committee on Medical Preparedness, of which Dr. Irvin Abell became general chairman. This committee was of great service in mobilizing the medical profession and all available medical and hospital facilities in preparation for the impending emergency. In the membership of this committee were two later presidents of the Association—Fred W. Rankin (1942) and James E. Paullin (1943).

Doctor Abell has been the recipient of many honors. He received the honorary degree Doctor of Science from the University of Louisville in 1937, from Georgetown University and Manhattan College of New York City in 1939. Marquette University conferred the degree Doctor of Laws in 1939. In 1938 Notre Dame University conferred on Doctor Abell the Laetare Medal. Up to that time this medal had been awarded to fifty-six recipients, including a former President of the Association, Dr. John B. Murphy.

Doctor Abell is a Fellow and Regent of the American College of Surgeons, and has had a prominent part in the development of the extensive postgraduate educational program of the College throughout the United States and Canada. He holds membership in the American Gastro-Enterological Association, the American Surgical, the Southern Surgical, and Southern Medical and the American Urological Associations.

Among other positions indicating his executive ability are Director of the Commonwealth Life Insurance Company, the Fidelity and Columbia Trust Company, and the Louisville Foundation. He is also a Trustee of the University of Louisville.

As chariman of the Ephraim McDowell Committee in 1936, he was instrumental in purchasing the McDowell home in Danville, Ky., and aiding in its restoration.

Dr. Abell delivered the William W. Root Alpha Omega Alpha Lecture in 1940, on "The Spirit of Medicine," and all who were privileged to hear it remember this gem of diction and eloquence with its fluency and charm of delivery.

This genial and highminded medical gentleman graced the office of president and will continue to add distinction and dignity to the sacred calling of medicine.

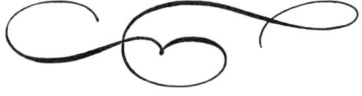

ROCK SLEYSTER, M.D.
Milwaukee, Wis.
1879–1942

*Ninety-third President, A. M. A.
St. Louis Session
May 15, 16, 17, 18, 19, 1939*

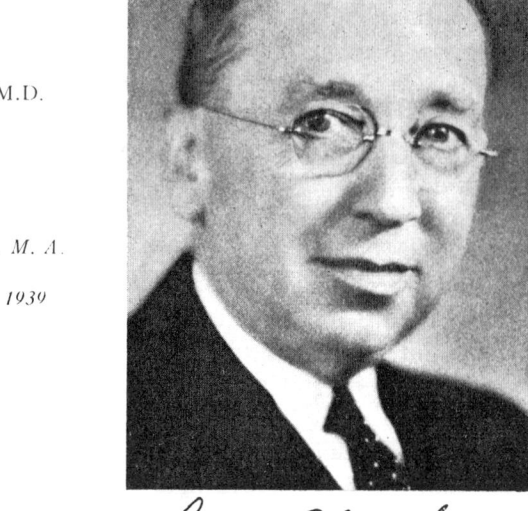

THE HONOR OF THE PRESIDENCY came to Dr. Rock Sleyster largely in recognition of thirty-five years of outstanding official service to the medical profession. It is further noteworthy that in this long period he was unanimously elected to every office which he occupied, having never been opposed by any other candidate.

He was born in Waupun, Wisconsin, June 14, 1879. After attending local public schools he entered the College of Physicians and Surgeons of Chicago, later University of Illinois School of Medicine, from which he graduated with the degree Doctor of Medicine in 1902. Soon after graduation he began to practice medicine in Kiel and Appleton, Wisconsin. Then he became physician to the prison for the criminal insane at Waupun, Wis., where he did creditable research work, much of which was later published. Here he first became interested in psychiatry, to which he devoted his life work in clinical medicine.

In 1903 he became Secretary of the Calumet County Medical Society, continuing for six years, and from that time forward was continuously associated with organized medicine and numerous medical societies. In 1910 he was appointed assistant secretary of the Wisconsin State Medical Society, serving four years, when he became secretary. In this post he continued until elected president of the State society in 1924. The following year he became treasurer, serving for many years. Doctor Sleyster was editor of the Wisconsin Medical Journal from 1918 to 1923.

His official connection with the American Medical Association began with his election from Wisconsin to the House of Delegates in 1913, and he served in the annual sessions of 1914, 1918 to 1926. During the last four years, 1922 to 1926, he served as vice-speaker. In 1926 he was elected to the Board of Trustees, serving until 1937, being chairman of the Board from 1935 to 1937. While President-elect he travelled extensively and delivered inspiring addresses in all parts of the country, but during the year as president his health became impaired and he had to limit his activities to a certain extent.

During World War I, Doctor Sleyster served as a Major in the U. S. Army Medical Corps, and was appointed medical aide to the Governor of Wisconsin. From 1916 to 1920 he served as Chief of the Bureau of Post-Graduate Medical Instruction at the University of Wisconsin, Extension Division.

Early in his professional career he became interested in institutional administration. From 1909 to 1919 he was Medical Director of the Central State Hospital for Insane at Waupun, and in 1919 he became the Medical Director of the Milwaukee Sanitarium at Wauwatosa, a suburb of Milwaukee. This hospital was devoted entirely to the diagnosis and care of nervous and mental conditions. Dr. Sleyster's ability as an organizer was specially exhibited in the creation of this model institution. The expression of Emerson, "An institution is the lengthened shadow of one man" is very applicable in this instance.

His presidential address in 1939 on "The Mind of Man and His Security" was a stimulating message, dwelling particularly on the vast expansion that has occurred in the field of nervous and mental diseases.

He was a member of the American Psychiatric Association, the Association of Research in Nervous and Mental Diseases, and the Central Neuro-psychiatric Association. Dr. Sleyster was a Fellow of the American College of Physicians and the College Governor for Wisconsin from 1926 to 1940.

It may well be said that Dr. Sleyster devoted his life to the service of his profession and to its members, giving freely of his time and energy for the advancement of medical organization. He was a gentle, modest thoughtful man, and a most cultured and genial gentleman. A host of devoted friends mourned his death, from heart disease, on March 7, 1942 at the age of sixty-two years.

NATHAN B. VAN ETTEN, M.D.
New York City
1866–

Ninety-fourth President, A. M. A.
New York City Session
June 10, 11, 12, 13, 14, 1940

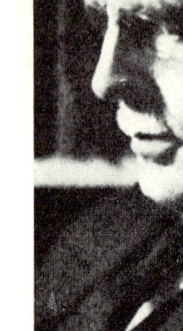

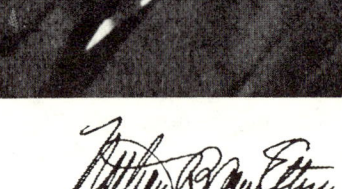

DR. NATHAN BRISTOL VAN ETTEN was the second Speaker of the House of Delegates to be honored with the presidency of the Association. It was equally a fitting recognition of his prominence as a general practitioner and a leader in medical affairs.

Doctor Van Etten was born in Waverly, New York, June 22, 1866. He received his degree Doctor of Medicine from Bellevue Hospital Medical School in 1890 and has practiced in New York City ever since. In 1906 he became visiting physician to the Union Hospital and has been constantly associated with that hospital. He has also been medical director of the Morrisania City Hospital since 1929, and president of the staff since 1932. He began as a general practitioner with surgical training, and further postgraduate work in this country and abroad, but an unusual experience with an epidemic of typhoid fever, and demands of other infectious diseases, gradually shaped his course into the field of internal medicine.

His quality of leadership is shown by the fact that he has been president of the Bronx County Medical Society, of the Bronx Borough Medical Society, of the New York Society of Medical Jurisprudence, of the Medical Alumni of New York University, of the Greater New York Medical Association, and also president and trustee of the Medical Society of the State of New York. Doctor Van Etten is a Fellow of the American College of Physicians.

In the American Medical Association he served as a member of the House of Delegates in 1920 and 1923, and continuously from 1926 through 1935, and also in the special session of 1935 which considered the Social Security Act. He was elected vice-speaker of the House of Delegates in 1933, and served in that position until he was elected speaker in 1935. While Speaker of the House in 1936, 1937 and 1938, he earned the respect and admiration of the delegates for his calm manner, his absolute justice, his parliamentary leadership and his unwavering fidelity to the principles of the Association.

It is fitting to quote from his address of acceptance of the office of President, in which he again dedicated himself to the work of the Association, and made a stirring plea for united action, "Yesterday, you adopted a report defining your position in relation to the proposed Wagner Health Act. It will have small value, however, unless the whole medical profession of the United States is educated to understand it. Every delegate must realize his official obligation as never before and carry home to every single practitioner in his state a full consciousness of the importance of this declaration of principles. That practitioner is potentially one of the most powerful persons in the democracy. If he can be made to see his duty to his country and educate his patients to a realization of the dangers of centralized control of medical practice, your action of yesterday will be sustained. In the name of welfare, gentlemen of the House, the practice of medicine as you know it and as you hoped it would become, is to be destroyed. The functions of the most highly educated group of professionals in the world are to be taken over by bureaus operated by adventurous amateurs. The time has come for the concerted action of every doctor in the United States."

In his address to the House of Delegates in 1940 he made a strong plea for a National department of health, and to coordinate all federal health functions under one agency. He expressed the conviction that this would be one way toward bringing the good offices of the Government into concert with the ideals of the American Medical Association.

In his inaugural address as President at the New York session in 1940, he spoke to the subject: "Better Health for America," which able presentation reflected the experience of the general practitioner in a large metropolitan community. He used the dictum "Better Health for America" as the objective of the organized medical profession, and stated "Organized medicine has been trying for the last ninety-four years to inspire all its members, who represent 85 per cent of the active practitioners in the United States with high ideals and with a sense of their responsibility for good public service." He again forcefully dwelt on the need of health education of the public, and made a plea for further change of educational procedure that would bring the physician earlier into practice; that the young doctor cannot begin at the top as a specialist, and that his education must be devised to prepare him to understand the average clinical problems which are presented by the average patients; he made the interesting comment—"Only competent physicians can succeed in country practice." He expressed the confidence "that the Association is moving consistently with conservation of real verities and real values, and that projection of new objectives promise to carry American medicine as a strong influence in the administration of the health programs of our country."

His record as president of the Association was in keeping with his fundamental concept of a physician's duty and responsibility to public service, to give unstintingly of himself to every medical and public effort to which he was called.

Doctor Van Etten continues his practice in New York City.

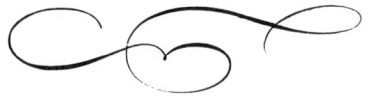

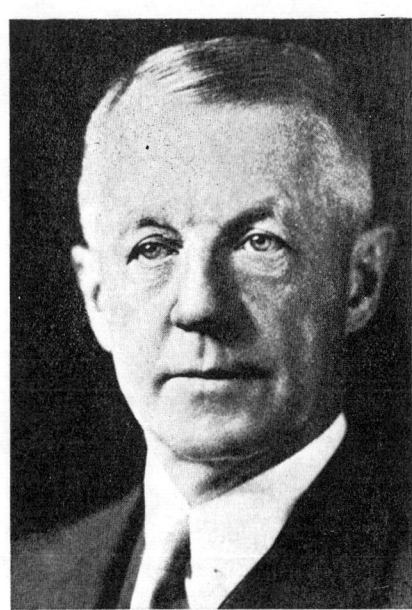

FRANK HOWARD LAHEY, M.D.
Boston, Mass.
1880–

Ninety-fifth President, A. M. A.
Cleveland Session
June 2, 3, 4, 5, 6, 1941

AT THE TIME OF THE ELECTION of Dr. Frank H. Lahey to the presidency of the Association, it is doubtful if any other surgeon in the United States was more widely known throughout the Nation. He had been the greatest single attraction in the field of graduate education for a number of years. His sixtieth birthday had occurred a few days previously, and his many friends, lay and medical, had presented him with a birthday volume, as a token of affection and testimony of his achievements in scientific medicine. This volume comprised fifty-five articles from leading physicians and surgeons of the United States. The last is "An Appraisal" by Dr. Arthur W. Booth, Chairman, Board of Trustees American Medical Association, from which is quoted: "I am particularly impressed that he accepts with such enthusiasm the broader responsibilities of his profession. To work within the close range of the doctor-patient relationship is obviously most essential and commendable, and by far too many excellent men essay no further. Fortunately, it is given to some to look beyond the narrow confines of the consultation room or the clinic to that broader horizon where loom the vital problems of the advancement of medical science and art, especially in the field of supervision and direction of the medical school and hospital."

Doctor Lahey was born in Haverhill, Mass., on June 1, 1880 of

Irish parentage. He received the degree Doctor of Medicine from Harvard University Medical School in 1904. After he served as intern and house surgeon in the Long Island Hospital in 1904 and 1905, and as surgeon in the Boston City Hospital from 1905 to 1907, he became resident surgeon of the Haymarket Relief Station in 1908, and instructor in surgery in Harvard Medical School during 1908 and 1909; this position he held from 1912 to 1915. He was assistant professor and later professor of surgery in Tufts Medical School from 1913 to 1917, and also served as professor of clinical surgery in the Harvard Medical School during the academic year of 1923–24.

During World War I, Doctor Lahey served as Major and also as director of surgery in Evacuation Hospital No. 30. After his return from military service he began practice in Boston, and started a private hospital, which gradually developed into the present Lahey Clinic. This has become a large institution and particularly distinguished for its contribution to medical education and medical investigation.

He has been for some time surgeon in chief of the New England Deaconess and New England Baptist Hospitals and director of surgery in the Lahey Clinic since its formation.

His chief literary contribution, in addition to many periodical articles, is the Lahey Clinic number of the Surgical Clinics of North America. He is a member of the editorial boards of Surgery, Gynecology and Obstetrics, and of the New England Journal of Medicine.

His particular contribution to postgraduate education has been in the form of well prepared lectures, always illustrated with slides and movies, delivered before medical societies, regional clinics, seminars, institutes and medical schools. He uses but few notes, and speaks entirely from his own experience, and the results obtained at the Lahey Clinic.

Doctor Lahey is a Fellow and member of the Board of Governors of the American College of Surgeons; a regent of the International College of Surgeons in Geneva, and a member of the American Surgical Association, the American Association for the Study of Goitre, and the Société des Chirurgiens de Paris. In 1941–2 he was president of the International Post-Graduate Assembly. Tufts College in 1927 conferred upon Doctor Lahey the Honorary Degree of Doctor of Science. He is a Harvard alumnus member of Alpha Omega Alpha Honor Medical Society.

In the American Medical Association, Doctor Lahey was secretary of the Section on Surgery, General and Abdominal, from 1926 to 1929, and Chairman the following year. He became a member of the Council on Scientific Assembly from 1927 to 1940, when he was elected president of the Association. He chose for the subject of his presidential address "Current Problems of American Medicine," which was largely concerned with the uncertain conditions prevailing at that time. He expressed gratification at the promptness at which the Association had offered its services and facilities to the Government in providing for medical personnel, better training for military service and continued preparedness for the emergency of war. When the Procurement and Assignment Service for Physicians, Dentists and Veterinarians, Office of Defense Health and Welfare Services, was authorized by President Franklin D. Roosevelt, on October 30, 1941, and an office established in Washington, D.C. Dr. Frank H. Lahey became the Chairman of the Directing Board, the other members being C. Willard Camalier, D.D.S., Harold S. Diehl, M.D., James E. Paullin, M.D., and Harvey B. Stone, M.D. The accomplishments of this service through scientific study and allocation of professional personnel in the war emergency, are among the outstanding achievements of the medical profession of the country.

Doctor Lahey has said frequently, that "he is devoting his life to the training of young physicians for better service in medicine and surgery" and therein will be his noblest monument.

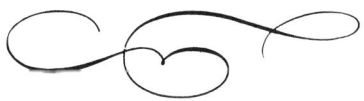

FRED WHARTON RANKIN, M.D.
Lexington, Ky.
1886–

*Ninety-sixth President, A. M. A.
Atlantic City Session
June 8, 9, 10, 11, 12, 1942*

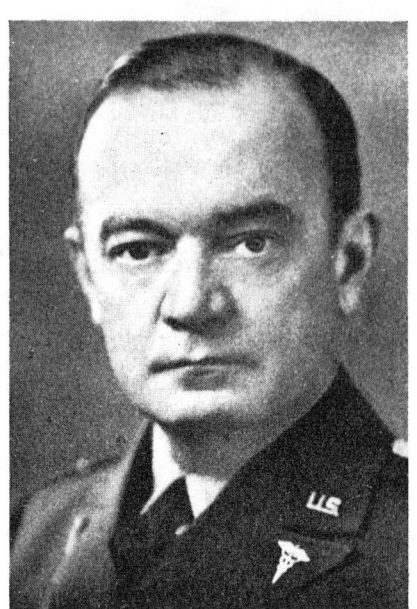

WITH THE ELECTION OF DR. FRED W. RANKIN as president of the Association, again a surgeon of international repute was accorded the highest honor in the province of scientific medicine. He had also participated notably in the affairs of the Association and other scientific bodies.

He was born in Mooresville, North Carolina, on December 20, 1886. After receiving his Bachelor of Arts degree from Davidson College in 1905, he entered the University of Maryland Medical School, Baltimore, and graduated with the degree Doctor of Medicine in 1909. He received the Master of Arts degree from St. John's College in 1913.

Following his graduation in medicine he became a resident surgeon at the University Hospital in Baltimore from 1909 to 1912, and served as assistant demonstrator of anatomy and associate in surgery at the University of Maryland Medical School from 1913 to 1916. He then joined the Mayo Clinic in Rochester, Minn., acting as assistant surgeon at St. Mary's Hospital from 1916 to 1923. For one academic year, 1922-23, he served as professor of surgery at the University of Louisville. In 1923 he married Miss Edith Mayo, a daughter of Dr. Charles H. Mayo. He was appointed surgeon to the Mayo Clinic and associate professor in the Graduate

Medical School, University of Minnesota and Mayo Foundation in 1926, remaining until 1933 when he removed to Lexington, Kentucky, for the practice of surgery.

He has been surgeon to St. Joseph's and the Good Samaritan hospitals of Lexington since January 1, 1934. Since 1941 he has been professor of clinical surgery at the University of Louisville.

In the first World War, Doctor Rankin served as a Major in the Medical Corps for seventeen months, and was attached to the First Army Corps, 4th and 26th divisions, in France, and as Commanding Officer of Base Hospital No. 26. At the close of the war he became a Colonel in the Medical Reserve Corps.

In the American Medical Association he was a member of the House of Delegates, representing the Section on Surgery from 1935 through 1940. In 1936 he was appointed to the membership of the Council on Medical Education and Hospitals, in which body he was very active until his election to the presidency in 1941. In 1940, the speaker of the House of Delegates appointed Dr. Rankin a member of the Committee on Medical Preparedness, and he was most assiduous in the duties of this committee, and specially for military preparedness in the Fifth Corps Area.

Doctor Rankin was ordered to active duty March 1, 1942 as Consulting Surgeon in the office of the Surgeon General, U.S. Army, with the rank of Colonel. He therefore appeared in uniform at the annual session in Atlantic City June, 1942. In his inaugural address he spoke of "The Responsibilities of Medicine in War Time," and referred to its being a quarter of a century since the Association met during war time to install a president. In 1917 the annual session was held in New York City two months after the opening of World War I. The president in 1917 was Dr. Charles H. Mayo, father-in-law of Doctor Rankin—an interesting coincidence. The title of President Mayo's address was "War's Influence on Medicine."

The address of President Rankin was an able, scholarly and serious analysis of the responsibilities that American medicine must assume in wartime. In 1943 Colonel Rankin was advanced to the rank of Brigadier General, Medical Corps, U. S. Army. As Chief Consulting Surgeon to the office of the Surgeon General he made journeys to the theaters of war in North Africa, Europe, the Pacific and the Far East.

At the session of the House of Delegates of the Association in Chicago in December 1945, a special ceremony was arranged for awarding the Distinguished Service Medal to Brigadier General Fred W. Rankin for "exceptional meritorious services from March 1942 to August 1945, which involved the responsibilities of the assignment of the highest type of surgical personnel and the selection of the most modern surgical supplies and equipment available."

Doctor Rankin has been honored by many medical organizations including the presidency of the Southern Surgical Association and the Southeastern Surgical Congress. He is a Fellow of the American College of Surgeons and member of the American Surgical Association, American Proctologic Society, Eastern and Western Surgical Associations, and Southern Medical Association. When the American Board of Surgery was organized in 1937, he was one of the founder members representing the Section on Surgery of the American Medical Association.

His contributions include a monograph on "Surgery of the Colon"; a work on "The Colon, Rectum and Anus" published in 1932 jointly with Drs. J. A. Bargen and L. A. Buie, and a work on "Cancer of the Colon and Rectum" published with Dr. A. S. Graham in 1939. He has also contributed chapters on these subjects in several systems of surgery. During the war period he published several interesting articles on "some current medico-military problems."

Doctor Rankin received the honorary degree Doctor of Science from Davidson College in 1937, and the University of Maryland in 1939. He is a member of Phi Beta Kappa and Sigma Xi societies. and honorary member of Alpha Omega Alpha Honor Medical Society.

His has been a career of distinction and of usefulness with the promise of further eminent service for human welfare in the years to come.

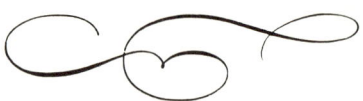

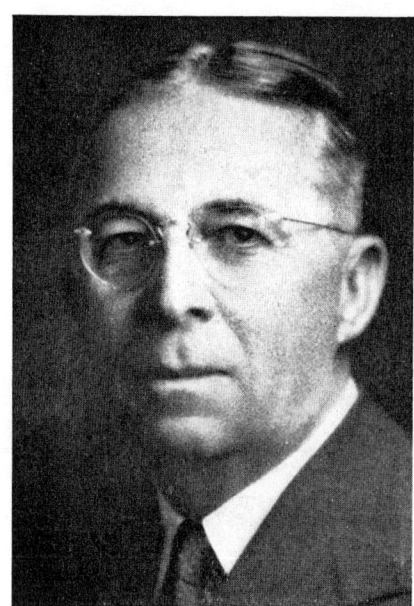

JAMES EDGAR PAULLIN, M.D.
Atlanta, Ga.
1881–

Ninety-seventh President, A. M. A.
Chicago Session
July 7, 8, 9, 1943

THE ELECTION OF DR. JAMES E. PAULLIN of Atlanta to the presidency of the Association was a merited recognition of a distinguished son of the South, and one of the foremost leaders in American medicine.

He was born in Fort Gaines, Georgia, November 3, 1881. After graduating from Mercer University with the degree of Bachelor of Arts in 1900, he continued as a graduate student throughout 1901, when he entered Johns Hopkins University School of Medicine, from which he received the degree Doctor of Medicine in 1905. He turned briefly to pathology, acting as resident pathologist of the Rhode Island Hospital at Providence from 1905 to 1906 in the Piedmont Hospital in 1906 and 1907, and as pathologist to the Georgia State Board of Health from 1907 to 1911. At the same time he was associate professor of pathology in the Atlanta College of Physicians and Surgeons. In 1909 he first became interested in internal medicine, being appointed associate visiting physician to Grady Hospital from 1909 to 1913. Then he was made visiting physician and chief of the Emory University Division, Grady Hospital. Two years later he became professor of clinical medicine at Emory University School of Medicine, which position he has held ever since.

With the outbreak of World War I, Doctor Paullin was commissioned a Major in the Medical Corps, U.S. Army, and served as chief of the medical service at Camp Shelby, Miss.

In the field of medical organization he had come up through all the ranks; first, as president of Fulton County Society in 1913; later as president of the Medical Association of Georgia; chairman of the Medical Section Southern Medical Association in 1920. In the American Medical Association he was chairman of the Section on Practice of Medicine in 1928, and member of the Council on Scientific Assembly from 1933 to 1942, the last five years serving as chairman. He was a member of the House of Delegates for six years from 1936 to 1942 as representative of the Section on Practice of Medicine.

With the beginning of preparations for World War II he became a member of the Committee on Medical Preparedness of the American Medical Association; at the same time he was a member of the Committee on Medical Sciences of the National Research Council. His principal contribution was the classification of specialists in internal medicine, as well as general practitioners specially in that field of practice. The functions of the Committee on Medical Preparedness were gradually taken over by the Procurement and Assignment Service for Physicians, Dentists and Veterinarians, and Doctor Paullin became a member of the Directing Board of this Service.

In his presidential address in 1943, while recognizing the heavy demands on the medical resources of the country, he urged early consideration of planning for postwar medical services, and his recommendation resulted in the creation of such a committee of which Dr. Paullin became one of the active members.

Doctor Paullin became a Fellow of the American College of Physicians in 1928, and served on its Board of Regents from 1932 to 1942, when he was chosen president-elect, and continuing as president to 1944, so that he had the distinct honor of serving at the same time as president of the largest medical association and the leading organization devoted to the special field of internal medicine. He was honored with the presidency of the American Clinical and Climatological Society in 1937, and holds membership in the Southern Medical Association, the Association of American Physicians, and is an alumnus member of Johns Hopkins University Chapter Alpha Omega Alpha Honor Medical Society.

Early in 1942 Doctor Paullin went to Cuba to aid in the organization of the Finlay Institute of the Americas for the securing of interchange of scientific medicine with the Latin American countries. He was decorated by President Batista with the Order of Carlos Finlay.

During the period of World War II he was Honorary Medical Consultant to the United States Navy. In 1945, by direction of Surgeon General Ross T. McIntire, he made an inspection tour of all naval stations in the Pacific area, covering 25,000 miles by air.

He was called as consultant during the last illness of President Franklin D. Roosevelt, and was with him when he died at Warm Springs, Georgia, April 12, 1945.

Doctor Paullin has collected a remarkable medical library, and is a lover of good books.

In addition to his extensive medical activities, he is interested in modern farming and the breeding of thoroughbred cattle.

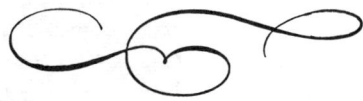

HERMAN L. KRETSCHMER, M.D.
Chicago, Ill.
1879–

Ninety-eighth President, A. M. A.
Chicago Session
June 12, 13, 14, 15, 16, 1944

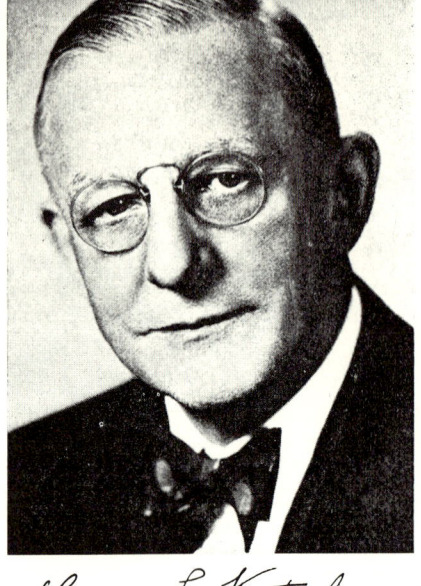

DR. HERMAN LOUIS KRETSCHMER was the unanimous choice of the House of Delegates for president of the Association, which was a distinct recognition of years of service devoted to its affairs.

He was the first specialist in urology to be elected to this high honor.

Doctor Kretschmer was born in Chicago on April 22, 1879. He was educated at Northwestern University, receiving the degree Graduate in Pharmacy in 1900, and that of Doctor of Medicine, cum laude, in 1904. In his senior year he was elected a member of Alpha Omega Alpha Honor Medical Society. He was granted the honorary degree of Doctor of Science from the University in 1942, and the same degree from Marquette University in 1943. Since 1904 he has devoted himself continuously to the practice and advancement of his profession. He has gained special distinction in the field of urology and genito-urinary surgery. In 1907 he became a member of Rush Medical College as professor of genito-urinary surgery until 1942, when he was appointed professor of urology.

During most of this period he has served as urologist at Presbyterian Hospital, and consultant at the Childrens Memorial Hospital, Chicago. He has been a keen investigator of pathologic conditions and special forms of treatment in his specialty of practice, and is the author of nearly 300 articles, published in numerous medical journals. Doctor Kretschmer has been honored by election to the presidency of many societies; Chicago Urological Society in 1915, the American Urological Society in 1925, the Clinical Society of Genito-Urinary Surgeons in 1931, the Chicago Medical Society in 1932, and the American Association of Genito-Urinary Surgeons in 1937.

He was a founder member of the American Board of Urology, and has been its president since 1935. Doctor Kretschmer is a member of the Chicago Pathological Society, the Illinois State Medical Society, the Western Surgical Association, the International Society of Urology, the American Radium Society, the National Research Council, and a Fellow of the American College of Surgeons. He is also a member of the Board of Honorary Consultants of the Army Medical Library, Washington, D.C., and of the editorial board of the American Journal of Urology.

In the American Medical Association he was Chairman of the Section on Urology in 1925, and Treasurer for ten years—from 1933 to 1943.

His address as President in 1944, "American Medicine and the War," reviewed the experience of the Association in the different wars since its organization in 1847. It brought forth in comparison the better state of health and nutrition of the military forces and that of the nation in World War II, and the greater degree of effort and opportunity on the part of the Association in the winning of the war. He deplored the efforts being made by forces outside the profession to promote the socialization and federalized control of the practice of medicine. In closing he spoke a high tribute to all physicians who had contributed so loyally to the war effort.

The Association was very fortunate to have the benefit of the experience and wisdon of Dr. Kretschmer during the critical years of the war period.

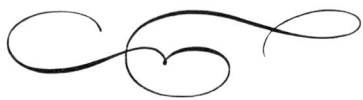

ROGER IRVING LEE, M.D.
Boston, Mass.
1881–

*Ninety-ninth President, A. M. A.
Chicago Session
(House of Delegates only)
December 3, 4, 5, 1945*

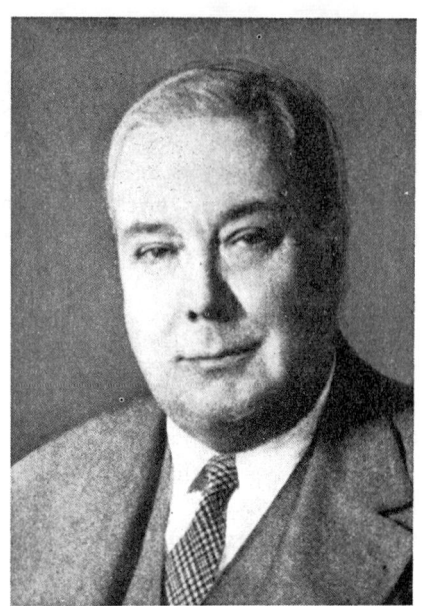

THE ELECTION OF DR. ROGER I. LEE was unique in the annals of the Association. In response to a general desire, he resigned as Chairman of the Board of Trustees, and then was summoned by a unanimous vote of the House of Delegates to accept the office of president-elect. It was a distinct recognition of many years of service in the Association and his leadership in the fields of education, public health, and the practice of medicine.

Doctor Lee was born in Peabody, Massachusetts, August 12, 1881. After attending Peabody High School, he entered Harvard University graduating in 1902 with the degree Bachelor of Arts (magna cum laude) and elected to Phi Beta Kappa Society in his senior year. He graduated from the Harvard Medical School in 1905, and began the practice of medicine in Boston. From 1907 to 1914 he served as assistant in medicine at the Harvard Medical School, and in 1912 he became visiting physician to the Massachusetts General Hospital continuing in that service until 1924. In 1914 he was appointed Henry K. Oliver Professor of Hygiene in Harvard University and this being a fulltime chair, it was necessary to give up medical practice. He continued in this protessorship for ten years, when he resumed private practice, mainly as consultant in internal medicine.

Doctor Lee was chosen an Overseer of Harvard University for

1930–1931, and since 1931 has been a Fellow of the Harvard Corporation, usually considered one of the highest honors for a Harvard graduate.

During the first World War he served as a Major in the Medical Reserve Corps, and was promoted to Lieutenant Colonel on June 6, 1918. He served in France as Chief Medical Officer with Base Hospital No. 5, and was consultant in medicine to the Third Corps of the American Expeditionary Forces. He was the recipient of a citation from General Pershing for "meritorious and conspicuous service" when discharged in February 1919. In World War II his three sons served as privates, their father saying—"there is distinction in being a private."

Aside from his professorship in Hygiene at Harvard University, he early became interested in public health activities. In 1910 he was Secretary of the Massachusetts Tuberculosis Commission. In 1917 he published a book on "Health and Disease." Doctor Lee was a member of the Public Health Council of Massachusetts from 1921 to 1934 and Treasurer of the American Public Health Association from 1919 to 1923. He is now a member of the National Advisory Health Council, and since 1941 a member of the Executive Committee, Division of Medical Sciences, National Research Council. He served as President of the Massachusetts State Medical Society in 1942 and 1943.

In the American Medical Association, Doctor Lee was Chairman of the Section on Pharmacology and Therapeutics in 1927 and 1928, and a member of the House of Delegates in 1911, 1926, 1928, and from 1930 to 1934. In 1934 he was elected a member of the Board of Trustees serving until 1945, being Chairman the last two years. In 1933 with Lewis W. Jones (now President of Bennington College) he published "The Fundamentals of Good Medical Care," as a part of the contribution to the Committee on the Cost of Medical Care, and some of the conclusions advanced at that time were incorporated in his presidential address in 1945 on "What is Adequate Medical Care?" This was a judicious analysis of the various reports and surveys published regarding inadequate medical care of a considerable portion of the people of the United States. He, however, regarded the advances in medical science and particularly the lessons learned in World War II, as the strongest influence in changing our concept of medical care, and therefore, there was need for continuous re-valuations in order to determine the place of the general practitioner and the specialist in any proposed plan of adequate medical care.

Doctor Lee is affiliated with other special societies, being a Fellow of the American College of Physicians, of which he has been a member of the Board of Regents and served as president in 1941.

In his presidential address to the American College of Physicians he stated in his platform—"a reasonable but not excessive specialism in medicine and an adequate appreciation of the efforts of the general practitioner."

He is a Diplomate of the American Board of Internal Medicine (Founders Group). Doctor Lee is also a member of the American Association of Physicians, the American Association for the Advancement of Science, the American Society for Clinical Investigation, a member of the American Academy of Arts and Sciences, and of Alpha Omega Alpha Honor Medical Society.

In the city of Boston he has been a member of the Committee on Health, the Boston Chamber of Commerce, and since 1934 has been a Trustee of the Boston Symphony Orchestra.

Doctor Lee is of large build and stature; a friend has described him as "big in body and big in mind"; another regards his greatest achievement "his capacity to make and retain friends—really true friends." Among the latter are many in other fields than medicine. In earlier days John Sargent, the painter; the former president of Harvard, Dr. A. Lawrence Lowell, and more lately Serge Koussevitsky, conductor of the Boston Symphony, and Winston Churchill —the resemblance to the latter having often been noted.

There is a further story that an old fisherman from Maine never comes to Boston without bringing the doctor a couple of fine lobsters, some oysters or scallops.

Thus at sixty-five, Roger Lee, the educator, disciple of public health, internist, lover of art and music, and cultured gentleman, exemplifies the best and noblest precepts of American medicine.

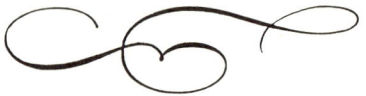

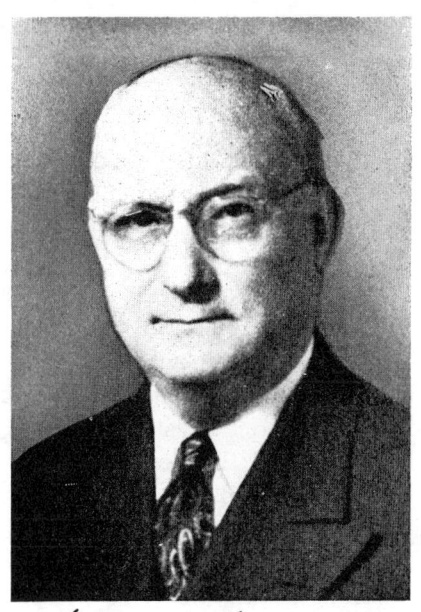

HARRISON H. SHOULDERS, M.D.
Nashville, Tenn.
1886–

One hundredth President, A. M. A.
San Francisco Session
July 1, 2, 3, 4, 5, 1946

DR. HARRISON H. SHOULDERS is the third Speaker of the House of Delegates who has been advanced to the presidency of the Association, and his election was also a distinct recognition of his important services to the cause of organized medicine. By a fortunate coincidence his election occurred on his twenty-third wedding anniversary.

Doctor Shoulders was born in Gainesboro, Tennessee, February 27, 1886. He was educated at Potter Bible College, Bowling Green, Kentucky, and received his degree Doctor of Medicine in 1909 from Nashville Medical College (later Vanderbilt University). He served an internship in St. Thomas Hospital, Nashville, 1909-1910, and was House Surgeon of Fonts Infirmary from 1910 to 1912. He then became assistant director of the Tennessee State Department of Health serving until 1917. Soon after the beginning of the first World War he was commissioned a Captain in the Medical Corps, United States Army and served from 1917 to 1919, mostly overseas. In 1920 he became Resident Surgeon at St. Luke's Hospital, and then House Surgeon in the Coley Service, Hospital for Ruptured and Crippled, New York City.

After completing these postgraduate studies he began the practice of surgery in Nashville, Tenn.

He was Secretary of the Tennessee State Medical Association and editor of its Journal from 1927 to 1945. From 1930 to 1938 Doctor

Shoulders served continuously as a member of the House of Delegates, representing the Tennessee State Medical Association. He was elected Vice-Speaker of the House in 1935, becoming Speaker in 1938, and serving in that position until his election as President in 1945. It became the privilege of Doctor Shoulders to preside at the first general assembly of the Association after the close of the hostilities, and his gracious presence added much to the pleasure and significance of the occasion.

In his address as president in 1946, entitled "Medical Progress in the United States under Freedom," he refers to the coming centennial of the Association and reviewed the achievements of American medicine during one hundred years under "freedom of action and thought." He referred to the American system of medical care that had developed over the years, and the need of constant vigilance to prevent the efforts to undermine the faith in American medicine. In closing he stated—"Not long ago our freedom was challenged by foes from without," "The situation that now exists calls for a rededication of all our strength and energy to the principles of the Association so that they shall be preserved for the benefit of mankind."

Doctor Shoulders was an organizer and the first president of the Nashville Surgical Society, and at present is assistant professor of clinical surgery in Vanderbilt University Medical School, and assistant visiting surgeon at Vanderbilt University Hospital. He is a member of the Southern Medical Association, a Fellow of the American College of Surgeons, and is certified by the American Board of Surgery (Founders Group). He served during the war period as Chief Surgeon of the Nashville Area, Office of Civilian Defense.

Doctor Shoulders has devised several new surgical procedures including a "new stitch for use in gastric surgery," published in Surgery, Gynecology and Obstetrics, and has otherwise been an extensive contributor to surgical literature.

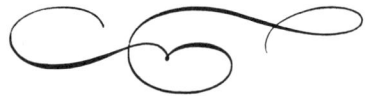

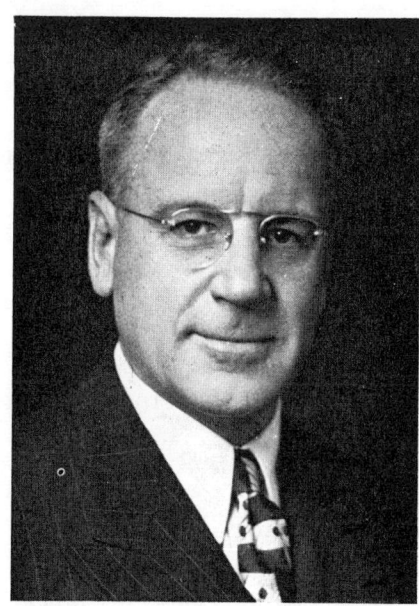

EDWARD L. BORTZ, M.D.
Philadelphia, Pa.
1896–

One Hundred and First President, A. M. A.
Atlantic City—Centennial Session
June 9, 10, 11, 12, 13, 1947

AT THE SAN FRANCISCO SESSION in July 1946, Dr. Olin West was unanimously chosen as president-elect, which was a fitting recognition of his quarter century service as general secretary and manager of the Association. There was a general regret when the announcement was made in March 1947 that because of continued ill health, Dr. West had decided to resign the office.

According to the Constitution and By-Laws of the Association Dr. Edward L. Bortz of Philadelphia, the vice-president elected in 1946, succeeded to the office of president-elect and inauguration as president at the Centennial session of the Association, Atlantic City, June 9–13, 1947. Thus for the third time in the history of the Association, the vice-president succeeds to the presidency.

Dr. Bortz was born in Greensburg, Pennsylvania, February 10, 1896. He received the A.B. degree from Harvard University in 1920, and the degree of M.D. in 1923. After his internship at Lankenau Hospital, Philadelphia, from 1923 to 1925, he pursued further studies at the universities of Berlin and Vienna in 1925 and 1926. After his return he carried on additional studies in pathology at the Mayo Clinic, and at the University of Illinois.

In 1930 he was appointed instructor in the department of pathology, University of Pennsylvania School of Medicine and the Graduate School of Medicine, serving for two years. Since 1932 he has been associate professor of medicine at the Graduate School of Medicine, University of Pennsylvania, as well as Chief of Medical Service B at Lankenau Hospital.

He has been a director of the Philadelphia County Medical Society, chairman of its committee on public relations, and president in 1940. He has also been chairman of the committee on scientific business of the College of Physicians of Philadelphia, and chairman of the committee for the study of penumonia control of the Pennsylvania State Medical Society. In 1939 he received the Meritorious Service Medal for distinguished service to the Commonwealth of Pennsylvania, the award being made by the then Governor George H. Earle.

Dr. Bortz became a Fellow of the American College of Physicians in 1929. At the present time he is a member and vice chairman of the Board of Governors. He is a Diplomate of the National Board of Medical Examiners, and of the American Board of Internal Medicine (Founders Group). He is also a member of the American Clinical and Climatological Association, and since 1929 has been assistant editor of the Cyclopedia of Medicine.

During World War II he was on active duty as Lieutenant Commander and later Captain in the Medical Corps of the United States Navy, serving from January 1942 to February 1, 1944.

In 1943 he was presented with the Founders Medal of the Association of Military Surgeons for exceptional services rendered in connection with the arrangements for its assembly in Philadelphia.

Dr. Bortz was made a member of the Council on Scientific Assembly of the American Medical Association in 1942, and became its chairman in 1945. He is also chairman of the Committee on National Emergency Medical Service of the Association. In 1945 he served as a member of the House of Delegates.

During his membership on the Council on Scientific Assembly he has shown high qualities of leadership, particularly in the arrangement of excellent programs for the general scientific meetings of the Association.

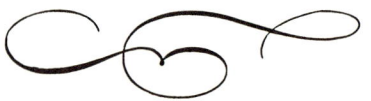

Councils and Bureaus of The American Medical Association

TRUSTEES OF THE AMERICAN MEDICAL ASSOCIATION

By Ernest E. Irons, M.D.

THE STORY OF THE ACTIVITIES of the Board of Trustees is essentially the record of the activities of the Association, of its growth in financial power and responsibility and of the expanding programs designed for the benefit of the medical profession and the public. Some only of the discussions of the Board will be included. By these were initiated new projects, accomplished often only after months and sometimes years of planning.

Today the Board of Trustees is charged with carrying on the business of the Association and of implementing between meetings of the House of Delegates the policies and instruction of the House. Some of the new projects were undertaken under instructions initiated by the House of Delegates; others originated in the Board as opportunities and requirements were recognized and were then brought to the House for consideration and approval. All actions by the Board are predicated on previous favorable action of the House of Delegates. The method of carrying out the instructions of the House has usually been left to the discretion of the Board. The Board of Trustees was originated to care for the property of the Association, acquired by reason of the establishment of the Journal. For many years the meetings and activities of the Association centered around the development of the Journal.

Prior to the establishment of the Journal of the American Medical Association, the proceedings of the annual meetings of the Association together with a few articles on medical subjects presented at the meetings were published in a volume called "The Transactions of the American Medical Association." As early as 1870, Professor Gross urged the Association to replace its annual volume of Transactions with a periodical medical journal. And again in 1872, Dr. Theophilus Parvin urged the same change "forcibly and at length." In 1879 Dr. Chaillé at the annual meeting in Atlanta in his address on State Medicine reviewed the activities of the Association and discussed what in his opinion should be done to bring the practice of medicine abreast of the then existing scientific knowledge. "State medicine is the application by the state of medical knowledge for the common weal; and embraces every subject for the apprehension of which medical knowledge and for the execution of which State authority are indispensable." He cited as an example of the lag of state medicine behind scientific knowledge the slowness with which vaccination against smallpox was being carried out as a prophylactic measure. The speech of Chaillé which initiated an expansion of policy of the American Medical Association was not planned for the promotion of personal interests of doctors, but for the improvement of the public health. This has always characterized the policies of the American Medical Association down to the present time. Committees were appointed which reported at the annual meetings of succeeding years. In 1881 Dr. John H. Packard read a report of the Committee on "journalizing the transactions" and at the annual meeting in 1883 after the final report of the Committee, it was resolved that there be adopted "the report of the Committee on Journalizing the Transactions and . . . that the journal be called the Journal of the American Medical Association."

THE FIRST BOARD

At this meeting in 1883 a Board of Trustees was appointed which organized with N. S. Davis as president and J. H. Packard as secretary. "The president of the Board was instructed to proceed with as little delay as possible to the printing of the report of the special committee on the subject of "journalizing the transactions of the Association." The first Board of Trustees included N. S. Davis of Illinois, E. M. Moore, New York, J. M. Toʳer, Washington; H. F. Campbell, Georgia; John H. Packard, Pennsylvania; L. Connor, Michigan; P. O. Hooper, Arkansas; A. Garcelon, Maine; L. S. McMurtry, Kentucky.

Previous to the establishment of the Journal, the Association had had little need for a Board of Trustees. The funds of the Association secured from dues were used in the publication of the transactions and for minor expenses. In 1879 the treasurer reported a balance of $1,245.66. The membership of the Association before this session was 2,100. "Undoubtedly a large number of these were centennial visitors of 1876 who attended the meeting of that year in Philadelphia with laudable but not wholly professional motives."

With respect to the editorial management of the proposed Journal, Dr. Chaillé had had this to say: "The editorial chair would not be a sinecure. It should be held by one who would neither shrink from theories nor shiver at thunder. He should be at once intelligent, conscientious and fearless; the elements of characteristics thus suggested combined in one individual would insure him ultimate success." For the next several years, the Trustees were referred to as the Trustees of the Journal and not of the Association. In 1883, also, Dr. Davis was chosen editor of the Journal and thereafter resigned as trustee.

THE INCORPORATION

In 1897 the American Medical Association was incorporated under the laws of Illinois and the by-laws suitably amended to meet the requirements of Illinois law. Reminiscent of the small beginnings and of the financial problems of the Board were such instructions as, "The treasurer was directed to secure a safety deposit box for the papers of the Association and to provide a security bond." "The resident trustees and editor are authorized to employ a clerk at $75.00 per month."

Under the new by-laws, passed April 8, 1898, three trustees were to be elected to serve three years each. The officers for that year were Alonzo Garcelon, president; Truman Miller, vice president; John B. Hamilton, secretary and editor, and Henry P. Newman, treasurer. In this year upon the death of Dr. Hamilton, Dr. Truman Miller, chairman of the Publication Committee of the Board and resident trustee, took charge of the Journal and the Trustees set about finding a new editor. After much discussion and search Dr. George H. Simmons of Lincoln, Nebraska, was chosen. One of the first requests of Dr. Simmons was for more printing equipment and thereafter there is no item which occurs with more frequency in the minutes of the Board in succeeding years than requests for new presses, folders and linotype machines. At this time circulation of the Journal was 13,672. The assets of the Association consisted of inventory of Journal property, $21,031.30 and securities and cash $27,368.80.

THE FIRST PERMANENT HOME

From these small beginnings the Journal began to grow under the able editorship of Dr. Simmons. Its circulation and earnings increased so that by June 1901 at the annual meeting at St. Paul the Board reported to the House of Delegates that "toward securing a permanent home for the Journal you now have invested in gilt edge securities $25,000 which yearly grows by the interest at least." By May, 1902, Holabird and Roche had completed plans for the Association building at 101–3 Dearborn Street, and here the Trustees met on February 11, 1903. The land and the new building had evidently been paid for out of current receipts for the $25,000 in securities was still intact.

Journal growth and expanding interest of the medical profession in problems of better medical care for the public multiplied the activities and obligations of the Board of Trustees as reflected in the minutes and in reports of the Board to the House of Delegates. From the management of a small organization and the direction of modest yearly expenditures, the Board found itself confronted with a rapidly growing business, later to involve millions in place of thousands in yearly turnover. Repeated reorganization of methods became necessary in order that the affairs of the Association might be kept on a sound basis, protected from the vicissitudes of the national business cycle. This involved the setting up of reserves commensurate with the yearly volume of business.

The necessity of improvement of quality of medical performance was increasingly recognized and the Trustees representing the Association concerned themselves more and more with standards of medical education and with the correction of frauds in medical advertising. Lively appreciation by each member of the Board of these problems is evident in the serious discussions of this early period of expansion. The new problems seemed unending, and it is probably as well that the Boards of those days could not look ahead to see the vast further increase of responsibility which was to come in subsequent years.

THE TURN OF THE CENTURY

The agenda for the annual meeting of the Board for 1903 included items concerning completion of the building; the setting up of a suitable financial system and deletion of proprietary advertising from the Journal; the proposed revision of the code of ethics; and a reconciliation of the bylaws with the provisions of the Illinois law governing corporations. A proposal had been made to obtain a national charter from Congress, but counsel advised that only a charter in the District of Columbia was feasible and that such a charter would not meet the requirements of the Illinois law. In this year membership in the Association was 12,540 and the weekly circulation of the Journal 25,321. A report of the Committee on Medical Education pointing out the serious defects in medical education and the low grade of instruction afforded medical students by the multiplicity of inferior medical schools was presented to the Board with a request for an appropriation of $5,000 for a survey of medical education. The report was approved in principle "but the appropriation was denied because the financial condition of the Association did not justify it."

In February 1905, the Board consisting of T. J. Happel, Chairman; E. E. Montgomery, A. L. Wright, H. L. S. Johnson, Philip

Marvel, William H. Welch, Miles T. Porter, M. L. Harris and W. W. Grant met at the headquarters building. Present also were Frank Billings, treasurer and George H. Simmons, editor and general manager. The total assets of the Association were $213,470.23 and the revenue for 1904, $43,465.03. The Board voted to sustain the action of the editor in his refusal of certain proprietary advertising. A proposal was made to add a fourth story to the building. Dr. Bevan again asked for an appropriation for the Committee on Education and received an appropriation of $4,000. "Dr. Simmons spoke on the subject of a Council on Pharmacy and Chemistry of the American Medical Association and of the advertisements in the Journal." He submitted a list of 26 companies whose advertising had been refused by reason of false claims or secrecy of formulae. . . . The Board approved the general plan of the editor to create a Council on Pharmacy and Chemistry and appropriated a sum not to exceed $3,000 to defray the expenses of this Council. Provisional rules for acceptance of medical products for New and Non-official Remedies were approved by the Board. Plans for the publication of a complete directory of legally qualified physicians for the United States were proceeded with.

THE ATTACK ON THE AMERICAN MEDICAL ASSOCIATION

The firm stand taken by the editor of the Journal against the acceptance of fraudulent and misleading advertising had had the whole hearted support of the Trustees, and the repeated approval of the House of Delegates. Dr. Simmons' plan for the organization of the Council on Pharmacy and Chemistry had been put in operation by the Board and the Council at the Portland meeting in 1905 had formulated its rules for the approval of medical products for which advertising would be approved for the Journal. By 1906 the effects of this insistence on clean advertising had aroused proprietary medicine interests to an attack on the Journal, the Editor and the Trustees in an attempt to disrupt the entire work of the Association. Damage suits for refusing objectionable advertising were threatened against the Association and the Trustees although the legal bases of such suits do not seem to have been clear.

Additional enemies of the Association came through the revelations of the Council on Medical Education concerning inferior proprietary medical schools; also the proposal of the Association to publish its own directory had incurred the active opposition of a large outside publishing interest.

The attack on the Editor and the Board evidently arose chiefly as a result of the clean advertising policy of the Journal, but the other groups no doubt lent encouragement. At this time the vicious personal attack on Dr. Simmons which later occasioned him so much suffering and was so universally resented by the Board and the profession in general, had not developed.

At Boston in 1906 a resolution was introduced in the House of Delegates, which charged the Trustees with making incomplete financial reports concealing essential information, alleging distrust of the management of the Journal and asking for an investigation by a committee of the House named in the resolution. The resolution was at once tabled without discussion by an almost unanimous vote of the House. There followed however a discussion of the entire situation in a series of letters to the Editor, published in the Journal.

In this post-mortem on the resolution, it was charged that: the Trustees had shown lack of tact in dealing with independent journals, which claimed to have clean advertising pages but continued to include false advertising in their magazines; that the Trustees should have printed the entire salary list of the Journal in their annual report; that the Board had failed to report the amount paid for the standard directory which was to be used as a beginning for our new directory; that the Board had accumulated reserves and that this was unnecessary.

These and other similar charges were answered by Dr. T. J. Happel, Chairman of the Board, who pointed out that independent medical journals were usually run for profit alone, and while "They claim not to want to publish unethical advertisements, they continue to do so for the money they receive. Their opposition is due to the fact that the Journal has shown up the fraudulent nature of these advertisements." "Some journals are doing noble work. The State Journals are rapidly becoming essentials in well organized medical associations." Further Dr. Happel showed that the complete financial report of the Board was printed and distributed to the delegates except an itemized statement of salaries, and of the expense account of the organizer. These two latter items are available for inspection by any member of the House. To pri t the salary payroll would expose the Association to raids on its personnel, and such a foolish procedure would certainly indicate that the Board lacked "common business sense." "It is an utter absurdity to suggest an investigation of a business of the magnitude of the Journal office by a committee of physicians who are not practical bookkeepers. The Board long since abandoned any such piece of folly and has the work done by expert accountants." With respect to the directory, a fight had been made at Portland in 1905 against publication of a directory by the Association, instigated by a rival directory, and the House by an almost unanimous vote directed the Trustees to proceed with publication. The price of the directory had been agreed on, but under an obligation binding both parties, it could not be given out until the House of Delegates had acted on it.

"Why should we accumulate stocks and bonds? Such a question by a business man would need no answer." No enterprise can be carried on in these days without money to tide over times of disaster. We have had several years of prosperity, but this will not continue, if we are permitted to judge the future by the past. A reaction must follow and if we have no money we must fail."

Other letters in support of the Board appeared, and then the clamor might have subsided, had it not been for a statement in an eastern medical journal in which among a number of other charges it was insinuated that the management of the American Medical Association was in the hands of a "ring or clique," that the "financial reports have been disquietingly analogous to those of insurance companies and have dealt in glittering generalities," that the accounts of the Association have been "juggled," that the Treasurer of the Association, referred to as "a prominent bank director and financier, is responsible for the investment of the surplus of the Association."

The statements in this magazine together with similar quotations by lesser satellites were appropriately disposed of in a scorching editorial by Dr. Simmons. And so the matter ended for the time.

THE FIRST SPECIAL JOURNAL

In 1907 the Board acted favorably upon a petition from a number of internists to establish a Journal of Internal Medicine which ultimately was named the Archives of Internal Medicine. Thus was begun the group of special publications which now number fifteen.

In 1908 the Board initiated a conference of the Council on Pharmacy and Chemistry with the U. S. Public Health and Marine Hospital service through the secretary of the treasury to investigate the use of drugs in patent medicines. From this conference there eventuated a revision of laws governing the use of drugs with a special reference to narcotics. Dr. W. H. Welch proposed that the Board recommend to the House of Delegates the creation of a Committee on the Defense of Scientific Research to meet the efforts of the anti-vivisectionists.

In 1911 the Board had under consideration the publication of a Journal of Surgery, but this project was violently opposed by the officials of other surgical journals and was postponed until 1923.

THE COOPERATIVE MEDICAL ADVERTISING BUREAU

In 1913 the Editor and General Manager and the Business Manager proposed the establishment of a cooperative medical advertising bureau. This the Board approved and appropriated $5,000 to establish the bureau. The membership of the Board in this year was W. T. Councilman, Chairman; M. L. Harris, Secretary; W. T. Sarles, Philip Marvel, F. J. Lutz, W. W. Grant, Philip Mills Jones, O. Dowling and Thomas McDavitt. The growth of the Association under efficient management of the Journal had increased the financial responsibilities of the Association. "The aims and financial interests of this Association demand the establishment of a reserve fund to meet any emergency that may arise." $125,000 was transferred from surplus to this reserve fund with the provision that each year, an increase of this fund be a first charge on surplus, the fund to be drawn on only by favorable vote by at least seven trustees.

In 1916 the Board approved a memorial to Congress on the necessity of the control of patent medicine and a committee consisting of W. L. Rodman, W. H. Welch, Alexander Marcy, George H. Simmons and W. T. Councilman was appointed to formulate the memorial.

FURTHER CRITICISMS

At the annual meeting of the Association in Los Angeles in 1911 under the presidency of Wm. H. Welch, there were again voiced criticisms of the Board and the editor, which again originated in certain interests excluded from the advertising pages of the Journal. The Board answered these criticisms as follows:

"In an association as large as this and extending over such a large territory, it is but natural that there should be honest differences of opinion among its members and diversity of interests due to local conditions which have a legitimate basis in fact, but these differences should not be permitted to interfere with the accomplishment of the real objects of the Association nor should they embitter anyone toward those who are conscientiously and diligently striving to obtain for all the fruition of these objects.

"That the accomplishment of some of these objects would injuriously affect certain interests outside of the profession which have profited by unscrupulous practices was self evident and it was therefore expected that their opposition, both direct and indirect, would be provoked, but the antagonisms of such outside interests, whether directed against the Association or against any of its representatives is harmless and can be withstood.

"The harmful attacks, however, are those which have their origin within the Association—harmful because an attack from within is a part arrayed against the whole, and the whole must certainly suffer as a result of the unharmonious action of its parts.

"A sharp distinction should be made between an attack, and an expressed difference of opinion. The former is an attempt to do violence, hence is always destructive in its tendency; the latter is an attempt to bring about a favorable change by showing wherein the thing sought to be changed is wrong, hence is constructive in its tendency; the former should be crushed, the latter encouraged."

WORLD WAR I

Our entry into World War I in 1917 entailed the solution of a number of new problems and in October a special meeting of the Board was called to consider a proposal of the War Department forwarded by the Provost Marshal General requesting the aid of the American Medical Association in organizing medical advisory boards to conduct examinations in connection with the draft. A committee consisting of Dr. Hubert Work, Speaker of the House; Dr. M. L. Harris and Dr. E. J. McKnight was appointed to cooperate with the War Department.

SOCIAL INSURANCE

In this year as in several preceding years, the question of social insurance was repeatedly discussed and extensive reports made on the working of social insurance in several European countries. In this discussion it was pointed out that if established it should be on a state level. The necessity was emphasized that in any law to provide social insurance there should be (1) adequate representation of the medical profession on administrative boards; (2) payment of physicians in proportion to the work done; (3) the maintenance of free choice of the physician; (4) the separation of the medical supervision from the professional care of the sick.

THE FIRST SPANISH EDITION

During the summer and fall of 1918 the Board discussed the details of the publication of a Spanish edition of the Journal with representatives of the Rockefeller Foundation. The project was undertaken and continued for several years, and at length was abandoned.

Shortly after the close of World War I an *ad interim* committee was appointed by the Board to cooperate with General Merritt W. Ireland, the Surgeon General of the Army, to inquire into methods and constructive suggestions for improving army medical service in the case of any later emergency.

THE EXECUTIVE COMMITTEE

The volume of activities of the Association and of the Journal had increased to a business of $1,500,000 per year and a net income of $60,000 so that it was felt unfair to the administrative officers not to have more frequent meetings of the Board of Trustees. The resident trustee had served as an active advisor at the headquarters during the preceding years and had contributed much to the safe conduct of the business of the Association. Of this group E. Fletcher Ingals, M. L. Harris and Frank Billings were outstanding. Three meetings of the Board of Trustees were then provided for with an executive committee of three which should meet each month and report to the full Board at their next meeting. In 1922 Dr. Olin West came to the Association as field secretary. Dr. Wm. C. Woodward was already in charge of the Bureau of Legal Medicine and Legislation and now moved to Chicago. Publication of the new popular journal, HYGEIA, was begun under the initial editorship of Dr. Victor C. Vaughan. Again consideration was given to developing a system of group insurance for employees. On the death of Dr. Craig, secretary of the Association, Dr. West was made general secretary to fill the vacancy until the next meeting of the House.

In 1923 with the continued growth of the business of the Association, further reorganization of the Board was found necessary. A survey of the membership of the Board of Trustees over the previous period of 40 years showed that in that time there had been 59 members of the Board of whom 23 had served from one to three years, 17 from four to six years, 8 from seven to nine years, five for twelve years, five for fifteen years and one for eighteen years—an average of six years service.

THE LENGTHENED TERM OF SERVICE

A committee was appointed to study the term of service of Board members and made the following report:

"The present three years period of trusteeship is too short to enable a member of the Board to gain the necessary knowledge and experience of the affairs of the Association to make his service of real value.

"To safeguard the interests of the Association, the term of service of a member of the Board should be long enough to insure from him a growing qualification for the duties and responsibilities of a trustee which is afforded by experience in the conduct of the affairs of the Association. At the same time the term of service of a trustee should not be so long as to promote a staleness of mind and interest and a tendency to fall into mechanical routine methods.

"It would promote harmony and give satisfaction to the fellows and members of the Association to provide a more equable geographical representation on the Board."

Three meetings of the whole Board were provided for, one at the annual session, one in October, and one in February with an executive committee meeting at approximately monthly intervals. The term of service of the members of the Board was increased from three to five years with the provision that no trustee should be reelected for more than one additional term.

SUBJECTS OF INTEREST

Illustrative of how the pattern of the work of the Board was dictated by national economic and social changes are some of the items considered by the Trustees during 1920. The passage of the Volstead act made necessary the issuance of regulations for the prescribing and dispensing of intoxicating liquor, some of which created much irritation in the medical profession, and the trustees were confronted by many problems in the correction or alleviation of unjust and unfair directives of those charged with the administration of an unenforceable law. Other live topics of discussion were a model state narcotic law, the Veterans Bureau and chiropractors, the Shepherd-Towner Maternity Act, an effort to obtain more just deductions for physicians under the federal income tax, the right of search of physician's records by the internal revenue department in the matter of estate taxes, animal experimentation and the protection of medical research, legislation to prevent accidents with lye.

At this time also the advertising and control of clinical laboratories was discussed and a report was made of a broadcasting program which had been established over one station and for which plans were formulated for other stations. The use of motion picture films and health exhibits was studied.

The annual meeting for 1923 was held at San Francisco, and W. A. Pusey was elected president elect. The new Board consisted of W. C. Phillips, Chairman; Frank Billings, secretary; O. Dowling, J. H. J. Upham, W. W. Williamson, C. W. Richardson, Thomas McDavitt, A. R. Mitchell, O. C. Brown. Dr. Simmons presented his resignation as Editor and General Manager to take effect in February, 1924.

By 1924 the circulation of Hygeia had increased to 23,687 and the net loss for the year was $38,990. It was not until 1940 that Hygeia had begun to pay its way and somewhat later was able to wipe out previous deficits. Its present circulation is 200,000.

DR. SIMMONS RESIGNS

On the resignation of Dr. Simmons, the Trustees appointed Dr. Olin West general manager and also secretary of the Association pending the annual meeting. Dr. Morris Fishbein was named Editor of the Journal.

National plans and issues continued to occupy the thought and plans of the Board. Membership in the United States Chamber of Commerce brought the Board into closer touch with national planning. The coordination of Federal health activities in a department of education and health with a secretary of Cabinet rank and an assistant secretary for health was again discussed in 1925 in conference with other agencies. The Board also considered the report of the Committee on Constitutional Rights. This Committee questioned the right of Congress, in passing the Volstead Act, to regulate the practice of medicine as indicated in the prohibition of the prescription of alcohol, holding that such regulation was a function of state governments. The committee maintained that this question had nothing to do with that of the therapeutic use of alcohol nor with the wisdom of the prohibition amendment.

The Supreme Court refused the appeal of the Committee, laying great stress on the resolution of the House of Delegates in 1917 which held in effect "that alcohol has no therapeutic value, and its use as a therapeutic agent should be discouraged." This resolution had been passed by the House in the closing moments of a war time session, and its implications had perhaps not been considered adequately by the House.

Many details of the proposed publication of the Index Medicus, combining it with the Quarterly Cumulative Index already published since 1919, were considered. Ultimately a series of steps was devised which resulted in union and under the name of the Quarterly Cumulative Index.

The story of the past 60 years of continued growth and expansion of the American Medical Association and its Journal is inspiring; it was made possible by the energy and devotion of great men of the past; its gains were consolidated from year to year by men who not only were great physicians, but who also exhibited a keen knowledge of business principles.

PRESENT-DAY ACTIVITIES

The Trustees who sacrificed and labored to conserve the interests of the Association in its early days would be astounded if they could see the volume of its present business and activities. And this expansion has required continuing rearrangement of business technics, and an increasingly complex operating organization. In considering new plans and policies the Trustees must look, in so far as they are able, beyond apparently desirable immediate results, to see what the later and perhaps unforeseen effects of an action may be. The recent war years presented an added load, about which but little properly could then be said. Time and geography add their share to the burden of the trustees and also of the officers who regularly attend Board and executive committee meetings. There are scheduled four regular meetings of the full Board, two of which extend throughout the annual and winter

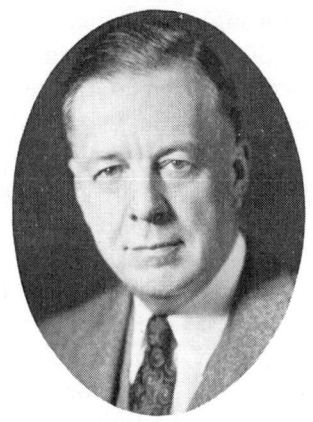

George F. Lull, M.D.
Secretary and General Manager, 1946.

meetings of the House, and also eight or nine meetings of the Executive Committee, making in all about 20 days of actual meetings with additional travel time of varying length depending on the residence of the members. The members of the Executive Committee also are frequently consulted in intervals between meetings, and members of the Board attend such Council and State society meetings as is possible and necessary, and to which they are invited.

Following the resignation of Dr. Olin West, the Board elected Dr. George F. Lull, formerly Deputy Surgeon General of the Army Medical Department, as General Manager. In 1946 he was elected Secretary by the House of Delegates.

THE OFFICE OF THE TREASURER

By Josiah J. Moore, M.D.

THE IDEALS OF THE AMERICAN MEDICAL ASSOCIATION: Better medical education, a more just system of licensure, better dissemination of medical knowledge through a national medical society and the formulation of a code of ethics, could not have been achieved without the realistic accumulation of the necessary funds. In the Report of the Committee on the Organization of the National Medical Association, as ordered by the National Medical Convention held in the city of New York in the month of May, 1846, the following offices were named: a president, four vice-presidents, two secretaries and one treasurer.

The report states, "The Treasurer shall have the immediate charge and management of the funds and property of the Association. He shall be a member of the Committee on Publications, to which committee he shall give bonds for safe keeping, and proper use and disposal of his trust, and through the same committee he shall present his accounts, duly authenticated, at every regular meeting." It should have been simple to fulfill these tasks in the early formative years, but even then difficulties were encountered in extracting the assessments from the delegates.

At 10:00 A.M., May 5, 1847, Dr. Isaac Hays, Chairman of the Committee on Arrangements from the Philadelphia delegation, opened the proceedings in Philadelphia which resulted in the formation of the American Medical Association. During the meeting he was elected the first Treasurer, which position he held for five years, until 1852, when his successor was elected. As one of his assignments was to be on the Committee on Publications, that committee very wisely selected him as chairman.

Dr. Hays was ably equipped to manage both these positions. He was then 51 years of age, an editor of medical journals, an ophthalmologist and a physician of repute. His father, a wealthy merchant in the East India trade, was eager that his son enter into his business, but Hays was not interested in mercantile life and in 1817 entered the medical department of the University of Pennsylvania, graduating in 1820. He was especially interested in ophthalmology, became an extensive contributor to ophthalmologic literature and was one of the first to detect astigmatism and to study color blindness. He was the first president of the Ophthalmological Society of Pennsylvania.

Hays' work as an editor extended over many years. In 1827 he was appointed to the staff of the "Philadelphia Journal of the Medical and Physical Sciences." He soon assumed the editorship and changed the title of the periodical to the "American Journal of the Medical Sciences." This position he held until his death on April 1, 1879.

In 1834 he projected, but completed only two volumes of, the "American Cyclopedia of Practical Medicine and Surgery." In 1843 he brought out a new monthly journal, "Medical News," which later became a weekly journal and which was published until 1906. He also started monthly abstracts of "Medical Science," which later merged with "Medical News."

Hays' interests were not confined to medical science. He edited "American Ornithology" (3 volumes, 1828); "Elements of Physics" in 1848 and other editions.

He was a member of the Academy of Natural Science of Philadelphia, serving as president from 1865 to 1869; an active member of the American Philosophical Society, and one of the founders of the Franklin Institute.

He was striking in appearance with gentle manners, and had a remarkably judicial mind, so that during all the years he managed the journals they never became known as organs of any party.

The first report of Dr. Hays as treasurer, in 1848, is as follows:

The Treasurer of the Association respectfully

REPORTS,

That he has received from Dr. J. Rodman Paul..................		$173 60	
The above sum is the balance of the amount received by him from one hundred and ninety-three members of the Convention of 1847, on account of assessment $3 00 each, four of the number having paid $5 00, (see G.—2,) making.............	$587 00		
Less cost of printing proceedings.....................	413 40		
		$173 60	
That he has received in account of assessment of members of Convention of 1847...		6 00	
			$179 60
That he has paid for printing memorial to the legislatures of the different states, as ordered by Convention of 1847...............		$6 00	
For Treasurer's book..		2 50	8 50
Leaving on hand a balance of...			$171 10

ISAAC HAYS.

Here we see that the major expenditure was for publications, and this relatively large expenditure extends through the entire history of the Association, in the early years for transactions of the Association and later for medical journals of varying types. This effort to advance knowledge of medicine to the profession, and later also to the public, should be a satisfactory answer to all present day critics of the organization as to its purpose and policy. Year after year reports accentuate the purpose of the Association in spreading medical knowledge. In 1851 Dr. Hays reported on the expenditure of $977.07 for publications, drawings and papers in Volume III of the Transactions, of a total expenditure of $1105.22. But $57.85 was spent for the expenses of the third meeting in Cincinnati. The next year the sum for publications was increased to $1873.00 of a total of $2022.00.

The treasurer had to carry on a voluminous correspondence with all delegates to collect their assessments and with the slowness of the mails in the middle of the 19th century and the lethargy of the delegates in paying their assessments, money did not flow too freely into the office. In 1849 forty-six had not paid the assessment of $3.00, while two hundred twenty-four had paid from $3.00 to $6.00. By 1850 the Treasurer and the Committee on Publicity were complaining about the restricted circulation of the Transactions and asking the delegates and their constituent societies to cooperate in diffusing information about the Transactions. The low price of the volumes did not permit of giving commissions or of paying for proper advertising.

In January 1852 "an extensive conflagration occurred in Philadelphia" which destroyed hundreds of copies of Volumes I to IV of the Transactions, leaving less than one hundred copies of each number on hand.

Indicative of mildly encouraging results is the fact that 137 copies of Volume I, 120 of Volume II, 194 of Volume III, and 448 of Volume IV had been sold up to the time of the fire. In 1852 after all expenditures, the balance on hand was $56.75. A balance of approximately $50.00 in the treasury of a national organization five years of age does not fit well with our modern mode of financial thinking. But the Treasurer at that time followed the instructions of Article VI of the report of the Plan of Organization for a National Medical Association, which reads:

"Funds shall be raised by the Association for meeting its current expenses and awards from year to year; but never with the view of creating a PERMANENT INCOME FROM INVESTMENTS. Funds may be obtained by an equal assessment of not more than three dollars annually on each of its members; by individual contributions for specific objects; and by the sale and disposal of publications or of works prepared for publication.

"The funds may be appropriated for defraying the expenses of the annual meetings; for publishing the proceedings, memoirs, and transactions of the Association; for enabling committees to fulfill their respective duties, conduct their correspondence, and procure the materials necessary for the completion of their stated annual reports; for the encouragement of scientific investigations, by prizes and awards of merit; and for defraying the expenses incidental to specific investigations under the instructions of the Association, when such investigations have been accompanied with an order on the treasurer to supply the funds necessary for carrying them into effect."

Our thinking changes over the years and much of the expenditure for research is now supplied from the permanent income from the investment of the Research fund.

In 1852 Dr. David Francis Condie of Philadelphia was elected treasurer and received the property of the Association. Since he had served on the Publications Committee with Dr. Hays for many years he was well informed on the work entailed in the office of Treasurer. He also was an alumnus of the University of Pennsylvania and of the same age as his predecessor.

While a general practitioner he wrote on many topics, in 1844 publishing "A Practical Treatise on the Diseases of Children" which went through six editions. Other books edited by him were Watson's "Lectures on the Practice of Physic"; Churchill on the "Diseases of Women"; Carpenter on the "Use and Abuse of Alcoholic Liquors" and Barlow's "Manual of the Practice of Medicine."

With John Bell he wrote a report of the College of Physicians to the Board of Health which contains "all the material facts in the history of epidemic cholera—and a full account of the causes, post mortem appearances and treatment of the disease."

He thoroughly believed in physical exercise, always visited his patients on foot, disapproving of a physician's driving. He declared that "those who rode in one horse carriages were physically deficient; those who rode in two horse carriages were mentally deficient." He died in March, 1875.

The report of the Treasurer in 1853 was discouraging. While Doctor Condie stressed the importance of scientific literature, the expenditure of over $1900.00 in publishing over nine hundred octavo pages left the Association $107.00 in debt to the Treasurer.

On April 20, 1854, in order to keep the treasury fluid and solvent, it was resolved that all delegates and permanent members be assessed $3.00 annually to defray the expense of printing the Transactions. This solved the difficulty for the year and Dr. Condie turned over $293.00 to his successor, Dr. Isaac Wood of New York, who served one year and accumulated over $1100.00 in the bank balance.

From American Medical Biographies we find that Samuel Wood, the father of Isaac Wood, opened a book store in New York and later, with four of his sons, established a publishing house which printed the American Edition of the Medico-Chirurgical Journal and the Medical Record. This firm in time became William Wood and Company.

Isaac preferred medicine to publishing and was licensed by the New York State Medical Society in 1815. He was especially interrested in anatomy, several times narrowly escaping danger in obtaining material for dissecting as a "resurrectionist." Rutgers University granted him the M.D. degree in 1816, his thesis being "Carditis and Pericarditis." In 1832, as a staff member, he helped treat the 2,000 victims affected with cholera in Bellevue Hospital, until weakened he joined the other sufferers. He had a high reputation as an ophthalmologist and for 25 years was an active manager of the New York Institution for the Blind.

He helped organize the New York Academy of Medicine and was twice its president. He also was a fellow of the College of Physicians and a member of the American Geographical Society.

The office was placed in the hands of Dr. Caspar Wister of Philadelphia in 1855, who had served as a delegate for the College of Physicians of Philadelphia to the Association in 1852 and subsequent years. Dr. Wister served the Association long and well, through the trying period of the Civil War and on through the reconstructive period.

As a youth he had a varied career. Withdrawn from Germantown Academy on request of the faculty because of his lack of restraint, he was entered at the age of 16 in the Institute for Young Gentlemen, a boarding school in Westchester, Pa. Here he remained for two years. Then he went to a school in New Jersey to study surveying, but after two years he decided that it was not a profitable profession. About this time there was a political disturbance in Harrisburg, and the Governor called for troops to quell a mob who were disputing the election. Wister joined a regiment and was made assistant to Dr. Thomas F. Belton, although he had no medical training. The episode was known as the "Buckshot War" because

Governor Retner ordered the troops to load their rifles with buckshot. Fortunately it was not necessary to fire the guns.

In 1839 he tried surveying in Texas but had little luck, so he became a general merchant until a severe fever followed by an accident compelled him to return home. Having recovered, he again returned to Texas in the latter part of 1841. Once there he joined the Army as a private when the Mexicans invaded Texas. He returned home in 1843 and began to study medicine under the preceptorship of Dr. George B. Wood. In March, 1846, at the age of 28, he received the degree of M.D. at the University of Pennsylvania. During the following years he devoted much time to charity, being physician for the "Indigent Widows and Single Women's Society" and the "Association for the Care of Colored Children," and a member of the Board of Managers of the House of Refuge. He also was a member of a score of societies of which only one-fourth were medical.

He was another Treasurer who was athletically inclined, enjoying walking ten miles to dine with a friend in the country and then walking home again. It is said of him that "no man was less bashful—few men so modest."

He had a delightful sense of humor. When the neighbors around 17th and Locust Streets complained about the new bell in the tower of St. Mark's Episcopal Church and brought suit to restrain the church from ringing it on Sunday morning, Dr. Wister wrote a poem about the law suit and distributed it to his friends.

Ailing for some time, anticipating death and not too sure of the diagnosis, he directed that an autopsy be performed on his body to determine the cause of death. He passed away peacefully in December, 1888.

In his first year in office, Dr. Wister had the Association pass a requirement that the delegates to the convention prepay their yearly assessment; therefore he retained a modest bank balance. The sale of transactions remained the black problem, as noted by this report in 1860. "It is still to be regretted that so great a want of interest prevails among the permanent members with regard to the annual publication, only some two hundred being annual subscribers to the Volume out of a list of two thousand names." In this report we also find this item, "By cash paid treasurer, for postage and stationery $11.49." Perhaps this accounts for the lack of sales of the Transactions.

A replica of what usually happens during the dark years of war is found in the reports of 1863. Because meetings were not held in 1861 and 1862 there was a lack of papers, so Dr. Wister writes

"That in consequence of the disturbed state of the country, the demands for the Transactions of this Association has literally ceased, two copies only having been sold within the last year. The expense of publishing has risen 30 per cent, since the last Volume was issued."

The sales decreased and the printing increased another 10 per cent in 1864, bringing forth another appeal from the Treasurer to use the utmost discretion in publishing only those papers of "unquestionable value to the profession" and to evade as much as possible illustrations by wood cuts and engravings and the introduction of tables. The entire income for 1864 had decreased to $1447.25, of which the Treasurer spent $3.50 for stationery and postage. In 1865 after the publication of a very small Volume of Transactions, there was but $300.00 in the treasury.

Finally the dark cloud of bankruptcy descended and engulfed the Association. Lack of desire on the part of the members for the Transactions left the Association in debt to the printer.

In 1868 the sunshine of solvency warmed the heart of Dr. Wister, but he raised his pen against the expenditure of one hundred dollars for an "essay of great worth" that "may deserve no such distinction" and which with illustrations and printing entails a heavy publication cost.

Over twenty-two years after its founding the Association takes an action which should have been the first order of business after the decision to publish the Transactions. He writes "The Treasurer has the honor to report that under the operation of the recent law, obliging permanent members to subscribe to the yearly Transactions or else suffer the removal of their names from the list of permanent members, the Association has been able to publish its volume of Transactions, pay all its debts, and have a surplus towards the expenses of the next year." The Committee on Prize Essays for that year decided that no essay offered was of great intrinsic merit.

However, the printing of great masses of worthless manuscripts with expensive illustrations and the giving of prizes to undeserving essays brings forth this admonition. "It is always with difficulty that the financial affairs of this Association are conducted, and the Treasurer desires this meeting to recollect that after it has adjourned and forgotten its heedless expenditure of money, the Treasurer remains to be responsible for its acts." And this was the year he had only $496.00 left from a gross income of $6614.00.

Finally in 1874 Dr. Wister, having a balance of $2000.00, which required nineteen years of hard personal service to accumulate, offered his resignation. This the Association, knowing his excellent qualities, refused to accept, but apparently it heeded his requests for abridging reports and manuscripts because he writes "The wisdom of the Association in publishing a more compact and abridged Volume of Transactions is a marked comparison with former years, and the Treasurer congratulates the Association upon the production of a more desirable Volume and a healthy condition of the Treasury."

In 1877 Dr. Caspar Wister resigned, after twenty-two years of service. It may have been induced owing again to the expenditure of $6000.00 in the publication of the prize essay, which left but a few hundred dollars in the Treasury.

The new Treasurer, Dr. Richard James Dunglison of Philadelphia had almost $2500.00 in the treasury at the end of his first year, due to the fact that the usual honorarium was not granted the Permanent Secretary. The son of Dr. Robley Dunglison, he graduated from Jefferson Medical College at the age of 22, in 1856. His father had accepted the invitation of Thomas Jefferson in 1824 to fill the chair of Anatomy, Physiology, Materia Medica and Pharmacy at the University of Virginia.

Although he practiced medicine, much of his time was devoted to writing and to activities in many societies. For a few years he was corresponding secretary of the State Medical Society of Pennsylvania and for many years was a member of many foreign, national, state and local societies. Among these he was honorary local secretary of the New Sydenham Society of London, for over 22 years president of the Musical Fund Society of Philadelphia, and assistant secretary of the International Medical Congress of 1876.

During the Civil War he was acting assistant Surgeon of the United States Army and on duty in various military hospitals in Philadelphia.

Numerous medical contributions came from his pen, among these being "Observations on the Deaf and Dumb" (1858), "Statistics of Insanity in the United States" (1860), "Reflections on Exanthemic Typhus" (1861), "Public Medical Libraries of Philadelphia" (1872) and "Letters of Medical Centennial Affairs" (1876). He edited his father's "History of Medicine" (1872) and the "Medical Dictionary" (1876).

Having acted as assistant secretary of the Association in 1876, he had some knowledge of the work of the Treasurer. He worked valiantly with those who had joined in 1876 as permanent members under the enthusiasm of the National Centennial to retain this enthusiasm, but many failed to pay their annual dues. The Association, however, went along on a fairly even keel, with a spurt in 1884 when it permitted membership by application, thereby receiving considerable funds from new members who did not have to attend the session. The income of $17,093.00 that year, the highest up to that time, was again used chiefly for educating the physician, as shown by the expenditure of almost $15,000.00 in publication expenses. A moderate growth during the next four years increased the income to $33,798.00, of which $29,000.00 was used for Journal Publications. The ever continuous melody in all the years of the Association is that all efforts will be made in dispensing medical knowledge to the medical profession. That policy still continues and has won worthy endorsement from all parts of the world. It is the major factor in making the American Medical Association the world leader in medicine.

In his seventeenth year as Treasurer, Doctor Dunglison asked to be relieved, stating "the labors of the Treasurership have now become so onerous that the giving of proper personal attention to the duties of this responsible office is a business of its own—I would suggest that hereafter the Treasurer should be a salaried officer, receiving annually a compensation commensurate with the amount of labor." The House of Delegates must have appreciated his efforts, since by resolution they granted him an honorarium of $300.00 for the fiscal year 1894.

The office of the Treasurer was moved to Chicago in 1894, and for the first time a Chicago physician, Dr. Henry Parker Newman, was elected to the office. Dr. Newman was born in New Hampshire, graduated from the Detroit Medical College, and spent two years in the leading universities of Germany, locating on his return in Chicago to specialize in obstetrics and gynecology. A member of all the local societies and his special national societies, he became president of the Chicago Gynecological Society. He was a founder of the International Congress of Gynecologists and Obstetricians and of post graduate medical education in Chicago. He was Professor of Obstetrics and Clinical Gynecology at the College of Physicians and Surgeons, Chicago, and at the Chicago Policlinic.

This sixth treasurer of the Association in the fifty years of its existence recommended that the fiscal year be changed from June to May, to coincide with the calendar year. This was accepted, and to the present the fiscal year of the Association has been the calendar year. Growth continued slowly, with 8000 members in 1898, a contrast to the 130,000 members of fifty years later. At the session in 1900 the House of Delegates passed a resolution presented by Dr. Donald Maclean of Detroit "that in the future the reports of the treasurer and secretary be printed from the Journal press and circulated in advance to the attending members." This became the

Handbook of each session. At this session the yearly honorarium of the Treasurer was raised to $1,000.00.

Prior to 1901 the Treasurer made his report to the delegates directly, but in 1901 the Board of Trustees announced in their report that "We desire to state that heretofore it has been customary for the Treasurer to submit his report direct to your body, but under our laws, it is made the duty of your Board of Trustees to 'annually audit and authenticate his accounts, and present a statement of the same in its annual report to the Association.' This duty we have performed and in our Journal report, that of the Treasurer is included." This custom has continued, but in 1946 the Treasurer was startled out of a complacent mood when the Speaker of the House called for the Treasurer's report after the President of the Board of Trustees had made his report and left the room. The Treasurer referred the delegates to the appropriate pages in the now published Handbook, as per the resolution of 1900.

Surplus funds, exclusive of the valuable Journal plant, were now accumulating to the extent of almost $32,000.00, $11,000 of which was invested in United States Government War Bonds. This speaks for conservatism of the finance committee of that time, which conservatism has continued and is still existent on the part of the present finance committee. That committee is also the executive committee of the Board of Trustees, and all investments and appropriations are endorsed by it before submission to the Board as a whole.

It was not until 1903 that the Treasurer discontinued the collection of dues. The Board of Trustees explained the new procedure in their report of 1905. "The consolidation of all bookkeeping of the Association under one head has resulted in greatly simplifying the business methods of the Association. The dues are no longer collected by the Treasurer, nor are any accounts kept by him against the individual member. Both members and subscribers pay directly to The Journal, and when the current funds are greater than is necessary the surplus is transferred to the Treasurer. The Treasurer of the Association is no longer a collecting agent but a Treasurer." They call attention also to one item in the Treasurer's report, namely $108.74 interest on the daily balance, indicating that the account is not lying idle.

Dr. Frank Billings of Chicago, who had already been President of the Association and who was familiar with all its activities, became Treasurer in 1904. This great leader, who had accomplished so much for medicine in all fields, again displayed his ability as an organizer in streamlining the Treasurer's office so that henceforth that official had little personal service to render. During his seven years as Treasurer, Dr. Billings acted as a most capable advisor to all departments of the Association. The Treasury continued to accumulate funds while the Association was following his many suggestions in the fields of medical education, pharmacy and other significant activities. A boundless energy drove him contantly to improve the practice of medicine. After serving as Treasurer, he was a trustee from 1918 to 1924. For a more complete history we refer to the Presidential Biographies.

Since the Treasurer for facilitating the official business had to be located in Chicago, the successor to Dr. Frank Billings was another outstanding figure in Mid-West Medicine, Dr. William Allen Pusey, professor of Dermatology at the University of Illinois. Dr. Pusey served as Treasurer from 1911 to 1922, was President of the Association in 1924-25 (see presidential biography) and continued in service to the profession as a member of the Committee on Medical Education from 1925 to 1932.

In 1922 Dr. Austin A. Hayden, a distinguished worker in the field of ophthalmology and otolaryngology, was elected by the delegates to assume the office. Born in Wisconsin, educated at Creighton University, the University of Chicago, Rush Medical College and New York Post Graduate Medical School, he selected Chicago as his residence and immediately became active in its medical activities, becoming an instructor at Rush Medical College and a hard working member in the medical societies. He became President of the Chicago Laryngological and Otological Society, of the Chicago Medical Society and of the American Association of Railway Surgeons; Vice-President of Alpha Omega Alpha, an honor medical society, and a member of many other societies. In his later years he gave much attention to the problems of the hard of hearing and served as President of the Chicago League of the Hard of Hearing.

While Treasurer of the Association he promoted the preparation of a motion picture which showed the activities of the different councils, bureaus and departments of the headquarters building. He wanted all members of the Association to become familiar with its projects and took great pleasure in showing the film to many of the state and local societies, thus attempting to infuse some of his own devotion for organized medicine into the hearts of his confreres.

Dr. Hayden was known for his cordiality, having his hand always extended in a warm courteous greeting, and for his intense activity and leadership in medical advancement.

Following his service as Treasurer, which ended in 1933, he became Secretary of the Board of Trustees, which position he held until his death in 1940.

Dr. Herman L. Kretschmer became treasurer in 1933. A native of Chicago, he received his degree of Doctor of Medicine from Northwestern University Medical School, then advanced to a leading position in his special field of urology, and became clinical professor at Rush Medical College. During his tenure of office he sat regularly with the Board of Trustees and gave invaluable advice in the field of investments, of which subject he made a special study. He resigned as Treasurer in 1943, to become President of the Association, under which title will be found a more complete biography.

Eleven Treasurers have served the Association in its first 100 years, their period of office being as follows:

Dr. Isaac Hays, Philadelphia	1847–1852
Dr. D. Francis Condie, Philadelphia	1852–1854
Dr. Isaac Wood, New York	1854–1855
Dr. Caspar Wister, Philadelphia	1855–1877
Dr. Richard James Dunglison, Philadelphia	1877–1894
Dr. Henry Parker Newman, Chicago	1894–1904
Dr. Frank Billings, Chicago	1904–1911
Dr. William Allen Pusey, Chicago	1911–1922
Dr. Austin A. Hayden, Chicago	1922–1933
Dr. Herman L. Kretschmer, Chicago	1933–1943
Dr. Josiah J. Moore, Chicago	1943–

While the first group were more or less general practitioners, yet Hayes specialized in diseases of the eye and ear, Wister in anatomy, Condie in pediatrics, Wood in surgery, and Dunglison in internal medicine.

Of those from 1900 to the present time, Newman was in obstetrics and gynecology, Billings in internal medicine, Pusey in dermatology, Hayden in otolaryngology, Kretschmer in urology and Moore in pathology. The group had one characteristic in common: All were very active in medical organizations and apparently when not satisfied with existing groups they became active in the formation of new ones. As a group they were prominent in establishing over twenty-five local, state or national societies. Therefore they were not the typical Treasurer pictured by the psychiatrist as an introvert but were the reverse, loving the companionship of their fellow physicians and enthused by conventions and assemblies.

In the later years, the work of the treasurers was made simple by the able comptroller, Mr. Edward Hoffman, who has served the Association faithfully for many years. For those financiers of the present and future who may desire more factual details, he has prepared the following report:

It may be expected that the responsibilities of the Treasurer have kept pace with the widening field of the activity of the Association and with the growth of the business departments, which now carry approximately 400,000 active accounts. Normal duties have become more arduous of late years by the impositions of Government, one of which places the Association under the provisions of the Social Security Act and requires the payment of Federal Old Age and Survivors Benefits Tax and of Unemployment Tax. Many other Governmental regulations pertaining to business operations require frequent reports and study by the Treasurer.

1. The large volume of cash receipts and disbursements is processed with the aid of specially adapted mechanical appliances.

2. Accurate accounts are maintained with each council, bureau, committee and periodical, and operational expenses and income are classified and reported thereon.

3. These records, together with other accounting records, are audited by Certified Public Accountants, whose report is published annually in the JOURNAL OF THE AMERICAN MEDICAL ASSOCIATION.

4. Insurance, ample in scope and amount, is carried on Association properties and in Association interests with approved risk companies.

Closer industrial relations with the headquarters' personnel, now numbering about 685 persons in plant, office and management, have been developed through the administration of employee group life and group hospital insurance and annuity plans.

A large fire resistant vault houses the financial, documentary and historical records of the Association.

Reserve Funds represented by investments in securities equivalent in value to the amount of each have been established from time to time for special purposes. As of December 31, 1946 Reserve Funds amounted to $3,325,000.00, in addition to the American Medical Association Research Fund of $1,500,000.00.

Land owned by the Association was acquired through various purchases at a cost of $328,773.98.

A modern fire resistant nine story building provides space for the printing of the many publications issued by the Association and office space for its large clerical staff. Completion of the last section in 1941 brought the total cost to $1,375,349.31. Annual depreciation allowances have reduced the building valuation to $763,415.54.

Machinery and printing equipment purchases dating from the time the Association set up its first shop total $521,317.80. The depreciated value after these many years is $164,958.16.

Office and Laboratory equipment costing the Association $221,126.08 is now valued at $84,807.55 on a depreciated basis.

The matter of investments has become somewhat of a problem. The purchase of suitable securities for the portfolio of the American Medical Association has been most difficult in recent years because of a scarcity in offerings of high quality bonds. Since security is of paramount importance, the portfolio is largely invested in Government bonds and notes. That the treasurers, finance committees and members of the Board of Trustees have fulfilled their trust and confidence of the membership in the management of the finances of the Association may be confirmed by an inspection of the Treasurer's report for the last fiscal year. It may be of interest to compare this last report with the first one in 1848.

TREASURER'S REPORT

Report of the Treasurer of the American Medical Association for the Year Ended December 31, 1946

Investments (at cost) as at January 1, 1946	$5,589,268.47	
Bonds Purchased (at cost)	3,960,952.66	
	$9,550,221.13	
Less:		
Bonds called, matured or sold $3,425,876.22		
Bonds transferred to American Medical Association Research Fund (at cost)... 1,499,512.50	4,925,388.72	
Investments as at December 31, 1946		$4,624,832.41
Balance for Investment January 1, 1946	126,824.36	
Interest Received on Investments in 1946	136,685.22	
	$263,509.58	
Transferred to General Fund	144,256.95	
Uninvested Funds at December 31, 1946		119,252.63
Invested and Uninvested Funds as at December 31, 1946		$4,744,085.04

American Medical Association Research Fund

Investments (at cost) as at December 31, 1946	$1,499,512.50
Uninvested Funds as at December 31, 1946	487.50
Invested and Uninvested Funds as at December 31, 1946	$1,500,000.00

Davis Memorial Fund

Balance in Fund January 1, 1946	$7,904.01	
Interest earned on Bank Balance in 1946	99.10	
Funds on deposit as at December 31, 1946		$8,003.11

JOSIAH J. MOORE, Treasurer.

HOME OF THE AMERICAN MEDICAL ASSOCIATION

By Morris Fishbein, M.D.

THE STORY HAS BEEN TOLD of some of the steps in the development of the home of the American Medical Association. During the early years of the American Medical Association when the membership was small and the cost of publishing the transactions practically exhausted the revenues of the organization, the Association had no headquarters except in the mind of the permanent secretary, Dr. William B. Atkinson. Except for the four days of the annual session, the Association was practically non-existent. Frequently presidents expressed the hope that some headquarters office might be developed but never were there sufficient funds or sufficient drive to take even the first steps toward accomplishing this objective.

When the Association decided in 1883 to publish its own journal, an editorial office became a necessity. Dr. N. S. Davis, as has been told, became the first editor and the editorial functions were carried on in his office. Soon it became necessary to purchase type and other printing equipment. The Journal moved successively on November 24, 1888, to 68 Wabash Avenue and on September 1, 1894, to 86 Fifth Avenue in Chicago. These changes in location were made necessary by the growth of The Journal. On May 1, 1896, the offices were moved to 61 Market Street. By this time the circulation had reached nearly 8,000 copies weekly. By 1902 it had increased to 25,000 copies weekly.

When the trustees met in 1902 they were told that the lease on the Market Street property would soon expire and that the editor had not been able to find sufficient room to accommodate the rapidly growing needs of The Journal. In March ,1902, under the leadership of Dr. E. Fletcher Ingals, property was purchased on the northeast corner of Dearborn Avenue and Indiana Street, a few blocks north of the Chicago River. This property, 100 feet on Dearborn Avenue and 80 on Indiana Street (now Grand Avenue) contained five two-story and basement houses. The property cost $42,000. Two of these houses were torn down and the first home of the American Medical Association erected. This was a three story building, 40 by 80 feet, with a high basement. The building was of brick with stone trimmings. Its cost was $35,000. The building was completely equipped and occupied December 1, 1902.

Almost immediately, however, that building became overcrowded. Some of the space in the adjacent houses was used. About this time opportunity arose to purchase at an extremely low price (approximately $15,000) the property which adjoined on the east. This was a lot 40 x 100 feet containing two three-story and basement houses.

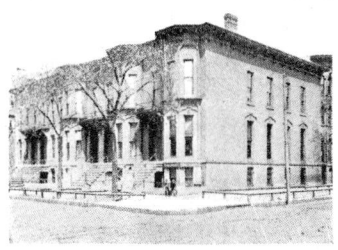

March, 1902

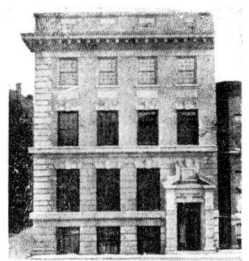

December, 1902

The trustees purchased the property in June 1903 and extended the ground space owned by the Association to 100 by 120 feet. In 1905 the old building was enlarged by extending it back 40 feet and by adding another story. Thus the Association had a four-story building with a high basement, 40 by 120 feet in dimension.

The circulation of The Journal continued to grow and its income correspondingly. In 1906 it had reached a circulation of 54,000

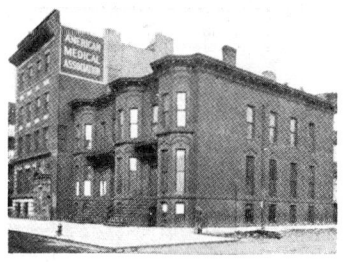

1905

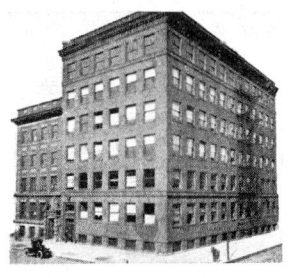

1911

weekly. It had increased its printing and publishing business and space was needed for the Councils on Medical Education, Pharmacy and Chemistry, by the Directory Department, and the Bureau of Medical Legislation. The Board of Trustees decided that the next step must be the erection of a first class building on the main corner of the Association's property. The original architects—Holabird and Roche (later to become Holabird and Root)—were instructed to provide provisional plans for a new building. These plans and an estimate of the cost were submitted to the House of Delegates by the Board of Trustees at the Atlantic City meeting in 1909. The Board of Trustees which made this report consisted of Drs. William H. Welch, chairman, Miles F. Porter, M. L. Harris, W. W. Grant, Philip Marvel, W. R. Townsend, Philip Mills Jones and W. T. Sarles. Dr. T. J. Happel, who had been chairman of the board for seven years and who also was a member, was present at the board meeting when the matter was discussed in February 1909, but he died on May 24, and his name was not attached to the report made by the Board of Trustees to the House of Delegates. The House of Delegates, with a reference committee headed by Dr. Alex. R. Craig as chairman,

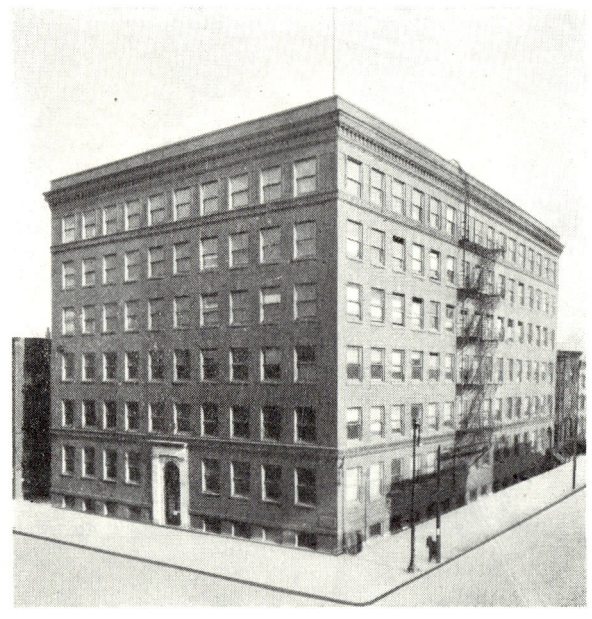

1923

recommended that the board be given full authority to proceed in erecting the proposed building.

Before five years had passed, it became apparent that this new structure would also be inadequate to meet the needs of the Association. But the war came in 1914 in Europe and the United States entered the war in 1916. With this came a rapid rise in the costs of labor and material so that the Board of Trustees postponed repeatedly the erection of additions to the building.

In the meantime, opportunity came to acquire 40 feet of ground to the east and it was decided to make the purchase. By May 1922 the Board of Trustees felt justified in authorizing completion of plans leading toward a final structure. A general contract was signed on May 29, 1922, for enlargement of the building northward on Dearborn Street to the alley, making a central entrance instead of a side entrance and including a six-story structure on the north side of the original building. Because of labor conditions progress in the erection of the building was extremely slow. The structure when completed covered ground of 160 by 100 feet. The building was of

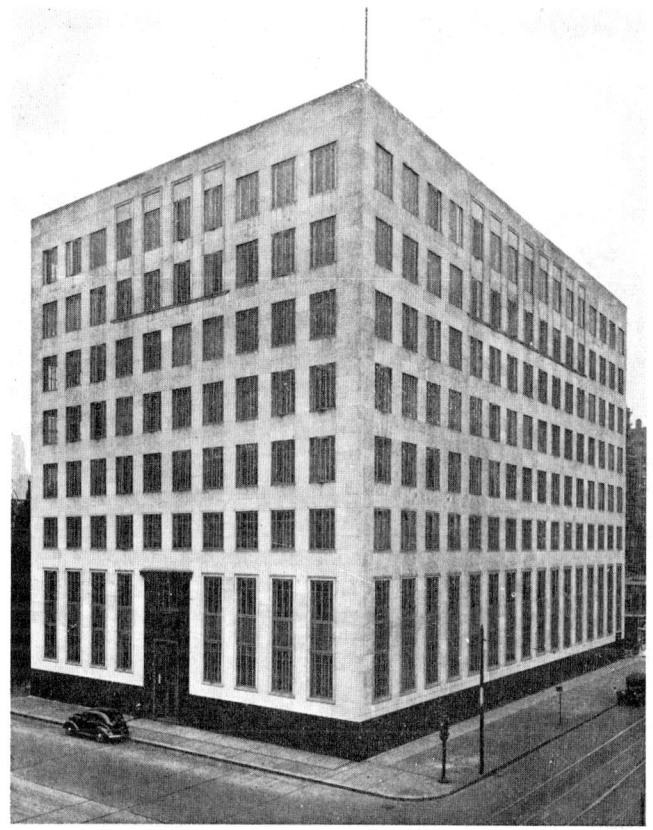

Present headquarters of the Association.

steel and concrete and provided a building which, while not ornate, was substantial, fireproof and adequate to the immediate needs of the Association. Wisely it was decided to construct the foundations so that additional stories could be added should increased space become necessary in the future.

As time went on, additional ground was purchased so that in 1947 the Association owns the ground from Grand Avenue north toward Ohio Street as far as the alley which separates the two halves of the block and from Dearborn Street east to State Street with the exception of a narrow strip on State Street.

This addition, it was thought, would be sufficient to accommodate the headquarters of the Association for many years to come, but by 1935 this building had become crowded. Now a committee of the trustees was appointed to look into the possibility of finding a suitable site elsewhere for the larger headquarters buiding or to work out some plan of expansion on the present site. After much consideration and many conferences with architects and others, it was decided to renovate the existing building thoroughly and to add two more stories and a penthouse. The entire structure was then modernized, the interior was redecorated and exterior on the Dearborn and Grand Avenue sides was veneered with granite and limestone. These extensive operations in 1937 produced the monumental building which is now the headquarters office of the American Medical Association.

Only a few years passed, however, before it became necessary again to expand. An additional three-story structure was developed to the east with sufficient foundations to permit enlargement—and as the 100th anniversary of the Association passes, the Board of Trustees has approved the addition of five stories to the three already constructed at the east end of the present property.

Space is still available on ground which is now used as a parking lot for employees of the Association. Negotiations are under way for the purchase of property to give the Association the entire block on Grand Avenue between Dearborn and State Streets.

THE PROPERTY OF THE ASSOCIATION

An inventory of the buildings and equipment of the Association indicates a worth of between $2,000,000 and $3,000,000. The printing equipment includes a great variety of presses, including a rotary press capable of printing 96 pages in a single operation. It will carry on its cylinders as many as 192 plates. There are flat presses and smaller rotary presses. There are binding and gathering machines, paper cutting machines, a stereotype room, 24 linotype machines, stitching, folding and sewing machines. Indeed the headquarters office is equipped for every type of printing: stationery, booklets, pamphlets, color plates, books and circular letters.

But the vast expansion in the circulation of The Journal, of Hygeia, of the special periodicals, the Quarterly Cumulative Index Medicus, and the vast amount of material created through the Councils and Bureaus has thrown such a tremendous burden on the printing equipment that it has become necessary to arrange for printing of much of the material by other agencies.

THE COUNCIL ON PHARMACY AND CHEMISTRY AND THE CHEMICAL LABORATORY

By Austin Smith, M.D.

IN OCTOBER, 1907, THE LATE Dr. George H. Simmons, then editor of THE JOURNAL, addressed the Kentucky State Medical Association. Speaking on "What the American Medical Association Stands For," he vowed that the Association is for "honesty and fairness and [is] unalterably and eternally against fraud and deception in all that relates to the health and physical welfare of the people."

In the same address Dr. Simmons declared: "From my standpoint, obtained from personal observation and from being brought into contact with actual conditions, the work being done by the Council on Pharmacy and Chemistry is the most important of all the good things with which the Association is to be credited."

One of the first questions that came before the preliminary convention of the American Medical Association in 1847 was the regulation of pharmaceutical matters and of "patent" and proprietary remedies. Even that long ago a resolution on this subject was offered by Dr. John B. Johnson of Missouri and adopted. In 1849 Dr. Thomas Wood presented a resolution which was adopted concerning drug adulteration, quack remedies and nostrums. The resolution called for an examining board which would analyze such remedies and report publicly its findings. The only reason why the work was not prosecuted at that time was that the Association was without funds for the successful undertaking of such a work. Other similar resolutions followed in 1850, in 1879, and in other years until finally the Council was created in 1905.

These resolutions indicated considerable protest by the members of the medical profession concerning certain commercial practices. Scarcely a year passed that the question was not brought up before the Association in some form or other. But, according to the late Dr. Simmons, "conditions . . . grew worse rather than better and finally the problem became very acute on account of the advertising pages of THE JOURNAL—to answer these questions the Council on Pharmacy and Chemistry was created. . . ." This statement by Dr. Simmons, which was made in 1914 while he was addressing the

Southern Medical Association, was offered in a review of the work of the Council and its effect on medical progress. He declared that the work of the Council appeared and proved to be stupendous but, he stated, "this much is certain: the Council's work has made it possible for the practicing physician of today to have a keener sense of the value and limitations of drugs. It has placed the allied arts and sciences of therapeutics and pharmacology on a sounder and more scientific basis than ever before." He said this at a time when the Council had been in existence only nine years, a fact which shows how progress can be made when the spirit is willing, the objectives sound, and the participants able and not subject to pernicious control.

MEMBERSHIP

The Council, which is a standing committee created by the Board of Trustees of the American Medical Association, was established immediately following a meeting of the Board on February 4 and 5, 1905, at which time such establishment was authorized. A number of outstanding scientists were invited to help form the Council and these men held their first meeting at the Hotel Henry in Pittsburgh, Pa., on February 11, 1905.

In attendance were Robert A. Hatcher, M. I. Wilbert, Lyman F. Kebler, Torald Sollmann, Arthur R. Cushny, J. O. Schlotterbeck, C. Lewis Diehl, William A. Puckner, C. S. N. Hallberg, and George H. Simmons. Dr. Simmons was elected Chairman; Professor C. S. N. Hallberg was elected Secretary.

There were also elected five additional members: J. H. Long, F. G. Novy, Samuel P. Sadtler, Julius Stieglitz, and H. W. Wiley.

Of these early members, fifteen in number, Dr. Torald Sollmann has offered a series of thumb-nail biographies which will serve to give an insight into the reasons for the Council's early success and immediate and general support. With men like these for charter members, any such endeavors as the activities of the Council were bound to succeed. In the words of Torald Sollmann:

ARTHUR R. CUSHNY, M.D., Professor of Pharmacology, University of Michigan Medical School. The outstanding representative of physiologic pharmacology in America; Trained at the Schmiedberg Institute in Strasburg he succeeded Abel at Michigan. An active investigator and author of a textbook on pharmacology, which went through many editions and survived his death. He transferred to his new post at University College, London, before the Council had its first meeting. He was then made an honorary member and continued as an active supporter of the Council. He was quiet, somewhat restrained, thoroughly conversant with pharmacology, a man of good judgment.

LEWIS DIEHL, Ph.M., Professor of Pharmacy, Louisville College of Pharmacy. An "apotheker" of the old school, prominent in U.S.P. revision work, possessing the full confidence of the pharmacists, and indeed of all who knew him.

C. S. N. HALLBERG, Ph.G., M.D., Professor of Pharmacy, University of Illinois School of Pharmacy. Primarily a pharmaceutical educator, and a virile power in pharmaceutical circles. A steady, fearless Scandinavian, sound if somewhat headstrong at times, ever ready to fight for his ideals, the promotion of honesty, science and efficiency in the drug business. As the first Secretary of the Council he organized the weekly bulletin system of transacting its business, which contributed materially to its successful work. He saw the Council off to a good start, but withdrew in February 1906 as he had other functions that occupied so much of his time that he felt he was unable to give the time necessary to serve as Secretary.

ROBERT A. HATCHER, Ph.G., M.D., Professor of Pharmacology, Cornell University Medical College. Starting as a retail pharmacist he passed through private practice, teaching in a pharmacy school, and finally to pharmacology, so that he has personally experienced the subject of drugs in all its branches. He was a meticulously conscientious worker and writer, industrious, exhaustive, precise, sometimes perhaps a little rigid. He was ever ready to pull more than his weight of work, and whatever he undertook was done thoroughly and exactly. He remained on the Council, doing not only the ordinary duties, but editing Useful Drugs and other Council publications until he felt that his years prevented him from giving full service. The Council then made him honorary member, a well deserved tribute. Until his death he continued to work with the Council.

LYMAN F. KEBLER, Ph.G., M.S., M.D., Chief of the Drug Laboratory, U. S. Department of Agriculture. A government official concerned with the Food and Drug Act, which was then making its bow to the public, none too sure of its welcome. He helped in working out mutual understanding and unification of effort wherever possible.

J. H. LONG, M.S., Sc.D., Professor of Chemistry, Northwestern University Medical School. Had served on the Food-Preservatives Referee Board. A competent chemist, with common sense, pleasant and cooperative; a man whom one trusted instinctively and found the trust confirmed by experience.

F. G. NOVY, M.D., Sc.D., Professor of Bacteriology, University of Michigan. A leader and pioneer in bacteriology, including its chemical aspects. An industrious and fertile worker, plain and to the point.

W. A. PUCKNER, Ph.G., Professor of Chemistry, University of Illinois School of Pharmacy. Succeeded Hallberg as Secretary of the Council until his death in 1931. Well balanced, even tempered, fair-minded and judicial, he kept the Council on an even keel during its formative and occasionally somewhat tempestuous days. He managed to organize affairs so well that the handicap of his increasing blindness was scarcely felt. He always heard all sides of the matter before he reached a decision, which he was always ready to change if more information became available.

SAMUEL P. SADTLER, Ph.D., Professor of Chemistry, Philadelphia College of Pharmacy. A chemist of skill and experience, possessing the confidence of manufacturers, and perhaps sometimes more inclined than other members to give them the benefit of any doubts. His fund of information was invaluable.

J. O. SCHLOTTERBECK, Ph.G., Ph.D., Professor of Pharmacognosy and Botany, and Dean of the School of Pharmacy, University of Michigan. An authority on botanical information and on pharmaceutical education, he supplied reliable data in this field.

GEORGE H. SIMMONS, M.D., LL.D., Secretary and General Manager of the American Medical Association and Editor of its Journal. Chairman and father of the Council, his favored child from its inception to his death—although his big heart had room for all the Association as well. He gave the Council the full benefit of his wide experience, his great ability, his power and his influence. The policies of THE JOURNAL, already the most powerful periodical in the profession, were in his keeping, and he employed them to interpret the Council to the physicians, to the House of Delegates and to the Trustees at a period when such interpretation and such support were vital. His enthusiasm was contagious, yet he was modest, self effacing, never opinionated, never officious; a wise father, ever helpful, never obtrusive.

JULIUS STIEGLITZ, Ph.D., Professor of Chemistry, University of Chicago. An all-around chemist with a consciousness for science in the service of the public and a deep sympathy for medicine. A mind that plumbed directly to the heart of every problem.

M. I. WILBERT, Ph.M., Assistant in the Division of Pharmacology, Hygienic Laboratory, U. S. Public Health and Marine Hospital Service, to which he came from what appears to have been the first full-time position as hospital pharmacist, which was at "German" Hospital in Philadelphia. He had an inexhaustible fund of pharmaceutical and miscellaneous information on science, trade and people. Genial, witty, warmhearted, unassuming—another man whom you would trust instinctively, and never find the trust misplaced.

H. W. WILEY, M.D., Ph.D., Chief of the Bureau of Chemistry, U. S. Department of Agriculture. The protagonist and obstetrician of the original Pure Food and Drug Act. A big man in every sense, equally strong as a practical political manueverer and as a scientist, and not to be despised in either function. His governmental work took up so much of his time that he was not as active in the Council as he would have liked, but when he was needed he was always available.

Thus has Torald Sollmann summed up fourteen of the original members of the Council. But what of the fifteenth man, Torald Sollmann, Professor of Pharmacology and Materia Medica, Western Reserve University Medical School? There is no need to describe him as a scientist; everyone knows of his contributions to medical knowledge in the field of pharmacological research. Nor is it necessary to describe him as an educator; as a teacher of pharmacology and materia medica and as Dean of Western Reserve University Medical School his name is widely known. As a writer, his contributions influenced profoundly the thinking of those interested in the subjects on which he wrote. His "A Manual of Pharmacology" will be known for years to come. The human side of Torald Sollmann may be less well known, but those who have been privileged to work with him will never forget him. Kindly, fair, determined to get the facts and see that justice was done, eager to learn of the new, possessed of a brilliant and discerning mind, this scientist's name became almost synonymous with that of the Council. As a coworker he is inexhaustible; as a social companion he is unsurpassable. His thinking is always up-to-date and his friends are forever being startled by some modern expression or bit of slang that perhaps does as much as anything else to make one realize the constant probing and the awareness of the modern world, its problems and its people, which is typical of Torald Sollmann. He was the youngest member of the Council when it was formed and has served continuously without thought of "thank you." He is one of those who have made people recognize the sincerity of the Council's motto "Non sibi sed medicinae (Not for ourselves but for medicine)."

In 1907 the Council membership was increased from fifteen to sixteen. In 1924 one more member was added, and in 1939 the membership was increased to eighteen. Membership has always been determined by the needs of the moment. It would have been impractical, perhaps impossible, to have representation of all fields of medical science. Instead the services of willing consultants were freely called upon.

In effect, the Council is a self-perpetuating body. When a member dies or resigns, the latter usually because of irresistible pressure of other work, each member proposes two names for a successor; two ballots are made, the last being a secret one, and the names of the two receiving the highest score in the last ballot are sent to the Board of Trustees of the Association, which appoints one of the two as a member. The term of Council membership is five years, and a member is usually re-elected unless he indicates his inability to serve another term, usually because of illness, or the demands of his regular professional work.

From 1905 until September 1946, when this article was written, there have been 64 members. The average age of these members on appointment was 44 years; the average age on retirement from Council membership 55 years. The average tenure of membership has been 11 years.

The names of the past and present members include:

Carl L. Alsberg, M.D., John F. Anderson, M.D., Edward M. Bailey, Ph.D., David P Barr, M.D., Stanhope Bayne-Jones, M.D., Kenneth D. Blackfan, M.D., J. Howard Brown, Ph.D., Joseph A. Capps, M.D., Anton J. Carlson, Ph.D., Samuel W. Clausen, M.D., Harold N. Cole, M.D., Arthur R. Cushny, M.D., C. Lewis Diehl, Ph.M., Eugene F. DuBois, M.D., Charles W. Edmunds, M.D., David L. Edsall, M.D., Morris Fishbein, M.D., Otto Folin, Ph.D., E. M. K. Geiling, M.D., C. S. N. Hallberg, Phar.D., Robert A. Hatcher, M.D., Robert P. Herwick, M.D., Alfred F. Hess, M.D., Albion W. Hewlett, M.D., John Howland, M.D., Reid Hunt, M.D., Ernest E. Irons, M.D., Treat B. Johnson, Ph.D., Lyman F. Kebler, M.D., Chester S. Keefer, M.D., Theodore G. Klumpp, M.D., Henry Kraemer, Ph.D., Eugene M. Landis, M.D., C. Guy Lane, M.D., James P. Leake, M.D., Paul Nicholas Leech, Ph.D., Robert F. Loeb, M.D., John Harper Long, Sc.D., Perrin H. Long, M.D., Warfield T. Longcope, M.D., Williams McKim Marriott, M.D., George W. McCoy, M.D., Lafayette B. Mendel, Ph.D., Stuart Mudd, M.D., Elmer M. Nelson, Ph.D., Frederick G. Novy, M.D., Oliver T. Osborne, M.D., Walter W. Palmer, M.D., Francis W. Peabody, M.D., William A. Puckner, Phar.D., William C. Rose, Ph.D., Leonard G. Rowntree, M.D., Samuel P. Sadtler, Ph.D., Julius O. Schlotterbeck, Ph.D., Elmer L. Sevringhaus, M.D., George H. Simmons, M.D., Austin E. Smith, M.D., Torald Sollmann, M.D., Isaac Starr, M.D., Julius Stieglitz, Ph.D., Soma Weiss, M.D.. Martin I. Wilbert, Phar.D., W. Barry Wood, Jr., M.D., Harvey W. Wiley, M.D.

At one time the Council had several "corresponding members": A. H. Cushny (Scotland), H. H. Dale (England), H. Thoms (Germany) and W. Heubner (Germany). There have been no corresponding members since 1937.

All of the members, with the exception of the Secretary, who is a full-time employee of the American Medical Association, have always served, and still do, without remuneration. They receive reimbursement only for expenses such as stationery, postage and attendance at Council meetings. The members of the Council have never accepted remuneration for the consideration of products which are included in its New and Nonofficial Remedies. Nor is the Council or its members influenced in the slightest by any proffer of advertising patronage for medical journals, including those of the Association. The cost of carrying on the work of the Council is borne entirely by appropriations made by the Board of Trustees of the American Medical Association.

RULES OF THE COUNCIL

At its first meeting the Council considered certain principles and finally adopted ten rules by which would be considered drugs and other articles for inclusion in New and Nonofficial Remedies. These rules were:

Rule 1.—No article shall be admitted unless its active medicinal ingredients and the amounts of such ingredients in a given quantity of the article be furnished for publication. The general composition of the vehicle, its alcoholic percentage, if any, and the identity of other preservatives, if present, must be furnished.

Rule 2.—No chemical compound will be admitted unless sufficient information be furnished regarding tests for identity, purity and strength, the rational formula or the structural formula, if known.

Rule 3.—No article that is advertised to the public will be admitted; but this rule will not apply to disinfectants, and food preparations, except when advertised in an objectionable manner.

Rule 4.—No article will be admitted whose label, package or circular accompanying the package contains the names of diseases, in the treatment of which the article is indicated. The therapeutic indications, properties and doses may be stated. (This rule does not apply to literature distributed solely to physicians, to advertising in medical journals, or to vaccines and antitoxins.)

Rule 5.—No article will be admitted or retained concerning which the manufacturer, or his agents, make false or misleading statements as to geographical source, raw material from which made, or method of collection or preparation.

Rule 6.—No article will be admitted or retained of which the manufacturer or his agents make unwarranted, exaggerated or misleading statements as to therapeutic value.

Rule 7.—Labels on articles containing "poisonous" or "potent" substances must show the amounts of each of such ingredients in a given quantity of the product. A list of such substances will be prepared.

Rule 8.—If the trade name of an article is not sufficiently descriptive of its chemical composition or pharmaceutical character, or is, for any other reason, objectionable, the Council reserves the right to include with the trade name a descriptive title in the book. Articles bearing objectionably suggestive names will be refused consideration.

Rule 9.—If the name of an article is registered, or the label copyrighted, the date of registration and a copy of the protected label should be furnished the Council. In case of registration in foreign countries, the name under which the article is registered should be supplied.

Rule 10.—If the article is patented—either process or product—the number and date of such patent or patents should be furnished.

These rules appeared in The Journal of the American Medical Association, in pamphlets for free distribution, and in the first issue of New and Nonofficial Remedies which was published in 1907. In the 1909 issue of New and Nonofficial Remedies may be found a modification of the rules, this modification consisting of the combining of the substance of Rules 9 and 10 relating to copyright and patent and the addition of another rule concerning unscientific and useless articles. This became Rule 10 and read as follows:

'Unscientific and Useless Articles.—No article will be admitted which, because of its unscientific composition, is useless or inimical to the best interests of the public or of the medical profession."

In New and Nonofficial Remedies 1924 may be found a new rule, Rule 11. This rule reads:

"Policies Dangerous to Public Health.—The evidence on which the Council may refuse recognition to the products of a firm shall consist: (1) the fact that but a small proportion of the firm's proprietary products are acceptable for New and Nonofficial Remedies; or (2) that a large proportion of the business of the firm is in products that are in conflict with the rules of the Council; or (3) that physicians who reply to the firm's advertisements of accepted products are supplied with advertising which features the use of products that are in conflict with the rules of the Council; or (4) that the firm makes claims that are seriously misleading; and especially if these claims tend to promote the use of products in any manner that would seriously endanger public health."

These rules were continued until 1946 and it is interesting to note that the principles set forth in 1905 were equally sound, and necessary, forty years later. From time to time editorial improvements were made and minor additions and explanatory notes added to clarify application of the rules.

After the Council rules had been in existence for several months and manufacturers had had opportunity to observe their application, a conference was held with representatives of the drug and pharmaceutic manufacturers when the Council held its second meeting, September 11, 1905, in Cleveland. These representatives entered fully into the discussion offering their comments and suggestions. Only minor changes seemed indicated and these were made.

In October 1945 a group of Council members met to study the rules and discuss any need for change. The results of the deliberations were considered by the Council at a general meeting in December when it was decided that the Federal Food, Drug and Cosmetic Act has made into legal requirements conditions which were formerly controlled only by the Council rules, and that some of these rules had thereby become superfluous. It seemed also desirable to revise or rescind certain other rules which had become more of a hindrance than a help in the Council's endeavor to provide guidance in the use of drugs and on other subjects. In May 1946 the new rules, seven in number, became effective. They are as follows:

Rule 1.—Composition.—The quantitative composition of preparations and articles submitted to the Council or considered by the Council for inclusion in New and Nonofficial Remedies must be made known and may be published.

Rule 2.—Identification.—Suitable procedures and criteria for determining the composition or standardization of the submitted preparation or article must be furnished.

Rule 3.—Advertising to the Public.—Preparations and articles promoted to the public for use in the treatment of disease will not be accepted except as specified in the following explanatory comments.

Rule 4.—Therapeutic Claims.—When an article is accepted, therapeutic representations by the manufacturers or their agents must be confined to those given in the N.N.R. or accepted by the Council between revisions of N.N.R.

Rule 5.—Protected Names.—Proprietary names for medicinal articles will be accepted if the Council deems the use of such exclusive names not to be harmful to health and if the proprietary names are not given greater prominence in labeling and other promotional activities than the official names or the nonproprietary names adopted by the Council.

Rule 6.—Patents and Trademarks.—If a preparation or product is patented as to process or product or both, the number of such patent or patents must be furnished to the Council. If the name of an article is registered or the label copyrighted, the registration (trademark) name and number and copies of the protected label must be furnished to the Council.

Rule 7.—Unscientific and Useless Articles.—A preparation or an article will not be accepted if in the opinion of the Council it will not be in the best interests of the medical profession and the public.

If further changes are needed in due time they will be made; the Council has been, and still is, ready to consider carefully any suggestions for the improvement of its rules or of any activity in which it may be engaged.

METHOD OF PROCEDURE

At its first meeting the Council outlined a plan for consideration of products. Briefly, it was: All information regarding a product would be obtained from the manufacturer and from other sources.

This information, together with samples of the article, were to be submitted to a sub-committee of experts who would examine critically the product, consider the claims made for it, and make its report. On the basis of this report the Council would accept, reject or hold for further consideration. If accepted, the information would be condensed and arranged somewhat on the plan of the U. S. Pharmacopeia but with the addition of brief pharmacologic and therapeutic data to be published in a book "New and Nonofficial Remedies" (N.N.R.). As fast as new articles were accepted, all information regarding them was to be published in The Journal of the American Medical Association and later be incorporated in the next edition of N.N.R.

There was at that time no book such as New and Nonofficial Remedies. The Council believed that the value of such a book would be proportionate to its completeness and "therefore proposed to be as liberal in approving articles for the book as is consistent with justice and honesty to the public, to the manufacturing pharmacist and chemist, and to the physician."

The Council also decided to examine preparations the usefulness of which was open to doubt. It stated that it did not "presume to dictate what preparations should be prescribed; nor is it the present intention to conduct an active campaign against fraudulent products; but merely to *supply information concerning those which it considers objectionable.*"

Today the plan of action is essentially the same, though perhaps more detailed. The firm must provide specimens of advertising material, specimens of the drug for laboratory examination, evidence in support of the efficacy and proposed claims, information on trade name and synonyms, definition, preparation, properties, tests, pharmacologic action, therapeutic indications, toxicology, dose, how supplied, manufacturer, patents and trademarks.

The Council office submits the firm's data with other information in its files to a Council member who serves as a referee. The referee prepares a report or puts in finished form a rough draft, which may have been prepared in the Council office by a consultant, and returns it to the Secretary who, every two weeks, transmits such material to the other Council members by a mimeographed bulletin. Accompanying this report are specimens of advertising material and other pertinent data which may aid the Council members in their decisions. Thus, each Council member has an opportunity to judge for himself the usefulness of the product, whether it complies with the Council's rules, and the report offered by the referee, who, incidentally, is an authority in the field of the subject which he is asked to consider.

In the next issue of the Bulletin appears the discussion by all members, which may elicit information not available to the Council office or the referee. In the following issue of the Bulletin appears the vote to accept the product, reject or hold in abeyance. A three-fourths affirmative vote of the voting members (a nonvoting member being one who may be ill, temporarily out of the country or otherwise occupied) is necessary for the acceptance or rejection of a product. If a product is accepted the firm is notified immediately of the outcome of the Council's consideration. If any advertising claims must be revised or deleted or more supporting evidence provided before the product stands finally accepted, the firm is so notified. On the removal of these conditions the product then becomes accepted and a description is submitted to the editor of THE JOURNAL for publication and subsequent transferral to New and Nonofficial Remedies. If insufficient evidence is submitted by the manufacturer to justify the acceptance of its product at the time of consideration, the manufacturer is notified so that he may submit the lacking information. If he refuses or is unable to do so the product may be held in abeyance for further investigation or be immediately rejected. The manufacturer always is given opportunity to argue the Council's decision and may at any time ask the Council to reconsider the status of a rejected product.

Occasionally there is brought to the attention of the Council a new product which shows promise of usefulness but on which the experimental work has not been sufficient to make it ready for general use by the medical profession. In order to assure proper and controlled clinical study of such a product the Council issues a preliminary report on identity and standards, on the experimental work that has been done and on the further study that may appear desirable.

With the exception of the continuance of acceptance of a drug, all the Council's actions, whether of acceptance, rejection or omission, are published in THE JOURNAL and later in New and Nonofficial Remedies or in the Annual Reprint of the Reports of the Council on Pharmacy and Chemistry. This gives full publicity for all the Council's decisions to manufacturers and physicians alike.

The Council insists that the manufacturer must supply evidence for therapeutic and other claims. The Council is not equipped to initiate a clinical investigation of every drug that is submitted for its consideration. It does have the facilities of seventeen Council members to draw upon, the members' associates and other outstanding authorities throughout the entire country, these men serving gladly as Council consultants. A chemical laboratory maintained at A.M.A. headquarters examines the chemical composition of every submitted product before it is admitted to New and Nonofficial Remedies.

An outline of the information required and of the Council rules can always be obtained simply by writing to the Secretary at A.M.A. headquarters.

RECEPTION AND COOPERATION

When the Council was formed manufacturing pharmacists and chemists of the United States were informed and invited to offer their comments. Practically all were favorable towards the organization and purpose. Some typical comments are:

The rules adopted governing the admission of articles are entirely reasonable and if carried out to the letter will elevate, energize and encourage manufacturing pharmacists to cater exclusively to the profession.

Everything contained in the announcement and circular is unqualifiedly and absolutely indorsed. Every rule is conducive to good and not one of the rules will, even in its strictest interpretation, harm any honest manufacturer.

We congratulate your Council on the initiation of this important work and hope that it will promote the interests of ethical medicine and pharmacy.

You have undertaken quite a contract but if it is carried out on the lines suggested, your book will be of invaluable service to the profession. There are, however, a great many products that are offered to the physician which in our judgment are not, strictly speaking, ethical and we would dislike to have our products appear in a book with some of these "so-called" remedies.

We do not hesitate to state that we approve very heartily of the movement. The ends you are striving for are very desirable indeed and it is our desire to cooperate with you.

We wish to congratulate you on this undertaking by the American Medical Association. Something of this kind has long been needed, particularly as there are a great many articles forced on the profession with absolutely no excuse except that of making money . . . I feel that it is the most important step taken in recent years in this country, as it holds out at least a ray of hope to the manufacturers who are trying to conduct an honest and ethical business.

We are heartily in accord with every movement which aims at the separation of the wheat from the chaff and indeed believe that with the issue of the book as proposed a pioneer and systematic step has been taken in the right direction. Desultory writings tending toward reformatory movements serve well as an initiatory purpose but fall short of ultimately obtaining its object. To accomplish this a systematic hammering is required and fathered and fostered as this movement is by the A.M.A., will make success a surety and in the end rid the Medical as well as the Profession of Pharmacy and in turn Therapy of the non-descripts.

We will do anything which you may wish in connection with this movement. The members of this concern are entirely in sympathy with you and will give you any information we have at hand. We are very glad to notice Rule number 1 and think it is very much to the benefit of the profession that this rule is carried out to the fullest extent.

Of course not every one was happy with this new regime. One manufacturer of a preparation which appeared in the advertising pages of THE JOURNAL wrote in part: "We don't recognize the right of any man or set of men to interfere with our property. We do not propose to submit any of our preparations to the so-called Council on Pharmacy and Chemistry. Furthermore, if we learn that the said Council on Pharmacy and Chemistry attempts to incorporate any of our preparations in the book referred to, we will ask for an injunction restraining any interference with our property." Needless to say, the Council and THE JOURNAL no longer needed to worry about accepting the product in question. In commenting on the foregoing letter one member wrote: "The legend that the scorpion when surrounded by fire and unable to escape, in its fury stings itself to death finds verification in the letter from. . . . If our Chairman can induce all the objectionable manufacturers to commit this form of suicide, he will indeed lighten the labors of the Council so that they may lie upon beds of roses. The wider the publicity given to the letter in contrast with those from reputable firms, the better will it show the true status of the (name of firm) concern."

At its July 1905 meeting the A.M.A. House of Delegates indorsed the action of the Board of Trustees in the creation of the Council on Pharmacy and Chemistry and requested the trustees to "devise a plan through which the Council may be made permanent." And thus was the Council urged to continue its efforts. (It discussed the necessary arrangements at its second meeting, September 11, 1905.)

At the same time the House urged the Trustees to "request the Secretary of Agriculture of the U. S. Government to give the Council on Pharmacy and Chemistry recognition by authorizing the Bureau of Chemistry to cooperate with the Council in its work." The Delegates also endorsed the work already performed by the Council and recommended the publication in book form of a list of the preparations that were accepted by the Council.

Subsequently the Secretary of the American Medical Association received a letter (dated September 29, 1905) from James Wilson, Secretary, Department of Agriculture, which stated:

"I beg to acknowledge the receipt of your communication of the 27th inst. containing the action of the House of Delegates of the American Medical Association at the meeting held in Portland, Ore., July 11–14, 1905.

In reply I will say that I have established in the Bureau of Chemistry of the Department under the authority of the Congress of the United States, a laboratory for the investigation of adulteration of drugs and medicines. I believe that the purpose of Congress included every possible avenue of useful activity for this laboratory.

It seems to me that the collaboration with the great body of American physicians who form the American Medical Association affords a splendid opportunity to carry out the work which Congress intended to be done.

It gives me pleasure, therefore, to inform you that I have authorized the Chief of the Bureau of Chemistry to cooperate with the Council on Pharmacy and Chemistry of the American Medical Association."

At the same time a copy of Mr. Wilson's letter to Dr. H. W. Wiley, Chief, Bureau of Chemistry, was received. About the same time a letter (dated September 26) was received by the Council from Dr. Philip Mills Jones, Secretary, Medical Society of the State of California, which read:

"At a recent meeting of the Publication Committee of the Medical Society of the State of California, it was unanimously decided to submit the advertising pages of the California State Journal of Medicine, published by the Society, to your honorable body, with the request that you indicate any advertisements of articles which do not conform to your rules, or which, in your judgment, should not be advertised by our Society.

"Under this Resolution, I am mailing you a copy of the last issue of our Journal, and will mail you a copy of the next issue as soon as it is published. In indicating such articles, if any, as in the judgment of your honorable body should not be advertised by our Society, I am instructed to request you to set forth reasons for such determination for the information and guidance of our Publication Committee. Such information to be regarded as confidential by us unless released by you. Obviously, in canceling any existing advertising contracts or in refusing to renew the same, we must have some reason for such conduct."

Although the Council had already received much support from medical and pharmaceutical journals, this was apparently the first request to consider the advertising pages of any periodical other than The Journal of the American Medical Association. Later, many journals were to exclude non-Council accepted drugs from their pages; state journal policies were even to be united through the formation of the Cooperative Medical Advertising Bureau.

As the years passed the prestige of the Council increased, and it became known around the world. Representatives of country after country sought information with a view to establishing similar organizations in their homelands. International correspondence with groups in several countries became a routine practice. Holland, Germany, England, France, Sweden, Norway, Switzerland and China are just a few of the countries represented, while from Central and South America the Council office has received a succession of visitors from many areas. As long ago as 1905 (see J.A.M.A., Sept. 9, p. 801) editorial comments on the Council appeared in the London *Lancet*, which contained the suggestion that an international working agreement might be effected with much benefit "through proper division of work and interchange of reports."

The Council has served as a pattern for the creation of the A.M.A. Council on Foods and Nutrition and Council on Physical Medicine, and for the A.D.A. Council on Dental Therapeutics. A number of people now in industry and elsewhere have received invaluable training in the Council office and in the Chemical Laboratory.

OTHER ACTIVITIES

As the Council passed through the years it took on new responsibilities and added duties as they seemed indicated. Today, the activities of the Council on Pharmacy and Chemistry include the preparation of special treatises, articles, status reports and books designed for the practitioner and medical student, the giving of grants-in-aid for therapeutic research, the securing of therapeutic trials of promising new preparations, the encouragement of basic research on fundamental therapeutic problems, and the answering of inquiries from the medical and allied professions.

The Therapeutic Trials Committee, a standing committee of the Council on Pharmacy and Chemistry, was established to encourage and aid sound research on medicinal agents and to promote therapeutics through an adequate understanding of the usefulness and limitations of drug products. It organizes impartial clinical trials of biological and pharmaceutical agents which offer promise in the prevention, treatment or diagnosis of disease. It provides this service without regard to size of manufacturer or sponsor and without charge for its part in organization of the trials. The cost of the trials are determined by the sponsor and the investigating center. Full details can be obtained from the Council office.

Some indication of the scope of activities of the Council can be gained from the annual report of the Board of Trustees to the House of Delegates. For example, the following excerpts are taken from the 1946 report:

MEETINGS

The Council held two meetings in 1945. The topics discussed included the promiscuous use of vitamins and the need for further studies on vitamin therapy, the consideration of cosmetic creams containing estrogens, the external use of sulfonamide preparations, the spread of infectious hepatitis by contaminated syringes and needles, acceptance of drugs for manufacturing use, the cooperative report on thiouracil, the Therapeutic Trials Committee, furtherance of the use of the metric system and revision of the Council's rules.

PUBLICATIONS AND REPORTS

During the year over 30,000 copies of New and Non-official Remedies, Useful Drugs, the Epitome of the U. S. Pharmacopeia and National Formulary, Annual Reprint of the Reports of the Council, and Glandular Physiology and Therapy were distributed.

Of this number New and Non-official Remedies comprised over 17,000 copies. One indication of the increasing popularity of this book is the frequency with which copies are requested for review purposes. The 1946 volume of New and Nonofficial Remedies is now being printed. Under the twenty-three general classes of preparations contained in the 1945 volume, approximately 1,000 brands of medicinal agents (exclusive of dosage forms and modifications) were listed and described. This number, of course, varies from year to year.

The Council also adopted for publication various reports concerning the use of drugs in the prevention and treatment of disease. Deserving special mention are reports on Dangers from the External Use of Sulfonamides; Dermatophytosis: Treatment and Prophylaxis; Dysentery Bacteriophage; Status of Cosmetics Containing Hormones; The Status of Passive Immunization and Treatment in Pertussis; Status of Poison Ivy Extracts. Many of the articles were requested in reprint form, a service available to physicians and to other interested scientists or organizations. These statements have been widely quoted and have been the basis of many references in periodicals and elsewhere.

RESEARCH

In addition to organizing the work of the Therapeutic Trials Committee and to initiating and sponsoring research resulting from certain phases of problems facing the Council in its considerations, the Council's Committee on Therapeutic Research issued twenty-two grants ranging from $100.00 to $3,000.00. Many articles have been published during the year as a result of work done under these grants.

PROFESSIONAL RELATIONS

The Council continued to enjoy cooperative relationship with many agencies of the federal government and with other bodies, and it supplied information and other assistance whenever possible. It encourages professional relations with agencies, associations and societies to promote helpful understanding of problems of mutual interest. An example of the Council's wide interest and its desire to be helpful is its cooperation with the Office of War Information in the preparation of a booklet on the Control of Communicable Diseases, a manual to be distributed for use in occupied countries. The Council provided assistance by appointing a committee to supply statements on treatment of the various diseases mentioned in the manual.

The Secretary of the Council attended a conference called under the auspices of the American Pharmaceutical Association to permit discussion of the sale of barbituric acid compounds and the steps that may be taken to effect control over this sale. It is apparent that the enforcement permissible under the present state laws and the Federal Food, Drug and Cosmetic Act is not preventing abuse of the barbiturates. There was representation at the conference from many interested organizations and the consensus seemed to be in favor of enforcing control at the state level, probably by means of a uniform state law and adequate personnel.

The Council and its office continued to be of assistance to other Council offices, bureaus and departments at A.M.A. headquarters and to work cooperatively on projects of mutual interest. For example, it considered with the Council on Industrial Health the status of the use of aluminum compounds in the modification and treatment of silicosis; for the Bureau of Health Education it provided information for replies to lay inquirers and assisted in the preparation of a number of radio programs. Such cooperation was given the editorial department, the business department, the Council on Medical Education and Hospitals, Council on Foods and Nutrition, Council on Physical Medicine, the Bureau of Investigation, the Bureau of Legal Medicine and Legislation, the Council on Medical Service and Public Relations, and other offices.

The Council also provided assistance for all medical and other journals interested in following Council policies, particularly the state medical journals. It has been especially interested in the problems of the state medical journals and societies and is working closely with the Cooperative Medical Advertising Bureau. The Secretary of the Council is ex-officio a member of the Advisory Council of the C.M.A.B.

OTHER ACTIVITIES

Other efforts to extend the usefulness of the Council and its office include the filing of data on patents for treatment measures, so that all possible approaches to drug therapy which have been studied will be available at the Council office; the collection of data on reactions to and deaths from drugs so that a repository of such information may be established; and the abstracting and filing of federal and state laws on research, the sale and distribution of drugs, and other problems of a similar nature. When pooled with the data now available at the Council office and the data accumulated under the auspices of the Therapeutic Trials Committee, this information should make the Council an outstanding source of information on the prevention, diagnosis and treatment of disease. The Council is even expanding its consideration of agents for inclusion in New and Nonofficial Remedies to include such products as insecticides, scabieticides, and cosmetic preparations creating a physiologic change in the body. All of this information will be freely available as fast as it can be released. Only lack of personnel created by the exigencies of war has prevented more rapid expansion of Council activities.

Inquiries directed to the Council office are encouraged, and during 1945 there was much correspondence concerning drugs used in this country and in other countries. The Council's files on foreign drugs, especially those sold in Latin-American countries, are rapidly increasing.

The Secretary addressed a number of scientific and non-scientifically trained audiences on varied subjects. He and his medical assistants in the Council office will continue to be available when invited and, furthermore, will be available with exhibits for scientific meetings. The Secretary also attended a number of meetings to represent the Council and present its views and information, and he worked particularly closely with the U.S.P. and N.F. committees.

During 1945 a new step in cooperation was undertaken by the Food and Drug Administration, the Council, and several representatives of the drug and pharmaceutic industry. Before thiouracil, a new drug for the treatment of hyperthyroidism, was released in interstate commerce, six manufacturers interested in this compound and the Food and Drug Administration prepared a survey by questionnaire of the toxicity of the drug. The study, which involved the results of use of 5,745 cases, was reported to the Council with a view to informing this body and through it the medical profession. The study was published in THE JOURNAL as a report to the Council and then was given wide distribution by reprint and by reproduction in a journal published by the American Pharmaceutical Association. Such cooperation is to be commended and manufacturers are urged to show a similar spirit in other therapeutic problems of common interest.

Representatives of the Council met with representatives of the Food and Drug Administration, United States Pharmacopeia and National Formulary to discuss ways and means of expediting the exclusive use of the metric system. Following consultation, several proposals were adopted which will encourage and hasten more extensive use of this system by industry, the medical and pharmaceutical professions and other groups.

Announcements of acceptance of new drugs by the Council are now being carried also in the Practical Pharmacy Edition of The Journal of the American Pharmaceutical Association, the American Professional Pharmacist, and the Journal of the National Association of Retail Druggists. All published Council statements are being circulated to all state medical journals for reproduction if they see fit.

OTHER COUNCIL PUBLICATIONS

In discussing the historical development of Council activities special mention should be made of a book that is not published now. Prior to 1911, reports of the Council on Pharmacy and Chemistry and the A.M.A. Chemical Laboratory, as well as articles dealing with so-called "patent medicines" prepared by THE JOURNAL's Propaganda Department (now the Bureau of Investigation) were published in the section of THE JOURNAL known as the "Pharmacology" department. In 1911 this section became "The Propaganda for Reform" department and it carried the following explanatory paragraph as a sort of sub-title: "In this department appear reports of the Council on Pharmacy and Chemistry and of the Association Laboratory, together with other matter tending to aid intelligent prescribing and to oppose medical fraud on the public and on the profession." During this period the Council's reports as well as those of the Laboratory received editorial attention by Dr. Arthur J. Cramp prior to publication.

In THE JOURNAL of May 30, 1925, p. 1644, there appears the following explanation of the change in the name of the "Propaganda Department" to "Bureau of Investigation" (the new name, however, was not used as a Journal heading until January 1928): "It will be noted that the name 'Propaganda Department' has been superseded by the more descriptive term, 'Bureau of Investigation.' This change was made because it was felt that the new name more accurately describes the activities of that department of the Association's work than the older term 'Propaganda Department.' At the time that the name 'Propaganda for Reform in Proprietary Remedies' was first applied, it fully and accurately described the functions of the department that bore the name. During those years, propaganda was truly needed. The acute need has passed and the work of the Bureau of Investigation covers a broader and a more general field in its attempt to give to the profession and the public information regarding nostrums, quacks, pseudomedicine and allied subjects."

For the convenience and ready reference of the profession many of the more important articles were originally published in THE JOURNAL in the "Pharmacology" and "Propaganda for Reform" departments. The book was originally issued in pamphlet form. There were nine editions of the first volume with the first eight of them appearing between 1907 and 1913. The ninth edition, now commonly referred to as Volume I, was issued in 1916, and the final book in this series, Volume II, came out in 1922. The "Propaganda for Reform in Proprietary Medicines" deals primarily with proprietary specialties advertised and sold to the medical profession. The so-called "patent medicines" advertised to the public are dealt with in another volume known as "Nostrums and Quackery."

COUNCIL SEAL

Special mention should also be made of the seal used by the Council. In 1929 the Council's committee on nonmedicinal foods proposed the use of an emblem to indicate acceptance of a product. In the same year the Council voted to adopt an insignia for all Council accepted products. In an editorial entitled "The Council on Pharmacy and Chemistry: A Twenty-Fifth Anniversary" (J.A.M.A., Feb. 8, 1930) The Journal of the American Medical Association called attention to the seal:

"This year the Council on Pharmacy and Chemistry has determined to make available to manufacturers whose products are accepted a

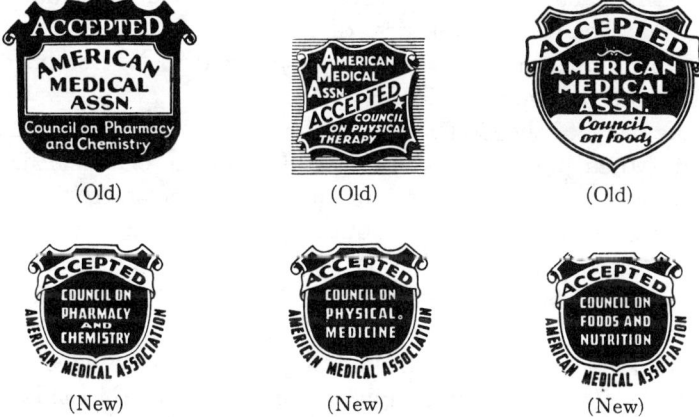

distinctive seal with which they may mark their products and their advertising, so that the purchaser may see at a glance that the product concerned has met the standards of science established by the Council. Manufacturers have welcomed this new step as an added advantage in promoting their preparations to physicians who wish to follow the Council's leadership."

The Journal of February 8, 1930, also contains an editorial discussion of the first acceptance by the Committee on Foods in which the following statement appears:

"Manufacturers have greeted with acclaim the permission to use on packages and in advertising the seal of the committee, reproduced herewith. It is reasonable to believe that both the medical profession and the public will cooperate by urging the manufacturers of food products to submit their material to the committee and to use the seal of the committee, so as to enable intelligent choice of foods by the public."

In 1946 the style of the seal was changed and made to conform to a new common pattern for the Councils on Pharmacy and Chemistry, Foods and Nutrition, and Physical Medicine.

The change in pattern permitted more emphasis on the name of the Council and conveyed to the observer a thought concerning the common purpose of the three Councils in their evaluating activities.

CHEMICAL LABORATORY

The early chemical examination of products submitted to the Council on Pharmacy and Chemistry was provided for by the Bureau of Chemistry, as explained elsewhere in this chapter. However, the Council, realizing the need for its own laboratory, suggested a central chemical laboratory in a report to the Board of Trustees in 1905. Laboratory space was provided soon and Prof. W. A. Puckner became the first director of the A.M.A. Chemical Laboratory. Subsequently the directors were Paul N. Leech, Ph.D. and Albert E. Sidwell, Jr., Ph.D.

As the work of the Council grew, the work of the Laboratory increased. Much pioneering was undertaken in the chemical field as the work of the Laboratory was unique—it was not merely a search for declared chemical substances but frequently an exhaustive search for undeclared, in fact, often carefully hidden, substances. Old technics had to be improved, new ones developed. As a result, the Laboratory was one of the foremost centers to recognize the value of and to make practical in the United States microanalytical examination and spectrographic determination of drugs. In 1924 the Laboratory was enlarged and established on the fifth floor of the headquarters building. An "air conditioned" room for microchemical work was installed in 1936, at which time equipment for spectrochemical analysis was also provided. Today the Laboratory can be regarded with pride as a well equipped, up-to-date "drug detective department" and as a leader in the setting of tests and standards, many of which are subsequently adopted in official compendia. Its staff is well trained and, of course, organized to meet practically any chemical problem relating to the determination and control of drugs, although it is faced as always with the need for enlarged quarters. The Laboratory is one of the oldest units at the headquarters of the American Medical Association and its usefulness has steadily increased as it gained experience and as it extended its contacts to other groups with mutual problems. It has been of particular help, in addition to the Council, to the Bureau of Investigation and to the Editorial Department. But its services have not been confined to these offices.

DIVISION OF THERAPY AND RESEARCH

And finally, a word about the Division of Therapy and Research is in order. In 1936 the Division of Drugs, Foods and Physical Therapy was established for purposes of administration. It consisted of the Councils on Pharmacy and Chemistry, Foods and Nutrition, and Physical Medicine and the Chemical Laboratory. In 1946 the name of the Division was changed to Division of Therapy and Research and the Bureau of Investigation was included in the group. The Secretary of the Council on Pharmacy and Chemistry was also appointed Director of the Division.

SUMMARY AND CONCLUSIONS

Until a few years ago, the work of the Council on Pharmacy and Chemistry, which was established in 1905, consisted essentially of evaluating drug products, preparing several books on the use of drugs, and answering inquiries from physicians. Of course, there were other activities such as the supplying of grants-in-aid for research, but the work of the Council seemed to revolve almost entirely around New and Nonofficial Remedies.

During the past few years the work has been expanded, new activities added and the older efforts re-directed so that the work can at this time be divided into: 1. Research; 2. Product Evaluation; 3. Education.

Thus, the Council promotes basic or fundamental research and research on the use of new products and technics; evaluates the laboratory and clinical evidence offered on behalf of products; and encourages the use of rational therapeutics, while discouraging the use of irrational preparations and technics. The latter is done in many ways, including the answering of inquiries, preparation of exhibits, and the preparation of status reports and books. The Council office now provides other help by, for example, making available professional men for lectures before lay and scientific groups, and to work with other A.M.A. offices and offices outside the A.M.A. on problems of mutual interest.

The Council promotes research by providing grants-in-aid, sponsoring the Therapeutic Trials Committee, and by working closely with other research agencies. It evaluates products by examining the proffered evidence, and that obtainable from other sources, and by subjecting the composition to close scrutiny in the Chemical Laboratory.

Included in newer work now being undertaken, and for which there is a pressing need, are the establishment of repositories on reactions to drugs, toxicity and identity of wetting agents, toxicity and identity of cosmetics, toxicity and identity of insecticides and rodenticides, and new chemicals developed for therapeutic investigation; closer relations with other agencies (within the U.S.A. and elsewhere) interested in problems of mutual interest; more exhibits and status reports; examination with a medical viewpoint of the laws regulating drugs, cosmetics, foods, insecticides, poisons, etc.; organization of therapeutic conferences; and encouragement and coordination of certain aspects of fundamental and applied research, including laboratory control and standardization.

THE COUNCIL ON MEDICAL EDUCATION AND HOSPITALS[1]

By Victor Johnson, M.D., Ph.D.

AT THE NEW ORLEANS MEETING of the American Medical Association in 1903, Arthur Dean Bevan, then chairman of the association's Committee on Medical Education, stated: "The American Medical Association was formed for the purpose of elevating standards of medical education in this country. . . . Your committee believe that this is still one of the important functions of the American Medical Association."[2] Dr. Bevan was referring to the wording of the original call of the Medical Society of the State of New York, which led to a preliminary national convention in 1846 and culminated in the organization of the American Medical Association in Philadelphia a year later. This call from New York commenced with this credo: "It is believed that a national convention would be conducive to the elevation of the standard of medical education in the United States." One of the first acts of the Philadelphia meeting was the establishment of a committee on education, which functioned for fifty-seven years before the formation of the Council on Medical Education, which continued and greatly expanded the pioneer work in education through the remainder of the first century of the Association's existence.

---

[1] Since this is a history of the Council rather than of medical education, emphasis is placed upon sources originating with the American Medical Association, while still recognizing that various other important influences have affected medical education. Excellent works on the state of medical education before the influence of the American Medical Association became markedly effective are the following: Davis, N. S.: Contributions to the History of Medical Education and Medical Institutions, Government Printing Office, Washington, D.C., 1877; Norwood, W. F.: Medical Education in the United States before the Civil War, University of Pennsylvania Press, Philadelphia, 1944; and Davis, N. S.: History of Medical Education and Institutions in the United States, S. C. Griggs and Co., Chicago, 1851. The latter volume is particularly enlightening regarding the educational motivation for the founding of the American Medical Association in 1847.

In the Appendix to this volume are to be found an alphabetical listing of all members of the Council since its origin with the dates of their service and also a list of important dates in the history of the Council.

[2] Bevan, A. D., Report of the Committee on Medical Education, J.A.M.A., $40{:}1372$ (May 16), 1903.

The first pronouncement of the Committee on Medical Education a hundred years ago read as follows:

> This Association considers defective and erroneous every system of medical instruction which does not rest on the basis of practical demonstration and clinical teaching; ... it is ... the duty of the medical schools to resort to every honorable means to obtain access for their students to the wards of a well regulated hospital.[3]

THE PIONEER YEARS

The lowly state of medical education at the middle of the last century is reflected in the frequent resolutions, discussions and recommendations dealing with the subject, usually as the principal topic, at the annual sessions of the Association. For example, about a decade after the Association was formed, the Committee on Medical Education recommended that "primary medical schools" should be encouraged. Yet the committee recognized that apprentice training would continue in volume for some time and urged physicians giving office instruction to provide for "demonstrations, illustrations and recitations," at the apprenticeship office, at a medical school or under a physician able to provide these "necessary advantages." It was recommended that professorships should number not less than seven, in the fields of anatomy and microscopy, physiology and pathology, chemistry, surgery, practical medicine, obstetrics and materia medica. It was considered desirable to lengthen the school term to six months, commencing in October and running until March. A "liberal primary education" was urged as an admission requirement, and it was recommended that there be "attendance upon a course of clinical instruction in a regularly organized hospital."[4]

In a pioneer country, with a rapidly increasing population and the continued westward migration, the demand for doctors, and therefore for medical schools, was great. There were virtually no legal restrictions on the establishment of medical schools. Many were decidedly inferior and were established primarily for the financial gain of the promotors and the faculty. The operation of a medical school was often a profitable enterprise and there was an intense competition for students. Besides the so-called medical schools and the apprentice training in physicians' offices, there arose "diploma mills" in all sections of the country. These sold diplomas with no pretense whatsoever of providing medical training of any kind.

The multiplication of medical schools was such that, by the end of

---

[3] Transactions of the American Medical Association, *1:*246 (1848).

[4] Report of the Committee on Medical Education. Transactions of the American Medical Association *11:*258 (1858).

the nineteenth century there were about as many medical schools in the United States as there were in all the rest of the world.

A few of these institutions were of good quality; even prior to 1800 there were four good colleges in operation which are still in existence: Pennsylvania (commencing as the "College of Philadelphia" in 1765), Columbia (first known as Kings College Medical Faculty, 1767), Harvard (in 1782) and Dartmouth (in 1797).

However, such exceptions were few and chaos was the rule. There was nothing resembling uniformity in the curriculum. Depending upon the interests of the professors, the time devoted to a given subject varied widely from school to school: anatomy, 200 to 1248 hours; bacteriology, 45 to 364 hours; pathology, 54 to 512 hours;

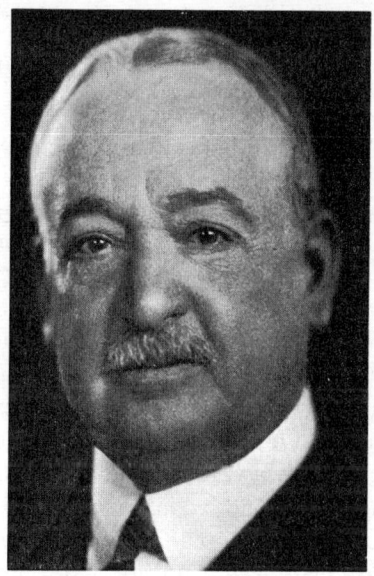

Dr. Arthur Dean Bevan
First Chairman, Council on Medical Education and Hospitals

surgery, 64 to 1168 hours; medicine, 140 to 1232 hours; and obstetrics, 67 to 320 hours. Admission requirements were usually non-existent. Often the ability even to read and write was not essential.[5]

Few annual meetings of the Association were held without discussions deploring conditions and resolutions aimed at their correction. The effects were limited. Simmons refers to the 1872 report of the Committee on Medical Education, which enumerated the evils of medical education and then regretted that

---

[5] Simmons, George H.: Medical Education and Preliminary Requirements, J.A.M.A. *42:*1205 (May 7) 1904.

"it seems much easier to show the defects in our present system than to advise a suitable and practical remedy."[6]

One reason given for this relative ineffectiveness was that the influence of medical college professors

> has always been so great in the Association as to prevent its doing what it should have done long ago, viz, establishing a national standard for medical teaching and demanding that the colleges shall accept it or not be recognized.[6]

There were those who would give up the struggle. After the first decade of hard work of the Committee on Medical Education resolutions were presented to the effect that:

> 1. The Association had not the power to control medical education. 2. The great objects of the Association were the advancement of medical science and the promotion of harmony in the profession. 3. The attempt on the part of the Association to regulate medical education had signally failed in its object and had introduced elements of discord, and . . . . any further interference on the subject would be useless and calculated to disturb the deliberations of the Association.[6]

Fortunately, such counsel did not prevail, and the struggle continued. Although the results did not seem great, and although

> Of all the resolutions adopted, and there were hundreds of them, not one can be regarded as resulting in any specific good. Of all the correspondence with, and appeals to, medical colleges, and there was an abundance of both, not a solitary bit of evidence is there of any practical compliance.[6]

Yet it cannot be concluded that nothing was accomplished by the American Medical Association and its allies, the American Academy of Medicine, the Association of American Medical Colleges and the state licensing boards. When the American Medical Association was established, colleges were awarding the M.D. degree for less than six months' attendance in addition to a period of apprenticeship. Such a degree admitted the holder to the practice of medicine in almost every state. There were no admission standards worthy of mention. Sixty years later, a four years' course of at least six months each was required for the degree. In almost every state, this degree admitted the graduate not the right to practice medicine, but to a licensure examination. A goodly number of schools exacted a high school diploma for admission and a few required two years of college.

The intangible effects of the repeated discussions and resolutions are hard to assess. Besides the modest tangible improvements in the medical course, public opinion was being molded, forces aimed at improvement were being mobilized and the stage was prepared for the revolutionary changes of the first two decades of the twentieth century.

---

[6] Quoted by Simmons, George H.: What the American Medical Association Stands For, J.A.M.A. *21*:1733 (Nov. 23) 1907.

CREATION OF THE COUNCIL ON MEDICAL EDUCATION

The early years of the present century saw changes in the American Medical Association and its work in medical education, of far-reaching consequence. Largely through the efforts of Dr. George H. Simmons, then Editor of the Journal of the American Medical Association, the basic structure of the Association was placed on a firm foundation at the turn of the century by the establishment and organization of the Association as a nation-wide representative body with a house of delegates meeting annually and a board of trustees and executive officers to carry out the policies and directives established by the house of delegates. This reorganization, in which the Association assumed essentially the organic structure we know today, was almost at once reflected in an important change in the Association's work in the field of medical education.

A year after the reorganization of the Association, in 1902, the president, Dr. John A. Wyeth, appointed the following committee to survey the problem of medical education in this country and make recommendations concerning the role which the American Medical Association should play in the improvement of medical education: Arthur Dean Bevan, Chicago, Chairman; C. A. Daugherty, South Bend, Ind.; R. A. Marmion, United States Navy, Washington; Rudolph Matas, New Orleans; and Floyd W. McRea, Atlanta. Two years later this committee reported as follows:[7]

> The American Medical Association was founded for the special purpose of obtaining a uniform and elevated standard of requirements for the degree of M.D.
> The American Medical Association has so far accomplished little toward this end. The existing standards are not satisfactory as compared to those of the other great powers.
> Our form of government makes it impossible, or improbable at least, to obtain national governmental control of medical education.
> In absence of national governmental control efforts to make uniform and elevated the standard of medical education can be made most effective through the agency of the organized medical profession of the entire country, and such a body we now have in the reorganized American Medical Association.
> The problem of using to the best purpose the weight and influence of the American Medical Association toward elevating medical education is a very large one and one which must be carefully worked out. This can best be done by a permanent committee. or council specially created for this purpose.
> We recommend the creation of such a council by the following addition to the By-laws, to be Chapter VI, Section 8.
> CHAPTER VI, Section 8.—The Council of Education shall consist of five members, to be appointed by the president and confirmed by the House of Delegates.
> Immediately after the adoption of this by-law, one member shall be appointed to serve for one year, one for two years, one for three years, one for four years and one for five years. Thereafter one member shall be appointed each year to serve for five years.
> The council shall organize, elect a chairman and secretary and shall adopt such

---

[7] Report of Committee on Medical Education to House of Delegates of the American Medical Association. J.A.M.A. *42:*1576 (June 11) 1904.

regulations for the government of its actions as it deems expedient. It shall expend money or contract financial obligations only as shall be authorized in writing by the Board of Trustees.

The functions of the Council on Medical Education shall be:

1. To make an annual report to the House of Delegates on the existing conditions of medical education in the United States.

2. To make suggestions as to the means and methods by which the American Medical Association may best influence favorably medical education.

3. To act as the agent of the American Medical Association (under instructions from the House of Delegates) in its efforts to elevate medical education.

The passage of this recommendation by the house of delegates conferred authority upon those entrusted with the responsibility for improving medical education and insured the desirable continuity in the work, by creating the permanent Council on Medical Education. The first council consisted of the following:

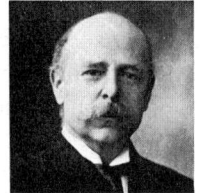
Dr. W. T. Councilman

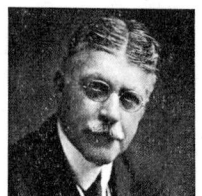
Dr. Charles H. Frazier

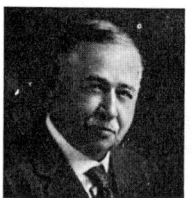
Dr. Victor C. Vaughan

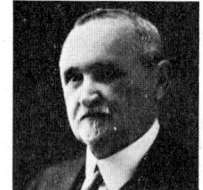
Dr. J. A. Witherspoon

The original Council on Medical Education, appointed in 1904.
The chairman was Dr. Arthur Dean Bevan.

Arthur Dean Bevan, Professor of Surgery, Rush Medical College (University of Chicago), Chairman; W. T. Councilman, Professor of Pathology, Medical School of Harvard University; Charles H. Frazier, Professor of Surgery, University of Pennsylvania School of Medicine; Victor C. Vaughan, dean, University of Michigan Medical School; J. A. Witherspoon, Professor of Medicine, Vanderbilt University.

The responsibilities placed on this new body were tremendous. Among the multitude of difficulties confronting it was that of financial support. When the Council was formed, the Board of Trustees found themselves unable to appropriate $5,000 for the work of the first year.[8] Today the annual budget of the Council for departmental printing alone exceeds this sum.

In the early years of the century immediately prior to the establishment of the Council, the intensified interest in medical education by the association was reflected in the initiation of new activities by the Committee on Medical Education. The first Educational Number of the Journal of the American Medical Association appeared,[9] and by the time the first Council was formed, medical school reports, including names of graduates, were being collected, and a file of medical school graduates was begun. The establishment of these records, culminating in the American Medical Directory, has been of enormous importance in the evolution of improved medical education and medical practice. In the field of licensure a department on "State Boards of Registration" was established and licensure laws, board rulings and reports were assembled and published.

The leading spirit in the resurgence of interest in medical education was the indomitable Arthur Dean Bevan, first chairman of the first Council, who continued in that capacity through 23 years, during which period medical education in the United States was transformed almost beyond recognition. In this work, the contributions of the first secretary of the Council, Dr. N. P. Colwell, were tremendous. Dr. Colwell commenced work with the American Medical Association in 1904 and became secretary in 1905. He personally participated in the early surveys, and visited every school with Dr. Abraham Flexner. He provided far more guidance in this famous survey than is generally known, and in every phase of the work of the Council for twenty-six years, the hand of Dr. Colwell is prominently in evidence.

MEDICAL EDUCATION IN 1905

In the first year of its life, the Council took stock of the status of medical education in this country, and made this the topic for discussion at its first conference on medical education in 1905.[10] The scene was not one to inspire satisfaction. By comparison with England, Germany and France, medical education in this country was decidedly inferior. Of the more than 160 medical schools in the

---

[8] Bevan, A. D., Cooperation in Medical Education and Medical Service, J.A.M.A. *90:*1173 (April 14) 1928. This paper was read at the twenty-fourth Annual Congress on Medical Education by Arthur Dean Bevan upon the occasion of his retirement as chairman of the Council. It is an excellent summary of the history of the Council to that time and is employed freely as source material for this chapter.

[9] Educational Number, J.A.M.A., *37:*744 (Sept. 21) 1901.

[10] First Annual Conference on Medical Education, J.A.M.A., *44:*1470 (May 6) 1905.

country at that time, many admitted students without a complete high school education, and there were only five requiring two or more years of college premedical work. Johns Hopkins had been the first school to establish this requirement twelve years earlier. The other schools with this requirement in effect were Harvard (since 1900), Western Reserve (since 1901), Rush-Chicago (since 1904) and the University of California (in 1905). Throughout the country, with far too few exceptions, academic standards were low, facilities and faculties were inadequate, financial support was lacking, students were poorly prepared, and failures in licensing examinations were many. One of the earliest of the criteria used in evaluating schools was the failure statistics in state board examinations, which had been published since 1902. In certain areas of the country conditions were especially bad. With characteristic vigor Bevan stated,

> It is evident from a study of the medical schools of this country and their work that there are five especially rotten spots which are responsible for most of the bad medical instruction. They are: Illinois with fifteen schools, Missouri with fourteen..., Maryland with eight..., Kentucky with seven... and Tennessee with ten.... That is, fifty-four medical schools in these five states and not more than six of these can be considered acceptable.[8]

These fifty-four schools in the five states mentioned have now been reduced in number to twelve approved four year institutions.

EARLY COUNCIL STANDARDS AND CLASSIFICATION

Employing the better schools of England, Germany and France as a yardstick, in 1905 the Council adopted as an "ideal standard" for the medical schools of this country, the recommendation that medical schools here ought eventually to require:

Preliminary education sufficient to enable the candidate to enter our recognized universities. A five-year medical course; the first year devoted to physics, chemistry and biology; the next two years to laboratory sciences of anatomy, physiology, pathology and pharmacology, and two years to the clinical branches, with close contact with patients in both dispensary and hospital. A sixth year as an intern in the hospital.[11]

This ideal now seems conservative, but in its day it was revolutionary. Its objective was to elevate medical education from the existing trade-school philosophy and practice to a true university level. Not only was it deemed desirable that a medical school should

---

[11] Report of Council on Medical Education to House of Delegates of American Medical Association. J.A.M.A., *45*:269 (July 22) 1905.

be part of an established university, but it was also felt that the year of physics, chemistry and biology preliminary to the medical studies proper should be taught in the scientific departments of universities rather than in the medical school. Two years of such work were thought to be preferable to one, to include also work in English and electives and the acquisition of a reading knowledge of French or German.

Although the first Council was determined that the goal defined in this "ideal standard," must be reached it wisely realized that this would have to be achieved gradually, and that an attempt to set standards too much higher than those in effect might well defeat the desired ends. Therefore, the Council advocated certain minimum requirements to be adopted at once as a temporary standard of acceptability. In the light of present-day requirements, they seem modest. In 1905, they represented a marked advance. The requirements were merely four years of high school for admission, a four-year medical course and satisfactory performance in a state licensing examination.

Performance of medical school graduates in the state licensure examinations as published in The Journal[12] was immediately recognized as a tangible and reasonably objective criterion of medical school performance. Consequently the Council published tables[13] in which the medical schools were placed into four classes based on the percentage of licensure examination failure:

Class 1, with less than 10 per cent of failures.
Class 2, with 10 to 20 per cent of failures.
Class 3, with more than 20 per cent of failures.
Class 4, unclassified colleges in which there were less than ten graduates or most of whose graduates were licensed by their own home state board or in which the evidence was insufficient to permit conclusions.

The publication of these tables was a stimulus to medical schools to improve themselves. However, the limitations of employing only the standard of licensure examination performance were fully appreciated and it became clear that a better evaluation of the schools necessitated inspections of the medical schools by Council representatives. The plans of the campaign were carefully drawn. A rating system was evolved to enable the Council to assign a grade to each school. Ten categories of qualifications were listed as a basis for the ratings, with each school to be graded in each category:

---

[12] State Board Examinations during 1904. J.A.M.A. *44:*1477 (May 6) 1905.
[13] State Board Statistics for 1907. J.A.M.A. *50:*1845 (May 30) 1908.

1. Showing of graduates before state boards.
2. Requirements of preliminary education and its enforcement.
3. Character of medical curriculum.
4. Medical school plant.
5. Laboratory facilities and instruction.
6. Dispensary facilities and instruction.
7. Hospital facilities and instruction. (These last three necessarily included the men giving this instruction.)
8. Extent to which the first two years are officered by men devoting entire time to teaching and also evidence of original research.
9. Extent to which the school is conducted for the profit of the faculty directly or indirectly, rather than for the teaching of medicine.
10. Libraries, museum, charts and teaching equipment.

It was determined that the medical school would be classified into three groups:[14]

Class A, those marked above 70, the acceptable class.

Class B, those marked from 50 to 70, the doubtful class.

Class C, those marked below 50, the nonacceptable.

Regarding the tremendous task of inspecting and classifying the schools we have the following understatement by Doctor Bevan:

> The country was divided into sections, and each one of the 160 or more schools was visited by some member of the Council or by the secretary, Dr. Colwell; in most instances by both the secretary and some member of the Council.[8]

The manner in which inspection problems were met, difficulties overcome and results achieved are well illustrated in the following:

> When we began our first inspection there were seven medical colleges in Louisville, Ky. I received a letter from one of my good friends in Louisville one day, telling me not to come to Louisville because all the medical schools had agreed not to allow themselves to be inspected by the Council. I wired at once that Dr. Colwell and I were leaving for Louisville that night and desired to inspect the schools the next day. With true Southern hospitality they received us and gave us every opportunity to inspect their schools. They gave us a luncheon at the Pendennis Club. We discussed the subject of consolidating all the medical schools of Louisville into one strong school, which might then secure the united support of the medical profession and the citizens of Louisville and secure the use of the Louisville Hospital as a hospital for teaching and research; this was finally agreed to and finally carried into effect, so that today Louisville has a single school much stronger than any of its predecessors and enjoys the benefit of excellent clinical material. The same story was repeated in many cities of the country.[8]

The inspections were begun in 1906 and the first classification was presented by the Chairman of the Council at the third annual congress in the following year.[15] Although "the Council was very lenient in its markings",[8] the 160 schools were placed in the following

---

[14] Although the A, B, C classification is no longer employed as such, these classes approximate the current designations for medical schools: Class A corresponds to the fully approved category; class B, to the approved schools on probation; class C, the unacceptable medical schools, which are no longer listed by the Council.

[15] Third Annual Congress on Medical Education. J.A.M.A., *48:*1701 (May 18) 1907.

groups: 82 in class A (above 70 per cent), 46 in class B (50 to 70 per cent) and 32 in class C (below 50 per cent and unacceptable).

In addition to this presentation to the third annual congress on medical education, the classfiication was presented by the Council to the American Medical Association in 1907. "That classification was not published, but each college was notified of the rating given to it."[16]

Even though this report was not published, the effect of its distribution to the colleges was profound. Dr. Bevan states:

> As a result of the report of this first inspection a great wave of improvement in medical education swept over the country. Fifty schools agreed to require by 1910, or before, at least one year of university physics, chemistry and biology and one modern language as a preliminary education before matriculating in medicine. Immediately a number of consolidations were arranged in many cities having several schools. A number of schools, as the result of state boards refusing examinations to their graduates, went out of business and it became evident that the 160 schools would be reduced within a short time to probably less than a hundred.[8]

Twenty homeopathic schools and ten eclectic schools were included in the survey and their work assessed in the same manner as that of the regular medical schools.

> It early became apparent that as soon as the one year, and then the two year university requirement of physics, chemistry and biology was generally adopted, homeopathy and eclecticism would die for the lack of students, and this proved to be the case. ... Today there is practically no strictly homeopathic school in this country. The one or two which have survived teach scientific medicine. The one remaining eclectic school is struggling to reorganize on a better basis.[8]

The latter school has since gone out of existence.

COOPERATIVE STUDIES WITH THE CARNEGIE FOUNDATION

Considerable resentment developed in the medical colleges from these reports, and

> it occurred to some of the members of the Council that, if we could obtain the publication and approval of our work by the Carnegie Foundation for the Advancement of Teaching, it would assist materially in securing the results we were attempting to bring about.[8]

This idea dominated the deliberations of the Council on Medical Education at its New York meeting in December of 1908. Excerpts from the minutes of that meeting read as follows:

> At one o'clock an informal conference was held with President Pritchett and Mr. Abraham Flexner of the Carnegie Foundation. Mr. Pritchett had already expressed, by correspondence, the willingness of the Foundation to cooperate with the Council in investigating the medical schools. He now explained that the Foundation was to investigate all the professions, law, medicine and theology. He had found no efforts being made by law to better the conditions in legal education and had met with some slight opposition in the efforts he was making. He had then received the letters from the Council on Medical

---

[16] Colwell, N. P.: Progress in Medical Education, in the Report of the Commissioner of Education, Bureau of Education, Department of the Interior, Chap. III, Vol. 1, 1913.

Education and expressed himself as most agreeably surprised not only at the efforts being made to correct conditions surrounding medical education but at the enormous amount of important data collected.

He agreed with the opinion previously expressed by the members of the Council that while the Foundation would be guided very largely by the Council's investigation, to avoid the usual claims of partiality no more mention should be made in the report of the Council than any other source of information. The report would therefore be, and have the weight of an independent report of a disinterested body, which would then be published far and wide. It would do much to develop public opinion.

It was considered wise to withhold publication of the list of satisfactory colleges until the Carnegie report comes out . . . (so that) . . . that report would make the Council's report at a later date more effective.

The Carnegie study was begun in 1908 by Drs. Abraham Flexner for the Carnegie Foundation and N. P. Colwell of the Council and their results were published two years later in what is commonly known as "The Flexner Report."[17] The Association was greatly strengthened in its struggle to improve medical education by this report from a neutral educational foundation of high standing. The report criticized medical education in this country even more severely than had the reports of the Council. It advocated reforms previously urged by the Council, including

the development of our medical schools as organic departments of our universities, the dictum that the proprietary school had no longer a right to exist, the necessity of university training in physics, chemistry and biology and modern languages before beginning the medical course, the necessity of having the laboratory sciences of anatomy, physiology, pathology and pharmacology taught by full-time men, the necessity of a teaching hospital and dispensary for the teaching of the clinical subjects, the importance of bedside instruction . . .

These intensive efforts were reflected in the ensuing decade in a considerable reduction in the number of medical schools, effected by the closure of very bad schools and the merger of other schools into institutions much stronger than the component parts. As compared with the 160 schools in 1905, the number was reduced to 95 in the following ten years, to 85 by 1920, and 80 by 1927. The accompanying table shows the classification of these schools.

Number of Medical Schools, 1905–1927

	1905	1915	1920	1927
Class A Schools (Approved)	82	66	70	62
Class B Schools (Probation)	46	17	7	3
Class C Schools (Unapproved)	32	12	8	6
Class A Schools of Basic Medical Sciences	. .	. .	. .	9
Total	160	95	85	80

[17] Flexner, Abraham. Medical Education in the United States and Canada, D. B. Updyke, Merrymount Press, Boston, 1910.

These results are amazing, when it is recalled that the Council had no legal powers, but had to depend upon results through the establishment of confidence in its findings on the part of government bodies (chiefly the licensing agencies), the better schools, the profession and the public at large. This confidence was established because of the fairness of the Council's studies, the objectivity and disinterestedness of its approach, and the staunch support of the licensing boards, the Carnegie Foundation and the Association of American Medical Colleges.

The important role of the Journal in establishing the wide influence of the Council cannot be over-emphasized. It was largely through Journal publications of state licensure examination statistics in the early years of the century that a demand was created for a thorough overhauling of medical education. Subsequently, the wide dissemination of the Council's findings, classifications, policies and recommendations in Journal publications were of inestimable value in making the Council's work an effective influence in the improvement of medical education.

CERTIFICATION OF HOSPITALS FOR INTERNSHIPS

The importance of hospital work by medical students was recognized from the very beginning of the American Medical Association a hundred years ago.[3] The necessity for a period of hospital internship training between medical school graduation and the licensure examination was suggested under the "ideal standard" of medical education adopted by the House of Delegates when the Council was formed. A realization of its value gained new impetus in the critical second decade of this century. In 1913 no medical school or state examining board required the internship for the M.D. degree or for licensure. Pennsylvania was the first state to require the internship for licensure (1914) and the University of Minnesota was the first school to require such training for the M.D. degree a year later. However, the value of the internship was widely recognized by students, physicians and medical schools. Before these first requirements were instituted, 70 per cent of the graduates elected to take internships voluntarily. Recognizing the need for improved standards at this level of medical education, the Council undertook its first survey (not always by actual inspections) of hospitals engaged in the training of interns in 1912 and two years later published the first list of approved internship hospitals. This list[18] designated 603 hospitals as suitable for the instruction of young graduates in the

[18] Provisional List of Hospitals Furnishing Acceptable Internships for Medical Graduates, a publication of the Council, 1914.

clinical branches of medicine and surgery. It included 508 general hospitals offering 2,667 internships and 95 special hospitals offering training to 428 graduates. This may be compared with 798 approved internship hospitals in 1946, offering a total of 8,584 internship positions.[19]

The internship as a formal requirement was adopted to an increasing degree following the first actions of the State of Pennsylvania and the University of Minnesota. For a time both medical schools and licensing bodies exacted this requirement in increasing numbers, so that by 1936 there were 15 medical schools and 19 states requiring an internship. Subsequently there was a reassessment of the relationship of the internship to the medical schools and to the licensing authorities. Medical schools began to be dissatisfied with the internship as a degree requirement, while still recognizing it as an essential in the education of a physician. Medical schools felt that there was little justification for requiring work in an institution not under the

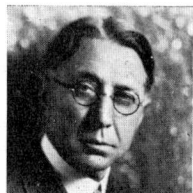　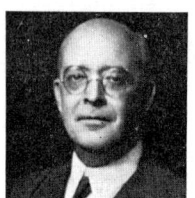

Dr. N. P. Colwell　　Dr. William D. Cutter

The first two secretaries of the Council. Dr. Colwell served from 1905 to 1931. Dr. Cutter was secretary from 1931 to 1942.

control of the university, and often located at a great distance, in partial fulfillment of requirements for the M.D., a university or medical school degree. There followed a period in which this requirement was abandoned by medical schools, so that today[19] there are only six such schools. Perhaps the current trend toward greater influence of medical schools upon the educational programs of affiliated and nearby hospitals may reverse this trend. Should this occur, it is probable that the quality of the internship will improve.

On the other hand, state licensing boards increasingly recognized that the internship is an experience indispensable for the best practice of medicine. The requirement of the internship for licensure continued to be demanded by more and more licensing boards throughout the years even after the decline in numbers of medical schools requiring such work. There are now 28 medical examining

---

[19] Johnson, Victor, Arestad, F. H., and Tipner, Anne, Medical Education in the United States and Canada, 1945–1946, J.A.M.A., *131:*1277–1354 (Aug. 17) 1946.

boards in the various states and the territories and possessions of the United States which require the applicant to complete an internship in an acceptable hospital.

Since 1928 the Council has maintained a staff of trained hospital inspectors who devote their entire time to improving educational standards in hospitals. These inspectors not only collect factual data necessary for evaluating educational services, but they interpret the standards of the Council to the hospital and confer with staffs and intern committees regarding ways and means of correcting deficiencies and fully employing every educational asset of the institution. This consultation service is one of the more important of the Association's many activities designed to promote the welfare of the sick by advancing the standards of medical education and hospital care. The service operates without cost to any hospital in the United States.

CONSOLIDATION OF GAINS

The "farewell address" of Arthur Dean Bevan in 1928,[8] upon his retirement from the Council, marked the end of an historic era of revolutionary improvement in medical education, following the pioneer decades before the Council was established. Tremendous changes for the better were effected during his chairmanship, in which the splendid work of the first secretary of the Council, N. P. Colwell, was always to be seen in the background. In the two decades following the Bevan-Colwell period, the leadership of the Council was continued by an equally great statesman of medical education, Dr. Ray Lyman Wilbur. The Wilbur era was one in which the great gains of the previous two decades were consolidated, medical education was further strengthened and improved, graduate medical education was vastly increased in volume and quality, the responsibilities and services of the Council greatly expanded, the "Weiskotten" survey was conducted and the trying problems of the war years were met.

When the results of the Council's early surveys began to take effect, and the number of medical schools decreased, considerable anxiety and even alarm were expressed in certain quarters. There was anxiety lest the diminution in numbers of schools would result in far fewer physicians being graduated and consequently an increasing dearth of physicians in the United States. This was probably the major concern expressed and came in some instances from people having no interest in the perpetuation of low standards in medical schools. They were undoubtedly sincere in their concern. Subsequent events seemed to provide a certain justification for this fear; however, the reduction in number of graduates proved to be of only a temporary nature. In the year 1905, when there were 160 medical schools, the graduates numbered 5,606. The year 1922 saw the low point in numbers of graduates. At that time there were 81 schools, approximately half the number operating seventeen years earlier, and there were 2,529 graduates—again about half the numbers graduating in 1905. Had this condition persisted there would undoubtedly have resulted a tremendous deficiency in physicians throughout the country since considerably more than 2,500 physicians die every year.

But this low graduation rate did not persist. In the twenty years from 1922 until 1942 the number of medical schools was still further decreased to 77. Yet the number of graduates gradually increased so that the number graduating in 1944 (5,163) was about double the number graduating in 1922 and approximated the number graduating from the 160 schools in 1905. In some instances the increased number of graduates from certain schools have not been justified by the equipment, facilities and faculties of the medical schools. On the whole, however, it is probable that much of this increase has been justifiable, since schools rather generally were strengthened financially and otherwise throughout the past two decades to an extent which warranted a larger student body and more graduates. Funds available to the schools have increased, faculties have been expanded and laboratory and clinical facilities increased. This development has fully justified the decrease in numbers of medical schools and all the efforts that were expended to eliminate the poorer schools. We now have about as many graduates from superior institutions as were produced forty years ago, many from decidedly inferior institutions.

Another fear which was expressed was that the increase in admission requirements and the lengthening of the medical school curriculum would make medical education unduly expensive and would tend to eliminate students from low income families from the study and practice of medicine. These fears also have been somewhat allayed since there are still many students today who earn much of their expenses while attending medical school. However it is fully admitted that this is now much more difficult than it may have been years ago. Yet there can be no compromise in facing the basic issue. Should medical education be organized so that even the poorest of students financially can carry out the course without regard to the quality of the education, or should the educational program be of high caliber even though it may eliminate certain qualified students from the profession? Put in this way there can be only one answer. The quality of medical education had to be increased to provide a higher type of medical care for the people of the country. The problem of financing students in their medical education is an independent one. However serious this problem is and however much still remains to be done in meeting the problem it should never be a factor in justifying an inferior type of medical education.

Medical education is never cheap either in terms of costs to the student, to the institution or to the state supplying the funds. Events have amply demonstrated that the reduction in number of schools and the increased expenditures for medical education have tremendously increased the quality of medical care in this country.

GRADUATE MEDICAL EDUCATION

In the first two decades of this century the work of the Council was properly concerned primarily with the improvement of undergraduate medical education. The ensuing two decades saw greater

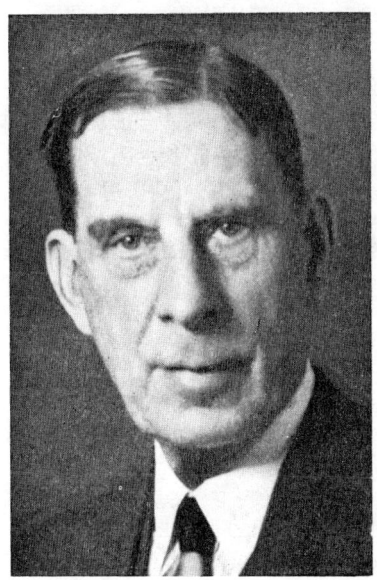

Dr. Ray Lyman Wilbur
Second Chairman, Council on Medical Education and Hospitals

emphasis placed upon an elevated quality of graduate medical education. There was a growing conviction that, in medicine, the learning process must continue throughout life. Dr. Ray Lyman Wilbur put this axiom aptly when he said, "The doctor who stops learning goes backward . . ." The rapidity with which change occurs and advances are made in medicine, make it imperative that the physician keep abreast of progress in medical research and progress, or he will rapidly become a poorer physician than he was at the time of his graduation. According to Wilbur:[20]

> Medicine is so avid for advance, so eager for new ways that are better to help the ailing or to stop suffering and pain, that those who practice it must be alert to research, must confer with their fellow physicians through societies and literature, and from time to time travel to see what others are doing or take up special studies or courses. Beyond the period of medical school training leading to the degree of Doctor of Medicine come years of graduate study if one is to perfect oneself for general practice or to become a specialist.
>
> These graduate years may come in the form of internships or residencies immediately following the course in medicine, or they may come later for a few months or years in sequence or on separate occasions.

Important beginnings were made in the field of education beyond the undergraduate medical school period with the survey of internship hospitals culminating in the first listing of approved internship hospitals in 1914,[18] and the survey of graduate schools and graduate education conducted in 1913–1915 under Council auspices. This survey, and a later one in 1919, revealed the existing facilities for advanced training were entirely inadequate, the demand for a high quality of training by physicians was not being met, proprietary schools and "postgraduate" schools of doubtful character were too plentiful, and there was lack of widespread interest in this field of education on the part of medical schools.

It became apparent from these studies that physicians seeking graduate medical studies fell into two distinct groups. In the words of Wilbur:[20]

> In 1919 there were two large groups of physicians seeking graduate study: those desiring continuation study for short periods and those desiring to fit themselves for special practice, the latter requiring a longer and more exacting preparation. It was estimated that 6,000 practicing physicians engaged in the short term study in 1919. Four thousand other graduate students were spending longer periods preparing themselves in special fields: a total of 10,000 medical graduates engaged in continuing their education.

Regarding the latter group, seeking to prepare themselves for practice in the specialties of medicine, the Council sought to provide the public and the profession protection against short cuts to specialty practice. Especially in surgery, abbreviated courses in special fields were condemned.

In 1920, by which time only one of the American Boards was functioning, in ophthalmology, the Council organized committees "to recommend what preparation was deemed essential to secure expertness in each of the specialties. . . ."[20] Fifteen committees of nine members each were appointed in the following special fields of

---

[20] Wilbur, Ray Lyman, Progress in Graduate Medical Education, J.A.M.A., *114:*1141 (Mar. 30) 1940.

medicine: internal medicine, pediatrics, neuropsychiatry, dermatology and syphilology, surgery, ophthalmology, otolaryngology, orthopedic surgery, urology and obstetrics and gynecology. There were also committees appointed in public health and hygiene, and, in the basic medical sciences, anatomy, pharmacology and therapeutics, physiology and pathology-bacteriology. It is significant to note that the ten clinical fields in the first of these groups became represented by American Boards by 1937, as was true also in the field of pathology. By 1940, four additional boards were organized in the fields of radiology, plastic surgery, anesthesiology and neurological surgery to complete the roster of fifteen American Boards operating today.

Thus the organization of these committees by the Council in 1920 set the pattern for the establishment of the specialty boards in the various fields of medicine and the committees were essentially the forerunners of the present American Boards. The recommendations of the committees regarding the minimum time for special training varied considerably, from one and one-half to three years, as contrasted with the usual board requirements at present, of three years of acceptable training beyond the internship, plus an additional two years of practice and/or training in the specialty. By 1923 standards had been adopted by the House of Delegates applying to specialty training, as regards admission requirements, supervision of the educational program, the qualifications of instructors, the necessary hospital, dispensary, laboratory, library and museum facilities, and the nature of the instruction, which was to include

(a) review courses in anatomy, pathology and the other basic preclinical sciences which apply to the respective specialties; (b) clinics in which students can have the opportunity personally to examine patients in hospital wards and outpatient departments and in which various therapeutic and operative procedures can be demonstrated; (c) courses of operative and laboratory technic, and (d)—to be assigned only when the student's previous training will warrant—assistantships in which, under the supervision of a physician who is recognized as an expert in the particular specialty, he can gradually assume responsibility in the diagnosis and therapeutic or operative treatment of the sick. Opportunity should be provided also for research work in the chosen specialty bearing on both the fundamental sciences and clinical fields.[21]

These standards have since been elaborated and redefined and are today incorporated into the documents of the Council, approved by the House of Delegates of the American Medical Association under the titles, "Essentials For Approved Examining Boards in Specialties" and "Essentials of Approved Residencies and Fellowships."

---

[21] Proceedings of the House of Delegates of the American Medical Association. J.A.M.A., *80:*1937 (June 30) 1923.

At the time of publication of the first list of approved internships, there were included 95 hospitals offering training in some specialized field of medicine.[18] It was in 1927 that the Council first listed hospitals specifically approved by it for residencies in the various medical specialties. That list contained the names of 270 hospitals providing 1,699 residencies.[22] This number may be compared with the most recent listing[19] which includes 887 hospitals offering 8,930 residency places.

The interest of the Council in elevating the standards of hospital education for the practice of the various specialties of medicine parallels the establishment and development of the American boards in these fields. The American boards have been organized by recognized leaders and national groups in the various specialties of medicine.

The American Board of Ophthalmology, the first of the examining boards in the specialties, was incorporated in 1917. Four additional boards were organized by 1933 (Otolaryngology in 1924, Obstetrics and Gynecology in 1930, Dermatology and Syphilology in 1932 and Pediatrics in 1933).[23]

In 1933 the House of Delegates of the American Medical Association adopted a resolution authorizing the Council on Medical Education and Hospitals "to express its approval of such special examining boards as conform to the standards of administration formulated by the Council" and providing for the employment of "the machinery of the American Medical Association, including the publication of its Directory, in furthering the work of such examining boards as may be accredited by the Council."

In 1933–34 the Advisory Board for Medical Specialties was organized with representation from each of the approved boards, to "act in an advisory capacity to such organizations as may seek its advice concerning the coordination of the education and certification of medical specialists."[24] The Council on Medical Education and Hospitals and the Advisory Board for Medical Specialties work in close collaboration through joint meetings and frequent conferences.

An American Board in a specialty is organized to assist in improving the quality of graduate education in that field, to establish minimum educational and training standards in the specialty, to

---

[22] Hospital Service in the United States, 1926. J.A.M.A., *88*:892 (Mar. 12) 1927.

[23] At this time the Council was itself publishing lists of competent specialists in Clinical Pathology and in Radiology. Such listings were discontinued when American boards in these fields were established.

[24] Constitution, Advisory Board for Medical Specialties.

determine whether candidates have received adequate preparation as defined by the Board, to provide comprehensive examinations to determine the ability and fitness of such candidates, and to certify to the competence of those physicians who have satisfied the requirements of the board, as a protection to the public and the profession.

The following branches of medicine at present are recognized as suitable fields for the certification of specialists. In each case, the symbol employed in designating specialists in the Directory of the American Medical Association is given (A.B.I., etc.). Certain of the boards also certify candidates in subspecialties, as indicated by footnotes:

	Name of Board	Year of Incorporation
A.B. 1.	American Board of Pediatrics[a]	1933
A.B. 2.	American Board of Psychiatry and Neurology	1934
A.B. 3.	American Board of Orthopaedic Surgery	1934
A.B. 4.	American Board of Dermatology and Syphilology	1932
A.B. 5.	American Board of Radiology	1934
A.B. 6.	American Board of Urology	1935
A.B. 7.	American Board of Obstetrics and Gynecology	1930
A.B. 8.	American Board of Internal Medicine[b]	1936
A.B. 9.	American Board of Pathology	1936
A.B. 10.	American Board of Ophthalmology	1917
A.B. 11.	American Board of Otolaryngology	1924
A.B. 12.	American Board of Surgery[c]	1937
A.B. 13.	American Board of Anesthesiology	1938
A.B. 14.	American Board of Plastic Surgery	1937
A.B. 15.	American Board of Neurological Surgery	1940

a. Also certifies specialists in allergy.
b. Also certifies specialists in allergy, cardiovascular disease, gastroenterology and tuberculosis.
c. Also certifies specialists in proctology.

A hospital seeking approval by the Council for the conduct of a residency in some specialty of medicine submits an application to the Council setting forth pertinent facts concerning the educational program. On the basis of the requirements set forth in the "Essentials for Approved Residencies and Fellowships" which regulations are formulated by the Council and approved by the House of Delegates, and supplemented by information contained in an actual survey of the institution, the Council may determine that the residency meets the desired educational standards. If the residency is in a field represented by a specialty board the conclusions regarding the hospital which were made by the Council are submitted to the proper American Board. In this way concurrence of the appropriate board is sought so that the Council's listing of approved residencies will name institutions offering work which will later be accepted by the American Board concerned to qualify the candidate for admission to the certification examination. The growing importance of the American boards and their certification in the specialties is indicated by the rapid growth in numbers certified. In the year 1940 there were 15,853 who had been certified by 14 boards. By 1946, the 15 boards in existence had certified a total of 26,108 physicians.[19] The growth in specialization under the auspices mentioned has unquestionably raised problems which are of great concern to many. While it has undoubtedly increased the quality of specialty practice it has probably also increased the costs of medical care and many feel that it has placed the general practitioner in an inferior position so far as prestige is concerned even though the general practitioner might well be competent to deal with the majority of patients seeking medical help.

POSTGRADUATE EDUCATION

In addition to the more definitive graduate educational programs in residencies and fellowships, preparing physicians to qualify to practice the various specialties, there has developed an educational category of courses now called "postgraduate continuation courses for physicians." In such courses the objectives are to keep physicians informed regarding advances in medicine, to assist them in reviewing for various special examinations, and, in general, to improve the practice of general practitioners and specialists. Such instruction tends to fall into one or another of the following: courses of instruction offered by institutions of high standing in large centers of population in which abundant clinical material is available, and "extension courses" brought to the physician in or near his home town by some such distant organization as a medical school, special scientific society or medical association.

The Council maintains contact with all organizations offering such courses. Semi-annually, in the Journal of the American Medical Association, it publishes classified lists of courses offered in this category during the ensuing six months. The listing for the last six months of 1946 included seventy-nine institutions and organizations offering 558 courses, some of which are given more than once in the period covered.[25] These listings are in great demand and are widely distributed. In the 1946 issue of the Educational Number of The Journal, it was reported that, during the previous year the attendance totaled 45,955. The courses offered varied in length from a few days to a year or more. There were 407 courses ranging in length from one to four months.[19]

---

[25] Postgraduate Continuation Courses for Veteran and Civilian Physicians. J.A.M.A., *131*:777 (June 29) 1946.

THE HOSPITAL REGISTER

With the expanding responsibilities of the Council, extending into the hospital field, the House of Delegates in 1920 changed the title of the Council to that of the Council on Medical Education and Hospitals. A need was recognized for the standardization and improvement of hospitals and for the collection and publication of data about hospitals generally, in addition to the hospitals offering internship and residency training. In fact, since 1906 the American Medical Directory carried a list of reputable hospitals in this country, periodic revision of which came to be a Council responsibility. Since 1928 the Council has maintained the Hospital Register which lists the names and pertinent statistical information of all acceptable hospitals in the United States which the Council judges to be operated with due regard to the public interest. The requirements which must be fulfilled by a hospital for inclusion on the Register are set forth in the Council's "Essentials of a Registered Hospital," which is an official document of the House of Delegates, and therefore of the American Medical Association. Adherence to the "Essentials" by a hospital is determined by inspection of the hospital by the professional staff of the Council. Annually the statistics on each of these hospitals are published in a special number of The Journal, under the title "Hospital Service in the United States," more commonly known as the "Hospital Number" of The Journal. In 1946, such information was published for 6,511 hospitals in this country, with a total bed capacity of 1,738,944.[26] This document is widely accepted as an authoritative hospital guide by government bodies, insurance companies, industry, hospital administrators, the medical profession and the public.

SURVEY OF MEDICAL EDUCATION, 1934–1936

In the early years of the Council, several "tours of inspection" of medical schools were carried out. The first was commenced in 1906, resulting in the first classification of schools a year later. The second "tour" culminated in the Carnegie report in 1910. Almost at once after this report a third series of surveys was conducted, to reinforce the Carnegie report findings and to lend additional weight to the recommendations of that document.

In the meantime, other valuable data on medical education were collected by the council, including a list of foreign medical schools (1907), a list of all medical schools, both existing and extinct (1908), descriptions of medical colleges based on surveys rather than the

---

[26] Arestad, F. H., and Westmoreland, M. G., Hospital Service in the United States, 1945. J.A.M.A., *130:*1073–1161 (April 20) 1946.

statements of the colleges (1908), and, in 1913 there were published life charts of medical colleges, showing the duration of their existence and a table of medical colleges whose standards did not meet those of the Council.

Throughout the ensuing years the Council's surveys were not always in the nature of complete "tours of inspection" of all medical colleges. In time, certain of the schools, especially those constituting integral parts of strong universities, were recognized as more competent to conduct high-quality programs than others, so that the attention of the Council inevitably became directed toward improving the weaker institutions, while still providing leadership in the broad field of medical education at all levels.

In the years following the Carnegie report such surveys of individual schools became a continuous process and were more common than complete "tours of inspection" of all schools. However, the desirability of another complete survey of all schools became apparent in the thirties. According to Wilbur:[27]

> The social and economic disturbances following the recent world-wide depression, however, retarded a great part of that steady progress which had been going on in medical education in America beginning with the early nineties. During and following the depression while certain institutions received large gifts and continued to advance, there was sufficient deterioration among some of the schools that had attained an approved rating to suggest the importance of a new nationwide study. Funds for this survey were authorized by the Board of Trustees of the American Medical Association. Every approved medical school was visited, each department was studied and its staff consulted and all of the institutions concerned were rerated. A score or more had failed to advance or had lapsed in their standards sufficiently to warrant either placing them on probation or withdrawing approval.

Therefore, in 1933 the Council decided to survey all the medical schools of the United States and (upon specific request) of Canada. In the survey The Council requested and received the whole-hearted assistance and cooperation of the Association of American Medical Colleges and the Federation of State Medical Boards of the United States. During the years 1934–1936 Dr. H. G. Weiskotten, Dean of Syracuse University College of Medicine (and now chairman of the Council) visited eighty-nine schools in the United States and Canada, which included all approved schools in both countries and two unapproved schools in the United States. At each school he was accompanied by a representative of the Council, of the Association of American Medical Colleges or the Federation of State Medical Boards.

[27] Weiskotten, H. G., Schwitalla, A. M., Cutter, W. D., and Anderson, H. H.: Medical Education in the United States, 1934–1939, American Medical Association, Chicago, 1940.

Schools were evaluated, department by department, and were told in detail wherein their program was strong and where weak. Although a public report of the survey was published,[27] there was no published statement regarding the defects of the various schools by name. Useful as such statements proved to be years earlier, when medical education was a sick infant in this country, it was felt that by this time medical education had more or less become of age. Regarding these two methods of reporting findings, Weiskotten states:[27]

In 1910, Mr. Flexner described in detail each of the medical schools he had visited. His incisive comment, reinforcing the efforts of the Council, was in large part responsible

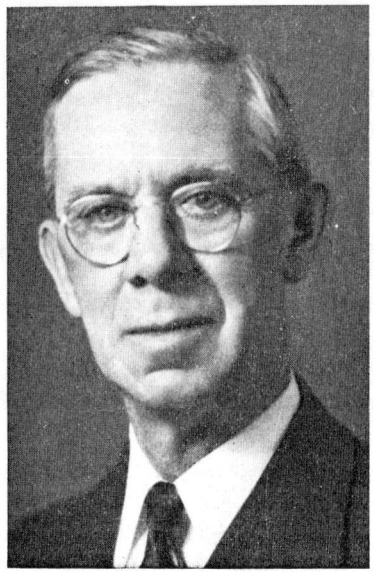

Dr. H. G. Weiskotten
Chairman, Council on Medical Education and Hospitals

for the discontinuance of many of the schools that were unworthy. In this report, however, individual comment was deemed undesirable. It deals instead with objectives and policies, organization and administration, physical and clinical facilities, teaching personnel and educational programs. In this way it is believed that faculties and administrative officers may learn what other schools are doing, emulating that which is good and avoiding that which experience has shown to be unprofitable.

The wisdom of this policy was confirmed by the beneficial results of the survey:[27]

Even the weakest of the medical schools at the time of this survey was a stable institution as compared with the numerous proprietary schools and diploma mills in existence at the time that the Council was created. Rather than to publish their deficiencies, therefore, it seemed wiser to give aid and encouragement to those schools which needed help, in the hope that within a reasonable period they would be able to conform to the current standards of medical education. This expectation has been justified by the achievements of the past three or four years during which the Council has been able to stimulate greater interest in medical schools on the part of their universities; to assist administrative officers in the solution of their problems of organization and personnel; to assist in securing satisfactory hospital relationships; to foster the development of more modern educational programs and stimulate curricular studies by faculty groups, and to secure greater financial and public support.

In all of these ways and many others the cause of medical education has been promoted, its standards advanced and its purposes more nearly achieved.

The acceptance of the Council's leadership, findings and recommendations by the profession, the public, and government units is no less remarkable than its acceptance by medical schools and hospitals. These educational institutions, while formerly sometimes considering the Council as a policing agency to be feared, have come to look upon the Council as a consulting agency to be sought when difficulties and problems arise. Today, instances in which the Council's advice is sought voluntarily as a guide are far more frequent than instances in which the Council initiates discussions with a school leading to a survey.

COOPERATION IN THE IMPROVEMENT OF MEDICAL EDUCATION

Throughout its efforts to improve medical education at all levels the Council was wise in seeking the cooperation of other interested organizations and fortunate in securing it. Much of the Council's work has been made doubly effective by collaboration with such groups as the Association of American Medical Colleges, the Federation of State Medical Boards of the United States, the National Board of Medical Examiners, and, as described earlier, the American Boards in the medical specialties and the Advisory Board for Medical Specialties. The history of the Council is in part a history of cooperative effort with these groups.

The Association of American Medical Colleges was organized in 1890 following a campaign conducted by Dr. John H. Rauch of the Illinois State Board of Health exposing many defects in medical education. For some years after its formation, the Association did not have a regular membership; any medical college could send delegates to the annual meetings. The proceedings of these meetings, with excellent treatises on the necessity for improved entrance standards and medical instruction, were similar to the discussions on medical education to be heard at the meetings of the American Medical Association. Very early medical school standards were formulated, adherence to which was required for representation in the Association, although initially the organization had to depend upon the published statements of the medical colleges, rather than direct inspections, to judge the degree of compliance with the regulations. The first published list of cooperating colleges containing 55 of the 155 schools, appeared in 1896, at which time the annual dues were $5.00.

In the early years of the century, with the increasing influence of the American Medical Association, there was a parallel improvement in the influence of the related Association. Coincident with the first A—B—C classification of medical schools by the newly created Council, the medical College Association conducted a vigorous campaign of inspections and the poorer colleges were required to raise their standards to retain membership.

For forty years the Association of American Medical Colleges has been controlled by the best elements in the medical schools of this country. A continuous leadership through these years has been provided by the present Secretary of the Association, Dr. Fred C. Zapffe. Increasingly, with the Council, the Association has wielded tremendous influence in the formulation and enforcement of entrance requirements, the development of a well-balanced medical curriculum and the establishing of improved methods of teaching.

An important landmark in the history of this collaborative enterprise was passed in 1942, when the Board of Trustees of the American Medical Association and the Association of American Medical Colleges established a liaison committee, with representation from the Council and from the College Association. This committee meets at least twice annually to discuss problems in medical education of mutual concern and to carry back to each organization the recommendations emerging from the discussions. In addition, it is now customary for a member or the secretary of the Council to attend the business meetings of the executive council of the College Association. That council, in turn, is usually represented at deliberations of the Council on Medical Education and Hospitals. Surveys of medical schools are conducted jointly. In recent years no important action pertaining to medical education has been taken without prior discussions with the other body, or without the concurrence of the other body.

In this manner the two organizations, seeking the same ends, present a solid front on all issues. Each strengthens the actions of the other, exerting a profound influence upon the improvement of medical education in this country.

The Federation of State Medical Boards of the United States is another of the several organizations with which the Council works in close collaboration. The annual Congress sponsored originally by the Council, is now held under joint auspices, so that it is called

"The Annual Congress on Medical Education and Licensure." The official organ of the Federation, the monthly "Federation Bulletin," is published, printed and distributed by the American Medical Association under the editorship of the secretary of the Federation and the managing editorship of the secretary of the Council. This journal is distributed widely to the members of the Federation and others interested in licensure.

The Council maintains licensure records utilized by the various licensing bodies virtually daily and publishes an annual compilation of licensing statistics in a special number of The Journal, "Medical Licensure in the United States," more commonly known as the "State Board Number."

The collaboration of the Council with the medical licensing bodies had its origin in the early hectic days of the Council's work. One of the first devices for calling the attention of the public to the poor quality of many medical schools in the early 1900's was the publication of statistics on licensure examination failures by graduates of those schools. Indeed, medical schools still scan the data of the "State Board Number" of The Journal, with an eager interest in the percentage of failures as tabulated by schools.

Graduation from a medical school once served to indicate who might practice medicine. But since many inferior schools came into being, an impartial measure of a physician's qualifications through examinations was deemed essential. This was a major factor responsible for the establishment of the various licensing boards of the states, territories and possessions.

The Federation of State Medical Boards of the United States was founded in 1912 as a voluntary organization of legally constituted licensing bodies.

Previously there were in existence two confederations of the boards, the "National Confederation of State Medical Examining and Licensing Boards" and the "American Confederation of Reciprocating Examining and Licensing Medical Boards." The first of these, which had held some twenty annual sessions, was primarily concerned with medical education. The second, which had held about ten sessions, was interested mainly in the technicalities and problems of licensure and reciprocity procedure. As a result of a good many conferences and discussions a union of the two groups was consummated and the present "Federation" emerged.

The Federation and the constituent licensing boards depend upon the Council for verification of the credentials of applicants for licensure. In general, they also depend upon the Council's evaluation of the applicant's education, by reference to the Council's listings of medical schools and hospitals maintaining acceptable educational programs. In some instances the medical practice act of the state makes the use of these lists mandatory. Elsewhere they are employed by regulation of the boards. Thus the "approved lists" of the Council have come to have the force of law, although neither the Council nor the American Medical Association was created by law.

The legality of this practice has been tested in the courts. In a recent case in an eastern state the plaintiff objected to the board's denial to admit him to the licensure examination. He charged that the board was not within its rights in failing to inspect the school of the plaintiff's graduation and in relying on the judgment of the Council regarding the inferior quality of that school. The court ruled that the licensing board had every right to seek advice from and rely on the opinion of any organization in which the board had confidence, whether or not that organization was a government body.

The National Board of Medical Examiners bears a relationship to the Council rather similar to that of the various state licensing bodies. The National Board was organized in 1915 by Dr. W. L. Rodman, then president of the American Medical Association. The aim was primarily to establish a comprehensive qualifying examination which would be rather generally acceptable to the legal agencies of the states. The board itself has no direct legal status except in so far as its examination findings have been acceptable to the states. This board consists of representatives of the three federal medical services, the Federation of State Medical Boards of the United States, the Council on Medical Education and Hospitals of the American Medical Association and the Association of American Medical Colleges. In addition it includes medical scientists and clinicians as well, selected for their high standing, with due regard for geographical distribution.

The prestige which has been achieved by this board, and the wide recognition granted the diplomates for licensure purposes attest the excellence of the work of the board in the thirty-odd years of its existence. Virtually all the states, territories and possessions of the United States accept the board's examinations in lieu of their own. Diplomates are also granted recognition by the qualifying boards in Great Britain and Ireland.

The National Board of Medical Examiners regularly reports its results to the Council; such records are incorporated into the directory's files of physicians, they are available to all state licensing bodies upon request, and with state board examination results, they become the basis for the statistics published annually by the Council in the "State Board Number" of The Journal. Since the formation of the National Board over 10,000 physicians have been licensed to practice medicine on the basis of board credentials, although more than this number have become board diplomates. Year by year there is a steady increase in numbers examined.[28]

MEDICAL EDUCATION IN CANADA

In the sphere of medical education there has developed a spirit of amity and good will between the Canadian medical schools and the Council, which is in the best tradition of friendship between the two countries. This spirit of understanding has been the product of years of close association, commencing with the original medical school surveys conducted by the Council. At present the Canadian schools are included in the official lists of the Council upon the request by the school, the schools provide the Council with the same enrolment and other statistics received from the schools in the United States and the Council offers survey and consultation facilities to the Canadian schools whenever these are requested. As is the case with hospitals and medical schools in the United States, no charges are made for such services, either for the consultation or for the expenses of conducting the survey. Within the past year, for example, requests for surveys from five Canadian schools were received.

THE TECHNICAL SCHOOLS

The Council's wide experience and recognized prestige in improving educational standards in medical schools and hospitals have led certain national organizations in fields ancillary to medicine to seek the Council's aid in the standardizing, surveying and accrediting of their schools. It is the policy of the Council to undertake such tasks only when requested to do so by the responsible national organizations through the medium of resolutions presented to and passed by the House of Delegates of the American Medical Association.

The earliest of the technical school groups to come under the guidance of the Council in this manner were the Physical Therapy Technicians and the Clinical Laboratory Technicians. "Essentials" for approved schools in these fields were adopted by the House in 1936. These documents outline the requirements for approval, aid the schools to achieve and maintain high standards, and serve as a basis for inspection surveys by the technical staff of the Council, upon which approval is based.

The "Essentials" in these fields were developed and are modified from time to time in collaboration with the American Registry of

---

[28] Johnson, Victor, and Tipner, Anne: Medical Licensure Statistics for 1945. J.A.M.A., *131:*109 (May 11), 1946.

Physical Therapy Technicians, the American Physiotherapy Association and the Council on Physical Medicine of the American Medical Association in the case of schools for Physical Therapy Technicians, and with the American Society of Clinical Pathologists and the Board of Registry of Medical Technologists in the case of schools for Clinical Laboratory Technologists.

This pattern has been repeated in the case of schools in other technical fields. "Essentials" were established for schools of Occupational Therapy in 1939, for Medical Record Librarians in 1943 and for X-Ray Technicians in 1944.

Annually these revised "Essentials" are reprinted in the "Hospital Number" of The Journal of the American Medical Association, as are also the list of approved schools which have been determined by actual Council inspections to adhere to these regulations and recommendations. In the most recent listing of these institutions,[26] the numbers of approved schools in these fields were as follows: X-Ray Technicians, 130; Medical Record Librarians, 10; Occupational Therapy Technicians, 18; Physical Therapy Technicians, 32; and Clinical Laboratory Technicians, 268.

The work of the Council in these technical fields has materially improved the education, and therefore the services of technicians, as a further contribution to the major goal of all the Council's efforts: an ever higher quality of medical care for the public.

Although the Council maintains no lists of approved nursing schools, it does maintain close liaison with the national accrediting bodies in this field, and has exerted considerable influence in the improvement of nursing education.

THE WAR YEARS, 1941–1945

During the war years, medical education joined wholeheartedly in the universal effort to mobilize all resources to defeat the enemy. Anticipating wartime needs for more doctors, the medical schools adopted the accelerated program in 1941, requiring the completion of the normal 36 months of medical instruction in three calendar years instead of four. Students were admitted every nine months and enrolments were increased. As a result of these policies, some 7,000 extra students were graduated by the time these emergency measures were discontinued, shortly after the war. The effects of this program were tremendous, since this number of graduates was sufficient to provide medical officers for nearly 1,500,000 extra troops.

Acceleration was very much overdone. Under the military college programs of the army and navy, premedical work was completed in about a year and a half. For two-thirds of the graduates, the internship was limited to nine months and only one-sixth of the able-bodied males were permitted as much as 27 months of hospital work. Thus the total program from the commencement of premedical work until the completion of the internship was scheduled to occur in just $5\frac{1}{4}$ years instead of eight years, although no student actually completed this entire sequence before the war ended. This acceleration was carried out in the face of considerable reductions in medical school and hospital teaching staffs, which were depleted by the departure of many for active duty.

To these handicaps were added the additional burden of repeated changes and lack of consistency in the military policies of the government. No sooner was the selective service deferment policy operating smoothly for medical students than they were enrolled in inactive reserve corps of the Army's Medical Administrative Corps and the Navy's Hospital Volunteers. This arrangement operated entirely satisfactorily, whereupon the military services decided to activate these men and place them in uniform in the Army Specialized Training and Navy V-12 programs. Students were provided with free tuition, had books and equipment purchased for them and received regular military base pay. To many this extremely costly policy seemed entirely unnecessary.

Interference with the medical curriculum was minimal, fortunately, although the military took great liberties with premedical education, chiefly by curtailing the time allotted for it. Premedical students also were on active duty assigned to studies by the army and navy.

With the war still far from won, and its duration an entirely unknown quantity in April of 1944 the Selective Service System, at the instigation of the War and Navy departments, abolished occupational deferments of premedical students. Meanwhile the army and navy had sharply reduced its premedical personnel. Soon thereafter all new army and navy assignments to premedical work ceased. Fortunately for those in authority, who completely disregarded informed counsel, the war ended sooner than was expected by anyone, including the military.

The wartime damage to medical education, and consequently to the quality of medical care, cannot now be assessed, but there is rather general agreement that some of the harm was unavoidable in a war of unprecedented wastefulness, and that some of it was due to the lack of vision of the military.[29]

---

[29] Discussions of wartime problems in medical education are to be found in the annual Educational Numbers of The Journal of the American Medical Association: *122:*1085–1125 (Aug. 14) 1943; *125:*1099–1145 (Aug. 19) 1944; *129:*33–75 (Sept. 1) 1945; *131:*1277–1354 (Aug. 17) 1946.

A study was inaugurated in 1946 into the use of medical personnel in wartime, by the Committee on National Emergency Medical Service of the American Medical Association. Wartime educational policies in medicine will be included in the study. Recommendations will be made by the committee for a more effective and efficient mobilization of all aspects of medicine in the event of another war emergency.

PROBLEMS OF THE FUTURE

The reconversion of medical education to a peacetime status presents problems which in many respects dwarf those of the recent war. Enrolments in the colleges of the country, largely because of the attendance of veterans benefiting from the educational pro-

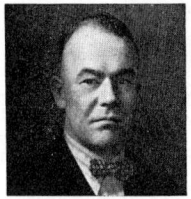
Dr. Reginald Fitz

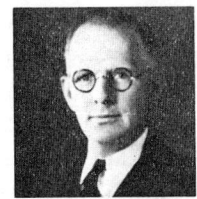
Dr. Russell L. Haden

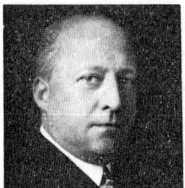
Dr. Charles G. Heyd

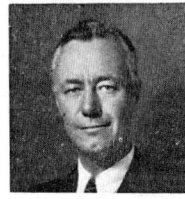
Dr. Victor Johnson

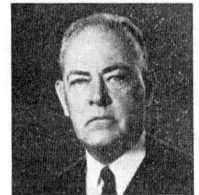
Dr. J. H. Musser

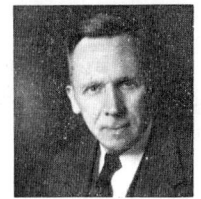
Dr. Harvey B. Stone

The present (1947) Council on Medical Education and Hospitals. The chairman is Dr. H. G. Weiskotten.

visions of the "G. I. Bill of Rights," is overwhelming, taxing to the utmost the educational facilities of faculties, classrooms and laboratories, as well as available housing facilities. On every important college campus of the country today there are improvised villages of trailers, reclaimed army barracks or temporary structures of any kind obtainable to house student veterans and their families. Academic performance, industry and motivation of these students appear to be good. The quality of medical student and physician eventuating from this emergency program is now a matter for conjecture. The years ahead hold the answer.

Many medical schools face critical times in the immediate future. Adequate financial support is a major problem. During the war the income from tuition sources was greatly increased. Acceleration and admissions every nine months, increased enrolments and the payment to state schools of out-of-state tuition fees for army and navy students swelled the income from student fees tremendously. With the termination of the war and the discontinuing of acceleration and the well-paying military programs, there was a sharp reduction in revenues from students. In a goodly number of schools this has precipitated a serious financial crisis. Financial support from other sources must be forthcoming in greatly increased amounts if medical schools are to continue at their former high level of performance in the training of doctors, the conduct of research and a superior grade of service to the community.

Related to the critical financial structure of many schools is the deficiency in qualified teachers, especially in the fields of basic medical sciences. Wartime government policies are involved here also, since virtually no science students were permitted to carry on advanced studies in this country during the conflict. Still, the major difficulty is the poor financial support of basic science instruction by medical schools, which have made no serious effort to meet the mounting competition for qualified scientists, from the government services, industry and the practice of medicine. Unless this problem is met and solved, the present high state of medical education in this country, unequalled anywhere, is sure to suffer.

There is again a distinct need for another complete survey of all medical schools, to determine the degree to which they are maintaining high standards, and to assist them in improving their programs. The Council provides survey and consultation services to medical schools continuously. Yet there is needed now, a systematic re-evaluation of the faculties, facilities, financing and operation of all medical schools in another comprehensive survey. This is now being planned by the Council on Medical Education and Hospitals and has been authorized by the Board of Trustees.

In the more advanced field of medical education, at the hospital residency level, the termination of the war has further multiplied the problems to be faced. At the very outset of the war the Council recognized that the curtailed hospital training of medical graduates during the war would result in an unprecedented demand for residencies after the war. Extensive studies were conducted to determine the postwar plans of medical officers[30] and every effort made in

---

[30]Lueth, Harold C., Results of Pilot Questionnaire to Physicians in Service, J.A.M.A. *125*:558 (June 24) 1944; Johnson, Victor and Arestad, F. H., Educational Facilities Required for Returning Medical Officers, J.A.M.A., *126*:253 (Sept. 23) 1944; Lueth, Harold C., Postgraduate Wishes of Medical Officers, J.A.M.A., *127*:759 (Mar. 31) 1945; Johnson, Victor, Lueth, Harold C. and Arestad, F. H., Educational Facilities for Physician Veterans, J.A.M.A., *129*:28 (Sept. 1) 1945.

collaboration with the specialty boards and the Advisory Board for Medical Specialties to stimulate hospitals to capitalize maximally on every possible educational asset, to increase the facilities for training physician veterans. Agreements and understandings with the Veterans Administration were also effected to facilitate the program.[31] As a result of these efforts, there were developed nearly 9,000 approved residency positions soon after the war's end, as compared with less than 6,000 before the war.[19]

The mobilization of educational facilities to meet the needs of physician veterans was a responsibility imposed not only by the desires of returning medical officers, but it was a necessary effort to offset the deficit in medical education created by the war. Uncorrected, this deficiency could spell a decreased quality of medical care in this country for many years to come.

The expansion of educational opportunities in our hospitals to provide for physician veterans must not be regarded as purely an emergency measure, to be contracted when the present acute demand subsides. Doubtless, the maintenance of high educational standards will necessitate a reduction in residency opportunities to somewhat less than the present supply.

Yet this country would be remiss in its world responsibility if it fails to recognize that these newly developed training facilities should be continued, when quality warrants, so that opportunities can be offered for many years, to provide advanced education for the physicians of foreign countries, which are looking to the United States in increasing numbers to exercise world leadership in medicine. The additional residency programs, of high quality, and positions which have been developed for veterans should be available later to the physicians of foreign countries who wish to carry back to their own lands a measure of the superior quality of medical practice in this country.

Problems in medical care in this country are inseparable from those of medical education. Are we educating too many specialists? Are we failing to provide sufficient numbers of general practitioners? Have we explored all possible opportunities to effect a better distribution of physicians as between rural and urban areas? Is the widespread desire to establish new medical schools sound, or is it merely an understandable reaction to wartime physician shortages? Should a new medical school be established on a university campus even in a small community with the handicap of a possibly inadequate quantity of clinical material? Since medical education has come of

---

[31] Hospital Residencies and Postgraduate Continuation Courses under the G. I. Bill, J.A.M.A., *130:*214 (Jan. 26) 1946.

age, and not a few medical schools lend scientific distinction to the parent university, rather than the reverse, does not the pronouncement of William Pepper a half-century ago assume new significance? He stated:

> There are branches of study, like Greek or Mathematics, which may be studied as well, granted a true teacher and the necessary books, in a small village as in a metropolis. But no excellence on the part of the teacher can atone to the student of mechanical engineering for the want of the fully equipped plant; and still less to the student of medicine for the want of the extensive and varied experience with all forms of disease and injury only to be acquired in the hospitals and dispensaries of a great city.[32]

These, and numberless other equally serious problems face the Council on Medical Education and Hospitals in the years ahead. In meeting the new tasks, the Council is fortunate in operating under the leadership of Dr. H. G. Weiskotten, elected chairman of the Council in 1946 to succeed Dr. Ray Lyman Wilbur, as the third chairman in over forty years of Council history. The problems to be met in the new era will be solved only by the application of the formula which has made medical education in this country thus far the best in the world: an idealistic and militant cooperation in the interests of improved medical education and medical care by every organization and individual possessing authority and influence coupled with medical knowledge and social wisdom. The accomplishments of the first 100 years of the American Medical Association have amply demonstrated the effectiveness of this formula.

---

[32] Quoted in Slayton, W. T.: Medical Education and Registration, United States and Canada, page 101, Hyde Park, Vermont, 1897.

THE COUNCIL ON PHYSICAL MEDICINE

By Howard A. Carter

THE COUNCIL ON PHYSICAL MEDICINE was created to protect the medical profession and the public against misleading and deceptive advertising of devices manufactured and sold for use in physical medicine, to aid in placing physical medicine on a sound scientific basis, and to disseminate trustworthy information about methods developed in this field of therapeutics.

The Council came into existence as the result of a resolution adopted by the House of Delegates in 1925. The members of the Council were appointed by the Board of Trustees. The first meeting was held in October. The Council has been active continuously since 1925.

In 1925, manufacturers were offering for sale to physicians and to hospitals many non-medicinal agents with unconfirmed claims of therapeutic value. Those products included electrical and mechanical contrivances, generators of ultraviolet and infrared radiation, and many other devices. Individual physicians, because of the lack of necessary technical knowledge and skill, were seldom able to evaluate such apparatus correctly. Often, as a result of misrepresentation members of the medical profession suffered great financial loss when buying these devices. The use of such machines, without adequate understanding and control, prevented proper therapy, thereby resulting in loss of time and money to the patients.

In the resolution passed by the House of Delegates in 1925, an important statement read as follows:

"Be it resolved, that the trustees of the American Medical Association be empowered to appoint a Council on 'Nonmedicinal Agents' similar to the Council on Pharmacy and Chemistry, consisting of at least two physicians, two physiologists, two pathologists and two clinicians, whose duty it shall be scientifically to investigate and report on the value and merits of all nonmedicinal apparatus and contrivances offered for sale to physicians and hospitals, and to publish in THE JOURNAL from time to time the results of its investigations."

This resolution, introduced by Dr. Joseph F. Smith, delegate from Wisconsin, was published in the Journal of the American Medical Association, June 6, 1925, was adopted and was referred to the Board of Trustees with a request for action.

An executive secretary was sought to organize and direct the work of the Council at headquarters. Technical and engineering knowledge was needed, and Mr. H. J. Holmquest, mechanical engineer, was appointed and served for five years.

Two essential problems had to be settled, namely, (1) the field and scope of the Council and (2) the selection of an appropriate name. After due consideration, the title "Council on Physical Therapy" was adopted. This name was retained until the nineteenth annual meeting of the Council, December, 1943, at which time a motion was passed to change the name to "Council on Physical Medicine," because the designation "physical medicine" is a more inclusive term.

Another major question before the Council was to formulate rules of procedure. Those first adopted were patterned after the rules of the Council on Pharmacy and Chemistry, but in 1931, the rules were revised to meet more fully the special problems created as the result of considering apparatus.

During World War I, physical medicine (then called physical therapy) was used to some extent for the rehabilitation of injured service men. Before that time, most members of the profession did not have a high opinion of physical medicine and many regarded it as having little value owing to the lack of fundamental information. A few years after the close of World War I, physical medicine was in a chaotic condition; this was especially true at the time the Council was organized by the Board of Trustees. By some of the profession, physical medicine was recognized as having many excellent attributes of therapeutic value, while at the same time it was discredited by many conservative physicians as being akin to quackery. At that time, only a few hospitals had adequate physical therapy departments and only a small number of physicians employed it solely for the welfare of their patients. The chaos was aggravated by the activities of salesmen and manufacturers who sold apparatus directly to physicians and to hospitals with assertions that the apparatus were the only therapeutic agents required for the adequate treatment of various conditions. Too much emphasis was placed on "machine therapy" and not enough on the intelligent management of the patient as a whole. A few manufacturers employed physicians of questionable repute who were being sent throughout the country to conduct clinics and to demonstrate apparatus claimed to be of therapeutic value. The profession had lost sight of the fact that true physical medicine consisted chiefly of intelligent handwork, such as the use of massage and exercise and simple therapeutic procedures for administering heat, radiation and certain forms of electrical energy.

As the Council viewed the field twenty years ago, its duty was to inform the profession that machines and apparatus played a minor part in physical medicine, in so far as the majority of the physicians was concerned. With the previously mentioned chaotic conditions confronting such a newly formed body, it can be readily understood that the first six or seven years of the Council's existence were devoted to the self-education of its members, to the formulation of rules of procedure and to the study of physical phenomena used in physical medicine before the Council could undertake seriously the work for which it had been created. In view of the conflicting claims advanced for many physical measures, the Council was obliged to move cautiously and conservatively if it wished its work to be permanent.

The aims of the Council on Physical Medicine may be expressed briefly as follows:

1. To inform the medical profession and the public about the efficacy of apparatus recommended for medical purposes.
2. To protect the medical profession against fraud and misrepresentation associated with the manufacture and sale of such apparatus.
3. To advise the profession regarding the content of curricula for both undergraduate and postgraduate education in physical medicine.
4. To promote research in physical medicine.

To the interested, loyal, sincere members of the Council and to its group of consultants, a great debt of appreciation and gratitude is due. These men, specialists in their chosen field, were and have been selected by the Board of Trustees for their proficiency. Members of the Council devote a considerable portion of their time holding meetings by mail every two weeks at no charge to the American Medical Association. The profession is fortunate in having this group of specialists who are willing to lend their services gratuitously for the benefit of humanity and the improvement of scientific medicine.

PERSONNEL

At the first meeting on October 16, 1925, the following were present: Drs. W. R. Bovie, Boston, biophysicist; Arthur Compton, Chicago, physicist; Ralph Pemberton, Philadelphia, internist; Harry E. Mock, Chicago, surgeon; George Miller MacKee, New York, dermatologist; Arthur U. Desjardins, Rochester, Minnesota, radiologist; W. B. Cannon (deceased), Boston, physiologist; A. S. Warthin (deceased), Ann Arbor, Michigan, pathologist; Francis Carter Wood, New York, pathologist. Drs. Olin West and Morris

Fishbein, ex-officio members, also attended. Dr. Mock was appointed chairman.

Three months after the first meeting in January, 1926, the following additional members were appointed: Dr. Frank Granger (deceased), Boston, physical therapist; and Dr. H. B. Williams, New York, physiologist.

In the course of the twenty-two years of the Council's existence, numerous changes in personnel have occurred. Dr. W. E. Garrey, Nashville, physiologist, in March 1927, accepted membership to the Council replacing Dr. Cannon, who had resigned in January. Dr. W. W. Coblentz, radiation physicist, Washington, D. C., accepted membership to succeed Dr. Compton, who had resigned in February, 1928. Dr. Granger died in October, 1928, and the term of Dr. Bovie expired in November, 1929. Dr. Robert S. Osgood, Boston, orthopedic surgeon, and Dr. John S. Coulter, Chicago, physical therapist, were elected in February, 1930, to succeed Drs. Bovie and Granger respectively. Mr. Holmquest resigned as Secretary of the Council in September, 1931, and Mr. Howard A. Carter, mechanical engineer, Chicago, was appointed. Mr. Richard B. Dillehunt, Portland, Oregon, was added to the Council in 1930, but he resigned shortly afterward. His place was filled by Dr. Frederick J. Gaenslen (deceased), Wisconsin, in March, 1931. Dr. Howard T. Karsner was elected to the Council in December, 1931, to succeed Dr. Warthin, who had died in May, 1931. Dr. Francis Carter Wood resigned in January, 1932. Because of the heavy schedule in his teaching program, Dr. Williams allowed his term to expire and in July, 1933, Dr. Yandell Henderson was appointed to succeed him. Dr. Frank H. Krusen, Philadelphia, physical therapist, was added to the Council in October, 1934. On the resignation of Dr. Henderson in July, 1935, Dr. H. B. Williams was again appointed to the Council in October, 1935. Dr. Frank Ober, Boston, orthopedic surgeon, accepted appointment in June, 1936, to succeed Dr. Osgood who had resigned that year. Dr. George C. Andrews, New York, dermatologist, accepted membership in December, 1936, to succeed Dr. MacKee, who had resigned in August. In September, 1936, Dr. Gaenslen resigned because of ill health and Dr. Frank Dickson, Kansas City, orthopedic surgeon, succeeded him. Dr. Andrews resigned in October, 1937, and was replaced by Dr. Anthony C. Cipollaro, New York, dermatologist, in March, 1938. Dr. Eben Carey, Milwaukee, Wisconsin, accepted membership to the Council in March, 1940, to succeed Dr. Karsner, who had resigned in November, 1939. Dr. Morris Bowie, Bryn Mawr, Pennsylvania, internist, and Dr. George M. Piersol, Pennsylvania, internist, succeeded Drs. Mock and Pemberton, whose terms had expired in February, 1942.

The present membership of the Council on Physical Medicine is: Dr. John S. Coulter, chairman; Dr. Morris A. Bowie; Dr. Eben J. Carey; Dr. Anthony C. Cipollaro; Dr. W. W. Coblentz; Dr. Arthur U. Desjardins; Dr. Frank D. Dickson; Dr. W. E. Garrey; Dr. Frank H. Krusen, vice chairman; Dr. Frank R. Ober; Dr. George M. Piersol; and Dr. H. B. Williams. Members of the Council are elected for a 3-year term.

At an early date, the Council on Physical Medicine found that it was necessary, in order to carry out its assigned duties, to appoint consultants to give advice on special problems. The following are standing committees of Consultants to the Council:

1. Consultants on Artificial Limbs: Drs. Henry H. Kessler, Harry E. Mock, S. Perry Rogers. Paul Klopsteg, Paul B. Steele, and Philip Wilson; Messrs. W. E. Isle, McCarthy Hanger, Sr., J. B. Korrady, Joseph A. Spievak, and David E. Stolpe.
2. Consultants on Medical Aspects of Atomic Energy: Drs. Kenneth C. Cole, L. F. Curtiss, Hymer L. Friedell, Shields Warren and Stafford L. Warren.
3. Consultants on Audiometers and Hearing Aids: Dr. Gordon Berry, Hallowell Davis, E. P. Fowler, W. E. Grove, Isaac H. Jones, Dean Lierle, Moses H. Lurie, Douglas Macfarlan, C. Stewart Nash, Paul E. Sabine, and B. R. Shurly.
4. Consultants on Contraceptive Devices: Drs. N. J. Eastman, William W. Greulich, Joseph Hughes, Andrew C. Ivy, Walter J. Meek, Ephraim Shorr, and Mr. R. R. Olin.
5. Consultants on Education: Drs. Frances Baker, Robert L. Bennett, Benjamin Boynton, Earl C. Elkins, F. W. Ewerhardt, Richard Kovacs, Fred B. Moor, William H. Northway, William H. Schmidt, Walter M. Solomon, Arthur L. Watkins, George D. Wilson, and Walter J. Zeiter.
6. Consultants on Electrocardiographs: Drs. A. R. Barnes, George Fahr, Harold E. B. Pardee, William D. Stroud, Carl J. Wiggers, and Frank N. Wilson.
7. Consultants on Electroencephalography: Drs. Percival Bailey, Edward J. Baldes, Stanley Cobb, Hallowell Davis and Frederic A. Gibbs.
8. Consultants on Occupational Therapy: Drs. Raymond B. Allen, Robert W. Johnson, Jr., Winfred Overholser, Howard A. Rusk, William D. Stroud, and Francis B. Trudeau.
9. Consultants on Ophthalmic Devices: Drs. Thomas D. Allen, S. Judd Beach, Conrad Berens, Frederick C. Cordes, Alfred Cowan, Walter B. Lancaster, William H. Luedde, Lawrence T. Post, Avery D. Prangen, and Kenneth C. Swan.
10. Consultants on Respirators: Drs. Edward L. Compere, Charles F. McKhann, and James L. Wilson.
11. Consultants on Roentgen Rays and Radium: Drs. William E. Chamberlain, Arthur C. Christie, Edwin C. Ernst, Gioacchino Failla, Fred M. Hodges, Robert R. Newell, Eugene P. Pendergrass, Ursus V. Portmann, Lauriston S. Taylor, and J. L. Weatherwax.

Many physicians and specialists in physical medicine and allied fields, too numerous to mention, have served as consultants to the Council. Each year, the Council has prepared a statement entitled "An Appreciation" and the physicians who have assisted the Council during the year are listed in that publication.

The Council recognized its need for standing committees and the following composed of members of the Council are in existence today: Committees on Advertising, Field Scope and Present Status, Education, High Frequency Electrical Currents, Nomenclature and Definition, Radiation, Rehabilitation, and Scientific Research.

ACTIVITIES

The Council has endeavored to demonstrate the value of physical medicine by: (1) publishing articles on physical medicine in the Journal of the American Medical Association; (2) publishing a "Handbook of Physical Medicine"; (3) preparing a booklet "Apparatus Accepted"; (4) suggesting speakers to state and county medical societies; (5) arranging for exhibits in physical medicine in conjunction with the Bureau of Exhibits and (6) providing information on physical medicine through correspondence, publications, and movies.

The first four years were largely devoted to organization and determination of field and scope and formulation of the rules of procedure. A summary of the major activities of the Council on Physical Medicine from 1929 to the present time follows:

1929—Dissemination of information on the merits and limitations of physical methods and therapeutic agents.
1930—Investigation of massaging and exercising machines and ultraviolet radiation devices.
1931—Investigation of sunlamps, ultraviolet and heat lamps, artificial respirators, and colonic therapy apparatus.
1932—Preparation and publication of "Handbook of Physical Therapy," consideration of anesthesia appliances, air conditioning, apparatus, oxygen therapy devices, respirators, resuscitation equipment, inhalators and pollen filters and ultraviolet and heat generators.
1933—Investigation of resuscitation equipment, exygen tents, diathermy apparatus, and ultraviolet and infrared generators.
1934—Investigation of ophthalmic instruments, study of physical characteristics and therapeutic efficacy of short wave diathermy.
1935—Intensification of its educational pursuits and encouragement of effective improvement of the curricula of courses for physical therapy, investigation of radiation and diathermy equipment.
1936—Consideration of positive and negative pressure resuscitators, diathermy apparatus, vaporizers, inhalators, ultraviolet and infrared devices and oxygen therapy equipment.
1937—Investigation of audiometers and hearing aids and advancement of Council's educational activities.
1938—Consideration of roentgen apparatus, artificial limbs, formulation of standards for audiometers, revision of "Handbook of Physical Therapy" and "Apparatus Accepted."
1939—Consideration of audiometers and hearing aids, inhalators and resuscitators, radium and radon, short wave diathermy equipment, galvanic generators, fever therapy appliances, and respirators.
1940—Promotion of education and active participation with other agencies in aiding

medical preparedness, study of the problem of radio interference in connection with diathermy apparatus.

1941—Renewal of emphasis on consideration of problems concerning artificial respiration, sponsored an exhibit on "Lame Backs," urging of the establishment of courses in physical medicine in medical schools.

1942—Concentration of its efforts on reviewing the field of physical therapy and on making available reliable information about physical therapy in the treatment and rehabilitation of men disabled in combat. Assisted in revising the curriculum for schools for physical therapy technicians, preparation of the "Handbook on Amputations," investigation of audiometers and hearing aids.

1943—Devotion of most of its energies to re-evaluation of physical therapeutic measures and to making this information available to the profession in civilian and military service. Unavailability of raw materials and curtailment of production restricted greatly the manufacture of equipment and therefore the Council's consideration of apparatus. The requirements for acceptance of contraceptive devices were formulated. The "Manual on Physical Therapy" and the "Manual of Occupational Therapy" were printed. The booklet "Apparatus Accepted" was revised. Artificial respiration, both manual and mechanical, were again studied. The Council prepared a set of slides designed for use at war-time medical meetings and in schools for physical therapy. Hearing aids and ultraviolet lamps for disinfecting purposes received attention.

One of the chief activities of the Council has been the publication in the columns of the Journal of the American Medical Association of a series of articles intended to elucidate the physical and physiologic bases on which various devices of physical medicine depend for their therapeutic efficacy. In these articles, emphasis has been placed on the fundamentals of the general effect of physical medicine, namely the use of heat, massage, exercise, passive motion and postural rehabilitation. Other activities of the Council have been concerned with the advertising of apparatus and methods alleged to be of value in various conditions.

The Council on Physical Medicine also has devoted time to the promotion of education in the field of physical medicine for premedical and medical students. The results of these studies have been incorporated and published in the "Handbook of Physical Medicine." This book is published by the AMA and is available for distribution by writing to the Secretary of the Council.

Another educational measure of vital importance to the profession and to the public has been the supervision over advertising of acceptable products. Although evaluating advertising may not, on first thought, be considered an "educational activity," it is virtually medical instruction but the other way around. One of the most important functions of the Council is its constant vigilance to insure accurate and truthful claims in the advertising of acceptable products.

Investigation of apparatus and physical methods for therapeutic purposes is conducted primarily for the medical profession but nearly half of the inquiries which come to the office of the Secretary requesting information on physical medicine are from laymen. Physical medicine covers a wide field. Recently, the Council was called upon to define physical medicine. The following definition was adopted: *Physical medicine includes the employment of the physical and other effective properties of ultraviolet and infra-red radiant energy, heat, cold, water, electricity, massage, manipulation, exercise and mechanical devices for diagnosis and for physical and occupational therapy. In one sense, physical medicine is really applied biophysics.*

Obviously, the aforementioned definition can be interpreted to embrace many appliances, contrivances and methods used in the practice of medicine. At the beginning, many products were investigated and reported on, which later were found to be unsuitable for consideration by this Council. In 1936, for the information of the Board of Trustees, the Council compiled a list of devices which it would consider, and also a list of those which were regarded as outside the Council's purview. In general, the active list includes equipment for diagnosis and treatment which in one way or another is applied directly to the patient, or the physical energy generated by the device is applied directly to the patient. For example, an ultraviolet lamp or a diathermy apparatus comes under the purview of the Council, whereas a blood calculator or an autoclave does not. The Council on Physical Medicine, at its last meeting, revised the list of devices which it will consider to include:

Anesthesia Apparatus	Infra-red Generators
Anti-Allergy Apparatus	Inhalators and Resuscitators
Atomizers and Assorted Sprayers	Metabolism, Basal, Test Apparatus
Audiometers	Oxygen Therapy Apparatus
Contraceptives	Passive Vascular Exercise Apparatus
Diathermy Machines	
Electrocardiographs	Radioactive Materials
Electroencephalographs	Respirators
Fever Therapy Equipment	Stethoscopes (Electrical)
Galvanic Generators	Ultraviolet Radiation Equipment
Hearing Aids	
Heat Applicators	Vaporizers

The Council is essentially a judicial body. It considers apparatus which is offered to the medical profession for diagnostic and therapeutic purposes. Although, according to the "Official Rules," the Council considers apparatus which is submitted voluntarily, it does at times, on its own initiative, investigate products which its members believe are detrimental to the public welfare.

Most of the deliberations of the Council are carried out by means of a confidential bulletin which is sent to the members from the office of the Secretary every two weeks. These bulletins are so prepared and the material so presented that they provide a means of holding a meeting by mail every two weeks. In the bulletins, as in parliamentary practice, opportunities are provided for discussion and vote. Supplementing the bulletins, the Council holds at least one meeting a year and sometimes more when the amount of work requires it. At these meetings are considered problems which are not easily solved in deliberations by mail. In investigating apparatus, the Council examines devices submitted and obtains information to determine whether these devices or methods are of therapeutic value, are free from unnecessary danger, and are manufactured and marketed in conformity with the rules of the Council. The Secretary of the Council cannot vote, and decisions are reached by a three-fourths majority.

Published reports are based in part on investigations made by, or under the direction of, the Council and in part also on evidence or information supplied by the manufacturer or his agent. Such essential data are examined critically and are admitted only when they appear to conform to the evidence. The Council may, at its discretion, refuse to consider a device because of lack of evidence of its therapeutic value. After the Council has thoroughly investigated a product or device, reports expressing the opinion of the Council are prepared and sent to the proponents of the devices or methods. When the final report recommends acceptance, it is sent to the manufacturer for his information and for the purpose of determining whether errors have been made. When the final report is a rejection, reasonable time is allowed the proponents to conform to the rules and principles of the Council before the report is published.

Seal of the Council. A product which has been investigated and accepted is listed in the booklet "Apparatus Accepted." Manufacturers are permitted to utilize the seal of the Council in advertising literature and on their devices. For at least 10 years, the Council did not have a seal, but permitted only the statement "Accepted by the Council on Physical Medicine" to be used. Since that time, the Council has adopted a seal which has been altered twice. The acceptance of a product is for three years; therefore, the seal may be used for that period, after which the product is re-examined and, if again found acceptable, is again listed in the booklet "Apparatus Accepted."

SIGNIFICANT PROBLEMS

The Council has studied many important problems, but some of them stand out more than others.

Ultraviolet Radiation (1929-1931). One of the first problems investigated was the value of ultraviolet radiation in the treatment of disease. Prior to the organization of the Council, ultraviolet equipment had been recommended for the treatment of a large number of diseases. Several years elapsed before the Council could launch its research program and could investigate the therapeutic value of ultraviolet radiation. Finally, this was accomplished and the results were published in a report "Therapeutic Value of Ultraviolet Radiation."[1] Needless to say, when compared with the glowing array of claims in some of the early advertising matter, the indications for ultraviolet radiation, as confirmed by the Council, were greatly diminished.

Sunlamps (1931-1933). Furthermore, the Council was confronted with the problem of investigating sunlamps. These devices were sold to the public, and in many instances, with unsubstantiated claims. Investigation revealed that these devices play an important role in deposition of calcium, may prevent rickets, and may be an effective aid in promoting the soundness of bones and teeth. Sunlamps are also used for producing a tan. The Council found that there was only limited evidence to support the claims that exposure to ultraviolet radiation increases or improves the tone of the tissues of the body as a whole, stimulates metabolism, acts as a tonic, increases mental activity or tends to prevent colds.

Short Wave Diathermy (1933-1935). For many years, high frequency current had been used for the treatment of diseases. At the time the Council was organized, the so-called "spark gap" diathermy apparatus was employed almost exclusively. With the advent of the vacuum tube, newer methods were devised for applying high frequency energy to the tissues of the body. With this new development, much higher frequencies were generated, and claims and counter claims of therapeutic value multiplied. When first placed on the market, short wave diathermy was claimed to be useful for applying heat to the tissues and for its selective bactericidal and physiological effects. The claim for heat was substantiated but the other claims were not. This and other information was compiled in an article entitled "Medical Diathermy."[2]

Artificial Respiration (1936-1945). One of the most controversial problems that ever confronted the Council dealt with artificial

---

[1] J.A.M.A. *120:*620 (Oct. 24) 1942.
[2] J.A.M.A., *112:* 2046 (May 20) 1939.

respiration. There was a wide divergence of opinion as to the relative value of manual and mechanical artificial respiration. An early product investigated by the Council was the respirator which consisted of a large tank into which the paralyzed patient was placed on a movable cot. In this apparatus, negative pressure alternating between zero and several inches of negative water pressure, is generated within the tank and expands the chest, thus distending the lungs and drawing air into the air passages and the alveoli. This appliance was found to be highly valuable for maintaining artificial respiration over long periods of time. Since patients with respiratory paralysis have been kept alive in these devices for as long as five or six years, their efficiency can hardly be doubted.

The aforementioned appliance is not to be confused with emergency life-saving equipment some of which has been severely criticized. In emergency situations, the question as to whether the manual or mechanical method is superior has been widely debated. Finally, in order to get at the facts, research grants were made available by the Board of Trustees and the problem has been thoroughly investigated by the Council. A survey of the records of several large fire departments in the United States has furnished considerable information. The solution finally narrowed down to the question whether a resuscitator providing negative and positive pressure at the mouth and nostrils was dangerous, and whether sufficient ventilation of the lungs could thus be accomplished. Research proved conclusively that the devices were not dangerous and that when handled correctly, were effective in providing ample ventilation of the lungs. However, the Council recognized that, in the case of an emergency, an apparatus is seldom available at the site of the accident and that much precious time may be wasted in waiting for the equipment to arrive. It was also recognized that, when a person in a state of apnea is allowed to go without exchange of air for a period of seven minutes, he seldom, if ever, survives. Hence, the investigations re-emphasized the importance of beginning artificial respiration immediately and of employing an approved method of manual artificial respiration. The Council is continuing its research in this field.

Education (1931–1946). Although the Council on Physical Medicine is a judicial body, it has at times undertaken promotional activities. Six years after the Council was organized, its members became aware that the profession was not utilizing the simpler methods of physical medicine such as heat, massage and exercise to the fullest extent. The Council decided to appoint a group of Consultants on Education. These were chosen for their interest in physical medicine and for their ability to speak before medical and lay groups. They came from widely separated localities. Several articles were published in the Journal and arrangements were made at the Secretary's office for establishment of an information bureau. When requests for speakers came to the Council, a list of available speakers was furnished. Furthermore, the results of the efforts of these men and of the consultants were widely felt, and many speaking engagements were made.

Hearing Aids (1936–1946). With the help of its Consultants on Audiometers and Hearing Aids, an extensive study of hearing aids and hearing testing equipment has been made by the Council. The Council members believe that their consideration and testing of hearing aids and instruments has given valuable assistance to the profession and to the hard of hearing. Another study has resulted in the compilation of a method for calculating percentage loss of hearing. This method was developed at the request of certain courts of law, insurance agencies and compensation boards. The Council has made available to the profession and to the public a list of accepted hearing aids.

Amputations (1942–1946). Through the Consultants on Artificial Limbs, a study of amputations and prostheses has been made (both artificial arms and legs). At the time of this study, the papers prepared were compiled and published in the volume "Handbook on Amputations." The Council was the first official body to recognize the refrigeration method for anesthesia, now being employed with notable success for operations on the extremities.

Exhibits (1928–1946). With the cooperation of the Bureau of Exhibits, the Council has presented a number of exhibits in widely separated parts of the country. Some have been presented at the annual meetings of the American Medical Association, and others at state, local and other medical society meetings. The purpose of these exhibits has been to acquaint the physician with physical therapeutic methods and procedures. The following are examples of the subjects covered: (1) History of Physical Medicine, (2) Simple Apparatus, (3) Plans for Departments of Physical Therapy, (4) Effects of Heat, (5) Demonstration of Massage and Therapeutic Exercises, (6) Physics of Electro-Medical Equipment, (7) Physics of Hearing Aids and Audiometers, (8) Demonstration of Lip Reading and (9) Amputations and Artificial Limbs.

The Council has sponsored more elaborate exhibits which have been financed by grants from the Board of Trustees on such subjects as: (1) Diagnosis, treatment and care of lame backs, (2) rheumatism, and (3) physical medicine with special reference to rehabilitation.

PUBLICATIONS

Although there are some one-hundred seventy reprints of Council articles, there are the following publications edited by the Council and available at the present time: 1. Handbook of Physical Medicine; 2. Official Rules of the Council on Physical Medicine; 3. Apparatus Accepted; 4. Manual of Occupational Therapy; 5. Manual of Physical Therapy; 6. Handbook on Amputations.

TRENDS

At the time the Council was organized, the machine age had made itself felt in the practice of medicine. Electrical and mechanical gadgets were promoted commercially, with intriguing, but mainly inaccurate and misleading therapeutic claims and were looked upon with suspicion. The discoveries of Franklin and Galvani had been employed for many years for the electrical stimulation of injured nerves and atrophied muscles. Though more claims were promulgated for these currents, the vast majority of the therapeutic indications for the electrical appliances were not substantiated by valid evidence. The discovery of x-rays by Roentgen in 1895 and the discovery of natural radioactivity by Becquerel in 1896 focused the attention of physicians and of the public on the value of physical agents in the practice of medicine. Furthermore, Tesla had discovered that high frequency electrical currents were capable of passing through the body without causing neuro-muscular response and that they generated heat within the tissues. The infamous "discovery" of Abrams that diagnosis and treatment of disease by electronics were possible, created marked interest. The excellent work of the Bureau of Investigation of the A.M.A. disproved the promotional claims of Abrams. Finally, an artificial method for producing erythema on the untanned skin comparable to the effect of the sun was discovered and ultraviolet lamps were sold to physicians and to the public on the basis of unsubstantiated claims.

The earliest efforts of the new Council, therefore, were directed toward advising the profession about the therapeutic efficacy of products sold commercially. As the Council's knowledge grew and one problem after another was solved, greater attention was placed on the promotion of simple physical therapeutic agents such as heat, massage and exercise, for use by general practitioners.

At the conclusion of World War II, the Council found itself vitally interested in rehabilitation, occupational therapy, radium, radon radiation and radioactive isotopes. The discovery of the release of the energy within the atom will undoubtedly be probed by the Council to determine its diagnostic and therapeutic values.

THE COUNCIL ON FOODS AND NUTRITION

By J. R. Wilson, M.D.

THE RAPID EXPANSION OF the science of foods and nutrition since 1900 has been spectacular and far reaching in its applications to human needs. Food manufacturers and advertising agencies early were alert to the widespread public interest in nutrition. Health claims appeared in the advertising of many food products; some of these claims were true, but many were inadequately supported by scientific evidence. Thus it seemed to the Board of Trustees of the American Medical Association that an authoritative body was needed to evaluate nutritional claims in the advertising of food products. In 1931 they created the Committee on Foods which since 1929 had been a subcommittee of the Council on Pharmacy and Chemistry. As time passed the size of the Committee grew and in 1936 it became the Council on Foods—still later the *Council on Foods and Nutrition, a standing committee of the Board of Trustees of the American Medical Association.*

The Council encouraged the development of processed foods of greater nutritive merit. It encouraged informative advertising and accuracy in labeling. Many of the good things in this field that have been accomplished with the Council's assistance have been the result of voluntary cooperation on the part of food processors and advertising agencies.

In his opening remarks at the 1946 Council meeting, Chairman James S. McLester, former president of the American Medical Association, said, "In the same manner that the English, little by little, have constructed their Constitution, so, gradually, we are perfecting our code of Rules and Regulations by making new rules from time to time and modifying old ones as circumstances demand." Thus the earlier "Rules and Regulations" and "Decisions" have been extended to better influence and evaluate the quality, labeling and advertising of foods.

The Council is now composed of eleven persons selected because of their knowledge of those branches of learning directly concerned with food composition, nutrition, and health. To assist the Council members and facilitate their work, a headquarters staff of technical assistants is maintained at the office of the American Medical Association. The members of the Council are not paid for their services; they contribute their time and information freely. The salaries of the full time secretary and other members of the headquarters staff are paid from the general funds of the American Medical Association; there are no fees in connection with the consideration or acceptance of foods or food advertising.

The work of the Council is carried on through consultation and correspondence and by the issuance of bi-weekly reports to each Council member and the annual meetings are held in Chicago. Summaries of the Council's opinions and decisions are published in *The Journal of the American Medical Association*. The experience and scientific integrity of the members of the Council make these reports authoritative in the field of foods and nutrition.

The original purpose of the Council was to consider foods and food advertising in the light of established knowledge or of the best authoritative opinion concerning food and nutritional values, and according to rules adopted by the Council in the interest and for the protection of public health and public welfare. The Council has expanded its usefulness as new knowledge and new problems have appeared and to its original objective it has added the study, the interpretation and the dissemination of nutrition information by means of Council reports or Council sponsored reports to the profession, and through them to the public.

The Council foresees new responsibilities created by advances in the science of nutrition and especially do they see the need for nutrition education to advance hand in hand with research in the field.

SERVICES AND ACTIVITIES OF THE COUNCIL

Various services are rendered by the Council through the following programs:

I. The Food Acceptance Program

The Council was created originally for the purpose of discouraging unwarranted, incorrect or false advertising claims in the promotion and merchandising of food products. Although this activity of the Council is still a definite part of its program, the necessity of policing has markedly diminished with progressively increasing cooperation of the food industry. Furthermore some of the Council's activities in this field have become unnecessary with the advent of the increased scope of the activity of the Food and Drug Administration. Gradually a transition is taking place to the positive phase—that is, the encouragement of good practices in the field of food advertising.

A Summary of Procedure in Consideration of Foods. It is often asked how the Council goes about consideration of food products. Briefly the rules specify that the Council be provided with the following information:

1. Name of product, name of both manufacturer and distributor and information relative to the extent of area of sales and advertising.
2. A complete list of ingredients and quantities thereof entering into the product.
3. Detailed information on the culture, harvesting, collecting, delivery, storage, freshness, selection, ripeness, quality, freedom from contamination and sanitation of the food itself.
4. Precise and detailed description of all steps of manufacture from the initial stages of the raw materials to the final packing operation or shipment from the factory.
5. A report of a complete chemical analysis made by a reputable laboratory. This should include: data on moisture, ash or mineral matter, fat, protein, sugar, crude fiber and total carbohydrates (other than crude fiber), and sometimes other ingredients. From the composition the calory or fuel value may be calculated.
6. Claims for sterility must be supported by reports of microscopic and bacteriologic examination by a competent laboratory or bacteriologist.
7. Claims for vitamins must be confirmed either by references to authoritative studies in scientific literature or by direct biologic or chemical tests by a competent laboratory or analyst.
8. Conformity of the food product to terms and provisions of the federal Food, Drug and Cosmetic Act or federal food regulations must be assured.

The market sample of the food product, which it is desired to have considered, is noted and its label and advertising carefully reviewed by each member of the Council. If the Council members are assured that the food is wholesome and complies with the requirements as to ingredients, composition or nutritional values prescribed by them or by the government under federal food statutes and if the label and advertising are considered truthful and proper for the food, acceptance is granted for two years. At the time of acceptance, the manufacturer or distributor of the food product must agree to maintain the food and all advertising subsequent to acceptance in complete accord with the rules and regulations of the Council. Firms are permitted to use new claims in their advertising provided such claims are first submitted to and accepted by the Council. At the end of each two years the product and its advertising are submitted to further review to determine whether acceptance can be extended.

A food product is not eligible for the list of accepted foods if the manufacturer or distributor is unwilling to disclose any facts regarding its preparation. The Council is of the opinion that the public deserves to know the ingredients of the food it purchases. There are no sound arguments justifying secrecy about the composition of foods.

A food product is not accepted if it does not comply with requirements of composition, standards and labels formulated by the United States Food and Drug Administration.

A food product is not accepted if its identification label is not properly informative or if the trade name is misleading or deceptive by implication. An acceptable food label has the common name of the food or a descriptive statement of the identity of its ingredients arranged in the order of their decreasing proportions by weight in the food and in easily legible type in proximity to the trade name on the label.

A food product is not accepted if the submitted advertising used in its promotion contains unwarranted nutritional or health claims, even though the composition, method of manufacture, and labeling of the food product appear in other respects to conform to the requirements of the Council.

If a food and its advertising do not comply with the requirements of the Council, the manufacturer or distributor is notified and allowed a reasonable time to make recommended changes in the advertising or in the composition of the food. If the manufacturer is unwilling to make these changes, notice of nonacceptability is published in *The Journal of the American Medical Association*. When rejected foods or advertising comply with Council requirements they may become eligible for acceptance.

If the manufacturer is willing to make the advised changes, the food product is accepted and notice of acceptance is published in *The Journal of the American Medical Association*.

All food products accepted by the Council are entitled to display the Seal of Acceptance on the label and in advertising. Thus, the Council hopes to institute a system of self control by which the food industry will be governed within itself by established knowledge. for the welfare of the public and the entire food industry.

Significance of Acceptance. The acceptance of a food is intended to signify that the food product is as represented and that its label and the nutritional claims made for it are consistent with established knowledge or the best authoritative opinion. The acceptance of general educational advertising is intended to signify that the information presented and the claims made are consistent with established knowledge or the best authoritative opinion. Acceptance is intended to signify further that the manufacturer, distributor or sponsor has complied and has agreed to continue to comply with the Rules and Regulations and the General Decisions of the Council on Foods and Nutrition.

The Seal. The Seal is not a recommendation, neither is it a certificate or guarantee of purity. The Seal does mean that the product on which it appears is produced by a manufacturer who has supplied all the information required by the Council and does not seem to be in violation of any Council rule. The Seal is, in a sense, a token which means that the product and its advertising are in harmony with the Rules, Regulations and General Decisions of the Council.

The appearance of the Seal on fabricated foods does not indicate that such products are to be preferred over nutritionally desirable products in their natural state. All foods which stand accepted are considered by the Council to be wholesome but not necessarily to be preferred to simple natural foods.

All food products accepted by the Council are entitled to display the Seal of Acceptance on the label and advertising.

A. *Special Purpose Foods.* Since November, 1943, emphasis has been given to the consideration of special purpose foods, defined as those having therapeutic value or others promoted for the health, growth or development of special groups of the population, such as infants, convalescents or invalids. Most general purpose foods were discontinued from acceptance at this time. A few general purpose foods, such as vitamin D fortified milks, iodized salt and processed juices, remained within range of the Council's program, and others may be added because of the need for education concerning their use. Among these are the following: 1. Vegetables—strained and chopped for the young and special diets. 2. Fruits—strained and chopped for the young and special diets. 3. Meats—strained and chopped for the young and special diets. 4. Cereals fortified with minerals and vitamins for the young. 5. Special formula foods for infants. 6. Diet supplements for adults. 7. Special food for the aged. 8. Special low carbohydrate yielding foods for diabetics. 9. Special foods for invalids or convalescents. 10. Foods with therapeutic usefulness.

Each of these products, when submitted by the processor for Council action, is subjected to consideration of information furnished relative to manufacturing methods, composition, packaging, labeling, methods of promotion and advertising claims. Acceptance with permission to use the Council's Seal is for a period of two years after which there is a reappraisal. During the interval the Council endeavors to check all advertising or radio copy used by the makers of such foods.

B. *General Purpose Foods.* Only those general purpose foods are considered which have a wide public health significance. The Council sponsors several programs in this field.

1. THE VITAMIN D MILK PROGRAM. For those who remember the frequency, the severity and the gross defects produced by rickets

twenty-five years ago the paucity of rickets as seen today is little short of miraculous. Factors contributing to the decline of rickets are many and well known but among them the contribution of vitamin D in milk is presumably considerable. The amount of vitamin D consumed in fortified whole, evaporated and powdered milks is large.

In the early 'thirties the Council began its encouragement of this program believing that milk, being a good carrier and a form of food taken daily by children in almost all economic and cultural strata, was perhaps the most suitable food to choose for fortification with vitamin D. Thus it came about, with the cooperation of many groups that vitamin D came to be so widely used and such an important factor in this aspect of the public health program. One of the considerable and difficult problems today is the constant checking that is required of the many vitamin D milks on which the Council's Seal of Acceptance is used.

2. THE IODIZED SALT PROGRAM. For a long time the Council has lent its support to this project. It grants its Seal of Acceptance to manufacturers who produce table salt, containing specified amounts of iodine, and who otherwise comply with the rules of the Council. The amount of iodine specified for incorporation with table salt is designed only to prevent the iodine deficiency condition characterized by simple goiter.

In order to support this program still further the Council has published reports or has sponsored reports on the subject. One of the most recent of such articles, "Iodized Salt for the Prophylaxis of Endemic Goiter" (J.A.M.A. *130*.80 [Jan. 12] 1946) was written by Dr. O. P. Kimball who with Dr. David Marine published their epoch making early research in a paper entitled, "The Prevention of Simple Goiter" (J. Lab. & Clin. Med., *3*:40 [Oct.] 1917).

3. THE FRUIT JUICE PROGRAM. The object of this program is to stimulate the production of juices containing high natural levels of vitamin C. The Council therefore recently proposed to grant the use of its Seal to those producers of orange, grapefruit and tomato juice who, through careful attention to selection and packing methods are able to produce juices which meet standards set by the Council.

The reasons for this program are numerous but one of the chief reasons is the persistence of some clinically recognizable frank scurvy and the assumption that there exists a very much larger number of cases of less severe deficiency of ascorbic acid.

All of the packers of Council accepted concentrated citrus juices have agreed to maintain a level of vitamin C which will give a reconstituted juice capable of meeting the vitamin C standards set up for whole juices.

II. *The Flour Enrichment Program*

The Council, one of the first groups to discuss and encourage flour enrichment, has participated in the inception and growth of this procedure which has become one of the notable public health movements of the past decade. The role played by the Council in this matter, briefly sketched, is as follows:

In Bulletin No. 110 (Nov. 1944) of the National Research Council, the following tribute is paid: "The Council on Foods and Nutrition of the American Medical Association provided early leadership in the movement to make proper use of vitamins and minerals to improve the nutritive quality of staple foods." At their March 12, 1936, meeting the Council (J.A.M.A. *107:*39 [July 4] 1936) discussed the question of fortified foods and announced a policy in these words: "If in exceptional cases a general need for vitamin (or inorganic salt) intake above that afforded by the usual mixed diet of common foods is indicated, the Council shall require (a) acceptable and convincing evidence that there is a need for enhanced amounts of vitamins (or inorganic salts) in the general food supply, and (b) that the food vehicles proposed for the distribution of such vitamins (or inorganic salts) are suitable and appropriate."

A joint committee of the Council on Foods and Nutrition and the Council on Pharmacy and Chemistry, in December, 1938, took important favorable action referable to the use of vitamins in certain staple foods including flour. At that time, as today, the Council regards as undesirable the indiscriminate fortification of foods with specialized food nutrients. On the other hand a standardized fortification of certain cheaper foods which are widely used was and is regarded as deserving encouragement.

Thus the Council on Foods and Nutrition proceeded to take action and appointed Dr. Cowgill to prepare a report on the evidence indicating the need for restoring lost thiamine to the American diet (Cowgill, G. R.: The Need for the Addition of Vitamin B to Staple American Foods (J.A.M.A. *113:*2146 [Dec. 9] 1939). Furthermore the Council adopted, with minor reservations (Mar. 18, 1939), the resolution of the joint committee and published it in the form of a report entitled, "Fortification of Foods with Vitamins and Minerals." (J.A.M.A. *113*.681 [Aug. 19] 1939). There were two notable qualifications, namely, (1) that only such vitamins and minerals should be added for which a wider distribution was considered desirable from the standpoint of public health, and, (2) that for general purpose foods the additions in the case of products not previously accepted (vitamin D milk, vitamin A fortified margarine, and iodized salt having already been accepted), should be related to the amounts naturally present in foods of the class. A sharp distinction was thus drawn between fortification and restoration. Encouragement was given to the restorative additions of thiamine, riboflavin and iron to cereal products such as flour and white bread.

Stimulated by this action, several millers tried the experimental restoration of thiamine to white flour. Bakers also began experimenting. Dr. Wilder, who has been actively interested in this movement since its inception and from whom most of this history was obtained, relates with Dr. R. R. Williams in "Enrichment of Flour and Bread—A History of the Movement" (Bul. Nat. Res. Council, No. 110 [Nov.] 1944) that, "Likewise the American Medical Association policy served as a guide to subsequent action by the Food and Nutrition Board of the National Research Council, and influenced later actions taken by the Food and Drug Administration of the Federal Security Agency in the matter of enriched flour and enriched bread."

Thus from its inception, as one of the great public health movements, the Council has been actively interested in this program as its numerous reports indicate. Among the more recent reports are, "Enriched 80 Per Cent Extraction Flour" (J.A.M.A. *131:*399 [June 1] 1946) and "Standards Established for Enriched Macaroni" (to be published).

III. *The Corn Enrichment Program*

Corn enrichment is more difficult but it likewise represents a problem which has wide public health implications in areas where corn is a principal article of diet. This project is an outgrowth of the flour enrichment program and is still in its infancy.

IV. *The Proteins, their Hydrolysates, and Amino Acids*

Growing general interest stimulated by current researches and perhaps other factors led to the publication of a series of articles prepared under the auspices of the Council in 1945. Collectively these articles constituted a small booklet called "Protein Nutrition in Health and Disease." It is hoped that in the near future this subject can be treated again and more extensively.

Early in 1946, a joint committee of the Council on Pharmacy and Chemistry and the Council on Foods and Nutrition was appointed and later met for the purpose of discussing means of evaluating the merits of protein hydrolysates and amino acid mixtures. Although these activities do not constitute the earliest interest of the Council in this subject it does give evidence of continued recognition of its responsibility in this field.

V. *The Nutrition Teaching Program*

Under this heading logically falls many of the present and contemplated activities of the Council. While not conducting classes or doing ward teaching as such, the Council has gathered and presented factual material in the form of reports, Council sponsored articles and scientific exhibits. Not only is factual material presented, but interpretations of new nutritional information are made by or obtained by the Council. This material, though slanted to the practitioner, is for the eventual benefit of his patients—the people of the United States. It is hoped that this material will also reach the medical student and the intern.

Not all of the efforts of the Council can be spoken of strictly as having an immediate bearing on the practitioner. Some of the work of the Council while apparently remote from this main objective, is none the less indirectly important to the doctor and his patient. Reference here is made to the stimulus that the Council has been in the field of improved, informatively labeled, and honestly advertised foods.

Some of the Council projects that contribute to its nutrition teaching program are:

A. Council Reports. Matters of concern or of interest in the field of nutrition are the subject of reports from the Council as a whole. In final form these reports are the result of the comments and criticisms of all of the Council members and represent the opinion of the Council as a whole. These reports are printed in the pages of the Journal just preceding the editorial pages.

B. Council Sponsored Reports. These are the reports of individuals or groups on matters of nutritional interest. The authors are chosen for recognized eminence in their given fields. Their papers too are reviewed by the Council members but are not as thoroughly revised as Council reports because it is recognized that these papers represent the interpretations of the authors and are not necessarily completely concurred in by the Council as a whole. A series of these reports when compiled and grouped have made such valued publications as: "The Handbook of Nutrition," "The Vitamins," and "Protein Nutrition in Health and Disease."

C. Scientific Exhibits. Scientific exhibits have been long recognized by the Board of Trustees of the American Medical Association as constituting a valuable method of showing the development of a field of scientific knowledge. The Council has concurred in this feeling and has prepared many exhibits with the help of the Committee on Scientific Exhibits for use at the Association's annual conventions. These exhibits are also loaned to state societies and to other organizations. The Council plans to continue to contribute its share of this form of teaching material. Material will also be provided for use by lay groups.

D. *Inquiries by Letter.* The central office of the American Medical Association receives numerous inquiries from physicians and laymen. The questions come from the United States mainly but many are from abroad. Those having a bearing on the subjects of foods and nutrition are referred to the Council office where a full answer is prepared as accurately and as quickly as possible.

E. *Informal Consultation Service.* Informal consultations are given whenever requested to persons visiting the Council office. The majority of these are held with representatives of industry who wish to secure the viewpoint of the Council on matters of foods, their utilization, their preparation, advertising etc. These consultations are regarded as important and are so treated because it is felt that here is another opportunity to exert some influence in the direction of improving the nutritional environment.

F. *Review of Educational Advertising Copy.* In addition to reviewing the advertising copy of foods and granting the use of its seal to those which it accepts, the Council reviews and grants the use of its seal to acceptable educational advertising. This may be regarded as a very important part of the service rendered by the Council. Among the organizations who have currently submitted such material in the form of published advertisements, booklets or books are: American Meat Institute, Cereal Institute, National Live Stock and Meat Board, American Can Company (The Canned Food Reference Manual), The Evaporated Milk Association, National Dairy Council, and National Association of Margarine Manufacturers.

G. *Review of Journal Advertising of Ineligible Food Products.* Certain foods which are ineligible for consideration by the Council because they do not come within its scope may advertise in Association publications but only if the advertising copy is acceptable. One of the added functions of the Council is to review these advertisements and to offer advice respecting their acceptability.

Thus in these several ways does the Association, through its Council help to favorably affect the advertising claims of food advertisers. The improvement is considerable as a perusal of food advertising now and of the 'twenties or earlier will demonstrate.

The cooperation of food manufacturers and advertising agencies with the work of the Council and their understanding of its motives are now of a high order.

VI. Nutrition Education in Schools of Medicine

"Teaching has not kept pace with the advancement of knowledge in the science of nutrition. This Council can well take upon itself, therefore, the additional function of promoting the teaching of nutrition in medical schools and hospitals. I should like at the outset, however, to offer objection, as have Dr. Wilder and Dr. Youmans, to the segregation of nutrition in a single water-tight compartment. The fundamentals should be taught, I assume, by the physiologist and the biochemist, but the practical application of this science should be integrated with the other teaching in all of the several clinical branches." These are the remarks of the Council chairman, Dr. James McLester, at the April, 1946 meeting. Thus at this time the Council renewed and intensified its interest in the subject of nutrition education. It has authorized a survey which is now in progress.

THE COUNCIL MEMBERS

When first in 1929, the Council, then a Committee on Foods of the parent Council on Pharmacy and Chemistry, had its inception the distinguished names of its members were: Dr. Eugene F. DuBois; Dr. Morris Fishbein; Dr. L. B. Mendel; Dr. McKim Marriott; Dr. H. C. Sherman.

Of this original group Dr. Fishbein has served continuously and is now contributing his generous share to the Council's many activities. Eight other members have served for nine or more years.

The fact that the Council on Foods and Nutrition has contributed to the stature of the American Medical Association can be attributed largely to the quality, the integrity, the energy and vision of these who have served as members. Their names, the date of their first affiliation with the Council, and the length of their service are as follows:

```
1929 Eugene DuBois.................................3 years
1929 Morris Fishbein..........................1929 to present
1929 Raymond Hertwig, Secretary.......................6 years
1929 Lafayette B. Mendel*.............................5 years
1929 McKim Marriott*..................................2 years
1929 Henry C. Sherman.................................1 year
1930 E. M. Bailey.....................................9 years
1930 Julius H. Hess*..................................4 years
1930 Grover Powers....................................9 years
1931 Philip C. Jeans..........................1931 to present
1931 Russell M. Wilder........................1931 to present
1933 Edwin O. Jordan*.................................4 years
```

1933 James S. McLester	1933 to present
1933 Mary Swartz Rose*	9 years
1934 Joseph Brennemann*	6 years
1934 Lydia J. Roberts	1934 to present
1936 Franklin C. Bing, Secretary	7 years
1937 Howard B. Lewis	1937 to present
1939 George R. Cowgill	1939 to present
1939 Irvine McQuarrie	6 years
1940 Culver S. Ladd	1940 to present
1940 Tom D. Spies	5 years
1941 C. A. Elvehjem	1941 to present
1943 George K. Anderson, Secretary	2 years
1944 John B. Youmans	1944 to present
1945 Ashley A. Weech	1 year
1946 Harold C. Stuart	1946 to present
1946 James R. Wilson, Secretary	1946 to present

* Deceased

The present membership of the Council on Foods and Nutrition, a standing committee of the Board of Trustees of the American Medical Association is as follows:

George R. Cowgill, Ph.D., Professor of Nutrition, Yale Nutrition Laboratory, Yale University, New Haven, Conn.

C. A. Elvehjem, Ph.D., Professor of Biochemistry, University of Wisconsin, Madison, Wis.

Morris Fishbein, M.D., Editor of THE JOURNAL of the American Medical Association, Chicago.

Philip C. Jeans, M.D., Professor of Pediatrics, University of Iowa School of Medicine, Iowa City.

Culver S. Ladd, B.S., Production and Marketing Administration, United States Department of Agriculture, Washington, D. C.

Howard B. Lewis, Ph.D., Professor of Biological Chemistry, Medical School; Director of College of Pharmacy, University of Michigan, Ann Arbor, Mich., Vice Chairman.

James S. McLester, M.D., Professor of Medicine, University of Alabama, Birmingham, Ala., Chairman.

Lydia J. Roberts, Ph.D., Department of Home Economics, The University of Chicago, Chicago.

Harold C. Stuart, M.D., School of Public Health, Harvard University, Boston, Mass.

Russell M. Wilder, M.D., Ph.D., Professor of Medicine, Mayo Foundation, Mayo Clinic, Rochester, Minn.

John B. Youmans, M.D., School of Medicine, University of Illinois, Chicago.

James R. Wilson, M.D., Secretary of the Council, American Medical Association, 535 North Dearborn Street, Chicago.

Through the Council as a focal point, new and pertinent nutrition information should be funnelled out in increasing volume to the physician in practice, to the teacher, to the medical student and through them to the people—our citizens. Likewise through the Council, the nutritional needs of the people as expressed by their physicians should be funnelled back to the producers and processors of foods and to interested government agencies.

JUDICIAL COUNCIL

By Morris Fishbein, M.D.

ONCE THE AMERICAN MEDICAL ASSOCIATION had adopted its "Principles of Medical Ethics," members began to be concerned with enforcement. In 1854 a motion was adopted that a committee be appointed charged with investigating charges "made against gentlemen in fellowship with this Association of sustaining proprietary medicines by certificate or otherwise." Apparently the committee was not appointed. However, in 1858 the first Committee on Ethics was appointed. It included:

> Dr. John Watson, New York
> Dr. John C. Dalton, Lowell, Mass.
> Dr. G. Everson, Philadephia, Pa.
> Dr. Frank H. Hamilton, Buffalo, N. Y.
> Dr. P. C. Gaillard, Charleston, S. C.

From that time onward the committees on ethics considered various problems with methods of practice. Then in 1860 the Committee on Ethics was asked to investigate the conditions demanded for a diploma of doctor of medicine in the various medical schools in the universities of Europe. In the ensuing years several such statements were published.

CASE OF DR. MONTROSE A. PALLEN

One of the most significant cases to come before the Committee on Medical Ethics was that of Dr. Montrose A. Pallen who was accused, following the Civil War, of having given aid to the enemy. The charges were found to be without foundation and he was restored to membership.

From time to time the Committee on Medical Ethics was asked to investigate the rise of specialization. In 1868 the committee was concerned with the entrance of women into medical practice. The committee, headed by Dr. Henry I. Bowditch of Massachusetts, strongly advocated the recognition of regularly educated and otherwise well qualified female physicians.

CULTIST PRACTICE

Next came the question of cultist practice, homeopathists and eclectics. In 1870 a committee, headed by Dr. Alfred Stillé of Pennsylvania, declared such cult practice "plainly in violation of the Code of Ethics."

The difficulties occasioned by such actions were to disturb the Association for many years. They resulted in the formation of two distinct medical societies in the state of New York and there was no compromising of the disturbance until the period following the reorganization in 1901.

These were the basic questions that disturbed the Committee on Medical Ethics until the reorganization. We find the committee considering the right of alumni associations to be represented by delegates, of certain medical schools of which a majority of the faculty are not members to be represented; certain hospitals and some medical colleges had on their staff men who had never been licensed to practice.

FORMATION OF JUDICIAL COUNCIL

Until 1873 it had been the custom of the president to appoint the Committee on Ethics. Then the By-Laws were amended so that the Committee on Ethics was to consist of nine members to serve for three years and until their successors were appointed. "Their duties shall be to examine and adjudicate all questions of a personal character, including complaints and protests, and all questions on credentials that may be referred to them by the Association. The decisions of the committee shall be final, until reversed by the Association, but no appeal from their decisions shall be brought before the Association until the following year."

After considerable debate, Dr. N. S. Davis offered as a substitute for this resolution the following amendment to the By-Laws:

XI. Judicial Council

"A Council, consisting of twenty-one members, shall be appointed by the Nominating Committee, whose duty it shall be to take cognizance of and decide all questions of an ethical or judicial character that may arise in connection with the Association. Of the twenty-one members of the Council first appointed, the seven first named in the list shall hold office one year, and the second seven named shall hold office two years.

"With these exceptions the term of office of members of the Council shall be three years, seven being appointed by the Nominating Committee annually.

"The said Council shall organize by choosing a President and Secretary, and shall keep a permanent record of the proceedings. The decisions of said Council on all matters referred to it by the Association shall be final, and shall be reported to the Association at the earliest practicable moment.

"All questions of a personal character, including complaints and protests, and all questions on credentials, shall be referred at once, after the report of the Committee of Arrangements or other presentation, to the Judicial Council and without discussion."

This substitute proposal was unanimously adopted. The first Judicial Council to be appointed included therefore, for the

Three Year Term:
- Dr. William Brodie, Michigan
- Dr. N. S. Davis, Illinois
- Dr. E. L. Howard, Maryland
- Dr. William O. Baldwin, Alabama
- Dr. H. W. Dean, New York
- Dr. J. P. Logan, Georgia
- (one vacancy)

Two Year Term:
- Dr. L. S. Joynes, Virginia
- Dr. R. N. Todd, Indiana
- Dr. H. F. Askew, Delaware
- Dr. J. E. Morgan, District of Columbia
- Dr. Samuel Lilly, New Jersey
- Dr. S. N. Benham, Pennsylvania
- Dr. D. Dunlap, Ohio

One Year Term:
- Dr. J. K. Bartlett, Wisconsin
- Dr. Edwin Powell, Illinois,
- Dr. R. H. Gale, Kentucky
- Dr. S. Gratz Moses, Missouri
- Dr. J. C. Hughes, Iowa
- Dr. S. M. Bemiss, Louisiana
- Dr. J. R. Bronson, Massachusetts

Few questions of great importance were referred to the Judicial Council during the years that followed. Most of their rulings involved determination of whether or not delegates were entitled to their positions in the representative body and the question of admission of homeopathists into medical societies. In 1881, however, business for the Judicial Council had so greatly accumulated that Dr. Nathan Smith Davis developed some rules for guiding the actions of the Judicial Council in the transaction of its business. Among these the following was of special interest:

"No more hypothetical questions asking for expressions of opinion shall be entertained by the Council, and no questions of any character shall be entertained, except such as are referred to the Council by action of the American Medical Association."

The years that followed still were primarily concerned with the admission of cultists. Then there came to plague the Judicial Council the problem of patents, copyrights and trademarks. In 1883 the Judicial Council was concerned with the question as to whether or not every delegate and permanent member should sign a pledge to support the Code of Ethics before admission to the Association. There was a case of one physician who had carefully erased certain portions of the pledge before signing.

In 1886 the Judicial Council was disturbed by advertising of physicians. From time to time it was requested to make revisions in both the Principles of Ethics and in the By-Laws which were routinely submitted to the House of Delegates for final approval.

Following the reorganization of the American Medical Association in 1901 and the adoption of the new Constitution and By-Laws, the functions of the Judicial Council became much more definitely established. Since that time many of the great leaders of the American Medical Association have held the position of chairman of the Judicial Council and under their leadership decisions of conduct have been made which have been vital to the maintenance of the highest standards in medical practice.

In the "Index and Digest of Official Actions of the American Medical Association" beginning with the year 1904 and published in 1942 there appears a complete subject index of the actions of the Judicial Council with digests of its special decisions.

REVISION OF COUNCIL

In 1911 an amendment to the By-Laws was introduced and adopted so that the Judicial Council from that time on included five members, nominated one each year by the president of the Association and confirmed by the House of Delegates. The Constitution and By-Laws have been amended from time to time but the section relating to the Judicial Council has been modified but little since 1911.

The first Judicial Council, after this amendment, included:

> Dr. Frank Billings, Illinois
> Dr. James E. Moore, Minnesota
> Dr. A. B. Cooke, Tennessee
> Dr. Alexander Lambert, New York
> Dr. Hubert Work, Colorado

The council organized at the meeting held in Los Angeles and elected Dr. Frank Billings, Chicago, as chairman. The Council at once drew up some rules for its functioning and they were adopted in the session in 1911 by the House of Delegates. They also prepared a redraft of the Principles of Medical Ethics.

In the meeting of 1912 the Judicial Council was asked to formulate amendments to the Constitution and By-Laws, to consider an invitation that had come from the Australian Medical Society, to consider a By-Law providing for a speaker for the House of Delegates and to investigate the secret division of fees and contract practice. In response to the first question, it presented an extensive series of amendments to the Constitution and By-Laws which clarified only the question of membership. It expressed its appreciation of the invitation to Australia. It did not consider it desirable that there be a speaker in the House of Delegates—an action which was, incidentally, changed by a later Council. On the question of division of fees and the giving of commissions, it spoke most wisely:

"It is interesting to note that in the replies given stating whether or not secret fee-splitting was justifiable, there was 77.3 per cent, who answered in the negative, 13.4 per cent who answered in the affirmative, and 9.3 per cent who were doubtful.

"By the term secret splitting of fees here used is meant the sharing by two or more men in a fee which has been given by the patient supposedly as the reimbursement for the service of one man alone. By secrecy is meant that the division of the fee is done without the knowledge of the patient or some representative of the family. It necessarily does not include any agreement between the patient or his representative made with one or more physicians or surgeons. It also does not include any payment to bona fide assistants with or without the knowledge of the patient or his representative. It does include, however, those cases in which the term assistant is used as a subterfuge to obtain a part of the fee which otherwise could not be rightfully claimed. The term commission here used refers to those rebates, 'rake offs,' or pro rata moneys sent for referring patients or favors received and not for medical and surgical services rendered to the donor by the receiver."

FEE SPLITTING AND CONTRACT PRACTICE

The following is a discussion of the reasons for and the growth of fee-splitting and its different forms, including percentage to hospitals, and contract practice:

"The remedies for the conditions here discussed lie partly in the hands of the American Medical Association, partly in the hands of the constituent state and county bodies and partly in the hands of the medical profession as individuals. The secret splitting of fees and the giving or receiving of commissions are best remedied by the profession announcing that it demands publicity in all transactions between patients and the members of the profession and refuses to sanction the retention on the roster of any of its organizations the names of those who are proved guilty of these practices.

"The replies received by the Judicial Council on the matter of contracts in mines and railroads and factories show that in some states the contracts are just and that the recompense to the physician is in ratio to services rendered and is adequate in amount for such services. On the other hand there are other replies which show the reverse. The Judicial Council believes the remedy for these evils resides in the county societies, that these societies should use their influence and power not to condemn the physician who must take the contract by ostracizing him, but to prevent underbidding for these contracts below what would give a fair reward for medical services rendered. So, too, in the matter of lodge practice, the Judicial Council believes it to be the duty of the local county societies to endeavor to reform and not alone to condemn the abuses of lodge practice."

The Judicial Council recommended for adoption by the House of Delegates the following resolutions:

"Resolved, That any member of the American Medical Association found guilty of secret fee-splitting or of giving or receiving commissions shall cease to be a member of the American Medical Association.

"Resolved, That the House of Delegates of the American Medical Association recommends to each constituent body that it endeavor through the action of its various county societies to reform the various abuses of lodge practice in their separate communities in order that the lodges may give an adequate service to its members and an honorable remuneration to the medical men."

In 1914 the Judicial Council investigated an appeal for funds from the Home for Widows and Orphans of Physicians.

Frequently it had to act on definitions, differences of opinion as to the significance of various statements in the Constitution and By-Laws and in the Principles of Medical Ethics.

ADVERTISING BY PHYSICIANS

In 1914 it discussed advertising in the public press as follows:

"In pursuance of its duty to investigate general professional conditions and all matters pertaining to the relations of physicians to one another and to the public, the Judicial Council calls the attention of the House of Delegates to the subject of advertising in the public press by physicians. The Judicial Council finds that the profession is restive under the flagrant misuse of the public press by certain members of the profession and certain prominent and nonprominent Fellows of the American Medical Association.

"The Principles of Ethics of the American Medical Association define clearly the methods which are objectionable for physicians to use to bring themselves into the public notice in their endeavor to gain a livelihood. They state clearly the methods by which a man may rise by honorable endeavor to the fame of a well-earned reputation, and suggest the different methods by which a man may gain an unsavory notoriety. The standards of the medical profession have always demanded that physicians shall not exploit their ability or achievement to the laity. The medical profession condemns such advertising as quackery. The refraining from or the employment of advertising is the clearly defined difference between a reputable physician and a quack—the physician, one who quietly, through his professional work and attainments, seeks by daily honorable dealings to spread the truth among his patients; the quack, one who endeavors to obtain his livelihood by playing on the credulity of the ignorant and the timid, imposing on the public statements known to be false, stopping at nothing in his effort to enhance his notoriety or fill his pocket."

At the same time it encouraged proper publicity for scientific medicine but hesitated to recommend that the names of physicians be used in connection with this publicity. Its discussions of the subject were extensive but the final resolution offered read:

"Resolved, That it is the sense of the House of Delegates of the American Medical Association that each county society should constitute a publicity committee whose duties shall be to give to the daily press accurate information on all medical matters of interest to the public, that this shall be freely given without the mentioning of names or from whence the information comes, and that this committee shall further act in an advisory capacity to all physicians of its society in questions relating to publications other than in the medical press. Be it further

"Resolved, That the Secretary of the American Medical Association be instructed to forward this resolution, with the reasons calling it forth, to the Secretary of each constituent state association, with the request that it be transmitted to each component society of that constituent association."

PATENTS AND COMMISSIONS

Of special concern in the years that followed were patents and commissions from the makers of instruments. In 1915 it drafted a By-Law for the election of a speaker in the House of Delegates. On another occasion the Judicial Council dealt with the eligibility of various candidates for the presidency of the Association. The Council spent a great deal of time studying the offer of the Mayo Clinic of the patent on thyroxin. From time to time it passed on the question of changing the number of the trustees of the Association.

CULTISM

When osteopathy began to be prominent, the Judicial Council spoke of the relationship of the scientific physician to the cultist. On this subject it said:

"In a communication received from a group clinic, inquiry is made as to the ethics involved in the admission of an osteopath into the clinic group. It seems that an osteopath had actually been admitted into this particular group and that a complaint had been registered with the county medical society. The Judicial Council is of the opinion that it is not in keeping with the Principles of Medical Ethics of the American Medical Association for members to associate themselves with osteopaths; that the by-laws of component societies not in conflict with by-laws of their state associations or of the American Medical Association cannot be ignored; that under the Principles of Medical Ethics, physicians cannot act with or support those who base their practice on an exclusive dogma or sectarian system; and that physicians associated with an osteopath in a clinic or otherwise cannot be debarred from membership in the American Medical Association in the absence of action by their component society.

"From another source, inquiry was made of the right of a county medical society to withhold membership or to withdraw the privileges of membership from a registered physician who graduated from an osteopathic school. This inquiry came from Texas, in which state a diploma from a high grade osteopathic school entitles the holder thereof to take the examination by the state board of medical examiners for a license to practice medicine. This examination must be in all respects the same as that to which a graduate of a medical school is required to submit, and the graduate of the osteopathic school who passes the examination successfully is granted the same kind of license to practice medicine as that granted to a graduate of a reputable medical school. The Judicial Council is of the opinion that a legally registered physician who has complied with the requirements of the law in securing a license by the state to practice medicine and who, having secured such license, has not practiced or claimed to practice sectarian medicine, but has conformed to the requirements of the Principles of Medical Ethics of the American Medical Association, and who has been accepted into membership in a county medical society, cannot be expelled therefrom without cause.

"It seems to be true that a concerted movement has been organized covering most of the states, to secure entrance to 'regular' hospitals for osteopaths and chiropractors, and possibly for followers of other sects and their patients. In response to several inquiries, received almost simultaneously, the Judicial Council formulated and submitted the following opinion:

"The board of control of any hospital (not maintained by general taxation) has the legal right for reasons sufficient to the board to refuse the privileges of the hospital at any time to any practitioner regardless of his so-called school of practice. The fact that the person applying for permission to bring to and treat in the hospital a particular patient is licensed by the state to practice does not alter the situation. The medical staff of a hospital likewise has the moral right to refuse to accept as an associate any person whom the staff may consider objectionable for reasons sufficient to the staff, and should insist on maintaining that right."

Later the Judicial Council was asked to define the difference between a sectarian and a physician, and evolved these two interesting definitions:

"In compliance with several requests received, the Judicial Council has formulated and adopted for purposes that may be served, the following definition of the term 'sectarian':

" 'A sectarian,' as applied to medicine, is one who in his practice follows a dogma, tenet or principle based on the authority of its promulgator to the exclusion of demonstration and experience.'

"Requests have also been received for the definition of 'physician,' and the following is submitted for consideration and for use in such purposes as may be served by such a definition:

" 'A physician' is one who has acquired a contemporary education in the fundamental and special sciences, comprehended in the general term 'medicine' used in its unrestricted sense, and who has received the degree of Doctor of Medicine from a medical school of recognized standing."

In connection with these definitions it discussed also the relationship of physicians and cultists as follows:

"Several communications addressed to the Council have raised various questions as to the relationships of physicians with cultists—the attitude that should be assumed by the physician called into a case under treatment by a cult practitioner, whether a pathologist in a hospital under the direction or regular physicians should refuse to examine material submitted by a cultist, and other questions of more or less similar nature. In the opinion of the Judicial Council, these are questions that are not sharply to be defined by words. In his relations with irregular practitioners, the physician should be bound by the Principles of Medical Ethics, Chapter II, Article I, Section 1, while bearing in mind the considerations set forth in Sections 6 and 7 of the same chapter and article, and with due consideration for the observations made in the Conclusion on Page 23 of the Principles of Medical Ethics of the American Medical Association. In such matters the policy must be governed largely by the circumstances governing the individual case; by the conditions existing in the special community; and by the realization that the first duties of the physician are the care of the sick and, at the same time, the upholding of the dignity and honor of the profession."

CORPORATION PRACTICE

Finally as there began to be formed commercial corporations selling the practices of physicians and large clinics with physicians employed on salaries, the Judicial Council was asked to determine the significance of the interference of a third party between doctor and patient. The question at issue involved specifically the Life Extension Institute which was examining patients in its offices and also rendering reports on specimens sent by mail. In brief, the Judicial Council said in 1925:

"At the last annual session of the Association, held in Chicago, the Judicial Council presented to the House of Delegates a supplementary report dealing with the specific question: Shall the medical profession vend its products directly to the consumer or shall it sell them to a middleman or third party? This question was discussed in the report of the Council from the standpoint of the independence of the physician, the interest of the invividual patient, the encouragement of medical progress, and from the standpoint of what is best for the public. The conclusion of the Council, which was endorsed and acciepted by the House of Delegates, was to the effect that the proper person to make pereodic examinations and to give advice relative thereto is the family physician, aided whtn necessary by local specialists; and that indirect medical service through a third party could not redound to the benefit either of the public or of the physician. In submiting that report to the House of Delegates, neither the Council as a whole nor any individual member of the Council was guided by any motive other than a desire to bring the questions considered in the report directly to the attention of the members of the American Medical Association and its duly elected delegates, in the hope that the best interests of the medical profession and of the public served by its members might be conserved. It was the purpose of the Council to discuss fundamental principles, and its supplementary report was offered on that basis. It was not the purpose of the Council to call into question the honesty or the sincerity of purpose of any person or group.

"The Judicial Council desires to express again its firm conviction that the benefits of scientific medicine cannot be adequately delivered to the individual through the medium of a third party, and that the communication of results of physical examination and the general advice with which it should be associated should go directly from the individual physician to his patients. As was stated in the report of the Council submitted at the Chicago session, the relation between the patient and the physician is an individual matter, and anything that disturbs this relationship is detrimental to the best interests of the patient.

"The Committee of the Whole recommends that the House of Delegates reaffirm confidence in the Judicial Council and that it endorse and approve their present report.

"It is the sense of this Committee of the Whole that every Fellow and member of the American Medical Association should live up to the spirit of the Report of the Judicial Council."

CONTRACT PRACTICE

By 1926 there arose the question of contract practice. For this the Judicial Council presented the following definition:

"Because of many inquiries received, it has been thought necessary to define the term 'contract practice.' The following definition, arrived at after very thorough consideration and prolonged discussion, is presented for the consideration of the House of Delegates:

"By the term 'contract practice,' as applied to medicine, is meant the carrying out of an agreement between a physician or group of physicians as principals or agents and a corporation, organization or individual, to furnish partial or full medical services to a group or class of individuals for a definite sum or for a fixed rate per capita."

In 1927 came a definition of the word "clinic":

"The Judicial Council has been asked to give a definition of the word 'clinic,' as used by those doing so-called group practice. Originally the word in its verbal form meant 'to lie down,' or 'to recline.' And in its nominal form it signified that on which one lies or reclines; namely, a bed. Owing to the fact that most persons who are really ill are confined to bed, the word acquired the somewhat specific meaning of a bed of sickness. With the recognition of the importance of practical instruction at the bedside in the teaching of medicine, the term 'clinique' was introduced in France to designate an insitution or school where students were taught by the examination and treatment of patients in their presence. Clinique was Anglicized into clinic, but its application to a teaching institution has always been retained up to very recent times. In a changing world words frequently acquire meanings not contained in their original significance. The term 'clinic' was adopted comparatively recently by a few physicians and by a greater number of groups of physicians to designate their offices or workshops, perhaps for want of a better term, perhaps for the purpose of conveying to the public mind the idea of greater importance or of institutional dignity. Whether or not the use of the term in this connection has come to stay cannot be predicted; but that its use in this way does not find justification in the original significance of the word is evident."

UNIVERSITY MEDICAL PRACTICE

As the universities and colleges began examining their students at a fixed fee per year, the Judicial Council was requested to investigate the matter as to the extent to which this practice prevailed. Later it was concerned with cooperative diagnostic laboratories and again, year after year, with questions of corporation practice.

SOCIALIZED MEDICINE

Following the report of the Committee on the Costs of Medical Care, the question of socialization of medicine was brought to the Judicial Council. Here is the pronouncement of the Council in 1933:

"During the past year, some of the basic beliefs and principles of the medical profession have been attacked and invaded more seriously and extensively than at any time before. An organized and financed campaign for a socialized system of furnishing medical care to a large proportion of the population has apparently crystallized its plans and begun its propaganda with the millions of certain foundations backing the effort. Practice of medicine by government in all the history of medicine in this country never has invaded the field of the private practitioner with his individual families as has the United States government through the Emergency Relief Administration. This is a complete and undisguised example of 'state medicine.' The avidity with which in general the government's offer was received can be explained only on the basis of an acute economic situation in the profession itself. The occurrence must be considered as a temporary expedient only, due to the unparalleled stress of the times, and must be discontinued as rapidly as the stress on the profession is relieved. A number of societies refused to enter into agreements whereby their members would be bound to provide services and accept compensation directly at the hands of the government. In some instances, official committees of state medical associations and county medical societies have strongly recommended to their members that they continue to provide medical service to all in need and refuse to accept compensation from the government for such services. One of the strongest holds of the profession on public approbation and support has been the age-old professional ideal of medical service to all, whether able to pay or not. That ideal is basic in our ethics. The abandonment of that ideal and the adoption of a principle of service only when paid for would be the greatest step toward socialized medicine and shortly state medicine which the medical profession could take. All our arguments as to better service to the people, freedom of choice of doctor, individual service, and maintenance of high grade medical service by highly qualified doctors would be as naught if such service were not available to a vast proportion of the people.

"There is no question that medical charity is badly abused and that the past two years of public support of vast numbers of unemployed have added thousands to that number of paupers we have always with us, people who never have worked and never will, who are content to live on public charity. It conceivably may be that this number may have become so great that the burden of their medical care should be borne by the community as are their other necessities of life. Perhaps the time has come when the profession should distinguish between the temporary and the chronic indigent and demand that the community relieve the private practitioner from furnishing free care to the chronically indigent. But the temporarily indigent, those who when able paid for medical care according to their ability to pay, should still be the charge of the medical profession in their period of distress.

"There have been widespread inquiries and complaints concerning the practice of medicine by hospitals, the division of fees between hospitals and doctors, the acceptance of commissions or rebates by ophthalmologists from opticians, the extensive unethical practice does not make it ethical. Ethics has to do with principles, not numbers or locality. A procedure unethical in one part of the country cannot be ethical under the same circumstances in another. Because the percentage of rebate is large in comparison, and in a year amounts to a considerable sum, and although many of the practitioners in a specialty may accept those rebates, the acceptance is no more ethical than for the general practitioner to accept a rebate on the occasional truss he may prescribe. The Judicial Council deplores such ignoring of ethical principles, not only because of the extent of the practices but because in may instances the plea of financial necessity cannot be offered as an excuse. The Council can only publicize the abuses and express its severe condemnation of them. It has no power in itself of control or correction."

As a result of this consideration a change was made in the Principles of Medical Ethics dealing with contract practice.

GROUP HOSPITALIZATION INSURANCE

By 1936 group hospitalization and individual hospital insurance plans required discussion. The Judicial Council said:

"Group hospitalization and individual hospital insurance plans have been rapidly spreading during the last few years as an effort on the part of hospitals to collect full payment for the hospitalization of people of low income groups who in the past have been and in the future will otherwise be unable to pay their hospital costs. This effort has been accentuated by the recent increase in the numbers of such cases combined with a great reduction in hospital income from endowment funds and public contributions. It is an effort at self preservation and secondarily to fix responsibility on a group that during the depression has been rapidly growing among those who have little sense of personal responsibility and rather expect government or charity to care for their needs.

"Hospital insurance as an economic device now exists almost nationally and is spreading. The American Hospital Association and various state hospital associations are actively promulgating it.

"Whether the scheme is or is not financially or economically sound is not the problem of our organization, but it is our business to see that the furnishing of medical service is not included in the sale of insured hospital accommodations. This can be done if a strong stand is taken and maintained by the organized medical profession, which must keep a watchful eye to see that medical care is not initially or later included when the usual sales efforts demand increased benefits to purchasers. It is well know that at the present time independently of the hospital insurance movement various hospitals are invading the field of the practice of medicine, sometimes at and sometimes against the desire of the members of our profession involved in such instances. It would seem that in this time of extensive changes in hospital economics the point had arrived at which further marriages between hospitals and staff physicians that make the doctor of medicine the servant of the hospital should be stopped and a series of attempts at divorce among marriages that have already taken place should be instituted. Our accepted ethical principles are adequate at the present time and the cooperation of the Council on Medical Education and Hospitals would be of invaluable assistance. It is not an impossible task but will need a militant local and national ethical spirit behind it and a frowning on those individuals in the profession who on personal grounds do not object to the gradual subjugation of the medical profession in the growth of hospital domination."

CULTISTS

At the same time the Council spoke again most severely on the question of contact with cultists:

"There are several general ethical principles underlying cult practice in its relation to medical practice as carried out by doctors of medicine. Primarily the basis for an ethical code is the well being of the people at large, who are dependent on the profession of medicine for their health. The profession of medicine is the custodian of the accumulated knowledge in medicine and should use it for the benefit of humanity. This knowledge, technical in nature and developed by experience, can be interpreted to the body of the people only by persons educated to understand it and trained to apply it. Of all those professing to heal the sick only the doctor of medicine has sufficient education and training to make use of the information already accumulated and keep abreast of that being developed continuously. We grant that even though this is true no one is compelled to choose only from this group in selecting his medical attendants. The individual may elect to receive his medical care from himself, his neighbor, osteopathy, chiropractic, naturopathy or Christian Science, but he is not entitled while under the care of such irregulars, to demand that the man educated in scientific medicine furnish opinion and advice to one so far deficient in education that he cannot so understand and apply that opinion and advice as to be able to make satisfactory use of it. Such degrading consultation would cheat the patient out of that which he might expect and the subsequent failure of results bring discredit on the science of medicine. If this is true of the occasional individual consultation, how much greater must it be in the case of repeated or conditional miscegenation!

"The Judicial Council is in receipt of much correspondence attempting to justify if not to advocate consultation between doctors of medicine and chiropractors, osteopaths, Christian Scientists and other cultists, and irregular practitioners; also appearance before their societies, teaching in their schools, and their admittance to hospital practice on a parity with the medical profession. The universal argument for all the procedures mentioned is based on the false premise 'to work them gradually into regular medicine.' One of our principles of ethics is as follows: 'The obligation assumed on entering the profession . . . demands that the physician use every honorable means to uphold the dignity and honor of his vocation, to exalt its standards and to extend its sphere of usefulness.' Such specious argument as mentioned above seems to the Council to lack substance and be unreal. It seems impossible that knowledge gained through years of scientific laboratory work and teaching can be assimilated by those of less preliminary training and use of scientific methods of investigation and practice ever to fit them to enter a profession the dignity and honor of which, the standards and sphere of influence of which, we are obligated to uphold, exact and extend for the service the profession can render to humanity. We further are of the opinion that it is just as unpractical to suggest that the small percentage of cult practitioners will through close relationship with the membership of our profession be raised to our professional standards as it is to expect the few rot-speckled apples in the apple barrel to become whole because of the preponderance of sound ones. We believe in continuous, complete separation between the true and the specious physician. Our traditional responsibility for the dissemination of sound scientific treatment for the people and for protection against the insidious influence of the weaker among our own is ever present. If and when the time comes that government through legislation places the cultists on the same legal plane with us, we must strive to maintain the aristocracy of learning and culture. A physical and professional separation as complete as is possible should be established and maintained."

RENTAL OF RADIUM

More recently the Judicial Council considered the question of the rental of radium:

"A widespread practice of renting radium for the treatment of patients by physicians not owning or being experienced in the use of radium has caused considerable discussion during the past year. Ordinarily instructions in the technic of the use of radium are sent by the person furnishing it. Sometimes the radium is furnished by a commercial concern, sometimes by a physician owning it. The advisability of the use of such a powerful agency by those not trained in its use and the ethics involved of prescribing and directing its use by a person who has not examined or seen the person on whom it is to be used has come before the Council. As a result of a rather extensive correspondence both from those favoring its use as described and those opposed, the Judicial Council is of the opinion that the prescribing and directing of its use in the case of a patient whom the prescriber has not examined or seen is an unethical medical procedure. The Council recognizes that advice and help in difficult cases is often furnished by those in a position to be of possible or probable assistance but it believes that the great dangers accompanying the use of radium removes that particular remedy from the field of advice without personal contact with the patient."

The membership of the Judicial Council since 1901 is included in the appendix. The important decisions made by the Judicial Council and some of their most important activities are reflected in the history of the Association in this volume.

COUNCIL ON INDUSTRIAL HEALTH

By Carl M. Peterson, M.D.

THE SECTION ON PREVENTIVE MEDICINE AND PUBLIC HEALTH in 1915 appointed a Committee on Industrial Sanitation. This committee promptly reported that the great mass of workers had been denied the enjoyment of healthful living and working and predicted great opportunities for satisfactory professional careers in the industrial medical field. Each year since, this Section in the Scientific Assembly has devoted a substantial part of its programs to industrial medicine, surgery and hygiene.

In 1915 also the Judicial Council, in recognition of the great social and medical implications of the workmen's compensation laws then beginning to appear on the federal and state statute books, prepared an extensive review of the whole subject. Subsequent developments in the field of industrial accidents and occupational diseases forcefully illustrate the vision of those who analyzed these laws and predicted their immense effect on future medical practice. Many other sections, committees, councils and bureaus have in one way or another made great contributions to the successful conduct of industrial health services. In more recent years, however, it became apparent that a single agency in the American Medical Association ought to be created as a point of reference, discussion, and report on all matters affecting the health of the employed population. For this reason the Council on Industrial Health was established.

The actual beginnings of the Council on Industrial Health date from the Kansas City session of the House of Delegates in May, 1936. Dr. A. R. McComas, a delegate from Missouri, introduced a resolution which called attention to the chaotic nature of workmen's compensation procedure and to the urgent need for better clinical and administrative care of occupational diseases. The Reference Committee on Hygiene and Public Health, after conferences with the sponsor of the resolution and others interested, submitted a substitute resolution approved by the House of Delegates as follows:

Resolved, That it be deemed essential that any active efforts by governmental agencies to study and to take measures tending to eliminate occupational diseases should be carried out under the supervision of the city, state or federal departments of health in this country and that this Association do all within its power to assist in this endeavor; and be it further

Resolved, That the Board of Trustees of this Association continue and enlarge its study of industrial hygiene, occupational diseases, and particularly silicosis, to the end that uniform legislation be put into effect in all the states to control these conditions.

At this same session in Kansas City the Committee on Industrial Dermatoses of the Section on Dermatology and Syphilology reported as follows:

Your committee met yesterday under the chairmanship of Dr. C. Guy Lane, Boston. Your committee recommends that a central clearing house be established for the recording and dissemination of information on industrial dermatoses. It recommends that its studies be continued, in cooperation with the Section on Preventive and Industrial Medicine and Public Health, with the United States Public Health Service and with the American Dermatological Association, for the purpose of establishing a cooperative approach to the problems of industrial skin diseases. It further recommends that the committee be empowered to appoint local subcommittees in various states or districts to gather information and to report operations to this central section committee.

In consideration of the resolution and the report, the Board of Trustees called a conference on March 12, 1937, which was attended by a group of physicians known to have given careful study to problems of industrial health. The recommendation of the conference was to the effect that a Council on Industrial Health should be established and maintained by the American Medical Association. At the Atlantic City session of the House of Delegates June 10, 1937, Dr. Rock Sleyster, Chairman of the Board of Trustees, presented the following report:

The Board of Trustees reports favorably on the creation of a Council on Industrial Health and, with the approval of the House of Delegates, will proceed with the organization of the Council as a committee of the Board.

This report was accepted, and acting on this authorization, the Board of Trustees promptly proceeded with the organization of the Council as one of its standing committees.

FIRST STEPS

Nine eminent physicians were chosen. Men were chosen who had demonstrated accomplishments in the field of industrial medicine, surgery and hygiene, with broad understanding of the field and with ability to provide as great a degree of integration as possible with the official agencies and medical specialties most concerned. Five of the original group are still serving on the Council. Their names as well as others who have been added since are listed in the accompanying table:

Name	Service Began	Terminated
Harvey Bartle, Philadelphia	September, 1937	....
Warren Draper, Washington, D. C.	September, 1937	....
Leroy U. Gardner, Saranac Lake, New York	September, 1937	1946
Morton R. Gibbons, San Francisco	September, 1937	November 1938
Henry H. Kessler, Newark, N. J.	September, 1937	....
Allen D. Lazenby, Baltimore	September, 1937	1939
Earl D. Osborne, Buffalo	September, 1937	1939
C. W. Roberts, Atlanta	September, 1937	1941
Stanley J. Seeger, Milwaukee	September, 1937	....
Leverett D. Bristol, New York	March, 1938	....
Anthony J. Lanza, New York	March, 1938	....
Clarence D. Selby	March, 1938	....
Robert T. Legge, Berkeley, Calif.	1939	1944
Philip Drinker, Boston	1941	1945
Raymond Hussey, Baltimore	1941	....
William D. Stroud, Philadelphia	1942	1944
William A. Sawyer, Rochester, N. Y.	1944	....
James S. Simmons, Washington, D. C.	1944	....
Paul Magnuson, Chicago	1945	....

R. L. Sensenich, from the Board of Trustees and Olin West Secretary and General Manager of the American Medical Association were appointed ex-officio members.

The first meeting of the Council on Industrial Health was held December 10, 1937, at the headquarters building of the American Medical Association in Chicago. Dr. Stanley J. Seeger of Milwaukee who had been nominated chairman of the Council, presided as he has at all succeeding meetings. Dr. A. D. Lazenby of Baltimore was elected vice-chairman, serving in that capacity until his death in 1939, at which time Dr. Raymond Hussey became vice-chairman. At this first meeting, attention was almost entirely given over to organizational details, in the furtherance of which a number of subcommittees were appointed to define scope and early activities, to elaborate a set of rules under which the Council could act, and to undertake the development of a system of nomenclature which would apply uniformly throughout the field. All subsequent activities have stemmed principally from the reports of these early committees.

Dr. Carl M. Peterson was appointed secretary of the Council by the Board of Trustees in February, 1938, and has served in that capacity since. Space was assigned in the headquarters building of the American Medical Association and facilities provided for the active promulgation of its meetings and program.

THE WAR YEARS

Almost the entire active career of the Council on Industrial Health has been influenced by the exigencies of preparedness or actual war. In 1939 and 1940 a mobilization program was developed, intended to be as helpful as possible to the Committee on Preparedness of the American Medical Association, and the Division of Industrial Hygiene of the National Institute of Health. All physicians engaged in industrial practice were identified and their special abilities cataloged for ready accessibility, an activity which was later of great usefulness to the Procurement and Assignment Service in the War Manpower Commission. Other phases of the early preparedness program dealt with location and control of dangerous occupational exposures through the use of local medical and health facilities, and the organization of intensive training courses under the sponsorship of medical societies, medical schools, or both. The Council took the position that industrial production is paramount in war, that industrial workers must be maintained at peak capacity to produce, and that as a consequence industrial physicians ought to be regarded as indispensable. As the war progressed, close cooperative relations sprang up with committees on industrial health and medicine in the Federal Security Agency, the National Research Council, and with special occupational health services set up in the medical departments of the Army, Navy, Air Forces, Maritime Commission, and the War Production Board. Many members of the Council served actively as officers of or advisory to these agencies.

During the later war years, primary emphasis shifted from professional mobilization to manpower conservation. Committees concerned themselves with the ordinary illnesses of factory workers, with nutrition and fatigue, with special problems of women and the aged, and with the uncountable health problems associated with keeping large numbers of substandard workers at high production levels. The proper utilization of the handicapped in industry through proper matching of job requirements and physical-mental ability was the subject of joint study by the Council on Industrial Health, the War Manpower Commission and official agencies dealing with compensation and rehabilitation. Certainly during the war industrial health rose to its highest level of recognition and acceptance.

GENERAL GROWTH AND DEVELOPMENT

In its nine short years the record of the Council on Industrial Health has been one of gradual expansion of functions, of growing realization of the vast scope of industrial health and welfare, and of sharpened focus on those medical relationships which stand out as of fundamental importance. The original Committee on Scope had emphasized that four major activities needed to be energetically pursued if industrial health services were to spread and if medical standards were to improve. These were, the creation of public interest and demand, the clarification of industrial health objectives, improved professional training and standards, and better medical organization for industrial health on the part of individual physicians and medical societies. These recommendations still govern the major activities of the Council.

Public interest deals particularly with management and labor. Good contacts were promptly established with the major trade and management associations and chambers of commerce, all of whom have been concerned with the expanding character of occupational health and more particularly its extension to the employees of small plants. Joint action has been taken with labor in the elaboration of industrial physical examinations standards, with many aspects of workmen's compensation coverage, and more recently with labor management cooperation for improved industrial health and safety. Other public relations activity has dealt with the place which industrial health and hygiene ought to occupy at international, inter-American, federal and state levels.

Better service to industry depends on professional education and organization, both of which have been regarded as primary obligations of the Council. All the available avenues for improvement have been used. Medical schools have been repeatedly urged to acquaint their undergraduates with the essentials of occupational health, and with tolerable success. Introductory and refresher courses have been conducted by medical schools and medical societies, frequently as joint enterprises. The active cooperation of the Council on Medical Education and Hospitals has been enlisted for guidance in all educational activities, and particularly to determine the desirability of embarking upon a specialty certification program. To further these efforts and for many other purposes, it was highly essential to develop proper cooperative agencies in state and local medical societies. These committees have been of great usefulness and the encouragement which they have given to the industrial health movement has been invaluable. In 1940 and 1941, the first efforts to develop active interest by the specialty groups was begun, using the Section on Dermatology and Syphilology as a pattern and stimulus. All specialty groups having direct relationship with industrial medical services have appointed liaison committees and the work accomplished by them has been one of the most valuable and fruitful phases of the Council's educational and organizational program. Nurses, hygienists, dentists and chemists have almost identical problems to solve and it has been the policy of the Council to work closely with these professional groups.

The Council has issued reports from time to time describing the objectives of industrial health, the physician's place in the industrial setting, the organization of industrial medical departments, the making of plant hygiene surveys, proper procedure for industrial nurses, and many others. It has worked closely with other councils, bureaus and sections of the American Medical Association in the elaboration of standards for industrial medicine and surgery and industrial hygiene, and in the fields of health education and legislation.

Medical relations in workmen's compensation have occupied the attention of the Council from its inception. Its range of interest includes effective relations with state medical societies, specialist organizations, with industrial commissions and compensation boards, and with the casualty and liability insurance companies. A National Conference Committee on Workmen's Compensation has been actively fostered, including representation from all official agencies dealing with compensation matters. It is confidently expected that through this means, administrative standards will be considerably improved and that great advances can be made in the simplification of report forms, uniform statistical methods, medical testimony, disability evaluation, and rehabilitation.

The Council on Industrial Health, confronted with a host of unsolved problems in the field of industrial health and welfare, rightly believes its career of useful activity has barely started.

THE COUNCIL ON MEDICAL SERVICE

By Louis H. Bauer, M.D., and George Cooley

THE COUNCIL ON MEDICAL SERVICE was established by the action of the House of Delegates in June 1943. Various groups within the Association felt that there should be better coordination of the activities within the States on the subject of medical care; that there should be more stress on public relations from the legislative angle; that there should be a more direct relation between this agency and the House of Delegates; and finally, many felt there should be representation of the Association in Washington, D. C.

In 1943, several resolutions on this general subject were brought before the House of Delegates. The meeting of the Reference Committee was attended by practically the whole House. After considerable discussion, followed by a referral of the matter to the Board of Trustees for clarification, the House established this Council. It consists of the President of the Association, the immediate Past President, the Secretary, a member of the Board of Trustees and six elective members, selected geographically, two elected each year for 3 years. The first Council was to be appointed by the Board of Trustees. Its duties as set forth in the By Laws are as follows:

"(1) To make available facts, data and medical opinions with respect to timely and adequate rendition of medical care to the American people;

"(2) to inform the constituent associations and component societies of proposed changes affecting medical care in the nation;

"(3) to inform constituent associations and component societies regarding the activities of the council;

"(4) to investigate matters pertaining to the economic, social and similar aspects of medical care for all the people;

"(5) to study and suggest means for the distribution of medical services to the public consistent with the principles adopted by the House of Delegates, and

"(6) to develop and assist committees on medical service and public relations originating within the constituent associations and component societies of the American Medical Association.

"In the exercise of its functions, this Council, with the Cooperation of the Board of Trustees, shall utilize the functions and personnel of the Bureau of Legal Medicine and Legislation, the Bureau of Medical Economics and the Department of Public Relations in the Headquarters Office."

The Council is also bound by the actions of the House of Delegates on the subject of medical care and its distribution, notably the platform adopted in 1937 as amended and amplified in subsequent years by the various resolutions and reference committee reports adopted by the House of Delegates.

The Board of Trustees appointed the first Council bearing in mind the geographic distribution of the members as provided in the By-Laws. The first Council consisted of the following:

James E. Paullin	as President
Fred W. Rankin	as Past President
Roger I. Lee	representing the Board of Trustees
Olin West	as Secretary
Louis H. Bauer	New York
Edward J. McCormick	Ohio
W. S. Leathers	Tennessee
A. W. Adson	Minnesota
James R. McVay	Missouri
John H. Fitzgibbon	Oregon

The first meeting was held in Chicago on July 21, 1943. It was an organizational meeting only with Dr. Bauer elected Chairman and Dr. McCormick, Vice-Chairman. Mr. J. W. Holloway, Jr., Director of the Bureau of Legal Medicine and Legislation, was appointed acting Secretary.

The second meeting of the Council was held on September 9 and 10, 1943. At this meeting a statement of general policies was adopted and referred to the Board of Trustees. The policies were:

1. The Council on Medical Service and Public Relations recognizes the desirability of widespread distribution of the benefits of medical science; it encourages evolution in the methods of administering medical care, subject to the basic principles necessary to the maintenance of scientific standards and the quality of the service rendered.

It is not in the public interest that the removal of economic barriers to medical service should be utilized as a subterfuge to overturn the whole order of medical practice. Removal of economic barriers should be an object in itself.

It is in the public interest that the standards of medical education be constantly raised, that medical research be constantly increased and that graduate and postgraduate medical education be energetically developed. Curative medicine, preventive medicine, public health medicine, research medicine and medical education all are indispensable factors in promoting the health, comfort and happiness of the nation.

2. The Council through its executive committee and secretary shall analyze proposed legislation affecting medical service. Its officers are instructed to provide advice to the various state medical organizations as well as to legislative committees concerning the effects of the proposed legislation. It shall likewise be the duty of its officers to offer constructive suggestions to bureaus and legislative committees on the subject of medical service.

3. The Council approves the principle of voluntary hospital insurance programs but disapproves the inclusion of medical services in those contracts for the reasons adopted by the House of Delegates at the 1943 meeting.

4. The Council approves voluntary prepayment medical service under the control of state and county medical societies in accordance with the principles adopted by the House of Delegates in 1938. The medical profession has always been strongly opposed to compulsory health insurance because (1) it does not reach the unemployed class, (2) it results in a bureaucratic control of medicine and interposes a third party between the

physician and the patient, (3) it results in mass medicine which is neither art nor science, (4) it is inordinately expensive and (5) regulations, red tape and interference render good medical care impossible. Propaganda to the contrary notwithstanding, organized medicine in general, and the American Medical Association in particular, have never opposed group medicine prepayment or group medical practice as such. The American Medical Association and the medical profession as a whole have opposed any scheme which on the face of it renders good medical care impossible. That group medicine has not been opposed as such is evidenced by the fact that there are many groups operating in the United States which have the approval of the medical profession, and members of these groups are and have been officials in the national and state medical organizations. That group medicine is the Utopia for the whole population, however, is not probable. It may be and possibly is the answer for certain communities and certain industrial groups if the medical groups are so organized and operated as to deliver good medical care.

5. The Council believes that many emergency measures now in force should cease following the end of hostilities.

6. The Council believes that the medical profession should attempt to establish the most cordial relationships possible with allied professions.

7. There is no official affiliation between the American Medical Association and the National Physicians Committee. However, since it is the purpose of the National Physicians Committee to enlighten the public concerning contributions which American medicine has made and is making in behalf of the individual and the nation as a whole, it is the opinion of the Council that the medical profession may well support the activities of the National Physicians Committee and other organizations of like aims.

8. American medicine and this Council owe a responsibility to our colleagues who are making personal sacrifices to answer the call of the armed forces. Therefore the Council expresses the desire to cooperate with the medical committee on postwar planning in order to assist our colleagues in reestablishing themselves in the practice of medicine and in the preservation of the American system of medicine.

The Council also presented a plan of operation to the Board of Trustees. This plan envisaged adequate sources of information, close contact with constituent associations and component societies, and a close relationship with other councils and bureaus of the American Medical Association. The provisions follow:

1. In carrying out the directive in the By-Laws as to relationship with the other Bureaus and Departments of the Association, the Council has established close collaboration (a) with the Bureau of Medical Economics, which has been asked and has expressed the willingness to do the research on many of the economic problems necessary for the Council's study, and which is well equipped to carry out such research; (b) with the Bureau of Legal Medicine and Legislation. Joint bulletins will be issued with that Bureau on legislative matters. Attempt will be made to effect wider distribution and, if necessary, more frequent publication of such bulletins; (c) with the Department of Public Relations. The Council shall utilize the sources of information of this department and joint bulletins may be issued from time to time with it, and if indicated with other bureaus of the American Medical Association. All planning will be to avoid overlapping of functions and duplication of effort.

2. The Council on Medical Service and Public Relations has extended the sources of information of the American Medical Association on problems with which the Council is specifically concerned. Through its membership and by cooperation with constituent associations and component societies and the utilization of other facilities, the Council will disseminate such information toward effecting its objectives. The Secretary of the Council, with its approval, will undertake such travel as may be necessary.

3. In order that constituent associations and component societies may be kept in-

formed of the activities of the Council, and of proposed changes in the status of medical care, and that the Council may be of assistance to those associations and societies, the Council has requested each State Association to designate an existing committee or create a new committee to function with the Council on a State level.

Each State organization has also been requested to contact each component society in the State and ask it similarly to designate or form a committee to function in connection with the programs of the Council. Where such organization is feasible, it has been suggested that committees be created along the lines of congressional districts.

Such State and county committees have been urged to keep the Council informed of their local problems and activities.

State organizations also will be requested from time to time to conduct experiments in the various methods of medical care and to inform the Council of their results so that the Council may study and evaluate the experiments and transmit the information acquired to all concerned.

4. The Council feels that under its directive it is its duty to endeavor to evolve such modifications of our present system of medical care as may be necessary to cover all the people and be in accord with the traditions of American Medicine as to high standards of medical care and the American tradition of free enterprise as already outlined in paragraph 1 of the Council's Policies previously published. To accomplish this, study must be made of all economic, social and similar aspects of such care.

5. In order that the above program may be effectively carried out, the Secretary of the Council, with the guidance of the Council in conformity with the above expressed relationships with other Bureaus and Departments, shall inform the profession through the various State organizations of all pending national legislation and bureau directives affecting the practice of medicine. It shall likewise be his duty with the guidance of the Council, to arrange for medical representation at meetings and hearings pertaining to medical care, collaborating in the representation with other Councils and Bureaus of the American Medical Association who have an interest in this same subject.

6. The Secretary is instructed with the supervision of the Council, and in collaboration with the Department of Public Relations, to disseminate information concerning the activities of the Council through the publications of the American Medical Association and the various state medical journals, and to prepare and release information on medical care.

This plan of operation was adopted by the Board of Trustees at its meeting on November 20, 1943.

The Council drafted a bulletin in opposition to the 1943 version of the Wagner-Murray-Dingell bill. All state societies were contacted and asked to designate committees to work with the Council. As the activities increased it became necessary to relieve Mr. Holloway of this additional load. As a result, in January 1944, Dr. G. Lombard Kelly was appointed Secretary of the Council. He served in that capacity until July 1, 1944.

In February 1944, conferences were held with representatives of the National Conference on Medical Service and with Dr. Martha Eliot. The Council studied the status of medical students and recommended to the Board of Trustees that a student membership be set up in the American Medical Association. A request was sent to the Council on Medical Education and Hospitals asking that steps be taken to see that medical schools include courses on medical sociology, medical economics, and medical ethics. A meeting was held in Washington, D. C., in May with representatives of the following present: American Dental Association, United States Public Health Service, Office of Vocational Rehabilitation, War Manpower Commission, Children's Bureau, American Federation of Labor, Committee on Industrial Organization, medical schools, National Physicians' Committee, Medical Society of Pennsylvania and Congress.

One of the important actions of the Council during its first year, was a revision of the Platform of the American Medical Association. It had been adopted originally in 1938, and at this time was brought up to date, with the revision approved by the House in June 1944.

WASHINGTON OFFICE

Another important step was the decision to open a Washington Office of the Council. This office was to serve as a bureau of information to Congressmen and department heads; to keep closer contact with legislative developments, and to keep State Societies informed of impending changes in the medical care situation. Dr. Joseph S. Lawrence of New York was appointed Director of this office which actually opened September 1, 1944.

At the meeting of the House in 1944, the first elected Council took office. The new Council consisted of:

Herman L. Kretschmer.................as President
James E. Paullin......................as Past President
Louis H. Bauer.......................representing the Board of Trustees
Olin West............................as Secretary

And the following elected members:

John H. Fitzgibbon...........................of Oregon for 3 years
James R. McVay..............................of Missouri for 3 years
Thomas A. McGoldrick.........................of New York for 2 years
Edward J. McCormick..........................of Ohio for 2 years
Alfred W. Adson..............................of Minnesota for 1 year
W. S. Leathers...............................of Tennessee for 1 year

The Council reorganized with Dr. Fitzgibbon as Chairman and Dr. McCormick as Vice-Chairman. Mr. Holloway again became acting Secretary. However, in February 1945, Mr. Thomas A. Hendricks of Indiana was appointed Secretary.

CLARIFICATION OF DUTIES

The first action of the new Council was to have its status with relation to other Councils and Bureaus of the Association clarified. This clarification follows:

1. To make available facts, data and medical opinions with respect to timely and adequate rendition of medical care to the American People.

This will require the services of the Bureau of Medical Economics in assembling statistical material, in making surveys and in preparing analyses of medical care plans for the Council's study. It will require the services of the Bureau of Legal Medicine and Legislation in preparing factual analyses of any legislative angles and it will require the services of the Department of Public Relations in spreading the information through the publications of the American Medical Association. The Council may also effect distribution of some of the information through its bulletins.

2. To inform constituent associations and component societies of proposed changes, affecting medical care in the nation.

This, of course, concerns legislation. It should be one of the functions of the Washington office. The information assembled by the Washington office, and other sources of information, should be transmitted to the states and by them to the counties unless the states have requested that the counties be notified direct. Under the plan proposed by the Council and approved by the representatives of those states sending representatives to conferences already held, there should preferably be one man designated by the state who will serve as the contact agent of that state with the Washington office. The information should be sent to the contact agent whose duty it will be to distribute this information as directed by his own state. In cases in which the proposed bill alone is to be sent, it may be sent direct from the Washington office, with copies going to the Council office in Chicago and to the other association bureaus and departments concerned in the Chicago headquarters, with request for advice from the department concerned. In case a factual analysis is to be made, this will be done in collaboration by the Washington director and the Director of the Bureau of Legal Medicine and Legislation, by mail when time permits, and when it does not, by telephone. The same will apply when the implications of the bill are to be included.

3. To inform constituent associations and component societies regarding the activities of the council.

This will be done by means of the Council's bulletins and, with the cooperation of the Department of Public Relations, by means of the Association's publications.

4. To investigate matters pertaining to the economic, social and similar aspects of medical care for all the people.

This will involve both the methods covered in 1 and 2, as there will be required both economic investigations by the Bureau of Medical Economics and the legislative aspects of the matter concerned by the Bureau of Legal Medicine and Legislation. The information received from the Bureau of Medical Economics, from the Washington office and a legislative analysis of the same by the Bureau of Legal Medicine and Legislation would be compiled in the Chicago office for submission to the Council for its study.

5. To study and suggest means for the distribution of medical service to the public consistent with the principles adopted by the House of Delegates.

Based on the results of the first four activities, the Council will prepare its recommendations for the approval of the Board of Trustees or, in case new principles are involved, for submission to the next session of the House of Delegates.

6. To develop and assist committees on medical service and public relations originating within the constituent associations and component societies of the American Medical Association.

To do this a field agent is necessary. Many of the representatives attending the conferences on June 11 and the meeting of the House of Delegates expressed their desire for an arrangement whereby conferences could be held with state representatives. It was also recommended in the Supplementary Report of the Council. The idea of the Council is that this field agent should spend some time in Chicago, familiarizing himself with all the activities of the Council and should keep in frequent touch with the Chicago office thereafter. However, he should act as a direct contact between the Washington office and the state agents mentioned. Under the direction of the Washington director and with the approval of the Council, invitations would be issued to groups of states to attend conferences in central areas. The states would be asked to send their contact agents and such others as they see fit to these conferences. The states would be asked to effect an organization within the state so that quick action could be had in emergencies in bringing to the attention of members of Congress the attitude of the medical profession on certain bills. The contact with the congressmen would be by these local units. The field agent would outline the plan to them and offer such assistance as the states desired. Contacts could be kept up then by correspondence with the state agents and only occasional personal contacts thereafter.

The Washington director would be responsible for obtaining information on legislative or government departmental matters and transmitting it to the proper persons outlined. He would have available all information possible on Association activities for the benefit of Congress and the government departments. He would see to it that both were informed that such a source of information was available for their use when desired. He would discuss bills with members of Congress when requested to do so by them or furnish them such information as requested by the congressman's constituents. He would never exert any pressure on any member of congress in an effort to influence his vote.

The director would develop sources of information gradually, and the Department of Public Relations would furnish him promptly with all information of a legislative nature which comes to it. The director would likewise keep the Department of Public Relations informed.

A part time legal counsel was recommended in the Council's Supplementary Report. The purpose of this counsel would be to give advice on the meaning of legal phraseology of bills and their legal implications, and the relationship of this bill to other legislation. For the present, at least, it would appear that this could be done by the Bureau of Legal Medicine and Legislation, although, in emergencies, some one on the ground would be essential.

There should also be a secretary to the director who should be a college graduate with secretarial training. A stenographer would also be necessary.

The director would function under the supervision of the Council or its executive committee.

NEWS LETTER

Early in its career the Council published special bulletins. These later evolved into News letters which now go to over 3000 persons. Bulletins on special subjects are also issued, including bulletins on the legislative situation, issued directly from the Washington office.

REGIONAL CONFERENCES

In order better to coordinate the activities of the State Societies it was decided to hold a series of regional conferences. Fifteen of these have been held at various points in the country and have resulted in a great deal of satisfaction and productive work.

The Council continued its contact with various groups and endeavored to help solve problems of Insurance Companies, the American Cancer Society and many other organizations. The Council was successful in arranging that all cancer detection clinics and medical service projects should be under the control of the County Medical Societies.

The Council adopted a fourteen point Constructive Program for Medical Care, which was approved by the Board of Trustees and by the House of Delegates which, however, suggested to the Board a rearrangement of the program in order to stress more particularly maternal and child welfare, medical research, and the medical care of the veteran as well as the part to be played by the voluntary health agencies. The restatement follows in the ten-point program later adopted:

NATIONAL HEALTH PROGRAM OF THE AMERICAN MEDICAL ASSOCIATION

1. The American Medical Association urges a minimum standard of nutrition, housing, clothing and recreation as fundamental to good health and as an objective to be achieved in any suitable health program. The responsibility for attainment of this standard should be placed as far as possible on the individual, but the application of community efforts, compatible with the maintenance of free enterprise, should be encouraged with governmental aid where needed.

2. The provision of preventive medical services through professionally competent health departments with sufficient staff and equipment to meet community needs is recognized as essential in a health program. The principle of federal aid through provision of funds or personnel is recognized with the understanding that local areas shall control their own agencies as has been established in the field of education. Health departments should not assume the care of the sick as a function, since administration of medical care under such auspices tends to a deterioration in the quality of the service rendered. Medical care to those unable to provide for themselves is best administered by local and private agencies with the aid of public funds when needed. This program for national health should include the administration of medical care, including hospitalization to all those needing it but unable to pay, such medical care to be provided preferably by a physician of the patient's choice with funds provided by local agencies with the assistance of federal funds when necessary.

3. The procedures established by modern medicine for advice to the prospective mother and for adequate care in childbirth should be made available to all at a price that they can afford to pay. When local funds are lacking for the care of those unable to pay, federal aid should be supplied with the funds administered through local or state agenices.

4. The child should have throughout infancy proper attention, including scientific nutrition, immunization against preventable disease and other services included in infant welfare. Such services are best supplied by personal contact between the mother and the individual physician but may be provided through child care and infant welfare stations administered under local auspices with support by tax funds whenever the need can be shown.

5. The provision of health and diagnostic centers and hospitals necessary to community needs is an essential of good medical care. Such facilities are preferably supplied by local agencies, including the community, church and trade agencies which have been responsible for the fine development of facilities for medi al care in most American com munities up to this time. Where such facilities are unavailable and cannot be supplied through local or state agencies, the federal government may aid, preferably under a plan which requires that the need be shown and that the community prove its ability to maintain such institutions once they are established (Hill-Burton bill).

6. A program for medical care within the American system of individual initiative and freedom of enterprise includes the establishment of voluntary nonprofit prepayment plans for the costs of hospitalization (such as the Blue Cross plans) and voluntary nonprofit prepayment plans for medical care (such as those developed by many state and county medical societies). The principles of such insurance contracts should be acceptable to the Council on Medical Service of the American Medical Association and to the

authoritative bodies of state medical associations. The evolution of voluntary prepayment insurance against the costs of sickness admits also the utilization of private sickness insurance plans which comply with state regulatory statutes and meet the standards of the Council on Medical Service of the American Medical Association.

7. A program for national health should include the administration of medical care, including hospitalization, to all veterans, such medical care to be provided preferably by a physician of the veteran's choice, with payment by the Veterans Administration through a plan mutually agreed on between the state medical association and the Veterans Administration.

8. Research for the advancement of medical science is fundamental in any national health program. The inclusion of medical research in a National Science Foundation, such as proposed in pending federal legislation, is endorsed.

9. The services rendered by volunteer philanthropic health agencies such as the American Cancer Society, the National Tuberculosis Association, the National Foundation for Infantile Paralysis, Inc., and by philanthropic agencies such as the Commonwealth Fund and the Rockefeller Foundation and similar bodies have been of vast benefit to the American people and are a natural outgrowth of the system of free enterprise and democracy that prevail in the United States. Their participation in a national health program should be encouraged, and the growth of such agencies when properly administered should be commended.

10. Fundamental to the promotion of the public health and alleviation of illness are widespread education in the field of health and the widest possible dissemination of information regarding the prevention of disease and its treatment by authoritative agencies. Health education should be considered a necessary function of all departments of public health, medical associations and school authorities.

A great deal of work has been done by the Council on voluntary prepayment medical insurance. All phases of the subject were studied by the Council. A survey of the various Medical Society Plans was conducted by Mr. George Cooley who has been added to the staff of the Council. Finally, the Council decided to establish a division of Medical Care Insurance. This was done because it seemed that stimulation of the formation and extension of Medical Society plans could be greatly helped by active participation on the part of the A.M.A. The House directed the Council in Dec. 1945 to endeavor to effect national coverage by these plans. Conferences were held with Medical Care Plan Directors and finally it was decided not to start a separate national plan, but to form an independent organization. The Medical Care Plans grouped themselves together in the Associated Medical Care Plans, Inc. This group works in close association with the Council. In fact, 3 members of the Council are on its governing board. Mr. Jay Ketchum, who has been so successful with the Michigan Society Plan, was appointed Director of the new Council Division on Medical Prepayment Insurance.

As a preliminary to this program, the Council appointed an Advisory Committee consisting of Directors of Medical Care Plans and adopted Rules and Regulations for acceptable plans. Any plan which is approved by the Council will be entitled to use a Council seal on its literature. It is expected that these plans will work out reciprocity among themselves and afford national coverage in a reasonable time.

In June 1945, Dr. Fitzgibbon resigned as Chairman, and Dr. McCormick was elected in his place. Dr. McVay was elected Vice-Chairman. Dr. Leathers resigned from the Council and the Board of Trustees appointed Dr. W. R. Brooksher of Arkansas to take his place.

In December 1945, the House elected Dr. A. W. Adson, to succeed himself for a three-year term; Dr. W. B. Martin of Virginia to succeed Dr. Brooksher for a three-year term; and Dr. Fitzgibbon having been elected to the Board of Trustees, resigned from the Council and Dr. Raymond L. Zech of Washington was elected to fill his unexpired term.

The new Council consisted of:

Roger I. Lee..........................as President
Herman L. Kretschmer................as Past President
Olin West............................as Secretary (later
                                    succeeded by Dr. George F. Lull)
Louis H. Bauer.......................representing the Trustees

And the following members:

A. W. Adson..of Minnesota
E. J. McCormick......................................of Ohio
J. R. McVay..of Missouri
T. A. McGoldrick.....................................of New York
W. B. Martin...of Virginia
R. L. Zech...of Washington

Dr. McCormick and Dr. McVay were continued as Chairman and Vice-Chairman respectively.

The executive committee, consisting of Dr. E. J. McCormick, Dr. J. R. McVay, Dr. A. W. Adson, and Dr. Louis H. Bauer, was reappointed and held its first meeting on January 11 in the Council office. The executive committee also met with the Board of Trustees of the American Medical Association to discuss the prepayment medical care program. A second meeting of the Council was held on February 13 and 14, and on February 14 another joint meeting was held with the Board of Trustees.

The Council with the cooperation of the Bureau of Medical Economics prepared a complete and up-to-date brochure entitled "Voluntary Prepayment Medical Care Plans." This was the first brochure published in which the material was organized and compiled in such a manner as to provide a means for comparison between various plans. The services of the Council staff were offered to state medical societies to assist them in the development of prepayment plans. Many conferences were held with state prepayment committees in an effort to stimulate active interest and to provide technical information. By July the Council was able to report that seventy-three plans were in operation in thirty-one states with an additional eight states in the process of developing programs.

The Council cooperated with Bureau of Information in arranging the First Annual Conference on Rural Health. The conference was sponsored by the Committee on Rural Medical Service of the American Medical Association and was participated in by the Farm Bureau, Farm Foundation, Grange, and other farm groups.

In July 1946, the House of Delegates deleted the Public Relations portion of the Council's name leaving it with its present title, Council on Medical Service.

The House of Delegates unanimously re-elected Dr. E. J. McCormick and Dr. T. A. McGoldrick; Dr. R. I. Lee, as past president, automatically moved into the place vacated by Dr. H. L. Kretschmer; and Dr. H. H. Shoulders became a member of the Council, taking the place of Dr. Lee. The Council met and re-elected Dr. E. J. McCormick, chairman, and Dr. J. R. McVay, vice chairman. The Council took under consideration and study a number of programs suggested by various state medical associations. Among these were a National Health Congress and a Speakers' Bureau. The Council proceeded to collect information on local health councils and concluded that a National Health Congress as a permanent body was not advisable because it would duplicate the efforts of and, to a certain extent would usurp the prerogatives of the House of Delegates and other bodies of the American Medical Association Instead it recommended the promotion of local health councils and the utilization of different interested groups whenever a matter pertaining to their specific fields was under consideration. Plans were evolved for setting up a briefing course at the American Medical Association headquarters for the purpose of providing a select group of doctors with sufficient background, information, and material so that they might return to their own states and organize county society speakers' bureaus.

In cooperation with the National University Extension Association the Council prepared a brochure containing pertinent articles expressing the views of those opposing compulsory sickness insurance. In connection with the national debate subject for the school year 1946–47, a large variety of material has been furnished to doctors, students, debate coaches, and libraries. Over 30,000 pieces of literature have been furnished by the Council office in reply to requests.

The staff of the Council was increased during 1946 by the addition of Mr. Howard O. Brower and Mr. L. S. Kleinschmidt. Mr. Brower came to assist in the technical aspect of insurance programs and to make more effective the cooperative efforts between the Council and the private insurance carriers. Mr. Kleinschmidt was added to facilitate the study and growth in the rural and community enrollment activities of prepayment plans.

Following recommendations of the House of Delegates, the Council has studied and followed the developments of the United Mine Workers Health Fund, the Taft-Smith-Ball proposed Health Bill, and the Hill-Burton Hospital Construction Act. Assistance and guidance have been given to state medical associations on all three programs, with specific recommendations included where advisable.

Much effort and study have been devoted to programs affecting particular aspects of medical care, such as those of the American Cancer Society, the U.S.P.H.S. and the Medical Cooperatives. Investigation and analysis have been made with the view of assisting state and county medical societies in evaluating such programs.

The Council, although only in existence for three years, has done a tremendous amount of work. It has had more than it could do and has been handicapped by difficulties in obtaining personnel, due to the war. Its Washington office has been most favorably received This Council will no doubt prove one of the most important and effective agencies of the American Medical Association in its relationship both to the profession and the public.

THE BUSINESS DEPARTMENT
OF THE AMERICAN MEDICAL ASSOCIATION

By Thomas R. Gardiner

JUNE 6, 1883, MAY BE CALLED the natal day of the Business Department. The thirty-fourth annual session of the Association was then being held in Cleveland, Ohio; one of the important items of business was consideration of plans for establishing The Journal of the American Medical Association. Dr. N. S. Davis, President of the Board of Trustees, gave full details of the proposed journal—thirty-two pages of reading matter, without advertising, issued weekly to the extent of 3500 copies per week at an aggregate cost for materials, printing, wrapping and mailing of $8000 per annum. Such an expenditure would leave "in the treasury only $4500 for editorial work and current expenses of the Association." Dr. Davis then proposed a procedure which proved to be of prophetic import to the material welfare of the Association. He said, "Such a journal reaching members of the Association and others in every State and Territory of the Union would constitute one of the best mediums for legitimate medical advertising, and under 'reasonably fair' business management the net proceeds from that source would not be less than $5000 per annum."

Even before the fourth issue of The Journal went to press, it became apparent that the projected 3500 copies per week would not be sufficient, and the press run was increased to 3800. Subscribers at that time were secured through recommendation of friends or colleagues, as the Association did not have an accurate list of physicians.

At this time advertising was solicited by a circular letter "explaining the merits of The Journal as an advertising medium." Letters were sent to the officers of medical colleges, drug manufacturers, instrument makers, etc., soliciting advertising patronage. The Journal was disappointed that medical college advertising for the coming year had already been placed and they were, therefore, tardy in applying for business from these institutions; however, a few of the larger and better class drug manufacturing firms promptly responded with page advertisements. "payments to be made at the end of each quarter." (Present terms, "payable monthly"). Many offers of advertisements were received from business firms, of such character that they were precluded from acceptance "by a rule adopted by the Association."

This rule had been laid down by the Board of Trustees at the very inception of The Journal as a weekly publication:

"Advertisements from all medical educational institutions and hospitals open for clinical instruction, from book publishers, pharmaceutists, instrument-makers and all other legitimate business interests. But all advertisements of proprietary, trade-mark, copyrighted or patented medicines should be excluded. Neither should any advertisements be admitted with one or more names of members of the profession as indorsers, having their official titles of positions attached. In other words, no advertisements should be admitted which fairly contravene, in letter or in spirit, the principles of the National Code of Ethics."

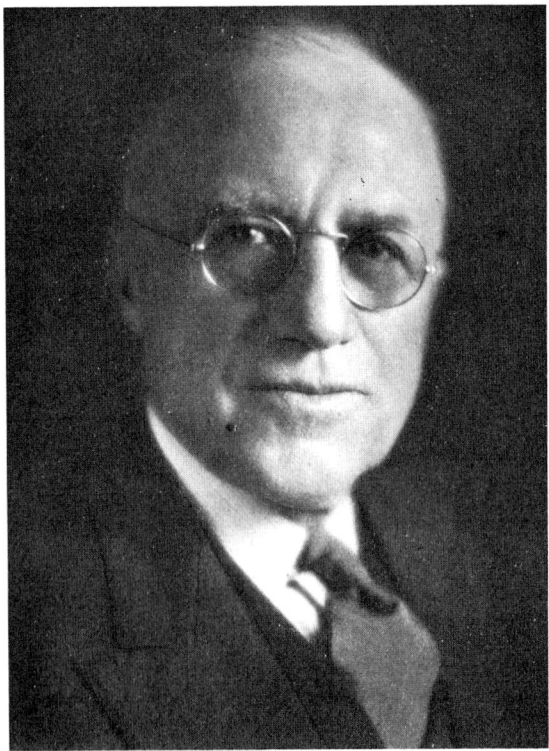

Will C. Braun

A realistic comment from the Board of Trustees states that: "This regulation is a wise restraint, tending to elevate the dignity of The Journal; but it, at the same time, deprives it of a considerable revenue."

For the first nine months in spite of the restrictions mentioned, the amount received on account of advertisements was $809.50, with $1000 "due on account." Though Dr. Davis' goal of $5000 income from advertising was not immediately achieved, later developments proved how sound his judgment had been.

The year 1891 brought a new personality to the business department of the American Medical Association—Will C. Braun of Ripley, Ohio. In 1891 he came to a dingy office at 68 Wabash Avenue, where editorial, circulation and advertising departments were situated in the center of the 30 x 60 foot typesetting room on a 10 x 12 foot platform, surrounded by a pine railing, illuminated by gas from two small jets, and by three windows facing an alley. Besides the typesetters, two men and two women worked in these crude quarters. From that time to 1946—fifty-four years later—when Mr. Braun turned over to his successor the Business Manager's desk on the seventh floor of the present building and assumed the title of Business Manager Emeritus, he had been an active promoter of The Journal's interests in both circulation and advertising. His first duties in the gas lit office were as bookkeeper and copy holder for the proofreader; in addition he was assigned to solicit subscriptions, which he did with enthusiasm and effect. Between 1890 and 1900, the circulation of the Journal sprinted from 3500 to 13,000. During this time, too, circulation was promoted by mail, often over the favorite conclusion, "Trusting you will lend us your assistance, with anticipated thanks, I am, dear Doctor, Faithfully yours."

By 1900, the combined circulation, advertising and accounting staff numbered eight persons. This included Miss Bertha C. Davy, who for 37 years—from 1900 to 1937—was given charge of the Membership and Fellowship Department and of the Fellowship registration at the annual A.M.A. sessions.

In 1900, the Board of Trustees reported: "The growth of The Journal for the past years has been steady. Every month has shown an increase of subscribers and the amount of advertising. Your Board of Trustees, in addition to the exclusions from the pages of The Journal already ordered, have decided that no proprietary medicines advertised in the public press shall be allowed space in The Journal's pages. This we felt was due to the medical profession, and less than that could not well be done." Advertising patronage showed a gratifying increase—close to fifty per cent in the year before 1900. Between ten and sixteen pages of advertising per issue were appearing at that time.

A forecast of the later growth of the technical exhibits sponsored by the advertising department appears in the following report to the Association made in 1900: "An effort is being made—and we are

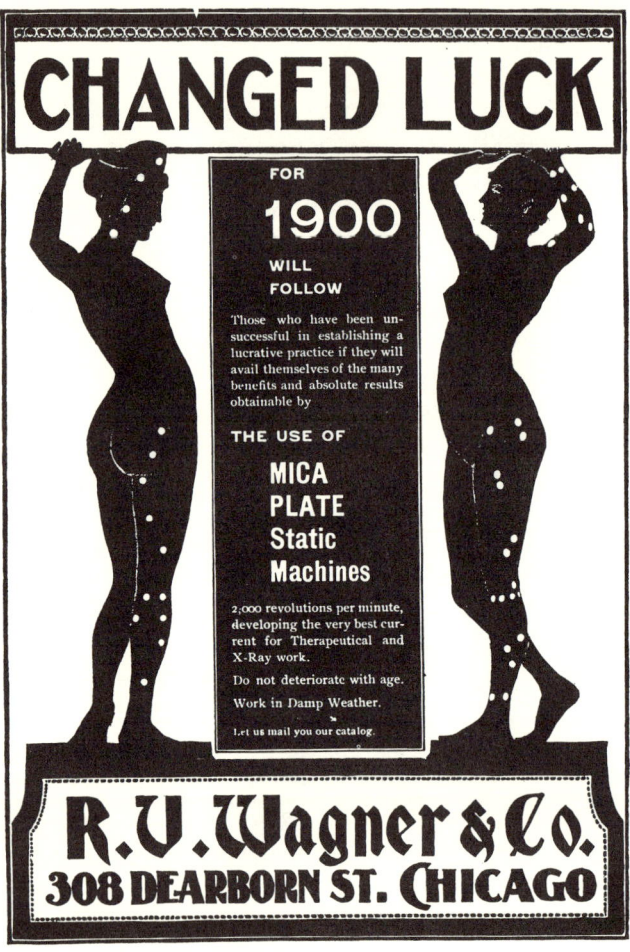

promised by the chairman of the Committee on Exhibits at the Atlantic City meeting that this will be carried out—to have The Journal advertisers receive preference in the allotment of space in the exhibit hall. If such an arrangement could be permanently effected, it would be a decided advantage; and, inasmuch as exhibit space at the annual meetings is under the jurisdiction of the Association, it seems practicable."

The efficient accounting department of today was beginning to take shape in 1900, when the annual session was told: "The board has attempted to reduce the affairs of The Journal to a business basis and to this end has had all of the books and papers gone over by expert accountants. New books have been opened and rearranged and the bookkeeping has been systematized. We believe your Journal to be on a firm basis." Even at that date, The Journal had built a sound foundation and become an advertising medium of recognized value.

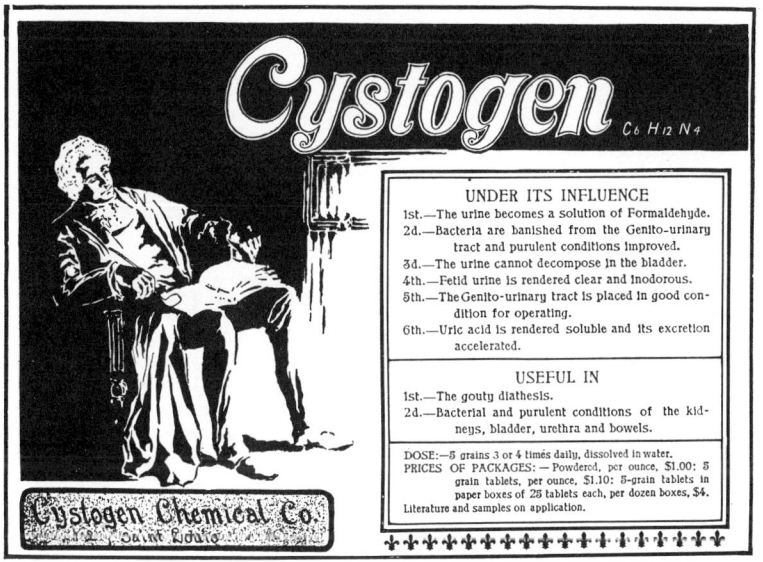

Furnishing a Fuel Fund.

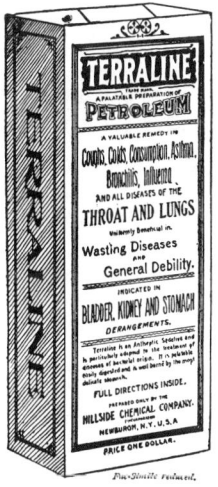

TERRALINE will prove equal to all demands of the economy when it requires heat and force. It is admitted by eminent Physiologists that the percentage of fat in the nerves is nearly twice that of the muscles, blood and brain combined, consequently, when it is essential to fortify the patient against the encroachments of diseases or against progressive retrogression of those subject to nervous diseases, **TERRALINE** is obviously of service.

Few other preparations have shown such satisfactory results in Coughs, Colds, Bronchitis and other Pulmonary diseases. **Terraline** has been used with particular benefit in catarrhal conditions of the alimentary mucous surfaces. Rapid recovery succeeds its employment. Its pleasant taste makes it an admirable vehicle for the administration of other remedies, and its high nutritive value indicates its efficiency in the treatment of Wasting Diseases.

Terraline is an ethical product advertised exclusively to physicians, to whom a liberal supply, together with literature, will be sent upon application to

THE HILLSIDE CHEMICAL CO.,
NEWBURGH, N. Y.

The Morton=Wimshurst=Holtz Influence Machine

Has received the highest commendations of the Medical Profession, and is admittedly

... THE BEST IN THE WORLD ...

Its generative power far exceeds that of any other Static Machine or coil, and being of double utility, it is available at all times

... FOR THERAPEUTIC PURPOSES OR X-RAY WORK ...

OZONE in limitless quantity is produced with this machine, and a new field of usefulness is opened with the advent of the recently devised OZONE INHALER of Dr. Cyrus Edson.

VAN HOUTEN & TEN BROECK
300 FOURTH AVENUE, NEW YORK
Makers of High-Grade Electro-Therapeutical Apparatus

MANUAL OF STATIC ELECTRICITY IN X-RAY AND THERAPEUTIC USES, by S. H. MONELL, M.D., Brooklyn, N.Y. Price, $6.30, prepaid to your address.

••• THE ••• SENSE ••• OF ••• STEAM •••

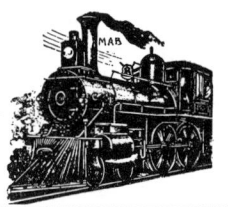

A LOCOMOTIVE is the lineal descendant of a Tea Kettle. As a motive power, steam has some rivals; as a germ destroyer none. Sterilization, to be perfect, must be complete. Tea-Kettle experiments are crude, primitive and incomplete. The...... **Rochester Combination Sterilizer** gives the operator the choice between Steam, Boiling Water and Hot Air. It is neat, portable, durable and effective. It combines simplicity with economy. Our Catalogue containing description and prices of many kinds of Sterilizers suitable for HOSPITALS, LABORATORIES and PRIVATE PRACTICE will be mailed free of charge to any physician on request.

WILMOT CASTLE & CO.,
5 ELM STREET,   ROCHESTER, N. Y.

THE ONLY NEBULIZER...

with which BALSAMS, OILS, IODINE, HYDROGEN DIOXIDE, OZONE, and all other agencies can be

APPLIED SUCCESSFULLY

in the treatment of all diseases of the nose, throat, middle ear, bronchial tubes and lungs.

Is superior to all others because metal parts are protected from contact with the fluids or vapor; has large globe with broad solid base, improved detachable pneumatic cushion mask, low pressure, non-clogging nebulizing tube, hard rubber mouth piece, nasal tip, etc. Can be used by hand or attached to any air receiver with cut-off. Send for Booklet.

Globe Nebulizer No. 6. Height 5½ in., diam. 3½ in.

THE GLOBE MANUFACTURING CO., Battle Creek, Mich.

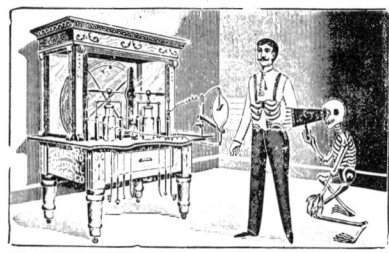

GREAT REDUCTION
In Price of High Grade

X RAY AND STATIC MACHINES
PORTABLE
DRY CELL
GALVANIC
FARADIC
COMBINATION **BATTERIES**

Cabinets, Wall and Table Plates, Switchboards, Cautery and Illumination Batteries, Rheostats, Meters and Electrodes.

Our new Catalogue No. 8 will be sent free on application.

ELECTRO-MEDICAL MANUFACTURING CO., 350 Dearborn St., Chicago, Ill.

In appearance, the advertising pages presented a rather dull picture. Aside from occasional pen drawings, much of the advertising consisted of rather monotonous arrangements of type, often ornamented with borders from the typographer's case. The copy is dated and characterized by such terms as "consumptives," "fetid," "the economy," "static machines." In the light of present day knowledge, too, some of the claims presented would be viewed with lifted brows:

"Changed luck for 1900 will follow those who have been unsuccessful in establishing a lucrative practice if they will avail themselves of the many benefits and absolute results obtainable by the use of Mica Plate Static Machines."

"Under the influence of (this product), the urine becomes a solution of formaldehyde."

"Passiflora Incarnata for insomnia. An invaluable aid in eradicating the morphine, opium, chloral, cocaine and whisky habits."

"It (an antiseptic) is indicated internally in all forms of dyspepsia and digestive

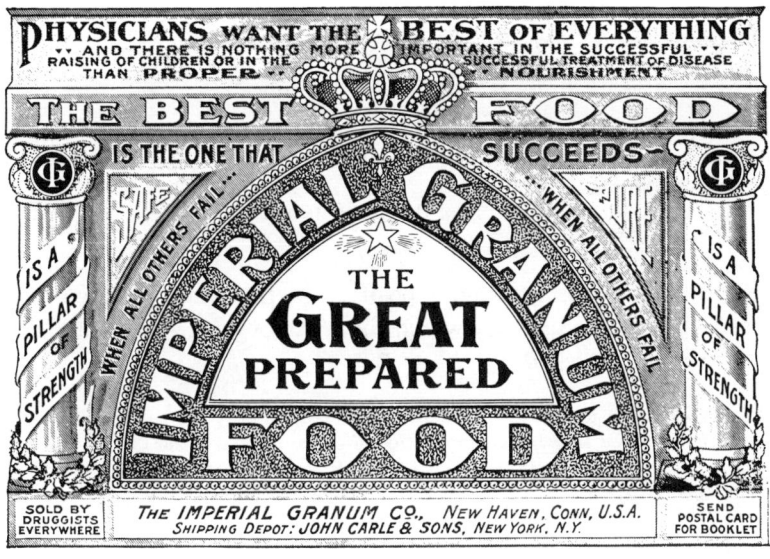

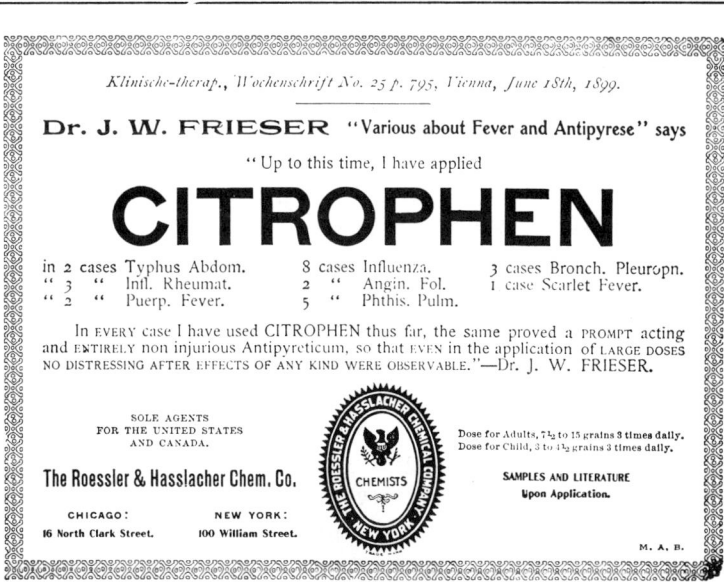

disturbances, butyric fermentation, gastric catarrh, gastric ulcers, etc., externally as a local application in the treatment of specific inflammations of the mucous membrane, chronic inflammatory conditions characterized by fetid discharges and wherever morbid conditions or foul secretions exist."

"Imperial Granum—The Best Food—Is the One that Succeeds—When All Others Fail ... A Pillar of Strength."

Superlatives appear frequently enough to foreshadow the measures for control of The Journal advertising which materialized just five years later. For instance, the advertisers of 1900 were claiming:

The Influence (x-ray machine) is "admittedly the best in the world."

"— is the original and only genuine Cascara Aromatic
— is the only full strength fluid extract of Cascara Sagrada that is not bitter and does not gripe.
— is the only Cascara Aromatic in the world that has made its own reputation; others have borrowed theirs.
— has never had a rival worthy of the name. As a tonic laxative it has never been equalled."

Another advertiser, though positive in his claims, forecasts the constructive procedures by which the truth of advertising claims was later to be established:

"We make the positive assertion—(and stand ready to prove it)—that (this product) actually *builds blood* in cases of anemia, etc. We can send you hosts of case reports, 'blood counts,' etc., as confirmatory evidence. If you want to prove it yourself, send for samples."

A food advertisement headed, "this is not a prescription. It is a food," appears to be forty years ahead of its time, for it states prophetically above the tabulated list of food elements contained:

"You will recognize in this combination essential constituents of a highly nutritious food, and you can prescribe it to your patients in the form of (cereal name)."

The decade between 1900 and 1910 saw a growth in the business enterprises of The Journal as conspicuous as that of publication headquarters, which was extended by building three times in ten years.

In ten years, The Journal circulation increased from 13,000 to 53,000, and advertising income more than quadrupled. A staff of eighteen worked in the business department, plus thirty who were engaged on the new Directory. The publication of the Directory, first , under management of Dr. Frederick R. Green and later under the supervsiion of Mr. Frank V. Cargill, added a new responsibility to those of the advertising department—the sale of space in this biennial reference. This, it appears, was no easy task, for it is recalled that solicitors were authorized to offer the advertiser who would purchase a full page in the Directory a bonus of a *free page* in the Journal.

A typical promotional letter of this time assures prospects for Journal advertising that: "Even though you were not an advertiser in The Journal during 1907, you will be interested in its steady increase in circulation. The year 1908 starts out equally promising. If you will advertise in The Journal you will be on the right track to get in touch with practically all of the more prominent physicians throughout the U.S."

In 1909, Thomas R. Gardiner joined the business staff of The Journal, to begin a period of service which now stands at 37 years and has brought him from the job of making up dummies, checking contracts and selling space, to the desk of Business Manager upon the retirement of Mr. Braun in December 1946. Early in his career, Mr. Gardiner spent three or four years in The Journal's circulation department. In 1913 he attended his first American Medical Association convention in Minneapolis. Since that time he has also been closely associated with the arrangement and promotion of the Technical Exhibition held in connection with the Annual Session.

Five years previously to 1910, the desire to raise the standards of advertising in The Journal and to reserve its pages for the drugs which represented real advances and deserved recognition, gave rise to the organization of a new department at American Medical Association headquarters—the Council on Pharmacy and Chemistry. This was followed later by two other organizations patterned after it—the American Medical Association Council on Foods and Nutrition and the Council on Physical Medicine. Although the story of the Council on Pharmacy and Chemistry appears elsewhere in this history, its influence on the character of Journal advertising through the years has been such that telling the story of the Advertising Department without mentioning the Council would be like disregarding the nerves when treating the muscle.

Announcement of the inauguration of the fifteen member Council brought forth hearty expressions of approval from many reputable manufacturing pharmacists and chemists, who believed that all ethical pharmaceutical houses would be fortified and protected from less desirable enterprises by the stand taken by the American Medical Association. Dissenters were in the minority.

By 1910, more illustrations were appearing in Journal advertising, and bold face type and many heavy borders were in evidence. One of the constructive features of present day medical advertising had already made its appearance in the full page advertisements of a large pharmaceutical house. The theme was asepsis in manufacture. Over

CARNOGEN

is the only preparation in which Red-marrow abounds in an absolutely vital and unaltered condition, and, being the most rapid producer of red corpuscles, it has established its position as the leading restorative and most active tissue builder obtainable.

Given in from one to four teaspoonful doses in plain cold or carbonated water, beer or wine, thrice daily, Carnogen has restored chlorotic patients when all else had failed.

We have some interesting reports which we shall be glad to send you.

American Therapeutic Company,
116 WILLIAM STREET, NEW YORK.

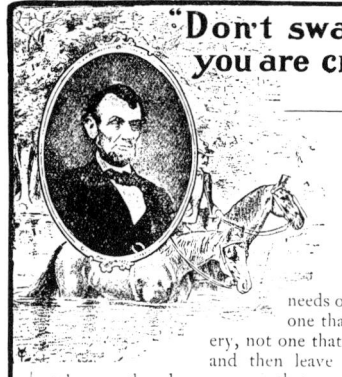

"Don't swap horses while you are crossing the stream"
—Abraham Lincoln.

In other words, do not give up a thoroughly tested, reliable remedy for something new and untried, something without a record; your reputation, possibly your success in life is at stake; prescribe what you KNOW is good, then you are safe.

If your patient needs a medicine, he needs one that you KNOW can be relied upon, one that will carry him steadily along to recovery, not one that will brace him up for a few moments, and then leave him nervous and exhausted until he takes another dose, nor one that goes all to pieces and has to be shaken up every time.

Scott's Emulsion is a smooth, perfect combination of Cod-Liver Oil, Glycerine and the Hypophosphites of Lime and Soda; **it does not separate**, it does not produce undue exhilaration, its action is steady and uniform, it is the STANDARD preparation of Cod Liver Oil.

All Druggists; 50c. and $1.00.   SCOTT & BOWNE, New York.

the caption, "Aseptic Hypodermatic Tablets," is shown a photograph of rows of white gowned and white capped women at neat work tables. The fact that the gowns favor the flowing lines of 1910 and the caps are quaintly frilled in no way detracts from the sincerity of purpose and performance expressed in the statements below:

"The mode of administering hypodermatic tablets makes it of the utmost importance that they come to the hand of the physician in an aseptic condition. In order that we may meet our obligations as manufacturers, all of our hypodermatic tablets are made in special apartments, under conditions of surgical cleanliness."

Another leading pharmaceutical house of today asserts in boldface type a principle of ethical manufacturing recognized from that day to this:

August 6, 1910

De Tamble

$650   **$1400**

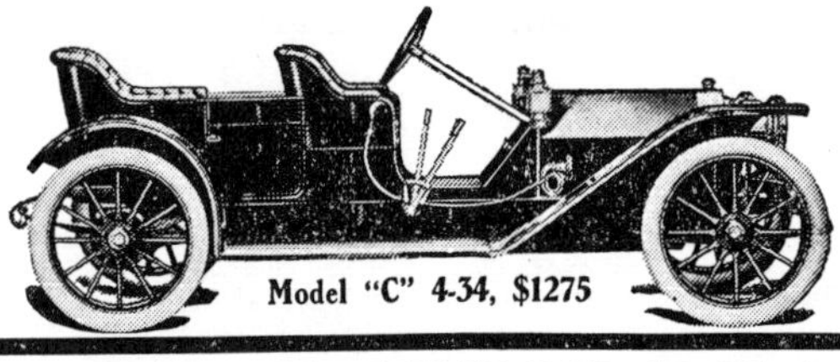

Model "C" 4-34, $1275

SIX COMMON SENSE REASONS
Why You Should Buy a De Tamble Automobile

1. **Power Plant**—Unit construction, 3 point suspension relieving same from all torsional strains and insuring perfect alignment between motor and rear axle at all times.
2. **Power**—Rated 34 h. p. because it develops that. Others claim it but fail on test.
3. **Wheel Base**—Unusual length in this price car—115"—the key to comfortable riding.
4. **Economical**—Light on fuel. Weight is distributed, making car well balanced.
5. **Cost**—It is a HIGH GRADE car within reach of all. There is nothing to compare with it below $1600.
6.—By reason of its simplicity in construction and method of operation, it is a car that assures the doctor of uninterrupted service when on his daily calls, taking him to his destination with the same comfort and satisfaction that he has only found heretofore in cars at three or four times the cost of the De Tamble. The reason for this is that Mr. E. S. De Tamble, previous to entering the automobile field, manufactured parts used in the higher priced cars identical with those now found in the cars bearing his name.

Specifications: 4-cyl. 34 h. p. unit construction; selective sliding gear transmission; multiple disc clutch; h. t. magneto; force feed oiling system; shaft drive; 34" wheels; 115" wheel base; five passenger straight line touring body.

Write to-day for catalogue and we will put you in touch with our nearest agent.

CAR MAKERS SELLING CO., 1256 Michigan Ave., Chicago, Ill.

YOUR HEALTH, COMFORT, SAFETY, CONVENIENCE AND PROFESSIONAL DIGNITY DEMAND THE COZY CAB

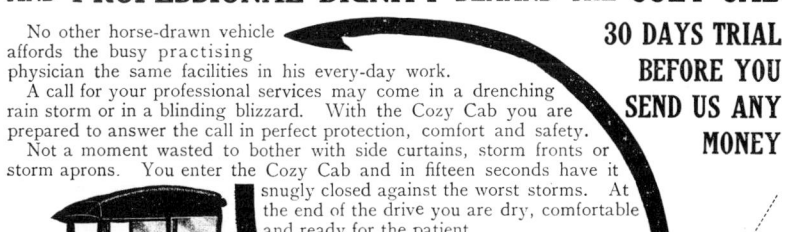

30 DAYS TRIAL BEFORE YOU SEND US ANY MONEY

No other horse-drawn vehicle affords the busy practising physician the same facilities in his every-day work.

A call for your professional services may come in a drenching rain storm or in a blinding blizzard. With the Cozy Cab you are prepared to answer the call in perfect protection, comfort and safety.

Not a moment wasted to bother with side curtains, storm fronts or storm aprons. You enter the Cozy Cab and in fifteen seconds have it snugly closed against the worst storms. At the end of the drive you are dry, comfortable and ready for the patient.

The impressive individuality of its appearance, its high grade finish and dignified style will add to the prestige and influence of any physician.

The quality of every piece of material and workmanship throughout is of Fouts & Hunter style and absolutely guaranteed

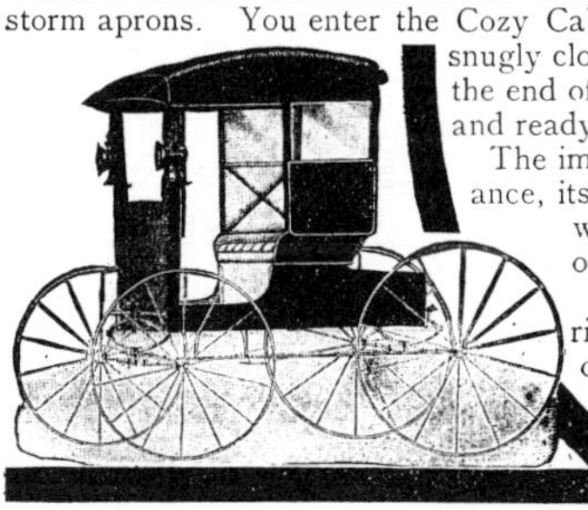

Our Cozy Cab catalog will give complete details and illustrations. The coupon or a card will bring it.

FOUTS & HUNTER CARRIAGE CO.
63 H THIRD STREET, TERRE HAUTE, INDIANA

Without placing myself under the slightest obligation, please send me your complete catalog and your TRY-BEFORE-YOU-BUY-PLAN.

FOUTS & HUNTER CARRIAGE MFG. CO.
63 H 3rd St.,   Terre Haute, Ind.

Name..............................
Town..............................
State.............................

"We make no dope for quackery."

Some dated therapeutic theories of the time are revealed in advertising captions which offer the profession:

"X-ray Treatment in Tuberculosis."
"Migraine Is an Auto-Intoxication."
"Perogen Bath (Sodium perborate with catalyzer) avoids the necessity of expensive trips to foreign watering places."

Medical "quizzing" was also frequently advertised—giving an interesting keyhole view of the medical student's life in 1910.

The vital issue of transportation in the practice of medicine is emphasized by advertisements such as:

"The Cozy Cab (a natty horse-drawn rig) will be shipped for 30 days trial before you send us one cent."

The earliest automobiles with all their shiny brass and startling exposure of mechanisim are advertised as follows:

"Enables you to cover more territory, handle more cases and reach patients in far less time than with horse and buggy—only $900.00."
"Rumble Seat $20 Extra."

"Holsman—Built high enough to travel the country roads like a carriage. Clears the center of the road by eighteen inches, and therefore has *twice the advantage* of the ordinary machine in muddy, rutty, rough or rocky roads. Has large wheels, solid rubber tires, and *rides like a carriage*. The Holsman exclusive patent marks an era in automobile building. It *does away with* all live axles, friction clutches, differential gears, water tanks, pipes, pumps, etc. Reverses without extra gears. *No water to freeze. No puncture troubles. No odor. New hill-climbing power.*"
"Rebuilt Thomas Flyers all *seasoned* cars—cars which have proven their reliability."
"With Solid or Pneumatic Tires—and for only $600 to $700."

Automobile goggles, "perfection non-skid climbers," auto tops and accessories and a book on "How to Run an Auto"—these and more transportation aids were continuously presented in The Journal at this period.

The circulation of The Journal had reached 74,000 by 1920, a fact which is at least partially responsible for the glowing report of the Board of Trustees on advertising revenue that year: "The advertising department makes an unusually good showing; this is due partly to the amount of advertising space sold, but more particularly to increased advertising rates. The past year has been one of great prosperity, and business firms have been very liberal in advertising. This must be kept in mind in planning for the future. It is needless to add that we are keeping our advertising up to the standard which has prevailed for many years; that if we cared to lower this standard there might be still a larger increase in the advertising income."

In spite of this increased income, the Board showed concern over higher expenses this year. It reported as follows in 1920: "The steadily increasing cost of production is likely to cause serious concern if it continues much longer. As an illustration we might refer to the price of paper used in The Journal. A reference to the auditor's report for 1918 will show that paper for The Journal that year cost approximately $162,000. Last year—1919—it was over $217,000—an increase over the preceding year of approximately $55,760. There was an increase in circulation, but this was small as compared with the increase in cost of paper. We entered this year with a still further increase; at the lowest estimate, our paper for the current year will cost in the neighborhood of $35,000 more than last year, even though there should be no further increase. Wages in the printing trade are still advancing; an increase that went into effect last February, 1920, adds at least $22,000 to the pay in the printing department. The increase in these two items alone—paper and labor in the mechanical department—will add at least $57,000 to the expense this year. In addition, there is a steady increase in the wages for all the other help—stenographers, typists, clerks, etc."

The personnel of the business department had more than doubled between 1910 and 1920, advancing from 18 to 39—a fact which may have contributed to the concern over rising costs.

In 1913, the Cooperative Medical Advertising Bureau was organized, representing the advertising interests of twenty-two state journals. Mr. Elwood W. Mattson was appointed director, a post which he held for 24 years.

The year 1917 had brought to the department another of the personalities who helped to build advertising in American Medical Association publications—Mr. Charles S. Mohler. In his capacity as advertising copy supervisor, Mr. Mohler helped to further the understanding of American Medical Association advertising principles among advertisers. Promotional minded, an able copywriter, he also had a hand in preparing much of the Association's advertising and circulation promotion literature from 1917 until his accidental death December 23, 1946.

Mr. Alfred J. Jackson, who had for some years been employed in the accounting department, joined the advertising department at this period, working on The Journal, Hygeia and the Special Journals.

By this time illustrations were profusely used and advertising had accordingly taken on additional interest; however, only an occasional advertiser revealed an awareness of the value of artistic design in layout. For the most part, space was filled with a *neat arrangement* of illustrations and profuse text. Many advertisements ran "T.F." (till forbidden)—the same text and picture appearing unchanged repeatedly. As might be expected, some of the limited number of advertisers whose promotion showed improvement then are leaders in their fields today. Copy showed a tendency to ingenuous statements such as:

> "Physicians, Hospital Executives and Health Officials *should be interested* in this new food product."
>
> "Hear the air rush in when you punch the vacuum cap on a bottle of —."
>
> "*Are you willing to be convinced* that electro therapy has a well defined and well established place in the practice of medicine?"

Advertising for radium (as well as for x-ray and electro therapy equipment), appears frequently during this period.

Transportation problems are still recognized in the advertising for an auxiliary transmission which is said to "assure complete confidence in the performance of your Ford, no matter what the weather or road conditions—snow, hills,—you may undertake on your country trips." Ankle length fur lined coats are also recommended—another reflection of the exigencies of medical practice then.

The circulation of The Journal had grown to 98,000 in 1930, and a staff of sixty carried forward the work of the circulation, advertising and accounting departments.

The Board of Trustees reported the increasing demand for advertising space with noteworthy modesty, as follows: "The volume of advertising secured through the efforts of the department established for the purpose during the year 1929 was entirely satisfactory, and the income derived from this source showed a considerable increase over that of the preceding year. It seems to be apparent that the publications of the Association offer a medium to the advertisers of worthwhile products that is attractive and satisfactory to their producers. The usual large amount of offered advertising matter was rejected, in keeping with the expressed determination of the Board of Trustees to maintan the same high standards that have characterized the advertising columns of the Association's periodicals in past years." An average of 67 pages of advertising per week was now appearing in The Journal.

The gratifying growth of the state journal organization is noted as follows: "The Cooperative Medical Advertising Bureau now serves thirty official publications of constituent state medical associations. Since the establishment of this bureau, more than $75,000 has been distributed to cooperating journals from its earnings."

The size of the mailbags also told a story of seemingly unbridled growth: "Indicative of the constantly increasing demands made on the offices of the Association, it is interesting to note that exclusive of first class mail, 213 tons of mailing matter went out from this department in 1929 as compared with 146 tons in 1928."

The auditors report, "We have pleasure in reporting that the books are maintained in excellent condition."

In 1924, Mr. Alfred W. Stack, present director of the subscription, membership and fellowship department had joined The Journal circulation staff, becoming director of the subscription department eight years later. Mr. Stack's previous work in building newspaper circulation provided the background for his efforts on Journal circulation.

By 1930, colored inserts had appeared in The Journal advertising section and occasionally color on inside pages. Both copy and layout had taken long strides forward. Today's trend toward predominant illustrations and small blocks of copy had asserted itself in only a small proportion of cases; type was still the favorite medium of expression. However, design had greatly improved and much of the copy was direct—its purpose, information.

In the light of subsequent therapeutic advances, physicians would be interested in such statements as the following:

"Don't whip a jaded appetite when there is a vitamin that will revive it. . . . Medical literature contains frequent references to this *peculiar* effect of Vitamin B deficiency."

"An *effective variation* in the treatment of pernicious anemia—Concentrated Liver Extract."

Advertisements for Creosote still appear frequently. Ultraviolet and Quartz Mercury lamps have taken possession of numerous pages in The Journal.

A popular soap which today bases its campaigns primarily on infant care exploited the romance motive in 1930, beginning a page ad in The Journal with the startling announcement, " 'Boo! We're engaged' announced Phyliss and Ben together." In the same advertisement, however, the manufacturer makes the prophetic statement:

"Advertising can never, perhaps, be as single-hearted as science, which has nothing to sell. But we have always believed that there need be no clash between the scientific attitude and the advertising of an honest product . . . and in that belief the —— advertisements have been designed."

Chemotherapy is still in the future, as evidenced by the advertising for Optochin Base—Ethylhydrocupreine in the treatment of pneumonia.

Although the decade between 1930 and 1940 encompassed a great national depression, The Journal circulation showed an increase—from 98,000 to 99,000. The personnel of the business department now stood at seventy.

In 1939, Hygeia, then going through a period of "advertising depression" was given extra impetus in promotion under the direction of Mr. Mohler. Within three years its advertising revenue had doubled, a growth which has continued steadily to the present day. The circulation of Hygeia, under the management of Mr. Cargill, had increased to almost 200,000 by the end of 1946.

The end of 1946, which marked the one hundredth year of the Association, saw a notable growth in the strength of the business department over the past years. The Journal circulation had mounted from 99,000 to 129,000 in six years. During the year 1946 an average of nearly 3200 new subscribers per month has been entered on the mailing list. Advertising volume has moved up to an average of seventy pages or more per issue. A staff of eighty-three persons carry on the work of the business department.

At the end of 1945, Mr. Harold L. Sandberg, who had been director of the Cooperative Medical Advertising Bureau for 8 years, was succeeded by Mr. Jackson of The Journal advertising department.

The sweeping improvement and refinement of general advertising since 1930 is reflected in the medical advertising now appearing in The Journal. The best efforts of a rapidly developing profession appear in the (1) improved attention-getting technics and (2) more interesting and informative content of Journal advertising—both in illustrations and text. Color—one of the most effective bids for reader attention—has become a commonplace in Journal advertising, running an average of 20 pages per issue, in addition to frequent four-color inserts. The strong psychological appeal of pictures is being exploited, and many excellent and authentic photographs are appearing, plus paintings by artists of recognized ability. Layout has become, at least comparatively speaking, a fine art. Taking cognizance of the tendency to hurried reading, The Journal advertising shows a trend toward brief copy—surrounded by ample white space further to enhance readability.

To convey maximum information to the professional man with a minimum expenditure of time, illustrations are made to assist text by *telling more* than formerly. Frequently now they show products *in use*, or show *the results of their use*. Copy is typically direct, factual, concise.

The roster of 1946 advertisers checked against those of 1930 would show the addition of numerous food and infant food manufacturers, with much of their promotion based on recently disseminated nutritional knowledge. The same body of knowledge is often tapped for the pharmaceutical maker's vitamin products copy. Medical book advertising has increased, and the pharmaceutical houses and equipment manufacturers of course claim many pages. Advertisements for drugs such as the sulfonamides and penicillin signify history-making advances. Cosmetic advertisements occur occasionally, and some cigarette advertising has been admitted. Although these additions to the advertising rolls indicate a broader coverage of products, claims are still controlled according to the principles laid down by the framers of The Journal in 1883.

On December 31, 1945, at the end of fifty-four years of service in the advertising and business department, Mr. Braun voluntarily retired and was named Business Manager Emeritus. The Board of Trustees reports the event as closing "a career of most useful and devoted service to the Association." The report continues: "The circulation of The Journal, which was one of Mr. Braun's primary responsibilities throughout the years, grew from 3,500 copies in 1899 to 112,510 in 1945. Mr. Braun's invaluable service in helping to keep the activities of the Association on a sound business basis has contributed immeasurably to the organization."

BUREAU OF HEALTH EDUCATION

By W. W. Bauer, M.D., Sylvia B. Martin and Audrey McKeever

AS AN EXAMPLE OF AWARENESS on the part of the American Medical Association and its membership of the importance of health education as a basic function of the profession, we find in the 1846 and 1847 proceedings of the Association a resolution introduced by Dr. Henry Carpenter of Lancaster, Pennsylvania, which pointed out difficulties arising among physicians in their attendance upon the sick and called for publication of the principles of medical ethics for the information of physicians, and then added this significant suggestion:

"That delegates request the editors of the public journals in their respective localities to publish the same as proper and useful information for the people."

This is health education in a modern form.

Further examination of these early proceedings reveals another interesting statement:

"Physicians as conservators of the public health are bound to bear emphatic testimony against quackery in all its forms, whether it appears with its usual effrontery or masks itself under the garb of philanthropy and sometimes of religion itself."

This also is a very modern form of health education. Doctors are still bearing testimony against quackery.

There could be no plainer statement of the obligations of the profession to the public in the field of health education than these words, which were contained in the 1847 report of the Committee on the Code of Medical Ethics:

"As good citizens it is the duty of physicians to be ever vigilant for the welfare of the community . . . they should also be ever ready to give counsel to the public in relation to matters especially appertaining to their profession, as on subjects of medical police, public hygiene, and legal medicine. It is their province to enlighten the public in regard to quarantine regulations,—the location, arrangement, and dietaries of hospitals, asylums, schools, prisons, and similar institutions,—in relation to the medical police of towns, as drainage, ventilation, etc.—and in regard to measures for the prevention of epidemic and contagious diseases; and when pestilence prevails, it is their duty to face the danger, and to continue their labors for the alleviation of the suffering, even at the jeopardy of their own lives."

From its very inception, medical organizations in the United States took a step toward the establishment of one of the fundamentals necessary for good public health work and for health education, namely, a knowledge of who died and where and why, who was born and where, and who was married to whom. The National Medical Convention, precursor of the American Medical Association, stating that upon the circumstances connected with the three important eras of existence—birth, marriage and death—are dependent to a very great extent the physical, moral and civil condition of the human family, appointed a committee to consider the expediency of urging upon the state governments the adoption of measures for a registration of civilian births, marriages and deaths.

At the same time another committee was charged with the duty of establishing the names of diseases and of assigning to these names, numbers by which death could be reported as to cause, and properly classified. This was the second step necessary for the establishment of proper recording of vital statistics. Such pioneer practice in health education was indeed forward-looking when considered as action taken only a few years after the discovery of anesthesia, and at least thirteen years before the beginning of the era of bacteriology and the work of Koch and Pasteur. In view of its available knowledge, the thinking of the profession in 1847 was no less clear and no less public spirited than it is today.

The problems which were foremost in public hygiene were expressed in the first report of the Committee on Public Hygiene in 1849: deficient drainage, street cleaning, water supply, ventilation, housing, and nuisances such as slaughter houses, factories, butcher shops, cotton mills, and other factories. Good ventilation was so rare that a special report was made of it when it was found to exist in the woman's wing of the Pennsylvania Hospital. Numerous other fundamental dangers to health existed, and the lay public was gradually turning to the medical profession for relief. Popular concern over conditions was aroused, and, as a consequence, studies on smallpox vaccination, epidemic control, diet, poisonous gases, and the possibility of poisoning from lead pipes were stimulated. These were the early gropings in the field of health education.

Meanwhile, the year previous, the American Medical Association had received a report on the physician in education. Proposed two-thirds of a century ago by the medical profession, the report resembles modern school health supervision at its best. It suggested that the physician be given authority in schools over all environmental factors in the school itself, such as sanitation and good lighting; periodical medical examination of the students; provision of facilities adjusted to best functioning of the sensory organs; daily medical survey of conditions; and courses in hygiene. Also at this time, humane societies came into the picture.

In 1907 the American Medical Association created its first organization for health education—a Board of Public Instruction. This Board, consisting of Drs. F. F. Simpson, Frank Billings, Charles Harrington, L. S. McMurtry, Howard A. Kelly, L. Emmett Holt, John G. Clark, Chairman, and R. Max Goepp, Secretary, proposed a program which was to begin with the preparation of popular articles by outstanding physicians. After the Board had approved the articles and they had been issued as publications of the A.M.A. Board of Trustees, they were to be offered to popular periodicals.

However, there was considerable debate as to whether the articles should be signed.

The Board of Public Instruction wisely recognized that an article in order to carry weight must be better identified than as the publication of a group, such as trustees. It must carry the name of the doctor who wrote it. We are still trying to persuade some medical societies that a radio speaker must be named if his speech is to carry weight.

The Board of Public Instruction then submitted an extensive outline of proposed topics on which the public was to be informed. In accordance with the general trend of the times, this outline read like the prospectus for a medical book. Public instruction by the medical profession at that time consisted largely of talking down to an audience. The technic had not yet been learned of speaking to the public in terms which the public could understand.

Other Board undertakings were a campaign for the prevention of blindness resulting from improper care of the eyes at birth and an attempt to have state medical societies establish committees similar to the Board. Many state medical societies now have such committees and much valuable work is being done through them.

In 1910, the section on hygiene and sanitary science asked the House of Delegates to create a permanent council that would merge the many committees concerned at that time with public health. The Council on Health and Public Instruction was appointed. The first members were Dr. H. M. Bracken, of Minneapolis, representing public health interest, Dr. W. B. Cannon, of Boston, representing medical research, Dr. Henry B. Favill, of Chicago, representing public instruction, Dr. J. N. McCormack, of Bowling Green, representing organization, and Dr. W. C. Woodward, Washington, D. C., representing legislation. It is from this Council that the present work of the American Medical Association in health education has grown.

An interesting reversal of modern tendencies appeared in the 1910 proceedings. The question was debated of whether boards of health might not object to encroachment upon their prerogatives by the American Medical Association; today, public health authorities are concerned about the resentment of the medical profession with respect to encroachment upon the field of medicine.

And in these same proceedings there was a resolution which reads: "Whereas the American Medical Association . . . stands committed to the education of the public with respect to the nature and prevention of disease, resolved, that the women physicians, members of the American Medical Association, take the initiative individually in their respective associations in the organization of educational committees to act through women's clubs, mothers' associations, and other similar bodies for the dissemination of accurate information touching these subjects among the people."

In 1911, the Council on Health and Public Instruction conducted a Press Bureau from which bulletins were sent weekly to approximately 5000 newspapers. Interestingly enough also at that time, the cartoons published in THE JOURNAL of the American Medical Association were an important feature in health education programs. They were reproduced on large cards for exhibitions, and made available to other publications through cuts and proof sheets. A Speakers Bureau was organized, and one or more speakers designated in each state who could be called upon to appear on behalf of the American Medical Association. A year later, when it was recommended that a lay health magazine be established by the Association, a great many speeches had been made and numerous educational pamphlets issued through the Council.

In 1912, at a meeting of representatives of the National Education Association and the American Medical Association, a resolution was adopted which led to one of the most significant and fruitful health education activities of the medical profession in the years to follow. The resolution authorized the undertaking by a joint committee of the two organizations of a "report on health aspects of school environment and equipment, and for promulgating other helpful suggestions." The work of the Joint Committee on Health Problems in Education was begun.

In 1914, the Council prepared and published a standard set of

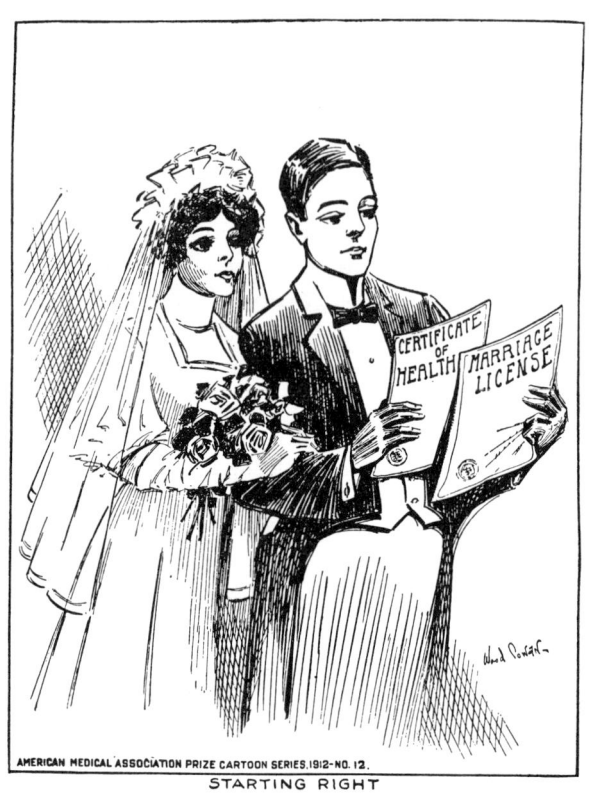

AMERICAN MEDICAL ASSOCIATION PRIZE CARTOON SERIES, 1912-NO. 12.
STARTING RIGHT

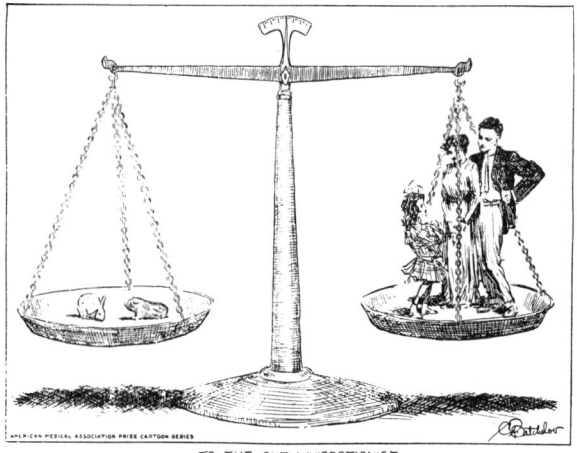

TO THE ANTI-VIVISECTIONIST
"AT HOW MANY RABBITS OR GUINEA PIGS DO YOU VALUE
YOUR WIFE, YOUR HUSBAND OR YOUR CHILD?"

Cartoons from 1912–1913 issues of J.A.M.A.

public health pamphlets for the use of state boards. The work of distributing pamphlets on numerous health subjects was continued. A special activity of the Council was a "Public Health Sunday" in

Philadelphia, participated in by the Philadelphia County Medical Society and other organizations, including churches. Although this form of promotion has fallen into disrepute, there was a place for it in that time.

In 1915, the Council issued plans for conducting a Baby Health Conference, a step to counteract prevalent baby contests in which babies were judged by lay persons solely on the basis of appearance. Many babies brought to these gatherings acquired communicable diseases, and there was no constructive outcome. Thus, when the Council had published record forms and instruction manuals for the holding of a Baby Health Conference, the Children's Bureau of the federal government commended the Council and referred to it inquiries for literature concerning the measuring and scoring of babies. This commendation stands in marked contrast to the present attitude of the Children's Bureau. It now seems to hold that there is little or no competence in the medical profession to care for the health of mothers and children, unless under the supervision of the Children's Bureau.

Also in 1915, one of the important pioneer publications of the Joint Committee on Health Problems in Education appeared: the pamphlet on "Minimum Sanitary Requirements for Rural Schools."

In the same year, the secretary of the Council served as consultant to a national newspaper syndicate which was preparing a health column for use in daily newspapers throughout the country. Material in the form of pamphlets, bulletins and reprints was furnished by the Council, and advice and suggestions were given freely. This cooperation, for which grateful acknowledgment was given by the editor of the syndicate, was a foreshadowing of the modern health column.

In 1918, Dr. Frank Billings, of Chicago, was Chairman of the Council. He was succeeded in 1919 by Dr. Victor C. Vaughan, of Ann Arbor, Michigan. The Council continued its work, steadily developing the health education phase. The result, stated in the 1919 report of the Council was this:

"Regarding the general plan of public education carried on for a number of years through press bulletins, Speakers Bureau, public meetings, distribution of pamphlets, leaflets, etc., these methods, while largely new at the time they were inaugurated, have been taken up by other organizations . . . It is . . . doubtful whether the purely educational activities of the Council can at present be enlarged to any great extent with any degree of success."

With that program on a firm basis, for several years the Council devoted increased attention to other phases of its health activities, that is, investigation of current health conditions and the adoption of laws commensurate with increased knowledge of disease prevention. A lay organization, the Women's Foundation for Health, became active, and a series of the Foundation's pamphlets were approved by the Council. The Joint Committee was also active in preparing additional literature on health improvement in rural schools.

In 1922, the lay health magazine was established. It was named HYGEIA, after the Greek goddess of health, with the subtitle "The Health Magazine, published by the American Medical Association."

The year 1923 marked the beginning of three outstanding features of health education by the American Medical Association. The first issue of HYGEIA appeared in April under the editorship of the Council.

Next, the Council was broken up into several groups, one being the Bureau of Health and Public Instruction.

And, third, the American Medical Association initiated radio broadcasting. Programs presenting information from HYGEIA and material furnished by the Propaganda Department of THE JOURNAL (nostrums, quackery and pseudo-medicine), were broadcast with the cooperation of Westinghouse Station KYW. These broadcasts marked the beginning of the present extensive radio coverage by the American Medical Association.

Dr. Olin West, Secretary of the Association, discharged the duties of Director of the new Bureau, but shortly Dr. John M. Dodson was made the Director on a full-time basis.

Using Bureau examination forms, the National Congress of Parents and Teachers in 1924 inaugurated the Summer Round-Up Campaign. Demand for examination forms and copies of the manual on periodic examinations increased steadily, as did distribution of a wide variety of printed matter on general health subjects. In addition, much health material was provided for national exhibits.

By 1925 local medical societies were having HYGEIA readings broadcast on local radio stations. Conduct of the Question and Answer column in that publication had devolved largely on this Bureau, and direct replies began to be sent. A questionnaire sent to medical societies revealed less than 5 per cent of those contacted making use of radio as a means of health education, approximately 80 per cent not actively promoting periodic health examinations.

The Bureau in 1926 provided height and weight charts for physical examinations of preschool children. And, because of the difficulty presented in securing free radio time, the Board of Trustees was considering the operation of an American Medical Association-owned broadcasting station. But such a step proved unnecessary, for in 1927 time for weekly health talks was obtained from Radio Station KYW and the sister Station KFKX.

In February, 1927, Dr. Rosco G. Leland accepted the position as Assistant Director of the Bureau of Health and Public Instruction. A new activity of the Bureau consisted of preparation of talks on medical subjects for lay audiences, these being made available to physicians. "Health education of the public," decided the Reference Committee on Reports of Board of Trustees and Secretary at the annual meeting, was "a most important function of modern medicine, and we urge the continuance of the work of the Bureau of Health and Public Instruction to meet this need." Health talks were being broadcast daily, and the Bureau was commended for its work in this field by the Board of Trustees.

The Bureau-inaugurated educational campaign, as well as the policy of cooperation with the National Congress of Parents and Teachers and the National Education Association, was reapproved in 1929.

Doctor Leland left the Bureau of Health and Public Instruction in 1930 to become Director of the newly-created Bureau of Medical Economics. In this same year the Summer Round-Up Campaign, was altered to make it more acceptable, emphasizing as its aim periodic health examinations by family physicians. One of the chief objections to the previous plans of this Campaign was expressed in the Report of the Reference Committee on Reports of Board of Trustees and Secretary this year: ". . . examination . . . en masse in clinics, health units and similar agencies . . . cannot be but perfunctory, superficial and unsatisfactory to physician and child alike."

By 1931 the broadcasts, now ranging from two to ten a week, had become for the medical profession a powerful counter-attack against the ill effects of advertising by charlatans. Hand in hand went an encouraging increase of health broadcasting by local medical societies.

Continued evidence of the important services rendered by the Bureau is found in the following quotation from the address of President-Elect E. Starr Judd, given at Philadelphia June 8, 1931:

"The Bureau of Health and Public Instruction has ever-increasing duties and associations. The American Medical Association must be the leader in preventive medicine and public instruction and in public health activities. Public health and preventive medicine are the most discussed subjects in medicine today, and influence and leadership in this work must be retained. . . . I make a plea that we not only continue our efforts but that we enlarge them and maintain our position."

On March 1, 1932, Doctor Dodson retired and Dr. W. W. Bauer succeeded him as Director of the Bureau. Radio work during this year suffered a temporary set-back when in June the health program over the Columbia System was discontinued. Distinct progress was being made toward the goal of examination of preschool children by family physicians.

In 1933 arrangements were made for the broadcasting of health talks over a coast-to-coast network of the National Broadcasting Company, and the program discontinued the previous year was resumed. Bureau cooperation with lay organizations was expanded to include the National Congress of Parents and Teachers, the National Committee for Boys' and Girls' Club Work, the General Federation of Women's Clubs, and the Joint Committee on Health Problems in Education of the National Education Association and the American Medical Association. The Director of the Bureau was appointed to membership on health education advisory boards of all these groups by the Board of Trustees. An added activity was assistance to the Bureau of Exhibits in its preparation for American Medical Association participation in the Century of Progress Exposition. A set of 145 questions and answers on health was made available by the Bureau for World's Fair visitors to the American Medical Association exhibit. The Director made numerous personal appearances before professional and lay groups, and wrote health articles which were published in national magazines. In addition, the Bureau began serving as a clearinghouse for health information to be distributed by local medical societies to the public.

In order to have wider distribution of health information by radio, the Bureau in 1927 had begun to have copies of the radio talks mimeographed, and so popular did these become that in 1934 there was a demand for 7,495 copies. With the problem of antivivisection becoming more prominent, the talks had been expanded to include matter on the necessity of animal experimentation, and pamphlets entitled "Animals in Research" were donated to graduating medical students.

In December, 1935, Dr. Paul A. Teschner was appointed Assistant Director of the Bureau. In that year a significant alteration in the character of the radio broadcasts was instituted. It was recognized that the days of monologue presentations of health topics were past, and that the general public, with so much from which to choose on the radio dial, would not listen unless health education could be given in a more attractive form. As a result, dramatization was introduced. That this offered successful competition to commercial presentations was evidenced by the fact that from all over the country and even abroad, where they might be heard on short-wave reception, commendation on them was received. In 1935 also the Director of the Bureau was elected Chairman of the Health Education Section of the American Public Health Association.

In 1937, a new type of radio program entitled "Your Health" was undertaken with the idea of reaching high school health classes. Printed material supplementary to these programs was provided in HYGEIA, and a workbook prepared by the Director and Assistant Director was published for use by the classes in coordination with the programs. Also in 1937, change of the Bureau name to its present title of Bureau of Health Education was proposed. Final action on this was not taken until 1938. In accordance with the long-established Bureau policy of cooperation with lay organizations, the Director became a member of the advisory committee of the Children's Bureau then in the U. S. Department of Labor. The year saw also the introduction of a new activity by the Bureau, a symposium on school health problems, held at Atlantic City during the annual A.M.A. meeting. Health education literature produced by the Bureau was more widely in demand than during any preceding year.

The second symposium on health problems in education was held in June, 1938, at San Francisco. It was at this American Medical Association session that special broadcasts were arranged by the Bureau of Health Education in connection with the scientific meeting. It was in this year that the Bureau's "Your Health" program received a first award for general excellence from the Institute on Radio in Education. Evidence of the Bureau's leadership in radio health education work is found in the fact its Director was now serving in an advisory capacity to outside radio programs dealing with health subjects. That basic principles were still being followed was demonstrated by the Bureau's preparation and distribution of three special sets of health posters during the year.

A new series of radio broadcasts under the title of "Medicine In The News" was begun in November, 1939, based on news contained in THE JOURNAL and HYGEIA. Indicative of activity by the Bureau was the ratio of this year's correspondence to that of 1925. A survey showed this had increased 325 per cent. As a result of this increase it had become necessary to set up a special department in the Bureau for handling health questions from the general public, separate from regular Bureau correspondence.

The following year, 1940, the radio network series was presented under the title "Doctors at Work." Three networks and ten radio stations were utilized for broadcasts from the New York American Medical Association session. The demand for prepared radio talks reached 6000. Approval in the Report of Reference Committee on Reports of Board of Trustees and Secretary cited ". . . a year of intense activity of the kind to bring credit on the American Medical Association and the American physician. The public relations value of this bureau is second only to its value as an authoritative health educational agency. . . ."

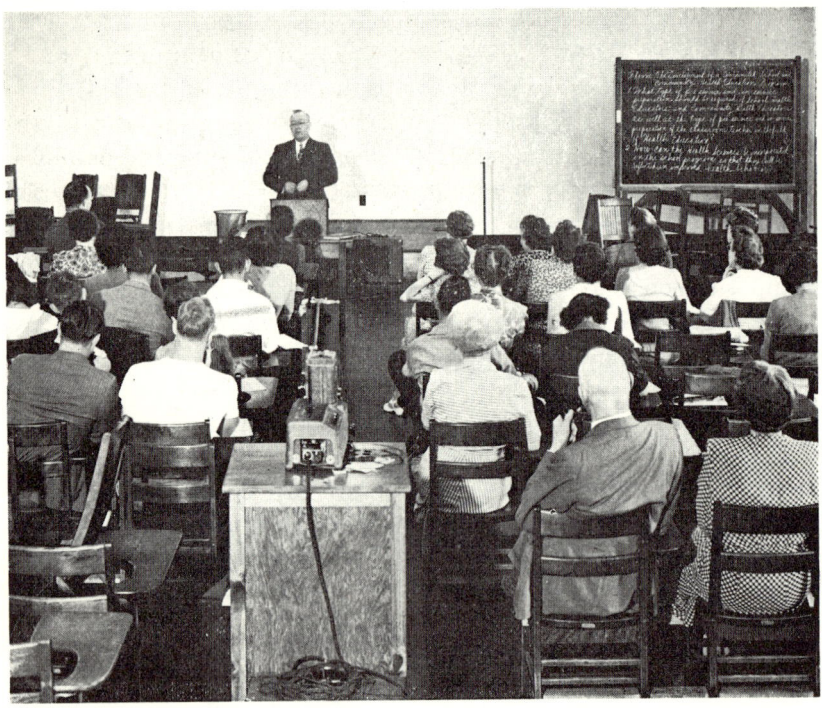

A typical Summer Workshop in Health Education. This one was under the auspices of the Pennsylvania State Department of Health.

The Bureau Director was assigned July 1, 1940, to supervision of office work for the Committee on American Health Resorts without actual membership on the committee.

The "Doctors at Work" network series was continued in 1941. Bureau exhibits were shown at the Cleveland Health Museum, the Chicago Museum of Science and Industry, the Milwaukee Midsummer Festival, and several state and county fairs. The Director was appointed by the Board of Trustees to membership on a Committee of The National Health Council for the Study of Voluntary Health agencies.

In 1942 war transportation difficulties curtailed extensive traveling on the part of the Director and Associate Director. The Director was assigned to cooperate with a new American Medical Association committee on student health, and also assisted in a review of literature relating to health and comfortable temperature for the Fuel Rationing Division of the Office of Price Administration.

From December, 1942, to June, 1943, a national radio series entitled "Doctors at War" was broadcast. The Director and Associate Director continued to contribute numerous book reviews and articles to both Association and outside publications. On July 1, 1943, the Bureau began preparation and distribution of electrical radio transcriptions. These, made in sets under various titles, were designed for use on donated radio station time by local medical societies or health agencies cooperating with medical organizations. Their immediate popularity both as an effective method of health education and as a favorable portrayal of American medicine, resulted in development of plans for greatly increasing this activity.

In 1944, the Bureau received a commendation on "Doctors at War" from the Surgeon General as an "excellent service to the Medical Department of the United States Army."

Popularity of the newly-developed electrical transcriptions for local radio use increased rapidly. Steady production of these sets was undertaken. As a further venture in the use of broadcasting material for school health education, a recorded series known as "Health Heroes" was prepared. This, intended for fourth and fifth grade levels, was available to schools having announcer systems.

A new venture in health education work was undertaken when the Bureau received a special group of post-graduate students from the U. S. Public Health Service and the Kellogg Foundation for a one-week course of instruction, and observation of educational activities of the American Medical Association. This activity is being continued, various groups being received each year.

A Joint Committee on Physical Fitness, authorized by the House of Delegates in June, 1944, to cooperate with the National Committee on Physical Fitness, ceased to function early in 1945 because insufficient funds were provided for operation of the latter body. The Board of Trustees then recommended development of a "Keep Fit" program.

Radio activities of the Bureau in 1945 remained at a continued high level. The network program entered its eleventh consecutive year of dramatized broadcasts on a nationwide network of the

National Broadcasting Company. Furnishing of radio scripts for local medical organization decreased, while demand for prepared electrical transcriptions for similar presentation increased greatly. During 1945, four new transcription series, including dramatization and interviews with physicians by professional radio workers, were prepared by the Bureau.

The death on May 25, 1945, of Dr. Paul A. Teschner, Associate Director, deprived the Bureau of a competent and conscientious

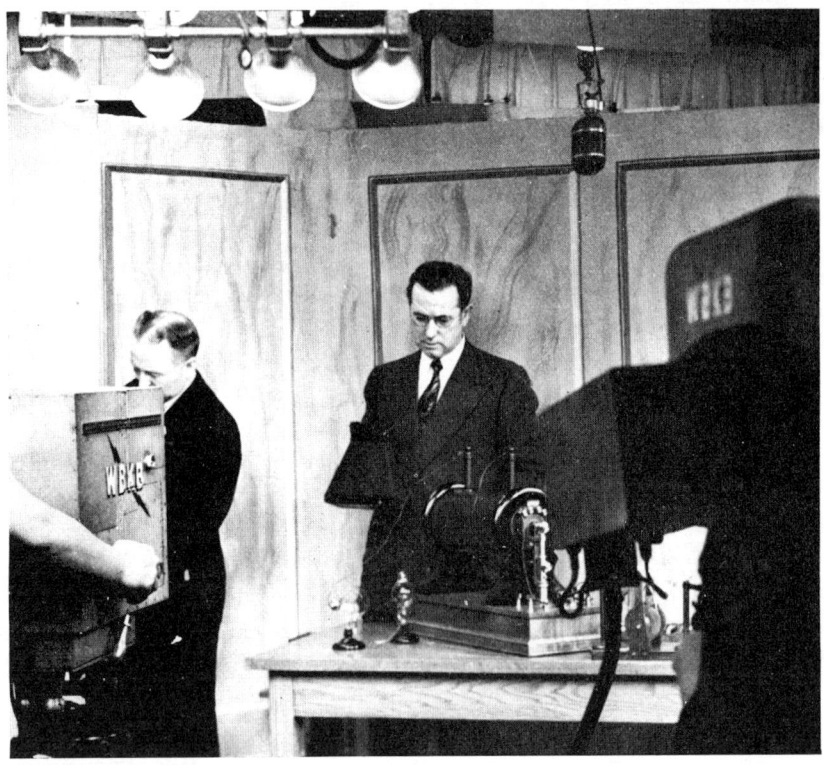

A telecast arranged by the Bureau of Health Education in cooperation with the Council on Physical Medicine.

worker. This position remained vacant until October 16 of that year, when Dr. William W. Bolton was appointed to it.

Cooperative relationships of the Bureau were continued with a wide variety of national organizations, including the Joint Committee on Health Problems in Education, U. S. Children's Bureau Advisory Committee, National Committee for Boys' and Girls' Club Work, National Congress of Parents and Teachers, American Public Health Association, National Conference for Cooperation in School Health Education, and various U. S. Government agencies.

Early in 1946 a new field of health education was entered by the Bureau. This consisted of presentation of health topics over television station WBKB, Chicago, a program being given once every two weeks under the general heading "Cavalcade of Medicine." This activity is being continued, and considerable helpful information is accumulating in the Bureau records on technics used in this relatively new method of reaching the public.

In furtherance of the recommendation of the Board of Trustees relating to a "Keep Fit" program, in 1946 the Bureau of Health Education undertook the organization of a Health and Fitness Program involving the setting up of a special department within the Bureau for the purpose of providing assistance to local organizations throughout the nation in the development of satisfactory health education programs. Shortly after the mid-year, this department began functioning following the appointment to it of two well known and ably qualified specialists in health education work, Dr. Dean F. Smiley, formerly Professor of Hygiene and Preventive Medicine at Cornell University, and Fred V. Hein, Ph.D., formerly director of health and physical education in the Oshkosh, Wisconsin, public schools. Activities of this department are expected to be widespread, and it is felt that assistance provided through it will bring about marked improvement in local health education programs.

As the 100-year anniversary of the American Medical Association dawns, health education activities of the profession may be said to have been established on a firm, long-term basis. The concepts enunciated a century ago still serve as guiding principles but at the same time the Bureau of Health Education has kept abreast of newer developments in teaching health to the public. This receptive, cooperative attitude will continue as the Bureau's fixed policy in all its future activities in promotion of health education under the guidance of the medical profession.

THE BUREAU OF LEGAL MEDICINE AND LEGISLATION

By J. W. Holloway, Jr.

THE CREATION OF THIS BUREAU a quarter of a century ago was the culmination of an interest that the Association had manifested from the beginning in medical legislation and in the various problems that fall in the medicolegal category. At its first meeting, held in May, 1848, the Association was addressed by Dr. T. O. Edwards, a member of Congress from Ohio, who was the chairman of a special committee created by the House of Representatives to consider the adulteration and misbranding of drugs. As a result of this address, the Association memorialized Congress to enact legislation providing for the appointment of a proper inspector at each chief port of entry to examine all imported drugs and medicines and to keep a record of such inspections, to be open for consultation to druggists and others concerned. Shortly after this action was taken by the Association, the Congress did, on June 26, 1848, enact a law to prevent the importation of adulterated and spurious drugs and medicines.

At its second meeting in 1849, a resolution was offered by Dr. A. H. Stevens, of New York, proposing the creation of a number of committees, including a committee on Forensic Medicine, of which Dr. Stevens was made chairman. The minutes of future meetings, however, do not reflect what activity, if any, was engaged in by this special committee.

At this same meeting, a report on Medical Education was submitted which contained a section outlining the laws in force in the several states regulating the practice of medicine. Very few states at that time had such regulatory laws. Four years later, in 1853, the situation as to medical licensure was vividly pictured by Dr. Beverly R. Wellford in his presidential address. He recommended that legislation be enacted in each state creating a state board of medical examiners to pass on the qualifications of persons undertaking to treat the sick.

Early consideration, too, was given to the unsatisfactory conditions surrounding expert testimony and to the desirability of including adequate instruction of medical jurisprudence in medical schools. In a report submitted to the seventh annual meeting, in 1854, by the Committee on Medical Education, this was said about medical testimony:

"All who have had an opportunity of observing the discreditable figure made by medical witnesses who are subjected, by ingenious barristers, to a searching cross-examination before courts of justice, need no other proof of the desirableness of ample and exact instruction in the principles and facts of medical jurisprudence, as a part of the collegiate training of medical students. Setting aside, then, the higher and more binding motives connected with the conscientious convictions of duty, the sense of disgrace attached to scenes in which, by a public exhibition of deplorable ignorance on the part of a witness, not only he, but the profession to which he belongs, is exposed to ridicule and contempt, should suffice to induce the members of this Association, collectively as well as individually, to use all legitimate means to reform this evil.

". . . Your Committee, therefore, regard it as essential to the welfare of society, and to the reputable standing of the profession, that medical graduates should be required to exhibit satisfactory proof of their acquaintance with the leading facts and principles of forensic medicine, and that they should be impressed, by the precepts of their teachers and by the example of their seniors in the profession, with a due sense of the solemn responsibilities of a medical witness."

THE CORONER SYSTEM

The following year, in 1855, a committee was appointed to report at the next annual meeting what measures should be adopted to remedy the evils then existing in the methods of holding coroner's inquests "by which the lives and liberties of the innocent may be jeopardized, and the ends of justice frustrated." This committee, composed of Dr. A. J. Semmes, Washington, chairman, Dr. Grafton Tyler, Washington, and Dr. D. F. Condie, Pennsylvania, did make the report at the tenth annual meeting, held in Nashville, in 1857. This report outlined the history and legal duties of coroners and pointed out the inadequacies existing in the system as operated in the United States. The committee recommended that the office of coroner be reorganized entirely on a new basis, that the person appointed to the office should in all cases be a competent and respectable doctor of medicine, to be selected by the criminal courts and that while the tenure of his office should be during good behavior, the incumbent should be liable to impeachment before the court for misdemeanors and derelictions of official duties. Other suggestions were made with a view of putting the office of coroner and its activities on a scientific basis, and the report concluded with the recommendation that committees of three be appointed in each state, territory and in the District of Columbia to be authorized in the name of the Association to memorialize their respective legislatures to pass such laws as would effectively carry into effect the objectives of the report submitted.

REGULATION OF POISONOUS DRUGS

At the thirteenth annual meeting, action was taken looking toward the prevention of the indiscriminate sale of poisonous drugs at retail. A resolution presented by Dr. L. A. Smith, of New Jersey, on behalf of the Essex Medical Union of that state, contained a recommendation that there be enacted in every state laws prohibiting the sale at retail of morphine, strychnine, arsenic, prussic acid or corrosive sublimate except on the prescription of a physician or on the personal application of a respectable inhabitant of adult age. It was recommended, too, that packages containing such substances be labeled "POISON" and that proper records be kept of sales. A committee was appointed composed of representatives from each state to present this matter to state legislatures, and Dr. Smith was designated as chairman of that committee.

LAWS RELATING TO CRIMINAL ABORTION

At the same meeting, a request was received from the Judiciary Committee of the Connecticut legislature for the appointment of a committee to frame a bill better to prevent criminal abortions, the bill to be introduced in Connecticut. Previously, the Association had recommended to each state that the laws by which the crime of procuring an abortion was attempted to be controlled be revised. The committee requested by Connecticut was appointed, consisting of Dr. Worthington Hooker, Connecticut, Dr. David L. Daggett, Connecticut, and Dr. D. Humphreys Storer, Massachusetts.

MEDICAL LICENSURE

Apparently the efforts of the Association to induce the states to enact medical licensure laws met with slight success for, in 1869, resolutions were adopted requesting each state medical society to appoint annually one or more boards to examine persons proposing to enter the practice of medicine. These resolutions further proposed:

"That each State medical society be requested to require its examining board or boards to exact of every applicant for examination adequate proof that he has a proper general education, is twenty-one years of age, and has pursued the study of medicine three full years, one year of which time shall have been in some regularly organized medical college, whose curriculum embraces adequate facilities for didactic, demonstrative, and hospital clinical instruction.

"That each State medical society be requested to act on the foregoing propositions at the next regular annual meeting after the reception of copies of the same, and, if approved and adopted by the State medical societies of two-thirds of the States, this Association shall deny representation from all organizations who longer refuse to comply with the same, and shall recommend the State societies to do the same; and all persons who after that date seek to enter upon the practice of medicine without first receiving a license from some State Board of Examiners, shall be treated ethically as irregular practitioners."

EXPERT TESTIMONY

The continuing interest of the Association in the subject of expert testimony was reflected in the following resolution adopted at the twenty-third annual meeting, presented by Dr. Henry Hartshorne, of Pennsylvania, on behalf of the Section on Chemistry and Materia Medica:

"*Whereas*, In all capital criminal trials involving questions of medical jurisprudence, there is an obvious disadvantage in the testimony of the scientific experts, being made to appear partial and antagonistic by their being engaged as witnesses upon one or the other side; therefore,

"*Resolved*, That it is the sense of this Association, that in important criminal cases requiring the evidence of medical or chemical experts, the cause of justice will be promoted by the appointment by the court, in every such case, of a commission of experts empowered to collect all purely scientific testimony bearing on the case, and report upon it to the court by which the case is to be tried.

"*Resolved*, That by the appointment of such scientific commission, the present system of summoning chemical and medical witnesses in criminal trials might be dispensed with to advantage.

"*Resolved*, That the same recommendation applies also to cases of accusation of surgical or medical malpractice.

"*Resolved*, That the State Associations be requested to bring this matter at an early date before their respective legislatures."

MEDICAL JURISPRUDENCE

In the minutes of the meeting held in New York City, in 1880, appeared an address by Dr. James F. Hibberd, of Richmond, Indiana, on Medical Jurisprudence, Psychology, Chemistry, State Medicine, and Public Hygiene. Dr. Hibberd stated that he had examined the Index Medicus and had found that during the year ending the preceding April, there were published on medical jurisprudence 15 books and reports, and 223 articles in periodicals. Not much of this literature, however, was in the English language. Possibly reflecting the beginning of the use of electrocution as a method of carrying out a death penalty, Dr. Hibberd reported an instance where a man was hung in Washington, D. C. during the preceding winter. When the trap fell, the shock severed the criminal's head, and thereafter the Congress, by resolution, asked the National Academy of Sciences if it knew of a better way of killing than hanging those who had forfeited their lives to the public by heinous crimes.

Another interesting comment in this address related to the day on which criminals had been sentenced to hang. A Judge Heller, of Indianapolis, had passed sentences on three murderers who had been condemned to be hung by a jury in his court. He fixed Wednesday, January 29, 1879, for the execution, "thus," in the words of the essayist, "breaking the almost universal custom of courts, in requiring capital punishment to be inflicted on a Friday, and by this means aiding in the maintenance of a superstition that ramifies through no inconsiderable portion of the industrial portion of all civilized countries. This act of Judge Heller's is a sample of jurisprudence, but its psychological bearings bring it within the pale of medical jurisprudence."

STATE BOARDS OF HEALTH

The minutes of the meeting held in 1883 and of other meetings reflect the activity of the Association looking toward the establishment of state boards of health. In this year, the chairman of the Section on State Medicine, reported the results of a survey he had made to ascertain what states and counties had health departments.

ANTI-VIVISECTION LEGISLATION

The activities of the anti-vivisectionists prompted the adoption of this resolution, presented by Dr. Henry H. Smith, of Pennsylvania, at the thirty-fifth annual meeting of the Association, in 1884:

"Whereas, It appears that an effort is being made to restrict, by legislative action, the practice of investigation in medical science by experiments on animals; and

"Whereas, In the opinion of this Association such restriction is not needed for the guidance of medical men in their investigations, and would be an injury and hindrance to the pursuit of medical knowlege and the improvement of the medical art; therefore

"*Resolved*, That a standing committee of seven be appointed by the President of the Association, to be known as the 'Committee on Experimental Medicine of the American Medical Association,' charged with the duty of opposing, by all legitimate means, any interference with the progress of medical science by unwise or ill-considered legislation."

The President appointed as members of this committee the following: Dr. H. C. Wood, Pennsylvania, Dr. William Pepper, Pennsylvania, Dr. James Tyson, Pennsylvania, Dr. C. Johnson, Maryland, Dr. J. C. Dalton, New York, Dr. A. Flint, Jr., New York, and Dr. J. S. Billings, United States Army.

MEDICAL RESEARCH

Resolutions relating to medical research were adopted at this same meeting. After referring to the fact that the Congress had theretofore made liberal appropriations for the scientific investigations relating to geology, natural history, the diseases of domestic animals, and other subjects, the Association by these resolutions petitioned the Congress:

"... to make available appropriations for the prosecution of scientific researches relating to the cause and prevention of the infectious diseases of the human race, to be expended under the direction of the National Board of Health, and that the permanent detail of one medical officer of the army, and one of the navy, be authorized for the prosecution of researches of this nature."

A committee was appointed with Dr. George M. Sternberg, U. S. Army, as chairman, to bring these resolutions to the attention of the Congress.

SECTION ON MEDICAL JURISPRUDENCE

Prior to 1886, there was no independent Section on Medical Jurisprudence, although the subject was included in other sections. In his presidential address delivered at the thirty-sixth annual meeting, Dr. Henry F. Campbell, of Augusta, Georgia, devoted considerable space to a discussion of the relationships of medicine and law with particular emphasis on expert testimony and malpractice. At the conclusion of his address, he made this recommendation:

"In conclusion, gentlemen, I would with great deference recommend that a committee —of which I would ask to form no part—be appointed to consider the expediency of organizing, or of rehabilitating a section of forensic medicine, for the reception and discussion of papers and reports on all subjects conversant about the important but at present anomalous, and little understood relations of the medical man to the tribunals of law.

"In time, may we not be able to prophesy of legal medicine, and in the words of the now almost mythic Seneca: the day will come, when those things which are now hidden shall be brought to light by true and persevering diligence—our posterity will wonder that we should have been so ignorant of that which is so obvious."

The President appointed the committee suggested by Dr. Campbell which in turn recommended the organization of a Section on Medical Jurisprudence, but since this necessitated an amendment to the by-laws, the matter was postponed for a year. The following year, in 1886, the by-laws were amended as suggested by the committee, and Dr. I. N. Quimby, of New Jersey, was selected as the first chairman of the new section and Dr. H. H. Kimball, of Minnesota, as its secretary.

COURSES IN MEDICAL JURISPRUDENCE

In his first address to the Association, following his appointment as chairman of the Section on Medical Jurisprudence, Dr. Quimby gave an interesting account of the development of medical jurisprudence and of the teaching of that subject in schools. He said:

"It is not a little remarkable that, while medical jurisprudence is but a new comer in the schools, and only one year ago received its first recognition as one of the legitimate subdivisions of the working scope of the American Medical Association, its origin may be traced to the very beginning of established governments. Among the Hindoos as, subsequently, among the Israelites, Greeks and Romans, jurisprudence appears to have engaged the attention of lawgivers from the earliest period of which there is any record. It is allied to and coordinate with medicine, but in the use of this comprehensive word medicine (preventive and curative), jurisprudence for the prevention of disease far antedates the use of remedies for curing it. Measures for the protection of health, long before they were codified, were first devised and intelligently applied—it scarcely seems necessary to say in this presence—by priests, who, in the exercise of their functions, laid the foundation of medical jurisprudence by a sacerdotal jurisprudence which, in some things has not been improved upon in the lapse of centuries.

"As a branch of special instruction in connection with medicine, medical jurisprudence appears to have been first organized into a science and taught in the medical schools of Germany, in the latter part of the eighteenth century. But the first professorships of the science were created in France, in 1792; and in 1803, the University of Edinburgh followed the example. But in England no similar chair was established in any college until 1820, sixteen years after it was first taught in a course of lectures in Columbia College, New York, by Dr. James S. Stringham, then Professor of Chemistry, and annually by the same professor until his death in 1817.

"He was succeeded by Dr. John W. Francis, who held the chair until 1826. Meanwhile, Dr. Charles Caldwell gave a course of lectures on the same subject in Philadelphia, 1812–13, and in 1815, Dr. Theodoric Romeyn Beck was called to fill a similar chair in the Western Medical College, and to him and his masterly work, first published in 1823, Forensic Medicine, in this country at least, is indebted for having been organized into a concrete science."

LIABILITY FOR MALPRACTICE

Some timely advice was contained in an address delivered at the thirty-ninth annual meeting by the then chairman of the Section on Medical Jurisprudence, Dr. E. M. Reid, of Baltimore, Maryland, entitled "The Status of Medical Jurisprudence as Affecting the Medical Profession and the Laity." After calling attention to the fact that a physician must confront the possibility that at any moment the aid of the law may be invoked to seek to hold him responsible for the consequences that may ensue, not only from the use of newly-discovered drugs, but from even the most intelligent administration of well established remedies, he continued:

"Therefore, when giving medicines, such as sodium salicylate, chloral, or others of like nature, which are liable to be followed by delirium, hallucinations, illusions, etc., it will be best to surround the patient with such safeguards as will prevent him from injuring himself or other persons. He must also bear in mind that many customs though founded on a humane basis, can no longer be followed with impunity; e.g., the physician cannot now safely conceal his lancet, and, without having given his patient warning, plunge it into an abscess; nor, even after the consent of the patient has been given to be anaesthetized, in order to have one eye removed, is it advisable for the oculist to remove both, no matter what grounds he may have for believing it necessary to do so. The consent of the patient to the removal of the second eye is as essential as it was to that of the first. After craniotomy and delivery should life remain in the child the accoucher may not on any grounds complete the work of destruction begun in utero, for the moment the safety of the mother is no longer involved the rights of the foetus, temporarily in abeyance, are restored, and the law recognizes the sanctity of that life no matter how feeble the existence or how monstrous the form. The time may not be far distant when the operation of craniotomy will have to be justified, not upon a mere assertion of impaction, but upon a basis of actual measurement, and the pelvimeter will have to precede the cranioclast. The physician should also know that the common law does not formally recognize the induction of premature labor, and when his State has failed to afford him protection by statutory provision, unless he exercise extreme caution he may find himself in a situation from which it might be difficult to escape creditably."

Incidentally, these annual addresses by the Chairmen of Sections were made pursuant to a by-law of the Association requiring such chairmen to "prepare an address on recent advancements in the branches belonging to his Section, including such suggestions in regard to improvements in methods of work, and present on the first day of its annual meeting, the same to the section over which he presides."

MORE ACTIVITY WITH RESPECT TO CORONERS

At this same meeting was submitted a report of the Committee Upon the Coroner System of the United States, which had been previously created. The committee recommended for earnest consideration in each of the several States the following propositions: (1) The abolition of the office of coroner; (2) The dispensing with the jury services in connection with the coroner's office; (3) The separation of the medical from the legal duties in all cases involving the examination into the causes of death where crime is suspected; (4) Entrusting the medical examination only to competent medical officers properly trained in their work; (5) Making the number of medical officers as small as consistent with the proper discharge of their duties; (6) Consigning all questions of law only to properly qualified legal magistrates; and (7) Removing the appointment of these officers entirely from the question of political consideration, and basing their appointment solely upon their possession of the requisite and proper qualifications. These recommendations are not materially at variance with those contained in the report of the Committee to Study the Relationships of Medicine and Law, under the chairmanship of Dr. Alan R. Moritz, Department of Legal Medicine, Harvard University Medical School, approved by the House of Delegates in 1945.

NATIONAL MEDICAL LICENSURE

Beginning with about 1887, the minutes of the annual meetings disclose accelerated activity on the part of the Association to obtain the enactment of uniform medical licensure laws. Special committees were created to promote such enactments and a draft of a uniform bill was formulated. But the Association refused to act favorably on the following resolution, unanimously adopted by the Medical Society of the State of California, in April, 1897, and presented at the forty-eighth annual meeting of the Association held in Philadelphia the same year:

"*Resolved*, That it is the sense of this Society that the American Medical Association take such action on the subject of medical legislation as will bring this matter to the attention of Congress and the President, and request the passage of such laws as will regulate by National examining boards the right to practice medicine in the United States; and, furthermore, we would urge that the delegates to the American Medical Association be instructed to make it their purpose to secure the adoption of such action by the American Medical Association."

A NATIONAL DEPARTMENT OF HEALTH

It was during this period, too, that greater interest was evidenced in the creation of a national department of health with a secretary at its head. At the annual meeting held in 1891, the President of the Association appointed a special committee of five to "memorialize Congress, at its next session, on the subject of creating a cabinet officer to be known as the medical secretary of public health." The following were appointed on this committee: Dr. C. G. Comegys, Ohio, as chairman, Dr. J. C. Culbertson, Ohio, Dr. W. T. Briggs, Tennessee, Dr. J. F. Hibberd, Indiana, and Dr. William B. Atkinson, Pennsylvania.

The following year, this special committee submitted a progress report on its activities, indicating that objection had been encountered to the establishment of a federal department of health from some members of the profession itself, referred to as "conservative members of our profession," who felt that the creation of such a department and a cabinet secretary "will expose us to the operation of low and disqualified political schemers in our profession." The committee discounted this possibility and submitted with its report a copy of a bill which apparently had been introduced in the Senate by Senator John Sherman and in the House of Representatives by Representative John A. Caldwell. The minutes for succeeding years reflected continuing efforts on the part of the committee to induce the Congress to create a federal department of health but indicated both a lack of interest on the part of the State medical societies and an inability to obtain sufficient funds to enable the committee to function effectively.

COMMITTEE ON NATIONAL LEGISLATION

While the Association had evidenced interest in federal legislation from its first meeting, and while special committees had been created to deal with special topics, it was not until 1899 that a Committee on National Legislation was created to represent the Association on the national front. At the meeting held during the preceding year, a communication was presented from the Ohio State Medical Society by Dr. William H. Humiston, Cleveland, recommending the creation of such committee, but this recommendation was not accepted.

Not discouraged by the refusal of the Association to act favorably on this recommendation, Dr. L. B. Tuckerman, Cleveland, presented another resolution at the meeting held in 1899 calling for the appointment of a special committee on legislation "to consist of three members, residing one in Washington, one in Philadelphia, and one in Baltimore, to whom shall be assigned the duty of representing this Association before the committees of Congress." Dr. Tuckerman also recommended that this special committee be authorized to invite, in the name of the Association, the Army medical service, the Navy medical service, the Marine hospital service, and each State Society of legally qualified practitioners of medicine, to send one delegate each to a conference to be held in Washington, D. C., at such time as the committee might determine; such conference to consider the medical and sanitary legislation then pending, and the members to report to their respective societies, such action as in their judgment ought to be taken. This time the recommendation was adopted and the following members were appointed on the first committee: Dr. H. L. E. Johnson, Washington, D. C., as chairman, Dr. William H. Welch, Baltimore, Maryland, and Dr. William L. Rodman, Philadelphia, Pennsylvania.

NATIONAL LEGISLATIVE COUNCIL

The first meeting of this special committee was held in Washington, November 10, 1899. As a result of this meeting, a communication was sent, under date of January 5, 1900, to each State medical society affiliated with the Association, requesting the appointment of one delegate by each to represent the society at a general conference to be held in Washington at a later date to consider (1) a federal department of health; (2) publication of the Index Medicus; (3) an anti-vivisection bill; (4) unification of medical practice acts; and (5) other "medical legislation of interest to your Society, now pending or to be proposed during the present session." A similar invitation was extended to the surgeons general of the Army, Navy and Marine hospital service.

A meeting of this legislative conference, which later became known as the National Legislative Council, was held in Washington May 1 and 2, 1900. The legislative matters included in the call for the conference were fully discussed and a special committee was appointed to convey to the Congress the results of the deliberations of the conference. A motion was adopted recommending to each State Society the creation of a committee on national legislation. These conferences were held annually for a number of years and current matters of medical interest as pertaining to legislation were discussed. Special committees were appointed to consider particular matters and a standing committee was created to represent the conference, ad interim, in all matters arising in Congress.

NATIONAL AUXILIARY CONGRESSIONAL AND LEGISLATIVE COMMITTEE

In 1903, further steps were taken to extend the framework of the organization that had been built up to consider legislation of medical interest. In its report to the House of Delegates in 1904, the Committee on National Legislation stated that there had been organized a national auxiliary congressional and legislative committee composed of official correspondents in practically every county in the United States. Nominations apparently were sent in by the several state associations which gave the Committee on National Legislation a list of some 1940 names and "commissions" were issued to these nominees.

The duties of the members of this group were described in this manner:

"It shall be the duty of each member of the N.A.C.L.C. to bring all and and only such matters of pending legislation as may be referred to him, either by the legislation committee of his respective state or territorial medical association, or by the Committee on Medical Legislation of the A. M. A. to the attention of the medical profession and the people of his respective county, and by every honorable means, personal and political, individual and professional, private and public, direct and indirect, secure desired action thereon by his representatives in both branches, as the case may be, of the state legislature or of the Congress of the United States. And it shall be his function and duty promptly to report all such efforts on his part, first relative to state legislation to the chairman of the committee on legislation of his state medical association, and secondly, relative to national legislation, to the chairman of the Committee on Medical Legislation of the American Medical Association."

A CENTRAL BUREAU OF MEDICAL LEGISLATION

The volume of activities engaged in by the Committee on National Legislation became so great that in 1905 it recommended to the House of Delegates the establishment of a Bureau of Medical Legislation at headquarters to function under the supervisory direction of the Committee. While this recommendation was approved by the House, the report of the Committee for the following year indicated that for some practical reason it had been found inexpedient to carry out the recommendation.

The Committee reported in 1906 further efforts in support of a National Department of Health, with representation in the cabinet. The Committee report reproduced resolutions adopted by the National Legislative Council at its meeting held in Washington, January 9–11, 1906, recommending that the Committee be instructed to proceed at once with the preparation of the necessary legislation and that the Board of Trustees be requested to appropriate $1,000 to be available to the Committee to employ competent counsel to draft a bill.

The requested appropriation, apparently, was not made available. In the report of the Committee submitted the following year, reference was made to a preliminary draft of a bill prepared by a physician member of the House of Representatives, Dr. Andrew Jackson of Pennsylvania, which had been considered by the Committee. Since the Board of Trustees had failed to make available the requested appropriation, however, the Committee felt disinclined to recommend specific legislation. About this time, the name of the Committee was changed to the Committee on Medical Legislation, the word national being dropped.

In the meantime, the American Association for the Advancement of Science had authorized the creation of a "Committee of One Hundred" to consider methods of establishing a national department of health, the committee being headed by Professor Irving Fisher of Yale University. The Chairman of the Committee on Medical Legislation became a member of the Committee of One Hundred and participated in its discussions.

HEADQUARTERS OF THE COMMITTEE ON MEDICAL LEGISLATION

At the 1907 annual session, the Board of Trustees in its report announced that the headquarters of the Committee on Medical Legislation would thereafter be the office of the Journal, "the point from which most of its work will be done in the future," and that the supervision of the work would remain in the hands of the chairman of the Committee on Medical Legislation but be carried on largely by one of the assistant secretaries in the headquarters office. The Committee also reported the establishment of a Bureau of Legislation at headquarters.

The Reference Committee on Legislation and Public Policy, in 1907, acted favorably on a recommendation of the Committee that an enlarged legislative policy be adopted, that attention be given not only to legislative matters of strictly national concern but to questions embracing the interests of the medical societies and of the profession in all of the states and municipalities. It recommended further that the Committee on Legislation, through the Bureau of Legislation, should "study the question of public policy in the different states and sections of the country, analyze and establish the principles which should govern the state and municipal legislative activities."

MODEL MEDICAL PRACTICE ACT

During the next several years, the official minutes of the meetings of the Association disclose further efforts—fruitless efforts—on the part of the Committee on Medical Legislation and the National Legislative Council to obtain action on federal legislation to create a federal department of health. In 1909, the calling of a general conference was authorized by the House of Delegates to discuss the essentials of a uniform medical practice act. To this conference were invited members of the Committee on Medical Legislation, of the National Legislative Council, the Council on Medical Education, all members and officers of state medical boards, all members of state committees on medical legislation, representatives of all medical colleges, and others who might be interested. The conference was held in Chicago, February 28, and adjourned on March 2, 1910. It was well attended—167 registering. After extended discussion of the subject which prompted the calling of the conference, a committee was appointed by the chair to formulate a uniform medical practice act, consisting of Dr. C. S. Bacon, chairman, of Chicago, Dr. S. D. Van Meter, Colorado, Dr. W. H. Sawyer, Michigan, Dr. F. J. Lutz, Missouri, and Dr. A. R. Craig, Pennsylvania. A draft of a model bill was submitted to this committee by Dr. Van Meter for consideration. Prior to this time, the Bureau of Legislation that had been established at the headquarters office had been working toward the formulation of a model medical practice act that could be recommended to the several states for adoption.

COUNCIL ON HEALTH AND PUBLIC INSTRUCTION

In 1910, the Council on Health and Public Instruction was given jurisdiction over legislative matters and the report of that council submitted to the House of Delegates in 1911 indicated that various bureaus had been established by it with one council member in charge of each. A Bureau of Legislation was established, of which Dr. William C. Woodward was put in charge, who later was to become the first director of the Bureau of Legal Medicine and Legislation.

An effort was made in 1912 to transfer the legislative work of the Council on Health and Public Instruction to a Council on Medical Legislation to consist of five members, to be elected by the House of Delegates. This recommendation, offered by the President of the Association, was concurred in by the reference committee of the House, but the House voted to have the recommendation referred to the Council on Health and Public Instruction for consideration and report at the next annual session.

The minutes for the 1912 meeting, too, reflected the early interest of the Association in securing the enactment of laws relating to the use of narcotics.

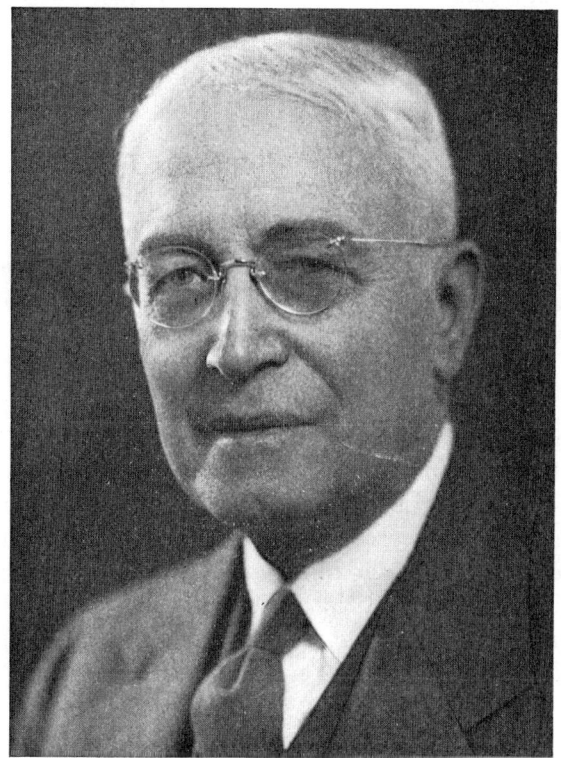

W. C. Woodward

MEDICOLEGAL BUREAU

At a meeting of the Council on Health and Public Instruction, October 19, 1912, the Secretary of the Association presented four propositions for consideration during 1913, including a recommendation for the establishment of a medicolegal bureau at headquarters in which could be collected under competent direction all material bearing on public health legislation and activities and which could formulate model laws, compile court decisions and make suggestions and recommendations for the benefit of state legislative committees. This recommendation was approved by the Council and by the Board of Trustees, and on January 1, 1913, such a bureau was created at headquarters and Mr. John Hubbard, a then recent graduate of Northwestern University Law School, became a member of the staff of the Council as the directing head of the new bureau.

This bureau proceeded with the assembling of material in the medicolegal field, including the collection, abstracting, indexing and digesting of all Supreme Court decisions relating to medical practice acts. The material thus assembled subsequently was published by the Council in a volume entitled "A Digest of the Case Law on the Statutory Regulation of the Practice of Medicine."

THE HARRISON NARCOTIC ACT

The report of the Council on Health and Public Instruction for 1914 reflected the fact that representatives of the Council participated in numerous conferences with respect to the legislation then pending which eventually became the Harrison Narcotic Act. The representatives appeared as witnesses in the Congressional hearings on the legislation and aided in framing its provisions.

MODEL LAWS

As a part of its activity in the field of legislation, the several reports submitted annually by the Council reflected the fact that much consideration was given to the preparation of model laws, including a model law providing for the registration of vital statistics, a model law providing for the reporting of ophthalmia neonatorum which was prepared in conjunction with the Committee on the Prevention of Blindness and a model law dealing with the organization of state boards of health.

BUREAU OF LEGAL MEDICINE AND LEGISLATION

In response to the suggestions made to the House of Delegates in 1922 by the President-elect, Dr. George E. de Schweinitz, by the Speaker, Dr. F. C. Warnshuis, and by the Council on Health and Public Instruction, the reference committee on Legislation and Public Relations submitted the following recommendation to the House:

"The committee recognizes in the several reports of officers, and in the report of the Council on Health and Public Instruction, a consensus of opinion that a central bureau should be established for the consideration of all legislative matters pertaining to medicine or the practice of medicine, and of the public health, relieving the Council on Health and Public Instruction of these duties, which must be carried out in view of the extension of the functions of the Council in the matter of public education, and it is recommended:

"1. That the trustees be memorialized to establish a bureau of this character, under whatever name, with such whole time assistance as may be necessary, the duties of which shall pertain to legislative matters and medicolegal problems in which the whole medical profession may be interested, and which shall be to (a) coordinate the activities of the several constituent state associations, (b) ascertain and crystallize the opinions of the medical profession and the said constituent state associations, and (c) represent the American Medical Association.

"In this connection, your committee desires to point to the desirability of the national organization reflecting the will of the great bulk of the medical profession, and that the bureau contemplated and these recommendations should act in matters of general policy, following instructions of the House of Delegates, or in emergencies following expression of opinion from the proper authorities of the several constituent state associations.

"In this connection, further, it is recognized that the details of organization and operation of the contemplated bureau may not be decided upon at this time. The discussion of this problem in the report of the Council on Health and Public Instruction is referred to."

The House of Delegates adopted the report of the reference committee. Acting on the authority of this action by the House of Delegates, the Board of Trustees immediately proceeded to establish at the headquarters a bureau on which could be devolved the functions referred to in the above resolution. The Executive Committee of the Board, on June 2, 1922, officially established the Bureau of Legal Medicine and Legislation and elected as its first director, Dr. William C. Woodward, who assumed office on June 9th. In reporting this action to the House of Delegates in 1923, the Board of Trustees, after referring to the authorization for the creation of the Bureau, said:

"In accordance with this authorization, the Board of Trustees established this Bureau, and elected as its Executive Secretary Dr. W. C. Woodward, formerly Commissioner of Health of the District of Columbia, and later of Boston. Dr. Woodward is especially qualified for this position, not only because of his active work in the past in public health and medicolegal matters, but also because, while a resident of Washington, he had much experience in connection with federal legislation as pertaining to the District of Columbia. He is further qualified because he has had legal training and holds a degree of Master of Laws."

In reporting the establishment of the Bureau, the Board of Trustees further elaborated on the functions to be exercised by it. These functions were outlined substantially as follows: (1) to keep in touch with federal and state legislation relating to medicine and public health; (2) properly and intelligently to advise interested state associations and component societies concerning medical legislation, and, so far as practicable, to cooperate with them in such proper action as they may take; (3) to study the circumstances under which actions for malpractice arise, with a view to devolving methods, if possible, of reducing the frequency of such action; and (4) to study and advise generally with respect to the legal and legislative matters of concern to the science of medicine and to the medical profession.

COOPERATION WITH SPECIAL COMMITTEES

During the next several years, the Bureau collaborated very closely with a number of special committees to help them obtain their objectives. In 1923, the House of Delegates adopted a resolution which called attention to the fact that the domestic use of concentrated lye and other caustic alkalies and corrosive substances was not an infrequent cause of death among children, or, if death did not ensue, of distressing disability. The House recommended that in the interest of public health and safety, the packing, labeling and distribution of concentrated lye and other caustic alkalies and corrosive substances should be regulated by law. A special committee on lye legislation was created by the Section on Laryn-

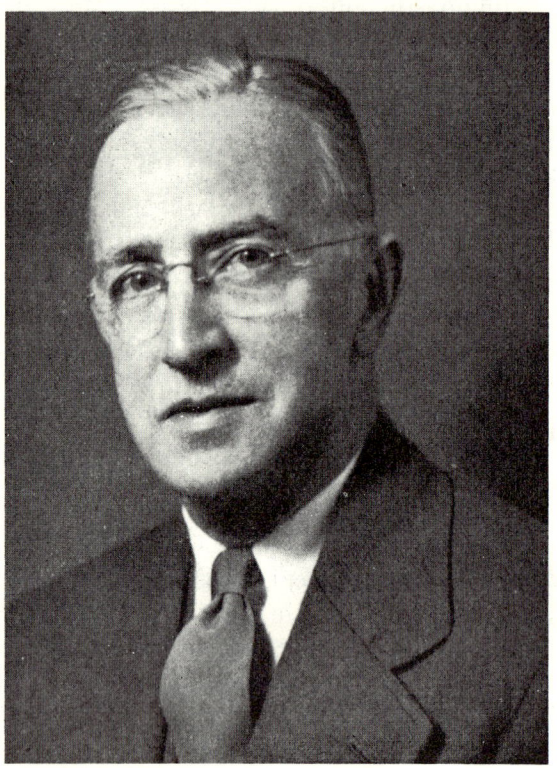

J. W. Holloway, Jr.

gology, Otology and Rhinology, under the able leadership of Dr. Chevalier Jackson. The Bureau collaborated with this committee to the fullest extent. It prepared a model state law and a bill for introduction in Congress and did all within its power to promote their enactment. The federal law was enacted, and the model state bill became a law in a considerable number of states.

The Bureau also collaborated with the special committee appointed by the Board of Trustees to investigate accidents arising from the use of zinc stearate dusting powders. As a result of this particular activity, the manufacturers of such powders agreed to market them in safe containers.

In 1924, the chairman of the Section on Dermatology and Syphilology appointed a technical committee to collaborate with the Bureau in connection with its activities under a resolution adopted by the House of Delegates recommending that the Association sponsor legislation placing cosmetic preparations under the Food and Drug Act and legislation prohibiting the use of paraphenylendiamine in hair dyes and dyes used for fur.

ENLARGEMENT OF THE BUREAU STAFF

On January 16, 1925, the personnel of the Bureau was increased by the addition of an assistant to the director, J. W. Holloway, Jr., a graduate in law from the University of Virginia and a member of the bar of that state. The following year, the services of another assistant were obtained, Goodwin L. Dosland, a member of the Illinois bar, who functioned with the Bureau from October 16, 1926, to May 15, 1928, at which time he became separated from the Bureau to engage in private practice. When Mr. Dosland left, Mr. T. V. McDavitt was employed to take his place, who became a member of the staff of the Bureau on November 1, 1928. He was a graduate in law from the University of Illinois and a member of the Illinois bar.

REDUCTION OF NARCOTIC TAX

One of the first matters that engaged the attention of the Bureau was the tax imposed on physicians under the Harrison Narcotic Act. Initially, physicians were required to pay $1.00 annually to register under the federal law. In 1918, this tax was increased to $3.00 and on numerous occasions the House of Delegates had voiced a protest over this increase, on the ground that the Harrison Narcotic Act was not supposed to be a revenue producing measure, but was enacted for the purpose of restricting the use of narcotics to legitimate medical needs. Fruitless efforts had been made to induce the Congress to reduce this tax to $1.00. Because of the renewed efforts of the Bureau it was able to report to the House of Delegates in 1927 that the revenue act of 1926 had reduced the tax payable under the Harrison Narcotic Act by physicians to its original amount, $1.00 a year. This reduction, it was estimated, effected a saving to the medical profession of probably more than $200,000.

MODEL STATE NARCOTIC LAW

At the suggestion of the Director of the Bureau, the National Conference of Commissioners on Uniform State Laws appointed a special committee to formulate a model state narcotic law. The Bureau collaborated in the preparation of this law which was subsequently submitted to the several states for enactment and was approved by the House of Delegates.

THE PRESCRIBING OF MEDICINAL LIQUOR

Following the passage of the National Prohibition Act and the Act supplemental thereto, many protests were made by physicians over the restrictions contained in these acts on the prescribing of medicinal liquor. The controversy finally reached the courts in a proceeding initiated by Dr. Samuel W. Lambert of New York, in 1922. Eventually, the case reached the United States Supreme Court which on November 29, 1926, by a five to four decision, upheld the constitutionality of the limitations imposed by the Prohibition Acts on the prescribing of medicinal liquor. This controversy is referred to in this history for the principal purpose of recording that the Bureau was authorized by the Board of Trustees to file a brief on behalf of the Association, as amicus curiae, when the case was before the Supreme Court. This brief was prepared and filed by Dr. Woodward.

MODEL BASIC SCIENCE LAW

In 1925, legislation was enacted in two states, Connecticut and Wisconsin, requiring all practitioners of the healing art to demonstrate their knowledge of the sciences basic to all forms of healing, the tests to be given by an impartial, nonsectarian board of examiners. Sensing the probability that this new type of legislation would be proposed in other states, the Bureau prepared a draft of a uniform bill and made it available to the several state medical associations.

NATIONAL LEGISLATIVE REPORTING SERVICE

In its report to the House of Delegates in 1927, the Bureau announced that arrangements had been made with a national legislative reporting service whereby it would receive promptly reports of all bills of interest to the medical profession introduced in the legislatures of the several states. This service has been continued and through it the Bureau is enabled to follow trends in medical legislation and to assemble factual material to assist it in aiding state medical associations which request assistance.

REPRESENTATION IN WASHINGTON

Reference has already been made to the activities of the National Legislative Committee, one member of which resided in Washington. Shortly before the beginning of World War I, Dr. Woodward, then residing in Washington, became the correspondent for the Association and kept it promptly informed of current developments. Later, the services of John F. Hayes were secured as a correspondent, and he has served the Association long and well in that capacity.

In its report to the House of Delegates in 1927, the Board of Trustees announced that in accordance with the wishes of the House as expressed at the Dallas, 1926, session, it had assigned a member of the staff of the Bureau to full-time duty at Washington during the sessions of Congress. Mr. Holloway was so assigned and functioned as the Washington representative of the Association from 1927 to 1932.

ABSTRACTS OF MEDICOLEGAL CASES

Prior to 1928, the abstracts of medicolegal cases that were published weekly in the Journal were prepared by a lawyer not associated otherwise with the Association, J. L. Rosenberger, Esq. All of these abstracts published since September 1, 1928, have been prepared by the staff of the Bureau.

In 1932, Dr. William R. Maloney, California, presented a resolution in the House of Delegates requesting that these medicolegal abstracts be published in book form. Such republication was authorized and volumes containing these abstracts are published at five year intervals.

FEDERAL INCOME TAXES

The reports of the Bureau for 1928 and 1929 told of the efforts made to secure for physicians the right to deduct, in connection with their federal income taxes, expenses incurred in attending medical meetings and in pursuing postgraduate study. Briefs and oral arguments were presented to appropriate congressional committees, but these committees assumed the position that until the decision of the Commissioner of Internal Revenue denying the deductibility of such expenses was contested in the courts, an appeal to the Congress was premature.

A case did later come before the then Board of Tax Appeals, now the U. S. Tax Court, involving the deductibility of traveling expenses and these deductions were allowed. The Board of Trustees authorized the Bureau to contest by appropriate proceedings the ruling in connection with postgraduate expenses but this was not done due to the inability to locate a physician with proper records who was willing to undergo the inconvenience of a test case even though all of the expenses were assumed by the Association.

MEDICAL DEFENSE OF MALPRACTICE SUITS

An early activity of the Bureau was concerned with the assembling of accurate data on the prevalence of medical malpractice, its underlying causes and the extent of the efforts made by state medical associations to reduce the incidence of such actions. These studies by the Bureau were the outcome of action taken at the Chicago session, in 1924, when the Reference Committee on Reports of Officers said:

> "We recommend continued and careful study of the proposed plan for the introduction of medical defense of malpractice suits with a view to determine what assistance can best be afforded by the central bureau to the several state associations maintaining or planning for medical defense."

COMMITTEE ON LEGISLATIVE ACTIVITIES

In 1930, the House of Delegates adopted a resolution authorizing the speaker to appoint a committee of five to function in cooperation with the Bureau in connection with legislation of medical interest. In pursuance of this resolution, the speaker appointed the following members of the committee: Dr. C. B. Wright, chairman, Dr. D. Chester Brown, Dr. E. H. Cary, Dr. Thomas S. Cullen, and Dr. J. H. J. Upham. Subsequently an auxiliary committee to this committee on legislative activities was created, composed of Dr. F. S. Crockett, Dr. Otho A. Fiedler, Dr. Angus McLean, Dr. Holman Taylor and Dr. H. H. Shoulders. This auxiliary committee concerned itself primarily with legislation relating to veterans and had numerous conferences with the American Legion and the Veterans' Administration in connection with the treatment of veterans for nonservice disabilities.

FEDERAL FOOD, DRUG AND COSMETIC ACT

The reports of the Bureau beginning with about 1934 reflected the growing agitation for the enactment of a more effective food and drug act. The Director of the Bureau took cognizance of this agitation and communicated with the then Assistant Secretary of Agriculture Tugwell, who had the matter in charge, informing him that the resources of the Association were at his disposal for use in connection with the drafting of a new law.

Subsequently, a bill was introduced which contained a number of objectionable features. On June 14, 1933, the Board of Trustees, after a careful study of this bill, adopted the following resolution:

> "Whereas, the American Medical Association has for years protested against the inadequacy of the National Food and Drugs Act of 1906, because of which inadequacy the officers of the government charged with the enforcement of the act have been and are unable effectively to protect the people against fraud and danger to health; be it

"*Resolved*, that the American Medical Association pledges its support toward procuring the formulation and enactment of effective national food and drug legislation adequate for the protection of the people."

During the next several years, the Director of the Bureau conferred with Senator Royal S. Copeland, of New York, chairman of the Senate Committee on Commerce, who was sponsoring the new legislation in the Senate, with the officials of the Food and Drug Administration, and with other interested parties in an effort to develop an effective bill. The new federal Food, Drug and Cosmetic Act was passed by the seventy-fifth Congress and approved by the President, June 25, 1938.

THE SOCIAL SECURITY ACT

The Bureau followed very closely the developments that led to the enactment of the Social Security Act in 1935. In a report submitted to the House of Delegates in 1935, the Bureau outlined the proposals that had been submitted to Congress, proposing the enactment of federal legislation for the establishment of a program for "the security of the men, women and children of the nation against certain hazards and vicissitudes of life," the quotation being from the message sent to Congress by President Roosevelt June 8, 1934. The initial bill that was sponsored in the Senate by Senator Wagner and in the House by Representative Doughton proposed "to alleviate the hazards of old age, unemployment, illness, and dependency to establish a social insurance board in the Department of Labor, to raise revenue, and for other purposes." This bill proposed to devolve on the Social Insurance Board, among other duties, the duty of "studying and making recommendations as to the most effective methods of providing economic security through social insurance, and as to legislation and matters of administrative policy concerning old age insurance, unemployment compensation, health insurance and related subjects." Subsequently, Representative Doughton introduced a redraft of the bill which passed the House on April 19 and eventually became law. This redraft omitted all references to illness in its title, changed the name of the administrative board to the Social Security Board and devolved no duty on the board to study and make recommendations with respect to health insurance.

THE PROMISCUOUS USE OF BARBITURATES

A resolution adopted by the House of Delegates at the Atlantic City, 1937, session called attention to the evils resulting from the promiscuous use of the barbiturates and recommended that these drugs be brought under proper control. This action taken by the House of Delegates was referred through the Board of Trustees to the Bureau with the suggestion that it take such steps as in its judgment were deemed proper to carry into effect the purpose of the resolution.

The Bureau did make a study of existing laws relating to the use of the barbiturates and prepared for publication in the Journal a statement embodying the results of the survey. Subsequently, communications were sent to state medical associations calling attention to the action taken by the House of Delegates and later the Director of the Bureau, with the Secretary of the Council on Pharmacy and Chemistry, met with the legislative committee of the American Pharmaceutical Association to formulate a uniform state bill placing the barbiturates on a prescription basis.

CHEMICAL TESTS FOR INTOXICATION

Since 1937, the committee created by the House of Delegates to study problems of motor vehicle accidents, of which Dr. Herman A. Heise, of Milwaukee, Wisconsin, is chairman, has studied carefully the relation of alcohol to traffic accidents. In this study it has collaborated closely with the Committee on Tests for Intoxication of the National Safety Council. It has on several occasions recommended definite borderline limits for alcoholic influence in terms of the amount of alcohol in the blood of the suspected drunken driver, and these limits have been approved by the House. In order to promote uniformity in state legislation in this field, the National Safety Council, through its Committee on Tests for Intoxication, and with the active collaboration of the Bureau, has formulated a draft of a uniform bill which embodies the borderline limits approved by the House. This draft has been approved in principle by the Board of Trustees and by the House of Delegates.

COMMITTEE ON MEDICOLEGAL BLOOD GROUPING TESTS

This committee submitted a report to the House of Delegates in 1937 in which it reviewed the dependability of blood grouping tests in disputed paternity cases and recommended that where necessary, laws should be passed which would authorize courts to order blood grouping tests in cases of disputed paternity, and to receive the results thereof in evidence. Dr. Ludvig Hektoen was the chairman of the committee that submitted this report, and the recommendation of the committee was approved by the House of Delegates.

THE RETIREMENT OF DR. WOODWARD

On January 1, 1940, at his own request, the retirement of Dr. William C. Woodward, Director of the Bureau, became effective. During his eighteen years as director of the Bureau, he devoted his fine abilities unselfishly always to the betterment of organized medicine and the House of Delegates on being advised of his retirement paid him a fine tribute in unanimously approving the following statement made by the Reference Committee on Reports of Board of Trustees and Secretary:

> "The retirement of Dr. William C. Woodward, who directed the activities of the Bureau of Legal Medicine and Legislation for eighteen years, deserves the attention of the House of Delegates. We are all familiar with the great work he has done in behalf of American medicine and your reference committee believes that it voices the sentiments of the House when it conveys to him a special message of appreciation and the wish that he may continue to enjoy good health for many years to come."

Mr. Holloway succeeded Dr. Woodward, first as Acting Director and then as Director of the Bureau.

George E. Hall, Jr. became a member of the staff of the Bureau on February 1, 1940. He is a graduate of the Chicago-Kent College of Law and a member of the Illinois Bar.

Another member of the staff of the Bureau, Dr. E. Ransom Koontz, resigned April 26, 1941, having been a member of the Staff since July 22, 1935 Dr. Koontz obtained his degree in medicine at the University of Michigan and was also a member of the Bar of that state and subsequently of the Illinois Bar.

IN CONCLUSION

During recent years, the introduction in the Congress of a wide variety of proposals relating to health has demanded the increased attention of the Bureau. The more important proposals have been carefully analyzed and physicians advised of their import through the Journal.

BUREAU OF INVESTIGATION

By Bliss O. Halling

THE AMERICAN MEDICAL ASSOCIATION, early in this century, began a campaign against the prescribing of proprietary medicines, an evil that existed within the medical profession itself. The custom, which has not entirely died out, was to introduce a nostrum to the public through such undiscerning, uncritical or even venal physicians as would prescribe it, or recommend it in testimonials calculated to impress the public. When it had cleaned its own house to a considerable degree, the Association extended its investigations to the more widely promoted "patent medicines" and other forms of outright quackery.

In 1906 Dr. Arthur J. Cramp came to the Association as an editorial assistant. Soon afterward he was put in charge of this new activity, which took the name: Propaganda Department. In 1925 the title was changed to the Bureau of Investigation.

Prior to the Association's entrance into this field, exposures of quackery by any other organization or publication had been few and scattered. Government agencies had given little if any attention to the subject, and medical journals had made only sporadic mention of it. There was no organized investigation of quackery in this country before the founding of the Propaganda Department.

In 1906, the Congress passed the first federal legislation in the "patent medicine" field. This was known as the federal Food and Drugs Act. It was a response to a series of articles in the *Ladies' Home Journal* and *Collier's Weekly* and to Upton Sinclair's book "The Jungle." Though it did not go far, at least, this was a start in the right direction. The law did not require declaration of any ingredients of a nostrum on the label, except alcohol and eleven narcotic drugs or their derivatives. Hence, under the new law the label did not reveal much about composition. It did, however, cover false and fraudulent claims on the label or carton and in accompanying circulars.

Of greater interest to the medical profession and the public, however, was the composition. This information became available through government chemists' reports on nostrums seized in interstate commerce under this new Act, and the Bureau prepared abstracts of these government reports (called Notices of Judgment) for THE JOURNAL. Time, of course, was required for government investigation of all labels whose claims violated the new law. Meanwhile the Bureau arranged to have many of the nostrums most widely advertised and inquired about examined in the Association's Chemical Laboratory, so that exposures of them could go into THE JOURNAL.

As the department grew and its activities increased, forms of quackery other than "patent medicines" also were investigated and exposed in THE JOURNAL. In those early days of the Bureau charlatans were advertising in huge headlines that they could "cure cancer without the knife," sexual weakness by means of "electric belts," rheumatism with "electric insoles," and anemia or general weakness with something that turned out to be essentially nothing but cottage cheese!

In that period, also, newspaper advertisements often ran to full-page or double spread, proclaiming the alleged virtues of Old Doc Somebody's "Tonic"—largely alcoholic, of course, to impart the requisite "kick," and a minimum of medicinal effects. These advertisements often carried photographs and testimonials of senators, congressmen, clergymen, actresses and opera singers who claimed to have been cured of this or that by Old Doc's "tonic." Also at that time "cures" for "catarrh," "female weakness," kidney and liver disorders and a wide variety of other ailments were common, and quacks often went so far as to claim cures for such serious conditions as cancer, diabetes and tuberculosis, nor have they yet entirely disappeared.

There seems to be no field of medicine that the quacks have not invaded. They have promoted some strange schemes. One sold an "anemia cure" that was essentially sand. Another offered a "secret," the substance of which would, he represented, cure just about everything. It was nothing but kerosene! The promoter of a "cancer cure" claimed that his treatment was "a radium-impregnated fluid," whereas examination showed it to contain nothing but a little quinine sulfate, some acid, alcohol and water, and to be utterly devoid of radioactivity. One "consumption cure" was practically nothing but a sugar solution, and its exploiter was stopped by the government and sent to prison.

To preserve the Bureau's reports of its investigations, those published up to 1912 were reprinted in "Nostrums and Quackery," the first volume of which was published in 1912, and ran into a second edition. Volume II came out in 1921 and Volume III in 1936, the latter with the longer title, "Nostrums and Quackery and Pseudo-Medicine." The second and third volumes are still in print (1947). Much of this material went into a series of pamphlets, each dealing with a separate phase of "patent medicines."

The Bureau also reprinted (with permission) and for many years issued the book "The Great American Fraud" by Samuel Hopkins Adams. This was a series of exposures of the "patent medicine" evil, originally published in *Collier's Weekly*. Further, the Bureau developed exhibit material, including a series of forty posters and a large collection of lantern slides. These slides were later reproduced in the form of a 35 mm. film strip, and this and the slides have for many years been lent to physicians and educators. The Bureau also has furnished speakers to medical societies and other organizations and has presented exhibits at the Association's annual meetings.

The early inquiries received by the Bureau came almost entirely from the medical profession, and some years were required to acquaint the general public with the service offered. Gradually, physicians encouraged patients to ask the Bureau about "patent medicines" and quacks that came to their attention. Further contact with the public resulted from the suggestion made in certain school and college textbooks on such subjects as general science, hygiene, biology and civics that the students write to the Bureau for its material. This suggestion has resulted in great numbers of inquiries. Similar ones have come from student nurses, Red Cross home-nursing classes, clubs and other groups.

Newspapers and magazines have sought information from the Bureau about medical advertising which had been offered them or which they were already carrying. In many cases members of clubs and lodges have inquired about doubtful advertising in their official publications, and sometimes their protests have resulted in a general cleaning up of the objectionable features.

Many medical and civic organizations have asked for reports on some alleged "medical authority," "food expert," "noted psychologist" or other highly-touted person who has been scheduled to address them, and on learning from the Bureau that the person is by no means an authority in his pretended field (and, in fact, is frequently an imposter), have canceled his engagement, gratified that they learned the truth in time to do this.

The Bureau has given generous cooperation to, and received it from, federal, state and municipal organizations and officials, and the numerous Better Business Bureaus. It has worked closely with the federal Food and Drug Administration which enforces the Food, Drug and Cosmetic Act of 1938; with the Federal Trade

Commission, which is empowered to eliminate unfair trade practices, including false or exaggerated advertising claims, and with the Post Office Department, which investigates transactions made through the mails and debars, by means of fraud orders, those, including medical ones, which are found to be swindles. The Bureau abstracts for THE JOURNAL the reports published by these federal agencies on their activities in the field of quackery.

Fashions change in this field, as in others. The old-time quack who drew throngs to his medicine shows by promising to heal them with some "miraculous touch," or by extolling the alleged wonders of his "snake oil" while sundry devenomized "rattlers" encircled his neck and arms, or by representing himself, in full-feathered regalia, as an "Indian Doctor" with "miracle herbs" which would cure all ills, is now seldom heard of. It can be said of him that he was at least picturesque, even if crude. In his place the public is now besought by another pied piper—the suave "lecturer" who poses as an "expert" on diet, "personality," love, sex and psychology and purports to be able to solve all individual problems. His name is legion and his "courses" are said to pay large profits. Vigilant medical societies and civic bodies, however, have succeeded in barring many of his kind from their localities when the impostor's true colors were obtained from the Bureau.

Fashions in nostrums also have changed. Though "cures" for cancer, tuberculosis, diabetes and some other serious conditions are still advertised—but to a lesser extent and with modified claims—the "patent medicine" trend of recent years has been toward nostrums capitalizing on the current interest in vitamins, minerals and the sulfa drugs. It is true that "fat cures" still hold their sway, chiefly over women, and range from glandular substances through laxatives and food substitutes to external preparations. "Tonics," which appealed to the previous generation because they usually were represented as cure-alls, have more or less had their day.

Cosmetics from the first came within the Bureau's field because of preposterous claims that they would correct skin disorders and beautify. A modern exploitation in the cosmetic field is the "rejuvenating cream" based on hormones. Hair dyes and "permanent wave" solutions have had a wide market in recent years and have been the subject of many complaints.

The enactment of a more effective federal law governing nostrums—the Food, Drug and Cosmetic Act, passed by the Congress in 1938—gave the public information about nostrums that the earlier law did not require. The new Act directed that the label must list the active ingredients and also carry warnings against taking the product in certain conditions, and proper precautions for use in some others.

The Bureau has for forty years been investigating and exposing the nostrum evil and quackery for the benefit of the medical profession and the public, and cooperating with many other agencies organized for public welfare. The inquiries coming to it have increased from a mere trickle to thousands of letters a year, until those from the public exceed those from physicians, and its collection of quack material has become voluminous.

Dr. Cramp retired as director of the Bureau in 1935 and was succeeded by Dr. Frank J. Clancy of Seattle. Dr. Clancy resigned in 1937 to pursue graduate work in his special field, urology. His successor was Dr. Paul C. Barton, a medical consultant on the staff of the Association's Council on Pharmacy and Chemistry. In 1942 he was called to Washington for special work with the Procurement and Assignment Service, and his duties then fell to Bliss O. Halling, A.B., who had been with the Bureau for many years.

BUREAU OF INFORMATION

By M. Virginia Shuler

THE HOUSE OF DELEGATES at its 1944 annual session in Chicago created and authorized the establishment of a Bureau of Information in the central office in Chicago. The activities of the Bureau were primarily to assist returning medical officers in their educational, licensure and placement problems. At the annual session of the House of Delegates in Chicago, December 1945, the Council on Medical Service recommended to the House:

"The Bureau of Information of the American Medical Association should be established in a permanent form and maintain adequate records of each physician in the United States from which county and state medical societies could obtain information. The Bureau of Information should also, by the establishment of a co-operative monthly reporting system with state societies, be kept informed of areas needing physicians, and from time to time seek information either directly or through state medical societies from individual physicians concerning location, type of practice, and other relative data.

"Each state medical society should be urged to establish an information service. This state information service should collect from various public and private agencies data relating to medical facilities, medical personnel, or medical needs, and other information concerning medical care within the state. This information service should at all times be in a position to furnish information concerning areas in need of physicians and a complete picture of the medical facilities, physical and economic aspects of any community within the state.

"The American Medical Association should be urged to provide advice or service to such state information services relating to methods of organization and procedure, and aid the state services in developing a usefulness to the medical profession and to the people of their states."

The Reference Committee on Postwar Planning of the House of Delegates recommended approval of the foregoing recommendations. The report of the Reference Committee was adopted.

The establishment of the Bureau of Information had a twofold purpose: first, to survey through the state and county medical societies the medical personnel, medical facilities and medical needs of every county in the United States; secondly, to be of service to the returning medical officer in choosing an area for the practice of medicine.

Pertinent data covering the economic and medical practice aspects for the 3,072 counties in the United States have been prepared.

Through the cooperation of the state medical societies, current listings are available for openings in general practice, specialties and associate positions throughout the country. Physicians requesting information regarding a specific area in a state are supplied with summary sheets covering the medical and economic features of the area, together with a listing of the communities in that state where there is a definite need for a physician.

Since V-J Day the Bureau of Information has had each week about 565 letters from medical officers and 110 physicians coming to the office for specific information regarding medical education, licensure, and re-location. Through the cooperation of the Council on Medical Education and Hospitals, the Bureau of Legal Medicine and Legislation, and the state medical societies, the Bureau has been able to give valuable information to the returning physicians to guide them in their adjustment to civilian life. An Information Bulletin for Medical Officers, designed to combine and abstract that information which would be most desired by medical officers, was published by the American Medical Association and sent to every doctor in the armed services.

Realizing that rural areas generally are not as well supplied with physicians as urban areas, the Bureau has been working closely with the Council on Medical Service and the Committee on Rural Medical Service of the American Medical Association in developing programs to arouse rural people to an appreciation of the benefits of modern medical science and to stimulate and coordinate the work of the various groups working for better rural medical service.

In cooperation with the Bureau of Health Education and the Council on Medical Education and Hospitals, the Bureau of Information gave a television program on rural health problems and the extension to needy areas of more adequate medical care through a better distribution of physicians.

The Bureau is working out a cooperative program with the Division of Hospital Facilities of the U. S. Public Health Service. It is hoped that through a coordinated system of rural, city and town hospitals medical service in farm communities will be improved. The Hill-Burton law, supporting the survey and construction of hospital, health and diagnostic centers throughout the nation, is one measure aimed at implementing this program in areas where the facilities are unavailable and cannot be supplied through local or state agencies. In order to attract physicians into areas where needed, there must be reasonable assurance not only of economic security and satisfactory medical facilities but also of an opportunity to conduct the highest type of medical practice.

In December 1946, the Bureau of Information began a survey through the local medical societies to determine the conditions and distribution of medical care in the rural areas of the country and the recent movements of physicians into rural areas. In developing this survey the Bureau sent a questionnaire to the state medical societies requesting specific information regarding the medical personnel, facilities and needs at present of every county in the United States.

BUREAU OF EXHIBITS

By Thomas G. Hull, Ph.D.

THE BUREAU OF EXHIBITS began in 1899, when a pathology exhibit was shown at the Columbus, Ohio, Session of the American Medical Association.

The function of the Bureau is graduate medical instruction, carried on through the Scientific Exhibit at each Annual Session of the Association, together with exhibits and motion pictures at meetings of state and county medical societies and other scientific groups. Health education is brought to the public by means of exhibits at fairs and expositions, at conventions and meetings of lay groups and by window displays.

THE SCIENTIFIC EXHIBIT

The Scientific Exhibit of the American Medical Association is the result of the initiative of two men—William N. Wishard, M.D. and Frank B. Wynn, M.D., of Indianapolis.

Pathology was coming into its own during the latter part of the Nineteenth Century. The Indianapolis Medical Society had been holding "case history" nights once a month with the presentation of pathologic specimens. Dr. William N. Wishard, president of the Indiana State Medical Society in 1899, requested Doctor Wynn to arrange a pathology exhibit at the state meeting held that year in Indianapolis. So successful was this venture that it was decided to show the exhibit at the meeting of the American Medical Association at Columbus, Ohio, the following week. Although nothing like it had ever been done before, a warehouse was rented in Columbus across from the Capitol Building and the major portion of the exhibit transported from Indianapolis. Dr. Wishard bore most of the expense personally. More than seven hundred specimens were shown, accompanied by demonstrations. Much favorable comment resulted, with an agitation for a continuation of the project. (J.A.M.A. *32:*1375 [June 17] 1899.)

In 1900, W. W. Keen, M.D., then president of the American Medical Association, in response to an action of the Columbus meeting, appointed two "unofficial" committees. The first, with

Joseph Stokes, M.D. as chairman, was assigned the task of arranging for a pathology exhibit at the coming meeting at Atlantic City. The other, of which Ludvig Hektoen, M.D. was chairman, was instructed to form a Section on Pathology. Dr. Wynn was secretary of both committees and the two projects were duly consummated. The pathology exhibit was "gratifying alike to the executive officers of the Association and to the committee in charge of the work." It was reported to be "the most instructive feature of the meeting" and "worth more than a thousand papers" (J.A.M.A., *35*:43–44 [July 7] 1900). The organization of the Section on Pathology and Bacteriology took place in the exhibit room. The pathology exhibit was

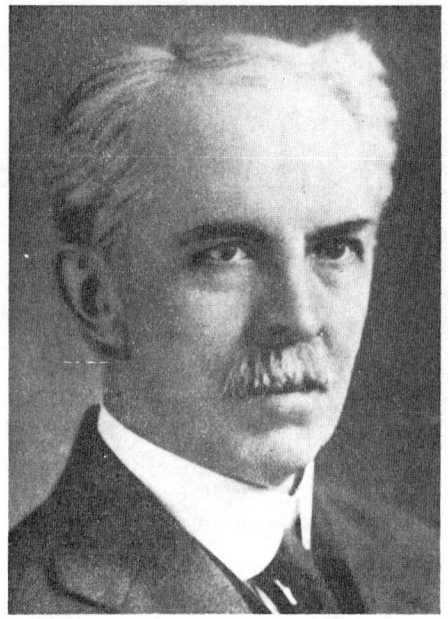

Frank B. Wynn, M.D., Director of the Scientific Exhibit, 1899–1916.

made a permanent feature of the Annual Session, under the auspices of this Section and the Association made an annual appropriation of $500.00 to defray expenses. This arrangement was continued for several years.

General policies were outlined by Doctor Wynn in his chairman's address to the Section on Pathology and Bacteriology in 1902 (J.A.M.A., *40*:350–352 [Feb. 7] 1903). His recommendations showed a masterly comprehension of the problems of such an exhibit; the policies which he outlined are still practical after nearly half a century of evolution. He proposed that the scope of the exhibit be broadened to include all of medicine instead of just pathology, and that the name be changed to the Scientific Exhibit. He likewise recommended that the Director of the Exhibit be appointed by the Board of Trustees and paid a salary; that the various sections develop their programs in correlation with the Scientific Exhibit; that the section secretaries constitute an advisory committee to the Scientific Exhibit; that exhibits be carefully chosen for their worthiness and that personal demonstrations by exhibitors be promoted. He made the suggestion that a medical museum be established—"a lasting monument to the work of the Association." From the first, he insisted that the exhibits be kept free from commercialism.

The recommendation made in 1902 that section secretaries develop their programs in conjunction with the Scientific Exhibit was agitated from time to time; by 1911 it reached a fair degree of success. In that year special mention was made of the efforts of W. A.

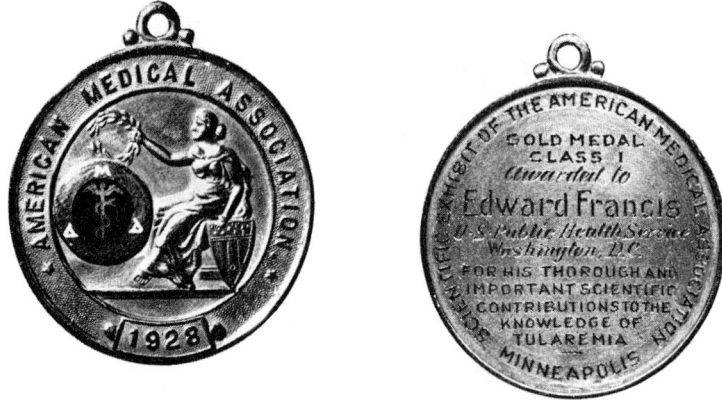

Medal used in Scientific Exhibit 1908 to 1929.

Evans, M.D., Chicago, in "persuading chairmen of sections to undertake this." (J.A.M.A., 57:87 [July 1] 1911.) Several of the sections later appointed exhibit committees and in 1936 this was changed to one representative to the Scientific Exhibit from each Section to assist and advise in the procurement of outstanding exhibits. The chairman of the Council on Scientific Assembly has been a member of the Advisory Committee of the Scientific Exhibit for many years.

Personal demonstrations by the exhibitor were encouraged but at first rarely accomplished. Often the exhibitor was not present at the meeting, his material being installed by the Director. In a letter written in 1942, Emanuel Libman, M.D., New York, states "In 1912, I introduced demonstrations of the exhibits at the American Medical Association meetings. I have always felt that was an important matter. It is strange, when one thinks back, to have to believe that for many years there was no demonstrating at the exhibits. In 1912, I induced Dr. E. C. Rosenow and Dr. Martin H. Fischer to demonstrate their exhibits (they were close to mine) and the Committee on Awards gave us all gold medals." Unfortunately another decade passed before the personal demonstration became general. The advantages are considerable. The visiting physician may talk personally to the exhibitor and ask as many questions as necessary. The exhibitor, on the other hand, benefits from contact with the many hundreds of visitors during the week, among whom are persons working in the same field of scientific activity.

Awards for creditable exhibits were first made in 1908 at the Chicago Session. The first year gold medals were offered for the best exhibit on original research and for the best exhibit on the subject of

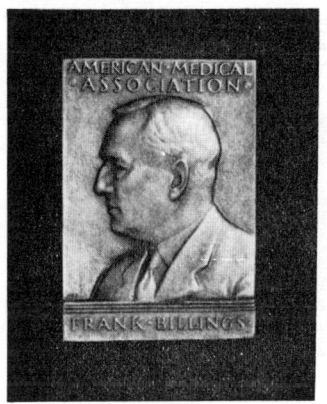 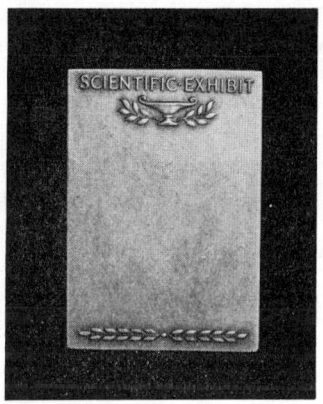

Medal used in Scientific Exhibit 1930 to 1947.

tuberculosis; the latter was not awarded, however. Certificates of Merit were given to other exhibitors. The medal for research has been continued from that time. In 1910, a medal for the best exhibit on clinical surgery was offered, but no exhibit on this subject was deemed worthy. In 1911 a medal was awarded for the exhibit showing the most care in preparation, completeness and instruction. For several years beginning with 1911, cash awards were offered for the best collection of health cartoons, $200.00 being the first prize and $100.00 the second prize.

One of the aims of the Scientific Exhibit, repeatedly emphasized from the beginning, has been the desirability of attracting the general practitioner of medicine, not only to come and observe the exhibit but actually to take part in it. On more than one occasion the exhibits of such individuals have been rewarded with medals.

It was felt, however, that the research worker in a large and well-endowed laboratory or institution had facilities at his command which were not available to the private practitioner and that the competition to the latter was unfair. Therefore, in 1916, and for several years thereafter, the system of awards was reclassified in such a way, as follows, that the physician in general practice would be encouraged to take part.

Class I   Institution Exhibits.
Class II   Research Exhibits.
Class III   Exhibits Relating to Methods of Laboratory Diagnosis.
Class IV   Public Health Exhibits.
Class V   Medical Society Exhibits.
Class VI   Practitioners' Exhibits.

The number of medals was extended to include silver and bronze, as well as gold, beginning in 1916. This policy has been continued

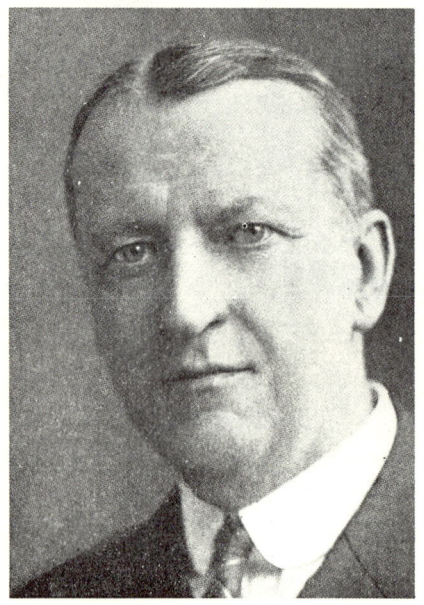

Dr. George Howitt Weaver, Director of the Scientific Exhibit 1917 and 1918.

to the present date—a gold, silver and bronze medal and several certificates of merit being given in each of two classes. Group I includes exhibits of individual investigation while Group II is composed of exhibits which do not exemplify purely experimental studies but rather the correlation of facts and excellence of presentation. Other awards include honorable mention and special citations at the discretion of the Committee on Awards.

Facilities were made available for showing lantern slides, accompanied by talks, in a theater adjoining the Scientific Exhibit in 1915. This was extended to include motion pictures and a continuous

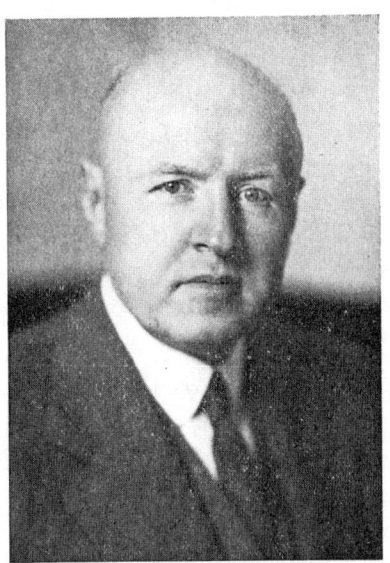

Kellogg Speed, M.D., Chairman, Special Committee on Fractures 1928–1947.

program of lectures was arranged for the entire week. So popular were these lectures and picture demonstrations that they were beginning to interfere with the section meetings, and in 1927 they were discontinued.

Motion pictures for many years were shown in exhibitors' booths. With the increasing use of 16 mm. film, however, motion pictures in the booths became quite a problem in clogging the aisles with visitors and interfering with the demonstration of exhibits. Beginning in 1941, arrangements were made for several motion picture theaters directly adjoining the Scientific Exhibit where films could be shown throughout the week on definite schedules and where the audiences could sit down in comfort to view them.

In addition to exhibits presented by individual physicians and investigators, the Board of Trustees in 1924 initiated special exhibits as leading features of the Annual Session. Fresh pathology and morbid anatomy have been shown on many different occasions under the direction of such outstanding pathologists as Ludvig Hektoen, Chicago; Allen G. Smith, Baldwin Lucke and Edward B. Krumbhaar, Philadelphia; Oscar B. Hunt, Washington; Frank R.

Menne, Portland; George T. Caldwell, Dallas; Frank W. Hartman, Detroit; Norbert Enzer, Milwaukee; Benjamin S. Kline, Cleveland and Harrison S. Martland, Newark, with numerous other pathologists assisting with the demonstrations.

The fracture exhibit, which has been a feature almost continuously since 1926, has been under the guidance of Kellogg Speed, M.D., Chicago. Other members of the committee have included Frederick J. Cotton, M.D., Robert J. Osgood, M.D., Charles L. Scudder, M.D., Nathaniel Allison, M.D., William Darrach, M.D., Frank D. Dickson, M.D. and Walter Estell Lee, M.D. Scores of orthopedic surgeons have assisted with demonstrations.

Biochemical diagnostic methods were presented several times under a committee of which Victor C. Myers, Ph.D. was chairman. Heart disease was featured in 1924 with Alexander Lambert, M.D. as chairman. Other special exhibits, with the chairman in charge, were as follows:

Public Health	W. A. O'Brien, M.D.
Immunology	H. R. Wahl, M.D.
Varicose Veins	Geza de Takats, M.D.
Cancer	Max Cutler, M.D.
Poliomyelitis	Ralph C. Williams, M.D.
Encephalitis	Ralph C. Williams, M.D.
Vaccines and Serums	Ralph C. Williams, M.D.
Physical Therapy	John S. Coulter, M.D.
Capillary Circulation	Irving S. Wright, M.D.
Nutrition	Reginald Fitz, M.D.
Prevention of Asphyxial Deaths	Chevalier L. Jackson, M.D.
Diabetes	E. P. Joslin, M.D.
Anesthesia	Ralph M. Waters, M.D.
Backache	Frank R. Ober, M.D.
Treatment of Burns	Stanley J. Seeger, M.D.
Chemotherapy and Infectious Diseases	Chester S. Keefer, M.D.
Rehabilitation	Carl M. Peterson, M.D. and Howard A. Carter
Physical Medicine	Frank H. Krusen, M.D.

In each of the above exhibits, most of which were repeated for several years, a large number of assistants took part in the demonstrations. On some occasions special lectures were given in conjunction with the exhibit, with exceedingly valuable results.

During the first several years of its existence, the Scientific Exhibit was the "handmaid of the Section on Pathology." Dr. Wynn was the moving spirit and acted as its director, with the exception of 1902, when, as chairman of the Section on Pathology, he appointed a committee consisting of F. M. Jeffries, M.D., New York, chairman; W. A. Evans, M.D., Chicago and Roger G. Perkins, M.D., Cleveland.

The House of Delegates assumed responsibility in 1903, appointing a Committee on Scientific Exhibit each year, of which Doctor Wynn was the chairman and director until his retirement in 1916. During the next five years, the responsibility was passed around, George H. Weaver, M.D., Chicago, being director in 1917–18 and then Fred-

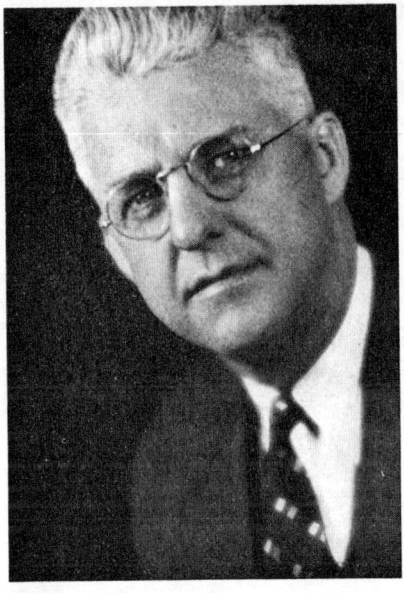

Thomas G. Hull, Ph.D., Director of the Scientific Exhibit since 1930.

erick R. Green, M.D., Secretary of the Council on Health and Public Instruction. The Board of Trustees, at the instigation of D. Chester Brown, M.D. and Frank Billings, M.D., assumed control in 1921, appointing three members of the Board as a Committee on Scientific Exhibit, with a Director acting under their guidance. Dr. Brown was Chairman of the Committee on Scientific Exhibit from 1921 to 1934; Allen H. Bunce, M.D. from 1935 to 1939; Thomas S. Cullen, M.D. from 1940 to 1941; Roger I. Lee, M.D. 1942; Elmer L. Henderson, M.D. from 1943 to 1945, and Charles W. Roberts, M.D. from 1945 to 1947.

The Scientific Exhibit from the first has been considered a course

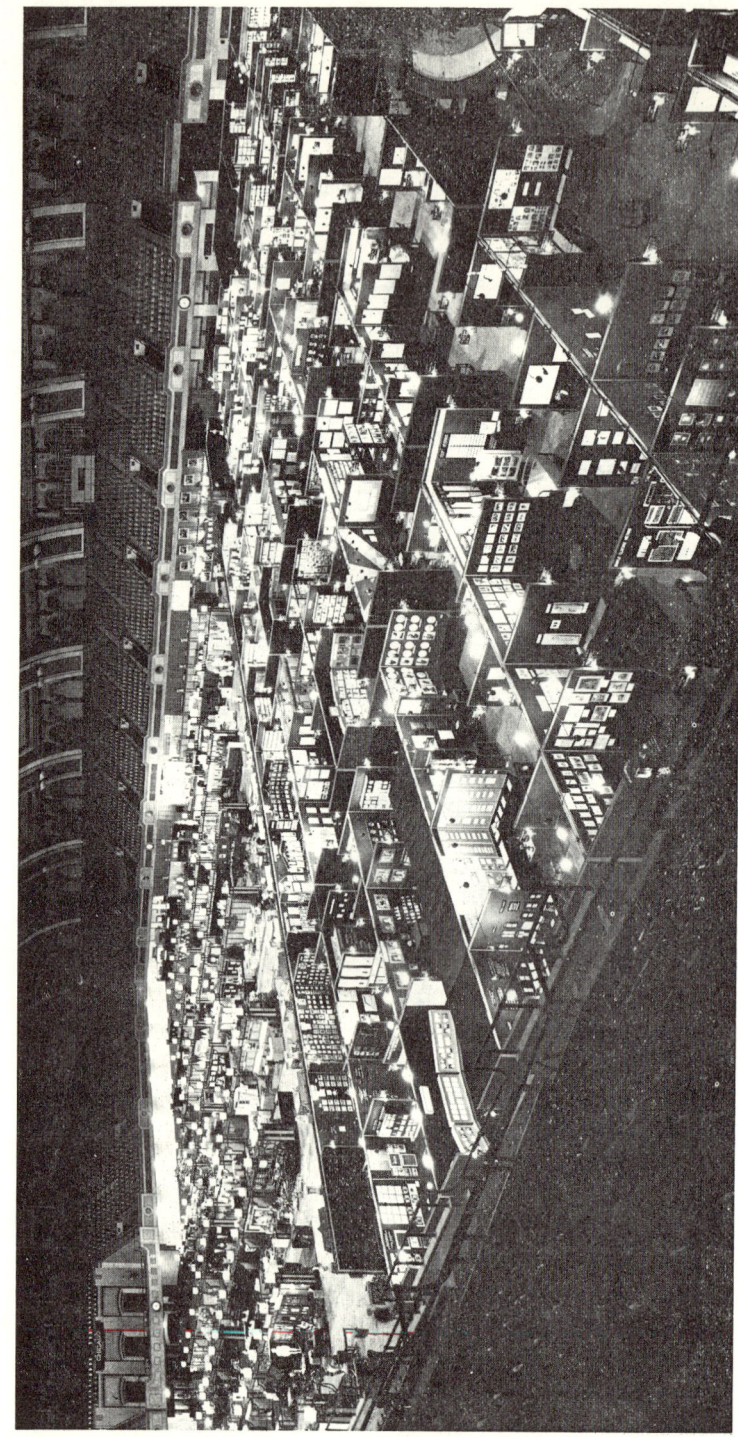

Scientific Exhibit in foreground, Technical Exhibit in background, Atlantic City Session, 1935.

in graduate medical instruction. As early as 1902 it attracted so much attention from the public that mothers were found wheeling baby buggies down the aisles to get medical advice from the world-renowned physicians who were demonstrating there. Guards were established first to keep out the public and later to limit the attendance to persons wearing the official badge or bearing guest cards.

The caliber of the exhibits has increased markedly over the years. In 1918 signed applications were required of all exhibitors. So numerous did the applicants become that nearly half of them were

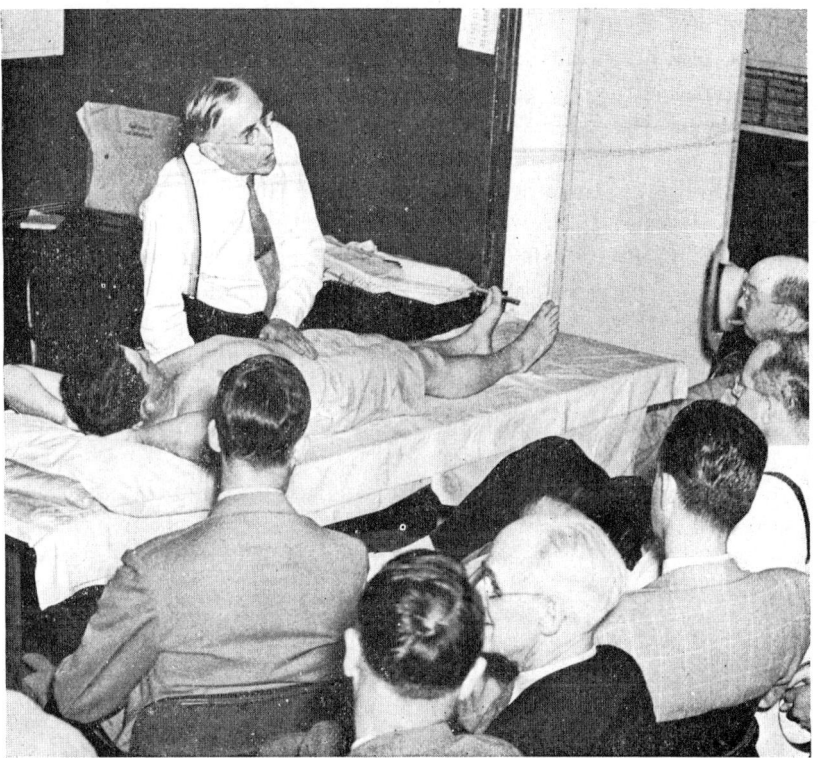

A demonstration in the Scientific Exhibit.

sometimes rejected for lack of space. This resulted in exhibits of exceptional quality being shown. The number of exhibits at a meeting has depended largely on the facilities available to accommodate them. The maximum number has been about two hundred and fifty. The subjects shown have included all of the medical sciences. Not only physicians, but dentists, veterinarians and scientists working in fields allied to medicine have participated. They have done this often at great personal sacrifice of time and effort and finances, without thought of personal gain, in order to give other physicians the benefit of their experience. As Hippocrates said "to teach them this art, if they should wish to learn it, without fee or stipulation."

EXHIBITS AT STATE MEDICAL MEETINGS

The success of the Scientific Exhibit at the Annual Session of the American Medical Association stimulated other groups to undertake similar exhibitions. Many state medical societies and other medical, dental and public health organizations present each year very creditable scientific exhibits, in which the American Medical Association often participates.

Previous to 1930, the different councils and bureaus of the Association presented exhibits occasionally at meetings of state medical societies. This was especially true of the Council on Medical Education and Hospitals, the Council on Pharmacy and Chemistry and the Bureau of Investigation. When the Bureau of Exhibits was established, this activity was greatly expanded. A series of thirty or more exhibits showed the work of the various departments of the American Medical Association, or subjects in which those departments were interested. Some of the displays which received awards in the Scientific Exhibit at the Annual Session were taken over and made available to state medical societies. New exhibits have been added each year to replace old ones that were out of date or worn out. An attendant from the American Medical Association has accompanied the exhibits whenever possible, but personnel was not available to cover the country, and demonstrators, in many instances, were supplied by the organization borrowing the exhibits.

HEALTH EXHIBITS

The demand for health exhibits for the public never ceases. The Bureau of Investigation, very early in its career, prepared exhibit material for such occasions. Not until 1930, however, was any concerted effort made to satisfy the demand.

Exhibits on such subjects as physiology, anatomy, medical economics, patent medicines, self diagnosis, communicable diseases, nutrition, posture, medical and hospital care and many others were prepared for loan to state and county medical societies or to organizations approved by those societies.

The exposition type of exhibit was used for state fairs and other occasions where many thousands of persons would view them. It is necessary for this type of exhibit to be well made in order to withstand repeated shipments; therefore, the exhibits were somewhat bulky and heavy. They were not practical for use in school rooms or at other small meetings.

World Fairs. The Bureau of Investigation prepared an exhibit on patent medicines for the San Francisco Exposition in 1915 which received an award. Beginning in 1933 there were six international expositions in which the American Medical Association participated.

At A Century of Progress Exposition in Chicago, 1933 and 1934, the material covered the progress of medical education, medical practice, the use of hospitals, health information for the public and the growth and activities of the American Medical Association. More than a million people viewed these exhibits.

The California-Pacific International Exposition at San Diego, California, had no medical exhibits the first year. The management realized its omission and the next year, 1936, not only asked the California Medical Association to take charge of such an exhibit, but furnished a liberal subsidy to carry out the plans. The American Medical Association presented exhibits on individual and community health, prevention of eye injuries and prevention of burns, danger of self diagnosis and periodic health examinations. An attendant was furnished with the cooperation of the San Diego County Medical Society.

The Texas Centennial Exposition in Dallas, 1936 and 1937, presented "The Story of Life" under the auspices of the United States Public Health Service. The American Medical Association contributed that portion of the "Story" dealing with the progress of medical care.

The Great Lakes Exposition at Cleveland, Ohio, in its first year had no health exhibits. In 1937, the second year, a liberal amount of space was donated to the Cleveland Academy of Medicine, in which the American Medical Association presented a group of exhibits on medical education and public health. So excellent were the exhibits arranged by the Academy that men instinctively took off their hats when coming into the Hall.

The Golden Gate International Exposition at San Francisco in 1939 contained an exhibit from the American Medical Association dealing largely with the requirements of medical education and the advancement of Pacific Medicine. The exhibit was unfortunately dismantled before arrangements were completed for continuing the Fair through 1940.

The New York World's Fair, 1939 and 1940, requested the American Medical Association to present an exhibit on medical education. A million and a half visitors viewed this exhibit during the two year period, while in another area of the Fair an exhibit on HYGEIA, The Health Magazine, was seen by many thousands more.

The cumulative effect of all these exhibits, shown in different parts of the country to many millions of visitors, was a tremendous factor in promoting health education.

State and County Fairs. Many of the state and county fairs held each year include health exhibits as special features. The American Medical Association, in cooperation with the local state or county medical societies, has participated in these on numerous occasions with great success. Such opportunities to reach rural groups of people have been accepted wherever possible, and the response received from such groups has been most gratifying. Among others, fairs in the following states have received exhibits: Alabama, California, Florida, Illinois, Indiana, Iowa, Kansas, Ohio, Oklahoma, Michigan, Minnesota, Mississippi, Missouri, Montana, Nebraska, Nevada, North Carolina, Ohio, Oklahoma, Oregon, Pennsylvania, Tennessee, Utah, Washington and Wisconsin. In some cases, the state medical society circulated the exhibits on a circuit through the county fairs until the end of the season.

Halls of Health. From time to time state and county medical societies have promoted health exhibits where the audience was not ready-made, but had to be assembled for the purpose. The American Medical Association has participated in several of these undertakings, with large groups of health exhibits. Especially successful were the Halls of Health sponsored by the Wisconsin State Medical Society in conjunction with the annual meeting of the Society in Milwaukee in 1937, and by the Sedgwick County Medical Society in conjunction with the meeting of the Kansas State Medical Society at Wichita in 1938. Similar undertakings were conducted by the Illinois State Medical Society in 1938, 1939 and 1940, the Minnesota State Medical Association in 1939, and the Tulsa County Medical Society at Tulsa, Oklahoma in 1940, to all of which the American Medical Association contributed. Among other similar projects was the Centennial Exhibit of the Scott County Medical Society at Davenport, Iowa, in 1936, to which a considerable number of exhibits were sent from the American Medical Association.

Museums. Museums offer ready-made audiences in receptive moods for health exhibits, and the American Medical Association has cooperated with several institutions in this endeavor. A large amount of material was installed in the Museum of Science and Industry, Chicago, following the Century of Progress Exposition in Chicago, and the Golden Gate Exposition in San Francisco. The Cleveland Health Museum in Cleveland, Ohio, and the Dallas

Health Museum in Dallas, Texas, have been the recipients of a considerable amount of material, while others which have taken advantage of this opportunity include the Toledo Museum of Science at Toledo, Ohio, the Cayuga Museum of History and Art at Auburn, N. Y., the Newark Museum at Newark, N. J., the Public Museum at Grand Rapids, Michigan, the Buhl Planetarium at Pittsburgh, Pennsylvania, and the Museum at Richmond, Va. At several of the museums, question boxes were installed, where visitors could leave questions for additional information. The questions were sent to the American Medical Association and answered by the Bureau of Health Education.

Health exhibits have been shown on other occasions too numerous to mention, at conventions and meetings wherever the public has gathered, and in store windows. The Women's Auxiliary, National, state and county, have been assisted with health exhibits in many areas.

CENTRAL SCIENTIFIC EXHIBIT

For many years there was an insistent demand that something be done to conserve the excellent material shown in the Scientific Exhibit at the Annual Session of the Association. In 1928 arrangements were made to install in the Headquarters Building each year several of the best exhibits presented at the Annual Session, in the hope that a creditable Central Scientific Exhibit could be built up. Part of one floor in the Headquarters Building was given over to the task and about thirty exhibits installed, which filled the room to capacity. The exhibit was used by visiting physicians and by classes from medical schools. In 1934, however, the demand for the space for other activities became so great that the exhibits were discontinued.

MOTION PICTURES

The growth of the motion picture industry included the utilization of motion pictures as adjuncts of medical teaching. By 1915 such films had become quite popular, confined however largely to surgical subjects. The early films were on 35 mm. stock, making them expensive to produce and cumbersome to show, because a fireproof booth had to be erected to protect against the fire hazard. Many of the films were made as hobbies to show a particular method of operation (not always so good) or even for self-exploitation of the producer. Because of the low standard to which motion pictures had fallen, the Committee on Scientific Exhibit in 1922 ruled that no motion pictures dealing with purely surgical technic could be shown in the Scientific Exhibit. (J.A.M.A., *87*:1563 [Nov. 6] 1926.)

In 1928 the House of Delegates "Resolved, That a committee on visual moving picture education be appointed by the Board of Trustees of the American Medical Association, who shall organize such methods of procedure as shall bring the ethical showing of medical and surgical moving picture films within the authority and approval of organized medicine." (Minutes of A.M.A. House of Delegates, 1928 Session, p. 52.) The committee, consisting of Irving S. Cutter, M.D., C. P. Emerson, M.D. and Carl Henry Davis, M.D., reported in 1929 that two meetings had been held and plans were under way with the Eastman Kodak Company for distribution of medical films. (Minutes, House of Delegates, 1929 Session, p. 17.) Apparently little was accomplished.

In 1930 the House of Delegates authorized "the Board of Trustees to appoint a special committee to investigate and study the subject and to take such action as may be necessary to give the American Medical Association leadership in this field." (Minutes, House of Delegates, 1930 Session, p. 31.) The new committee, consisting of Drs. Emerson, Davis and A. B. Luckhardt, held one meeting at which time it requested the Director of Exhibits to make a survey of the field of motion pictures in medical and public health teaching and to submit a report. No further meetings were held.

The Bureau of Exhibits established a small film library at the headquarters building in 1930, which included motion pictures on various medical subjects for medical meetings and other scientific groups. The films were lent without charge to hundreds of medical societies, hospitals, universities, and during World War II to the Army and Navy. In addition, a source file of other motion pictures was maintained to answer thousands of inquiries for information about the availability or suitability of films on certain specified subjects.

Numerous problems on the distribution and utilization of medical films continued to arise, however, many of which were discussed at a conference during the Atlantic City Session of the American Medical Association in 1942. In 1945, the Board of Trustees appointed a Committee on Medical Motion Pictures to study the problem further and report back to the Board. In 1946, the Trustees made the committee permanent, with the following members: Morris Fishbein, M.D., Dean Smiley, M.D., W. L. Benedict, M.D., Thomas S. Jones, John G. Bradley and Ralph P. Creer, with C. W. Roberts, M.D., Victor Johnson, M.D. and Thomas G. Hull, Ph.D., as ex-officio members. Mr. Creer was engaged on a full-time basis to take charge of the work. A policy was established whereby the American Medical Association would not produce films, but would promote a more effective utilization of those already available by expanding its source file, publishing critical reviews on medical motion pictures and enlarging its film library.

PUBLICATIONS

Each year pamphlets have been prepared for distribution at the Annual Session in connection with the special exhibits or with exhibits presented by the different departments of the Association. Some of these have proved extremely popular and have required many reprints to meet subsequent demands. The pamphlets from the Special Exhibit on Fractures were collected into a book, entitled "Primer on Fractures" (1930) which is now in its fifth edition. Similarly the material shown in the Special Exhibits on Anesthesia was published in book form, "Fundamentals of Anesthesia" (1942), two editions of which have been printed.

MEDALS AWARDED IN SCIENTIFIC EXHIBIT, 1908–1946

1908 Dr. H. R. Ricketts, Chicago.
GOLD MEDAL for research exhibit on tick fever.
1909 New York Lying-In Hospital, New York.
GOLD MEDAL for research work.
Indianapolis Medical Society.
GOLD MEDAL for tuberculosis exhibit.
1910 Dr. Claude A. Smith, Stockbridge, Ga.
GOLD MEDAL for exhibit bearing on experimental researches on hookworm disease
1911 Hendryx Laboratory, Los Angeles.
GOLD MEDAL for pathologic exhibit.
U. S. Public Health and Marine Hospital Service.
GOLD MEDAL for exhibit of preparations and material concerning research in plague and leprosy.
1912 Dr. Martin H. Fischer.
GOLD MEDAL for research exhibit on experimental nephritis.
Dr. Emanuel Libman, New York.
GOLD MEDAL for the best exhibit of general nature, series of hearts showing bacterial endocarditis.
Dr. E. C. Rosenow, Rochester, Minn.
GOLD MEDAL for research exhibit on experimental endocarditis.
1913 Dr. C. C. Bass, New Orleans.
GOLD MEDAL for exhibit on the Cultivation of Malarial Plasmodia in Vitro.
1914 Miss Maude Slye, Chicago.
GOLD MEDAL for exhibit of charts, diagrams, specimens and tables on the transmission of hereditary cancer and other diseases in mice.
1915 Pathological Department of Stanford University, San Francisco.
GOLD MEDAL.
Pathological Department of the University of Michigan, Ann Arbor, Michigan.
GOLD MEDAL.
1916 Dr. Edward C. Rosenow, Rochester, Minn.
GOLD MEDAL for exhibit on elective localization of organisms.
Dr. Martin H. Fischer, Cincinnati.
SILVER MEDAL for exhibit on fatty degeneration and allied biological problems.

Dr. Edward C. Kendall, Rochester, Minn.
SILVER MEDAL for exhibit on active principle of the thyroid.

1916 Dr. C. V. Weller, Ann Arbor, Mich.
BRONZE MEDAL for exhibit on the blastophthoric effects of lead.
Dr. J. Shelton Horsley, Richmond, Va.
BRONZE MEDAL for exhibit on reversal circulation in the leg, and reconstruction of the common bile duct.

1917 Dr. B. S. Oppenheimer, New York.
GOLD MEDAL for electrocardiographic exhibit, illustrating pathological physiology of the cardiac mechanism.
Dr. Victor Lespinasse, Chicago.
SILVER MEDAL for exhibit on obstructive sterility.
Department of Obstetrics, Yale University Medical School, New Haven, Conn.
BRONZE MEDAL for an exhibit on placental pathology.

1918 Fort Riley Sanitary Laboratory, Fort Riley, Kansas.
GOLD MEDAL for exhibit of fifty models of Army Sanitary apparatus.
Dr. David J. Davis, Chicago.
SILVER MEDAL for exhibit of investigations of sporotrichosis, including specimens, cultures and pictures.
Mayo Foundation, Rochester, Minn.
SILVER MEDAL for exhibit of work of the Mayo Clinic.

1919 Dr. H. S. Warthin.
GOLD MEDAL.
Dr. Hideyo Noguchi, New York.
SILVER MEDAL.

1920 Dr. Edmond Souchon.
GOLD MEDAL for admirably prepared anatomic specimens.
Medical Department, U. S. Army.
SILVER MEDAL for an exhibit of pathologic preparations, excellent in appearance and highly instructive.

1921 Dr. Kenneth M. Lynch, Charleston, S. C.
GOLD MEDAL for exhibit of photographs and microscopic preparations illustrating investigation of ulcerative granulomata.

1922 Drs. Frank Hinman, D. M. Morison, A. E. Belt, and R. K. Lee-Brown, San Francisco.
GOLD MEDAL for exhibit of a study of renal circulation.
Mr. Robert A. Hodges, University, Alabama.
SILVER MEDAL for a study of certain culture-medium characteristics of ringworm fungi.

1923 Dr. Frank Hinman, San Francisco.
GOLD MEDAL for exhibit on hydronephrosis.
Dr. Benjamin T. Terry, Nashville, Tenn.
SILVER MEDAL for the demonstration of instructive specimens of pathologic anatomy.

1924 Mr. E. L. Judah, Rochester, Minn.
GOLD MEDAL for exhibit thoroughly demonstrating the pathology of gallbladder disease.
Dr. W. W. Duke, Kansas City, Mo.
SILVER MEDAL for completeness of the exhibit on "allergy."
Dr. Benjamin T. Terry, Nashville, Tenn.
BRONZE MEDAL for the effort involved in his personal demonstration of pathologic material carrying a message to the mass of physicians.

1925 Dr. C. Latimer Callander, San Francisco.
GOLD MEDAL for exhibit on surface capillaries in health and in disease.
Drs. H. N. Cole and L. J. Karnosh, Cleveland.
SILVER MEDAL for presentation of the effect of syphilis on the teeth.

Drs. Benjamin S. Kline and Samuel S. Berger, Cleveland.
SILVER MEDAL for originality of exhibit on spirochetal pulmonary gangrene.
Drs. Thomas A. Menees and H. C. Robinson, Grand Rapids, Mich.
BRONZE MEDAL for study on oral cholecystography.
Dr. Alexander Randall, Philadelphia, Pa.
BRONZE MEDAL for demonstration of gross pathology of prostatic obstruction.

1926 Dr. Aldo Castellani, New Orleans, La.
GOLD MEDAL for exhibit on some tropical mycoses and their causative agents.
Dr. Francis Carter Wood, New York.
SILVER MEDAL for the introduction of an experimental method and for studies of sarcoma and for excellence of presentation.
Drs. F. W. Hartman, Adolph Bollinger and H. P. Doub, Detroit, Mich.
SILVER MEDAL for exhibit showing the development of a promising experimental method and studies of nephritis.
Dr. Russell L. Haden, Kansas City, Kans.
BRONZE MEDAL for bacteriologic study of periapical dental infections.
Drs. Montrose Burrows, Louis H. Jorstad, Charles Johnson, G. Payling Wright and Edwin C. Ernst, St. Louis, Mo.
BRONZE Medal for work showing the relation of vitamins to cancer.

1927 Drs. F. W. Hartman, Adolph Bollinger and H. P. Doub, Detroit, Mich.
GOLD MEDAL for exhibit on cardiorenal and cardiac studies, illustrated with specimens showing the heart and kidney lesions produced by deep roentgen rays.
Dr. Hideyo Noguchi, New York.
SILVER MEDAL for exhibit illustrating studies of Oroya fever and trachoma.
Dr. Chevalier Jackson, Philadelphia, Pa.
SILVER MEDAL for exhibit of household accidents to children and prevention.
Drs. W. M. James, L. B. Bates, L. Getz and J. J. Valarino, Medical Association of the Isthmian Canal Zone, Ancon, Santa Tomas and Panama Hospitals.
BRONZE MEDAL for exhibit illustrating the diagnosis, etiology and pathology of infection with Endomeba histolytica.
Dr. V. P. Blair, St. Louis.
BRONZE MEDAL for exhibit on plastic surgery dealing with the retracted upper lip and nose.

1928 Dr. Edward Francis, U. S. Public Health Service, Washington, D. C.
GOLD MEDAL, Class I, for his thorough and important scientific contributions to the knowledge of tularemia, illustrated by his exhibit.
Dr. Eben J. Carey, Milwaukee.
SILVER MEDAL, Class I, for an exhibit showing the results of excellent experimental work on the dynamics of origin, structure and repair of bone.
Drs. Adelbert Ames, Jr. and Gordon H. Gliddon, Hanover, N. H.
BRONZE MEDAL, Class I, for exhibit showing significant application of physics to ophthalmology.
Dr. Walter M. Simpson, Dayton, Ohio.
GOLD MEDAL, Class II, for exhibit of the gross and microscopic changes in tularemia and for excellence of presentation.
Dr. Arthur J. Bedell, Albany, N. Y.
SILVER MEDAL, Class II, for an instructive exhibit of stereophotographs of the living eye.
Dr. O. E. Denny, Carville, La.
BRONZE MEDAL, Class II, for excellent exhibit of color photographs illustrating various manifestations of leprosy.

1929 Drs. Eugene P. Pendergrass and Temple Fay, Philadelphia, Pa.
GOLD MEDAL, Class I, for exhibit on encephalography.
Dr. Frank W. Hartman, Detroit, Mich.
SILVER MEDAL, Class I, for exhibit showing experimental work on the pathology of the kidney.

Drs. Howard D. Haskins and Edwin E. Osgood, Portland, Oregon.
BRONZE MEDAL, Class I, for exhibit on hematologic methods.
Drs. Olof Larsell, N. W. Jones and B. I. Phillips, Portland, Oregon.
BRONZE MEDAL, Class I, for exhibit on original experimental work on the treatment of anemia with nuclear extractives.
Dr. P. E. Truesdale, Fall River, Mass.
GOLD MEDAL, Class II, for exhibit showing experimental demonstration of the mechanism of transposition of abdominal viscera following rupture of the diaphragm.
Dr. A. V. Hardy, Iowa City, Iowa.
SILVER MEDAL, Class II, for exhibit of various aspects of undulant fever.
Drs. W. T. Cummins, San Francisco, Joseph K. Smith, Kern General Hospital, Bakersfield, California, and C. H. Halliday, Baltimore, Md.
BRONZE MEDAL, Class II, for exhibit of various aspects of coccidioidal granuloma.

1930 Dr. R. R. Spencer, U. S. Public Health Service, Washington, D. C.
GOLD MEDAL, Class I, for original work in preparation of vaccine for Rocky Mountain spotted fever and excellence of presentation.
Drs. William Duane, Jr. and Rubin M. Lewis, Philadelphia.
SILVER MEDAL, Class I, for original method of estimating physiologic pressures and excellence of presentation.
Drs. Cyrus C. Sturgis and Raphael Isaacs, Ann Arbor, Mich.
BRONZE MEDAL, Class I, for original work in the treatment of pernicious anemia and excellence of presentation.
Drs. M. H. Soule, F. G. Novy and P. B. Hadley, Ann Arbor, Mich.
GOLD MEDAL, Class II, for excellence of presentation of studies on respiration and dissociation of micro-organisms.
Dr. Russell S. Rowland, Detroit, Mich.
SILVER MEDAL, Class II, for excellence of presentation of studies on lipoid metabolism.
Drs. Vincent W. Archer and Charles H. Peterson, University, Va.
BRONZE MEDAL, Class II, for excellence of presentation of original work on intestinal ascariasis.

1931 Dr. Jacob Furth, Philadelphia, Pa.
GOLD MEDAL, Class I, for exhibit on experimental leukemia.
Drs. Bedford Shelmire and W. E. Dove, Dallas, Texas.
SILVER MEDAL, Class I, for original work on spread of typhus fever by the tropical rat-mite and excellence of presentation.
Drs. Eliot R. Clark, E. L. Clark, J. C. Sandison, R. G. Williams, H. T. Kirby-Smith, R. O. Rex, W. J. Hitschler, J. H. Smith and R. G. Abel, Philadelphia, Pa.
BRONZE MEDAL, Class I, for original work on the growth of living tissue as seen in artificial chambers introduced into the rabbit's ear and excellence of presentation.
Drs. J. Parsons Schaeffer and Warren B. Davis, Philadelphia.
GOLD MEDAL, Class II, for excellence of presentation of model specimens illustrating embryology, development and anatomy of the paranasal sinuses.
Drs. Harrison S. Martland, A. V. St. George, Alexander O. Gettler and Ralph H. Muller, Newark, N. J.
SILVER MEDAL, Class II, for excellence of presentation of exhibit illustrating the effects of radium poisoning in the watch dial industry.
Drs. Walter M. Freeman and Karl H. Langenstrass, Washington.
BRONZE MEDAL, Class II, for excellence of presentation of specimens illustrating diseases of the brain with clinicopathologic correlation.

1932 Drs. Frank A. Hartman, C. W. Greene, J. J. Maisel and G. W. Thorn, Buffalo, N. Y.
GOLD MEDAL, Class I, for original investigative work on the development and use of a hormone from the adrenal cortex and excellence of presentation.

Dr. C. W. Emmons, New York.
SILVER MEDAL, Class I, for original work on the variations in ringworm fungi and excellence of presentation.
Drs. J. A. Bargen, P. W. Brown and H. M. Weber, Rochester, Minn.
BRONZE MEDAL, Class I, for original investigation of diseases of the colon and excellence of presentation.
Drs. Max Ballin and Plinn F. Morse, Detroit, Michigan.
GOLD MEDAL, Class II, for excellence of presentation of exhibit on parathyroidism.
Drs. L. G. Rowntree and C. H. Greene, Rochester, Minn.
SILVER MEDAL, Class II, for excellence of presentation of exhibit of comprehensive study on Addison's disease.
Dr. Ernest Carroll Faust, New Orleans, La.
BRONZE MEDAL, Class II, for excellence of presentation of exhibit on human helminth infections.

1933 Dr. Moses Swick, New York.
GOLD MEDAL, Class I, for original investigative work on intravenous and oral urograms demonstrating various urologic conditions by means of sodium iodohippurate, developed by him.
Dr. L. F. Badger, Washington, D. C.
SILVER MEDAL, Class I, for original work on the differential diagnosis of Rocky Mountain spotted fever and endemic typhus, both of which occur endemically in some sections of the United States.
Drs. John W. Towey, Powers, Michigan, Henry C. Sweany, Chicago, and Willis H. Huron, Iron Mountain, Michigan.
BRONZE MEDAL, Class I, for original investigation of a form of pneumonitis produced by spores of a fungus (Coniosporium corticale) in maple bark.
Dr. Elliott P. Joslin, Boston, and Mr. Herbert H. Marks, New York.
GOLD MEDAL, Class II, for excellence of presentation of exhibit illustrating the prevention of diabetes mellitus and certain of its complications.
Dr. F. P. McNamara, Dubuque, Iowa.
SILVER MEDAL, Class II, for excellence of presentation of an exhibit illustrating the activities of the pathologic laboratory in a hundred bed hospital.
Dr. Plato Schwartz, Rochester, N. Y.
BRONZE MEDAL, Class II, for excellence of presentation of an exhibit illustrating the electrobasographic methods of recording the gait of man.

1934 Dr. Gregory Schwartzman, New York.
GOLD MEDAL, Class I, for original investigation of skin reactivity to bacterial filtrates, its role in immunology and its practical applications.
Dr. Timothy Leary, Boston.
SILVER MEDAL, Class I, for original work on the relation of cholesterol to atherosclerosis.
Dr. Charles C. Higgins, Cleveland.
BRONZE MEDAL, Class I, for original work on experimental production and solution of urinary calculi.
Drs. William M. James, Lewis B. Bates, Lawrence Getz, and Ernesto Icaza, Panama, R. of P.
GOLD MEDAL, Class II, for excellence of presentation of an exhibit illustrating diagnosis and pathology of human amebiasis.
Dr. Claude S. Beck, Cleveland, Ohio.
SILVER MEDAL, Class II, for excellence of presentation of exhibit illustrating circulatory failure produced by compression of the heart and curable by operation shown.
Dr. William P. Murphy, Boston.
BRONZE MEDAL, Class II, for excellence of presentation of exhibit illustrating the therapeutic effects of intramuscular injections of liver extract in pernicious anemia and in secondary anemia.

1935 Drs. M. Edward Davis and F. L. Adair, Chicago.
GOLD MEDAL, Class I, for original investigations in the development of ergot as a therapeutic agent and especially of a new active principle isolated in crystalline state from ergot, together with its pharmacologic and medicinal properties.
Drs. L. G. Rowntree, J. H. Clark, Arthur Steinberg and A. M. Hanson, Philadelphia.
SILVER MEDAL, Class I, for original investigations on the biologic effects of thymus and pineal extracts.
Drs. Jane Sands Robb, J. G. Fred Hiss and R. C. Robb, Syracuse, N. Y.
BRONZE MEDAL, Class I, for original investigations on cardiac muscle-bundle physiology and experimental coronary lesions.
Drs. Stuart W. Harrington and Willis S. Lemon, Rochester, Minn.
GOLD MEDAL, Class II, for excellence of presentation of exhibit illustrating the surgical treatment and clinical manifestations of various types of diaphragmatic hernia and intrathoracic tumors.
Drs. David W. MacKenzie and Alexander B. Wallace, Montreal, Canada.
SILVER MEDAL, Class II, for excellence of presentation of exhibit on lymphatic studies, particularly relation of the lower urinary and genital tracts to renal infections.
Dr. James Harold Mendel, Miami, Fla.
BRONZE MEDAL, Class II, for excellence of presentation of exhibit on ear drums and their interpretation.
1936 Drs. Charles B. Huggins, W. J. Noonan and B. H. Blocksom, Chicago.
GOLD MEDAL, Class I, for original investigation on the distribution of red and yellow bone marrow and the reticulo-endothelial system in the bone marrow.
Drs. G. C. Supplee and S. Ansbacher, Bainbridge, N. Y.
SILVER MEDAL, Class I, for original investigation on the development of pure lactoflavin an entity of the water soluble vitamin B complex.
Dr. Alvan L. Barach, New York.
BRONZE MEDAL, Class I, for original investigation on the role of helium and oxygen in various types of dyspnea.
Drs. Rudolf Schindler, Marie Ortmayer and John F. Renshaw, Chicago.
GOLD MEDAL, Class II, for excellence of presentation of exhibit on chronic gastritis as studied by gastroscopy.
Drs. John O. Bower, J. C. Burns and H. A. Mengle, Philadelphia, Pa.
SILVER MEDAL, Class II, for exhibit illustrating the treatment of spreading peritonitis complicating acute appendicitis.
Dr. Hamilton Montgomery, Rochester, Minn.
BRONZE MEDAL, Class II, for excellence of presentation of exhibit illustrating the histopathology of various types of cutaneous tuberculosis.
1937 Drs. L. G. Rowntree, Arthur Steinberg, N. H. Einhorn, J. H. Clark, George M. Dorrance, E. F. Ciccone, and A. M. Hanson, Philadelphia, Pa.
GOLD MEDAL, Class I, for exhibit illustrating original investigation on normal and abnormal growth associated with the development of sarcoma in albino rats from the ingestion of a crude wheat germ oil made by ether extraction.
Dr. Eben J. Carey, Milwaukee, Wis.
SILVER MEDAL, Class I, for exhibit illustrating original investigation on intrinsic wave mechanics of the nervous and muscular systems.
Dr. Louis Gross, New York.
BRONZE MEDAL, Class I, for an exhibit illustrating experimental studies on the blood supply to the heart in relation to coronary occlusion.
Drs. M. S. Henderson, H. W. Meyerding, R. K. Ghormley and H. B. Macey, Rochester, Minn.
GOLD MEDAL, Class II, for excellence of presentation of exhibit illustrating fractures, a potential source of deformity and disability.

Dr. Frank W. Hartman, Detroit, Michigan.
SILVER MEDAL, Class II, for exhibit on oxygen therapy with the use of liquid oxygen and air; a new efficient low cost oxygen tent.
Drs. Franklin F. Snyder, Morris Rosenfeld, Baltimore, Md.
BRONZE MEDAL, Class II, for exhibit illustrating intrauterine respiration of the fetus and its relation to respiratory failure at birth.

1938 Drs. A. C. Ivy, R. R. Greene and M. W. Burrill, Chicago.
GOLD MEDAL, Class I, for exhibit illustrating experimentally produced intersexuality in the rat.
Dr. Hermann Sommer, San Francisco.
SILVER MEDAL, Class I, for exhibit illustrating plankton and paralytic shellfish poisoning.
Dr. H. J. Corper, Denver, Colorado.
BRONZE MEDAL, Class I, for exhibit illustrating immunity in tuberculosis: historical and experimental.
Drs. Frank W. Konzelmann, Edward Weiss, Lawrence W. Smith, Walter I. Lillie and Edwin S. Gault, Philadelphia, Pa.
GOLD MEDAL, Class II, for exhibit illustrating cardiovascular-renal disease, clinical and pathologic correlation.
Dr. Philip Lewin, Chicago.
SILVER MEDAL, Class II, for exhibit illustrating newer concepts and methods of teaching orthopedic surgery.
Drs. R. J. Reitzel, S. P. Lucia and Karl F. Meyer, San Francisco.
BRONZE MEDAL, Class II, for exhibit illustrating clinical and epidemiologic demonstration of various infectious diseases.

1939 Drs. George W. Thorn, R. Palmer Howard, Kendall Emerson, Jr. and Warfield M. Firor, Baltimore, Md.
GOLD MEDAL, Group I, for exhibit illustrating studies on desoxycorticosterone (a synthetic adrenal cortical substance).
Drs. George P. Robb and Israel Steinberg, New York, N. Y.
SILVER MEDAL, Group I, for exhibit illustrating visualization of the chambers of the heart, the pulmonary circulation and the great blood vessels in man.
Drs. J. F. Fulton, Margaret A. Kennard and Carlyle F. Jacobsen, New Haven, Conn.
BRONZE MEDAL, Group I, for exhibit illustrating functions of the frontal lobe with particular reference to the motor and premotor areas (areas 4 and 6 of Brodmann).
Drs. Elmer L. DeGowin, John E. Harris and E. D. Plass, Iowa City, Iowa.
GOLD MEDAL, Group II, for exhibit illustrating the preservation of blood for transfusion.
Dr. Philip Lewin, Chicago, Illinois.
SILVER MEDAL, Group II, for exhibit illustrating backache and sciatica.
Dr. Morris Moore, St. Louis, Mo.
BRONZE MEDAL, Group II, for exhibit illustrating mycotic infections of man.

1940 Drs. Charles B. Huggins, Philip Clark and W. W. Scott, Chicago, Illinois.
GOLD MEDAL, Group I, for exhibit illustrating experimental benign hypertrophy of the prostate in the dog.
Drs. John R. Paul and James D. Trask, New Haven, Conn.
SILVER MEDAL, Group I, for exhibit illustrating a rural epidemic of poliomyelitis; clinical and geographic features.
Drs. Charles F. Nelson and Roland C. Nelson, Beverly Hills, Calif.
BRONZE MEDAL, Group I, for exhibit on bone metabolism.
Dr. Norman Treves, New York.
GOLD MEDAL, Group II, for exhibit illustrating the significance of the bleeding nipple.

Drs. A. H. Logan, P. W. Brown, J. A. Bargen, H. M. Weber, L. A. Buie, H. H. Bowing, A. H. Baggenstoss, C. F. Dixon, J. deJ. Pemberton and C. W. Mayo Rochester, Minn.
SILVER MEDAL, Group II, for exhibit on polyps of rectum and colon and illustrating what can be done about them.
Dr. W. H. Wright, National Institute of Health, Washington, D. C.
BRONZE MEDAL, Group II, for exhibit illustrating the public health aspects of trichinosis.

1941 Drs. Alvin L. Berman, F. S. Grodins and A. C. Ivy, Chicago, Ill.
GOLD MEDAL, Group I, for exhibit on the rationale of bile salt therapy.
Drs. Harold Thomas Hyman, William Leifer, and Louis Chargin, New York.
SILVER MEDAL, Group I, for exhibit illustrating massive dose chemotherapy of early syphilis by the intravenous drip method.
Drs. Walter M. Boothby, W. R. Lovelace, C. W. Mayo and A. H. Bulbulian, Rochester, Minn.
BRONZE MEDAL, Group I, for exhibit illustrating physiologic problems in aviation medicine.
Drs. Waltman Walters, Howard K. Gray and James T. Priestley, Rochester, Minn.
GOLD MEDAL, Group II, for exhibit illustrating malignant lesions of the stomach; importance of early treatment and end results.
Drs. Grover C. Penberthy and Charles N. Weller, Detroit, Mich.
SILVER MEDAL, Group II, for exhibit illustrating the treatment of burns.
Dr. G. V. Brindley, Temple, Texas.
BRONZE MEDAL, Group II, for exhibit illustrating carcinoma of the colon; factors affecting its cure.

1942 Drs. Eben J. Carey and Leo C. Massopust, Milwaukee, Wis.
GOLD MEDAL, Group I, for exhibit on experimental ameboid motion of motor end plates.
Drs. Deryl Hart and Samuel E. Upchurch, Durham, N. C.
SILVER MEDAL, Group I, for exhibit on air disinfection with bactericidal radiant energy.
Dr. O. V. Batson, Philadelphia, Pa.
BRONZE MEDAL, Group I, for exhibit on the vertebral vein system as a mechanism for the spread of metastases.
Drs. John C. Bugher and Manuel Roca-Garcia, Bogota, Colombia.
GOLD MEDAL, Group II, for exhibit on the epidemiology of jungle yellow fever.
Dr. Emanuel Libman, New York.
SILVER MEDAL, Group II, for exhibit illustrating endocarditis and "Libman-Sack's disease."
Drs. L. M. Randall, M. C. Piper, L. A. Brunsting and M. B. Dockerty, Rochester, Minn.
BRONZE MEDAL, Group II, for exhibit on kraurosis and allied lesions of the vulva and certain neoplasms of the ovary.

1943 (Meeting Cancelled)

1944 Drs. William H. Feldman, H. Corwin Hinshaw and Frank C. Mann, Rochester, Minn.
GOLD MEDAL, Group I, for exhibit on chemotherapy of tuberculosis.
Dr. Robert H. Williams, Boston, Mass.
SILVER MEDAL, Group I, for the exhibit on thiouracil in thyrotoxicosis.
Drs. J. A. Roth, A. C. Ivy and A. J. Atkinson, Chicago.
BRONZE MEDAL, Group I, for the exhibit on the effect of caffeine on the stomach.
Dr. Armand J. Quick, Milwaukee, Wisconsin.
GOLD MEDAL, Group II, for exhibit on determination of prothrombin.
Dr. Keith S. Grimson, Durham, N. C.

SILVER MEDAL, Group II, for the exhibit on paravertebral sympathectomy for hypertension.
Drs. Leo G. Rigler, Henry S. Kaplan and Captain Daniel L. Fink, Minneapolis, Minnesota.
BRONZE MEDAL, Group II, for the exhibit on pernicious anemia, benign polyps and carcinoma of the stomach.

1945 (Meeting Cancelled)
1946 Dr. A. D. Ruedemann, Cleveland, Ohio.
GOLD MEDAL, Group I, for the exhibit on a permanent plastic eye.
Drs. Bert R. Boone, Fred G. Gillick, George C. Henny, Morton J. Oppenheimer, and W. Edward Chamberlain, Philadelphia, Pa.
SILVER MEDAL, Group I, for the exhibit on the electrokymograph: a recorder of cardiovascular motions.
Drs. Kurt Lange, Linn J. Boyd and David Weiner, New York.
BRONZE MEDAL, Group I, for the exhibit on frostbite—functional and morphologic pathology and the prevention of subsequent gangrene.
Dr. Herbert M. Evans and Associates, Berkeley, Calif.
GOLD MEDAL, Group II, for exhibit on hormones of the anterior hypophysis.
Dr. Frederick H. Falls and Charlotte S. Holt, Chicago.
SILVER MEDAL, Group II, for exhibit on toxemias of pregnancy.
Drs. Elmer C. Bartels and George O. Bell, Boston, Mass.
BRONZE MEDAL, Group II, for exhibit on use of thiouracil in preparation of patients with severe hyperthyroidism for thyroidectomy.
Dr. Thomas G. Hull, Director, Scientific Exhibit, American Medical Association, Chicago, Ill.
GOLD MEDAL for his notable contribution through the years to the scientific exhibits of American medicine.

BUREAU OF MEDICAL ECONOMICS

By Frank G. Dickinson, Ph.D.

WHEN THE BUREAU OF MEDICAL ECONOMICS was established in 1931, there was practically no printed material prepared by the medical profession on the economic phases of medicine. The Committee on the Costs of Medical Care was just completing its studies. Almost the entire administrative staff of that committee were persons out of sympathy with the point of view of the medical profession.

The Bureau of Medical Economics proposed to become a source of thoroughly reliable facts on the economic problems of medicine. Although the Bureau has continuously published much material based largely on its own research, the accuracy of its factual material has not been challenged.

The problems that confronted the medical profession when the Bureau was organized varied greatly from those today. The research and reports of the Bureau reflect the changing character of these problems. The first publication in 1931 was the "Cost of Medical Education," followed by "Incomes from Medical Practice" and "Some Phases of Contract Practice" which appeared the next year.

During the first year of the Bureau's existence the most frequent request from physicians concerned the practices of commercial collection agencies. The pamphlet, "Collecting Medical Fees," issued in 1932, revised in 1934 and again in 1938 with numerous reprints, seems to have practically ended the abuses of collection agencies. Letters of complaint are rarely received now.

"Group Practice," in 1933 and later revised in 1940, discussed another problem. By 1933 experiments were being conducted in hospital insurance, and an examination of "Prepayment Plans for Hospital Care" and "New Forms of Medical Practice," issued in 1933, and "Group Hospitalization" in 1938 reveals something of the struggle to control the abuses that existed in the early days of hospital insurance.

During this same period there were many experiments with methods of payment for medical care which were described in "New Forms of Medical Practice," issued in 1933, and revised in

1934, in "Medical Service Plans" in 1935 and "Organization of Medical Services" in 1936. The experience in this field was summarized in "Organized Payments for Medical Services" in 1939, revised in 1940, and finally in "Medical Service Plans" in 1943. These studies provide a continuous history of the experiments that finally culminated in the organization of medical society prepayment plans.

Early in 1933 sickness insurance, which had been recommended by the Committee on the Costs of Medical Care, became a live political question. "A Critical Analysis of Sickness Insurance," first published in 1934, has passed through nine editions. The "Handbook of Sickness Insurance," first issued in 1930, before the establishment of the Bureau, was revised by the Bureau in 1934, since which there have been five editions and a revision in 1939. "Health Insurance in England" in 1934 passed through five editions and was revised in 1938. Five smaller pamphlets on sickness insurance were issued during 1934 and 1935. In 1934 much material was supplied to schools debating state medicine.

The first draft of the Social Security Bill included provisions for sickness insurance. Representatives of the Bureau spent much time in Washington working with the president's commission to discuss such legislation; finally sickness insurance was omitted from the Social Security Bill.

Other problems which concerned the Bureau and which also have more or less bearing on the development of present prepayment plans are suggested by the publication of "Medical Relations under Workmen's Compensation" in 1933, which was revised in 1935 and 1938. Most of the suggestions contained in the first edition were found to have been adopted by the time of the latest revision of this study. The "Care of the Indigent Sick," published in 1935 and revised in 1936, summarized experience, much of which has been used in the later experiments of prepayment plans.

More general studies issued in the same period were "University and College Student Health Service," 1935; "Economics and the Ethics of Medicine," of which there have been nine editions since 1936; "Cooperatives and Medical Services," 1936, and "Medical Directories," 1937, which seems to have terminated a type of annoying exploitation of physicians. "Rural Medical Service" was published in 1937, and in 1939 "Factual Data on Medical Economics," which was revised in 1940, presented the most complete compilation of statistics yet issued bearing directly upon medical economic problems. The "Distribution of Physicians in the United States" in 1934, revised in 1936, has been the standard work in that field since it was issued. The Bureau also directed extensive studies of "Medical Care in the United States" in 1939 and issued the "Basic Principles of Medical Economics" in 1941. Another task which bore less directly on medical economic problems, but which required a great amount of time and work, was the preparation of the "Index and Digest" of the proceedings of the House of Delegates from 1904 to 1941.

In June 1940 the Bureau of Medical Economics undertook a census of physicians for medical preparedness. This census was conducted in conjunction with the Committee on Medical Preparedness of the American Medical Association, and the Procurement and Assignment Service for Physicians, Dentists and Veterinarians of the Federal Security Agency, until fall of 1943, at which time activities were transferred from the Bureau.

In response to a request in 1942 from the Metropolitan Life Insurance Company for information on the death rate of physicians, data and figures were compiled and submitted for statistical surveys.

At the end of 1943, approximately 1,932,000 copies of Bureau publications had been published and distributed. This distribution was not a forced one; on the contrary, a majority of the copies were sent not only on direct request from medical societies, but also from schools, universities and a wide variety of other institutions and individuals.

At its September 1946 meeting the Board of Trustees changed the name of this Bureau, established in 1931, from the Bureau of Medical Economics to the Bureau of Medical Economic Research. The Board also announced the appointment of Frank G. Dickinson, Ph.D., as the new Director of the Bureau, succeeding Dr. R. G. Leland. The Board also stated that the Bureau would be reactivated and expanded and that research would be stressed.

Dr. Dickinson resigned his position as associate professor of economics at the University of Illinois, where he had taught economics since graduation in 1921 except for the school year in 1922–23, when he was instructor in economics at the Pennsylvania State College. He also received his A.M. degree at the end of that year. He received his Ph.D. degree at the University of Illinois in 1927. His principal fields of study and teaching were insurance and statistics. He had served as president of the American Association of University Teachers of Insurance during 1944 and 1945. He was first informed of the post by his family physician.

The Director works in close cooperation with the Council on Medical Service, attending its meetings and being a member of its

Subcommittee on Cooperation with Insurance Industry in the Development of Prepayment Medical Care Plans and of its Committee on Rural Problems on Medical Care Insurance.

The staff operating the International Business Machines equipment at Association headquarters was transferred to the Bureau in September. The Bureau has been called on to furnish information for several agencies, including the Coal Mines Administration in Washington. This information could not have been furnished without the I. B. M. equipment. It should be stressed that for the most part the Bureau in this capacity acts as a service agency for the

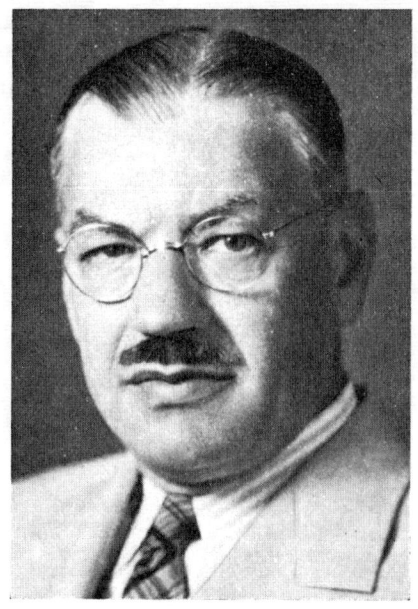

Dr. R. G. Leland
Director, Bureau of Medical Economics 1931-44

Councils at American Medical Headquarters, especially the Council on Medical Service and the Council on Medical Education and Hospitals, and for local and state medical societies.

Research work, almost completed by Dr. Leland, for the preparation of a life table for physicians which will be presented at Atlantic City by the Statistical Bureau of the Metropolitan Life Insurance Company has been continued.

The Director has observed that the studies made here and elsewhere on the supply of medical service use county data; that is, the population of a county is divided by the number of physicians in that county, and this ratio is called the physician-population ratio. Economic data do not follow county boundary lines, although the county may be an excellent unit for organizing a professional society. A physician is not a county coroner, and his patients often reside outside the county. The accessibility of medical service has undergone many changes in the last generation, and a study of the supply of medical service must recognize the changes wrought by hard roads and other improvements in transportation. Hence the Bureau is attempting to develop medical service areas which cut across county boundary lines and circumscribe the area served by the physicians in the community. These physician-population ratios for medical service areas, when completed, will indicate the actual supply of medical service to the people in all sections of the United States. It is estimated that it will require at least two years to mark out the entire map of the United States into medical service areas as has been done for retail trading areas by several research organizations.

THE LIBRARY OF
THE AMERICAN MEDICAL ASSOCIATION

By Marjorie H. Moore

THE EARLIEST RECORD OF PLANS to establish a library of the American Medical Association is to be found in a resolution introduced by Dr. N. S. Davis of Illinois at the 19th Annual Meeting held in Washington, D. C., May 5–8, 1868, which read[1]: "Resolved, That the Chair shall appoint a committee of three, to report at the next session, on the practicability of establishing a library of American medical works, including books, monographs, and periodicals. Committee: Drs. J. M. Toner, of District of Columbia, N. S. Davis, of Illinois, and D. F. Condie, of Pennsylvania." Accordingly in 1869[2] at the 20th Annual Meeting in New Orleans the committee so appointed to report on the practicability of establishing a library of American medical works including books, monographs, and periodicals submitted its report which included in part the following:

"After carefully viewing the project in all the relations in which it has presented itself to us, we deem it not only practicable but exceedingly desirable that a library of the character suggested be established under the auspices of the American Medical Association, and commend the measure to the patronage of the medical profession of the United States.

"The value of books to the medical man cannot be overestimated. They are the inexhaustible fount of knowledge from which the discoveries of the day, and the accumulated experience of ages may be drawn.

"The physician whose studies lead him to consult early American medical literature must be painfully struck with the perishable character of our professional literature, and the meagre or fragmentary collections which have been made.

"There is no city or library in our country that can boast of anything like completeness in the works of American authors. Indeed, it is to be feared that the combined collections of all the libraries in the country would not now produce a complete list of the various contributions to the science of medicine by local practitioners since the settlement of this continent.

"It is to be hoped that national pride will, in this direction, aid our professional requirements, and that this body may, at its present session, inaugurate measures that will lay the foundation of a great national medical library, or repository of all American medical works, including books, pamphlets, periodicals, journals, transactions, reports, addresses, circulars, catalogues, etc., that are in any way connected with the history and

---

[1] Tr. Am. Med. Assoc. *19*:39, 1868.
[2] Tr. Am. Med. Assoc. *20*:117, 1869.

practice of medicine, and such other medical works as may be contributed to the collection.

"Much of the material that is desirable for such a library, and which is so intimately connected with the most interesting period in the history of the medical profession in America, is now almost irrevocably lost, and further delay but adds to the danger of its complete destruction, or enhances the difficulty of recovering copies for preservation. We should aim to make the collection absolutely complete in all that has been contributed to the literature of medicine by American physicians, from the settlement of the country to the present time.

"Such a collection would interest the whole medical profession, and the inquisitive, not less than the curious student of our own and foreign countries."

The committee also considered it their duty to include in their report suggestions as to the steps necessary to be taken to effect the object, the location of the library, and the preservation of a collection. Among the plans included in their report were the following:

"First. Let the American Medical Association, by resolution, affirm its purpose to found a library of American medical literature, and request for it contributions of books, pamphlets, periodicals, and money, from the profession of the United States, for whose benefit the collection is designed.

"Second. Let the Association, by resolution, request every American medical author or publisher now living to present a copy of all their medical publications to the library of the American Medical Association, to be preserved and catalogued with the name of the donor and kept in condition to be readily consulted.

"Third. Let the Association request, by resolution, physicians and others throughout the United States having duplicate copies of early American medical publications that are scarce and out of print to present a copy to the library, to be catalogued with the name of the donor and preserved for reference.

"Fourth. Let the Association place annually a small sum, say one or two hundred dollars, at the disposal of the librarian to invest as opportunity may offer in books of the character indicated, and to pay postage, expenses of packages, etc.

"Fifth. Let the Association instruct the Librarian to exchange, at a fair valuation, as opportunity may offer, such duplicates as may accumulate in the library for desirable works not in the collection, and to report yearly to the Association the expenses, and the annual increase and condition of the library.

"Sixth. A book-mark, engraved or printed, should be adopted, which would display prominently the name of the Library of the American Medical Association, having on it a blank for the insertion of the name of the donor, and the number of the volume. One of these should be pasted on the inside of the cover of each book, as evidence of ownership and protection against loss."

After some discussion, on motion of Dr. James F. Hibberd, Indiana, the report was accepted and an amendment to the constitution was adopted which read as follows: "The librarian shall receive and preserve all the property in books, pamphlets, journals, and manuscripts presented to or acquired by the Association, record their titles in a book prepared for the purpose, acknowledge the receipt of the same, and he shall also be a member of the Committee of Publications." The housing of the proposed library was considered carefully by the committee. Included in the report are two letters written by Dr. Toner, as chairman of the Library Committee, to Dr. Thomas Miller, president of the Medical Society of the District of Columbia, and to A. R. Spofford, Esq., Librarian of Congress, discussing this point. In the letters Dr. Toner inquires if the library of the Medical Society of the District of Columbia and the Library of Congress would consent to receive any collection the American Medical Association might make as a special deposit and catalogue and keep them in a condition to be readily consulted. It appears that Dr. Toner feared that the Association might raise an objection to housing the collection in the library of the Medical Society of the District of Columbia because the building was not fireproof and that physicians having copies of rare and early medical works would not feel like parting with them unless they were placed in a fireproof repository. He therefore approached both libraries with the idea of having an alternative choice should the Association reject the offer of the Medical Society of the District of Columbia for the reason mentioned above. Favorable answers were received from Mr. Spofford of the Library of Congress and from Dr. J. W. H. Lovejoy, corresponding secretary of the Medical Society of the District of Columbia. Mr. Spofford of the Library of Congress stated in his reply that in so far as he was able to act in the premises, he would heartily welcome such an accession to the stores of the national library, provided the books were of the nature of a public deposit and therefore available for the consultation of readers in the library. A portion of his letter seems interesting enough to record here: "The fact that there is already a collection of over 6000 volumes of works relating to medical science here, adds to the importance of your enterprise, which, as I understand, contemplates the gathering into a central and fireproof repository, all the stores of early medical books and pamphlets which the liberal contributions of members of your Association and of the public may bring together. This may justly be considered as an object of national importance, aside from its professional value to your Association; and I know of no other method so likely to accumulate the early pamphlets and books relating to medical science into a comprehensive library for universal public reference, as the zealous cooperation of the members of your Association towards the completion of such a collection.

"It would give me pleasure to set apart an alcove in the medical department of this Library, which, with its present accumulation of 176,000 volumes, is a literary repository worthy of the American people, whose contributions it represents, for your collection. I would suggest that each book should have a distinctive label, printed for the purpose, and identifying it as the property of your Association. I have no doubt that the Joint Library Committee of Congress would concur in such regulations as might be agreed upon relating to the reception and care of this special collection." Dr. Davis of Illinois offered a resolution "that the proposition of the librarian of the Congressional Library be accepted," and the resolution was adopted.

Readers will note perhaps that the bookplate prepared for the collection bears the following notation: "This collection of Books is a special deposit in the Library of Congress." Since the collection was never at any time so deposited in the Library of Congress, an explanation of this discrepancy is needed. In Dr. Reyburn's library report read at the 21st Annual Meeting of the

LIBRARY OF THE
AMERICAN MEDICAL ASSOCIATION.

Chap
Shelf
No
of
Donor.

This collection of Books is a special deposit in the LIBRARY OF CONGRESS.

Early bookplate prepared for Library of the American Medical Association.

American Medical Association in Washington, D. C., 1870, there was incorporated the text of a circular prepared by the library committee and transmitted to the medical journals, officers of medical societies, and colleges, as well as to many of the prominent physicians of the United States. The circular was for the most part an appeal for contributions to the library. It was stated, however, in the circular, that "the Librarian of Congress has kindly consented to receive and preserve as a special deposit, in the Government fireproof building any collection of medical works the American Medical Association may make, and will catalogue, and keep them in condition to be readily consulted." Obviously the committee, at the time of the preparation of the circular, believed that all arrangements had been completed to house the book collection of the American Medical Association in the Library of Congress and had had the bookplates prepared with that arrangement in mind. Later on in Dr. Reyburn's report, however, he expressed regret that the Congressional Library Committee had not as yet authorized the Librarian of Congress to receive the books belonging to the American Medical Association as a special deposit. He stated that: "In order to obviate the embarrassment thus caused, Dr. J. M. Toner (chairman of the Library Committee) applied to Professor Henry, who very kindly and courteously fitted up a room in the Smithsonian Building for their safe-keeping and preservation." We may assume that the original bookplate was corrected, deleting the notation "This collection of Books is a special deposit in the Library of Congress," for a revision of the bookplate of the American Medical Association is reproduced in Dr. Morris Fishbein's comphrehensive article, Medical Bookplates, Bull. Soc. Med. Hist. of Chicago

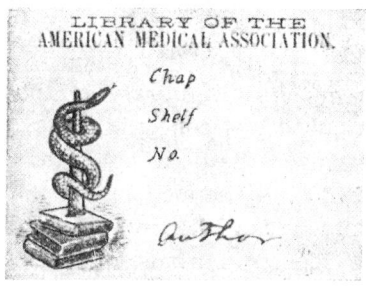

Medical book label at one time employed by the American Medical Association.

2:303–320, March 1922, and the misleading words above quoted are conspicuously absent from the bookplate as revised.

In 1870, arrangements were made, through the courtesy of Professor Henry of the Smithsonian Institution, to house and preserve books collected by the Association in a room provided in the Smithsonian building. Dr. Robert Reyburn of Washington, D. C. was the first appointed librarian, 1869. He was succeeded by Dr. F. A. Ashford, Washington, D. C. in 1871. Dr. William Lee of Washington, D. C. was appointed librarian in 1873 and retained the appointment until 1883. Dr. C. H. A. Kleinschmidt, Washington, D. C. became librarian in 1883 and was succeeded in 1891 by Dr. George W. Webster, Illinois.

It appears from a study of the reports made by the early librarians that the main objective for the establishment of the library was not to provide library service to members of the American Medical Association but rather to provide an "American Medical Repository where the whole medical literature of this country and continent might be preserved and owned by the representative Association of the new world." That this plan on the grand scale fell far short of its goal is only too well evidenced by the printed lists of the titles collected, which can be found in various issues of the Transactions of the American Medical Association, i.e., volumes 22 through 32, 1871–1881. In twenty-five years, from 1870 to 1895, only 3,781 volumes and 3,708 pamphlets were collected; these are the figures for the American Medical Association library collection that was turned over to the Newberry Library of Chicago in 1895.

In 1892, the librarian, Dr. George W. Webster, Illinois, suggested, in his report to the Board of Trustees, that the book collection which had been accumulating for twenty-four years in the Smithsonian Building of Washington be turned over to the Newberry Library of Chicago. The following is quoted from Dr. Webster's report[3] of that year: "About twenty-four years ago, when there were no large medical libraries in Washington, and when it was expected that the American Medical Association would probably have a permanent home there, Dr. Toner of Washington was instrumental in organizing the library of the American Medical Association for the purpose of collecting books, journals, etc. to be a safe depository for even the perishable literature of medicine, to be a library of reference for the members of the medical profession, and to be a library in fact as well as in name. For a period of twenty-four years the books, reports, journals, etc., have been accumulating, and have been tied up in bundles and placed in the garret of the Smithsonian Institution at Washington, and at no time in the history of the Library has it been accessible; at no time has any part been utilized by the members of the American Medical Association or the medical fraternity. In view of the foregoing, your Librarian recently had an interview with the trustees of the Newberry Library, at Chicago. At that interview, and more recently in writing, the trustees of said Newberry Library agreed that, if the American Medical Association shall decide to place its books, journals, etc., in the medical department of the Newberry Library, the trustees of said Library, agree to pay for transportation, receive, arrange, catalogue, bind and make them readily accessible to the entire profession, whether resident or non-resident of Chicago. Such books, journals, etc., to be held in trust until called for by the Association." Dr. R. Harvey Reed of Mansfield, Ohio, moved that the report be adopted. The motion was seconded and carried. It was some time, however, before a mutual understanding could be reached between

---

[3] J.A.M.A., *18*:804, June 25, 1892.

the American Medical Association and the trustees of the Newberry Library, but in 1894, at the 45th Annual Meeting in San Francisco, an agreement was reached between the parties for the transfer of the American Medical Association book collection from the Smithsonian Building in Washington to the Newberry Library in Chicago, under the circumstances and conditions named in the contract, reading in part as follows[4]: "That the said books and pamphlets shall be treated by the Newberry Library in all respects as its own, and as it treats its own books, except that in labeling, stamping, or otherwise marking them they shall, when received, be so marked as to show that they belong to the collection received from the American Medical Association; and the said Association shall never thereafter have any right to remove said collection of books or any part thereof from the custody and control of the Newberry Library. That the American Medical Association shall hereafter continue to deposit in the Newberry Library all the books, journals, etc., donated or contributed to it from any and all sources; except those given to reviewers for writing the reviews, and such journals as are needed to keep complete files in the office of the Journal of the American Medical Association."

In what we may surmise was a compliance with the terms of the contract above mentioned, a deposit of the American Medical Association's entire book collection with the Newberry Library was carried out in 1895. With this transfer of the collection came the end of the first effort sponsored by the Association to establish a library of American medical works. The American Medical Association collection remained in the Newberry Library until August, 1907, when the entire medical collection of that library was transferred to the John Crerar Library of Chicago. There is no record respecting the agreement on the part of the American Medical Association for such a removal of the collection, but perhaps legal sanction for such a removal is contained in those generous words of the contract to the effect that "The said books and pamphlets shall be treated by the Newberry Library in all respects as its own." The bookplates originally inserted in each book belonging to the American Medical Association collection were covered over with the Crerar Library bookplate, and today no identification of the books belonging to the early collection of the Association can be made. Looking back upon the ambitious early plans of the men who blazed the trail for an Association Library, we can readily see the difficulties which faced the pioneers in the establishment of such a library and have some understanding why such a worthy project,

---

[4] J.A.M.A., *22:*945, June 23, 1894.

in its beginning, failed. Among other things, the Association was without a headquarters office to house a library; it was without the services of a professional librarian to care for and administer the collection; and it was dependent solely upon the generosity of the profession for the acquisition of books and pamphlets.

From 1895, the date the Association's book collection was transferred to the Newberry Library, until 1903, when the first building ever owned and maintained by the Association was erected, no attempt was made to maintain a library or to furnish any type of library service. In 1903, however, with the completion of the first American Medical Association headquarters building in Chicago, a single room was set aside and maintained as the library. In this room were kept a few reference books, bound volumes of the Journal, and other periodicals received through exchange arrangements. There was no librarian in charge and no library service offered to members of the Association.

The actual history of the library department begins only thirty-five years ago (in 1911) under the impetus and enthusiasm of Dr. George Simmons' leadership. Miss Helen Hutchinson of Chicago, who later became the wife of Dr. Frederick R. Green, Secretary of the Council on Health and Public Instruction, came to the Association in September, 1911, as the first professional librarian of the American Medical Association. Miss Hutchinson was one of the first students to receive a diploma in librarianship from the then newly organized Wisconsin Library School. Upon the completion of the required library school course at that institution in 1908, she accepted a position with the Michael Reese Hospital of Chicago to classify for the first time their records and to become the medical record librarian. She also had charge of the Physicians Library of Michael Reese Hospital, which was at that time a small and informal department of the hospital. In the fall of 1910, she became librarian of the Washington University School of Medicine in St. Louis. Through Miss Meta Loomis, formerly librarian of the University of Illinois School of Medicine, Miss Hutchinson learned that Dr. Simmons was looking for a librarian to organize the library department of the American Medical Association. Miss Hutchinson, wishing very much to return to Chicago and her own home, arranged for an interview with Dr. Simmons, after which she was immediately employed as the Association's first librarian. The room which housed the first library department was on the fifth floor of the present headquarters building, constructed in 1910. The room was an attractive one with fine wood paneling, about forty by forty feet in size. By action of the Board of Trustees it was dedicated as the Nathan S. Davis Memorial Hall. It is occupied today by the Bureau of Health Education. Steel shelving was installed to house the small book collection, and wood shelving with glass doors along two of the side walls housed the periodical collection. One of the first duties of the librarian was the preparation of the Index to The Journal of the American Medical Association. Formerly this work had been done by the Editorial Department, but from that day in January 1912, when Miss Hutchinson first assumed the responsibility of indexing The Journal to the present time, The

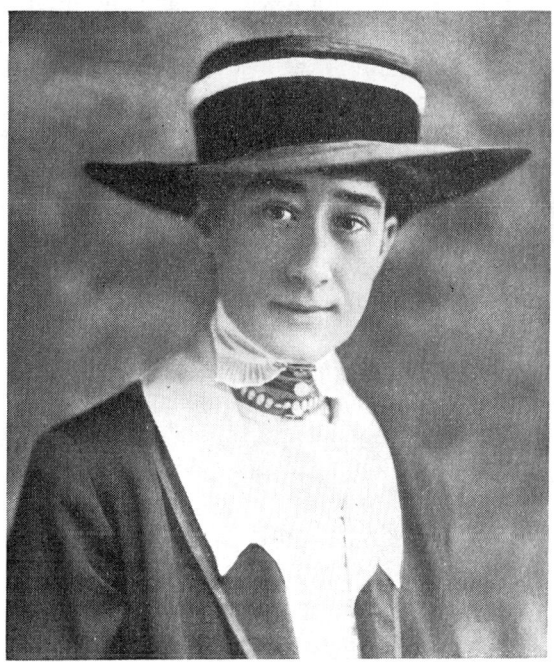

Helen Hutchinson Green.

Journal Index has been prepared in the Library Department. Apparently Miss Hutchinson did an excellent job on the Index and must have pleased Dr. Simmons with her work, because she was eventually given all of the Association's publications to index. In those early years, all of the titles listed in the current literature section of The Journal, not merely those articles abstracted, were indexed meticulously in The Journal Index by author and subject. This scheme gave the practicing physician an excellent over-all picture of current medical literature twice a year, i.e., June and December, when the volume indexes were published. The index to the current literature section was bound and sold in separate form from The Journal Index proper and soon became a popular guide to current medical literature. From this modest venture developed the Quarterly Cumulative Index to Current Medical Literature, in 1916, which was destined to have world wide recognition thirty years later. A more detailed description of the Quarterly will be discussed later in this paper. The work of the library department from 1911 to 1923 covered general reference work for staff members, publication of the Quarterly Cumulative Index to Current Medical Literature, bibliographic asssistance for the preparation of the Query and Minor Note Section of the Journal, maintaining records of books received and reviewed in The Journal, lending foreign periodicals, indexing The Journal and other publications of the Association, maintaining an employees' library of popular literature, and various types of routine library work. By 1918 there had developed gradually a periodical lending service covering foreign publications only. Because of limited filing space available in the library department at that time, it was not possible to keep a periodical collection covering many years. Approximately two or three years' collection was available for lending. It was the beginning, however, of the extensive periodical lending service carried on by the library today.

EMPLOYEES' LIBRARY

In 1921 an employees' library was established for all employees of the American Medical Association and was conducted in the library department during the noon hour only. A deposit of several hundred popular books was secured from the Chicago Public Library as a basis for the collection. Each employee contributed 25 cents a year which entitled him to borrowing privileges. The Association also contributed generously toward the fund, and with these funds new books were purchased. Later the fee for employees was increased to 50 cents which enabled us to subscribe to many popular magazines. The employees' library was maintained from 1921 to 1943, when it became impossible to conduct it any longer due to an acute shortage of personnel in the library department. It is an activity of the department which we hope will be resumed without too much delay.

COVER INDEX

A cover index for each weekly issue of The Journal was instituted in 1923, the preparation of which became a logical assignment for the library department. Unfortunately, during the recent war years, it was necessary to discontinue this popular feature of The Journal, but it is hoped that it will be restored upon return to normal times.

PACKAGE LIBRARY

Upon Miss Hutchinson's resignation in 1923, to be married, Dr. Florence Johnston, a practicing physician of Cedar Rapids, Iowa, was appointed librarian. She assumed her duties July 1, 1923, and resigned in 1925. Dr. Johnston received her library degree from the New York Public Library School in 1914 and her medical degree from the medical school of the University of Pennsylvania in 1919. Very soon after her appointment as librarian, Dr. Johnston established (in 1924) a package library service which is today one of the most popular and important services offered by the library department. She conceived the idea of detaching tear sheets from great numbers of duplicate copies of special journals of the American Medical Association press which were on hand, as a basis for the package library collection. Each article was classified by subject, following closely the subject headings used in the Quarterly Cumulative Index. The collection was, of course, not extensive at first but grew rapidly. Once the impetus to collect and classify reprints was started, there was a phenomenal development of the collection in a few years. This service was established primarily to meet the needs of members located in rural communities and isolated from medical libraries, but because of its popularity it ultimately came to serve physicians in the larger cities in the United States in spite of the excellent library facilities therein. Records indicate that the greatest number of requests for this service come from New York, Pennsylvania, Illinois and Ohio. The package library service is available to members of the American Medical Association and to subscribers to its scientific publications. A nominal fee of 25 cents is made to cover postage and the material is supposed to be returned six days after receipt. Foreign publications are not included in the package libraries unless specifically requested. About a year after Dr. Johnston's appointment as librarian, she became assistant editor of The Journal and divided her time between that position and director of the library. In 1925, she resigned her position with the American Medical Association and was succeeded by Miss Marjorie Hutchins, the present librarian, now Mrs. Marjorie Moore.

THE LIBRARIAN

Mrs. Moore, a graduate of the University of Illinois, came to the Association as an assistant to Miss Hutchinson in 1920. She had been an assistant in the Urbana Public Library from 1917 to 1919, and had been employed as an indexer in the Bureau of Educational Research of the University of Illinois from 1919 to 1920. Soon after her appointment as librarian, the library department, by direction of the Board of Trustees, was put under the supervision of Dr. Morris Fishbein, then the newly-appointed editor of The Journal. Dr. Fishbein's absorbing interest in all things pertaining to literature has had a profound influence on the development of the library department to the important position it holds today in the conduct of the work of the Association.

THE QUARTERLY CUMULATIVE INDEX MEDICUS

Under his leadership plans were started in 1925 for the consolidation of the Index Medicus and Quarterly Cumulative Index. In 1926 the final plans were completed for a joint sponsorship of these two publications to cover a trial period of five years. This venture increased the work of the library department and created an urgent need for additional floor space. The assembly room on the fifth floor adjacent to the library was assigned to the library in 1932 for a stack room to house its rapidly expanding periodical collection. The floor space thus acquired, 2400 square feet, enabled the establishment of a five year collection of more than 1000 periodicals, which were available for lending to members and subscribers. The demands for the periodical lending service increased immediately. In 1923 only 475 periodical loans were requested; in 1926, 2,651; in 1936, 10,852; in 1938, 13,012; in 1941, 12,833; in 1944, 10,836. In 1936, four years after the Association assumed complete control of the publication of the Index Medicus, the library department moved to new quarters on the eighth floor of the remodeled and present building. The department was assigned 8560 square feet of floor space for the rapidly expanding services. There was at last adequate stack space to house a ten years' collection of more than 1400 periodicals and adequate space to house our package library collection and staff members. Provision was also made for additional stack space should any be needed in the future.

The floor space occupied by the library department for the past twenty years portrays significantly its rapid expansion—1600 square feet in 1925 and 8560 square feet in 1946! Today, in 1946, we have in the library a book collection of approximately 4500 volumes. The book collection includes leading texts in the special fields of medicine, books on history of medicine, and various encyclopaedias and reference works. As all books reviewed in The Journal become the property of the reviewers, as the only payment for their services, they are not available in the department library. Occasionally staff members review books which are needed for the library department. No attempt has been made to build up an extensive book collection or to maintain a book lending service.

When the library was first established in 1911, it was Dr. Simmons' idea and has continued to be that of Dr. Fishbein that with such excellent medical libraries already established in Chicago and elsewhere, there was no need for the American Medical Association to establish or maintain an extensive book collection. It was felt that since most of the important medical research is reported first in periodicals, the Association library should concentrate on the building up of an outstanding periodical collection. We have on hand a ten-year collection of approximately 1400 medical periodicals. They are not bound but are housed in black cardboard boxes specially designed for that purpose so that single issues are available at all times for lending. As we are frequently asked by visitors being shown through the library department what we do with our discarded periodicals, it seems fitting here to explain that for many years previous to 1929 it had been our custom to give them to the Crerar Library of Chicago. The periodical discards covering the years 1929 to 1931 were offered to the Medical Library Association exchange service for distribution. The 1932 discards, however, were presented to the Army Medical Library. Upon an appeal from that library in 1943 the Board of Trustees agreed to present to the Army Medical Library in the future all of the periodicals discarded yearly by the Association library. The Army Medical Library will use them to fill gaps in their own collection and also as a basis to establish reciprocal exchanges with foreign periodicals and libraries.

A brief summation of the work of the library department today follows:

1. The Package Library Service. This service is available to the members of the American Medical Association and subscribers to its scientific publications. Collections of reprints, reports, etc. on all phases of clinical medicine are loaned on request for the small sum of twenty-five cents. To insure fair and prompt service for all members regardless of their geographic location, written requests are required for this service. This requirement enables the physician located in Seattle, for example, to secure service as promptly as the physician in Chicago. Packages may be retained six days after receipt, or renewed thereafter upon request. A nominal fee of 25 cents is made to cover postage. Approximately 100,000 reprints on all phases of medicine form the basis for this service. The reprints cover essentially the past ten years only.

2. The Periodical Lending Service. Approximately 1400 periodicals covering a period of ten years are available for lending to members of the Association and to individual subscribers to its scientific publications. A charge of six cents per periodical is made to cover postage. The collection is in unbound form and represents the most important part of our library holdings.

3. Special Indexes. The preparation of THE JOURNAL Index which includes three volume indexes per year is one of the major responsibilities of the department. Before the recent war many indexes were prepared in the library for books published by various bureaus and councils of the Association. Because of the personnel shortage during the past six years, however, no special indexes have been prepared, with the exception of the index for the latest edition of *Standard Classification and Nomenclature of Disease* which was prepared in 1941 by Miss Doherty of the library staff.

4. The Journal Book Reviews. Copy for the Books Received column appearing in THE JOURNAL each week is prepared in the library department. All books sent to THE JOURNAL for review are received in this department and the maintenance of all records covering books received for this purpose is the responsibility of the library.

5. Reference Work. The library answers all types of reference questions, prepares recommended lists of books, compiles short bibliographies on various subjects, locates and verifies references for hundreds of requested articles.

6. Quarterly Cumulative Index Medicus. One of the most important functions of the library department is the publication of the Index Medicus. This work includes a quarterly compilation of new books in the field of medicine and the indexing by author and subject of more than 1100 medical periodicals. All titles in the foreign periodicals appear under subjects in translated form in the Index Medicus. As an indexing guide for the library staff a volume of standardized subject headings for medical literature was compiled and published (but not for sale) in 1932. Because of popular demand a revised edition was brought out in 1940 and offered for sale. The compilation of this volume was done under the supervision of Miss Magdalene Freyder, assistant librarian.

Thus is shown that the library maintains a unique type of library service which we believe is not duplicated either in scope or in minimal cost by any other organization. It emphasizes and specializes, as it were, in current medical literature.

Among the staff members who have served the Association long and faithfully in the library should be mentioned Miss Harriet Wilson, a graduate of the University of Nebraska, in charge of the package library service and reference librarian since 1923, Miss Margaret Doherty, a graduate of the University of Illinois, in charge of the preparation of The Journal Index since 1925 and also assistant reference librarian, Miss Magdalene Freyder, assistant librarian, a graduate of the University of Iowa, who joined the library staff in 1924, and who has had charge of the editing of the Quarterly Cumulative Index Medicus since 1926.

Of the 25 persons on the library staff today, twelve or forty-eight per cent have been with the department for ten or more years. It is fitting to record here our grateful appreciation for their faithful service: Magdalene Freyder, Harriet Wilson, Margaret Doherty, Clara Ricketts, Minnie Bagus, Arlene Hipple, Thelma Smith, Laura Brich, Mildred Lund, Eloise Murray and Ann White. The names of others who have joined the staff more recently from 1939 to date are: Inez Wicklund, Geraldine Osuch, Marion Linn, Virginia Cyboran, Jeannette de Bruyn, Mabel Benton, Helen Marshall, Marie Kelly, Rose Stawarz, Isabel Turnbull, Ellen Haskell, Irene Nilsen, Garnet Snowberger.

THE COMMITTEE ON SCIENTIFIC RESEARCH

By Ludvig Hektoen, M.D.

AT THE MEETING OF The American Medical Association in 1898 it was resolved "that a committee be appointed by the President, at his leisure, to cooperate with similar committees from other bodies to consider the desirability of formulating plans for dissemination of knowledge of the value of experimental research in the progress of the science and art of medicine." A committee was appointed,[1] but there is no record of any report by it. Two years later, in his presidential address, Dr. W. W. Keen made this statement:[2]

"It is not, I trust, too much to hope, if not now, that in the near future the American Medical Association will set a fruitful example by giving each year 'Scientific Grants in Aid of Research.' The first object of the Association must be, necessarily, to place itsef on a strong financial basis. It should own its own building, its printing and publishing plant, and, as soon as possible, should have a reserve fund of considerable proportions Nothing conduces to the stability and conservativeness of any institution like a good. bank balance. The British Medical Association has today an excess of assets over liabilities of nearly $380,000, chiefly invested in its building at 429 Strand, London. The American Medical Association has made a fair start with a surplus of over $27,000 last January, and, with its large, and, let us hope, rapidly increasing membership, it will before long assume a rank second only to the British Medical Association. Last year the Scientific Grants Committee of the British Association allotted £741, or somewhat more than $3,500, for research work, distributed to three research scholarships, the holders of which were paid $750 each year, and thirty-three grants in aid of research work, varying in amounts from $25 to $100. Among those to whom grants were made occur the well known names of Beevor, Vaughan Harley, Kanthack, Luff, Manson, Noel Payton, and Risien Russell. I should hope that the American Medical Association might even now begin by a modest appropriation, say of $500 a year, which should be allotted by the trustees, or by a special committee on scientific grants, after a careful investigation of the merits and the character of the person to whom such grants were made. No grant should exceed $100, or possibly even, at first, $50 in amount. The results of such grants would be not only absolute additions to our knowledge, but the cultivation of a scientific spirit which would permeate the whole profession and elevate its objects and aims."

The Association decided[3] "that the suggestion of the president be adopted, namely, that the Trustees set aside the sum of $500 annually for the encouragement of scientific research, with the further recommendation that, as our financial condition will permit,

---

[1] J.A.M.A., *34:*701 (March 17) 1900.
[2] Keen, W. W.: The President's Address, J.A.M.A., *34:*1445, 1900.
[3] J.A.M.A., *34:*1557, 1900.

in the future, the sum be increased to as great extent as possible. Also that the manner in which this sum is to be expended be left to the Committee on Scientific Research, provided, however, that sums given to individuals do not exceed $50 to $100 at one time."

The members of the committee, a pioneer agency in its field, were H. C. Wood, Philadelphia, chairman; Wm. J. Mayo, Rochester, Minn.; Wm. H. Welch, Baltimore; J. F. Fulton, St. Paul; C. A. Powers, Denver. The committee announced[4] "that it has available the sum of five hundred dollars for the assistance of researches to be undertaken in the next six months, and that the money will be appropriated if applications be received within the month of January, 1901. Applicants should state clearly the character of the research to be undertaken, and the facilities at their command. Address Dr. H. C. Wood, chairman, 1925 Chestnut Street, Philadelphia." But, on account of illness of its chairman, no other actions were taken by the committee, as explained by Dr. Welch in his letter[5] to Dr. Simmons:

"Baltimore, June 1, 1901

"Dear Doctor:—I regret that it is impossible for me to be present at the meeting of the American Medical Association this year.

"I do not suppose that Dr. Wood has been able, on account of illness, to send a report in behalf of the Committee on Scientific Research. I cannot learn that there was any organization, and certainly there has been no meeting of the Committee. Dr. Wood, however, inserted notices in the medical journals calling attention to the existence of the grant by the Association, and requested that applications for appropriations from the fund be sent to him before a specified date. Ten such applications were received, and Dr. Wood communicated with the members of the Committee by letter regarding the selection of applicants and the amounts to be appropriated to each. A decision in this matter had not been reached when Dr. Wood became so ill that he could give no further attention to it. He then asked me to take the matter in hand. You may recall that I then communicated with you, and that you suggested that in view of the lack of previous organization and of meeting of the Committee, and the lateness of the season remaining for action, it might be well to postpone further action until after the meeting of the Association. I have followed your suggestion. There have been ten applications for appropriations from the funds, several of which at least were eminently deserving.

"While I regret that the initiation of this important undertaking on the part of the Association has not led to results during the first year, I sincerely trust that the grant will be continued. If the $500 appropriated by the Association last year could be added to an additional $500, making $1000 for the coming year, I believe that much good would result. If this is not deemed best, I hope that at least the appropriation of $500 will be continued for another year. I should suggest that the Committee be not limited as now to the granting of sums not exceeding $100 to a single individual. It would be well, I think, in selecting the Committee to consider somewhat the ease with which the members can be brought together for conference.

"Hoping that the Association will continue these grants for research, I am,

Very truly yours,
WILLIAM H. WELCH."

---

[4] J.A.M.A., *35*:1658, 1900.
[5] J.A.M.A., *36*:1648, 1901.

The appropriation of $500 was continued[6] for another year and in March, 1902, a new committee was appointed, consisting of Alfred Stengel, Philadelphia, Chairman; Wm. H. Welch, Baltimore; and James B. Herrick, Chicago. At the 1902 meeting of the Association Dr. Stengel reported[7] that, owing to the recent appointment of the committe, no steps could be taken during the past year "to encourage scientific research by the utilization of the generous appropriation of the Association. The chairman and members of the committee appreciate the opportunity afforded them to influence wholesome, scientific work, and desire especially to make it clear to the members of the House of Delegates that the failure of the committee to act has been unavoidable. Through the illness of the chairman of the committee before the appointment of the present one, no action could be taken last year. The appointment of the present committee dates from March 21, 1902. It is hoped that next year through early advertisement in the columns of the Journal applications may be received by the committee for participation in the grants established by the Association. There will doubtless be sufficient applications to permit a careful selection of scientific workers."

The appropriation of $500 was again renewed. Dr. Stengel was continued as chairman, the other members being Wm. Osler, Baltimore, and Ludvig Hektoen, Chicago. In 1908 Wm. Osler, Baltimore, was replaced by L. F. Barker, Baltimore; otherwise there was no change in the committee until 1912, since when Ludvig Hektoen has served as chairman. In 1912 and 1913 the other members were Graham Lusk, New York, and Eugene L. Opie, St. Louis; in 1914 Wm. Litterer, Nashville, and Simon Flexner, New York; in 1915 Frederick G. Novy, Ann Arbor, and C. C. Bass, New Orleans. During World War I the committee remained dormant but was reestablished in 1919 with J. W. Churchman, New Haven, H. C. Moffitt, San Francisco, F. F. Russell, Washington, D. C., and G. N. Stewart, Cleveland, as the new members. During the last war the grant-aided research was slowed up much; in several cases work under way had to be given up and only few applications were received for new grants.

FUNDS

As stated, the first appropriation by the Trustees in support of research under the auspices of a special committee was made in 1900, in response to the appeal by Dr. W. W. Keen in his presi-

---

[6] J.A.M.A., *36*:1917, 1901.
[7] J.A.M.A., *38*:1657, 1902.

dential address.[2] Annual appropriations have been made since then, except in 1915, 1916, 1917, 1945 and 1946. The annual amounts appropriated have risen from $500 at first to $1,000 in 1909, then to $2,000 and in 1926 to $13,200. After the first few years the appropriations have been treated as cumulative, and so far all refunds and balances have been used for grants.

Private donations have been received as follows:

Charles A. Brant Fund from unnamed donor..........................	$3,640.51
For aid of medical research..	
Dr. Cornelius van Zwalenburg, Riverside, California...................	1,000.00
For study of hydraulic abdominal factors	
Cardiac Research Fund from unnamed donor..........................	1,000.00
For work on cardiac problems by young physicians in practice	
For research on cancer by unnamed donor............................	114.90
	$5,758.41

The receipts and disbursements of the committee may now be summarized:

Receipts

American Medical Association......................	$276,468.40	
Donations..	5,758.41	
Refunds of balances of grants.......................	18,327.78	$300,554.59

Disbursements

Grants for research...............................	$276,856.03	
Administrative expenses...........................	18,006.58	294,862.61
Balance on hand, December 31, 1946...........................		$ 5,691.98

GRANTS

The first effective grant was awarded in 1903 to Gustav F. Ruediger in support of work on the mechanisms of streptococcus infections, which yielded noteworthy results.[8] At the end of 1946, 707 grants have been awarded, in most cases in sums of $500 or less, on the basis of formal applications stating the qualifications of the applicant, the problem to be studied, and why aid was needed.

Almost without exception, the committee itself has not developed or organized projects for research. At the instance of the committee on the recommendation of Dr. George H. Simmons, Dr. Edwin O. Jordan, professor of bacteriology in the University of Chicago, was induced (grant 39) to review the literature on the influenza epidemic of 1918–19. This review, published in book form by the Association, is an outstanding contribution to the literature on influenza. In the report of the committee for 1924,[9] which

---

[8] Grants for Scientific Work, J.A.M.A., *41:*969 (Oct. 17) 1903.

[9] Report of the Committee on Scientific Research, J.A.M.A., *84:*1646 (May 30) 1925.

includes a list of the grants to that time and also of papers on the results of work aided by the grants, it is stated that "in some cases grants were made to the director of a laboratory for use as he saw fit in aiding research; in most cases, however, the grants were made to individual workers on application stating the problem to be investigated and why aid was needed." Many of the papers referred to in the 1924 report were read before the Section on Pathology and Physiology at meetings of the Association. The grants to R. M. Pearce, while professor of pathology in Albany Medical College and later at the University of Pennsylvania, are examples of grants to the director of a laboratory for support of research under his direction.

Since 1927 grants, as the rule, have been made for needed supplies and expenses, which could not be provided easily, if at all, from the means at hand, for the conduct of promising individual research in various fields of medical interest. The two exceptions to support of individual research are grant 171 (1929), $2,500, to the National Research Council for study of brucelliasis under the auspices of the Council's committee on infectious abortion and grant 650 (1942), $1,000, to the tuberculosis committee of the Minnesota State Medical Association toward its tuberculosis survey of Meeker County, Minnesota.

The committee early adopted the policy of not granting money for the purchase of permanent equipment and apparatus. Whatever articles of permanent nature have been purchased by means of grants remain the property of the Association. With the changes in working methods, more and more requests for support of technical assistance have been granted, with the understanding that so far as possible preference be given to service by medical students and assistants.

With few exceptions, the responses to requests at intervals for reports on the work and expenditures by grantees have been prompt and satisfactory. So far as possible, grants have been paid to the financial officers of the institutions with which the grantees were connected, with the understanding that the money would be subject to the orders of the grantees at the same time as accurate accounts were kept of the expenditures.

The annual reports of the committee to the trustees and published in The Journal of the American Medical Association, which give the main facts in regard to the individual grants as well as to the articles by the grantees on the results of their work, show that the grants have been used to good purpose. In most cases the research undertaken has been carried out at least to the extent that results deemed worthy of publication in standard medical periodicals have been obtained. The articles listed in the annual reports of the committee do not necessarily cover all the grant-aided research designated as completed. Further results may have been published in later years—in some cases reports have appeared years after the financial account was settled.

As complete a set as possible of reprints of articles on the results of grant-aided research has been maintained.

In the case of certain closed grants the records do not show that any results have been published. Publication of results is, of course, the most immediately tangible return from a grant but not necessarily always the most important. Failure of publication has been caused in various ways. One grantee died soon after he had started his work. Certain grantees have had to give up their research because of changes in position and work. War has forced several to stop research. Again, in other cases, the work failed to yield results worthy of publication, which may be the outcome of the best conducted research. "Research may lead to closed doors as well as to open corridors." In some such cases the results of the research may prove of value in other work. It should be noted that the grants were given in support of what seemed to be promising individual work on concrete problems but not always under favorable conditions. Nevertheless, only very few failures in the work have been due to incompetence or lack of interest on part of the grantee. Here again the significance of a grant as stimulus not only to the grantee but to the institution with which he was connected should not be overlooked, especially in the early years of the committee.

The grants have influenced the advancement of knowledge favorably by the results of aid to research and also by stimulating the spirit of research, the development of investigators, and improvement in medical teaching. Certain grantees whose early efforts at research were aided by the committee have risen to distinction in medical science and education. And in several cases foundations have taken on the larger support of research at first carried on by the help of small grants. During the last war grant-aided projects were taken over by governmental agencies and carried forward on greatly expanded scales. As stated elsewhere, small grants may help to produce results far in excess of what might be expected from the amount of money involved, as for example the establishment of the rickettsial infections on the basis of the pioneer work of Howard T. Ricketts which was promoted by small grants from this committee. Small grants have sometimes brought spectacular achievement of which the Rockefeller grant of $1,280 which started the penicillin development is only a recent example.

MEMBERS OF THE COMMITTEE ON SCIENTIFIC RESEARCH

L. F. Barker, Baltimore	1905–1911
C. C. Bass, New Orleans	1914–1919, 1923–1939
J. W. Churchman, New Haven	1919–1923
Martin H. Fischer, Cincinnati	1925–
Simon Flexner, New York	1913–1919
Charles A. Frazier, Philadelphia	1923–1928
E. W. Goodpasture, Nashville	1939–
Ludvig Hektoen, Chicago	1903–
James B. Herrick, Chicago	1902–1903
Noble Wiley Jones, Portland	1924–
William Litterer, Nashville	1914–1915
Graham Lusk, New York	1912–1913
H. C. Moffitt, San Francisco	1919–1923
John J. Morton, Rochester	1928–
F. G. Novy, Ann Arbor	1915–1919
Eugene L. Opie, St. Louis	1912–1913
William Osler, Baltimore	1902–1905
F. F. Russell, Washington, D. C.	1919–1923
Alfred Stengel, Philadelphia	1902–1912
G. N. Stewart, Cleveland	1919–1925
William H. Welch, Baltimore	1900–1902
H. C. Wood, Philadelphia	1900–1901

THE SCIENTIFIC SECTIONS OF THE AMERICAN MEDICAL ASSOCIATION

By Morris Fishbein, M.D.

FOR THE FIRST TWELVE YEARS of its existence the American Medical Association held only large general meetings. The attendance was never great. Neither were the contributions so considerable in number as to require breaking up the general meeting into several smaller meetings.

In 1859, at the meeting of the Association in Louisville, a resolution was offered by Dr. J. B. Lindsley of Tennessee:

> That a committee of three be appointed by the Chair to inquire into and report upon the propriety of dividing the Association into Sections for the purpose of performing such parts of its scientific labor as may relate to practical branches of medicine and surgery.

The resolution was adopted and a committee of three was appointed to prepare the report. This committee, of which Dr. Lindsley was chairman, recommended a division of the association into the following sections:

1. Anatomy and Physiology
2. Chemistry and Materia Medica
3. Practical Medicine and Obstetrics
4. Surgery

This report was adopted, but later the same day two additional sections were added—one on Meteorology, Medical Topography and Epidemic Diseases and another on Medical Jurisprudence and Hygiene. At the meeting in 1860 all except the Section on Chemistry and Materia Medica reported the manuscripts read to them, and their reports were referred to the Committee on Publication.

In 1869 the By-Laws of the American Medical Association were amended to make the election of the chairmen and secretaries of the sections by the general meeting on nomination by the Committee on Nominations. From that time on a new chairman and secretary were elected each year. Then in 1884 Dr. Foster Pratt offered an amendment which empowered the sections to elect their own officers. This, however, did not prevail until the meeting two years later in

St. Louis. Some years ago the By-Laws were changed to read "that each section may elect its secretary to serve a longer time at its discretion."

In 1943 and in 1945, during World War II, a scientific assembly was not held; consequently the sections did not hold meetings.

PRACTICAL MEDICINE AND OBSTETRICS

The Section of Practical Medicine and Obstetrics has a continuous record since 1859, but from time to time the title has been modified by the breaking off of various branches, the first being obstetrics. Then in 1873 the name was changed to the Section on Practical Medicine, Materia Medica and Physiology. In 1890 "Materia Medica" was dropped because of the creation of a Section on Materia Medica, and in 1891 "Physiology" was dropped with the establishment of a Section on Physiology and Dietetics. In 1946 the name of the section was changed to Section on Internal Medicine.

SECTION ON PHYSIOLOGY AND DIETETICS

The Section under this name was somewhat short-lived. It was a development from the Section on Practical Medicine and Obstetrics, which was established in 1859, and the title of which was changed in 1873 to Section on Practical Medicine, Materia Medica and Physiology. In 1890 "Physiology" was separated from that section and a new section was formed under the title "Section on Physiology and Dietetics." In 1901 that Section and the Section on Pathology and Bacteriology were combined under the title "Section on Pathology and Physiology."

ANATOMY AND PHYSIOLOGY

The Section on Anatomy and Physiology was one of the four sections originally recommended by the committee in 1859. Apparently, however, this section was never organized. At a later date there are references to papers that were referred to this section, but in the sixteenth volume of the Transactions of the Association, published in 1865, the Permanent Secretary reported that a meeting of this section had never been held, and the section was abolished. "Anatomy" was then added to the Section on Surgery, and "Physiology" was added to the Section on Medical Jurisprudence and Hygiene, making it read "Section on Medical Jurisprudence, Physiology and Hygiene." In 1873, when the sections were reorganized, the name was changed to Section on Medical Jurisprudence, Chemistry and Psychology.

SECTION ON METEOROLOGY AND EPIDEMICS

This Section was established in 1859 by resolution. The name was changed in 1870 to the Section on Climatology and Epidemics, and in 1871, to "Section on Meteorology and Epidemics." This section was abolished in the reorganization of the sections which occurred in 1873.

SURGERY AND ANATOMY

The Section on Surgery was first organized June 7, 1860. It has held meetings regularly since that time except in 1861 and 1862, when annual sessions were not held because of the Civil War. The word "Anatomy" was added to the title in 1865. In 1909 the word "Anatomy" was deleted, so that it again became known as the Section on Surgery, and at the meeting in Atlantic City in 1914 the name was changed to the Section on Surgery, General and Abdominal.

OBSTETRICS AND DISEASES OF WOMEN AND CHILDREN

A Section on Obstetrics and Diseases of Women and Children was created in 1873. Then in 1880 "Children" was dropped from that title and the section was called the Section on Obstetrics and Diseases of Women. At the meeting of the Association in 1911 the name of the section was changed to the Section on Obstetrics and Gynecology, and in 1912 it was changed to the Section on Obstetrics, Gynecology and Abdominal Surgery. That name prevailed until 1938, when it was changed to the Section on Obstetrics and Gynecology. The record of changes in the various Section titles corresponds closely to the gradual development of specialization in the practice of medicine.

OPHTHALMOLOGY, LARYNGOLOGY, OTOLOGY AND RHINOLOGY

One of the earliest sections to be organized was that on Ophthalmology, Otology and Laryngology, which was created in 1878. Then in 1888 this was divided into two sections, one known as Ophthalmology and the other as Laryngology and Otology. At the meeting in 1912 to the name of the latter was added "Rhinology," making it the Section on Laryngology, Otology and Rhinology.

SECTION ON PEDIATRICS

When the Section on Obstetrics and Diseases of Women and Children was split in 1879, one portion was known as the Section on Diseases of Children. In 1933 this name was changed to the Section on Pediatrics.

SECTION ON EXPERIMENTAL MEDICINE AND THERAPEUTICS

In 1890 the words "Materia Medica" were removed from the Section on Practical Medicine and a new section, known as Materia Medica and Pharmacy, was formed. In 1895 the name was changed to Materia Medica, Pharmacy and Therapeutics; in 1904, to Pharmacology; in 1905, to Pharmacology and Therapeutics, and in 1941, to Experimental Medicine and Therapeutics.

SECTION ON PATHOLOGY AND PHYSIOLOGY

This section was organized in 1900 as the Section on Pathology and Bacteriology. In 1901 the Section on Physiology and Dietetics was combined with it and the section became the Section on Pathology and Physiology.

DERMATOLOGY AND SYPHILOLOGY

In 1886 a Section on Dermatology and Venereal Diseases was organized. The title was changed in 1887 to Dermatology and Syphilography; in 1897, to Cutaneous Medicine and Surgery; in 1909 to Dermatology; in 1919, to Dermatology and Syphilis, and in 1920 to Dermatology and Syphilology.

SECTION ON NERVOUS AND MENTAL DISEASES

The subject of conditions affecting the nervous system and the brain was considered first as a portion of the Section on Medical Jurisprudence, formed in 1885. The section held its first meeting in 1887. Then in 1890 the name was changed to Medical Jurisprudence and Neurology, and in 1900, to the Section on Nervous and Mental Diseases.

SECTION ON MEDICAL JURISPRUDENCE, CHEMISTRY AND PSYCHOLOGY

A Section on Medical Jurisprudence and Hygiene was established in 1859 and existed, with various changes in name, until 1880. In 1865, when the Section on Anatomy and Physiology was abolished, "Physiology" was incorporated in this section and the title was changed to Section on Medical Jurisprudence, Physiology and Hygiene. In 1873 there was some reorganization of the sections and it was combined with the Section on Psychology to make the Section on Medical Jurisprudence, Chemistry and Psychology. In 1879 two sections were again combined and the title was changed to "Medical Jurisprudence, Chemistry, Psychology, State Medicine and Public Hygiene." In 1880 a resolution was adopted providing that the name be changed to State Medicine. In 1885 a resolution offered by the President for the establishment of a Section on Medical Jurisprudence was adopted. This resolution laid over until 1886, at which time the section was created. The report on the Section on Preventive and Industrial Medicine and Public Health indicates the changes in the name of the Section from 1900 to date.

SECTION ON PREVENTIVE AND INDUSTRIAL MEDICINE AND PUBLIC HEALTH

By resolution a Section on State Medicine was established in 1872, and a formal definition of state medicine was accepted which included the whole subject of public health. In 1873 this section became known as the Section on State Med cine and Public Hygiene. In 1879 the Section on Medical Jurisprudence, Chemistry and Psychology was combined with it, making a Section on Medical Jurisprudence, Chemistry, Psychology, State Medicine and Public Hygiene. The unwieldiness of this title resulted promptly in a return to "State Medicine" as the name of the section in 1880. In 1900 the name was changed to Hygiene and Sanitary Science; in 1908, to Preventive Medicine, and in 1909, to Preventive Medicine and Public Health. Then in 1922, when industrial medicine began to loom large on the horizon, the name of the section was changed to the Section on Preventive and Industrial Medicine and Public Health.

ORTHOPEDIC SURGERY

In 1912 the Association organized a Section on Orthopedic Surgery, which has had but the one name.

SECTION ON UROLOGY

At the meeting in 1910 a Section on Genito-Urinary Diseases was formed and held its first meeting in 1912. Since 1919 this section has been known as the Section on Urology.

SECTION ON GASTRO-ENTEROLOGY AND PROCTOLOGY

The Section on Gastro-Enterology and Proctology was organized in 1916 and has had no other name.

SECTION ON RADIOLOGY

The Section on Radiology was organized in 1925 and has had no other name.

SECTION ON PSYCHOLOGY

By resolution a Section on Psychology was created in 1865, but in 1873 it was combined with other groups to make the Section on

Medical Jurisprudence, Chemistry and Psychology. The evolution of this section is reported under the Section on Preventive and Industrial Medicine and Public Health.

SECTION ON STOMATOLOGY

For awhile it seemed that dentistry would be incorporated with medicine into a single organization. In 1881 the Section on Dentistry was organized in the American Medical Association, which became known in 1882 as the Section on Dental and Oral Surgery, and in 1897, as the Section on Stomatology. By 1925 dentistry had grown so greatly in its own right as a profession that it was decided to eliminate the Section on Stomatology and to incorporate papers on dental surgery in the other surgical sections.

SECTION ON HOSPITALS

The relationship of the hospital to the medical profession was such that it seemed desirable in 1911 to organize a Section on Hospitals. However, hospital management and the problems of the hospital differentiated by 1916, at which time this section was abolished.

SECTION ON MISCELLANEOUS TOPICS

In 1917 the Section on Miscellaneous Topics was established, and various sessions have been held under the auspices of that section from time to time since that date. For instance, there was a Session on Reclaiming and Reeducation of War Injured and one on Selective Service Regulations in 1918. A Symposium on The Scope of Industrial Medicine and Surgery and one on Some Future Aspects of Industrial Medicine and Surgery were held in 1919, and there were sessions on Anesthesia in 1921, 1922, 1924, 1933, 1935, 1939 and 1940.

A Symposium on Ethylene was held in 1924 and there were sessions on Radiology in 1924 and 1925.

A Session on Forensic Medicine and one on Nutrition were held in 1934; a Session on History of Medicine and one on Military Medicine, in 1935; a Session on Tuberculosis, in 1936; a Session on General Practice and a Session on Legal Medicine, in 1942, and a Session for the General Practitioner, in 1944.

SECTION ON ANESTHESIOLOGY

The sessions on Anesthesia developed into a Section on Anesthesiology at the New York Session in 1940, and the first meeting of that Section was held in Cleveland in June 1941.

SECTION ON GENERAL PRACTICE OF MEDICINE

The Session on General Practice held in 1942 and the Session for the General Practitioner held in 1944 developed into the creation of a Section on General Practice of Medicine in 1944. The first meeting of that Section was held in 1946.

THE WOMAN'S AUXILIARY TO THE AMERICAN MEDICAL ASSOCIATION

By Mrs. Jesse D. Hamer

THE WOMAN'S AUXILIARY to the American Medical Association was organized in St. Louis, Missouri, May 26, 1922, as a logical outgrowth of state and county auxiliaries which were already in existence. Such organizations had been created in Minnesota, Oklahoma, South Dakota and Texas. Maine and Montana had organized, but had not been active. The idea of a National Auxiliary originated with the Woman's Auxiliary to the State Medical Association of Texas. In 1922 Mrs. Samuel Clark Red, president of the Texas Auxiliary, solicited the assistance of Dr. Edward H. Cary of Dallas, in introducing the following resolution to the House of Delegates of the American Medical Association:

"The Woman's Auxiliary to the State Medical Association of Texas respectfully requests the approval of the American Medical Association of a movement to organize a Woman's Auxiliary to the American Medical Association, the object of which shall be, 'To extend the aims of the medical profession through the wives of doctors to the various women's organizations which look to the advancement in health and education, to assist in entertainment at all medical conventions and to promote acquaintanceship among doctors' families so that closer fellowship may exist.'"

This resolution was adopted and the Woman's Auxiliary to the American Medical Association was organized. Twenty-four women from nine states attended the organization meeting. In 1932, ten years later, there were thirty-eight states and the District of Columbia organized with a membership of 13,351. In 1942, twenty years later, forty-one auxiliaries were organized with a membership of 27,532.

Today, twenty-five years later, there are forty-three auxiliaries organized with a membership of approximately 30,000, and auxiliaries are in the process of being organized in two other states. There are 625 county auxiliaries. To facilitate the work of the organization, the states have been equally divided into four geographical sections: Eastern, North Central, Southern and Western, with a Vice President from each section responsible for the organization of Auxiliaries in her district.

MEMBERSHIP

There are three types of membership: active, associate and honorary. Honorary membership has been bestowed on the following seven members, six of whom are Past Presidents: Mrs. Samuel Clark Red, Houston, Texas, Mrs. Franklin P. Gengenbach, Denver, Colorado, Mrs. John O. McReynolds, Dallas, Texas and Mrs. Willard C. Bartlett, St. Louis, Missouri in 1941; Mrs. James Blake, Hopkins, Minnesota and Mrs. J. Newton Hunsberger, Norristown, Pennsylvania in 1942; Mrs. James F. Percy, Los Angeles, California in 1946.

THE PLEDGE

The members repeat the following pledge at the opening of the Annual Convention, the Conference and many of the meetings of the State and County Auxiliaries:

"I pledge my loyalty and devotion to the Woman's Auxiliary to the American Medical Association. I will support its activities, protect its reputation and ever sustain its high ideals."

GIFTS

The Mother State of Texas presented its gavel made of oleander wood from the Galveston Coast to the Auxiliary and it is still in use at its meetings. At the Annual Convention in 1937 a beautiful silver cup was presented to the Auxiliary "to be passed yearly to the State Auxiliary showing the largest increase in membership" but in 1939 it was decided that instead of using the cup as a membership award, it be used for flowers at the Memorial Service held each year at the Annual Convention. Upon the death of the donor it was resolved that it be called after her the "Mrs. Philip Schuyler Doane Memorial Cup." In 1932 Mrs. Walter Jackson Freeman, President of the Auxiliary, died in office and there was established in her memory the "Corinne Keen Freeman Memorial Fund," gifts in money that were sent for floral tributes from the State Auxiliaries being used as the nucleus around which it was built. For a period the fund was available as a loan to the incoming administrations, but the present financial status of the Auxiliary making this use of it no longer necessary, the money is now kept in a special fund pending a decision as to its future use.

THE PRESIDENT'S PIN

Since 1928 at the Annual Convention the Auxiliary has presented the incoming President with a pin having the design of one half of the Medical Caduceus and the letters W.A.—A.M.A. engraved on it. The pin is worn during her term of office, at the termination of which it is handed down to her successor, while she, as retiring President, is presented with a pin of like design in appreciation of her service. From the design of the President's pin the official seal was evolved and adopted.

THE NEWS LETTER

In order to keep the members informed of the activities of the Auxiliary a quarterly "Newsletter" was started in 1931. This gave place in 1939 to a quarterly Bulletin which has since been the official publication of the Woman's Auxiliary. The Bulletin is in printed form and each issue deals, more or less, with some specific phase of the program and activities of both the national and state organizations. The American Medical Association has published the Minutes and Reports of each Annual Convention of the Auxiliary since 1930. From that time it has also published news of the Auxiliary, first in the Bulletin of the American Medical Association and after its discontinuance, in the Journal of the American Medical Association.

POLICIES

As this organization is an auxiliary to the American Medical Association, its basic policies are determined by that organization, one being that it shall not affiliate with other federated organizations, nor have represented on its Board of Directors representatives of other organizations, nor be represented officially on the Board of other organizations. The Auxiliary is also instructed not to endorse any commercial interest nor any candidate for public office. Although the Auxiliary may take the initiative in proposing its projects, they must be approved by the Advisory Council. The Advisory Council consisted of five members of the Board of Trustees and the Secretary of the American Medical Association and the Editor of the Journal of the American Medical Association until 1946 when it was enlarged to include all nine members of the Board of Trustees, the Secretary and the Editor of the Journal. At the Annual Convention in San Francisco at which this change was made, the Board of Trustees also proposed that the Advisory Council should meet with the Board of Directors of the Woman's Auxiliary twice a year, at the time of the Mid-Year Board meeting and immediately preceding the Annual Convention. The first such meeting was held in Chicago in December 1946. In addition to the Advisory Council and the Board of Directors of the Woman's Auxiliary, there were present also the Chairmen of Standing Committees of the Auxiliary and the following officers of the American Medical Association: the President, the President-Elect, the Vice President, the Treasurer and the Vice Speaker of the House of Delegates. It was a remarkably inspiring meeting and everyone felt it was the beginning of an era which will be characterized by a closer working relationship that will prove beneficial to both organizations and enable them to be of greater service to the American people.

THE CENTRAL OFFICE

During the first twenty years of the organization of the Auxiliary, the Presidents performed not only the routine work of the office but also many other time-consuming tasks, such as checking membership cards, sending out the President's packet to the State and County Auxiliaries, assisting in the preparation and editing of the Newsletter and later, the Bulletin. In 1942, however, the Auxiliary opened a Central Office in Chicago and employed an Executive Secretary who has since assumed many of these responsibilities. At the Annual Meeting of the Board of Trustees in 1946 plans were made to house the Central Office of the Auxiliary in the American Medical Association's Headquarters Building in Chicago.

CONVENTIONS

The regular Annual Conventions of 1943 and 1945 were cancelled because of the war, although in 1943 there was a meeting of the House of Delegates and in 1945 a meeting of the Board of Directors. Since there is no provision in the Constitution or By-Laws for the election of officers without an annual meeting, the women who were in office in 1944–1945 served for a second year.

Up to 1944 the State Presidents had automatically been members of the Board of Directors of the Woman's Auxiliary to the American Medical Association, but at the Annual Convention held in Chicago in that year there were changes in the Constitution and By-Laws which resulted in the discontinuance of this practice. The New Constitution and By-Laws provided instead for a Conference of State Presidents, State Presidents-Elect and Chairman of Standing Committees to be held at the time that the Board of Directors of the Auxiliary holds its annual Mid-Year meeting. An amendment passed in 1946 provided that the President-Elect preside at the Conference.

The Convention meets annually at the same time and at the same place as the Annual Session of the American Medical Association. The voting body at this meeting consists of the President of each constituent Auxiliary and one additional representative for every hundred members or a major fraction thereof, each State Auxiliary being entitled to at least one voting delegate besides the President. All Auxiliary members are entitled to attend the sessions of the Convention.

OBJECTIVES

The objects of the Auxiliary as stated in the Constitution are:

1. To extend the aims of the medical profession to all organizations which look to the advancement of health and health education;
2. To cultivate friendly relations and promote mutual understanding among physicians' families;
3. To participate in any endeavor on the request of the American Medical Association;
4. To coordinate and advise concerning the activities of constituent auxiliaries; and
5. To assist in the entertainment at all conventions of the American Medical Association.

The social side has played an important part in the development of the Woman's Auxiliary, not only from the entertainment angle but in cultivating friendly relations and promoting mutual understanding on the County, State and National levels. On a basis of friendship and common interests it has been possible to work effectively toward the carrying out of the other objectives of the organization.

The first request made of the Auxiliary by the American Medical Association was that it promote interest in Hygeia, the only authentic health periodical in the country for the laity. In 1931 the House of Delegates of the American Medical Association passed a resolution urging the Woman's Auxiliary, including the County, State and National organizations, to promote the distribution of Hygeia through Parent-Teacher Associations, Boards of Education and similar bodies interested in education. In compliance with this request the Auxiliary members have endeavored to place the magazine in as many places as possible where the lay public may have access to it, realizing that the promotion of health education is a valuable community service. It has been a source material which has been widely drawn upon in the writing of essays on health subjects, in classroom work, in contests etc. The most spectacular appreciation of the value of Hygeia was that shown by the legislatures of two states which appropriated several thousand dollars each in order to put it into the schools of the state; in one case, in the elementary schools; in the other case, in the Junior and Senior High Schools. Every year the American Medical Association gives $400 in cash awards to the Auxiliaries obtaining the largest number of subscription credits to Hygeia in proportion to their membership. The names of the winners of the Hygeia Contest each year will be placed on a Memorial Plaque which was presented to the Auxiliary by Dr. Herman L. Kretschmer of Chicago in memory of his wife, Lucy

Barnett Kretschmer. The plaque is large enough to have inscribed on it the names of the contest winners for twenty years.

The second request made of the Auxiliary by the House of Delegates of the American Medical Association was to help in the dissemination of knowledge both to its members and to the public concerning the hazards of some of the current medical legislation.

The Woman's Auxiliary has done its utmost to inform its members of the practical workings of politics and to keep them informed concerning the current health legislation. Many State Auxiliaries have been given credit for materially assisting in bringing about the enactment of Basic Science Laws, for defeating laws which would jeopardize the public health by allowing charlatans and quacks to engage in the art of healing, and for preventing the passage of Anti-Vivisection Bills. The implications of politically sponsored medicine have been repeatedly called to the attention of the State and County Auxiliaries over a period of several years as has also been the need of being thoroughly informed on other important issues. The members of the State and County Auxiliaries have been encouraged to become familiar with the National Health Program of the American Medical Association, as well as with the Prepayment Medical Care Plans of their own states as alternatives to the Compulsory Health Insurance Plans. The various County and State components of the Woman's Auxiliary have worked constructively and effectively for the passage of legislation designed to improve the public health.

HEALTH EDUCATION

Perhaps the outstanding accomplishment of the Woman's Auxiliary to the American Medical Association has been in connection with health education and the furthering of health measures. Its members work closely with the Anti-Tuberculosis Association, the American Cancer Society and the National Foundation for Infantile Paralysis; in certain states they actively participate in the campaign against Rheumatic Fever; and at the present time they are vitally interested in the survey that is being conducted by the American Academy of Pediatrics. In addition they carry on many other activities. These are quite varied because of the fact that the work of the organization is done largely through the State and County units which adapt the suggestions of the National Auxiliary to the particular needs of their communities. A Handbook prepared by the National Auxiliary is in constant use by the component auxiliaries and has proved a valuable tool in carrying on their work.

A few illustrations may give a glimpse of the scope of the work done by the State and County groups. They have worked extensively with the State, County and City Health Departments, the American Red Cross, and also such Women's groups as the Parent-Teacher Association, the Federated Women's Clubs, the Young Women's Christian Association, the American Association of University Women and the Junior League.

One effective medium for health education has been the Public Health Institute which is conducted annually by many of the State Auxiliaries. An interest in these has been manifested alike in cities and rural communities, in the larger cities a three day institute being sometimes held, and in the smaller communities usually a one day institute. Recently in a sparsely settled rural community, as an experiment, they planned to have a one day program, not knowing whether or not there would be anyone in attendance, but to the delight of those who sponsored it, six hundred came. In addition to the Institute they have fostered public health meetings and talks and distributed health literature. In many places the Auxiliary has a Speakers' Bureau through which speakers may be obtained for civic groups. In one state in which the cities and towns are of moderate size thirty-five talks were arranged during one season, which is fairly typical. Radio programs and health films some of which are furnished by the Bureau of Health Education of the American Medical Association are often provided for interested groups.

Considerable work has been done in connection with Clinics of various types. The members have assisted in the County Clinics with the immunization programs by personally aiding in its administration and by carrying on preliminary educational work. They have also given material and personal assistance to the Crippled Children's, the Prenatal and Maternity, and the Nutrition Clinics.

In practically every state the Auxiliaries work for the hospitals, the type of work differing according to the local needs. Their work has consisted of such activities as entertaining children in the Pediatric wards and furnishing toys for them, redecorating and maintaining nurseries, supplying materials for occupational therapy in Veterans' Hospitals and State Hospitals for Nervous Diseases, and buying equipment of different types. One County Auxiliary, for instance, contributed $400 for an orthopedic chair and others have given beds, tables, wheelchairs, etc. At the present time one state group is working in cooperation with other Women's organizations for the enactment of a "Child Colony Bill" which, if passed, will provide an institution for the care of the mentally deficient children of the state.

Realizing that the health of children means the health of the future citizens of the country, the women of the organization have supplemented the health work in the schools by conducting Dental Clinics, by providing for physical examinations and the correction of physical defects, and by contributing to funds for the employment of County school nurses, for furnishing milk and hot lunches for needy children, as well as for the purchase of glasses and other necessities. One State Auxiliary bought portable players and through them and through films, stories on good health were brought to rural schools, making it possible for three thousand children who would not otherwise have obtained this health information to benefit by them. Several other states have sent children to summer camps. This year one of them has made plans for sending ten girls and ten boys to such camps.

Contributions of money and of books have been made to medical association libraries, to the permanent and circulating libraries of hospitals, and to the libraries of state institutions. In addition, shelves in public libraries have been supplied with books and literature on medical subjects. One County Auxiliary put two juvenile health publications called "Jimmy Microbe Books" in all the libraries of its district and the librarians report that they are in constant use. One allied project is the collection of historical data and supplies pertinent to medicine, such as books, letters, medical and surgical instruments and general equipment; and another is the collection by the Southern Auxiliaries of historical data concerning the lives and achievements of Southern physicians and the medical profession. It is known as "The Research and Romance of Medicine."

Throughout the entire history of the Auxiliary there has been a continuous and wide interest in the prevention and eradication of Tuberculosis, particularly among children. Besides the regular Christmas Seal sales, the endowment of rooms in preventoria and sanatoria, the promotion of early diagnosis clinics, the giving of Radio programs, the encouragement of essays and contests relative to the subject, a number of specific things have been done by individual auxiliaries that are worthy of note. In one city fifty thousand pamphlets on Tuberculosis were distributed with the gas and water bills. Several years ago one Auxiliary aided in giving skin tests to five thousand children, the value of which was proved by the fact that three hundred out of each thousand tested showed a positive reaction. At the present time the members are helping with the Chest X-Ray programs which are being conducted in a number of communities by the United States Public Health Service, by the State and County Health Departments, and by other Health Agencies.

The Auxiliaries are manifesting a similar interest in the activities of the American Cancer Society. They are assisting in the educational program by distributing literature, by paying for exhibits to be brought to different centers in connection with the membership campaign, and by soliciting memberships in order to raise funds to carry on the work of the Society. One County unit raised over $800 for the membership campaign in 1946.

SCHOLARSHIP AND BENEVOLENCE FUNDS

A large percentage of the Auxiliaries maintain some type of a Scholarship Loan Fund. Some of these are available to the sons and daughters of doctors; some, to nursing students; and some, to medical students. One known as the "Jane Todd Crawford Memorial Fund" will in the future be available to postgraduate medical students. In some states the Auxiliaries have accumulated a Benevolence Fund to be used for physicians and their families where there is need of assistance due to illness or other adversities. In 1945 one State Auxiliary added $7000 to its Benevolence Fund.

WAR SERVICE

It is impossible to tell the true story of the time given by the Auxiliary members to the war effort because of the intangible nature of much of their work. However, the report turned in accounts for 1,291,564 hours or 63,325 days. Bonds and stamps were sold to the amount of $4,700,972. Their war service included all phases of Red Cross work, assisting Draft and Ration Boards, Nurse Cadet Corps Recruiting, Salvage Drive, General Duty and Operating-Room work in Hospitals, and work in connection with O.C.D. and U.S.O., Blood Banks and the Doctors' Aide Corps.

A QUARTER CENTURY

During the twenty-five years of its history the Woman's Auxiliary to the American Medical Association has laid a sound foundation which enables it to face new problems and responsibilities. It aims to take as conscientious and active a part in the activities of the post war period as it did during the years of the war emergency, and with increased interest and devotion to maintain the high standards and ideals for which it was organized.

PAST PRESIDENTS OF THE WOMAN'S AUXILIARY TO THE AMERICAN MEDICAL ASSOCIATION

1922–1925 Mrs. Samuel Clark Red, Houston, Texas
1925–1926 Mrs. Seale Harris, Birmingham, Alabama
1926–1927 Mrs. F. P. Gengenbach, Denver, Colorado
1927–1928 Mrs. John O. McReynolds, Dallas, Texas
1928–1929 Mrs. Allen H. Bunce, Atlanta, Georgia

1929–1930	Mrs. George H. Hoxie, Kansas City, Missouri	
1930–1931	Mrs. J. Newton Hunsberger, Norristown, Pennsylvania	
1931–1932	Mrs. A. B. McGlothlan, St. Joseph, Missouri	
1932–1933	Mrs. Walter Jackson Freeman, Philadelphia, Pennsylvania	
	Mrs. James F. Percy, Los Angeles, California	
	Mrs. Freeman served as President from May 13, 1932, until her death on October 27, 1932. She was succeeded by Mrs. Percy, First Vice President.	
1933–1934	Mrs. James Blake, Hopkins, Minnesota	
1934–1935	Mrs. Robert W. Tomlinson, Wilmington, Delaware	
1935–1936	Mrs. Rogers N. Herbert, Nashville, Tennessee	
1936–1937	Mrs. Robert E. Fitzgerald, Wauwatosa, Wisconsin	
1937–1938	Mrs. Augustus S. Kech, Altoona, Pennsylvania	
1938–1939	Mrs. Charles C. Tomlinson, Omaha, Nebraska	
1939–1940	Mrs. Rollo K. Packard, Chicago, Illinois	
1940–1941	Mrs. V. E. Holcombe, Charleston, West Virginia	
1941–1942	Mrs. Roscoe E. Mosiman, Seattle, Washington	
1942–1943	Mrs. Frank N. Haggard, San Antonio, Texas	
1943–1944	Mrs. Eben J. Carey, Wauwatosa, Wisconsin	
1944–1946	Mrs. David W. Thomas, Lock Haven, Pennsylvania	
1946–1947	Mrs. Jesse D. Hamer, Phoenix, Arizona, President	
	Mrs. Eustace A. Allen, Atlanta, Georgia, President-Elect	

ANNUAL CONVENTIONS OF THE WOMAN'S AUXILIARY

Year	Place	Registration
1922	St. Louis, Missouri	26
1923	San Francisco, California	18*
1924	Chicago, Illinois	23*
1925	Atlantic City, New Jersey	27*
1926	Dallas, Texas	924
1927	Washington, D. C.	1,304
1928	Minneapolis, Minnesota	1,296
1929	Portland, Oregon	724
1930	Detroit, Michigan	413
1931	Philadelphia, Pennsylvania	1,103
1932	New Orleans, Louisiana	918
1933	Milwaukee, Wisconsin	974
1934	Cleveland, Ohio	1,426
1935	Atlantic City, New Jersey	1,910
1936	Kansas City, Missouri	1,589
1937	Atlantic City, New Jersey	1,964
1938	San Francisco, California	1,246
1939	St. Louis, Missouri	1,526
1940	New York City, New York	1,321
1941	Cleveland, Ohio	1,577
1942	Atlantic City, New Jersey	1,326
1943	Chicago, Illinois	196**
1944	Chicago, Illinois	520
1945	No Annual Convention	
1946	San Francisco, California	1,140
1947	Atlantic City, New Jersey	

* Roll call by states, no registration of attendance.
** House of Delegates Meeting only.

Publications of the American Medical Association

ARCHIVES OF INTERNAL MEDICINE

By N. C. Gilbert, M.D.

THE ARCHIVES OF INTERNAL MEDICINE, sponsored and published by the American Medical Association, celebrates the fortieth anniversary of its foundation in 1947. In 1906, the question of publishing a special journal devoted to internal medicine was brought before the trustees of the Association on two occasions, once by Dr. Simmons, then General Secretary, and again by Dr. Malcolm L. Harris, then one of the trustees. Definite steps were not taken at that time. How much influence this had on future events is not known. Records are not available of what transpired prior to the June meeting of the trustees at Atlantic City in 1907. At this meeting a petition was presented to the trustees requesting that the Association undertake the publication of a journal devoted to the more important researches made by American students in clinical medicine—a journal conducted on the general plan of the ZEITSCHRIFT FÜR KLINISCHE MEDIZIN and the DEUTSCHES ARCHIF FÜR KLINISCHE MEDIZIN. Among the signers of the petition were Dr. Frank Billings of Chicago, Dr. Henry A. Christian of Boston, Dr. David L. Edsall of Philadelphia, Dr. William S. Thayer of Baltimore, Dr. Lawrence Litchfield of Pittsburgh, Dr. Warfield T. Longcope of Baltimore, Dr. Joseph H. Pratt of Boston, Dr. Hugh T. Patrick of Chicago, Dr. Philip King Brown of San Francisco, Dr. George Dock of Ann Arbor, Dr. Richard C. Cabot of Boston and Dr Alfred Stengel of Philadelphia.

The petition found immediate favor with the trustees; a motion was adopted that Dr. George Dock, Dr. W. S. Thayer, Dr. Joseph L. Miller, Dr. David L. Edsall, Dr. Theodore Janeway and Dr. Richard Cabot be appointed to act as a committee to consider the publication of such a journal and to report to the trustees at the October meeting. A motion was also adopted that "it is the sense of the Board of Trustees that the above mentioned gentlemen will constitute the editorial staff of the proposed journal, should the same be started, for a period of six years, the term of one to terminate each year, and his successor to be elected for six years by the Board of Trustees, on the nomination of the Editorial Staff."

In August, Dr. George H. Simmons, as General Secretary of the

American Medical Association, wrote to all the members, formally notifying them that they were a committee to formulate plans for the new journal, and advising Dr. Dock that he was to act as chairman. In this letter, Dr. Simmons referred to the general objectives of the new journal and the need for such a journal to bridge the gulf between purely scientific research and its application to practical clinical medicine. The committee was requested to report to the trustees at the October meeting, not only on the general objectives but on the

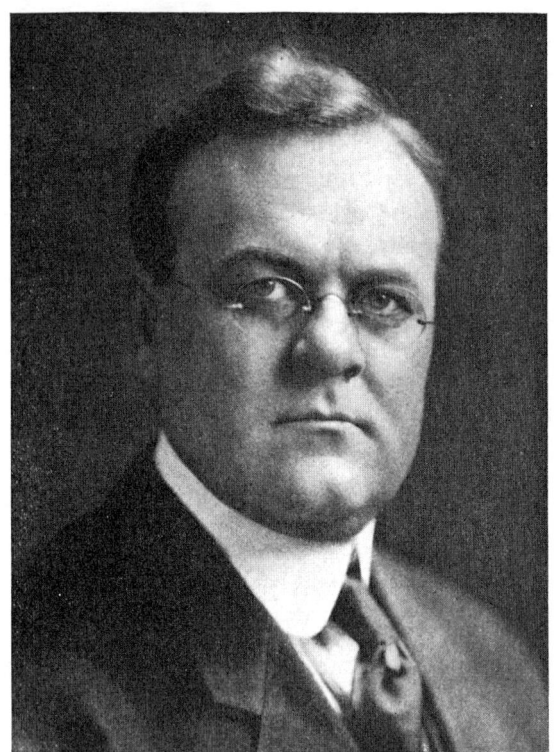

Joseph L. Miller, M.D.
Editorial Board, Archives of Internal Medicine.

size of the journal, its mechanical make-up and whether or not it was to be a monthly journal. "The appearance of the journal," wrote Dr. Simmons, "will have something to do with its reception and success. Personally I think there should be nothing cheap about it. It should be gotten up in good form on high class paper, and should not carry advertisements." Again, "the facilities of the Journal office for doing first class work are ample. In fact we have at the present time a perfectly equipped printing establishment, even including an up-to-date rotary press."

The committee, largely through correspondence among themselves, and with Dr. Simmons' help, considered every aspect of the new journal in detail. Dr. Cabot, as a true Bostonian, wrote that the size should be that of the *Atlantic Monthly*. He was particular, also, as regards the type. "Small differences are what count in type, as in the cast of a man's countenance." There was also considerable discussion as to whether or not the edges were to be cut, especially the first few copies. Dr. Cabot considered uncut edges an affectation. The other editors were, for the most part, more easily satisfied. Dr. Janeway's only comment on the setting of the title page was that he thought the price should be less conspicuous and the date more so. Besides the typography, the quality and texture of the paper were considered, and samples of the cover were referred to each of the editors. It was decided to have the cover reproduced on the title page of the journal, just preceding the text, in case the cover should be torn off. In all of this, Dr. Simmons was of the greatest possible help, and the reader of the correspondence is certain to be impressed by the thoughtfulness and kindly spirit of helpfulness shown by him. His guidance and attention to detail did a tremendous amount to assure the immediate success of the ARCHIVES, and this guidance continued throughout his life. Certainly the profession owes a debt of gratitude to him for the establishment of this splendid periodical.

Early in October, the committee sent a report to Dr. Simmons. The name suggested in this report was THE JOURNAL OF CLINICAL MEDICINE. The form and size of the journal were recommended, as well as the objectives, which were previously covered. There were to be no abstracts, no editorials and no advertising. The journal was to be issued monthly and published by the press of the American Medical Association of Chicago. Dr. Joseph L. Miller was chosen as Editor-in-Chief, with the stipulation that the other members of the Board were also to pass on the manuscripts submitted. The report was approved with the exception of the name, which was considered too similar to the name of a proprietary journal published as the advertising medium of a drug firm. Accordingly, it was decided to use the present name.

The first meeting of the editorial board was called for November 9 in New York City, at which time Dr. Cabot, Dr. Edsall, Dr. Thayer and Dr. Janeway were to be in New York for a meeting of the Clinical Interurban Club. Dr. Dock suggested that the Chicago members take the Wolverine, which went through Ann Arbor. It would be strange if the new journal were not discussed en route. The new editorial board spent the morning at the Rockefeller Institute, with the Eastern Interurban Club. After lunch with Dr. Janeway, they met at the New York Academy of Medicine for their first formal meeting.

Shortly after, the editorial Board published an announcement in The Journal of the American Medical Association, stating that "the Board of Trustees of the American Medical Association has taken steps to the foundation of the ARCHIVES OF INTERNAL MEDICINE. It will be devoted to the publication of original studies carried on at the bedside, or in the laboratory, on clinical medicine and of all the physiological and pharmacological researches that relate to the diagnosis or treatment of this class of conditions. Scholarly, thorough work, well abreast of the present position of medical science is what is desired of the ARCHIVES OF INTERNAL MEDICINE. All technical details and protocols necessary to prove the thesis, will be welcome, although unnecessary details must be avoided. Articles that summarize what is already known on a topic, to which is added something new, are typical of what it desires, as are also short, critical reviews of important subjects and short, original communications on matters of internal medicine." This was signed by each of the editors. These principles are reproduced just as they appear, because they have continued to be the guiding principles of the Editorial Board through all the changes that have occurred and they are still closely followed.

The first number of the new Journal appeared in January, 1908, with the following table of contents:

CONTENTS OF VOLUME I

January, 1908, Number 1

The Nervous Affections of the Heart. Friedrich Muller, M.D., Munich, Germany.
The Hemolytic Reactions of the Blood in Dogs Affected with Transplantable Lymphosarcoma. Richard Weil, M.D., New York City.
Trichomonas Hominis Intestinalis: A Study of its Biology and its Pathogenicity. Hugo A. Freund, M.D., Detroit, Michigan.
An Experimental Study of the Action of Oil on the Gastric Acidity and Motility. David Murray Cowie, M.D., Ann Arbor, Mich., and James Frederick Munson, M.D., Sonyea, N. Y.
Experimental and Clinical Investigation of the Pulse and Blood Pressure Changes in Aortic Insufficiency. Hugh A. Stewart, M.D., Baltimore.

The ARCHIVES has appeared each month since that initial number. With such sponsors and so distinguished an Editorial Board, the success of the new periodical was assured from the first. The circulation has steadily increased until it is nearly ten thousand copies. There have been minor fluctuations in the circulation because of World War I and the depression of the early thirties, but these were only temporary and the increase has been consistent. The rise in

1945 was due in part to government subscription for the Army and Navy personnel, but even without this the circulation remained over 8,000. The circulation in Europe and in Latin America and the Far East was at first small, but following World War I it rose steadily until the increase was temporarily interrupted by World War II. The distribution of the foreign circulation has naturally varied with world conditions.

The subscription price was initially $4.00, or $3.00 if the Archives was taken in conjunction with The Journal of the American Medical Association. It has been necessary to advance the price of subscription from time to time in an attempt to approximate the cost of production. In 1913, after consideration by members of the board, advertisements began to appear.

The editorial staff remained unchanged until 1911, when Dr. Edsall was succeeded by Dr. Longcope. In 1913, Dr. Hamman of Baltimore succeeded Dr. Janeway, and he was succeeded by Dr. Walter W. Palmer of New York in 1924. In 1931, Dr. George Dock was succeeded by Dr. James H. Means of Boston. THE ARCHIVES was indebted to this distinguished group of former editors for its continued success and its high standing in scientific medicine. Dr. Joseph L. Miller remained as Editor-in-Chief of the ARCHIVES from the time of its inception until 1932. An especial debt of appreciation is due to him. He carried throughout more than his share of responsibility. In addition to this, he showed to young investigators and authors the same kindly interest and spirit of helpfulness which characterized him in his relations with others throughout his life.

In 1932, a new Editorial Board was selected by the trustees, consisting of Dr. Arthur Bloomfield of San Francisco, Dr. Reginald Fitz of Boston, Dr. John H. Musser of New Orleans, Dr. Russell M. Wilder of Rochester, Minn., and Dr. N. C. Gilbert of Chicago. This Board, which has continued until the present time, has endeavored to follow as closely as possible the ideas of its predecessors.

Each manuscript submitted to the Editorial Board is passed from one member to another, and the opinion of each is recorded on a card which accompanies the manuscript. No effort is made to refer manuscripts to an editor whose primary interest covers the field of the article which is to be considered. It is felt by the Board that a better cross section of opinion is gained when several men with different points of view review the paper and that the interests of the reader are better served in this manner. No paper is ever accepted which does not have the approval of at least three members of the Board. If any one editor has a very strong or clear-cut objection to a paper, that paper is rejected. It is a rather trying ordeal for any manuscript and the mortality is high. But the editors are certain that this plan has resulted in a superior selection of material, and it is one reason why there are more references to articles appearing in the ARCHIVES than in any of the other American journals except The Journal of the American Medical Association.

No editor expresses an opinion on any paper submitted from his own university or his own city. This is not because he might possibly be influenced by personal considerations. On the contrary, the experi-

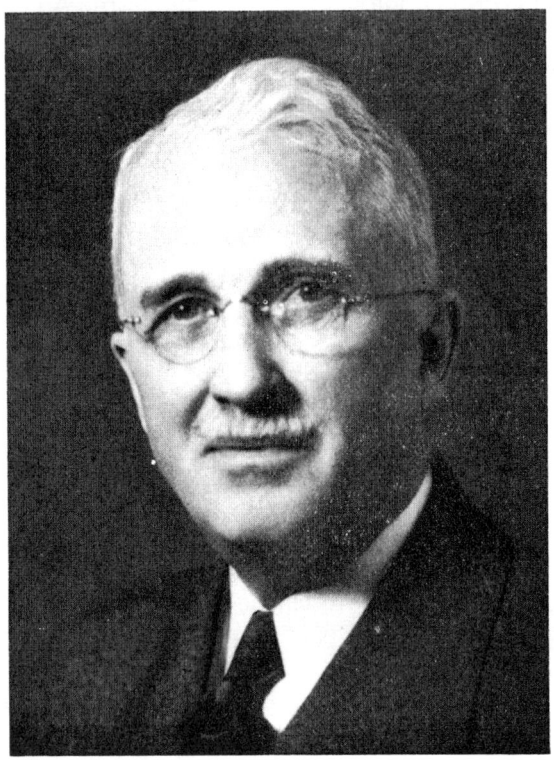

N. C. Gilbert, M.D.
Editorial Board, Archives of Internal Medicine.

ence has been that he is more apt to lean backward in his desire to be impartial.

Until the annual meetings of the Association of American Physicians and of the American Medical Association were interrupted by the war, the Editorial Board met at least once, and usually twice, a year. At these meetings the Board reviewed the opinions noted on the record cards on all of the manuscripts received since the last meeting and the reasons for acceptance or rejection. The views expressed were discussed and any sins of omission or commission were considered jointly. Such meetings proved to be of great help to the Board in developing policies and common points of view. The meetings are now being resumed.

The policy of the present Board is exactly that set forth in the preliminary announcement of the first Board. Manuscripts should be as short as is consistent with clear exposition. There is only a moderate limit on illustrations. With respect to colored illustrations: part of the extra expense of reproduction is usually borne by the author. The manuscripts are edited by trained editorial readers and it is essential that the papers conform to certain rules of English usage which have been adopted as the policy of the A.M.A. press. The editorial procedure is sometimes a little trying to the author, who sees his favorite expressions altered by the editorial readers, but the wisdom of this is usually readily granted.

The actual responsibility for the publication of the magazine is borne by the managing editor, Dr. Morris Fishbein, and his assistant, Miss Jewel Whelan. Just as much of the early success of the ARCHIVES was assured by the friendly advice and cooperation of Dr. Simmons, so now it is to Dr. Fishbein and Miss Whelan that the present editorial Board is indebted for the welfare of the magazine.

During the paper shortage occasioned by the war, it was necessary to alter the format of the ARCHIVES and to reduce its size somewhat to conserve paper, but the old format has been resumed and is that outlined by the original Board.

In 1934, a series of general reviews was instituted at the suggestion of Dr. Russell M. Wilder. Twelve general subjects in the field of internal medicine were chosen for review, such as Diseases of the Blood, Infectious Diseases, and Allergy. The writing of such reviews was assigned to a representative leader in each field, who was selected for his special knowledge. He was asked not merely to write a summary of the work produced during the year, but to present a critical evaluation for the benefit of the reader who possesses no special knowledge of that particular field and who looks to him for guidance.

The individual book reviews are prepared by men who are especially fitted to pass judgment on the subject to be reviewed. It is hoped that each review will be so written as not only to afford the reader some idea as to the contents of the book but to give him an impartial expression in regard to its value. The book reviews are not necessarily prepared by the editors; they frequently are assigned to other men. The book reviews are not signed, in order that the reviewer may be freely critical.

Throughout its forty years of existence, the ARCHIVES has steadily maintained the objectives enunciated by the original Board and has striven to adhere to the same high ideas and conservative scientific standards.

THE AMERICAN JOURNAL OF DISEASES OF CHILDREN

By Clifford G. Grulee, M.D.

THE DECEMBER ISSUE, 1946, was the last of the seventy-first volume of the American Journal of Diseases of Children. The first volume appeared in 1911.

When the Board of Trustees of the American Medical Association met on February 4, 1910, Dr. Isaac Abt and F. S. Churchill, on behalf of a number of pediatricians, presented the following communication requesting the publication by the Association of a periodical devoted to pediatrics:

"Appreciating the need in America of a journal of pediatrics published and entirely controlled by the medical profession; impressed, moreover, by the high character and success of the Archives of Internal Medicine established by your Board two years ago, we respectfully request that you establish a journal of pediatrics on somewhat similar lines.

"There is at present no journal in the English language devoted to this important branch of medicine, which at all corresponds, for example, to the *Jahrbuch für Kinderheilkunde* published in Germany. The large and increasing number of articles relating to pediatrics which are constantly appearing in *The Journal of the American Medical Association* and other general medical journals is evidence of the amount of creditable work in pediatrics which is being done in this country, and of the abundance of material which is available for such a publication as we propose. Such a journal would command the support of all who are engaged in pediatric practice, teaching and research in the United States, and would make a strong appeal to the general practitioner much of whose practice is of necessity among children.

"Such a journal should give prominence to articles embodying research in pediatrics, but should include, as well, good articles of a practical character including even clinical memoranda—abstracts of important discussions in the pediatric societies, all carefully selected and edited, and, finally, carefully prepared abstracts of the pediatric literature of the world. It should carry no advertisements.

"It is suggested that if this request be favorably considered by you, that you select an Advisory Committee of ten or twelve pediatrists, representatives of the leading medical centers, which committee shall consider and report to your Board, as soon as practicable, upon the essential details of this proposed journal such as the name, frequency of issue (a bimonthly has been suggested), size, subscription price, character and arrangement of contents, etc., and to nominate an editorial board of four to six pediatrists, who shall have editorial control of the journal, in a manner similar to that of the Editorial Board of the Archives of Internal Medicine.

"Should the proposed journal be established we pledge our earnest and continued support as contributors and subscribers."

In response to that petition the Board of Trustees appointed a committee of eleven to secure information in regard to the publication by the American Medical Association of a periodical devoted to pediatrics. The committee consisted of Drs. Abraham Jacobi, L. Emmett Holt, Thomas Southworth and G. R. Pisek of New York; T. M. Rotch of Boston; Edwin E. Graham and J. P. C. Griffith of Philadelphia; and W. J. Butler, Isaac A. Abt, J. N. Dodson and Frank Spooner Churchill of Chicago.

At the meeting of the Board of Trustees on June 6, 1910, the following letter was presented from the Section on Diseases of Children.

Gentlemen:

At a meeting of the Section on Diseases of Children, June 7, 1910, it was moved and after due discussion carried, that the Section approve the recommendation to the Board of Trustees for the publication of a special journal devoted to the diseases of children and that the matter be referred to the Executive Committee of the Section with power to act.

A meeting of the Executive Committee of the Section on Diseases of Children was held June 8, 1910, at 8:30 a.m., in conjunction with the Committee appointed by the Board of Trustees.

Doctor Snyder, Chairman of the Executive Committee, first called to order a meeting of that Committee.

Doctor Graham moved, and the motion was carried, that the Executive Committee transmit to the Board of Trustees the action of the Section in approving the establishment of a special journal.

The Executive Committee then adjourned.

Doctor Abt, Chairman, called to order a meeting of the joint committees.

A motion was made, and carried, to accept the report of a subcommittee on names of the proposed journal and to recommend to the Trustees that it be called *The American Journal of Diseases of Children*.

The following recommendations were also adopted: That the periodical should contain original articles, abstracts and occasional complete reviews by men appointed by the Editorial Board; that it should begin as a bi-monthly of approximately 64 pages an issue; that it should be about the size of the *Archives of Pediatrics;* that the Editors shall choose their own chairman, and that the subscription price be referred to the Trustees.

The joint meeting then adjourned.

The Executive Committee of the Section on Diseases of Children reconvened at 9:30 a.m., and voted to submit the following names to the Board of Trustees for selection of an Editorial Board:

Dr. Abraham Jacobi, New York
Dr. John Lovett Morse, Boston
Dr. Edwin E. Graham, Philadelphia
Dr. Frank Spooner Churchill, Chicago
Dr. J. H. M. Knox, Baltimore
Dr. G. R. Pisek, New York
Dr. Isaac A. Abt, Chicago
Dr. W. J. Butler, Chicago
Dr. J. R. Snyder, Birmingham
Dr. J. P. C. Griffith, Philadelphia
Dr. H. M. McClanahan, Omaha
Dr. L. Emmett Holt, New York

Respectfully submitted,

Executive Committee { J. Ross Snyder
Section on Diseases { Edwin E. Graham
of Children { Thomas S. Southworth

At that meeting—June 6, 1910—the Board of Trustees authorized the publication of a periodical to be known as the American Journal of Diseases of Children. The selection of men to constitute the Editorial Board, however, was postponed until October, at which time the following Board was elected:

Drs. Abraham Jacobi of New York and W. Fitch Cheney of San Francisco—each for two years.

Drs. John Howland of New York and John Lovett Morse of Boston—each for four years.

Drs. F. S. Churchill of Chicago and Edwin E. Graham of Philadelphia—each for six years.

Dr. George H. Simmons was appointed managing editor to represent the Board of Trustees.

The edict of the Board of Trustees at this time was that the periodical was not to carry any advertisements.

The introduction of Volume I was written by Abraham Jacobi and the first articles were by Fitterolf and Gittings, the latter of whom was subsequently an Editor of the Journal. Of the original Editorial Board not a single one is now alive, Dr. Churchill having died recently.

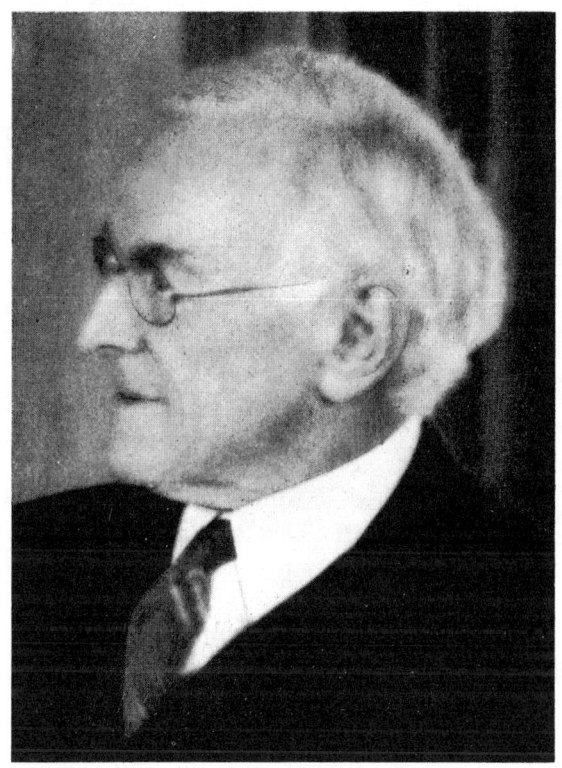

Frank Spooner Churchill, M.D.
Chief Editor, The American Journal of Diseases of Children, 1910.

In the first volume appeared names of physicians who have made pediatric history—L. Emmett Holt, Sr., Martha Wollstein, I. A. Abt, Kerley, Schloss, Brenneman, Alfred Hess, Morse and Talbot. Most of the articles were clinical. However, the pace for future volumes was set by the scientific articles of Schloss, Courtney and Gittings. In this first volume an article in Progress in Pediatrics provided selected abstracts.

Volume II which appeared in July, 1911, had added such names as Fife, Veeder, Thomas Morgan Rotch, Howland, Koplick, J. H. M. Knox, Harry Shaw, Sedgwick and Schlutz and Julius Hess, in his first article in the Journal on prematurity. News notes appeared in August, 1911, for the first time and Progress in Pediatrics was changed to composite reviews. This first year set the type of the future Journal and although at times there was a change in the composition of the Journal it reverted in time to this arrangement consisting of original papers, Progress in Pediatrics, abstracts and news notes. Later other features were added.

In 1911, Dr. Cheney resigned from the Editorial Board and was replaced by Dr. David M. Cowie.

In 1912, Volume III, the first article by a foreign contributor appeared. This was by E. Plauchu, Professor of Obstetrics of Lyons, France, and was on "Resuscitation of Asphyxiated Infants by the Insufflation Method of Meltzer and Auer." In February of this year appeared the index of current literature which was not continued for long and in March there was an article by Ad Czerny on the "Atrophy of Infants." The first of May Michael's most comprehensive résumés on tuberculosis appeared in this volume, and others appeared for many years until her death. They were at the time an outstanding feature of the Journal. An article by Churchill in this volume was the first that the Chief Editor had contributed. In the Fall of 1912 the name of Kenneth Blackfan as a contributor first appeared, a man who was to become later one of the outstanding figures in American pediatrics. There also appeared at this time the outstanding article by Benedict and Talbot on Metabolism which was the forerunner of Talbot's fundamental studies on this subject. For the first time in this number there occurred an article by John Ruhräh.

Dr. Abraham Jacobi was replaced by Dr. L. Emmett Holt, Sr. on the Editorial Board in 1913. In Volume V occurred the names as contributors of such well-known figures in pediatrics as H. C. Carpenter, La Fetra, Richard M. Smith, De Buys, Josephine Baker and Maynard Ladd and in the May number was the first of the Latin-American contributions by Melilo Leitao of Rio de Janeiro. In the Fall of that year we notice the names of Langley Porter, Northrup, Blackader, Alan Brown and Zahorsky.

The first World War had not yet affected conditions in this country and seemed far away and the work in pediatrics continued to advance. It was in Volume VII of 1914 that observations on stomach, pylorus and the use of the duodenal catheter by Alfred Hess first appeared and Philip Van Ingen contributed an article on "Progress in Infant Welfare Work."

In Volume VIII of the same year Benedict and Talbot began their series of articles on respiratory exchange. In this year for the first time Chapin, Faber and Jeans appeared and two outstanding articles, one by Alfred Hess on "Infantile Scurvy" and the second by Dandy and Blackfan on "Internal Hydrocephalus" were published. For the first time in Volume VIII appeared obituaries, those of Rotch, Putnam and Forchheimer.

Volume IX, 1915, began to show more intensive interest in chemical and biochemical problems. Murlin and Hoobler published an article on "Energy Metabolism" and Holt, Courtney and Fales began their series of articles (which were to continue for several years) on the chemical composition of stools. Here, too, first appeared an article by Gamble.

Volume X had articles by Helmholz and Gerstenberger. Volume XI contained an article by Howland and Marriott on "Acidosis in Diarrhoea." This is the first time that these two eminent pediatricians appeared jointly as authors of an article.

In the next volume in 1916, Helmholz began his study on pyelitis. Edwards A. Park first appeared in a review and A. Graeme Mitchell as a contributor. During 1917 and 1918 the effect of the war apparently made a great deal of difference. There did appear a number of papers on chemical subjects in Volume XIII, 1917, but the size of the Journal was reduced and the effect of the war is shown by the fact that in Volume XVI, 1918, there were several articles in the October issue dealing with the work of the Children's bureau of the American Red Cross in France.

In 1919, Dr. Churchill left Chicago to take up his home in Massachusetts and was replaced on the Editorial Board by Dr. Henry F. Helmholz who became the Chief Editor. In November of this year in Volume XVIII, there appeared the first monograph by Park and McClure on the thymus. In 1920, John L. Morse was replaced by Fritz B. Talbot on the Board and in Volume XX of that year there appeared the first article by Grover Powers.

In 1921, Volume XXII, occurred two articles which were definitely to influence the practice of pediatrics. The first was by Cooke on the "Ammoniacal Diaper" and the second was by Brenneman on "Abdominal Pain." These two articles have shown their practicality throughout the years and have resulted in much benefit to pediatrics. In 1922 Volume XXIV appeared the first book reviews and at this time Dr. E. E. Graham was replaced by Dr. W. McKim Marriott. In 1923 Volume XXV appeared for the first time the names Toomey and L. Emmett Holt, Jr.; and in Volume XXVI, Weech and James Wilson, who are at present on the Editorial Board.

In 1924, Dr. Helmholz went to the Mayo Clinic and Dr. L. Emmett Holt, Sr. died. Dr. David M. Cowie was succeeded by the author and Dr. L. Emmett Holt, Sr., by Oscar M. Schloss. At this time the Trustees of the American Medical Association requested a change, an enlargement of the scope of the Journal. The résumés were continued but unfortunately those on tuberculosis ceased due to the death of May Michael. Book reviews, News and Comment, and Society Transactions began to appear and abstracts of current literature were stressed. An attempt was made to cover the current literature on pediatrics, an attempt which was fairly successful be-

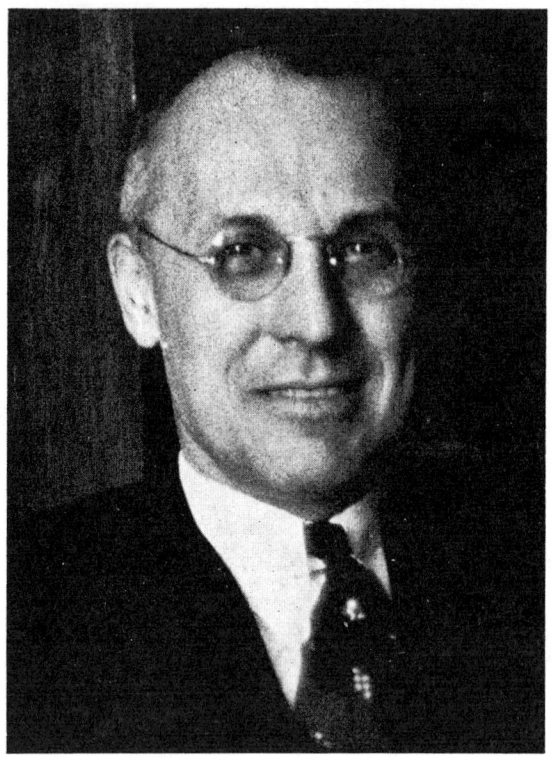

Henry F. Helmholz, M.D.
Chief Editor, The American Journal of Diseases of Children, 1919.

cause of the active cooperation of many of the younger men going into pediatrics and of the older men who could find the time for abstracting.

In October of 1924 Volume XXVIII, for the first time appeared the transactions of the American Pediatric Society. These had previously appeared in the Archives of Pediatrics but owing to a change in policy on the part of the Society it was decided to publish the papers in abstract together with the discussions in the American Journal of Diseases of Children. In this number it is interesting to note that W. H. Parke and Zingher published an article on "Diphtheria Immunization in New York City" which was most timely and it is probably due to these two authors that there has been such an extensive use of immunization procedures in this country. Immunization procedures which are now adopted by all the armies of the world have not been used as extensively in any other country as they have in the United States. Apparently the period of adolescence had gradually been outgrown and the Journal was beginning to take on

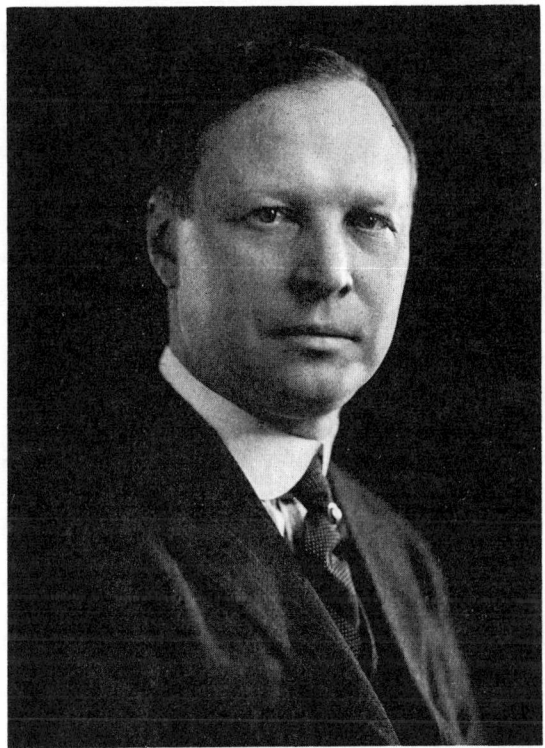

Clifford G. Grulee, M.D.
Editorial Board, The American Journal of Diseases of Children.

its full maturity. It is doubtful whether this meant that more outstanding articles were to appear since many of the articles already mentioned may be regarded as some of the milestones in American pediatrics. However, from now on the Journal took a more scientific turn. Following the war and the resulting prosperity, more time and money were devoted to scientific investigation. This was taken advantage of by pediatricians and most of the scientific articles were published in the American Journal of Diseases of Children. For instance, the respiratory metabolism studies of Sam Levine and his co-workers appeared in 1926, Volume XXXI, and in 1926, Volume XXXII, Hartmann began his chemical studies, Aldrich his work on nephritis, Powers his work on intestinal intoxication and the name of Joseph Stokes first appeared and in that year, too, the pediatric profession had a grave loss. John Howland who had meant so much to American pediatrics died before his time but not before he had made a profound impression on American pediatrics and founded a new school really in that branch of medicine. It was in this year that L. R. DeBuys came on the Editorial Board.

In 1927, Volume XXXIII Sanford's first studies on the newborn appeared and Lynne A. Hoag who started with so much promise first appears here. His untimely death unfortunately occurred not much later. In 1927 Volume XXXIII appeared first in the March number the Directory of Pediatric Socities. In Volume XXXIV of the same year occurred the outstanding article by Thomas Cooley of Detroit on "Anemia in Children." This was the original article on the so-called Cooley's anemia. In this volume, too, appeared for the first time MacIntosh, Casparis and McQuarrie. In the beginning of 1928 in Volume XXXV Ruhräh started his pediatric biographies which carried through for several years and in the second volume for that year appeared the article by Clara Davis on the "Self Selection of Diets for Children" and Wallgren's first article on tuberculosis. Darrow appeared for the first time. John C. Gittings was taken on the Editorial Board in this year. In 1929 Volume XXXVIII McQuarrie's article on water metabolism in epilepsy has received a great deal of attention.

Soon after this the Journal began to expand in size so that it became almost unwieldy. By Volume XLIX, 1935, it had reached 1692 pages. This was the largest volume that was published.

The first of Icie Macy's human milk studies occurred in 1931 Volume XLII and the succeeding years were marked by the presentation, by her and her co-workers, of many different subjects, especially on chemical analysis. The first report of the American Board of Pediatrics occurred in Volume LI in 1936. In 1937 McKim Marriott died and his unexpired term was filled by Dr. A. G. Mitchell. In 1938 appeared in Progress in Pediatrics an outstanding article by Dorothy H. Andersen on "Cystic Fibrosis of the Pancreas," and in the next year Volume LVII the article by McIntosh and Donovan on the "Disturbances of Rotation of the Intestinal Tract." Following this, in Volume LIX in 1938 was the article by Hilde Bruch on "Obesity." All of these three articles have been most stimulating. In 1939 Horton Casparis replaced L. R. DeBuys on the Board and in 1940 Dr. F. S. Smyth succeeded Dr. John C. Gittings. In 1942 appeared the obituary of Kenneth Blackfan and this volume, too, marked our first year in World War II.

The Journal by this time had reduced to 1,200 pages per volume. In the latter part of this year the obituary of Casparis appeared. 1943 was marked as a year of the beginning of shortages and the format of the Journal was changed to a larger page with smaller print. This later was changed again to a double column page. The paper was much thinner than had been used previously. Of course during this period the abstracts were reduced in number due to the fact that there was almost a cessation of scientific work in the rest of the world. In Volume LXV of 1943 appeared the first of Warkany's articles on "Malformation Induced by Diet," and in LXVI the last of Brenneman's articles. In Volume LXVI, too, in this year appeared the outstanding contribution of Hattie E. Alexander on the "Treatment of Influenzal Meningitis." Brenneman's obituary appeared in Volume LXVIII in 1944 and in 1945 Volume LXIX appeared the first of the series of articles on the celiac syndrome by Dorothy H. Andersen. In 1943 Dr. James L. Wilson had succeeded to the Board on the death of Dr. Casparis and in the same year Dr. A. A. Weech had replaced Dr. Mitchell who had died in that year.

This is the chronicle of the American Journal of Diseases of Children. There are other names such as those of Bret Ratner and the Bakwins whose outstanding contributions have been much appreciated and it is altogether likely that the judgment of the author might not be upheld by some of his colleagues and perhaps by the future of pediatrics. Judgments differ and it is oftentimes hard to tell what will and what will not be of outstanding importance.

The Editorial Board is at present constituted as follows:

Dr. A. A. Weech	1946	Dr. Clifford G. Grulee	1948
Dr. Francis Scott Smyth	1946	Dr. Oscar M. Schloss	1949
Dr. H. F. Helmholz	1947	Dr. Fritz B. Talbot	1950
	Dr. James Leroy Wilson	1951	

The American Journal of Diseases of Children has not been, in one sense, a national journal. In looking through the numbers one finds contributions from all over the world: In addition to many contributions from Canada, England, France, Germany, Russia, Italy, Holland, Sweden, Denmark, Norway, Spain, Greece, Poland, Japan, China, Netherlands East Indies, Brazil, Argentina, Chile, Cuba and Mexico, are among the nations whose pediatricians have contributed to the success of this Journal. Throughout the years it has maintained a high standard, accepting only those articles which were of high scientific value or definite clinical import. It has attempted to cover the literature of the world in its abstracts and has, now and then, had articles of a definitely cultural value such as Ruhräh's articles on pediatric biographies and on pediatrics in art. For the last several years with the growth of American medicine it has probably held the outstanding position in pediatrics in the world. Repeatedly I have been told so by foreign observers. It has come through two World Wars without lowering its standards and while it has at times been reduced in size it has never accepted material which could be regarded as "padding." There have been times when the criticism has been raised that the Journal was not sufficiently scientific and that it should contain only scientific articles. Those who maintain such a position probably forget that the value of a journal depends to a certain extent not only upon the articles which are contributed to it but upon the people who read it and that only where there are sufficiently large numbers of readers in the main does the average contributor of excellent articles wish to publish his contribution. The few advertisements which have been published with the Journal have always been of high order and carefully scrutinized by the American Medical Association. It has published from time to time the transactions of the American Pediatric Society, the American Society of Pediatric Research and of many of the local societies, notably those of New York City, Philadelphia and Chicago. Withal, while it has been essentially a scientific Journal it has had appeal to the higher type of practitioner of pediatrics. He has not had to go through the literature of several journals to be able to obtain the gist of pediatric thought in the world. It has always maintained, so far as I can determine, a very fair editorial judgment. Its Editorial Board has looked on the contributions without bias or favor. They have usually been constructively critical and this without exception during the period when I have acted as its Chief Editor. All articles are submitted to at least two members of the Editorial Board and these two members must not reside in the city from which the articles come. Every attempt has been made to judge every contribution on its merit and, rarely has an article appeared which has suffered criticism from the standpoint of scientific inadequacy. On the whole the Journal may be said to have become a leader in American and, therefore, world pediatrics and it is to be hoped that down the years it may maintain the high standard which has been part of its being.

ARCHIVES OF OTOLARYNGOLOGY

By George M. Coates, M.D.

THERE WERE TWO AMERICAN journals devoted to otolaryngology in 1923, well established and popular with the profession. For many years previously other journals had appeared, prospered for a few years and disappeared, leaving only a memory among the older otolaryngologists. In the year above mentioned, however, there was a growing sentiment among the members of the profession interested in diseases of the ear, nose and throat that the time was ripe for the introduction of a new journal, not privately owned, in which advertising should be strictly ethical according to the standards of the American Medical Association, in which only council accepted products could be advertised and the pages of which should be open especially to research reports, although also containing enough clinical material to make it acceptable to the average reader.

In accordance with these views, at the business meeting of the Section on Laryngology, Otology and Rhinology of the American Medical Association held in Boston in June 1923, the following resolution was introduced by Dr. Charles W. Richardson of Washington, D. C.:

Resolved: By the Section on Laryngology, Otology and Rhinology of the American Medical Association in session assembled that the Board of Trustees of the Association be requested to establish a monthly journal pertaining to the specialty of otology and laryngology.

Dr. Richardson moved adoption of this resolution; after due discussion the motion was seconded by Dr. Wendell C. Phillips of New York and Dr. Robert Levy of Denver and unanimously carried. It is understood that the petition to the Board of Trustees was signed by a large majority of those attending the session. This petition was received by the Board at this same meeting and it was unanimously decided to concur with the petitioners' request at the earliest feasible date.

At the meeting of the Board of Trustees in February 1924, the following physicians, all distinguished men and leaders in the profession, were elected to constitute the Editorial Board of the Archives of Otolaryngology: Dr. George E. Shambaugh, Chicago, Chairman; Dr. Isidore Friesner, New York; Dr. Chevalier Jackson, Philadelphia; Dr. Robert C. Lynch, New Orleans; Dr. Greenfield Sluder, St. Louis, and Dr. Eugene A. Crockett, Boston. According to the recollection of the writer, an informal canvass of the members of the two senior societies, namely the American Otological Society and the American Laryngological Association, was made to obtain suggestions for appointments to this Editorial Board. It is probable that the Trustees acted in accordance with the information thus obtained. At all events the situation met with the entire approbation of the profession, and the new journal was launched under favorable auspices. All of the members of the Editorial Board were among the best known American specialists; all were active in the deliberations of the national societies, and their writings and research had made their names "household words": Isidore Friesner, co-author of two widely read books on the Labyrinth and Brain Abscess, head of the department of otolaryngology at Mt. Sinai Hospital, New York City, and later secretary and president of the American Otological Society; Chevalier Jackson, internationally known for his pioneer work in broncho-esophagology, author of many textbooks and monographs, at various times professor of broncho-esophagology in Jefferson Medical College, University of Pennsylvania Medical School and Graduate School of Medicine, Temple University Medical School and Woman's Medical College of Pennsylvania, of which later he became president; Robert Clyde Lynch, New Orleans, an original member of the American Board of Otolaryngology and head of department in Tulane University, one of the popular writers of the day; Greenfield Sluder of St. Louis, author of Lower Half Headaches, inventor of new systems of tonsillectomy, ethmoidectomy, treatment of middle ear disease and appropriate instruments, who was president of the American Laryngological Association and professor of otolaryngology in Washington University Medical School; Eugene A. Crockett, professor of otology in the Medical School of Harvard University and president of the American Otological Society, one of the best known otologists in America. It is of record that it was understood by the Board of Trustees that the Chairman of the Editorial Board would endeavor to promote further action by all the special societies of otolaryngology throughout the country in regard to the proposed journal of otolaryngology. The subscription price was fixed at $6.00 a year and has remained so until the present time.

With this able Board behind him, Dr. Shambaugh, as Chairman

or Chief Editor, drew up plans for the new venture and prepared to begin publication early in 1925. To Dr. Shambaugh belongs all the credit for perfecting the organization of the Archives and making it the successful publication that it has been from the first issue. The format has been unchanged except for a short period during World War II and all of the departments inaugurated by him have been maintained. On the third cover of each issue appears the following announcement:

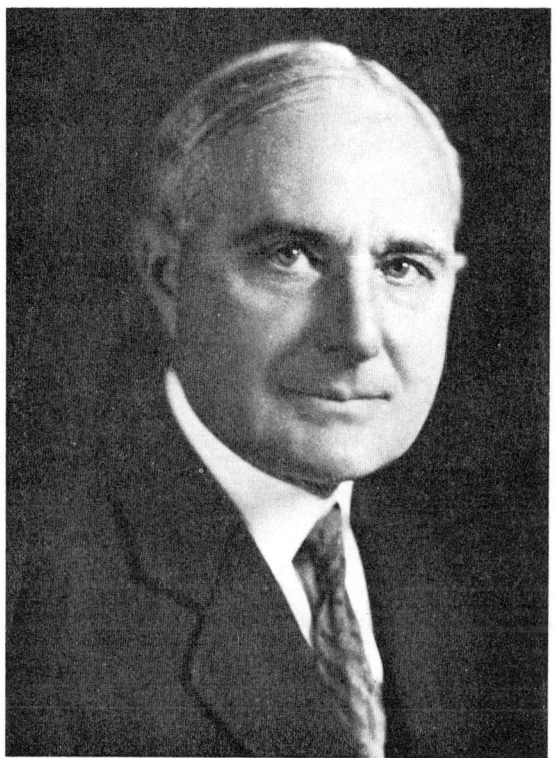

George E. Shambaugh, M.D.
Chief Editor, Archives of Otolaryngology.

"The Archives of Otolaryngology is published by the American Medical Association to stimulate research in the field of otology and laryngology and to disseminate knowledge in this department of medicine.

"Manuscripts for publication, books for review and correspondence relating to the editorial management should be sent to the Chief Editor or to any other member of the Editorial Board. Communications regarding subscriptions, reprints, etc., should be addressed to the Archives of Otolaryngology, American Medical Association, 535 N. Dearborn St., Chicago 10, Ill."

Then follow some rules for the preparation of manuscripts, footnotes and bibliography. These rules were established by the Board of Trustees for all journals published by or under the auspices of the American Medical Association. The actual editing of manuscript is done in the offices of the Association in Chicago by an able and well trained corps of assistants, under the direction of Miss J. F. Whelan, to whom the present Chief Editor wishes to make grateful acknowledgment for their invaluable assistance.

The first issue of the Archives of Otolaryngology was in January 1925 and consisted of 130 pages. Dr. Shambaugh had obtained papers from a distinguished group of writers for the first issue, and the other departments had been developed much as they are today. Besides the original articles, there was printed each month a summary of all available literature for the past year on one of twelve subjects, as follows: Functional Examination of Hearing, originally written by Dr. Robert Sonnenschein and now by Dr. Alfred Lewy; Physiology of Ear Including Vestibular Reactions, by Dr. Philip E. Meltzer and now by Drs. John Richardson, Edgar M. Holmes and Werner Mueller; Endoscopy, by Dr. Louis Clerf; Tonsils and Adenoids, Dr. Arthur W. Proetz and Dr. French K. Hansel, now by Dr. J. D. Singleton; Benign and Malignant Growths, Dr. Gordon B. New; Otosclerosis and Labyrinth Disease, Dr. J. K. M. Dickie, of Canada, now by Dr. George E. Shambaugh Jr.; Intracranial Complications, Dr. Wells P. Eagleton; Accessory Sinuses, Dr. Samuel Salinger; Suppurative Otitis Media and Complications, Dr. S. J. Kopetzky, now by Dr. Ben R. Dysart; Plastic Surgery, Dr. J. Eastman Sheehan, now by Dr. Lyndon A. Peer; Hay Fever, Allergy and Allied Conditions, Dr. W. W. Duke and E. L. MacQuiddy; and Tubercular Diseases, by Dr. George B. Wood, now by Dr. George E. Wilson. News and comments of interest to subscribers, book reviews, abstracts from current literature, transactions of national and local societies, clinical notes, case reports, descriptions of new instruments and a directory of national societies, giving the names and addresses of their officers and the meeting dates, also are published monthly.

The following table of contents of the first issue will be of interest:

CONTENTS OF VOLUME 1

January 1925. Number 1

The Relation of Endocrine Glands to the Disorders of the Ear, Nose and Throat.. 1
    A. J. CARLSON, M.D., CHICAGO

The Technic of Operations for Abscess of the Brain.......................... 14
  CHARLES A. ELSBERG, M.D., NEW YORK
The Treatment of Brain Abscess: A Surgical Technic in Which the Usual Drainage
  Methods Are Avoided... 26
  JOSEPH E. J. KING, M.D., NEW YORK
The Present Status of the Intranasal Ethmoid Operation...................... 42
  JOHN A. PRATT, M.D., MINNEAPOLIS
Results of Treatment of Carcinoma of the Esophagus by the Combined Use of
  Radium Emanations and the Deep Roentgen Ray: Report of Sixteen Patients
  Treated at the Massachusetts General Hospital and Huntington Memorial
  Hospital... 51
  D. CROSBY GREENE, M.D., BOSTON
Further Statistics on Chlorin Gas as a Treatment for Respiratory Diseases....... 58
  MARVIN F. JONES, M.D., and CHARLES GAROFALO, M.D., NEW YORK
Bacteriologic Study of the Nasopharynx in Patients Treated with Chlorin Inha-
  lations.. 64
  MARJORIE B. PATTERSON, NEW YORK
The Treatment of Papilloma of the Larynx by Fulguration and Diathermy...... 70
  THOMAS HUBBARD, M.D., and EVAN G. GALBRAITH, M.D., TOLEDO, OHIO
Some Aspects of the Problem of the Testing of Audition, with Demonstration of a
  New Portable Apparatus.. 79
  FREDERICK W. KRANX, PH.D., GENEVA, ILL.
The Functional Examination of Hearing. Annual Summary on the Problems of the
  Deaf, Papers Relating to Deaf-Mutism and Education of Deaf Children, Me-
  chanical Devices for Hearing, Lip Reading and so forth................... 89
  ROBERT SONNENSCHEIN, M.D., CHICAGO

News and Comment:
  American Board of Otolaryngology....................................... 109
  American Federation of Organization for the Hard of Hearing............. 109
  Postgraduate Course in Otolaryngology in Bourdeaux...................... 110
Abstracts from Current Literature 111
Society Transactions 116
Book Reviews 129

Under News and Comments, the following description of the formation of the American Board of Otolaryngology is given. It will be noted that Dr. Shambaugh was the prime mover in the establishment of the Board (the second of the national boards, that of ophthalmology having preceded it by some years) and presided at the first meeting, but that he declined membership after the Board was favorably organized:

NEWS AND COMMENT

The American Board of Otolaryngology, for whose organization Dr. George E. Shambaugh was responsible, met at his invitation, on November 10 at the University Club of Chicago, for the purpose of organizing a board of directors.

The American Board of Otolaryngology was organized, with the following as members of the first Board of Directors: Dr. H. P. Mosher, Boston, president; Dr. F. R. Spencer, Boulder, Colo., vice-president; Dr. H. W. Loeb, St. Louis, secretary-treasurer; Dr. J. C. Beck, Chicago; Dr. T. E. Carmody, Denver (absent); Dr. T. H. Halsted, Syracuse,

N. Y.; Dr. R. C. Lynch, New Orleans; Dr. B. R. Shurly, Detroit; Dr. R. H. Skillern, Philadelphia, and Dr. W. P. Wherry, Omaha.

The Board of Directors are the representatives of the five national otolaryngological associations: The American Otological Society, the American Laryngological Association, The American Laryngological, Rhinological and Otological Society, The American Academy of Ophthalmology and Otolaryngology and the Section on Laryngology, Otology and Rhinology of the American Medical Association.

The object of the Association is to elevate the standard of otolaryngology; to familiarize the public with its aims and ideals; to protect the public against irresponsible and unqualified practitioners; to receive applications for examination in otolaryngology; to conduct examination of such applicants; to issue certificates of qualification in otolaryngology, and to perform such duties as will advance the cause of otolaryngology.

The first examination will be held at the time of the meeting of the American Medical Association.

The work of the Board, examination into the qualifications of those who desire to be recognized as specialists and the issuing of certificates, will, it is believed, have a wide-reaching effect. In the first place, it will have the effect of educating the medical public to a better appreciation of what should be undertaken in the way of preparation by those who take up this line of work. The certificate should aid the public in much needed discrimination between the man properly prepared to practice the specialty and those who without sufficient preparation are willing to pose as specialists. Hospital managements should welcome the movement, as it will aid them not only in determining the selection of men to serve in the Department of Otolaryngology but in determining what men shall be allowed to bring patients into the hospital for nose and throat operations. Hospital managements who desire to make their institutions places in which patients can be assured of receiving competent service in matters relating to otolaryngology can do so by insisting that the men who are to practice otolaryngology in the hospital hold the certificate from the American Board of Otolaryngology.

The names of the abstractors for the first volume are given below, as well as those serving at present. All available literature, foreign and domestic, came under their observation and that of sufficient interest was ably abstracted. None of the original abstractors has continued this arduous work until the present time.

Dr. Robertson, Chicago
   Schulhof, Chicago
   McNally, Montreal
   Snapf, Grand Rapids
   Amberg, Detroit

Dr. Vail, Cincinnati
   Connor, St. Paul
   Bort, Chicago
   Lewy, Chicago
   Lepidus, Chicago

At the present time the corps of abstractors includes:

Dr. M. Valentine Miller, Philadelphia
   A. H. Persky, Philadelphia
   Wm. J. Hitschler, Philadelphia
   William Gordon, Philadelphia
   A. P. Seltzer, Philadelphia
   George E. Lieberman, Philadelphia
   Edw. H. Campbell, Philadelphia
   Francis W. Davison, Danville, Pa.
   Stanton A. Friedberg, Chicago
   Robert L. Goodale, Boston
   W. E. Grove, Milwaukee
   H. James Hara, Los Angeles
   Milton L. Jennes, Waterbury, Conn.

Dr. Karsten Kettel, Denmark
   Francis L. Lederer, Chicago
   F. E. LeJeune, New Orleans
   Robert B. Lewy, Chicago
   Romeo A. Luongo, Philadelphia
   Albert F. Moriconi, Trenton
   Leroy A. Schall, Boston
   Ernest M. Seydell, Wichita, Kansas
   J. D. Singleton, Dallas, Texas
   Pierre Viole, Los Angeles
   Irving W. Voorhees, New York
   Earl L. Wood, Newark, N. J.
   E. W. Palmer, Wichita, Kansas

Having established the Archives of Otolaryngology in 1925 and guided it most successfully for the first twelve years of its existence, Dr. Shambaugh retired in 1937. He had done a magnificent piece of editing and made his journal, almost single handed, one of the outstanding publications of the world. It was due to his wise planning, foresightedness, hard work and acquaintance with the leading members of the profession. To his eminence in all other lines of otolaryngologic endeavors, to his ability and skill, the Archives will always remain as a monument. An editorial in the Archives on the occasion of his retirement expresses the feeling not only of the American Medical Association and of the Editorial Board of the Archives but of the otolaryngologic branch of the medical profession as well:

EDITOR OF THE ARCHIVES

"With the current issue, Dr. George Elmer Shambaugh, Editor of the Archives of Otolaryngology since its establishment in 1925, retires as Editor-in-Chief, to be succeeded by Dr. George M. Coates of Philadelphia. Under the editorship of Dr. Shambaugh, the Archives has assumed a special position in the field of otolaryngologic literature. Established by the Board of Trustees primarily with the purpose of advancing the specialty of otolaryngology and of making available a periodical not in any way dependent on the advertising and promotion of products disapproved by the Council on Pharmacy and Chemistry, the Archives has been concerned largely with the publication of reports of research, some of them monographic in scope, in the otolaryngologic field. As a leader in the advancement of the highest scientific ideals in his field, Dr. George Elmer Shambaugh, as editor, has been instrumental in defining this position. His association with the certifying board in the field of otolaryngology is generally well known. Dr. Shambaugh has been professor of otolaryngology and head of that department in Rush Medical College since 1916, and also otologist and laryngologist of the Presbyterian Hospital since 1902. His eminence has been attested by his being elected president of the American Otological Society and of the American Laryngological Association, and by his membership in every other important special group in this field.

"Among other contributions to his field are his articles entitled 'Investigation of Blood Supply of the Internal Ear' and 'Embryology and Histology of End Organs in Labyrinth of Ear.' In 1912, he was awarded the Lenval prize for his research on the internal ear. In making this acknowledgment of his services, the Board of Trustees of the American Medical Association tenders to Dr. George

Elmer Shambaugh its utmost appreciation for his contribution to the advancement of the Archives of Otolaryngology."

Other changes have taken place in the Editorial Board.

On the death of Dr. Sluder in 1928, Dr. George Fetterolf of Philadelphia was elected to fill the unexpired term of one year. Dr. Fetterolf was professor and head of the department in the University of Pennsylvania. He was reelected for a six year term in 1929 but died in 1932, and was succeeded by Dr. George M. Coates

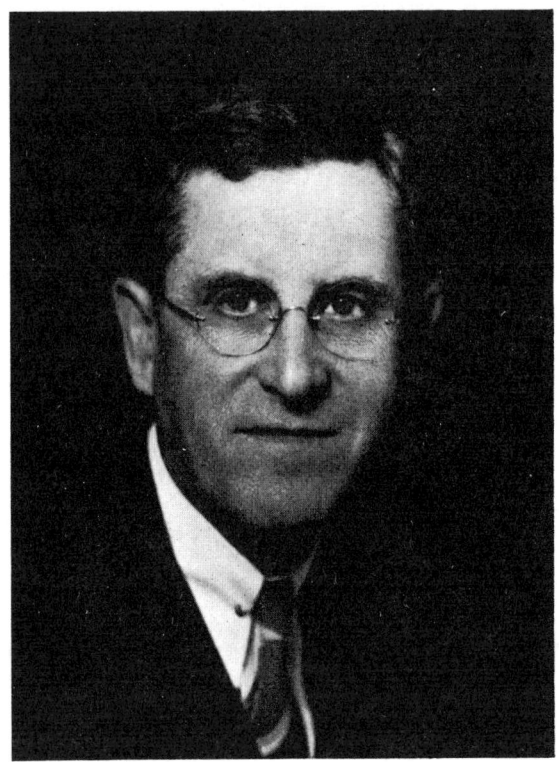

George M. Coates, M.D.
Chief Editor, Archives of Otolaryngology.

of Philadelphia. Dr. Crockett served for five years and was succeeded in 1930 by Dr. Ralph A. Fenton of Portland, Ore., a Trustee of the American Medical Association, a director of the Board of Otolaryngology and professor of otolaryngology in the University of Oregon. Dr. Robert Clyde Lynch died in 1931 and his unexpired term of three years was filled by Dr. John F. Barnhill, professor and head of the department of the University of Indiana School of Medicine, author of textbooks and past president of the

American Laryngological Association, the American Academy of Ophthalmology and Otolaryngology and the American Laryngological, Rhinological and Otological Society. Dr. Shambaugh was succeeded in 1937 by Dr. William P. Wherry of Omaha, Nebr., secretary-treasurer of the American Board of Otolaryngology, executive secretary of the American Academy of Ophthalmology and Otolaryngology and professor of otolaryngology in the University of Nebraska Medical School. He died in 1942 and was succeeded by Dr. Ernest M. Seydell, Wichita, Kansas, former president of the American Otological Society and a director of the American Board. In 1939 Dr. James A. Babbitt, Philadelphia, was elected an additional member of the Board and served until his death in 1944. He had been clinical professor of otolaryngology in the Medical School and Graduate School of Medicine, University of Pennsylvania, the secretary, treasurer and president of the American Laryngological Association, and president of the American Laryngological, Rhinological and Otological Society and of the American Academy of Ophthalmology and Otolaryngology. He was succeeded by Dr. Robert L. Goodale, Boston, a distinguished member of the Boston profession. On the death of Dr. Barnhill in 1943, Dr. Carl H. McCaskey was elected in his place. Dr. McCaskey holds the chair in the University of Indiana formerly occupied and made famous by Dr. Barnhill and is a director of the American Board. In 1941, Dr. J. Mackenzie Brown, Los Angeles, was elected an additional Board member. Dr. Brown is professor and head of the department in the Medical School of the University of Southern California and is a former president of the American Laryngological, Rhinological and Otological Society. Dr. Friesner, a member of the original Board, died in 1946 and was succeeded by Dr. Westley M. Hunt, New York City, a director of the American Board; otologist to St. Luke's Hospital; professor of clinical otology, New York University; president of the New York League for the Hard of Hearing, and member of all the national special societies.

The present Editorial Board of the Archives is composed as follows (figures in brackets denote the date of expiration of the present 6 year term):

Dr. George M. Coates, Chief Editor (1952)   Dr. Ernest M. Seydell (1949)
    Carl H. McCaskey (1946)   Westley M. Hunt (1950)
    J. Mackenzie Brown (1952)   Chevalier Jackson (1951)
    Ralph A. Fenton (1948)   Robert L. Goodale (1951)

ARCHIVES OF DERMATOLOGY AND SYPHILOLOGY

By Howard Fox, M.D., Sc.D.

WITH REMARKS BY MEMBERS OF THE EDITORIAL BOARD

DUE TO HIS FORESIGHT, Dr. William Allen Pusey conducted negotiations whereby the former Journal of Cutaneous Diseases was taken over by the American Medical Association, thus relieving its sponsors of a heavy financial burden. The name of the former Journal was then changed to the Archives of Dermatology and Syphilology. It has continued to be the official journal of the American Dermatological Association, an organization regarded as the most select body of dermatologists in this country (founded in 1876).

AN APPRECIATION OF DR. WILLIAM ALLEN PUSEY

In 1937, a series of 7 articles occupying 60 pages appeared in the Archives paying tribute to the many phases of Dr. Pusey's life. The authors of these tributes were Drs. Olin West, Morris Fishbein, D. J. Davis, James B. Herrick, Herbert Rattner and Mr. Rufus C. Dawes. It is rare that a man has the opportunity to read so many complimentary remarks about himself, all of which were richly deserved.

The article by Dr. Fishbein was entitled "William Allen Pusey, the Editor" from which the following is quoted: "The Archives of Dermatology and Syphilology under his [Dr. Pusey's] editorship has come to occupy a place in the very forefront of dermatologic literature throughout the world. Indeed there is probably no other single dermatologic publication anywhere else in the world so completely meeting the needs of the dermatologist for announcements of research in his field, clinical reports, news, editorial comment, the proceedings of dermatologic societies and abstracts of the significant dermatologic literature."

Dr. Pusey was a scholar, a born leader, a gifted writer, a forceful speaker and a public spirited citizen. He was of course a great dermatologist as well. Dr. Pusey was a courageous man who was never afraid to express his honest opinion. He had an unusual combination of forcefulness and tact, and he was a kindly man, especially with inexperienced and young colleagues. As editor, he occasionally accepted papers which were not quite up to his standard of excellence because the authors were young men who needed encouragement or perhaps lacked opportunities afforded by large medical centers.

That Dr. Pusey was a scholar was natural for a man who had been valedictorian of his class at Vanderbilt University. As a leader in organized medicine, he became president of the Chicago Medical Society and later President of the American Medical Association, the only dermatologist who has ever held this great honor. In writing of Dr. Pusey's presidency Dr. Olin West said "The Association has had no more faithful, no more intensely earnest, active and efficient officer than he."

Among his civic activities was membership in the executive committee of the National Research Council. He also was proud of being one of the 11 members of the executive committee of the Board of Trustees of the Century of Progress Exposition in Chicago. During World War I, he did his part by serving as chairman of the Committee on Venereal Diseases in the Surgeon General's Office.

Dr. Pusey's ability to make friends was greatly aided by his delightful sense of humor. It was his influence for good, which he exerted over his colleagues, which made him great. Probably the greatest thing he did for the dermatologic profession was his aid in establishing the Archives of Dermatology and Syphilology in 1920.

THE EDITORIAL BOARD

The Editorial Board should really be called the Advisory Board; until recently its members have functioned largely in an honorary capacity. This was true of the Editorial Board of the Journal of Cutaneous Diseases, when practically all the work was done by the editor. It was also largely true of Dr. Pusey's regime on the Archives, as most of the work was done by him and his former assistant, Dr. Herbert Rattner, who had charge of the abstracts and society transactions. At least it can be said that all who have served on both boards were distinguished dermatologists whose names added prestige to the publication they represented.

In recent years the specialty of dermatology has become more and more complex and technical, with the advancements in physical therapy, histopathology, mycology, allergy and syphilis. I have therefore often submitted original articles of extreme technicality at times to members of the Board who were especially versed in these subjects. I have received prompt and invaluable help, especially from Drs. Cole, MacKee and Weidman and recently also from Dr. O'Leary. Although I appreciated the knowledge of Dr. Lane, I spared him as much as possible on account of his time consuming work as secretary of the American Board of Dermatology and Syphilology from its inception until this year. I might add that all the present members of the Editorial Board except one and also two former members, Drs. Schamberg and Dennie, were members of the American Board of Dermatology and Syphilology. Dr. Herbert Rattner has had charge of the abstract department during my regime and has done excellent and painstaking work.

I would also like to express my thanks to several New York men who were not members of the Editorial Board but on whom I have called at times for opinions. These included Drs. George M. Lewis, Emanuel Muskatblit, H. Victor Mendelsohn, David Bloom, Maurice J. Costello, Herman Sharlit and Fred Wise.

Dr. William T. Corlett is the only living member of the original Editorial Board of both the Journal of Cutaneous Diseases in 1904 and the Archives of Dermatology and Syphilology in 1920. He retired from the latter board in 1935, his place being taken by Dr. Harold N. Cole. He served for years, with distinction, as professor of dermatology in the Western Reserve University. He is now the oldest living dermatologist in the United States and one of the most respected and beloved. He makes the following remarks about the Archives: "I have before me a list of the Editorial Board of the Journal of Cutaneous Diseases Including Syphilis in 1904 and of the Archives of Dermatology and Syphilology in 1920. I know all the men who served on both boards and I regard them as outstanding in the profession. They were the younger men, as I recall it, of the older American Dermatological Association."

The other original members of the Editorial Board of the Archives of Dermatology and Syphilology were Drs. Martin F. Engman of St. Louis, Milton B. Hartzell of Philadelphia, George M. MacKee of New York, William Allen Pusey of Chicago (Chief Editor) and Charles J. White of Boston.

Dr. Engman, like practically all who served as members of the Editorial Board, was a professor of dermatology and leader in his community. One of his outstanding accomplishments was the founding of the Barnard Free Skin and Cancer Hospital, of which he has been the chief for many years. Dr. Engman is also one of the few dermatologists in this country whose son has followed in his father's specialty. Dr. Engman retired as a member of the Board in 1939, his place being taken by Dr. Charles C. Dennie.

Dr. Milton B. Hartzell was professor of dermatology in the University of Pennsylvania, but unfortunately did not hand his talents to posterity, as he was a bachelor. After his death in 1927, he was replaced by Dr. Jay Frank Schamberg.

Dr. Schamberg served on the Board until his untimely death in 1934, when he was replaced by Dr. Frederick Weidman. In addition to his scientific work of the highest class, Dr. Schamberg took an active interest in organized medicine and served as president of the Philadelphia County Medical Society and was a charter member of the American Board of Dermatology and Syphilology.

Dr. Charles J. White followed in the footsteps of his illustrious father, Dr. James C. White, by becoming professor of dermatology in Harvard University. Dr. White's son has become a distinguished surgeon. Unfortunately for us, he did not take up dermatology and thus carry the famous name of White into the third generation of dermatologists. Dr. White retired from the Board in 1936, his place being taken by Dr. Howard Fox. Dr. White has written the following complimentary remarks about the Archives and its editors: "As a faithful and admiring reader of the Archives of Dermatology and Syphilology, it gives me great pleasure to feel that the editors of this old journal have given us in the past, and especially in the last decade, a worthy medical volume quite the equal of the former preeminent German Archives and the French Annales. Now we can surely say that our American Archives is at the top and we owe this preeminence to the large number of American workers and to the able editors who assemble this work of modern research in so compact and presentable a form."

Dr. George M. MacKee not only has served on the Editorial Board of the Archives since its inception but had previously been editor of the Journal of Cutaneous Diseases from 1909 to 1920. Dr. MacKee's knowledge of x-rays and other physical modalities has made him an invaluable member of our Board. He was a charter member of the Council on Physical Medicine of the American Medical Association and has been a member of local and national societies dealing with x-rays and radium. His book on "X-Rays and Radium in the Treatment of Diseases of the Skin" is now in its fourth edition and has no equal. He served under Dr. Fordyce at the New York University as clinical assistant and later at Columbia University as chief of clinic, assistant and finally full professor. He went to the New York Post-Graduate Medical School as full professor in 1933 and later, when the Skin and Cancer Hospital was taken over, he became director and has held this position to the present.

Dr. MacKee's many honors include the presidency of the American Dermatological Association and of numerous other societies. He is now president of the American Academy of Dermatology and Syphilology. He has written 4 books and 13 chapters of other books and is a corresponding or honorary member of 7 foreign dermatologic societies.

Perhaps Dr. MacKee's greatest achievement was to create the largest and most important department in the country for graduate teaching of dermatology, where he has a staff of 117 physicians and 70 nurses, technicians and clerks. He has directed an enormous amount of investigational activity and yet has found time to write and collaborate on books in dermatology and radiology. He has a keen analytic mind and has the happy faculty of supervising a large group of workers, of keeping them all busy, happy and satisfied.

Dr. MacKee's long editorial experience adds to the value of the following remarks he makes about the Archives: "The American Medical Association should be given credit for a generous and exceedingly important contribution to dermatology in taking over the publication of the indispensable Journal of Cutaneous Diseases. In spite of a global war, which has caused a shortage of manpower and paper and in spite also of social unrest, which has caused strikes, the Archives has not missed an issue and at no time has its size been injuriously reduced.

"The Archives has been and is the most important dermatologic journal in this country. Years ago, the articles published in the German and French dermatologic journals were, on the whole, superior to those published in this country. That is no longer so. At present, the Archives is probably the best dermatologic periodical in the world. There are a number of reasons for this change: Some of these are (1) Two world wars, social unrest and global chaos. (2) American dermatology has advanced tremendously in the last 2 or 3 decades and along scientific lines. Now, there is a large percentage of articles by dermatologists based on creative research, involving all the basic medical sciences. This is of the utmost importance, because it brings medicine into dermatology rather than having medicine absorb our specialty. (3) The present Chief Editor has used excellent judgment in accepting only articles of merit, whether clinical or based on laboratory or other research.

"The first Editor-in-Chief, Dr. Pusey, was a pioneer in roentgen therapy. His book, with Caldwell, was an important contribution at the time. You know his other books and articles. I remember him mostly because of kindness to young men, geniality and common sense."

In every way, the standard of the Archives has been high: ethics, literary style, typography, paper, binding and illustrations. Always, the men on the Editorial Board have been among the outstanding dermatologists of the country. In recent years the members have been selected with care. The Board is probably the best yet and of definite service to the Editor.

Dr. Frederick D. Weidman became a member of the Editorial Board in 1934, replacing Dr. Schamberg, who died in that year. Dr. Weidman's value to the Archives is due to his expert knowledge of both dermatology and pathology. He spent 10 years in the department of pathology of the University of Pennsylvania, half of this period on a full time basis. He also spent years of work in the laboratory of comparative pathology of the Philadelphia Zoological Gardens. He not only is a general pathologist, but is a cutaneous histopathologist and mycologist of the highest rank. He is frequently consulted by dermatologists from all over the country regarding puzzling histopathologic problems. In the Third International Congress of Microbiology in 1939, he was a co-president. On the death of Dr. Schamberg, he became professor of dermatology and vice dean in dermatology and syphilology in the Graduate School of Medicine.

Although a full time laboratory man, he has served since 1920 as visiting dermatologist to the Philadelphia General Hospital and president of the Society of Investigative Dermatology in 1945. During the past war he served as consultant to the Secretary of War in tropical medicine.

Dr. Weidman makes the following remarks about the Archives: "Editor Fox has discharged his responsibility splendidly in all respects. He may be regarded as one of the deans in American dermatology.

"The other members of the Editorial Board are naturally men of the highest caliber; the dignity which the Archives enjoys is commanding, and membership confers an honor which is promptly grasped as the opportunity arises. Six of the seven members have been or are presidents of the American Dermatological Association, are professors in their respective universities and most of them have been presidents of the outstanding national organizations in dermatology."

Dr. Harold N. Cole became a member of the Board in 1935, taking the place of Dr. Corlett. Dr. Cole not only is an able dermatologist but is one of the outstanding syphilologists in this country. His knowledge of syphilis has made him an invaluable member of the Board. He has been clinical professor and head of the department of dermatology and syphilology in the Western Reserve University since 1936, having served previously for years as associate and assistant professor. He is also head of the dermatologic departments of the University, the Cleveland City and the United States Marine Hospital No. 6. He is a member of the American Association of Pharmacologists and Experimental Therapeutists and a consultant to the Penicillin Panel of the United States Public Health Service.

Dr. Cole was a former Chairman of the Section on Dermatology and Syphilology and a former member of the Council on Pharmacy and Chemistry of the American Medical Association, and a member of the Surgeon General's Cooperative Clinical Group. He is a corresponding or honorary member of 7 foreign dermatologic societies.

Dr. Cole expresses his opinions of the Archives and members of the Editorial Board as follows: "The Archives of Dermatology and Syphilology, under the aegis of William Allen Pusey and of his successor Howard Fox, has become one of the most important, if not of the best known, journals of dermatology in the world. This is particularly true since the last years before and during the second World War. More and more writers from Australia, England, Holland, the Scandinavian countries and more particularly Cuba and the South American countries have been turning to the Archives for publication of their work. This is due to a variety of circumstances:

"It is true that due to Hitlerism, with all that this has entailed, for 10 years or more publication in a European journal has often been either difficult or even impossible. This is by no means the complete answer. Other reasons are quite obvious. More and more medical men are reading the Archives. It has a broad circulation both here and abroad. It contains the latest developments in its line, much experimental work and reports on society proceedings that have no peers anywhere. Even the second World War did not cripple the journal too much.

"The Archives has been headed during the past decade by an editor who goes all out to make it a success. It is rare that such a publication is edited by such an erudite scholar, linguist and well trained physician. Moreover, there is probably no dermatologist in the United States who has such a broad acquaintance among dermatologists of the world. No one realizes more than a member of the Editorial Board the immense amount of personal work that has been taken over by the Editor himself.

"We men grouped around the Editor on the Editorial Board are a well grounded group, favoring no particular region, party or clan.

Men have been selected to include various aspects of dermatology and syphilology as related to chemistry, mycology, bacteriology, histopathology, pharmacology, radiology and internal medicine."

Dr. C. Guy Lane became a member of the Editorial Board in 1937 when Dr. Pusey retired to become Editor Emeritus of the Archives. Dr. Lane has also had a good deal of editorial experience as a member of the editorial board of the New England Journal of Medicine. He received his M.D., cum laude, in 1908 from Harvard University. During World War I, he served in the Medical Corps from January 1918 to April 1919. He served in the department of dermatology of the Massachusetts General Hospital from 1919 to the present, and in the department of dermatology of Harvard Medical School from 1925 to the present. During the past decade, he has been head of both of these departments. He has served as president of the American Dermatological Association and the New England Dermatological Society.

One of the most outstanding and unselfish services that Dr. Lane performed was to act as secretary of the American Board of Dermatology and Syphilology from its inception in 1932 to 1944, when he became president. In addition to this onerous duty, he found time to serve for two years as secretary of the Advisory Board of Medical Specialties.

Dr. Lane expresses the following opinions about the Archives: "The outstanding accomplishments of the Archives of Dermatology and Syphilology have been achieved by the able leadership of the two chief editors of the past 25 years, Drs. William Allen Pusey and Howard Fox. Since Dr. Pusey in 1920 persuaded the American Medical Association to assume the responsibilities of the Journal of Cutaneous Disease, these two leaders of American dermatology, selected by the Trustees of the American Medical Association, have by their inspiring leadership brought the Archives to its present position in the medical publishing world as the principal dermatologic journal. Scientific accuracy has been insisted on, as well as correct methods of expression and the proper use of words. Both these editors have done much to stimulate young investigators and inexperienced writers. They have displayed a readiness to call on outside authorities to evaluate the contents of manuscripts. It is difficult to express in words all that these two leaders have done for the Archives, but to their energy, their careful selection of material and their guiding hands is due in large measure the success of the Archives.

"The dissemination of progress in cutaneous medicine is the outstanding accomplishment of the Archives. In its pages have appeared a wealth of dermatologic investigation and experience which has been a most important contribution to cutaneous medicine.

"The publication of reports on patients exhibited at national and local dermatologic societies and the discussions of their conditions are widely read and are considered as one of the most valuable features of the present Archives. The careful selection of advertising material has also been a distinct contribution and adds to the pleasure of the average reader. Book reviews and indexes, while perhaps not outstanding, fulfill their purposes."

Dr. Herbert Rattner became a member of the Editorial Board in 1935, having served since 1931 as abstract editor, a position which he has admirably filled. Before studying medicine, he entered the Northwestern University in the student army training corps during World War I. After finishing his internship at Cook County Hospital, he went directly into Dr. Pusey's office as an assistant, where he remained for 10 years. He is now associate professor of dermatology at the Northwestern University Medical School and attending dermatologist at the Cook County and Michael Reese hospitals. He is a former president of the Chicago Dermatological Society. His long, close association with Dr. Pusey made him an ideal person to write the charming sketch entitled "Pusey at Close Range." He is so widely read that he is indispensable in supervising the abstracts of the world literature which appear in the Archives.

Dr. Rattner writes in regard to accomplishments of the Archives: "I would think that it is largely responsible for the high position that dermatology enjoys today in this country."

Dr. Charles C. Dennie became a member of the Editorial Board in 1939, replacing Dr. Engman. Dr. Dennie is an outstanding syphilologist as well as dermatologist and is the author of an excellent book on congenital syphilis. He has been professor of dermatology at the Medical School of the University of Kansas since 1938 and is attending dermatologist at the principal hospitals in Kansas City. He was vice-president of the American Dermatological Association and is now a member of the American Board of Dermatology and Syphilology. He is a corresponding member of the French Society of Dermatology. During World War I, he served as major in the Medical Corps, during 1918–1919, most of the time in France.

Dr. Paul A. O'Leary became a member of the Editorial Board in 1944 replacing Dr. Dennie. Dr. O'Leary is one of the foremost syphilologists in this country and his position as a dermatologist is shown by his election for the coming year as president of the American Dermatological Association. He was president of the

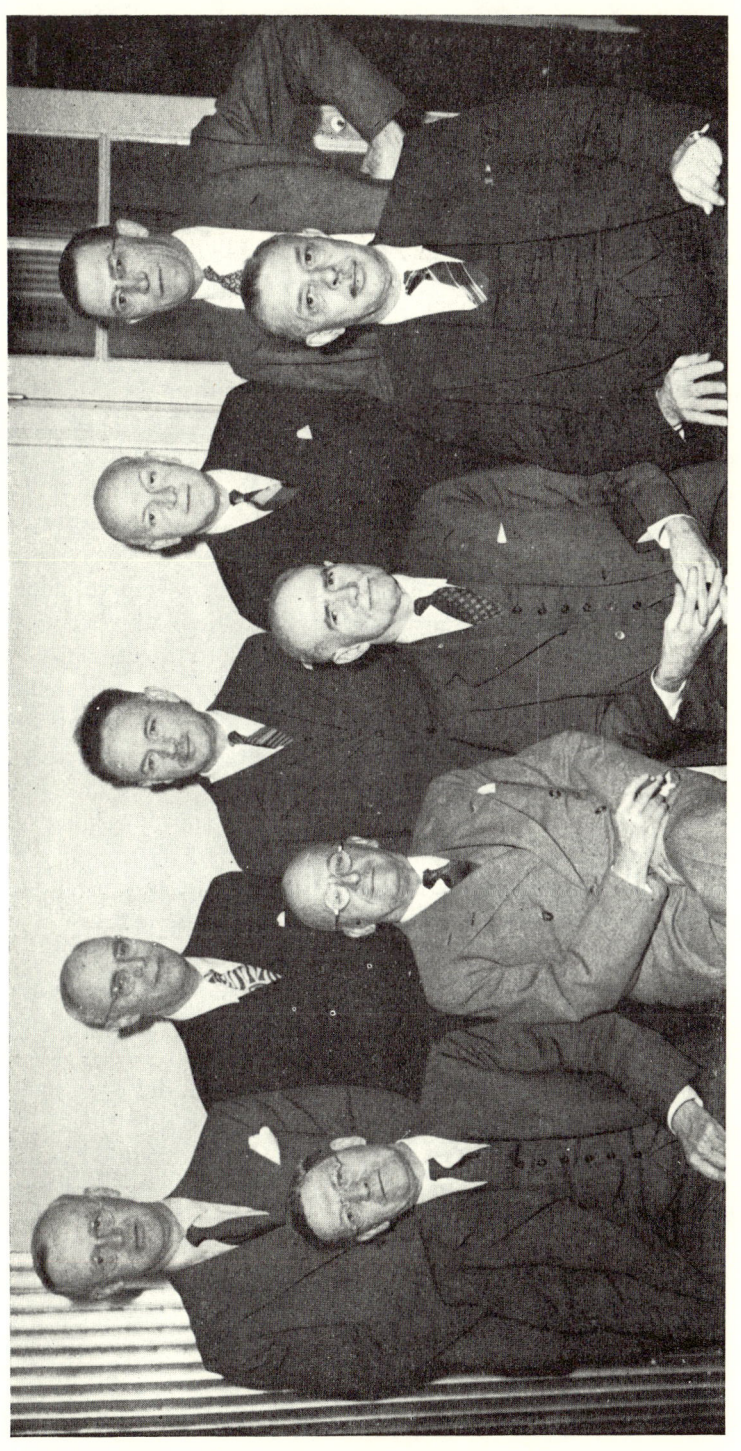

American Board of Dermatology and Syphilology, June 7, 1945, Waldorf-Astoria, New York City. *Top Row*—Left to right: O'Leary, Michelson, Lewis, Senear, Shelmere. *Front Row*—Weidman, Fox, Lane, Dennie.

American Academy of Dermatology and Syphilology in 1939, and has been for years head of the Section on Dermatology and Syphilology of the Mayo Clinic and professor at the University of Minnesota Graduate School. Dr. O'Leary is secretary-general of the Tenth International Congress of Dermatology to meet in the future in the United States. He is a member of 7 foreign dermatologic societies, has written or collaborated in writing over 300 articles and served for 4 months in World War I in the Medical Corps of the Army.

Dr. O'Leary makes some constructive criticisms as follows: "I am definitely in sympathy with the plan to encourage younger dermatologists, especially in isolated communities. However, I believe it is more important to maintain a high standard of publication by requiring that their literary standards approach our standards rather than that we seek their level. The lack of articles dealing with fundamental investigative procedure is probably due to the war, and is a criticism of the dermatologists of this country, rather than of the Editor. I do not believe that the Archives should discourage the publication of reports of technical investigations, even though they are involved and uninteresting to the dermatologic practitioner. I see no objection to the publication of articles which may have a controversial trend. I believe the Editor has done a marvelous job under trying circumstances in putting the Archives at the head of the list."

After the foregoing praise of the Archives and the complimentary remarks about myself, I would be ungrateful indeed if I did not fully appreciate the honor of being Editor of this fine journal. My work has been a pleasure; I read every word that is printed in the Archives, except the advertisements. My hardest duty has been to reject 352 of the 3003 articles submitted for publication in the past decade.

I feel grateful to my colleagues on the Editorial Board and to the authors who have almost invariably treated me kindly and shown a spirit of complete cooperation.

In closing, it is a pleasure to acknowledge the invariable kindness and many helpful suggestions given to me by Dr. Morris Fishbein and his assistant, Miss J. F. Whelan. Without such help, I could not have accomplished my duties.

ARCHIVES OF NEUROLOGY AND PSYCHIATRY

By Louis Casamajor, M.D.

BEFORE THE ADVENT OF *The Archives of Neurology and Psychiatry* America had seen the rise and fall of a number of journals devoted to nervous and mental disease. Two have persisted to the present day: The American Journal of Psychiatry, founded as The American Journal of Insanity in 1844, for which the present title was adopted in 1921, and the Journal of Nervous and Mental Diseases first published in 1874. Over the years and up until the first World War these two sufficed for the publication of what neurologic and psychiatric articles were produced in this country. For years the Journal of Nervous and Mental Diseases was the official journal of the American Neurological Association. In the early days of the first World War the membership of this association began to be dissatisfied with their "official journal"; not the least among their complaints was that of the difficulty in having papers published. Now more neurologic and psychiatric articles are being produced than could find outlet in only two journals. The need for a new journal of neurology and psychiatry was pressing.

Up to 1918 there was little that was constructive in the American Neurological Association meetings, but a real start was made at the 44th annual meeting on May 9, 1918. At this meeting, according to the minutes, "Dr. Patrick read a letter from Dr. George H. Simmons, who on behalf of the American Medical Association offered to publish a journal of neurology representing the interests of the American Neurological Association, provided a sufficient number of members of the latter association requested the publication of such a journal. The proposal received free discussion and was referred to the next executive meeting for further action."

At the next meeting a motion was made by Dr. Patrick and seconded by Dr. M. Allen Starr, that the Association be circularized with a petition in order to obtain a number of signatures of members of the American Neurological Association sufficient to assure the Trustees of the American Medical Association of proper support of their undertaking. This petition must have been satisfactory, for when it was presented at the June 1918 meeting of the American

Medical Association "the board took the matter under advisement until its October meeting."

At a meeting of the Council of the American Neurological Association on June 3, 1918, Drs. Weisenburg and Tilney were appointed a committee to select the names of twelve members of the American Neurological Association to be submitted to the Trustees of the American Medical Association from which number an editorial board might be chosen. There is no record of who the twelve were, but in the minutes of the Board of Trustees of the American Medical Association, Oct. 25, 1918 this notation occurs: "It was duly moved, seconded and carried that the Association publish a journal of neurology and psychiatry and that the following constitute the editorial board:

Dr. E. E. Southard, Boston
Dr. Hugh T. Patrick, Chicago
Dr. Frederick Tilney, New York City
Dr. Pearce Bailey, New York City
Dr. August Hoch, Montecito, Calif.
Dr. T. H. Weisenburg, Philadelphia

Further that this editorial board of the American Journal of Neurology and Psychiatry shall be regarded as an ad interim board until our annual meeting in February 1919. . . . Dr. Hugh T. Patrick shall be chairman of the editorial board." This ad interim board immediately got to work and the first number of the Archives of Neurology and Psychiatry, consisting of 8 articles and occupying 143 pages, appeared in January 1919. This was not at all a poor start for a new journal and clearly showed the need for it. In the minutes of the Board of Trustees meeting of Feb. 7, 1919 the journal was designated the Archives of Neurology and Psychiatry, the same editorial board was appointed permanently, the length of the term of the editors was established and Dr. Weisenburg was elected as editor-in-chief.

The "Editorial Announcement" in the first number is worth quoting:

"About 100 leading neurologists and psychiatrists formally requested the Board of Trustees of the American Medical Association to undertake the publication of a new journal devoted to nervous and mental diseases. After due consideration the Trustees granted the request and this first number of the Archives of Neurology and Psychiatry is the result.

"We must all recognize that during the last twenty-five years there have been great, at times startling, advances in neurology and psychiatry. It is not so well recognized that in the recent war the neurologist and psychiatrist at the front has probably been of more importance than the internist. And we believe it will be generally admitted that the mass of the medical profession is not so well informed on nervous disease and mental disorders as on most other branches of medical science.

"The Trustees agreed with the petitioners that there was need of a publication which would at once stimulate the efforts of the best neurologists and psychiatrists of the country and serve as an adequate medium for reports of the fruits of their labors; which would keep its readers in touch with the best work in all countries, and which would help to elevate the general standards of knowledge of the nervous system and its diseases. Just at this time the need is greater than ever before. The war has been a great school but many of the lessons taught need to be—must be—more generally known. The complexities of civil life are increasing, changes are rapid and more are impending. The enormous industrial development of the United States has involved and will involve injuries and diseases of the nervous system, psychoneuroses and psychoses. All of these things demand research, report, education. In short the need is for a scientific publication which shall not only serve the purpose of the research man and technical expert, but which shall also be of immediate practical value to the clinician. This need *The Archives of Neurology and Psychiatry* aspires to meet.

"Owing to many difficulties and delays the editorial organization is not complete and the board is keenly alive to the defects of this first number. The unexcelled facilities of the American Medical Association press will leave nothing to be desired in the way of illustrations: colored and black and white. It may be proper to add that the Archives is published for the benefit of the medical profession and in the interests of scientific medicine and not for monetary gain. It will be as ethical, as independent and helpful as the editors can make it. In return they hope for the sympathy and support of their colleagues." These promises have been more than met.

One need not dilate on the material published in the Archives, which soon took its place as the foremost journal of neurology and psychiatry in the world—a position which it holds today. Starting with a paid circulation of 797 in April 1919, in 1943 there were 2378 paid and 2504 complimentary subscriptions. In 1946 the circulation was 3620 paid; 3837 complimentary. Under the able leadership of Theodore Weisenburg, who made for himself an enviable reputation as a medical editor, the scientific reputation of the Archives kept pace with its circulation. We have published and continue to publish each year more articles than any other similar journal in the world. Papers come to the editorial desk from many countries in both hemispheres. Vol. I (January to July 1919) consisted of 804 pages. This number rose steadily, reaching over 1000 in 1927, with a peak of 1514 pages in 1932. From then on until 1942 the volume size fluctuated between 1200 and 1500. With the advent of the second World War the number of pages per volume dropped to a little over 1000. Then came the shortage of paper and this, together with the fact that many of our contributors were in the services and not writing papers, reduced our pages successively below 1000 until Vol. 34 (July to December 1945) contained but 442 pages—a little more than half of the number in Vol. I. With the end of the war restrictions, the Archives rapidly began to pick up to its normal size.

The original Editorial Board functioned well but unfortunately they did not remain together long. Dr. Hoch died in 1919, Dr. Southard in 1920 and Dr. Bailey in 1922. Their places on the Board were filled by Dr. Samuel T. Orton, Dr. A. H. Barrett and Dr. E. W. Taylor. In 1924 Dr. Barrett retired and Dr. H. Douglas Singer took his place; 1926 saw the retirement of Dr. Patrick, who might with propriety be called the father of the Archives. He was succeeded by Dr. Stanley Cobb. A seventh member was added to the Editorial Board in 1929 in the person of Dr. Adolf Meyer. Dr. Orton resigned in 1930 and Dr. Louis Casamajor was elected. In 1932 Dr. Taylor died and no one was appointed to succeed him. In 1934 the Board suffered a severe loss in the death of Dr. Weisenburg, who had acted as Chief Editor from the start. Dr. B. J. Alpers was appointed in his place and Dr. Singer was elected as Editor-in-Chief. 1931 saw the election of Dr. Wilder Penfield as contributing member. Dr. Tilney resigned in 1935 and Dr. Tracy J. Putnam took his place. In 1940 Dr. Singer died very suddenly and the Archives lost its second Chief Editor. Dr. John Whitehorn was elected to fill this vacancy and Dr. Putnam became Editor-in-Chief. In 1941 Dr. Percival Bailey was elected as an additional member of the Board. Dr. S. W. Ranson, who had been named as an additional member of the Editorial Board in 1933, died ten years later and Dr. Charles D. Aring joined the Board.

To-day the Editorial Board is composed of the following members:

Chief Editor

Dr. Tracy J. Putnam   New York

Associate Editors

Dr. Bernard J. Alpers   Philadelphia
Dr. Charles D. Aring   San Francisco

Dr. Percival Bailey   Chicago
Dr. Louis Casamajor   New York
Dr. Stanley Cobb   Boston
Dr. Adolf Meyer   Baltimore
Dr. John Whitehorn   Baltimore

Contributing Member

Dr. Wilder Penfield   Montreal

The Editorial Board of the Archives of Neurology and Psychiatry is proud of the Archives and the part it plays for neurology and psychiatry of the world. Neurology and psychiatry owe and pay a debt of gratitude to the American Medical Association for its foresight in founding the magazine and its scientific spirit in supporting it.

ARCHIVES OF SURGERY

By Waltman Walters, M.D., and Morris Fishbein, M.D.

AFTER THE AMERICAN MEDICAL ASSOCIATION had established the Archives of Internal Medicine in 1910, came requests for the publication of periodicals devoted to pediatrics and to surgery. Both the House of Delegates and the Board of Trustees agreed to proceed at once with the journal of pediatrics but there were some misgivings about the undertaking of a publication in the field of surgery. These were related no doubt to the fact that there were already available in the United States several excellent publications devoted to the surgical specialty. The agitation for such a publication continued, however; in the following year—1911—a motion was passed that a periodical, to be known as the American Archives of Surgery, be published beginning with 1911. Nevertheless the time was still apparently not ripe. Two groups began to assume form in relationship to this venture. One hundred of the most prominent surgeons of the country sent to the Board of Trustees in 1912 a request that they proceed with the publication of a surgical periodical. At the same time, however, the board received a letter signed by Drs. Lewis S. Pilcher, Philadelphia, editor of the Annals of Surgery, and Franklin H. Martin, Chicago, editor of Surgery, Gynecology and Obstetrics, protesting against the publication of the Archives of Surgery. They asserted that it would result in serious damage to the publications of which they were editors and stated that it would result in the destruction of independent surgical journalism.

After the Board of Trustees had given careful consideration to these two presentations, the board decided to proceed with the publication of the Archives of Surgery. However, there was much delay before action was finally taken. Eight more years passed before medical opinion consolidated sufficiently to enable the trustees to proceed with the publication. When the periodical did appear in July 1920, it was published with an editorial board that included Dr. Dean Lewis, Chicago, as chief editor, and Drs. Evarts A. Graham, St. Louis; Hugh Cabot, Ann Arbor; Thomas Cullen, Baltimore; William Darrach, New York City, and William J. Mayo, Rochester,

Minn. The first number contained a wise editorial signed by William J. Mayo in which he said, in part:

"For a number of years the trustees of the American Medical Association have purposed the establishment of an Archives of Surgery similar in character and scope to the Archives of Internal Medicine, The American Journal of Diseases of Children, the Archives of Neurology and Psychiatry, and other comparable publications. Delays of various kinds have arisen, among others those resulting from the war, which have prevented the fulfilment of this purpose. The fact, too, that there were already in this country two great journals of surgery, the Annals of Surgery, and Surgery, Gynecology and Obstetrics, has made this delay of less consequence.

"The Journal of the American Medical Association has the largest circulation of any medical journal in the world, and represents the activities of the American medical profession. The Journal, therefore, must carry contributions which will cover all the different fields of medicine. Contributions to its surgical section are so numerous as to make it difficult to publish them all in The Journal, especially since many of these contributions are too technical to be of interest to the entire profession.

"The Trustees in establishing the Archives of Surgery have wisely determined that it shall not enter into competition with the journals of surgery now in existence. They believe that it should, besides lessening the burden of The Journal's publication, establish a sphere of its own. They believe, and again rightly, that another journal of clinical surgery is not warranted, and the task of the editor, Dr. Dean Lewis, and of the editorial board is to develop an organ which will in no way interfere with the justly earned successes of the existing publications, and yet establish a journal which will be creditable to the great organization that it represents, and sufficiently useful to the profession to warrant its entering the field.

"In the growing period of surgery, it was not possible to train surgeons in the true sense. Only a few men had the opportunity to work as assistants to experienced surgeons. This is no longer the case. In the future, the surgeon will serve an apprenticeship; and three-year courses of instruction in which such training can be given are now being offered for those graduates in medicine who have served their hospital internship. It is the hope of the editorial board that the Archives of Surgery may be one of the organs of expression in this growing field of surgical education, and that it may furnish an opportunity for the publication of original articles pertaining to research and investigation in those subjects which lay the foundation for sound surgical progress. American surgery has developed unevenly. Many competent observers are of the opinion that clinical and operative surgery and surgical technic have advanced faster than the growth of knowledge with regard to the fundamental but less attractive branches would warrant. It may be said that the philosophy of surgery has lagged, and operations based on unsupported opinions as to their wisdom or their necessity are too frequently advocated.

"The Archives of Surgery will attempt at least to enlarge the surgical horizon and assist in establishing surgery on a sounder basis. Unpleasant as it may be, the editors will not hesitate to comment editorially on the papers published in its columns in order that both sides of a moot question may be considered. The reader will be given an opportunity to peruse surgical fads and fancies if such be presented, but if the subject matter introduces questionable material it will not be allowed to go unchallenged."

The first article in the first number was a joint contribution by Dr. Harvey Cushing, Professor of Surgery in the Medical School of Harvard University, and Dr. W. G. MacCallum, Professor of Pathology at Johns Hopkins University Medical Department. It dealt with splenic anemia. The following is the table of contents of the first number:

EDITORIAL ANNOUNCEMENT. William J. Mayo, Rochester, Minn.

TWO CASES OF SPLENECTOMY FOR SPLENIC ANEMIA: A Clinical Lecture, Jan. 21, 1920, to Third-year Students, Telling an Old Story. Harvey Cushing, M.D., Boston.

A REPORT ON THE PATHOLOGIC CHANGES IN SPLENIC ANEMIA (Written in 1900, but not Published). W. G. MacCallum, M.D., Baltimore.

DIAPHRAGMATIC HERNIA. Arthur Dean Bevan, M.D., Chicago.

ESOPHAGEAL DIVERTICULA. E. S. Judd, M.D., Rochester, Minn.

MANAGEMENT OF DIRECT INGUINAL HERNIA. William A. Downes, M.D., New York.

A REVIEW OF EIGHT YEAR'S EXPERIENCE WITH BRAIN TUMORS. Ernest Sachs, M.D., St. Louis.

AMPUTATION NEUROMAS: THEIR DEVELOPMENT AND PREVENTION. G. Carl Huber, M.D., Ann Arbor, Mich., and Dean Lewis, M.D., Chicago.

POSTOPERATIVE PULMONARY COMPLICATIONS. Elliott C. Cutler, M.D., and Alice M. Hunt, R.N., Boston.

THE SECOND GREAT TYPE OF CHRONIC ARTHRITIS: A LABORATORY AND CLINICAL STUDY. Leonard W. Ely, M.D., San Francisco.

A COMPARATIVE STUDY OF SODIUM IODID AS AN OPAQUE MEDIUM IN PYELOGRAPHY. Donald F. Cameron, M.D., Fort Wayne, Ind.

This was a galaxy of American surgical talent sufficient to establish the Archives of Surgery at once as one of the leading periodicals in its field. At first the periodical was published bi-monthly. It was not long, however, until the accumulation of surgical material made necessary its monthly publication.

Among the most distinguished of its contributions was a memorial number of the Archives of Surgery dedicated to Dr. Harvey Cushing. This was published in 1929 at the time of Dr. Harvey Cushing's sixtieth birthday. Following the publication there was an interchange of correspondence between Dr. Elliott C. Cutler (who was acting as editor on this special issue), Dr. Harvey Cushing and Dr. Morris Fishbein, which we are privileged to quote from the biography of Dr. Harvey Cushing by Dr. John F. Fulton:

H. C. TO MORRIS FISHBEIN (by hand)   9 April 1929

"Dear Brother Fishbein. I am simply bowled over, flabbergasted, dumbfounded, by that Birthday Book you have seen fit to publish. I suppose you must have thought: now the only way to get rid of, to wholly and effectually eliminate, that pestiferous Cushing who behaves as though he was in the manor (Boston) born but wasn't, is to allow his cubs to get out this book after which the only decent thing he can do is to resign and I'll no longer be troubled by his hyphens, dyphthongs (sic), P.B.B.H. surgical numbers, his Oljenicks (Ign.) and other crotchets. . . .

Anyhow I am much beholden to you for the trouble you must have taken over this book. . . . I am enclosing a sketch which I am sure represents, in the foreground, a meeting between you and E. C. C.'[1]"

---

[1] Comic sketch entitled "The Head Proofreader in the Educator Cracker Factory Discovers a Typographical Error"—one of the holes in the cracker is found to be missing.

To this letter Fishbein replied:

"Dear Dr. Cushing: I am placing your note of April 9 among my highly prized personal documents. Who knows, some day it may enter into a history of American Medicine. My unbounded respect for your position in your chosen field, and for the unusual number and the quality of your students and assistants, as well as for your literary attainments, made me assent without a moment's hesitation to the suggestion of a birthday volume. I am not going so far as to say that every moment of the process was a pleasure, but it was indeed highly instructive. I have seldom met so delightful and accomplished a personality as E. C. Cutler."

Elliott Cutler then wrote to H. C.

"I am getting a great kick out of the Birthday Book. Thanks for this note from Fishbein which I am returning. I did not know before I started—and this opinion is not constructed since seeing his letter—that Fishbein really had such high ideals. Of his intelligence I was long ago assured but the constant turmoil of this recent publication led me to respect his ideals, his generosity, his patience and his ability. . . . " H. C. sent this letter to Fishbein with the following note written across the top:
"Dear Fishbein—In these fallen times when more brickbats than bouquets are handed out, it is sometimes consoling to learn, even if indirectly, of the commendation of occassional people. You will therefore not take it amiss if I send you this letter of Cutler's which has just come over my desk."

Dr. Waltman Walters of Rochester, Minn., became chairman pro tem of the editorial board of the Archives of Surgery in Feb. 1939 and chairman in June 1939 when Dr. Dean Lewis became editor emeritus. The remainder of this history of the Archives of Surgery is by Dr. Waltman Walters.

It had been Doctor Dean Lewis' practice to review personally every paper being considered for publication in the Archives of Surgery. As a result, during his illness there was an accumulation of papers of which the new chairman of the Editorial Board had to dispose. At this time, also, the earliest publication that could be assured to any paper was six months, and sometimes publication was delayed from nine months to one year. Following Doctor Lewis' death and the appointment of a new Chief Editor, who asked to be designated as the Chairman of the Editorial Board, a plan was devised by which all members of the Editorial Board would participate in reviewing an equal number of papers. As these papers were received by the Managing Editor's office, they were equally divided, each paper being reviewed by two members of the Board, who would indicate whether or not in their opinion the papers were acceptable for publication and then, following this, the paper was sent to the Chairman of the Board for final decision. Following this plan, a review of every paper could be assured within a period of one month and the delay in publication was decreased to usually not more than three months. In order to stimulate a more participating interest in the journal by a larger group of American surgeons, it was decided to change the policy governing type of papers to be presented from those dealing principally with experimental surgical problems to those dealing with clinical problems as well, and authors of papers containing outstanding contributions to the advancement of surgery were given priority and early publication of their papers. It was thought, too, that it might make each issue more interesting to a larger group of surgeons if several papers dealing with related subjects be published as a symposium. The most noteworthy of these was that on cancer of the stomach which occupied the entire issue of June, 1943. Letters were written to the heads of the departments of general surgery and surgical specialties of the various medical schools and hospitals in this country, calling their attention to the fact that the Archives of Surgery was the surgical journal of the American Medical Association, that it was founded at their request to provide a place for the publication of papers dealing with research problems, which, because of the nature of the research or the length of the papers, were not thought to be suitable by the other surgical journals of the time. Attention was called also to the change in the policy of the Archives to include papers dealing with clinical surgery as well. To further stimulate and elicit support, similar announcements were made at the business session of the Section on Surgery, General and Abdominal, of the American Medical Association.

The circulation of the Archives of Surgery increased thirty-three per cent in the following year and one-half, and this increase was maintained during the war period.

During the war, because of the fact that the chairman of the Editorial Board was called to active duty in the Medical Corps of the United States Navy, in July 1942, at his suggestion, Dr. Lester Dragstedt, one of the very active members of the Editorial Board, was appointed as Chairman, pro tem. Under his guidance the same policies were carried out until the release from active duty of the Chairman of the Board in December, 1945, when he again resumed the chairmanship. During the war period because of the additional duties acquired, Dr. Evarts Graham, Chairman of the Surgical Committee of the National Research Council, who had been a member of the Board since the founding of the journal in 1920, asked to be relieved of his duties on the Board. He was persuaded to postpone his resignation until the termination of the war, at which time the place which he held with great credit to himself and value to the Archives was filled by the appointment by the Board of Trustees of the American Medical Association of Dr. Robert Elman, Associate Professor of Surgery at Washington University in St. Louis. When the Chairman of the Editorial Board contacted members of his

Board for nominations to fill the vacancy caused by Dr. Graham's resignation, Dr. Darrach, also one of the founder members who had contributed greatly to the development of the Archives, expressed his desire to be relieved of his duties, in order to give way, as he said, to a younger man to help develop the journal in the years to come. His vacancy was filled by the appointment of Dr. Gustaf Lindskog, Associate Professor of Surgery at Yale. The sudden and unexpected death of Dr. Walter E. Dandy left another vacancy on the Editorial Board. This was filled at the July, 1946 meeting of the Board of Trustees by the appointment of Dr. Cobb Pilcher, Associate Professor of Neurosurgery at Vanderbilt University. During Dr. Dandy's tenure as an editor, he displayed enthusiastic and conscientious interest in reviewing all papers dealing with his specialty and gave the Board the benefit of his advice as to their suitability for publication.

In order to defray postage, as well as other small miscellaneous expenses attendant upon sending the various papers for review among the members of the Editorial Board, the Board of Trustees yearly sets aside the sum of six hundred dollars, which is given to the Chairman of the Editorial Board and, in turn, by him passed on to the members of the Board to meet such expenses. Since 1939, it has been the custom of the Chairman, after payment of these expenses, to divide the remainder into equal parts and purchase some small gift for each of the editors.

Since 1940 the yearly meetings of the Editorial Board have been held at the time of the meeting of the American Medical Association or the meeting of the American Surgical Association. At these meetings suggestions as to policies tending to improve the value of the Archives have been discussed, and suggestions and criticisms made to further such a program. The previously stated policies of the Archives continue, the editors regarding themselves as trustees and servants of the American surgeons in assisting them to publish at an early date important contributions tending toward the advancement of surgery in all of its aspects, and receiving in turn from the managing editor, Dr. Morris Fishbein, and his assistant, Miss J. F. Whelan, most excellent cooperation to make the Archives of Surgery one of the best surgical journals. Evidence of this is the fact that the papers published in the Archives of Surgery were republished in abstract in foreign journals in greater percentage than those from any other American journal.

ARCHIVES OF OPHTHALMOLOGY

By Francis H. Adler, M.D.

THE ARCHIVES OF OPHTHALMOLOGY is a relatively new journal published by the American Medical Association, but its roots go back to the early days of ophthalmology in this country and had much to do with the high level of scientific and scholarly thinking which early characterized the literature of those days. The magazine from which the Archives grew was the Archives of Ophthalmology and Otology, first published in 1869. After seven volumes of this magazine had been issued a division was made between the ophthalmologic and otologic contents for the convenience of the increasing number of men who were by that time limiting themselves to the practice of one or the other specialty and not both. The first issue of the Archives of Ophthalmology is numbered Volume 8 and appeared in 1879.

From the start the Archives had two editions, one in English and one in German, with an editorial board headed by Dr. Herman Knapp of New York and Dr. J. Hirschberg of Berlin. The associate editors were men prominent in their fields in America and abroad, including England, Germany and Austria-Hungary. All papers were translated into either English or German for the two editions, but some of the papers were abridged when the editors thought they were too long. It is interesting to note that emphasis was laid on practical aspects of ophthalmology, for the preface of the first issue states that "In their selections the editors will give preference to those original papers in which speculation and theory are subordinate to direct observation and fact. Their greatest satisfaction will be to hear their readers continue to say 'What we read in your journal, we can make use of.'"

Dr. Herman Knapp, who had founded the Archives of Ophthalmology and Otology, continued as the Editor-in-Chief of the Archives of Ophthalmology until his death in 1911. His son, Dr. Arnold Knapp, who was then professor of ophthalmology at Columbia University, became his worthy successor, and the publication of the fortieth volume is identified with Dr. Arnold Knapp and Dr. W. A. Holden of New York, together with Dr. C. Hess of Wurzburg, as editors. By 1924 with the appearance of the fiftieth volume the name of C. Hess had been dropped from the list of editors, and Drs. Knapp and Holden continued as the sole Editorial Board until 1928.

There were at that time several other publications in this country devoted exclusively to ophthalmology. The American Journal of Ophthalmology had been founded in 1883 and in 1896 an announcement appeared in its editorial column that "as stated in the last number, it, furthermore, is from now on under the sole and absolute control of its editor." This was signed by the editor, Adolf Arlt of St. Louis. In 1904 the Ophthalmic Yearbook made its appearance, being a digest and review of the literature of ophthalmology for each current year, edited by Edward Jackson.

We have reason to believe that by 1928 the number of journals devoted exclusively to ophthalmology had about reached the saturation point and in order to maintain the standards already set and to eliminate wasteful repetition serious consideration was being given to combining some of these separate efforts. That this sentiment was quite general throughout the country is testified to by a petition which was presented to the Board of the Trustees of the American Medical Association in May 1928, as follows:

"We, the representatives of the American Ophthalmological Society, the American Academy of Ophthalmology and Oto-Laryngology, and the Ophthalmic Section of the American Medical Association, and the present Editors of the Archives of Ophthalmology, the American Journal of Ophthalmology and the Ophthalmic Yearbook, believe that in the interests of Ophthalmology and American medicine in general, the above named three publications should be continued under the direction of the Board of Trustees of the American Medical Association and therefore respectfully request that the Board of Trustees of the American Medical Association consider taking over these publications.

APPROVED BY
American Ophthalmological Society
  W. E. Lambert, Preident
Ophthalmic Section of A.M.A.
  Arnold Knapp
American Academy of Ophthalmology
  and Oto-Laryngology
  Luther C. Peter
American Ophthalmological Society

SIGNED BY
William Campbell Posey
John Green
Arnold Knapp
Harry S. Gradle
George S. Derby
Edward Jackson
Walter R. Parker
W. H. Wilmer

April 30, 1928"

The Chairman of the Board of Trustees stated that he had met in Washington with a committee composed of representatives of the three periodicals mentioned and several other individuals and that the committee had suggested that Drs. Arnold Knapp, Edward Jackson, Harry S. Gradle and William Henry Crisp meet with the

Board in Minneapolis to discuss the subject. The Chairman stated that he felt that if the Archives of Ophthalmology and the American Journal of Ophthalmology were taken over by the American Medical Association and combined, another journal of ophthalmology probably would be established by outside parties. He was, therefore, in favor of the Association's taking over the Archives of Ophthalmology and the Ophthalmic Yearbook and leaving the American Journal of Ophthalmology to be published as it was at that time. After some discussion the entire matter was referred to the June meeting of the Board of Trustees. At that meeting a committee, consisting of Drs. Knapp, Gradle, Crisp and Jackson, was present and entered into the discussion of the subject. They were then invited to attend the meeting of the Board of Trustees in September. Drs. Crisp and Jackson were unable to accept the invitation, but Drs. Knapp and Gradle were present and gave their views. After the discussion the Board of Trustees voted to establish a periodical to be known as the Archives of Ophthalmology and elected Dr. Knapp as Editor-in-Chief. Dr. Knapp expressed his willingness to serve in this capacity and the desire that the periodical be a perpetuation of the journal founded by his father. To carry on this idea it was suggested that for the first year the new journal carry "Volume 1" on the cover and "Volume 1 (old series Volume 58)" on the inside. It was further suggested that in selecting members for the editorial board, one be chosen to procure and handle the abstracts; another, the reviews; another, society proceedings, and the others for such assistance as the Editor-in-Chief might find it necessary to call on them. Drs. George S. Derby, Boston; Francis Heed Adler, Philadelphia; Sanford R. Gifford, Omaha; John Herbert Waite, Boston, and William Zentmayer, Philadelphia, were elected to serve with Dr. Knapp as the Editorial Board. The first issue was published in January 1929.

Dr. Derby, whose term was to expire in 1933, died in 1931, and Dr. Walter R. Parker was elected to fill his unexpired term. Dr. Parker was then reelected for a term of six years, but resigned in 1937 and was succeeded by Dr. W. L. Benedict. Dr. J. H. Waite resigned in 1941 and Dr. David G. Cogan was elected to fill his unexpired term of two years. Dr. Cogan was reelected in 1943 for a period of six years. Dr. Sanford R. Gifford died in 1944, shortly after being reelected, and Dr. Frederick C. Cordes was elected to succeed him.

Dr. Arnold Knapp has carried on the policy established by his father of maintaining a high standard in the quality of papers published. He has broadened the scope of the journal in many ways.

He has believed that one of the functions of the Archives was to present articles from border line fields of medicine and the first issue began with an important article on Meningiomas by Harvey Cushing. A number of outstanding articles on medical and neurosurgical ophthalmology have appeared over the years and the inclusion of articles from authors in other parts of the world has made the journal an international one. A new feature was the inclusion each month of a review article which would bring up to date the knowledge on any chosen subject. Some of these reviews have been valuable contributions to current literature by collecting our knowledge on a subject from various sources of medical literature which would otherwise not have become available to the average ophthalmologist.

Reports of American and foreign ophthalmologic meetings were included, so that the American reader might be kept informed on what was going on in the rest of the ophthalmologic world.

The growth of the Archives has been steady and wholesome. It owes its present standard of excellence to the wise leadership of its Editor-in-Chief and the loyal cooperation of the members of the Editorial Board, who have been untiring in their efforts to keep this an outstanding scientific journal in its field.

ARCHIVES OF PATHOLOGY

By Ludvig Hektoen, M.D.

THE FIRST NUMBER OF the Archives was issued in January 1926. It contained the following introductory statement by the Editorial Board:

"The establishment of a periodical for pathology by the American Medical Association has been urged from various sources for many years with increasing insistence. The general need for such a periodical was voiced formally in resolutions by the Section on Pathology and Physiology that received the endorsement of the House of Delegates. After thorough consideration the Board of Trustees decided to publish Archives of Pathology and Laboratory Medicine in order: (1) to meet the present need in this country for increased facilities in publication of results of scientific work in the field of pathology in the broad sense, and (2) to serve as a medium for information, for physicians and others, of progress in pathology and in the practical use of all clinicopathologic procedures that for want of a better term may be referred to collectively as 'laboratory medicine.' In other words, the purpose of the Archives is to serve the growth and to promote the spread of scientific knowledge of the nature and causes of disease as the basis for rational and successful methods of prevention and treatment. Accordingly, conducted at a high level and in the spirit of scholarship, the Archives will contain articles on the results of new work in all departments of pathology; general reviews of subjects of special interest; technical notes and descriptions of new and modified laboratory methods; matters of significance in the medicolegal application of pathology; abstracts of current pathologic literature in all its phases; reports of meetings of pathologic and other scientific societies; notes and news of personal and general interest, and competent reviews of appropriate books."

Since then two volumes, each of 6 monthly numbers, have been published yearly, the number of pages in a volume as the rule varying from 900 to 1300. Before long the subtitle "and Laboratory Medicine" was omitted. A few years ago the number of acceptable articles submitted became so large that it seemed best to omit abstracts of current pathologic literature as well as reports of meetings of pathologic societies. Here are listed the members, past and present, of the editorial board:

Granville A. Bennett, Chicago	1944–	Frank R. Menne, Portland	1934–
James Ewing, New York	1926–1943	William Ophüls, San Francisco	1926–1934
Wiley D. Forbus, Durham, N.C.	1945–	Oscar T. Schultz, Evanston, Ill.	1927–1945
Ludvig Hektoen, Chicago	1926–	Alfred Stengel, Philadelphia	1926–1939
Victor C. Jacobsen, Albany	1933–1935	George H. Whipple, Rochester	1940–
Wm. G. MacCollum, Baltimore	1926–1933	S. B. Wolbach, Boston	1926–

The number of subscribers has grown to 2600 in 1946. Of this number 2225 are domestic and 375 are foreign subscribers.

QUARTERLY CUMULATIVE INDEX MEDICUS

By Marjorie H. Moore

THE QUARTERLY CUMULATIVE INDEX MEDICUS is one of the most important publications issued by the American Medical Association, as an aid to the progress of scientific medicine. The first volume was published in 1916.

Soon after his appointment as editor in 1899, Dr. George H. Simmons inaugurated a "current literature section" in each weekly issue of The Journal. In this section was recorded by title and author the contents of each issue of the more important medical periodicals of the world. Some of the articles were abstracted but all of the American titles were indexed meticulously by author and subject. These entries were included in the volume indexes to The Journal but were published as a separate section. This separate section containing the index to the American medical current literature was available for sale in separate form; it provided the practicing physician with a ready and valuable guide to the important medical literature (American) of his day. This publication was known as the Guide to Current Medical Literature. The first such index appeared in The Journal, vol. 33, covering the material published from July-December, 1899. This venture was an immediate success.

Within a short time, because of popular demand, titles in the foreign medical periodicals as well were included in the index to the current literature section. The first such index covering both the American and foreign medical literature titles appeared in the index to The Journal for vol. 38, 1902. An editorial in The Journal June 28, 1902, page 1692, states:

"The readers of The Journal will note that the Index of Current Medical Literature in this, the concluding number of the volume, contains not only the American, but also the European titles. Heretofore this has been—since the discontinuance of the publication of the Index Medicus—the most complete index of papers in the medical publications of this country. With the present additions, which nearly double its size, it affords an index also of most of the leading foreign journals, sufficient, it is thought, for many purposes, for the consultors of foreign medical literature. With the abstracts given, The Journal reader should be kept well posted as to what is being done in medical science abroad. There is a utility in this which we believe will be appreciated by American workers, as the Bibliographia Medica, the successor to the Index Medicus, is not readily available to many in this country and its continuance is, moreover, an uncertainty. Unless we have evidence which has been wanting heretofore that the efforts of The Journal in this direction are not appreciated by the profession, its index of current literature will continue to appear with each volume and such features as may seem to increase its value will be added from time to time."

No doubt Dr. Simmons was influenced in his decision to establish such an index by the fact that the Index Medicus was forced to suspend publication just at that time (1899) because of lack of funds. Several years later, realizing the importance to the general practitioner of this index to current medical literature, he conceived the idea of developing it into a more useful guide. He felt that the style of the original Index Medicus did not meet the needs of the majority of practicing physicians. Therefore, in 1916, about five years after the establishment of the library department and the appointment of Miss Helen Hutchinson as librarian, he suggested that she devise a style for an index to medical literature that would replace the subject index to the current medical literature section of The Journal. The plan was to issue an index to medical literature each quarter in paper bound form and to cumulate thereafter each year references covering the succeeding quarters into a final yearly volume. The final volume for the year was to be bound in cloth for permanent use. To Miss Hutchinson (now Mrs. Frederick Green) all credit should be given for devising the style of the first Quarterly Cumulative Index to Current Medical Literature. She had the entire responsibility of preparing and editing the first eight volumes of this publication as an extra-curricular duty, as it were, to the management of the library department. Moreover, she accomplished this seemingly impossible task with one assistant the first few years and never more than four in the later years. In his article "The Quarterly Cumulative Index; What It Stands For and How to Use It" (J.A.M.A. July 2, 1927) Dr. Fielding H. Garrison had this comment to make about the first volume of the Quarterly Cumulative Index to Current Medical Literature:

"Here intact was a new departure and along lines for which the world had long waited; viz, an automatic system of self-indexing which dispensed with the cumbersome index to an index, whether of authors or subjects or both. The gain in checks on accuracy through the full time service of a large personnel was also of moment. The only drawback to the new publication was the relatively small number of periodicals indexed, 157 in 1916, 326 in 1926."

As soon as the Quarterly Cumulative Index to Current Medical Literature was issued, in 1916, the Guide to Current Medical Literature which had been published in each volume index to The Journal since vol. 33, 1899, was discontinued. The dictionary plan of the new index had a great appeal to reference workers. In a short time it was recognized by the medical profession as a most valuable guide to current medical literature. In contrast to the style of the original Index Medicus published under the auspices of the Army Medical Library, the new Quarterly Cumulative Index to Current Medical Literature contained in one alphabet subject and author references. All entries from foreign periodicals appeared in translated form under subject headings. For ten years, the Quarterly gradually increased the number of periodicals indexed until in 1926 it was covering 326 periodicals. The original Index Medicus had resumed publication in 1903 with the financial aid of the Carnegie Institution of Washington.

FUSION OF THE QUARTERLY CUMULATIVE INDEX WITH THE INDEX MEDICUS

As both the Index Medicus and the Quarterly Cumulative Index were being published at a loss it was natural that some plan of fusion of these two similar publications should be discussed. It was not until 1926, however, soon after Dr. Morris Fishbein's appointment as editor of The Journal, that constructive steps were taken to combine these two valuable publications. The original agreement for the fusion of the two indices provided that it should be published under the title of Quarterly Cumulative Index Medicus combining, as can be seen, the titles of the two previous publications. It was agreed that for a period of five years after the consolidation the library staff of the Army Medical Library would provide the American Medical Association Library with index cards covering a certain number of periodicals and that the American Medical Association Library would be responsible for the remainder. The Carnegie Institution agreed to contribute $10,000 toward the loss on the Index for a period of five years. In 1927, therefore, the library staff of the American Medical Association assumed responsibility for the editing and printing of the Index Medicus under the terms mentioned.

Soon it was felt that many errors occurred in the Index due to the widely separated indexing staffs. Delays were occasioned by the necessity of writing to Washington frequently to verify questionable references; it was impossible to maintain accurate records of issues indexed. The five year experiment proved forcibly to the editing staff that every periodical indexed in the Quarterly should be available in the office of publication for consultation when editing so many thousand entries. Therefore, when, at the termination of the five year contract in 1932 the Carnegie Institution withdrew its financial support, the American Medical Association assumed the entire responsibility of indexing and publishing the Index Medicus.

SUBJECT HEADINGS

During the period of 1927 to 1932, great strides were taken by the Index Medicus staff towards the establishment of standardized subject headings for medical periodical literature; the first volume of Subject Headings, Quarterly Cumulative Index Medicus was published in 1931 under the supervision of Miss Magdalene Freyder, Assistant Librarian. No thought was given to the sale of copies as the work had been published originally as a guide for Index Medicus staff members. However, many requests were received for copies. Without public announcement or any advertising, all of the one hundred copies first printed were soon sold. In 1940 a second edition of the Subject Headings was published containing many changes and additions and was offered for sale. A third edition is one of the goals to be attained in future years.

THE WAR YEARS

The number of periodicals covered in the Index Medicus reached over 1200 in 1939 when the plans for gradually expanding the list of periodicals indexed which had been progressing so satisfactorily were abruptly halted by the war in Europe. The receipt of periodicals from Europe dropped considerably. Fortunately arrangements were made early in 1942 to index much of the European literature from microfilm copies of various French, German and Scandinavian periodicals which were supplied us through a governmental agency in Washington. A complete coverage of the medical literature for the war years has not been possible and such coverage must, of necessity, be a gradual process. The Index Medicus had, until the war years, always been published as a quarterly but for the first time in its history, the paper bound issue of July-September, 1944 had to be cancelled. The paper issue for the corresponding period in 1945 was also omitted. Shortage of paper, lack of personnel, printers' strikes, etc., had been responsible for this unfortunate situation. The efficient staff which had taken years to train was suddenly disrupted. Wives left to join their husbands in service, many younger staff members left to be married, others to enter war work.

The Quarterly Cumulative Index Medicus is valuable to the profession not only as a tool for reference but as a record of trends in medical development and interest. Many diseases appear, others are realigned and reclassified, new drugs are synthesized and new treatments are introduced. Some of these subjects become firmly established in the literature, others die as quickly as they are popularized. These trends can be followed closely through the subject headings in the Quarterly Cumulative Index Medicus. From 1927 to 1936 a guanidine preparation "synthalin" commanded attention as a new treatment for diabetes. Volume 3, 1928 of the Quarterly contains 24 references to the subject. At present it is not even mentioned in the literature.

Recently the Kenny method in treating poliomyelitis attracted wide spread attention with 25 articles listed in volume 32, July-December, 1942. In volume 39, January-June, 1946, only one article is listed. Early volumes of the Quarterly Cumulative Index Medicus contained few articles on sex hormones. For example: thirteen articles were recorded in vol. 3, 1928. In the following years, the articles on sex hormones in the literature increased to such an extent that separate subject headings had to be established for the androgens, estrogens and gonadotropins. A total of 244 articles appeared under all of these classifications in vol. 39, January-June, 1946.

The Quarterly Cumulative Index Medicus is a means for the systematization of medical knowledge. Its publication gives permanence to the medical literature of today, carrying forward the knowledge of this generation to the workers of the ages to come. The Board of Trustees has considered the loss sustained in the publication of the Index Medicus well worth while as a contribution to the progress of medicine.

THE AMERICAN MEDICAL DIRECTORY

By Frank V. Cargill

THE DESIRE AND NEED FOR a reliable medical directory was often expressed at official meetings of the American Medical Association. Even as early as the 1846 convention, a resolution was adopted to ascertain the number of licensed practitioners and the "number who practice medicine without any authority whatever." Apparently no action was taken, for in 1849 a similar resolution was adopted.

In 1868 a committee was appointed to report on the subject of an annual register of the regular profession in the United States. Three years later, this committee reported adversely and was discharged. The subject of a register of physicians recurs in the minutes of annual meetings, but during these early years such schemes were chimerical, and all called for a greater expenditure of money than was then available.

In the report of the Board of Trustees for 1904, reference was made to the Plan of Reorganization discussed at St. Paul in 1901, stating that "One of the objects to be accomplished in the near future was the publication by the Association of a complete directory of registered physicians of the United States." There was one proposal to make the directory only a blue book of the members of the American Medical Association. This plan was rejected. The report of 1904 further states, "The Board recommends that the so-called blue book be not published but instead of it a complete directory be published and that the names of members of the organization, that is, the members of constituent organizations and their component branches, be printed in said directory in large type and those of nonmembers in ordinary type."

RESOLUTION TO PUBLISH A MEDICAL DIRECTORY

Finally, at the annual meeting of the American Medical Association in Portland, Oregon, in 1905, the House of Delegates proposed the establishment of a biographical record of physicians and the publishing of a medical directory. It was decided that the directory should differ from other directories in three particulars:

1. It should be a directory of the American medical profession, published and owned by the physicians themselves;
2. Information regarding college and year of graduation and date of licensure and society membership should be verified from official sources;
3. The directory should furnish the same information regarding each physician whether a subscriber to the directory or not.

No information was to be inserted for pay. The book was to contain the names of all members in good standing of the constituent state associations and to indicate membership in the American Medical Association. The information on each physician was to include his name in full, year of birth, medical school and year of graduation, year in which he received his license, residence and office addresses, and office hours.

The need of an authentic directory of physicians was obvious. It was recognized that a permanent biographical card index of American physicians would be of inestimable value to the profession and to the public.

PREVIOUS MEDICAL DIRECTORIES

The only national medical directories published up to this time were those in which a physician could, on payment of a small fee or by purchasing the directory, have from one to four inches of information printed about himself. Often the most pretentious advertisement was that of the faker or quack, who made extravagant or fraudulent claims regarding his medical education, teaching positions, hospital connections, and society affiliations, and gave his past and present history along with his future aspirations. With the exception of the information concerning the school of graduation, apparently the data submitted were not verified. In many instances, only the name of the physician appeared, or the name with a symbol indicating that information had not been received. Occasionally the names proved, on investigation, to be those of veterinarians, ministers, lawyers, druggists, or dentists. The display advertisements were undesirable, such as those of alcoholic cure-alls, institutions of doubtful character, and questionable proprietary medicine.

GATHERING BASIC RECORDS FOR THE DIRECTORY

The gathering of this basic material and the compiling of a directory was under the direction of Dr. Frederick R. Green. The fundamental and most important work was that of securing a list of those physicians who were legally entitled to practice in each state. A card index was made from records of 37 states, including not only the regular licensing boards but also the homeopathic and eclectic boards. A few states had printed reports from which cards were later made. Difficulties were encountered in states such as Pennsylvania, which had only county registration, making it necessary to secure data from each prothonotary of its 67 counties. In Texas and Oklahoma, physicians were required to reregister under a new medical practice act, while in Georgia the Association helped by writing a set of licensing cards.

All this work stimulated the licensing boards to realize the importance of accurate registration. The spirit of cooperation shown by the officers of the boards was extremely gratifying. A list of legally qualified practitioners of medicine in the United States, derived from official records, was gathered and made available to the medical profession and to the licensing boards. In many cases, it was the first time a complete list of licentiates of a state was available, for, although in a few states the records had been kept in excellent condition, in many others the official records of the licensing boards had been apparently considered more a matter of form than a means of determining an individual's legal right to practice medicine. In a number of cases, the secretaries had no idea of the number of names on their records. In three instances, after having completed what they thought to be a copy of the entire records of the board, they found a forgotten register containing one or two thousand additional names in the back of the vaults or in obscure corners of the clerk's office.

An incomplete list of graduates up to 1902 was obtained from the "Standard Directory" which was taken over in 1905 from G. P. Engelhard & Company. This purchase included a set of eight books which purported to contain the names of all graduates of medical schools in the United States from 1860 to 1901. After 1901, the list was supplemented yearly by the data received from the colleges and the licensing boards of the various states.

STARTING THE FIRST EDITION

In the period from September 1905 to April 1906, letters containing biographical blanks were sent to approximately 90,000 physicians. Besides the blanks sent directly to the physicians, similar information blanks were inserted in the advertising pages of The Journal on several occasions. From these sources, about 65,000 personal biographical reports were received from physicians. A complete list of members (later referred to as Fellows) of the Amercan Medical Association was on file at the headquarters.

During 1905, a card index of members of constituent state associations (which included members of county, district, and state societies) was set up, so that there was on file a complete list of the membership of the branches of the American Medical Association.

A reporting system was also instituted in 45 states so that regular reports regarding changes of membership would be received.

To supplement the information on file, a staff of correspondents was organized for directory purposes, with one physician in each of the 2,830 counties and one physician in each town having ten or more physicians, making a total of approximately 5,000 correspondents.

Lists of physicians, based on Engelhard's "Standard Directory," with other information added, were sent to these correspondents for revision and correction. When the lists were returned, the information was checked with the four office files—the personal information blanks, the list of graduates from medical colleges, the reports of secretaries of state medical societies, and the list of members of the American Medical Association. The completed copy was then compared, name by name, with the list of legally qualified physicians obtained from the various state licensing boards, and the date of license inserted as an evidence of qualification. All names not found on the state board lists were referred to the Secretary of the board, and, unless O.K.'d by him, were stricken off the proof. As this was the first time that information from all of these sources had ever been carefully and systematically compared, a large number of discrepancies were found. Names intended for the same individual were spelled differently; varying Christian names and initials were reported for the same individual; a physician would be reported on separate lists as a graduate of two different colleges or as having graduated in two different years; many physicians, among them members of county and state societies, were not reported as licensed.

To settle these discrepancies as far as possible, letters were sent (1) to all physicians reported as practicing but not reported as licensed; (2) to all physicians reported as licensed but not reported as graduates of any medical college; (3) to all physicians whose names appeared as members of the American Medical Association but who were not reported as members of either their county or state society, and (4) a special blank to physicians who were reported as practicing but concerning whom we had no adequate information.

Composition on the Directory was begun on March 1, 1906. As fast as a state was completed, revised and corrected, a complete proof of the state by counties was made and sent to each correspondent according to the territory he covered. A proof of the entire state was sent to the secretary of the state society and also to the secretary of the licensing board. The work of compilation, writing copy, composition, and correction was carried on simultaneously, taking the states in alphabetical order. As soon as the list of physicians by states was in pages, the alphabetical index to the Directory was compiled.

FIRST EDITION COMPLETED

Late in 1906, the First Edition of the American Medical Directory finally came from the press. A total of 8,500 copies were printed, to satisfy the 7,300 advance orders for the book which had been entered at the list price of $5.00. For the first time in the history of American medicine, a directory was issued which was owned, compiled, and published by the medical profession for its own use and purposes. The book was published in the hope that it would prove of value to the medical profession, hospitals, colleges, licensing boards and other allied organizations interested in the practice of medicine.

The 1906 Edition of the Directory listed the name of the physician in full, year of birth, sectarian initial or American Medical Association symbol (H for homeopath, E for eclectic, P-M for physiomedical), medical college and year of graduation, year of license, street and number with office hours in towns of sufficient size to make this information necessary. In addition, membership was indicated by listing physicians' names in capital letters; the symbol of a cross in a circle was used to indicate membership in the A.M.A. As far as possible, symbols and abbreviations were used so as to include as much information in as small a space as possible and still keep the book in one volume. The First Edition contained information on 121,484 physicians in the United States and 6,689 in Canada and United States dependencies, or a total of 128,173 names. The Directory was arranged in three general sections—(1) general information in the front of the book; (2) a geographical section in which the names of physicians were listed alphabetically by state and city; and (3) an alphabetical index listing the names of the physicians followed by city and state, so that the subscriber could locate the physician and his data in the body of the Directory if he knew only the name.

The Directory also included, under each state, a copy of the medical practice act, a list of the officers of the state board of health, the various licensing boards, the officers of the state and county medical organizations, as well as a list of hospitals and sanatoriums. The book also contained information on the officers of the American Medical Association, with its constitution and by-laws, the officers of national special societies, medical officers of the Army, Navy, Pension Service, and a list of medical colleges and medical journals.

In compiling the First Edition, however, it had been impossible, without delaying the book, to obtain official information regarding all alumni of many colleges and complete licensing records previous to 1901. The lack of this material was sorely felt, since without it, official data were missing as to the graduation of quite a large percentage of physicians. Accordingly, as soon as the first edition had been issued, efforts were continued to get more complete lists of graduates of all existing medical colleges. From these complete lists alumni record cards were made for those physicians who had graduated subsequent to 1865; thereby enabling this department to verify the record of graduation for those physicians whose names already were listed in our files and for those who were to be added to the Directory. Out of the 161 schools, complete lists were promptly received from 146. Of the 15 remaining, only six were unable to supply the information; in one case the college records had been destroyed by fire. When it was considered that these alumni lists were the only records of graduation and that when a college went out of existence the records were lost, the value of the duplicate lists in the Directory Department became apparent.

To ascertain the improvements needed in the Directory, a circular letter and report blank were sent to each subscriber, during 1907, asking him to express an opinion as to the advisability of including in subsequent editions information on medical college positions, hospital appointments, life insurance positions, as well as to offer general suggestions and criticisms. About 2,000 replies were received, and, as a result of the information supplied by the subscribers, several improvements and additions were made to the Second Edition.

THE SECOND EDITION

When work was begun on the Second Edition in September, 1906, one of the improvements was the enlargement of the college historical matter, with a new college key table for quick reference. A list of medical libraries was added to the book. Additional personal information regarding individuals was obtained so that college professorships and specialties could be indicated. To condense this material, titles of positions were abbreviated and the colleges indicated by the key number. Although some specialties were listed, it was admitted that the list of specialists was merely a beginning, as there was no recognized standard to distinguish these men. A plan was arbitrarily adopted to list as specialists, upon request of the physician, all members of special societies (local as well as national), teachers in medical colleges and physicians registered in special sections of the A.M.A., thus basing the recognition of specialists on society membership and positions held rather than only on the statements of the individuals concerned.

The Second Edition was completed and offered for sale in October,

1909, at a price of $7.00, with a discount of $1.00 on orders placed before publication. It was more complete than the First Edition, with a total of 142,070 names of physicians. There were 6,250 copies of this edition printed.

ESTABLISHMENT OF THE TWO MASTER CARD SYSTEMS

After publishing the Second Edition of the Directory it was realized that compilation of a more accurate book would make necessary the establishment of a unit card system—a card for every name in the geographical section (the body of the book) and a card for the names in the index. Mr. Frank V. Cargill was made director of the Department and was given authority to make up a biographical card from the information on file for every physician. This card, which was 4″ by 6″, was to include the full name, place and year of birth, premedical education, medical school and year of graduation, a record of all licenses, internship or special training, and a record of the physician's changes of location. About 75 per cent of the cards were written direct from the personal information reports, and the basic information verified from our official records. It was necessary to write biographical cards for the other names and later fill in the data as it was obtained.

The second, 3″ by 5″ master card included the printed information that had appeared in the geographical section of the Second Edition of the Directory. The compilation of the Third Edition was not started until these card indexes were completed. The use of these cards simplified the work of preparing copy for the Directory, as they offered a unique way to correct the previous edition. New cards were made up for recent graduates and the cards of physicians who had died were dropped. For those previously entered in the Directory it was necessary only to change the location on the two cards and refile the geographical card under the new location. The geographical card was later used as copy for the printer. After the geographic section of the book was put in galley form, the geographic cards were filed alphabetically and checked against the alphabetical cards so that it was possible to produce a very accurate book.

THE THIRD EDITION

The Third Edition was compiled and printed in 1912 from the two master-card records. It was considered the most accurate, up-to-date medical register of physicians yet published, and was practically free from duplications. More than 20,000 new names were added to the Third Edition, and over 30,000 membership changes were made, as organized medicine was growing at a rapid pace.

There was a definite change in type face, and a special paper imported from Belgium was used. A valuable new feature was a separate list, in the front section of the book, of members of special societies. This membership was also included in the personal data under each physician's name. For the first time, the Directory included a new section known as "Physicians Whose Addresses Are Unknown." This list helped greatly because many new addresses for these physicians were furnished by users of the Directory.

THE FOURTH EDITION

Special effort in this edition was made to make the Directory more usable for subscribers. In the index, wherever a surname was listed that commonly had more than one spelling, the variations were listed for the guidance of the user, as, under the name "Cain," the reader was referred to "Caine, Cane, Kane, Kean, Keane, Keen, Keene." The Directory was now firmly established and widely used by the medical profession, hospitals, and commercial firms. The Fourth Edition was printed in 1914, at a price of $7.00 charged for advance orders and $10.00 for orders received after publication.

SUBSEQUENT EDITIONS OF THE DIRECTORY

The Fifth Edition was issued in April, 1916, and 7,000 copies were printed, with no change in price over that of the Fourth Edition.

The supreme test of the value of the biographical records and Directory files came shortly after the United States entered World War I, for it was from these records that the Association greatly aided the War Department in verifying the records of 35,000 physicians who entered military service. Information concerning medical education and society affiliations was especially desirable; the Biographical Department of the Association was the only central place where such data were on record.

The publishing of the Sixth Edition in 1918 was exceedingly difficult because so many physicians, moving about in military service, had no permanent address. Because of rising costs, the price was set at $10.00 for advance orders and $12.00 for orders received after publication. About 6,000 copies were printed.

To follow the biennial pattern of the Directory, a new edition should have been issued in 1920, but the Seventh Edition was not completed until 1921, partly because of the difficulty of securing up-to-date addresses of physicians, but principally because of the lack of available satisfactory help to compile the book. Costs of paper and clerical labor had increased enormously over those of 1918, but the circulation of the book also spurted upward, with over 8,000 advance orders for the Seventh Edition as compared to 4,100 prepublication subscriptions for the Sixth Edition. It was necessary to increase the prepublication price of the Seventh Edition to $12.00 and the price for orders received after publication to $15.00.

Partly because there had been a longer interval between the issuance of the Sixth and the Seventh Editions, but also because of the unsettled social conditions there was an unusually large number of changes of location—at least thirty per cent of the physicians in the country having changed their addresses during this period.

There was a growing need on the part of some of the subscribers to the Directory to get a list of corrections as they occurred in the interval between Directories. This need was particularly felt by advertisers in The Journal, medical book publishers, pharmaceutical houses, insurance companies, and addressing companies. A supplement to the Directory, called the "Directory Report Service," was established in 1921, in which were listed the names of new physicians, changes of address, and the names of physicians who had died. This was simply a record of the changes we had made in our master card system. The Service was first offered monthly and later was issued twice a month. It was a means of bringing in additional revenue to help support the work of keeping up corrections in the biographical file. This Service has greatly helped to round out the functions of the Biographical and Directory Departments.

It might be mentioned here that it was not until 1923, five years after the war, that the entire profession had actually returned to the practice of medicine, with many physicians having given up rural practice and moved to urban locations; many having taken postgraduate courses were now limiting their practice to a specialty. The Eighth Edition was published in this year.

Beginning with the compilation of the Ninth Edition, which was issued in 1925, a special letter and a new type of information card were sent before publication to each physician to provide an opportunity to supply up-to-date information as to his location and current practice. Various other sources of information had been developed to insure continued accuracy in the book. Proofs of pages were cut, pasted and sent to city and county correspondents for correction and additions. Telephone directories for cities throughout the United States were checked for addresses as well as used for other reference purposes.

It had been found that it was necessary to verify all information, as many times a physician was reported to have moved or died, but he was later found to be practicing at a new address. At least fifteen per cent of the reports of deaths of physicians received from correspondents were false. In many instances, new names listed proved on investigation not to be physicians. All information, therefore, was checked and rechecked unless received direct from the physician.

Immediately after the publication of one edition, preparations were made for the next edition, so that the Directory was a biennial publication. After the publication of the Twelfth Edition in 1931, however, economic conditions made it necessary to forego issuance of a new edition for a year, and the Thirteenth Edition did not appear until 1934. To bridge the gap between the two editions, a special mimeographed supplement was issued in 1933, listing the names of new physicians and the names of physicians who had died.

With the Fifteenth Edition, in 1938, the price was increased from $12.00 to $15.00 before publication and from $15.00 to $18.00 after publication. The indication of certification of specialists by examining boards became a feature of the Directory, and the diplomates of twelve boards were indicated by special abbreviations. The number of examining boards has increased until the diplomates of fifteen boards are now indicated. The Sixteenth Edition appeared in 1940. In the Seventeenth Edition, issued in 1942, a special symbol was used to designate physicians on extended active duty with the military forces as the result of the national emergency proclaimed in 1941.

With the outbreak of World War II, the biographical files of the Directory Department again proved invaluable to the War Department in expanding the small group of medical officers into a peak mobilized force of about 60,000 physicians for the armed forces. Through the establishment, in the Association headquarters building, of a liaison office between the Surgeon General's Office and the Association, records and facilities were made available to the War Manpower Commission, the state Procurement and Assignment Service chairmen, and the various medical service committees.

Because of wartime restrictions, it was necessary to postpone the publishing of a Directory in 1944 and 1946. With the ending of hostilities, there was a rapid demobilization of the medical profession, which occasioned an enormous number of changes of address, as the majority of these physicians took postgraduate courses or finished their internships or residencies. Because of the accurate record kept of the physicians in the medical reserve corps, there will be available a valuable record to help the thousands of veterans who make inquiry regarding physicians to prove disability claims. The lack of complete information of this type proved a great handicap after World War I.

At present, the shortage of clerical help, labor in the printing department, and paper, makes impossible accurate prediction as to when a new Directory will be available.

WAR MEDICINE

By Morris Fishbein, M.D.

WITH THE BEGINNING OF WORLD WAR II, the Board of Trustees authorized the editor of The Journal to cooperate with the Division of Medical Sciences of the National Research Council in the publication of a periodical to be entitled "War Medicine" and issued bimonthly. The first issue appeared in January 1941 as a publication edited by the Committee on Information, Division of Medical Sciences, National Research Council, with the following editorial board:

Morris Fishbein, Chief Editor, Chicago
J. J. Bloomfield, Washington, D. C.
John F. Fulton, New Haven, Conn.
Richard M. Hewitt, Rochester, Minn.
Ira V. Hiscock, New Haven, Conn.
Sanford V. Larkey, Baltimore, Md.
Robert N. Nye, Boston, Mass., in cooperation with
Charles S. Stephenson, Commander, U. S. Navy Medical Corps
R. R. Spencer, United States Public Health Service

Thus the editor of The Journal of the American Medical Association, who was at the same time chairman of the Committee on Information of the Division of Medical Sciences of the National Research Council, became editor of the publication. The associate members of the editorial board were editors of other publications in the field of medicine, librarians familiar with medical literature, medical historians and representatives of the various governmental services.

Each of the original contributions was considered by an expert in one of the numerous special committees in the Division of Medical Sciences of the National Research Council. Thus the material was authentic. The first number of War Medicine included the following content:

EDITORIAL:
War Medicine
INDUSTRIAL HYGIENE AND THE NAVY IN NATIONAL DEFENSE. Ernest W. Brown, M.D., New York.

AMPHETAMINE (BENZEDRINE) SULFATE: A REVIEW OF ITS PHARMACOLOGY. A. C. Ivy, M.D., Ph.D., and L. R. Krasno, Ph.D., Chicago.

AVIATION MEDICINE IN THE UNITED STATES NAVY. Frederick Ceres, M.D., Pensacola Florida.

MARCH FRACTURE: REPORT OF THREE CASES. Prentice L. Moore, M.D., and Allen N Bracher, M.D., Schofield Barracks, Territory of Hawaii.

OFFICIAL STATEMENTS:
Chemotherapy for Infectious Diseases and Other Infections: Circular Letter No. 81

THE HEALTH AND MEDICAL COMMITTEE. E. H. Cushing, M.D., Cleveland.

ACTIVITIES OF THE MEDICAL DEPARTMENT IN AUGMENTATION OF THE ARMY. Official, Statement from the Office of the Surgeon General of the United States Army.

THE NATIONAL RESEARCH COUNCIL AND MEDICAL PREPAREDNESS. Sanford V. Larkey, M.D., Baltimore.

A CENSUS OF PHYSICIANS FOR MILITARY PREPAREDNESS. Rosco G. Leland, M.D., Chicago.

PREPAREDNESS WITH DRUGS AND MEDICINAL CHEMICALS. S. De Witt Clough, Chicago.

ABSTRACTS FROM CURRENT LITERATURE.

BOOK REVIEWS.

As the war progressed and the need for information became more and more apparent, it became necessary to make War Medicine a monthly publication. At the end of the war, War Medicine had reached a circulation of many thousands and had invariably been published with a small profit. At the end of the war it seemed desirable to discontinue publication of War Medicine and to substitute for it a new periodical to be called "Occupational Medicine." The editorial board on the final issue follows:

Morris Fishbein, Chairman of the Committee and Chief Editor, Chicago.
John F. Fulton, New Haven, Conn.
Robert N. Nye, Boston, in cooperation with
    Brig. General James S. Simmons, United States Army
Captain E. H. Cushing (MC), U. S. N.
Assistant Surgeon General R. C. Williams, United States Public Health Service

EDITORIAL BOARD:
    Dr. Robert F. Loeb, New York
    Dr. W. W. Palmer, New York
    Dr. Clarence D. Selby, Detroit
    Dr. Chester S. Keefer, Boston
    Dr. Winfred Overholser, Washington, D. C.
    Dr. O. H. Perry Pepper, Philadelphia
    Dr. Frederick A. Coller, Ann Arbor, Mich.
    Dr. Milton C. Winternitz, New Haven, Conn.

The Contents of the last issue, dated December 1945, follow:

PUBLIC HEALTH IN FRANCE FROM THE INVASION TO THE LIBERATION. L. Justin Besançon, Paris, France.

WAR INJURIES OF THE EYES AND VISUAL PATHWAYS. Lieutenant Colonel Gilbert C. Struble and Major Alfred J. Kreft, Medical Corps, Army of the United States.

QUINACRINE HYDROCHLORIDE AS A MALARIA-SUPPRESSIVE AGENT FOR COMBAT TROOPS. Colonel George Garfield Duncan, Medical Corps, Army of the United States.

EXPERIENCES WITH AMEBIASIS IN AN EVACUATION HOSPITAL. Major Alton G. Brown, Medical Corps, Army of the United States.

NUTRITIONAL DISEASES IN CABANATUAN. Captain Merle M. Musselman, Medical Corps, Army of the United States.

THE PROBLEM OF HEMOLYTIC STREPTOCOCCUS CARRIERS IN HOSPITAL PERSONNEL. Colonel Francis F. Harrison and Lieutenant Colonel John K. Miller, Medical Corps, Army of the United States.

A PSYCHIATRIC PROGRAM FOR A NAVAL RECEIVING STATION. Lieutenant Commander John B. Dynes (MC), U. S. N. R.; Lieutenant Commander N. Norton Springer (S), U. S. N. R., and Lieutenant F. Howard Thomas (MC), U. S. N.

PSYCHIATRIC CASUALTIES IN COMBAT. Major H. H. Garner, Medical Corps, Army of the United States.

REACTIVE DEPRESSION: A STUDY OF ONE HUNDRED CONSECUTIVE CASES. Captain Henry J. Myers, Medical Corps, Army of the United States, and Corporal Sigtrid Von Koch, Medical Department, Army of the United States.

PSYCHOGENIC DISORDERS OF THE UPPER GASTROINTESTINAL TRACT IN COMBAT PERSONNEL. Major Edwin A. Weinstein and Captain Martin H. Stein, Medical Corps, Army of the United States.

DISEASES AND DEFECTS IN AIRCREW TRAINEES: III. VISUAL SYSTEM. Major Oscar M. Marchman Jr., Medical Corps, Army of the United States.

EARLY TREATMENT OF OPEN HEAD WOUNDS. Major Jerome F. Grunnagle, Medical Corps, Army of the United States.

FAMILIAL PERIODIC PARALYSIS: REPORT ON FATHER AND SON IN WORLD WARS I AND II. Major Joseph W. Johnson Jr., Medical Corps, Army of the United States.

THE HISTAMINE FLARE IN THE EVALUATION OF PERIPHERAL NERVE LESIONS. Captain Bernard Tolnick and Lieutenant Colonel William C. Beck, Medical Corps, Army of the United States.

TYPES OF SHIGELLA ISOLATED FROM MILITARY PERSONNEL IN NORTH AFRICA. Major Charles C. Randall, Medical Corps, Army of the United States, and First Lieutenant H. O. Dunn, Sanitary Corps, Army of the United States.

ABSTRACTS FROM CURRENT LITERATURE.

BOOK REVIEWS.

GENERAL INDEX.

OCCUPATIONAL MEDICINE

By Morris Fishbein, M.D.

THE INCREASED INTEREST in industrial health caused the Board of Trustees at the end of World War II to transform the periodical called War Medicine into a new publication known as Occupational Medicine. The first editorial board of Occupational Medicine included:

William A. Sawyer, Chief Editor, Rochester, N. Y.
A. J. Lanza, New York
Arthur L. Watkins, Boston
Willard Machle, New York
Winfred Overholser, Washington, D. C.
Clarence D. Selby, Detroit
Rexford L. Diveley, Kansas City, Mo.

The contents of the initial number in January, 1946, was:

PHYSICAL CAPACITY FOR WORK: PRINCIPLES OF INDUSTRIAL PHYSIOLOGY AND PSYCHOLOGY RELATED TO THE EVALUATION OF THE WORKING CAPACITY OF THE PHYSICALLY IMPAIRED. Verne K. Harvey, M.D., and E. Parker Luongo, M.D., Washington, D. C.

SPONTANEOUS COMA DUE TO HYPOGLYCEMIA IN UNDERNOURISHED PERSONS. Hughes Gounelle and Jean Marche, Paris, France.

GROUP PSYCHOTHERAPY FOR NEUROPSYCHIATRIC PATIENTS BEING DISCHARGED FROM THE ARMY. Major Joseph J. Michaels, Medical Corps, Army of the United States and Second Lieutenant Emmette O. Milton, Adjutant General's Department, Army of the United States.

LATENT NEUROLOGIC MANIFESTATIONS FOLLOWING DECOMPRESSION: REPORT OF A CASE OF SEVERE REACTION FOLLOWING ASCENT TO 38,000 FEET. D. W. Lund, M.D.; J. H. Lawrence, M.D., and L. B. Lawrence, M.D., Berkeley, Calif.

PENICILLIN LOZENGES IN TREATMENT OF ORAL INFECTIONS. Captain Robert O. Levitt, Medical Corps, Army of the United States, and Captain William W. Leathen, Sanitary Corps, Army of the United States.

ABSTRACTS FROM CURRENT LITERATURE AND BOOK REVIEWS.

In 1947 the periodical was expanded by the addition to the editorial board of Dr. Carl M. Peterson, secretary of the Council on Industrial Health, and the planning of a new section to be devoted to complete abstracting of the periodical literature in the field of occupational disease and occupational medicine.

HYGEIA, THE HEALTH MAGAZINE

By Morris Fishbein, M.D.

AS IS RECORDED IN THE HISTORY of the American Medical Association, health education for the public was an early concern of many of its leaders. Not until 1920, however, did this concept begin to take practical form in the minds of the physicians who constituted the Council on Health and Public Instruction of the American Medical Association. Through a recommendation by this council, the House of Delegates of the Association at the Boston session in 1921 authorized the publication of a health magazine. The Board of Trustees at that time considered the Council on Health and Public Instruction the logical source for the development of such a publication. From June 1921 until June 1922 this council cooperated with the Board of Trustees in the development of the periodical.

At the meeting of the House of Delegates in St. Louis in June 1922, the Board of Trustees was authorized to proceed. The first issue of this magazine appeared in April 1923. The name Hygeia was selected after consideration of many other possible titles because it was a symbol of medical science and preventive medicine and also because it would be a name distinctive and not likely to be used by any other publication. Hygeia was the mythical daughter of Aesculapius, the father of medicine, and the Greeks revered her as the Goddess of health.

Attempts were made to find a suitable editor for the publication but without conspicuous success, so that the board authorized Dr. Victor C. Vaughan, at that time director of the Council on Health and Public Instruction, to be editor of Hygeia. He asked at once for assistance and the Board of Trustees established an advisory group, including Dr. Morris Fishbein, then assistant to the editor of The Journal of the American Medical Association; Dr. John M. Dodson, secretary of the Bureau of Health and Public Instruction, and Dr. Arthur J. Cramp, Director of the Bureau of Investigation.

After a brief period when it became apparent that the publication was not successful under such an arrangement, the board of editors was discontinued and Dr. Morris Fishbein became editor of Hygeia, with authority to appoint such assistants and members of the staff as seemed necessary. A group of other employees in the headquarters office, including Dr. Arthur J. Cramp, the director of the Bureau of Investigation and Dr. W. W. Bauer, director of the Bureau of Health Education, were authorized to assist. The Bureau of Health Education has had charge since that time of the section on Questions and Answers. The Bureau of Investigation was authorized to contribute popular material on nostrums and quackery.

The first issue of Hygeia was 25,000 and for several years it had great difficulty in maintaining that circulation. Indeed for several years the periodical was published at a considerable loss. Within the last ten years, however, it has continued to gain in circulation so that it has in 1947 a circulation in excess of 200,000 copies per month. Moreover, it has within the last five years shown continuously a considerable profit on its operation—in fact, sufficient in that period of time to have repaid all the previous losses.

The associate editors included at various times Jane Pine, Mildred Whitcomb, Leola J. Harris, Sibyl Johnston, William Siegel, Robert M. Cunningham Jr. and Betty L. Eckersall. In 1947 Mr. Ellwood Douglass was employed as managing editor under the direction of Dr. Morris Fishbein as editor.

The policy of the magazine was outlined in the first issue of Hygeia in April 1923. The success of Hygeia as a periodical for health education of the public is fully established. Hygeia prints authentic information and gives it in clear, concise and simple terms that even a school child can understand. It supplies reliable information regarding quacks, faddists and cultists and thus safeguards the public. Its articles lead to the formation of intelligent health habits.

In addition Hygeia has served as a voice of the medical profession to the public in emphasizing the point of view of medicine on questions relating to social and economic problems. Hygeia is probably the most quoted periodical in the United States. Following the appearance of each monthly issue, from twenty to thirty requests are received for republishing articles from Hygeia in other publications. Hardly an issue of the popular digest magazines appears, including Scientific Digest, Reader's Digest, Fact Digest, Read, Reader's Scope, This Month, and The Woman, that does not contain a reprint from Hygeia.

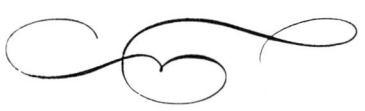

Appendices

APPENDIX 1

SESSIONS AND PRESIDENTS OF THE ASSOCIATION

No.	Year	Place	President	State
1	1847	Philadelphia	Nathaniel Chapman	Pennsylvania
2	1848	Baltimore	Alexander H. Stevens	New York
3	1849	Boston	John C. Warren	Massachusetts
4	1850	Cincinnati	Reuben D. Mussey	Ohio
5	1851	Charleston, S. C.	James Moultrie	South Carolina
6	1852	Richmond	Beverly R. Wellford	Virginia
7	1853	New York	Jonathan Knight	Connecticut
8	1854	St. Louis	Charles A. Pope	Missouri
9	1855	Philadelphia	George B. Wood	Pennsylvania
10	1856	Detroit	Zina Pitcher	Michigan
11	1857	Nashville	Paul F. Eve	Tennessee
12	1858	Washington, D. C.	Harvey Lindsly	District of Columbia
13	1859	Louisville	Henry Miller	Kentucky
14	1860	New Haven	Eli Ives	Connecticut
	1861	No session held		
	1862	No session held		
15	1863	Chicago	Alden March	New York
16	1864	New York	N. S. Davis	Illinois
17	1865	Boston	N. S. Davis	Illinois
18	1866	Baltimore	D. Humphreys Storer	Massachusetts
19	1867	Cincinnati	Henry F. Askew	Delaware
20	1868	Washington, D. C.	Samuel D. Gross	Pennsylvania
21	1869	New Orleans	William O. Baldwin	Alabama
22	1870	Washington, D. C.	George Mendenhall	Ohio
23	1871	San Francisco	Alfred Stillé	Pennsylvania
24	1872	Philadelphia	D. W. Yandell	Kentucky
25	1873	St. Louis	Thomas M. Logan	California
26	1874	Detroit	Joseph M. Toner	District of Columbia
27	1875	Louisville	W. K. Bowling	Tennessee
28	1876	Philadelphia	J. Marion Sims	New York
29	1877	Chicago	Henry I. Bowditch	Massachusetts
30	1878	Buffalo	T. G. Richardson	Louisiana
31	1879	Atlanta	Theophilus Parvin	Indiana
32	1880	New York	Lewis A. Sayre	New York
33	1881	Richmond	John T. Hodgen	Missouri
34	1882	St. Paul	J. J. Woodward	U. S. Army, D. C.
35	1883	Cleveland	John L. Atlee	Pennsylvania
36	1884	Washington, D. C.	Austin Flint	New York
37	1885	New Orleans	H. F. Campbell	Georgia
38	1886	St. Louis	William Brodie	Michigan
39	1887	Chicago	E. H. Gregory	Missouri
40	1888	Cincinnati	A. Y. P. Garnett	District of Columbia
41	1889	Newport, R. I.	W. W. Dawson	Ohio

No.	Year	Place	President	State
42	1890	Nashville	E. M. Moore	New York
43	1891	Washington, D. C.	W. T. Briggs	Tennessee
44	1892	Detroit	H. O. Marcy	Massachusetts
45	1893	Milwaukee	Hunter McGuire	Virginia
46	1894	San Francisco	James F. Hibberd	Indiana
47	1895	Baltimore	Donald MacLean	Michigan
48	1896	Atlanta	R. B. Cole	California
49	1897	Philadelphia	Nicholas Senn	Illinois
50	1898	Denver	George M. Sternberg	U. S. Army, D. C.
51	1899	Columbus	J. M. Mathews	Kentucky
52	1900	Atlantic City	W. W. Keen	Pennsylvania
53	1901	St. Paul	C. A. L. Reed	Ohio
54	1902	Saratoga Springs	John A. Wyeth	New York
55	1903	New Orleans	Frank Billings	Illinois
56	1904	Atlantic City	J. H. Musser	Pennsylvania
57	1905	Portland, Ore.	L. S. McMurtry	Kentucky
58	1906	Boston	W. J. Mayo	Minnesota
59	1907	Atlantic City	Jos. D. Bryant	New York
60	1908	Chicago	H. L. Burrell	Massachusetts
61	1909	Atlantic City	Wm. C. Gorgas	U. S. Army, D. C.
62	1910	St. Louis	Wm. H. Welch	Maryland
63	1911	Los Angeles	John B. Murphy	Illinois
64	1912	Atlantic City	Abraham Jacobi	New York
65	1913	Minneapolis	John A. Witherspoon	Tennessee
66	1914	Atlantic City	Victor C. Vaughan	Michigan
67	1915	San Francisco	William L. Rodman	Pennsylvania
68	1916		Vice-President—Albert Vander Veer	New York
69	1916	Detroit	Rupert Blue	U.S.P.H.S., D. C.
70	1917	New York	Charles H. Mayo	Minnesota
71	1918	Chicago	Arthur D. Bevan	Illinois
72	1919	Atlantic City	Alexander Lambert	New York
73	1920	New Orleans	W. C. Braisted	U. S. Navy, D. C.
74	1921	Boston	Hubert Work	Colorado
75	1922	St. Louis	George E. de Schweinitz	Pennsylvania
76	1923	San Francisco	Ray Lyman Wilbur	California
77	1924	Chicago	William Allen Pusey	Illinois
78	1925	Atlantic City	William D. Haggard	Tennessee
79	1926	Dallas	Wendell C. Phillips	New York
80	1927	Washington, D. C.	Jabez N. Jackson	Missouri
81	1928	Minneapolis	William S. Thayer	Maryland
82	1929	Portland, Ore.	Malcolm L. Harris	Illinois
83	1930	Detroit	William Gerry Morgan	District of Columbia
84	1931	Philadelphia	E. Starr Judd	Minnesota
85	1932	New Orleans	Edward H. Cary	Texas
86	1933	Milwaukee	Dean D. Lewis	Maryland
87	1934	Cleveland	Walter L. Bierring	Iowa
88	1935	Atlantic City	James S. McLester	Alabama
89	1936	Kansas City, Mo.	James Tate Mason	Washington
90	1936		Vice-President—Charles Gordon Heyd	New York
91	1937	Atlantic City	J. H. J. Upham	Ohio
92	1938	San Francisco	Irvin Abell	Kentucky
93	1939	St. Louis	Rock Sleyster	Wisconsin
94	1940	New York City	Nathan B. Van Etten	New York
95	1941	Cleveland	Frank H. Lahey	Massachusetts

No.	Year	Place	President	State
96	1942	Atlantic City	Fred W. Rankin	Kentucky
97	1943	Chicago	James E. Paullin	Georgia
98	1944	Chicago	Herman L. Kretschmer	Illinois
99	1945	Chicago	Roger I. Lee	Massachusetts
100	1946	San Francisco	H. H. Shoulders	Tennessee
101	1947	Atlantic City	Edward L. Bortz	Pennsylvania

APPENDIX 2

BOARD OF TRUSTEES

ALONZO GARCELON—Lewiston, Maine
1882 to 1901
Chairman: 1892 to 1901
P. O. HOOPER—Little Rock, Ark.
1882 to 1892
Chairman: 1890 to 1892
H. F. CAMPBELL—Augusta, Ga.
1882 to 1887
J. M. TONER—Washington, D. C.
1882 to 1890
Chairman: 1883 to 1888
E. M. MOORE—Rochester, N. Y.
1882 to 1889
1890 to 1891
L. S. MCMURTRY—Danville, Ky.
1882 to 1889
1893 to 1894
Secretary: 1882 to 1883
J. H. PACKARD—Philadelphia
1882 to 1887
Secretary: 1883 to 1884
LEARTUS CONNOR—Detroit
1882 to 1890
1892 to 1894
N. S. DAVIS—Chicago
1882 to 1883 (Chairman)
(Resigned to become Editor)
J. H. HOLLISTER—Chicago
1883 to 1891
Secretary: 1884 to 1889
E. O. SHAKESPEARE—Philadelphia
1887 to 1890
WILLIAM T. BRIGGS—Nashville, Tenn.
1887 to 1890
W. W. DAWSON—Cincinnati
1890 to 1893
ISAAC N. LOVE—St. Louis, Mo.
1889 to 1892
1895 to 1901
JOHN B. HAMILTON—Washington, D. C.
(later Chicago)
Secretary: 1890 to 1893
(Resigned to become Editor)
J. V. SHOEMAKER—Philadelphia
1890 to 1893

D. E. NELSON—Tennessee
1890 to 1893
JOHN H. RAUCH—Chicago
1891 to 1894
D. C. PATTERSON—Washington, D. C.
1892 to 1894
P. H. MILLARD—St. Paul, Minn.
1892 to 1895
E. FLETCHER INGALS—Chicago
1893 to 1896
1900 to 1903
E. E. MONTGOMERY—Philadelphia
1893 to 1908
Secretary: 1902 to 1904
JOHN E. WOODBRIDGE—Youngstown, Ohio
1894 to 1896
J. W. GRAHAM—Denver, Colo.
1894 to 1895
JOSEPH EASTMAN—Indianapolis, Ind.
1894 to 1900
J. T. PRIESTLEY—Des Moines, Iowa
1894 to 1900
D. W. GRAHAM—Chicago
1894 to 1897
J. E. REEVES—Chattanooga, Tenn.
1895 to 1896
C. A. L. REED—Cincinnati
1896 to 1900
Secretary: 1899 to 1900
G. C. SAVAGE—Nashville, Tenn.
1896 to 1898
JOSEPH M. MATHEWS—Louisville
1896 to 1898
1900 to 1902
TRUMAN W. MILLER—Chicago
1897 to 1900
H. L. E. JOHNSON—Washington, D. C.
1898 to 1908
Secretary: 1901 to 1902
T. J. HAPPEL—Trenton, Tenn.
1898 to 1909
Chairman: 1901 to 1908
W. L. RODMAN—Philadelphia
1900 to 1903

BOARD OF TRUSTEES (Continued)

MILES F. PORTER—Fort Wayne, Ind.
1900 to 1909
JOHN F. FULTON—St. Paul, Minn.
1901 to 1904
W. W. GRANT—Denver, Colo.
1901 to 1916
Chairman: 1911 to 1913
A. L. WRIGHT—Carroll, Iowa
1902 to 1908
WILLIAM H. WELCH—Baltimore
1903 to 1909
Chairman: 1908 to 1909
M. L. HARRIS—Chicago
1903 to 1918
Chairman: 1909 to 1911
Secretary: 1904 to 1909; 1911 to 1918
PHILIP MARVEL—Atlantic City, N. J.
1904 to 1910
1911 to 1920
Chairman: 1919 to 1920
W. T. SARLES—Sparta, Wis.
1908 to 1923
Chairman: 1921 to 1922
PHILIP MILLS JONES—San Francisco
1908 to 1917
WISNER R. TOWNSEND—New York City
1908 to 1911
Secretary: 1909 to 1911
W. T. COUNCILMAN—Boston
1909 to 1917
Chairman: 1913 to 1917
C. E. CANTRELL—Greenville, Texas
1909 to 1913
C. A. DAUGHERTY—South Bend, Ind.
1909 to 1913
FRANK J. LUTZ—St. Louis, Mo.
1910 to 1916
OSCAR DOWLING—Shreveport, La.
1913 to 1925
Chairman: 1922 to 1923
THOMAS MCDAVITT—St. Paul, Minn.
1913 to 1926
Chairman: 1917 to 1919
A. R. MITCHELL—Lincoln, Nebraska
1916 to 1933
Chairman: 1920 to 1921 and 1932 to 1933
E. J. MCKNIGHT—Hartford, Conn.
1916 to 1918
H. BERT ELLIS—Los Angeles
1917 to 1920
WENDELL C. PHILLIPS—New York City
1917 to 1924
Chairman: 1923 to 1924

FRANK BILLINGS—Chicago
Secretary: 1918 to 1924
D. CHESTER BROWN—Danbury, Conn.
1918 to 1934
WALTER T. WILLIAMSON—Portland, Ore.
1920 to 1925
Chairman: 1924 to 1925
C. W. RICHARDSON—Washington, D. C.
1920 to 1929
J. H. J. UPHAM—Columbus, Ohio
1923 to 1935
Chairman: 1933 to 1935
J. H. WALSH—Chicago
Secretary: 1924 to 1933
E. B. HECKEL—Pittsburgh
1924 to 1932
Chairman: 1925 to 1932
E. H. CARY—Dallas, Texas
1925 to 1929
JOSEPH A. PETTIT—Portland, Ore.
1925 to 1935
ROCK SLEYSTER—Wauwatosa, Wis.
1926 to 1937
Chairman: 1935 to 1937
ALLEN H. BUNCE—Atlanta, Ga.
1929 to 1939
THOMAS S. CULLEN—Baltimore
1929 to 1941
ARTHUR W. BOOTH—Elmira, N. Y.
Member: 1932 to 1937
Chairman: 1937 to 1942
CHARLES B. WRIGHT—Minneapolis
1933 to 1940
AUSTIN A. HAYDEN—Chicago
Secretary: 1933 to 1940
ROGER I. LEE—Boston
Member: 1934 to 1944
Chairman: 1942 to 1944
JAMES R. BLOSS—Huntington, W. Va.
1935 to 1945
Chairman: 1944 to 1945
RALPH A. FENTON—Portland, Ore.
1935 to 1945
R. L. SENSENICH—South Bend, Ind.
Member: 1937 to present
Chairman: 1945 to present
E. L. HENDERSON—Louisville, Ky.
1939 to present
WILLIAM F. BRAASCH—Rochester, Minn.
1940 to present
ERNEST E. IRONS—Chicago
Secretary: 1940 to present
CHARLES W. ROBERTS—Atlanta, Ga.
1941 to present

BOARD OF TRUSTEES (Continued)

EDWARD M. PALLETTE—Los Angeles
 1942 to 1944
LOUIS H. BAUER—Hempstead, N. Y.
 1944 to present
ROBERT A. PEERS—Colfax, Calif.
 1944 to 1945

JAMES R. MILLER—Hartford, Conn.
 1945 to present
JOHN H. FITZGIBBON—Portland, Ore.
 1945 to present
DWIGHT H. MURRAY—Napa, Calif.
 1945 to present

APPENDIX 3

MEMBERSHIP OF COUNCIL ON MEDICAL EDUCATION AND HOSPITALS SINCE THE ORIGIN OF THE COUNCIL

ARNOLD, HORACE D. Harvard Medical School Courses for Graduates Boston, Massachusetts	1913–1919
BEVAN, ARTHUR DEAN Rush Medical College Chicago, Illinois	1904–1917 1919–1928
COFFEY, ROBERT C. Clinic and Hospital, Portland, Oregon	1915–1920
COUNCILMAN, WILLIAM T. Harvard Medical School Boston, Massachusetts	1904–1909
DOCK, GEORGE Washington University School of Medicine St. Louis, Missouri	1910–1915
DODSON, JOHN M. Rush Medical College Chicago, Illinois	1918–1919
DONALDSON, WALTER F. Medical Society of the State of Pennsylvania Pittsburgh	1925–1932
DYER, ISADORE Tulane University School of Medicine New Orleans, Louisiana	1919–1921
FITZ, REGINALD Harvard Medical School Boston, Massachusetts	1928–
FRAZIER, CHARLES H. University of Pennsylvania School of Medicine Philadelphia	1904–1907
HADEN, RUSSELL L. Cleveland Clinic Cleveland, Ohio	1941–
HAGGARD, WILLIAM D. Vanderbilt University School of Medicine Nashville, Tennessee	1912–1921

HEYD, CHARLES GORDON 1937–
  New York Postgraduate
  Medical School
  New York, New York

HOLLAND, JAMES W. 1907–1917
  Jefferson Medical College
  Philadelphia

HUMISTON, CHARLES E. 1930–1937
  University of Illinois
  College of Medicine
  Oak Park, Illinois

IRELAND, MERRITTE W. 1921–1930
  Surgeon General, U. S. Army
  Washington, D. C.

JOHNSON, VICTOR 1946–
  University of Chicago
  School of Medicine
  Chicago, Illinois

LAHEY, FRANK H. 1938–1940
  Lahey Clinic
  Boston, Massachusetts

LEWIS, DEAN 1931–1932
  Johns Hopkins University
  School of Medicine
  Baltimore, Maryland

MCLESTER, JAMES S. 1929–1934
  Medical College of Alabama
  Birmingham, Alabama

MOORE, FRED 1934–1941
  Iowa Methodist Hospital
  Des Moines, Iowa

MUSSER, JOHN H. 1934–
  Tulane University
  School of Medicine
  New Orleans, Louisiana

NORTH, EMMETT P. 1927–1934
  St. Louis University
  School of Medicine
  St. Louis, Missouri

PEPPER, WILLIAM 1917–1927
  University of Pennsylvania
  School of Medicine
  Philadelphia

RANKIN, FRED W. 1936–1941
  University of Louisville
  School of Medicine
  Lexington, Kentuky

SOUTHARD, ELMER E. 1909–1910
  Boston Psychopathic Hospital
  Boston, Massachusetts

STONE, HARVEY B. 1941–
  Johns Hopkins University
  School of Medicine
  Baltimore, Maryland

VAUGHAN, VICTOR C.   1904–1913
   University of Michigan
   School of Medicine
   Ann Arbor, Michigan
WASHBURN, F. A.   1932–1938
   Massachusetts General Hospital
   Boston, Massachusetts
WEISKOTTEN, H. G.   1940–
   Syracuse University
   College of Medicine
   Syracuse, New York
WELCH, S. W.   1921–1929
   State Board of Health
   Montgomery, Alabama
WELLS, H. GIDEON   1917–1919
   University of Chicago
   School of Medicine
   Chicago, Illinois
WILBUR, RAY LYMAN   1920–1923
   Stanford University   1925–1946
   Stanford University, California
WILSON, LOUIS B.   1923–1930
   Mayo Foundation
   Rochester, Minnesota
WITHERSPOON, JOHN A.   1904–1912
   Vanderbilt University
   School of Medicine
   Nashville, Tennessee

Chairmen of Council on Medical Education and Hospitals

BEVAN, ARTHUR DEAN   1904–1917
   Rush Medical College   1919 1928
   Chicago, Illinois
WILBUR, RAY LYMAN   1928–1946
   Stanford University
   Stanford University, California
WEISKOTTEN, H. G.   1946–
   Syracuse University
   College of Medicine
   Syracuse, New York

Secretaries of Council on Medical Education and Hospitals

COLWELL, N. P.   1905–1931
CUTTER, WILLIAM D.   1931–1942
WEISKOTTEN, H. G.   1942–1943
JOHNSON, VICTOR   1943–1947
ANDERSON, DONALD G.   1947–

APPENDIX 4

DATES IN THE HISTORY OF THE COUNCIL ON MEDICAL EDUCATION AND HOSPITALS

1847

American Medical Association organized.
Committee on Medical Education appointed.

1901

Annual Educational Number of THE JOURNAL begun.

1902

Reports from medical schools and names of graduates filed.
Graduate file begun.
Department "State Board of Registration" begun in THE JOURNAL.
Reports of individual State Board examinations published in THE JOURNAL, later called the Annual State Board Number.

1903

Publication of booklet of laws and board rulings regulating the practice of medicine in the United States and abroad begun.

1904

Creation of the Council on Medical Education.

1905

Beginning of Annual Conferences on Medical Education and Licensure.
Reports from State Licensing Boards including names of candidates recorded.
Licensure file begun.

1906

First publication of Educational Standards for Medical Schools: "Standard now Recommended" and "Ideal Standard."
American Medical Directory first published, containing biographies, index and hospitals.
First inspections of Medical Schools begun.

1907

First classification of Medical Colleges completed.
First list of foreign Medical Schools published.

1908

First complete list of all medical schools, existing and extinct, published.
Publication of descriptive lists of colleges based on first hand information.

1909

"Essentials of an Acceptable Medical College" published.
Report of Committee of 100 on Medical Curriculum.
Second tour of inspection of Medical Schools begun.

1910

Second classification published ("Carnegie" Report issued).
Student register established.
Medical educational standards abroad published.

1911

Third tour of inspection of Medical Colleges.

1912

First survey of hospitals for the training of interns.

1913

Life chart of medical colleges published.
First positive knowledge of exact number of medical colleges existing in each year since 1765.
First published table of non-recognized colleges.

1914

One year college work required of Class A Medical Schools.
First list of approved internships published.

1918

Two years of college work required for admission to Class A Medical Colleges.

1919

Establishment of essentials for approved internships.

1920

Hospital Bureau established. Name of Council changed to include ". . . and Hospitals."

1921

First publication of Hospital Number of THE JOURNAL.

1927

Beginning of certification of hospitals for residencies.

1928

Establishment of essentials for registered hospitals and for approved residencies and fellowships.
"A–B–C" classification of medical colleges discontinued.

1934

Approval of examining boards for the certification of specialists. Establishment of standards for the formation of American Boards in the specialties.

1934-1936

Survey of all medical schools in the United States and Canada by H. G. Weiskotten.

1936

Establishment of essentials for approval of schools for physical therapy technicians and also for clinical laboratory technicians.

1939

Establishment of essentials for approved schools of occupational therapy.

1940

Publication of volume "Medical Education in the United States, 1934-1939."

1942

Formation of liaison committee with Association of Amerian Medical Colleges.

1943

Establishment of essentials for approved schools for medical record librarians.

1944

Establishment of essentials for approved schools for x-ray technicians.

APPENDIX 5

SESSIONS AND ATTENDANCE OF THE ASSOCIATION

1900	Atlantic City	2,019
1901	St. Paul	1,806
1902	Saratoga Springs	1,425
1903	New Orleans	2,006
1904	Atlantic City	2,890
1905	Portland	1,680
1906	Boston	4,722
1907	Atlantic City	3,713
1908	Chicago	6,446
1909	Atlantic City	3,273
1910	St. Louis	4,086
1911	Los Angeles	2,153
1912	Atlantic City	3,598
1913	Minneapolis	3,243
1914	Atlantic City	3,998
1915	San Francisco	2,307
1916	Detroit	4,581
1917	New York	5,147
1918	Chicago	5,553
1919	Atlantic City	4,929
1920	New Orleans	3,681
1921	Boston	5,506
1922	St. Louis	5,174
1923	San Francisco	3,726
1924	Chicago	7,819
1925	Atlantic City	4,861
1926	Dallas	4,179
1927	Washington	6,273
1928	Minneapolis	4,876
1929	Portland	3,061
1930	Detroit	5,104
1931	Philadelphia	7,006
1932	New Orleans	2,778
1933	Milwaukee	4,601
1934	Cleveland	6,293
1935	Atlantic City	8,469
1936	Kansas City	6,824
1937	Atlantic City	9,764
1938	San Francisco	6,034
1939	St. Louis	7,412
1940	New York	12,864
1941	Cleveland	7,269
1942	Atlantic City	8,238
1944	Chicago	7,284
1946	San Francisco	7,746

There were no records before 1900 and no meetings in 1943 and 1945.

APPENDIX 6

MEMBERS OF THE JUDICIAL COUNCIL

WHILE THE JUDICIAL COUNCIL was in evolution, its membership varied considerably. The group was chosen in many instances at the session during which they were to function. Hence from 1901 to 1911 a varying number of members appears. After 1911, however, a change in the Constitution and By-Laws established the membership at five and the secretary of the Association as ex officio member.

1901–1902
   Term expires 1902:
     J. D. Griffith
     P. H. Bailhache
     J. E. Cook
     J. P. Lewis
     F. H. Wiggin, Secretary
     J. W. Irwin
     Waltman Wyman
   Term expires 1903:
     James R. Guthrie
     G. P. Gillespie
     R. C. Moore
     Ida J. Heiberger
     John B. Roberts
     Charles S. Rodman, Chairman
     S. L. Jepson
   Term expires 1904:
     George Cook
     H. H. Grant
     John B. Murphy
     Philip Marvel
     Louis H. Taylor
     John L. Dawson
     N. Fred Essig

1902–1903
   Term expires 1903:
     F. H. Wiggin
     G. B. Gillespie
     D. C. Peyton
   Term expires 1904:
     T. C. Martin
     J. B. Roberts
     Christopher Tompkins
   Term expires 1905:
     Philip Marvel
     George Cook
     N. S. Davis, Jr.

1903–1904
   Term expires 1904:
     T. C. Martin
     J. B. Roberts
     Christopher Tompkins
   Term expires 1905:
     Philip Marvel, Chairman
     George Cook
     N. S. Davis, Jr.
   Term expires 1906:
     F. H. Wiggin, Secretary
     G. B. Gillespie
     D. C. Peyton

1904–1905
   P. Maxwell Foshay
   D. C. Peyton
   George Ben. Johnston
   W. B. Russ
   F. H. Wiggin

1905–1906
   P. Maxwell Foshay
   D. C. Peyton
   George Ben. Johnston
   W. B. Russ
   W. S. Foster

1906–1907
   D. C. Peyton
   P. Maxwell Foshay
   W. B. Russ
   W. S. Foster
   George Ben. Johnston

1907–1908
   C. E. Cantrell
   R. C. Cabot
   G. W. Guthrie
   Thomas McDavitt
   Charles J. Kipp

1908–1909
  C. E. Cantrell
  R. C. Cabot
  G. W. Guthrie
  Thomas McDavitt
  Charles J. Kipp
1909–1910
  C. E. Cantrell
  J. H. Wilson
  Harold Gifford
  C. S. Sheldon
  H. A. Christian
1910–1911
  John H. J. Upham
  Lawrence M. Shaw
  Louis A. Hahn
  Charles S. Huffman
  George K. Angle
1911–1912
  Frank Billings, Chairman
  A. B. Cooke
  Alexander Lambert
  James E. Moore
  Hubert Work
  Alexander R. Craig, Secretary, ex off.
1912–1913
  Alexander Lambert, Chairman
  A. B. Cooke
  James E. Moore
  Hubert Work
  George W. Guthrie
  Alexander R. Craig, Secretary, ex off.
1913–1914
  Alexander Lambert, Chairman
  A. B. Cooke
  James E. Moore
  Hubert Work
  George W. Guthrie
  Alexander R. Craig, Secretary, ex off.
1914–1915
  Alexander Lambert, Chairman
  A. B. Cooke
  James E. Moore
  Hubert Work
  George W. Guthrie
  Alexander R. Craig, Secretary, ex off.
1915–1916
  Alexander Lambert, Chairman
  James E. Moore
  Hubert Work
  A. B. Cooke
  Randolph Winslow
  Alexander R. Craig, Secretary, ex off.
1916–1917
  Alexander Lambert, Chairman
  Randolph Winslow
  A. B. Cooke
  James E. Moore
  Herbert A. Black
  Alexander R. Craig, Secretary, ex off.
1917–1918
  Alexander Lambert, Chairman
  A. B. Cooke
  H. A. Black
  Randolph Winslow
  James E. Moore
  A. R. Craig, Secretary, ex off.
1918–1919
  M. L. Harris, Chairman
  H. A. Black
  Randolph Winslow
  William S. Thayer
  James E. Moore
  A. R. Craig, Secretary, ex off.
1919–1920
  M. L. Harris, Chairman
  I. C. Chase
  H. A. Black
  Randolph Winslow
  William S. Thayer
  A. R. Craig, Secretary, ex off.
1920–1921
  M. L. Harris, Chairman
  I. C. Chase
  H. A. Black
  Randolph Winslow
  William S. Thayer
  A. R. Craig, Secretary, ex off.
1921–1922
  M. L. Harris, Chairman
  Randolph Winslow
  William S. Thayer
  I. C. Chase
  J. N. Hall
  A. R. Craig, Secretary, ex off.
1922–1923
  M. L. Harris, Chairman
  W. S. Thayer
  I. C. Chase
  J. N. Hall
  J. H. J. Upham
  Olin West, Secretary, ex off.
1923–1924
  M. L. Harris, Chairman
  W. S. Thayer
  I. C. Chase
  J. N. Hall
  F. W. Cregor
  Olin West, Secretary, ex off.
1924–1925
  M. L. Harris, Chairman
  W. S. Thayer

I. C. Chase
J. N. Hall
F. W. Cregor
Olin West, Secretary, ex off.
1925–1926
M. L. Harris, Chairman
J. N. Hall
F. W. Cregor
W. S. Thayer
G. E. Follansbee
Olin West, Secretary, ex off.
1926–1927
M. L. Harris, Chairman
F. W. Cregor
W. S. Thayer
G. E. Follansbee
J. N. Hall
Olin West, Secretary, ex off.
1927–1928
M. L. Harris, Chairman
F. W. Cregor
George E. Follansbee
J. N. Hall
Donald Macrae, Jr.
Olin West, Secretary, ex off.
1928–1929
George E. Follansbee, Chairman
James B. Herrick
F. W. Cregor
J. N. Hall
Donald Macrae, Jr.
Olin West, Secretary, ex off.
1929–1930
George E. Follansbee, Chairman
J. N. Hall
Donald Macrae, Jr.
F. W. Cregor
James B. Herrick
Olin West, Secretary, ex off.
1930–1931
George E. Follansbee, Chairman,
J. N. Hall
Donald Macrae, Jr.
Frank W. Cregor
James B. Herrick
Olin West, Secretary, ex off.
1931–1932
G. E. Follansbee, Chairman,
Donald Macrae, Jr.
F. W. Cregor
J. B. Herrick
Walter F. Donaldson
Olin West, Secretary, ex off.
1932–1933
George E. Follansbee, Chairman
Frank W. Cregor

James B. Herrick
Walter F. Donaldson
Edwin P. Sloan
Olin West, Secretary, ex off.
1933–1934
George E. Follansbee, Chairman
Walter F. Donaldson
James B. Herrick
John H. O'Shea
Edwin P. Sloan
Olin West, Secretary, ex off.
1934–1935
George E. Follansbee, Chairman
Walter F. Donaldson
Edwin P. Sloan
John H. O'Shea
Emmett P. North
Olin West, Secretary, ex off.
1935–1936
George E. Follansbee, Chairman
Walter F. Donaldson
John H. O'Shea
Lloyd Noland
Emmett P. North
Olin West, Secretary, ex off.
1936–1937
George E. Follansbee, Chairman
Lloyd Noland
John H. O'Shea
Edward R. Cunniffe
Walter F. Donaldson
Olin West, Secretary, ex off.
1937–1938
George E. Follansbee, Chairman
Edward R. Cunniffe
Walter F. Donaldson
John W. Burns
John H. O'Shea
Olin West, Secretary, ex off.
1938–1939
George E. Follansbee, Chairman
Edward R. Cunniffe
Walter F. Donaldson
John W. Burns
John H. O'Shea
Olin West, Secretary, ex off.
1939–1940
George E. Follansbee, Chairman
Walter F. Donaldson
Holman Taylor
John H. O'Shea
Edward R. Cunniffe
Olin West, Secretary, ex off.
1940–1941
George E. Follansbee, Chairman
Walter F. Donaldson

Holman Taylor
John H. O'Shea
Edward R. Cunniffe
Olin West, Secretary, ex off.

1941–1942
George E. Follansbee, Chairman
Holman Taylor
John H. O'Shea
Edward R. Cunniffe
Walter F. Donaldson
Olin West, Secretary, ex off.

1942–1943
George E. Follansbee, Chairman
John H. O'Shea
Edward R. Cunniffe
Walter F. Donaldson
Lloyd Noland
Olin West, Secretary, ex off.

1943–1944
George E. Follansbee, Chairman
Edward R. Cunniffe
Walter F. Donaldson
Lloyd Noland

John H. O'Shea
Olin West, Secretary, ex off.

1944–1945
Edward R. Cunniffe, Chairman
Walter F. Donaldson
Lloyd Noland
John H. O'Shea
Olin West, Secretary, ex off.

1945–1946
E. R. Cunniffe, Chairman
Walter F. Donaldson
Lloyd Noland
John H. O'Shea
Louis A. Buie
Olin West, Secretary, ex off.

1946–1947
Edward R. Cunniffe, Chairman
Lloyd Noland
John H. O'Shea
Louis A. Buie
Walter F. Donaldson
George F. Lull, Secretary, ex off.

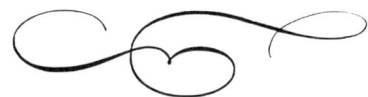

Indices

INDEX OF PERSONS

Abbott, W. C., 249, 256
Abell, Irvin, 430, 436, 439, 442, 446, 450, 454, 460; biography, 805
Abrams, Albert, 269
Abt, Isaac A., 261, 363, 390, 477, 483, 1118
Acuna, Miguel, 461
Adams, Samuel Hopkins, 132, 280, 1036
Adler, Francis Heed, 1162
Adson, A. W., 976
Agramonte, Aristides, 709
Ahart, Mabel D., 440
Allen, J. Adams, 129
Alpers, Bernard J., 1152
Ambruster, Howard W., 383, 393
Anderson, Charles P., 302
Anderson, R. B., 416
Andrews, Edmund, 110
Angell, James R., 264
Anthony, Susan B., 204
Aring, Charles D., 1152
Arlt, Adolf, 1161
Arnold, Richard D., 24, 27, 35
Arnold, Thurman W., 534
Asher, Leon, 424
Ashford, F. A., 1075
Askew, Henry Ford, biography, 609
Atkinson, William B., 84, 106, 170, 171, 188, 191, 860
Atlee, John Light, 110; biography, 641
Atlee, Washington L., 93
Atwater, D. F., 180, 183

Babbitt, James A., 1137
Bach, John L., 481
Bache, Franklin, 590
Bacon, C. S., 1022
Baehr, George, 373, 430, 462
Bailey, Pearce, 1150
Bailey, Percival, 1152
Bailey, William, 187
Baker, Frank, 193
Baker, Norman, 383, 392, 501, 517–525
Baldwin, William Owen, 77, 78; biography, 614
Balsinger, William E., 530
Bancroft, George, 140
Barker, L. F., 1087
Barnes, Joseph K., 96
Barnhill, John F., 1136
Barrett, A. H., 1152
Barringer, Emily D., 467
Barton, Edward H., 51
Barton, Paul C., 472, 1038
Barton, Thomas, 710
Bauer, Louis H., 490, 968, 976
Bauer, W. W., 393, 421, 422, 1004, 1185
Baxter, George E., 363
Beardsley, C. D., 148

Beck, T. Romeyn, 5, 1016
Bedford, Gunning S., 24
Belfield, W. T., 265
Bell, A. N., 102
Bell, Alexander Graham, 119
Bell, John, 24, 35, 37, 46
Belton, Thomas F., 850
Benedict, W. L., 1162
Benjamin, Harry, 406
Bennett, Granville A., 1164
Bernard, Claude, 647
Betts, Helen L., 133
Bevan, Arthur Dean, 227, 295, 302, 308, 393, 736, 759, 887, 891, 892, 893, 901; biography, 741
Bierring, Walter Lawrence, 404, 407, 413, 418; biography, 792
Bigelow, Henry J., 44
Bigelow, Jacob, 607
Billings, Frank, 247, 281, 299, 306, 317, 403, 497, 606, 775, 797, 998, 1049; activities at AMA sessions, 195, 225, 232, 235, 238, 255; attacks on, 324; biography, 688; chairman of Council on Health, 296, 1001; chairman of Judicial Council, 268, 271, 951; member of Board of Trustees, 307, 316, 321, 842; president of AMA, 224, 226, 227; treasurer of AMA, 230, 855; work on Rush monument, 237
Billings, John Shaw, 57, 87, 99, 103, 104, 106, 119, 122, 124, 139, 196
Billroth, Theodor, 119
Bishop, W. T., 189
Bloodgood, Joseph Colt, 518
Bloomfield, Arthur, 1115
Blue, Rupert, 295; biography, 735
Blumer, George, 599
Bobbs, John S., 240
Bolton, William W., 1008
Booth, Arthur W., 440, 442
Bortz, Edward L., 492, 494; biography, 829
Bowditch, Henry I., 75, 77, 93, 97, 629, 948; biography, 630
Bowling, William K., 615; biography, 625
Braasch, William F., 439, 448
Bracken, Henry M., 267, 998
Bradley, Omar, 492
Brainard, Daniel, 10, 44, 60, 601
Braisted, William C., 302, 314, 318; biography, 748
Branner, John Casper, 759
Braun, Will C., 214, 218, 276, 319, 344, 349, 481, 489, 981, 995
Brice, Fannie, 500
Briggs, William T., biography, 657
Brinkley, John R., 346, 383, 392, 399, 503–516
Brinton, John K., 679

[1209]

Broders, Albert C., 518
Brodie, William, 91, 102, 103, 107, 127, 151; biography, 648
Bronson, J. R., 102, 103
Brook, J. D., 439
Brooksher, W. R., 976
Brower, D. R., 204
Brower, Howard O., 978
Brown, D. Chester, 348, 1030, 1049
Brown, J. Mackenzie, 1137
Brown-Séquard, Charles-Édouard, 74, 140
Browning, Peaches, 500
Bruce, Herbert, 302
Brunson, Asa, 530
Bryant, Joseph Decatur, 158, 222, 253, 680; biography, 702
Buchanan, A. H., 27, 31
Buck, Gurdon, 43
Buel, William P., 24
Buie, Louis A., 476
Bulkley, L. Duncan, 187, 237
Bulson, Albert E., 403
Bunce, Allen H., 1049
Bunting, C. H., 227
Bunts, F. E., 316
Burke, E. M., 461
Burnet, Waldo J., 60
Burns, Robert, 72
Burnsworth, Mrs. Z., 240
Burrell, Herbert Leslie, 256; biography, 704
Butler, S. W., 171

Cabot, Hugh, 282, 287, 434, 545, 1154
Cabot, Richard C., 1111
Caldwell, Charles, 1016
Caldwell, John A., 1018
Camalier, C. Willard, 815
Campbell, Henry Frazer, 108, 122, 834, 1015; biography, 646
Campbell, Robert, 647
Cannon, Walter B., 258, 267, 998
Cargill, Frank V., 986, 1176
Carlson, Anton J., 483, 488; biography, 565
Carpenter, George A., 497
Carpenter, Henry, 996
Carroll, James, 709
Carstens, J. H., 245
Cary, Edward H., 392, 395, 402, 448, 485, 1099; biography, 785
Casamajor, Louis, 1152
Cash, M. H., 6
Chaillé, S. E., 100, 833
Chapin, Charles V., 291, 311
Chapman, Nathaniel, 31, 36, 41, 110, 589, 616, 642; biography, 573
Chatfield, Daniel, 5
Cheney, W. Fitch, 1120
Chittenden, Russell H., 744
Christopher, W. S., 150
Churchill, F. S., 261, 1118, 1120
Churchill, Winston, 826
Clancy, Frank J., 1038
Clark, A., 35
Clark, Daniel, 3, 4, 604
Clark, John G., 998
Clark, Percival Lemon, 392, 502
Cleveland, President Grover, 156, 158, 166, 680, 703

Coates, George M., 1136
Cobb, Stanley, 1152
Coe, H. W., 252
Cogan, David G., 1162
Cole, Harold N., 1143
Cole, R. Beverly, 104, 106; biography, 668
Collins, Frederick, 358
Colwell, N. P., 893, 898, 901
Comegys, Cornelius G., 147, 1018
Condie, David Francis, 849, 1011, 1071
Connor, Leartus, 108, 117, 169, 177, 245, 834; biography, 184
Cooke, A. B., 268, 951
Cooley, George, 975
Cooley, Thomas B., 434
Coolidge, President Calvin, 773
Cooper, Astley, 593
Cooper, E. S., 622
Cordes, Frederick C., 1162
Corlett, William T., 146, 1140
Cortelyou, George B., 254
Coulter, John M., 302, 927
Councilman, William T., 286, 775, 840, 892
Cowgill, George R., 942
Cox, G. C., 76
Craig, Alexander R., 251, 267, 269, 280, 298, 304, 309, 334, 862, 1022
Cramp, Arthur J., 282, 335, 354, 410, 423, 450, 882, 1034, 1184, 1185
Crane, R. T., 294
Crawford, James E., 505
Crile, George W., 316, 418, 421, 464
Crisp, William Henry, 1161
Crockett, Eugene A., 1130
Crockett, F. S., 1030
Crothers, T. D., 147, 148, 150, 178
Crowder, Enoch H., 304
Crownhart, George, 434
Culbertson, H., 90
Culbertson, John C., 142, 145, 150, 157, 159
Cullen, Thomas S., 271, 280, 283, 313, 380, 483, 1030, 1049, 1154
Cummings, Homer S., 412
Cunniffe, E. R., 483
Cushing, Emily, 176, 464
Cushing, Harvey, 413, 791, 794, 1155, 1156
Cushny, A. H., 870
Cushny, Arthur R., 866
Cutler, Elliott C., 1156
Cutler, Max, 518
Cutter, Ephraim, 103
Cutter, Irving S., 1056
Cutter, William D., 463, 900
Cutting, Charles S., 302
Czerny, Vincenz, 119

DaCosta, Jacob M., 679
Daggett, David L., 1012
Dale, H. H., 870
Dalton, John C., 948
Dandy, Walter E., 1159
Darrach, William, 1154
Darwin, Erasmus, 36
Daugherty, C. A., 891
David, Vernon C., 791

[1210]

Davis, Anna Maria Parker, 6
Davis, Carl Henry, 1056
Davis, Frank Howard, 11
Davis, Frank Howard, II, 15
Davis, Jefferson, 651
Davis, Michael M., 406, 415, 450
Davis, Nathan Smith, 160, 162, 179, 193, 210, 215, 601, 645, 696; activities at AMA sessions, 52, 54, 60, 65, 67, 76, 80, 87, 93, 96, 97, 102, 104, 106, 107, 108, 117, 156, 170, 585, 949, 950, 1071; attendance at British Medical Association meetings, 13; attendance at fiftieth jubilee of AMA, 14; biography, 3-16, 603-606; death, 14; editor of Journal of AMA, 12, 109, 116, 118, 120, 122, 124, 125, 126, 128, 130, 134, 136, 142, 860; efforts toward organizing AMA, 7, 22, 23, 25; History of AMA written by, 9, 21; medal honoring, 88; memorial to, 239, 253, 264, 269, 299, 358; portrait, 203; president of American Association of Medical Editors, 110; president of AMA, 10, 69, 73; president of Board of Trustees, 834, 979; president of International Medical Congress, 127; Principles and Practice of Medicine written by, 12; tributes to, 108, 129, 183; vice president of AMA, 9; views on function of AMA, 58
Davis, Nathan Smith, Jr., 11, 131
Davis, Nathan Smith, III, 15
Davy, Bertha C., 981
Dawson, William Wirt, 102, 139; biography, 653
Dayton, George L., 184
Delafield, Edward, 24
Delafield, Francis, 713
Delameter, John, 5
DeLee, Joseph B., 138, 497
Delphey, E. F., 324
Demarest, A., 795
Dennie, Charles C., 1146
Derby, George S., 1162
de Schweinitz, Edmund, 754
de Schweinitz, George E., 329, 335, 337, 1024; biography, 754
Dickinson, Frank G., 491, 1068
Dickinson, R. C., 366
Didama, Henry D., 156, 163
Diehl, C. Lewis, 866
Diehl, Harold S., 815
Doane, Mrs. Philip Schuyler, 1100
Dock, George, 247, 333, 477, 1111; biography, 562
Dodson, John M., 336, 338, 393, 1002, 1184
Doherty, Margaret, 1084
Donaldson, Walter F., 483
Dosland, Goodwin L., 1027
Doughton, Robert, 1031
Douglass, Ellwood, 1185
Dowler, B., 65
Dowling, Oscar, 285
Dragstedt, Lester, 1158
Drake, Daniel, 46, 52, 53, 57, 77, 579, 587, 598
Draper, Warren F., 436, 483
DuBois, Eugene F., 379, 946
Dunbar, J. R. W., 31

Dunglison, Richard James, 106, 163, 853
Dunglison, Robley, 853
Dunham, George C., 454
Dunn, T. C., 35
Dunster, E. L., 96

Eagleton, Wells P., 340
Earle, George H., 830
Eastman, Joseph Rilus, 190, 193
Edsall, David L., 1111
Edwards, T. O., 1010
Eggleston, William G., 130, 131
Eiselsberg, Anton von, 741
Ellis, H. Bert, 175, 228
Eliot, Charles William, 10
Eliot, Martha, 970
Elman, Robert, 1158
Emerson, C. P., 1056
Emerson, G., 35
Engman, Martin F., 1140
Erdman, John F., 703
Eshner, A. A., 200
Evans, William A., 272, 279, 1044
Eve, Joseph, 646
Eve, Paul F., 646; biography, 593
Everson, G., 948
Ewing, James, 264, 455, 459, 1164; biography, 557

Falk, Isidore, 415
Favill, Henry B., 267, 289, 998
Fenger, Christian, 559, 606, 672, 688, 698
Fenton, Ralph A., 1136
Ferguson, Burr, 514
Ferguson, E. D., 170, 188
Fernel, Edna Purdy, 530
Fernel, Jean Paul, 428, 526, 531
Fetterolf, George, 1136
Fiedler, Otho A., 1030
Finlay, Carlos J., 675, 708
Finney, John M. T., 355, 791
Fischer, Martin H., 1045
Fishbein, Morris, 379, 381, 411, 430, 436, 440, 490, 1082; activities in World War II, 456, 462, 463, 465, 476, 1180; assistant to editor of Journal, 280, 343, 353; editor of Hygeia, 335, 1184; editor of Journal, 344, 349, 415, 438, 844, 1117, 1156; libel suits against, 499-533; member of Council on Foods and Nutrition, 946
Fisher, Irving, 1021
Fitz, Reginald, 1115
Fitzgibbon, John H., 971
Fletcher, Robert, 196
Flexner, Abraham, 893, 898
Flexner, Simon, 436, 459, 477, 775
Flint, Austin, 12, 13, 31, 38, 46, 52, 55, 66, 114, 127, 713; biography, 643
Flint, Austin (younger), 643
Flint, Austin, VI, 643
Flint, J. B., 248
Flynn, James M., 448
Follansbee, George Edward, 385
Foote, John G., 363
Forbus, Wiley D., 1164
Foshay, P. Maxwell, 190, 198, 201, 205, 214, 223, 352

[1211]

Fouts, Roy W., 488
Fox, Howard, 1141, 1143
Fox, W. W., 197
Francis, John W., 585, 1016
Frazier, Charles H., 892
Freeman, Mrs. Walter Jackson, 1100
French, S. H., 8
Freyder, Magdalene, 1084, 1168
Friesner, Isidore, 1130
Fulton, John F., 148, 197, 1086
Furnas, J. C., 515
Furno, Giovanni. See *Fernel, Jean Paul.*

Gaillard, P. C., 948
Garcelon, Alonzo, 108, 110, 175, 193, 834, 835
Gardiner, Thomas R., 986
Gardner, E. J., 159
Garfield, President James A., 161
Garnett, Alexander Y. P., 134; biography, 651
Garrison, Fielding H., 365, 1166
Garrison, William Lloyd, 631
Gayle, John, 707
Gearing, Charles, 519
Gerhard, W. W., 54, 617
Ghadiali, Dinshah P., 531
Gifford, Sanford R., 1162
Gihon, Albert L., 181, 194
Gilbert, N. C., 1115
Giles, Roscoe C., 441
Goepp, R. Max, 998
Goin, Lowell S., 488
Goldwater, S. S., 313
Goodale, Robert L., 1137
Goodrich, Charles H., 416
Goodwin, E. J., 280, 293
Gorgas, Josiah, 707
Gorgas, Marie C. Daughty, 708
Gorgas, William Crawford, 261, 302, 304, 355, 747; biography, 707-711
Gould, George M., 190
Gradle, Harry S., 110, 157, 1161
Graham, Edwin E., 1120
Graham, Evarts A., 1154, 1158
Graham, J. A., 181
Grant, David N. W., 474
Grant, W. W., 286
Graves, John Temple, 175
Green, Frederick R., 244, 262, 267, 296, 312, 328, 358, 986, 1049, 1078, 1171
Green, J. S., 102
Gregory, Elisha H., 130; biography, 650
Griffith, J. P. C., 261
Griscom, John H., 25
Gross, Samuel D., 94, 171, 588, 594, 598, 612, 632, 644, 656, 833; activities at AMA sessions, 10, 79, 89, 97, 100, 102, 105, 126; biography, 610; death, 115; president of AMA, 77; report on medical literature, 63; tributes to, 122, 149, 172
Grosvenor, J. W., 252
Grulee, Clifford G., 1127
Gunn, S. M., 278

Haggard, William D., 339, 347, 361, 366, 766; biography, 766
Hahn, Eugen, 119

Hahnemann, Samuel C. F., 172
Hale, Enoch, 46
Hall, George E., Jr., 1033
Hall, J. Basil, 360
Hall, Marshall, 647
Hallberg, C. S. N., 235, 867
Halling, Bliss O., 1038
Halsted, W. S., 713, 789
Hamilton, Edwin S., 486
Hamilton, Frank H., 42, 948
Hamilton, John B., 13, 127, 136, 137, 157, 159, 163, 165, 168, 173, 189, 835
Happel, T. J., 191, 222, 239, 245, 256, 836, 838
Hardie, T. Melville, 193
Harding, President Warren G., 342, 753
Hare, Hobart A., 157, 188, 193
Harper, William Rainey, 689
Harrington, Charles, 998
Harris, E. Eliot, 222, 227, 238, 239
Harris, Malcolm L., 229, 230, 252, 261, 286, 299, 313, 1111; biography, 778; chairman of Board of Trustees, 262, 269, 280; chairman of Judicial Council, 320, 370; member of Board of Trustees, 842; president elect of AMA, 375, 377; president of AMA, 384
Harrison, John, 27
Hart, Ernest, 103, 156, 158
Hartshorne, Henry, 1013
Hartzell, Milton B., 1141
Hastings, Daniel H., 182
Hatcher, Robert A., 867
Hawley, Paul R., 483, 484
Hayden, Austin A., 328, 406, 415, 441, 456, 856
Hayes, John F., 1029
Hays, Isaac, 25, 27, 31, 35, 36, 47, 110, 642; first treasurer of AMA, 846
Heberden, William, 36
Hein, Fred V., 1009
Heise, Herman A., 1032
Hektoen, Ludvig, 171, 190, 200, 281, 302, 307, 354, 436, 455, 459, 464, 1032, 1043, 1087, 1164; biography, 559
Helmholz, Henry F., 1123
Henderson, E. L., 490, 1049
Henderson, Yandell, 271, 381
Hendricks, Thomas A., 971
Henrotin, Fernando, 159
Herrick, James B., 158, 4847, 1087; biography, 554
Hershey, General Lewis B., 464
Hess, C., 1160
Heubner, W., 870
Heyd, Charles Gordon, 426, 428, 430, 492; biography, 801
Hibberd, James F., 162, 1013, 1072; biography, 663
Hines, Frank T., 342
Hirschberg, J., 1160
Hirschman, L. J., 431
Hoch, August, 1150
Hodgen, John T., 104; biography, 638
Hoffman, Edward, 857
Holden, W. A., 1160
Hollister, John H., 110, 138, 142, 144, 148, 151
Holloway, J. W., Jr., 440, 968, 1027, 1033
Holmes, Bayard, 154, 157, 190

[1212]

Holmes, Oliver Wendell, 46, 120, 137, 165, 607
Holmquest, H. J., 924
Holt, Luther Emmett, 177, 261, 998
Holt, Luther Emmett, Jr., 434
Hooker, Worthington, 1012
Hooper, P. O., 108, 110, 639, 834
Hoover, President Herbert, 380, 716, 756, 759, 760
Hopkins, Harry L., 412, 432
Hopkins, Joel, 28
Horder, Lord, 422, 424
Horlick, A. J., 94
Horsley, J. Shelton, 298
Hough, Charles A., 147
Hough, W. M., 497
Howland, John, 1120, 1126
Hoxsey, Harry M., 501, 518, 523
Hoxsey, John C., 501
Hubbard, John, 1023
Huber, G. Carl, 789
Hughes, C. H., 150
Hull, Thomas G., 384, 1049
Humiston, Charles E., 313
Humiston, William H., 1018
Hunt, Westley M., 1137
Hunter, John, 36, 642
Hurty, J. N., 217, 279
Hussey, Raymond, 963
Husted, N. C., 102
Hutchinson, Helen, 1078, 1166
Hutchison, Ralph Cooper, 492
Hutter, Charles G., 460
Hyde, Edward Everett, 280, 353

Ingals, E. Fletcher, 169, 193, 220, 842, 860
Ireland, General Merritt W., 317, 841
Irons, Ernest E., 457, 474
Ives, Eli, biography, 599

Jackson, Alfred J., 991
Jackson, Andrew, 1021
Jackson, Chevalier, 117, 447, 455, 1026, 1130; biography, 556
Jackson, Edward, 155, 164, 189, 447, 757, 1161
Jackson, J. M., 685
Jackson, Jabez N., 247, 370, 373; biography, 772
Jackson, James, 630
Jackson, John Wesley, 772
Jackson, Thomas, 4, 604
Jackson, General Thomas J., 661
Jacobi, Abraham, 103, 247, 261, 274, 276, 713, 1120; biography, 721
Jacobsen, Victor C., 1164
Jaggard, W. W., 138
Janeway, Theodore, 1111
Jarvis, W. C., 110
Jeffries, F. M., 1049
Jewell, Wilson, 601
Johnson, Charles B., 94
Johnson, H. L. E., 203, 221, 1019
Johnson, Hugh S., 299
Johnson, John B., 31, 180, 183, 865
Johnson, Victor, 488
Johnston, Albert Sidney, 619

Johnston, Florence, 1081
Jones, Philip Mills, 227, 244, 252, 296, 877
Jones, R. Watson, 430
Jordan, David Starr, 758
Jordan, Edwin O., 427, 1089
Josephson, Emanuel M., 426
Joslin, Elliott P., 464, 470; biography 561
Joslyn, L. B., 387
Judd, E. Starr, 298, 390, 698, 1003; biography, 782

Kales, Albert Martin, 15
Kales, Francis Henry, 11, 15
Kales, John Davis, 14, 15
Kales, William Robert, 15
Kean, Jeffeson R., 734
Keen, W. W., 183, 199, 205, 264, 381, 703, 1042, 1085; biography, 679
Kehler, Lyman F., 867
Kelleher, Grant, 545
Kelly, Aloysius O. J., 693
Kelly, G. Lombard, 970
Kelly, Howard A., 713, 998
Kelly, T. Henshaw, 420
Kendall, E. C., 294
Kennedy, Walter L., 488
Kerr, John W., 295, 736
Ketchum, Jay, 975
Kilgore, Eugene S., 432
Kimball, H. H., 1015
Kimball, O. P., 941
Kingsbury, John, 406
Kirk, Norman T., 471
Kleinschmidt, C. H. A., 1075
Kleinschmidt, L. S., 978
Klumpp, Theodore G., 462, 463
Knapp, Arnold, 1160, 1162
Knapp, Herman, 1160
Knight, Jonathan, 24, 27, 31, 60, 73, 567; biography, 585
Koch, Robert, 119, 675, 713
Koch, William F., 426
Koenig, A., 169
Koontz, E. Ransom, 1033
Kopetzky, Samuel J., 430
Koussevitsky, Serge, 826
Kreider, George N., 210
Kretschmer, Herman L., 415, 475, 477, 479, 483, 857, 976, 1103; biography, 822

LaGarde, Louis A., 795
Lahey, Frank H., 455, 460, 461, 463, 465; biography, 813
Lambert, Adrian S., 744
Lambert, Alexander, 268, 289, 295, 302, 709, 736, 951, 1048; biography, 744; chairman of Judicial Council, 278; president elect of AMA, 308; president of AMA, 317, 319; reports on sickness insurance, 286, 292, 296, 306, 307, 313
Lambert, Edward W., 744
Lambert, Samuel W., 744, 1028
Landon, Alfred, 425
Lane, Arbuthnot, 282, 302
Lane, C. Guy, 962, 1145
Lape, Esther E., 423, 428, 430

Lawrence, Joseph, 476, 971
Lazear, Jesse W., 709
Lazenby, A. D., 963
Leahy, William E., 546
Lee, Edward W., 717
Lee, General Robert E., 661
Lee, Roger I., 479, 483, 486, 488, 490, 976, 1049; biography, 824
Lee, William, 1075
Leech, Paul Nicholas, 344, 383, 436, 457, 884
Leidy, Joseph, 755
Leland, R. G., 368, 372, 389, 415, 464, 1003, 1068, 1069
LePrince, Joseph L., 709
Levy, Robert, 1129
Lewin, John Henry, 544
Lewis, Dean D., 399, 403, 407, 743, 784, 1154, 1157; biography, 788
Lewis, Denslow, 200
Lewis, F. Park, 255
Lewis, J. Hamilton, 429
Libman, Emanuel, 1044
Liebman, Joshua, 492
Lim, Robert Kho-sheng, 479
Lindskog, Gustaf, 1159
Lindsley, J. B., 1092
Lindsly, Harvey, biography, 595
Lister, Joseph, 637, 658, 680
Lloyd George, David, 360
Logan, Joseph P., 98
Logan, Thomas Muldrop, biography, 621
Long, J. H., 867
Loomis, Meta, 1078
Louis, Antoine, 630
Love, I. N., 144, 170, 175, 177, 181, 187
Lovejoy, J. W. H., 1073
Lowell, A. Lawrence, 826
Lower, W. E., 316
Luce, Henry, 406
Luckhardt, A. B., 789, 1056
Lueth, H. C., 472
Lull, George F., 476, 482, 489, 494, 845, 976
Lutz, F. J., 1022
Lydston, G. Frank, 157, 159, 190, 199, 266, 281, 305
Lynch, Kenneth M., 800
Lynch, Robert C., 1130

Macatee, Henry C., 404, 416
McCall, John, 21
McCaskey, Carl H., 1137
McClellan, George, 110
McClellan, Samuel, 171
MacCollum, William G., 1164
McComas, A. R., 961
McCord, Carey, 381
McCormack, Arthur T., 256, 746
McCormack, J. N., 267, 272, 999; organizer for AMA, 224, 225, 226, 227, 230, 231, 236, 238, 243, 244, 254, 255, 310; tributes to, 331, 361, 362; work in reorganization of AMA, 201, 205, 210, 211, 214, 352
McCormick, Edward J., 968, 971, 976
McDavitt, T. V., 1027
McDowell, Ephraim, 641, 677
McDowell, Joseph N., 588, 677
McGoldrick, T. A., 976

McGuire, Hugh Holmes, 660
McGuire, Hunter H., 156, 226; biography, 660
McGuire, Stuart, 661
McIntire, Ross T., 455, 821
MacKee, George M., 1141
McKenna, Hugh, 497
Mackenzie, James, 302
McKinley, President William, 181, 182, 217
McKnight, E. J., 299, 841
McLean, Angus, 384, 1030
Maclean, Donald, 168, 175, 200, 698, 854; biography, 665
McLester, James S., 410, 418, 423, 424, 936, 946; biography, 796
McMillan, J. A., 280
McMillan, R. J., 514
McMurtry, Lewis S., 108, 110, 241, 253, 834, 998; biography, 695
McNaughton, James, 5, 7, 22
McNutt, Paul V., 466
McRea, Floyd W., 891
McVay, J. R., 976
Macy, Mary Sutton, 263
Maloney, William R., 1029
Manley, Thomas H., 147
Manners, Lady Diana, 500
March, Alden, 6, 22; biography, 601
March, Allen, 75
Marcy, Alexander, 840
Marcy, Henry O., 146, 152, 239; biography, 658
Marine, David, 941
Marmion, R. A., 891
Marriott, W. McKim, 379, 946
Marris, M. L., 841
Marshall, General George C., 462
Martin, Franklin H., 270, 300, 303, 304, 336, 339, 346, 355, 366, 418, 1154
Martin, Newell, 675
Martin, W. B., 976
Mason, A. S., 799
Mason, Claiborne Rice, 799
Mason, James Tate, 421, 423, 424, 426; biography, 799
Massey, G. Betton, 157
Mastin, Claudius H., 149
Matas, Rudolph W., 193, 436, 891; biography, 553
Mathews, Joseph M., 193, 280; biography, 677
Mattson, Elwood W., 991
Mayo, Charles H., 293, 294, 304, 305, 355, 697, 782, 816, 817; biography, 738
Mayo, Hattie N. Damon, 698
Mayo, William J., 197, 239, 249, 300, 355, 686, 738, 779, 1086, 1154, biography, 697-701
Mayo, William Worrall, 697, 738
Medin, Oscar, 150
Mendel, Lafayette B., 354, 379, 946
Mendenhall, George, 634; biography, 616
Menne, Frank R., 1164
Merkel, S. B., 83
Merriam, J. C., 365
Meyer, Adolf, 1152
Miller, Bruce, 501, 523
Miller, Henry, 67, 634; biography, 597
Miller, Joseph L., 253, 394, 690, 1111, 1113

[1214]

Miller, Thomas, 1073
Miller, Truman W., 190, 191, 835
Miller, W. H. H., 500, 527
Miller, Watson B., 412
Minot, George R., 483; biography, 564
Mitchell, A. R., 280, 316, 348, 349, 403
Mitchell, S. Weir, 680, 700, 755
Moffett, E. D., 148
Mohler, Charles S., 991
Moll, A. A., 303
Monihan, Berkeley, 718
Monson, Eneas, 599
Montgomery, E. E., 163
Moore, Edward M., 108, 834; biography, 655
Moore, Fred, 431
Moore, James E., 268, 951
Moore, Josiah J., 857
Moore, Marjorie Hutchins, 1081
Morehouse, George R., 680
Morgan, Hugh J., 434
Morgan, William Gerry, 378, 384, 387, 389; biography, 780
Morgenthau, Henry, Jr., 412
Moritz, Alan R., 1017
Morris, George M., 471
Morris, Roger S., 298
Morris, W. W., 35
Morse, John Lovett, 1120
Morton, Rosalie Slaughter, 263
Morton, William T. G., 44, 70, 578
Mott, Valentine, 73, 142, 585
Moultrie, James, 31; biography, 581
Moyer, Harold N., 146, 157, 174, 177, 190
Mundt, G. Henry, 403
Munn, W. P., 189
Murdock, Thomas P., 483
Murphy, John B., 158, 270, 279, 289, 672, 673, 806; biography, 717
Murphy, William P., 565
Murray, Dwight H., 207, 281, 321, 322
Musser, Benjamin, 692
Musser, John H., Sr., 193, 232, 237, 775; biography, 692
Musser, John Herr, II, 693, 1115
Musser, Martin, 692
Musser, Milton B., 692
Mussey, Reuben D., 5, 51, 634; biography, 579
Mussey, Robert D., 580
Myers, Victor C., 1048

Neisser, Albert, 119
Newell, A. J., 109
Newman, Henry Parker, 835, 854
Nicholls, Annie E., 351
Noguchi, Hideyo, 374
Nordbye, Gunnar H., 517
Norris, William F., 754
Novy, F. G., 727, 867

Ochsner, Edward H., 306, 324
O'Connor, Basil, 335, 492
O'Fallon, John, 588
Ogier, Thomas L., 621
O'Leary, Paul A., 1146
Ophüls, William, 1164
Orton, Samuel T., 1152

Osgood, Robert S., 434
Osler, William, 54, 168, 170, 171, 190, 662, 710, 713, 774, 775, 1087
Otis, George A., 639
Ozias, Charles O., 518

Packard, Francis R., 641
Packard, John H., 104, 105, 106, 108, 116, 834
Paget, James, 593
Paine, Martyn, 23
Pallen, Montrose A., 72, 948
Palmer, G. S., 80
Palmer, George T., 727
Pancoast, W. H., 102
Park, William H., 745
Parker, Painless, 418, 525
Parker, Walter R., 1162
Parker, Willard, 636
Parkes, Charles T., 671
Parran, Thomas, 424
Parsons, Usher, 60
Parvin, Theophilus, 97, 99, 620, 833; biography, 634
Pasteur, Louis, 119, 172
Patrick, Hugh T., 1149, 1150
Patten, John A., 495
Patten, Zeboim C., Jr., 495
Patterson, R. U., 395
Pattison, G. S., 24
Paullin, James E., 467, 469, 471, 472, 475, 477, 806, 815; biography, 819
Payne, Clarence H., 441
Peabody, Francis, 374
Pearce, R. M., 1089
Pederson, James, 265
Pelley, William Dudley, 515
Penfield, Wilder, 1152
Pennington, J. R., 203
Pepper, William (elder), 618
Pepper, William (younger), 90, 140, 627, 692
Percival, Thomas, 35, 36
Perdue, E. M., 521
Perkins, Frances, 411, 412, 794
Peters, John P., 432, 434
Peterson, Carl M., 963
Phillips, Wendell C., 307, 321, 362, 366, 368, 843, 1129; biography, 769
Physick, Philip Syng, 110, 142, 642
Pierson, Clarence, 313
Pilcher, Cobb, 1159
Pilcher, James E., 142
Pilcher, Lewis S., 270, 1154
Pitcher, Zina, biography, 591
Plauchu, E., 1122
Pope, Charles Alexander, biography, 587
Powers, C. A., 197, 1086
Pratt, Foster, 102, 1092
Prentis, H. W., Jr., 492
Priestly, J. T., 190
Proctor, James M., 535, 539, 546
Prudden, T. Mitchell, 713, 744
Puckner, W. A., 344, 867, 884
Pusey, William Allen, 164, 299, 328, 339, 344, 349, 358, 359, 843, 856, 1138; biography, 762
Putnam, Tracy J., 1152
Putnam-Jacobi, Mary, 722

[1215]

Quimby, I. N., 170, 1015
Quine, William E., 672

Rankin, Fred W., 461, 465, 467, 470, 472, 740, 806; biography, 816
Rankin, W. S., 324
Ranson, S. W., 1152
Rappleye, Willard C., 434, 794
Rattner, Herbert, 1139, 1146
Rauch, John H., 912
Red, Mrs. Samuel Clark, 332, 1099
Redman, John, 123
Reed, Charles A. L., 150, 193, 202, 205, 214, 227, 232, 234, 251, 256, 263, 264, 497; biography, 683
Reed, R. Harvey, 147, 157, 158, 1076
Reed, Walter, 226, 237, 676, 709
Reese, D. M., 65
Reese, David M., 66
Reid, E. M., 1016
Reid, W. W., 655
Reyburn, Robert, 161, 1075
Reynolds, Edward, 607
Richardson, Charles W., 348, 365, 380, 1129
Richardson, Tobias G., 97, 226, 614; biography, 632
Ricketts, Howard Taylor, 265, 1090
Ridlon, John, 171, 305
Rist, Edouard, 302
Roberts, Carl G., 441
Roberts, Charles W., 1049
Roberts, John B., 183
Roberts, Kingsley, 435
Robertson, John Dill, 328, 358
Roche, Josephine, 436, 438, 446
Rockefeller, John D., 204
Rockefeller, Nelson, 458
Rodman, James, 730
Rodman, John, 730
Rodman, W. B., 730
Rodman, William L., 203, 223, 234, 237, 239, 288, 795, 840, 915, 1019; biography, 730
Rolleston, Humphry, 795
Rooney, James F., 324
Roosa, D. B. St. John, 38
Roosevelt, Eleanor, 423
Roosevelt, President Franklin D., 399, 412, 446, 455, 740, 815, 821
Roosevelt, President Theodore, 132, 234, 709, 747, 749
Rosenberger, J. L., 157, 1029
Rosenow, E. C., 1045
Roussy, Gustave, 795
Routley, T. C., 471
Rubinow, I. M., 281, 287, 291, 318
Ruediger, Gustav F., 1088
Rush, Benjamin, 573, 575, 642; monument to. See *Rush monument* in Subject Index.

Sadtler, Samuel P., 867
Salter, Lawrence C., 481
Sand, René, 302
Sandberg, Harold L., 994
Sargent, John, 826
Sarles, W. T., 316
Sawyer, C. E., 336, 339

Sawyer, W. H., 1022
Sawyer, William A., 1183
Sayre, Lewis A., 100, 104, 106; biography, 636
Sayre, Reginald Hall, 636
Schamberg, Jay F., 1141
Schereschewsky, J. W., 321
Schireson, Henry J., 359, 379, 499
Schloss, Oscar M., 1127
Schlotterbeck, J. O., 867
Schultz, Oscar T., 1164
Schurz, Carl, 722
Scofield, T. J., 496
Scott, X. C., 188
Seeger, Stanley J., 963
Seip, J. W., 522
Selden, W., 46
Semmes, A. J., 1011
Senn, Nicholas, 14, 147, 163, 179, 186, 222; biography, 670
Sensenich, R. L., 426, 474, 476, 488, 963
Seydell, Ernest M., 1137
Shambaugh, George E., 1130, 1135
Shattuck, G. G., Jr., 46
Shaw, Anna, 204
Sheen, Msgr. Fulton J., 492
Shelly, E. C., 424
Sherman, Henry C., 379, 946
Sherman, John, 1018
Sherman, General William Tecumseh, 128
Shoemaker, John V., 145
Shoulders, Harrison H., 425, 434, 442, 446, 452, 483, 488, 489, 492, 977; biography, 827
Sidwell, Albert E., Jr., 884
Silliman, Benjamin, 586
Simmons, George H., 187, 276, 280, 294, 298, 319, 326, 370, 690, 840, 843, 867, 1078, 1089, 1120; activities at AMA sessions, 194, 200, 203, 252, 267; appointed editor and secretary, 190, 191; attacks on, 242, 243, 256, 260, 261; biography, 350-357; chairman of Council on Pharmacy and Chemistry, 235; death, 431; editor of Journal, 219, 230, 274, 315, 334, 340, 352-354, 835, 837, 865, 891, 1149, 1165; publication of American Medical Directory, 248; resignation, 337, 348; secretary of AMA, 221, 262, 266, 1111; tributes to, 249, 255, 257, 338, 362; work on reorganization of AMA, 201, 205, 214; work in World War I, 300, 301, 304, 355
Simons, A. M., 415
Simonton, A. C., 172
Simpson, Burton T., 518
Simpson, Frank F., 300, 998
Sims, J. Marion, 56, 88, 90, 92, 94, 122, 637, 686; biography, 627
Sinai, Nathan, 406, 415
Sinclair, Upton, 132
Singer, H. Douglas, 1152
Sleyster, Rock, 415, 439, 442, 446, 449, 452, 962; biography, 808
Slocum, Charles E., 194
Slosson, Edwin E., 333, 334
Sluder, Greenfield, 1130
Small, W. B., 321
Smiley, Dean F., 1009
Smith, Austin E., 463, 492

[1216]

Smith, Charles Emory, 181
Smith, F. G., 55
Smith, Henry H., 1014
Smith, Joseph F., 923
Smith, L. A., 1012
Smith, Nathan, 586
Smyth, Francis Scott, 1127
Solis-Cohen, J., 75
Solis-Cohen, Solomon, 146, 152, 161, 168, 200
Sollmann, Torald, 488, 497, 868
Soule, Herbert Edwin, 520
Southard, E. E., 1150
Speed, Kellogg, 1048
Spofford, A. R., 1073
Squibb, E. R., 91, 95, 185
Stack, Alfred W., 993
Stahl, Frank, 193
Starr, M. Allen, 1149
Stengel, Alfred, 197, 1087, 1164
Sternbergh, George M., 186, 200, 316, 708, 731, 1015; biography, 674
Stevens, Alexander H., 27, 31, 42, 1010; biography, 575
Stevens, J. Thompson, 531
Stevenson, Sarah Hackett, 91
Stewart, F. Campbell, 27, 58
Stewart, F. E., 173, 228
Stewart, G. N., 193
Stewart, J. Q. A., 730
Stieglitz, Julius, 868
Still, George A., 333
Stillé, Alfred, 24, 27, 31, 53, 54, 57, 80, 82, 179, 493, 949; biography, 617
Stokes, Joseph, 197, 1043
Stone, Harvey B., 472, 815
Stone, Richard French, 187, 196
Storer, David Humphreys, 1012; biography, 607
Storer, H. R., 80
Stringham, James S., 1016
Stroud, William D., 477
Summers, S. Lewis, 392, 399, 516
Swart, Charles, 492
Swift, Joseph K., 610
Sydenstricker, Edgar, 292
Syme, James, 665

Taft, William H., 747
Tait, Lawson, 155, 683
Talbot, Fritz B., 1127
Taylor, E. W., 1152
Taylor, Holman, 1030
Teschner, Paul A., 1004, 1008
Thayer, Ezra, 774
Thayer, James Bradley, 774
Thayer, William Sydney, 228, 371, 374, 376, 1111; biography, 774-777
Thomas, W. G., 650
Thompson, Alexander, 22
Thoms, H., 870
Thrash, E. C., 385
Ticknor, Luther, 23
Tilney, Frederick, 1150
Toner, Joseph M., 87, 88, 108, 622, 834, 1071, 1075; biography, 623
Trask, James D., 61
Trendelenburg, Friedrich, 700
Trudeau, E. L., 264

Truman, President Harry S., 485
Tuckerman, L. B., 1019
Tugwell, Rexford B., 1030
Turner, Mary, 519
Tyler, Grafton, 1011
Tyler, Moses Coit, 554

Upham, John H. J., 415, 426, 428, 436; biography, 803

Van Buren, Peter, 7, 22
Vander Veer, Albert, 289, 290; biography, 733
Van Etten, Nathan B., 409, 424, 428, 436, 449, 452, 455, 459; biography, 810
Van Meter, S. D., 1022
Van Sickle, F. L., 313
Vaughan, Henry F., 427, 727
Vaughan, Victor C., 154, 365, 698, 705, 708, 775, 795, 892, 1001; biography, 726; chairman of Council on Health, 312; editor of Hygeia, 334, 335, 842, 1184; president of AMA, 280, 285, 288; work in World War I, 355
Vaughan, Victor C., Jr., 728
Vaughan, Warren T., 729
Veeder, Borden S., 363, 434
Vest, Walter E., 453
Virchow, Rudolf, 611, 658, 680
Vohs, Carl F., 442

Wadley, James, 5
Wadlow, Robert, 432, 529
Wagner, Robert F., 445, 450, 1031
Waite, John Herbert, 1162
Walker, H. O., 210, 233
Walker, Norman, 795
Wallace, Henry A., 412
Walters, Waltman, 1157
Ware, John, 631
Waring, Holbert, 795
Warnshuis, Frederick C., 207, 328, 337, 344, 359, 368, 376, 418, 422, 423, 1024
Warren, B. S., 292
Warren, John, 577
Warren, John Collins, 42, 48, 53, 607; biography, 577
Warren, Jonathan Mason, 50
Warren, Joseph, 577
Warren, Joseph H., 103
Watkins, Robert Lincoln, 159
Watson, John, 948
Weatherby, J. S., 105
Weaver, George Howitt, 1049
Webster, George W., 157, 1075
Webster, J. Clarence, 497
Weech, A. A., 1127
Weidman, Frederick D., 1143
Weisenburg, T. H., 1150
Weiskotten, Herman G., 463, 910, 922
Welch, William H., 33, 185, 203, 238, 365, 383, 708, 709, 839; activities at AMA sessions, 222, 227, 231, 234, 267; biography, 712-716; chairman of Board of Trustees, 862; chairman of Rockefeller fund, 204; member of Board of Trustees, 256; member of committee

on legislation, 1019; member of Committee on Scientific Research, 1086, 1087; president of AMA, 260, 272, 840; work in World War I, 355
Wellford, Beverly R., 55, 59, 1010; biography, 583
Wells, Horace, 44, 84
West, Olin, 372, 383, 440, 976, 1002; activities in World War II, 465; biography, 493-494; field secretary of AMA, 326, 334; general manager of AMA, 344, 349, 390, 844, 963; president elect, 489; retirement, 482, 489; secretary of AMA, 335, 364, 384, 415, 417, 842
Whalen, Charles J., 192, 321
Whelan, Jewel F., 1117, 1132, 1148, 1159
Wherry, William P., 1137
Whipple, George H., 565, 1164
White, Charles, 36
White, Charles J., 1141
White, J. Harrison, 130, 148
White, James C., 1141
Whitehorn, John, 1152
Whitford, William, 176
Wiggin, F. H., 197
Wilbert, M. I., 868
Wilbur, Dwight L., 466
Wilbur, Ray Lyman, 302, 342, 380, 388, 742, 776; biography, 758; chairman of Committee on Costs of Medical Care, 371; chairman of Council on Medical Education, 385, 391, 439, 448, 901, 903, 922; president of AMA, 337, 338, 346
Wilder, Russell M., 943, 1115, 1117
Wiley, Charles R., 526
Wiley, Harvey, 233, 868, 877
Williams, L. R., 365
Williams, R. R., 943
Willoughby, Westel, 5
Wilson, Harriet, 1084
Wilson, J. C., 237
Wilson, James, 876
Wilson, James Leroy, 1127
Wilson, William, 648

Winston, C. K., 64
Wishard, William N., 1042
Wistar, Caspar, 110, 642
Wister, Caspar, 88, 850
Withering, William, 36
Witherspoon, John A., 226, 274, 282, 892; biography, 724
Witte, Edwin E., 412
Wolbach, S. B., 1164
Wood, Casey A., 193
Wood, Francis Carter, 488, 518
Wood, George B., 27, 639, 642, 851; biography, 589
Wood, H. C., 95, 197, 1086
Wood, Isaac, 850
Wood, Thomas, 51, 865
Woodbury, Frank, 157, 170
Woodhull, Alfred A., 186
Woodward, Joseph J., biography, 639
Woodward, W. C., 267, 279, 333, 338, 343, 390, 430, 431, 450, 842, 999, 1022, 1025, 1029, 1033
Work, Hubert, 253, 274, 299, 335, 841; biography, 751; member of Judicial Council, 268, 951; president of AMA, 321, 322, 329; Secretary of Interior, 362; speaker of House of Delegates, 207, 295, 304, 314, 319
Wragg, W. T., 42
Wright, Charles B., 391, 403, 415, 456, 1030
Wyckoff, R. M., 150
Wyeth, John A., 164, 221, 891; biography, 685
Wynn, Frank B., 195, 197, 244, 1042, 1043

Yandell, David W., 85, 730; biography, 619
Young, Hugh, 265

Zapffe, Fred C., 913
Zech, R. L., 976
Zentmayer, William, 1162
Zobel, A. J., 280

INDEX OF SUBJECTS

Abortion, criminal, prevention of, 1012
Abstracts in Journal of AMA, 218
Advertising Committee, 341
Advertising in Journal of AMA, 163, 164, 168, 231, 979–995; formulation of principles, 109; use of color, 381
Advertising in medical periodicals, 168, 198, 220, 837
Advertising by physicians, 953
Advisory Board for Medical Specialties, 906
Aims of medical profession, 1938, 439
Alcohol, therapeutic use of, 321, 326, 330, 331, 339, 364, 371, 378, 394, 1028; traffic accidents and, 1032
Amebiasis, Chicago epidemic, 406
American Archives of Surgery, 267. See also *Archives of Surgery.*
American Association for Advancement of Science, Committee of One Hundred, 1021
American Bar Association, 471
American College of Surgeons, 283; attitude on compulsory sickness insurance, 421; plan for medical care, 418
American Foundation Studies in Government, report, 432
American Journal of Diseases of Children, 1118–1128; first editorial board, 1120; founding of, 261, 1119
American Medical Association, activities of: 1918, 303; 1919, 306; 1922, 326; 1924, 343; 1925, 358; 1928, 372; 1930, 381; 1931, 388; 1932, 392; 1933, 399; 1934, 405; 1935, 415; 1936, 423; 1937, 427; 1938, 433; 1939, 444; 1941, 457; 1942, 463; 1943, 468; 1944, 476; 1945, 481; 1946, 487; 1947, 491; attacks on, 245, 260; Board of Trustees, 833–845. See also *Board of Trustees;* book publication by, 394; Bulletin, 327; Bureaus, 832; business department, 979–995; conception, 19; Constitution adopted, 30; Constitution revised, 155, 156, 229; Councils, 832; crusading activities of, 240, 243; expanding activities of, 388; fiftieth jubilee meeting, 14; first meeting, 8, 27; first officers, 31; first property purchased, 220; history, 19–492; home of, 176, 860–864; income of, effect of Journal, 121; indictment under Sherman Act, 441, 444, 447, 534–550; insignia of, 265; Journal of. See *Journal of AMA;* libel suits of, 456, 495; Library, 1071. See also *Library of AMA;* national health program of, 488, 973; national incorporation of, 237; organization, 27; presidents of, biographies, 567; presidents of, list, 1189; Principles of Ethics, adoption, 37; publications of, 1109; reorganization of 1901, 201, 204, 213; representation in, 32, 125, 128, 141; secretary, 170, 175, 262; Sections of, 1092–1098; semicentennial, 179; sessions of, list, 1189. See also *Sessions of AMA;* Transactions, 42; treasurer. See *Treasurer, office of;* trial, 458, 544; Woman's Auxiliary to, 332, 1099–1108; World War II and, 465, 471
American Medical Directory, 242, 243, 248, 470, 986, 1170–1179; basic records for, 1171; card index system, 1176; first edition of, 1174; origin of, 1170; report service, 319, 1178; second edition, 1175
American Pediatric Society, 1124
American Red Cross, health functions, 335
American Surgical Association, 119
Amputations, study by Council on Physical Medicine, 934
Andrology, 149
Anesthesia, 264; report of 1848 session, 44
Anesthesiology, American Board, 907; Section on, 1097
Animal experimentation, 155, 178, 183; resolution of 1884 session, 115
Anti-trust laws, indictment of AMA under, 534–550
Anti-vivisection legislation, 1014
Apparatus, therapeutic, considerations by Council on Physical Medicine, 930
Archives of Dermatology and Syphilology, 316, 764, 1138–1148
Archives of Internal Medicine, 394, 397, 1111–1117; first issue, 1114; founding, 253, 839
Archives of Neurology and Psychiatry, 1149–1153; first editorial board, 1150
Archives of Ophthalmology, 372, 1160–1163; founding, 1160; taken over by AMA, 1162
Archives of Otolaryngology, 340, 1129–1137; abstractors, 1134; first issue, 1132
Archives of Pathology, 363, 1164
Archives of Surgery, 269, 316, 1154–1159; first number, 1155, 1156
Army Medical Museum, 122
Army, physicians in, rank of, 68, 90, 96
Artificial respiration, investigations of Council on Physical Medicine, 932
Associated Medical Care Plans, 488
Association of American Medical Colleges, founding, 11, 912
Association of Medical Editors, founding, 11, 78; 1883 meeting, 110
Atlanta, 1879 session, 98; 1896 session, 174
Atlantic City, 1900 session, 200; 1904 session, 232; 1907 session, 249; 1909 session, 256; 1912 session, 269; 1914 session, 281; 1919 session, 307; 1925

session, 359; 1935 session, 418; 1937 session, 428; 1942 session, 464; 1947 session, 492
Attendance at AMA sessions, 1201
Automobile number of Journal of AMA, 260

Baltimore, 1848 session, 41; 1866 session, 74; 1895 session, 168
Barbiturates, control of, 1031
Befsal, libel suit on, 392, 516
Bicycle, effects of, 178
Birth control. See *Contraception*.
Blood grouping tests, legal aspects, 1032
Board of Public Instruction, 254; organization of, 998
Board of Trustees, 833–845; attacks on, 837, 840; executive committee of, 315, 316, 842; financial control by, 131; first members, 108, 834; functions of, 241; meetings of, 315; members of, 1192; reorganization in 1923, 336, 842; responsibility of, 219
Boards, examining, for specialties, 906
Book publication by AMA, 394
Book reviews in Journal, 167
Boston, 1849 session, 48; 1865 session, 71; 1906 session, 240; 1921 session, 322
British Medical Journal, 160; discussion at 1880 session, 100; discussion at 1881 session, 103
British physicians, visit to U.S., 406, 422
Buffalo, 1878 session, 96
Bulletin, AMA, 327
Bureau of Exhibits, 1042–1065; medals awarded, 1057; publications, 1057; work of, 1052
Bureau of Health Education, 996–1009; adoption of title, 1005; Health and Fitness Program, 1009
Bureau of Health and Public Instruction, organization, 1002
Bureau of Information, 1039
Bureau of Investigation, 1034–1038
Bureau of Legal Medicine and Legislation, 333, 1010–1033; establishment, 1025; first report, 338
Bureau of Medical Economic Research, 1068
Bureau of Medical Economics, 384, 386, 389, 1066–1070; publications, 1066; report on sickness insurance, 409
Bureau of Medical Legislation, 234
Bush Committee, 462
Business department of AMA, 979–995

California, health insurance in, 420
Calomel, report of 1863 session, 68
Campaigns of Journal of AMA, 427
Canada, medical education in, 916
Cancer, Coffey-Humber treatment of, 388; "cures," 518
Carnegie Foundation study of medical education, 897
Centennial, AMA, plans for, 482, 492
Charlatanism. See *Quackery*.
Charleston, 1851 session, 53

Chattanooga Medicine Co., 285, 495
Chicago, 1863 session, 67; 1877 session, 93; 1887 session, 130; 1908 session, 253; 1918 session, 302, 304; 1924 session, 344
Chicago Medical College, 10
Children's Bureau, health activities of, 382; liaison with, 422
Cigarette advertising, 405
Cincinnati, 1850 session, 51; 1867 session, 75; 1888 session, 134
Cleveland, 1883 session, 108; 1934 session, 407; 1941 session, 459
Clinic, definition, 956
Clinic, diagnostic, definition, 447
Coffey-Humber treatment of cancer, 388
College of Physicians and Surgeons of Western New York, 5
College of William and Mary, Medical Department, 20
Columbia University Medical School, founding, 20
Columbus, 1899 session, 693
Commission on Medical Education, 794
Committee on Costs of Medical Care, 371, 372, 377, 760, 1066; report of, 398
Committee on Defense of Medical Research, 258, 264
Committee on Economic Security, appointed by President Roosevelt, 412; Medical Advisory Committee to, 412, 413
Committee on Foods, 379
Committee on Hygiene and Public Health, 251
Committee on Legislative Activities, 389
Committee on Medical Legislation, 1021
Committee on Medical Motion Pictures, 1056
Committee on Medical Preparedness, 454, 455, 806; 1941 report, 460
Committee on Mental Hygiene, 389
Committee on Military Affairs and National Defense, 381
Committee on National Legislation, 1018. See also *Committee on Medical Legislation*.
Committee of Physicians, 433, 444; Principles and Proposals of, 432
Committee on Scientific Research, 1085–1091; funds, 1087; grants, 1088; membership list, 1091
Committees, standing, appointment of, 48
Compensation for eye injuries, 362
Congress of American Physicians and Surgeons, 149, 152
Contraception, 371; committee on, 422; control by AMA, 429; resolution on, 328
Contract practice, 952; definition, 956
Cooperative Medical Advertising Bureau, 280, 281, 475, 991; origin of, 276
Corn enrichment program of Council on Foods and Nutrition, 948
Coroner system, 149; reform of, 1011, 1017
Corporations, practice of medicine by, 385, 955
Council on Foods and Nutrition, 424, 936–947; activities of, 937; membership list, 946; Seal of Acceptance, 939
Council on Health and Public Instruction, 267, 273, 278, 282, 291; discontinuation

of, 336; formation, 998; legislative activities, 1022; 1919 report, 309
Council on Industrial Health, 961–966; formation, 962; growth and development, 964; membership, 963; war activities, 963
Council, Judicial. See *Judicial Council*.
Council on Legislation, Health and Publicity, 265
Council on Legislation, Organization and Publicity, 261
Council on Medical Education and Hospitals, 689, 742, 887–922; change of title, 909; cooperation with other groups, 912; dates in history of, 1198; first members, 237, 892; formation, 232, 891; membership list, 1195; 1934–1936 survey, 910; origin, 227; standards of 1905, 894
Council on Medical Service, 967–978; duties, 967, 971; first members, 968; formation, 475; news letter, 973; origin of, 440; plan of operation, 969; policies, 968; Washington office, 971
Council on National Defense, World War I, 300
Council on Pharmacy and Chemistry, 235, 865–886, 988; first members, 866; formation of, 837, 866; membership list, 869; origin, 226; procedure of, 872; publications, 878; rules, 870; rules, 1946 revision, 872; seal, 883
Council on Physical Medicine, 923–935; activities, 928; aims, 925; committees, 928; consultants to, 927; formation, 923; membership, 925; publications, 935; seal, 931
Council on Physical Therapy, 364. See also *Council on Physical Medicine*.
Council on Scientific Assembly, 298; formation, 288
Coxey's army, 162
Crerar Library, transfer of AMA Library to, 1077
Cultism, medical, 322, 345, 949, 954, 959; resolution of 1878 session, 96

Dallas, 1926 session, 366
Dartmouth College Medical School, founding, 20
Daylight Saving Time, 314
Deaths of physicians, summary of, 231
Denver, 1898 session, 186
Dermatology and Syphilology, American Board, 906, 907, 1147; Section on, 1095. See also *Archives of Dermatology and Syphilology*.
Detroit, 1856 session, 62; 1874 session, 86; 1892 session, 152; 1916 session, 289; 1930 session, 384
Diagnostic clinic, definition of, 447
Diathermy, short wave, investigations of Council on Physical Medicine, 932
Diphtheria, antitoxin for, 177; prevention, 132
Directory, American Medical, 1170. See also *American Medical Directory*.
Directory, medical, 229. See also *American Medical Directory*.

Diseases of the Interior Valley of North America, 57
Distinguished Service Medal, 425; 1938 award, 436, 553; 1939 award, 447, 554; 1940 award, 455, 556; 1941 award, 459, 557; 1942 award, 464, 559; 1943 award, 470, 561; 1944 award, 477, 562; 1945 award, 483, 564; 1946 award, 488, 565; recipients of, 553–566
Division of Therapy and Research of AMA, 885
Dress reform, 133
Drugs, resolution of 1879 session, 99. See also *Proprietary medicines*.

Economics, medical, 384. See also *Bureau of Medical Economics*.
Education, health. See *Bureau of Health Education*.
Education, medical, 161, 258, 268; Committee on, early work of, 887; Council on. See *Council on Education and Hospitals;* early history of, 888; effect of World War II, 917; first conference on, 894; full time vs. part time clinical teaching in, 323; future problems, 919; graduate, 903; National Commission on, 364; postgraduate, 908; postwar problems, 484; remarks at 1884 session, 114; wartime, 469
Education, nursing. See *Nurses, education of*.
Education, nutritional, 944
Education, preliminary, for medical students, first resolution of AMA, 28
Educational Number of Journal, 178
Electrocution, 149
Electrophone Corporation, libel suit by, 502
Emergency Relief Administration, 407
Endocreme, 530
Ergot, advertising of, 383
Ether anesthesia, 53
Ethics, Committee on, early activities, 35, 948; first members, 948
Ethics, medical, Percival's code, 36. See also *Principles of Medical Ethics* and *Judicial Council*.
Ethylene anesthesia, 789
Examining boards for medical specialties, 448
Executive committee, appointment of, 315
Exhibits, Bureau of. See *Bureau of Exhibits*.
Experimental Medicine and Therapeutics, Section on, 1095
Expositions, scientific exhibits at, 1053

Fairs, scientific exhibits at, 1054
Federal health department. See *Health, national department of*.
Federation of State Medical Boards of the United States, 913
Fee splitting, 277, 952
Ferrell, Jean, Inc., 531
Flexner report on medical education, 898

Flour enrichment program of Council on Foods and Nutrition, 942
Food acceptance program of Council on Foods and Nutrition, 937
Food and drug legislation, 151, 1034
Food, Drug and Cosmetics bill, 405, 431, 1030, 1036, 1037
Foods, Committee on, 379
Foods and Nutrition, Council on. See *Council on Foods and Nutrition.*
Foods, proprietary, advertising of, 375
Foods, special purpose, acceptance by Council on Foods and Nutrition, 940
Fourth of July accidents, 196, 225
Fruit juice program of Council on Foods and Nutrition, 941

Gallstones, first operation for, 240
Gastro-enterology and Proctology, Section on, 280, 1096
General practice as specialty, 314, 491
General Practice of Medicine, Section on, 1098
Genitourinary diseases, section on, 265
Georgia Warm Springs Foundation, 422
Goat-gland rejuvenation, 507
Gorgas Memorial Institute, 336, 339
Graduate medical education, 903
Great American Fraud, 1036
Great Britain, health insurance in, 360
Group Health Association, 430, 432, 534
Group practice, advertising and, 331; definition, 330
Guide to Current Medical Literature, 1165

Halls of Health, 1054
Handbook of Physical Medicine, 929
Harrison Antinarcotic Act, 288, 1024, 1027
Harvard University Medical School, adoption of AMA recommendations, 10; founding, 20
Health education, conference on, 445. See also *Bureau of Health Education.*
Health insurance in Great Britain, 360. See also *Insurance, sickness,* and *Social insurance.*
Health, national department of, 132, 151, 166, 279, 325, 339, 844, 1018, 1020
Health program of AMA, 488, 973
Hearing aids, study by Council on Physical Medicine, 934
Hill-Burton bill, origin, 455
Hirestra Laboratories, libel suit by, 530
Home of AMA, 176, 860-864
Home Owners' Loan Corporation, cooperative medical service of, 430
Homeopathy, resolution of 1855 session, 62; resolution of 1878 session, 96
Hospital insurance, 958
Hospital internships, requirement of, 899
Hospital Register, 909
Hospital residencies, 906
Hospital staff meetings, 374
Hospitalization, group, problems of, 435
Hospitals, construction of, 454
Hospitals, Council on. See *Council on Education and Hospitals.*
Hospitals, practice of medicine by, 474

House of Delegates, committee on legislative activities, 1030; executive sessions, 392; first proposal of, 202; functions of, 215; representation in, 207; 1943 session, 470; 1944 session, 477; 1945 session, 483; speaker, 207, 216, 291, 295; special session on sickness insurance, 415; special 1938 session, 441
Howard University, barring of delegates from 1870 session, 80; barring of delegates from 1872 session, 84
Hoxide Cancer Institute, libel suit, 501
Hygeia, 343, 358, 843, 994, 1103, 1184; editing of, 335, 340; founding of, 333, 842, 1002; organization of, 334
Hygiene and Public Health, Committee on, 251

Immigrants, health conditions among, 55
Income tax deductions by physicians, 341, 387, 1029
Index Catalogue, 119
Index of Journal of AMA, 195, 1079
Index Medicus, 155, 193, 196, 294, 365, 1166. See also *Quarterly Cumulative Index Medicus.*
Indigent physicians, 370
Industrial health. See *Council on Industrial Health.*
Infant foods, proprietary, advertising, 363
Information, Bureau of, 1039
Insignia of AMA, 265
Inspection of medical schools, 909
Insurance, hospital, 958
Insurance, sickness, 281, 286, 289, 292, 296, 306, 312, 313, 320, 321, 409, 410, 475, 841; California report on, 420; special sessions of House of Delegates on, 415; ten fundamental principles, 409
Interim committee on emergency problems, 306
Internal Medicine, American Board, 907; Section on, 1093. See also *Archives of Internal Medicine.*
International League of Medical Practitioners, 364
International Medical Congress of 1887, 13; battle over, 124
Internship, requirement of, 899
Investigation, Bureau of. See *Bureau of Investigation.*
Iodized salt program of Council on Foods and Nutrition, 941

Johns Hopkins University, 119; School of Medicine, 714
Joint Committee on Health Problems in Education, 999
Journal of AMA, accomplishments of, 248; advertising in, 163, 164, 168, 231, 979-995; automobile number, 260; Board of Trustees, and, 106, 834; book reviews in, 167; campaigns of, 427; contents of volumes: 1884, 113; 1885, 120; 1886, 123; 1887, 129; 1888, 131; 1889, 136; special 1889 issue, 139; 1890, 142; 1891, 145; 1892, 150; 1893, 154; 1894, 160; 1895, 167; 1896, 173; 1897, 178; 1898,

[1222]

185; 1899, 190; 1900, 197; 1901, 201; 1902, 220; 1903, 224; 1904, 231; 1906, 245; 1910, 260; early advertising in, 979; editorial board, 1890, 142; editorship of George H. Simmons, 352; Educational Number, 178, 893; first convention issue, 139; first editor, 109; first issue, 109; founding, 12, 100; Hospital Number, 909; index, 195, 1079; progress in first volume, 112; proposals for: 1880, 100–103; 1881, 104, 105; 1882, 106; removal to Washington, controversy on, 144–149; resolution of 1870 session, 79; Spanish edition, 303, 368, 373, 458, 467, 841; State Board Number, 914; World War I and, 300
Journal of Biological Chemistry, 237
Journal of Cutaneous Diseases, 316. See also *Archives of Dermatology and Syphilology.*
Journal of Laboratory and Clinical Medicine, 727
Journals, medical, 272; free, 411, 446; typical of 1847, 46
Judicial Council, 268, 277, 948–960; first members, 950; formation, 85, 949; members of, 1202
Jurisprudence, medical, 1013; Section on, 1015

Kansas City, 1936 session, 424
Keeley cure, 151, 153
Kings College Medical School, founding, 20

Labor, anesthesia during, report of 1848 session, 45
Laboratory, chemical, of AMA, 874, 884
Laboratory technicians, clinical, educational standards for, 916
Laryngitis, oedematous, Buck treatment, 43
Laryngology, Otology and Rhinology, Section on, 1094
Latin American physicians, attendance at 1942 session, 467
Laymen, journal for, 321, 327. See also *Hygeia.*
Lecture Bureau of AMA, 327
Lectureships: Frank Billings, 690; George de Schweinitz, 757; William Sydney Thayer, 777
Legislation, Bureau of, establishment, 1021. See also *Bureau of Legal Medicine and Legislation.*
Legislation, medical, 203, 251, 263; committee on, 234; early efforts of AMA, 1010; See also *Bureau of Legal Medicine and Legislation.*
Legislation, public health, 279
Legislative activities, committee on, 389
Libel suits of AMA, 295, 456, 495–533; Baker case, 517; Brinkley case, 503; Fernel case, 526
Librarians, medical record, educational standards for, 917
Library of AMA, 163, 172, 1071–1084; first report, 1870 session, 81; founding, 1071; 1882 report, 108; work of, 1083

Library of Congress, deposit of AMA library in, 1073
Licensure, medical, 1017; control of, 1012; examinations for, educational standards and, 895; illegal, 345
Lind University Medical Department, founding, 10
Literature, medical, report of 1848 session, 46; report of 1856 session, 63
Litigation against AMA, 358, 426. See also *Libel suits of AMA.*
Lobbying, 362
Los Angeles, 1911 session, 267
Louisville, 1859 session, 66, 90
Lye, legislation on, 1026

Malpractice, liability for, 1016; suits for, 1030
Mayo Foundation, 701, 740
Medal, president's, 375
Medals awarded in Scientific Exhibit, 1057–1065
Medical care, program for, 442, 484, 488
Medical education. See *Education, Medical.*
Medical Record, attacks on AMA, 245
Medical Repository, founding, 19
Medical schools. See *Schools, Medical.*
Medical societies, early history, 19
Medicine, state. See *State medicine.*
Medicines, proprietary. See *Proprietary medicines.*
Medicolegal bureau, establishment, 1023
Meetings of AMA. See *Sessions of AMA.*
Mental hygiene, committee on, 389
Metric system, resolution of 1879 session, 98
Middlesex College of Medicine and Surgery, 342
Milk, purity, resolution of 1854 session, 60
Milwaukee, 1893 session, 156; 1933 session, 402
Minneapolis, 1913 session, 275; 1928 session, 373
Miscellaneous Topics, Section on, 1097
Motion pictures, Committee on, 1056; scientific exhibits by, 1055
Museums, scientific exhibits in, 1054

Narcotics, control of, 320, 381; tax on, 1027
Nashville, 1857 session, 64; 1890 session, 143
National Auxiliary Congressional and Legislative Committee, 1020
National Board of Medical Examiners, 288, 293, 731, 915
National Commission on Medical Education, 364
National Conference on Planning for War and Postwar Medical Services, 469
National Health Conference, 440; program of, AMA stand on, 443
National League of Medical Freedom, 260
National Legislative Council, 1019
National Medical Association, 441
National medical convention, early efforts toward, 21–24; first meeting, 7, 24

[1223]

National Physicians Committee for the Extension of Medical Service, 451, 485
National Science Foundation, 488
Negro delegates, resolution of 1870 session, 81
Negro physicians, 478
Nervous and Mental Diseases, Section on, 1095
Neurological Surgery, American Board, 907
Neurology and psychiatry, journal of, 303. See also *Archives of Neurology and Psychiatry*.
New and Nonofficial Remedies, rules for inclusion, 870, 872
Newberry Library, transfer of AMA Library to, 163, 172, 1076
New Haven, 1860 session, 67
New Orleans, 1869 session, 78; 1885 session, 122; 1903 session, 226; 1920 session, 318; 1932 session, 395
Newport, 1889 session, 140
New York, 1853 session, 58; 1864 session, 69; 1880 session, 100; 1917 session, 294; 1940 session, 452
New York Medical Journal, 153
New York Polyclinic Medical School and Hospital, 686
New York State medical society, amalgamation, 227; early efforts toward national medical convention, 21–23; exclusion from AMA, 107, 113, 188, 238
Nomenclature of diseases, 397, 421
Northwestern University Medical School, founding, 10
Nostrums and Quackery, 271, 1035
N.R.A., 404
Nurses, education of, 361, 370; resolution of 1868 session, 78
Nurses, shortage of in World War I, 305
Nutrition, national conference on, 458; teaching program of Council on Foods and Nutrition, 944. See also *Council on Foods and Nutrition*.

Obstetrics and Gynecology, American Board, 906, 907; Section on, 1094
Occupational Medicine, 1183
Occupational therapists, educational standards for, 917
Ophthalmia neonatorum, 255, 258
Ophthalmology, American Board, 906, 907; Section on, 1094. See also *Archives of Ophthalmology*.
Ora-Noid, libel suit, 503
Organizer, traveling, for AMA, 224
Orthopaedic Surgery, American Board, 907
Orthopedic Surgery, Section on, 271, 1096
Osteopathy, 179, 954; challenge by, 333
Otolaryngology, American Board, 906, 907, 1133
Otolaryngology, journal of, 276. See also *Archives of Otolaryngology*.

Package library service, 1081
Pan American Medical Congress, 1893, 159
Panama Canal, 709
Patent medicines. See *Proprietary Medicines*.
Patents, medical, 185, 294, 305, 379, 400, 954
Pathology, American Board, 907
Pathology, Archives of. See *Archives of Pathology*.
Pathology and Bacteriology, Section on, 1043
Pathology and Physiology, Section on, 1095
Patient, physician's duties to, 38
Pediatrics, American Board, 906, 907
Pediatrics, journal of, 1118. See also *American Journal of Diseases of Children*.
Pediatrics, Section on, 1094
Pharmacopeia, National, proposed at 1876 session, 91; report at 1877 session, 95
Pharmacy and Chemistry, Council on. See *Council on Pharmacy and Chemistry*.
Philadelphia, 1847 session, 27; 1855 session, 61; 1872 session, 83; 1876 session, 90; 1897 session, 179; 1931 session, 390
Physical fitness program, AMA participation in, 476
Physical Medicine, Council on. See *Council on Physical Medicine;* definition, 930
Physical Therapy, Council on, 924. See also *Council on Physical Medicine;* technicians, educational standards for, 916
Physician, definition, 345, 955; duties of, 38
Physicians, advertising by, 953; directory of, 1170; Latin American, attendance at 1942 session, 467; service in World War II, 466
Plastic Surgery, American Board, 907
Poisonous drugs, regulation of, 1012
Poliomyelitis, 150; Crane prize for work on, 299
Porter narcotics control bill, 382, 383
Portland, 1905 session, 235; 1929 session, 376
Postgraduate medical education, 908
Postgraduate schools, commercial, 363
Practice, medical, uniform legislation on, 1022
Prescription writing in English, 1849 resolution, 50
Presidents of AMA, biographies, 567; list of, 1189; summary of, 568
Preventive and Industrial Medicine and Public Health, Section on, 1096
Principles of Medical Ethics, 35, 37, 38, 155, 156, 162, 222, 332, 437, 948; contract practice and, 408; enforcement, 948; 1903 revision, 227; violations of, 289
Procurement and Assignment Service for Physicians, Dentists and Veterinarians, 463, 815; origin, 461
Prohibition. See *Alcohol, therapeutic use of*.
Propaganda Department of AMA, 1034
Proprietary medicines, 233, 1034; advertising of, 161, 163, 169, 198, 199; attacks on AMA, 240, 243, 837; crusade against, 246; resolution of 1879 session, 99
Protein hydrolysates, activities of Council on Foods and Nutrition, 943
Psychiatry and Neurology, American Board, 707. See also *Archives of Neurology and Psychiatry*.

Public health, early efforts toward by medical profession, 997
Public Health Education Committee of Women, 263
Public Instruction, Board of, 254
Public, physician and, 39
Public relations of AMA, 486, 487. See also *Council on Medical Service.*
Publications of AMA, 1109
Puerperal fever, 138
Pullman cars, 217

Quack cures, 1035
Quackery, first resolution of AMA, 31
Quacks, libel suits by, 495–533
Quarterly Cumulative Index Medicus, 365, 844, 1080, 1082, 1156–1169
Quinine, memorial by 1870 session, 81

Radio broadcasting by AMA, 421, 1002; health education by, 1005
Radiology, American Board, 907; Section on, 1096
Radium, rental, 960
Railroads, free passage to AMA members, 61; special rates on, 186; special trains on, 173, 174, 176
Reference committees of AMA, 222, 251
Reforestation, 274
Refugee physicians, 391; numbers of, 419
Rejuvenation, 140
Research, Scientific, Committee on, 1085
Reserve corps, medical, 306
Residencies, hospital, 906
Richmond, 1852 session, 55; 1881 session, 103
Ross-Loos Clinic, 424
Rural medical service, 1040; conference on, 435
Rush monument, 122, 131, 134, 140, 143, 153, 168, 172, 178, 181, 188, 194, 225, 226, 233, 237
Rutgers College, Medical Department, founding, 19

St. Louis, 1854 session, 60; 1873 session, 85; 1886 session, 126; 1910 session, 260; 1922 session, 328; 1939 session, 446
St. Mary's Hospital, Rochester, 698
St. Paul, 1882 session, 105; 1901 session, 201
Sanatology, 502
San Francisco, 1871 session, 81; 1894 session, 162; 1915 session, 285; 1923 session, 336; 1938 session, 436; 1946 session, 488
Saratoga Springs, 1902 session, 221
Schools, medical, 293; classification, 896; early history, 19; inspection of, 250; number of graduates, 902; rating of, 265; See also *Education, medical.*
Scientific Exhibit, 272, 1042–1052; awards, 1045; medal winners, 1057; origin of, 194, 1042; permanent, 371
Scientific Sections of AMA, 1092–1098
Secretary of AMA, 170, 175, 191; payment of, 1872 session, 84; payment of, 1873 session, 86

Sectarian, definition, 344, 955
Section on Anatomy and Physiology, 1093
Section on Anesthesiology, 1097
Section on Dermatology and Syphilology, 1095
Section on Experimental Medicine and Therapeutics, 1095
Section on Gastro-Enterology and Proctology, 280, 281, 293, 1096
Section on General Practice of Medicine, 1098
Section on Hospitals, 1097
Section on Internal Medicine, 1093
Section on Laryngology, Otology and Rhinology, 1094
Section on Medical Jurisprudence, 1095; formation of, 1015
Section on Meteorology and Epidemics, 1094
Section on Miscellaneous Topics, 332, 1097
Section on Nervous and Mental Diseases, 1095
Section on Obstetrics and Gynecology, 1094
Section on Ophthalmology, 1094
Section on Orthopedic Surgery, 1096
Section on Pathology and Physiology, 1095
Section on Pediatrics, 1094
Section on Physiology and Dietetics, 1093
Section on Practical Medicine, 1093
Section on Preventive and Industrial Medicine and Public Health, 1096
Section on Psychology, 1096
Section on Radiology, 1096
Section on Stomatology, 1097
Section on Surgery, 1094
Section on Urology, 1096
Sections, unit system for, 298
Selective Service, development of, 443
Sessions of AMA, attendance at, 1201; list of, 1189; 1847, 27; 1848, 41; 1849, 48; 1850, 51; 1851, 53; 1852, 55; 1853, 58; 1854, 60; 1855, 61; 1856, 62; 1857, 64; 1858, 66; 1859, 66; 1860, 67; 1863, 67; 1864, 69; 1865, 71; 1866, 74; 1867, 75; 1868, 76; 1869, 78; 1870, 79; 1871, 81; 1872, 83; 1873, 85; 1874, 86; 1875, 90; 1876, 90; 1877, 93; 1878, 96; 1879, 98; 1880, 100; 1881, 103; 1882, 105; 1883, 108; 1884, 115; 1885, 122; 1886, 126; 1887, 130; 1888, 134; 1889, 140; 1890, 143; 1891, 148; 1892, 152; 1893, 156; 1894, 162; 1895, 168; 1896, 174; 1897, 179; 1898, 186; 1899, 193; 1900, 200; 1901, 201; 1902, 221; 1903, 226; 1904, 232; 1905, 235; 1906, 240; 1907, 249; 1908, 253; 1909, 256; 1910, 260; 1911, 267; 1912, 269; 1913, 275; 1914, 281; 1915, 285; 1916, 289; 1917, 294; 1918, 302, 304; 1919, 307; 1920, 318; 1921, 322; 1922, 328; 1923, 336; 1924, 344; 1925, 359; 1926, 366; 1927, 368; 1928, 373; 1929, 376; 1930, 384; 1931, 390; 1932, 395; 1933, 402; 1934, 407; 1935, 418; 1936, 424; 1937, 428; 1938, 436; 1939, 446; 1940, 452; 1941, 459; 1942, 464; 1943, 470; 1944, 477; 1945, 483; 1946, 488; 1947, 492
Shadid Clinic, 424
Sheppard-Towner Act, 331, 384

[1225]

Sherman Antitrust Act, indictment of AMA under, 441, 444, 447, 458, 534–550
Sickness insurance. See *Insurance, sickness*.
Skyscrapers, 179
Smithsonian Institution, housing of AMA library in, 1075
Social insurance, 286, 296. See also *Insurance, sickness*.
Social Security Act, 1031; Medical Advisory Board for, 794
Socialized medicine, 374, 384, 398, 408, 433, 434; pronouncement of Judicial Council on, 957. See also *Insurance, sickness*.
Solicitation of patients, ethics of, 331
Solicitation of votes for AMA offices, 224; rule on, 419
Spanish-American war, 186
Spanish edition of Journal of AMA, 303, 368, 373, 458, 467, 841
Specialization, reports of 1866 session, 74
Specialties, medical, certifying boards for, 387, 448; education for, 904; organizations for, 135
Standard Medical Directory, purchase of, 237
Standard Nomenclature of Disease, 373, 421
State boards of health, 1014; establishing, 83; remarks at 1878 session, 97; resolution of 1877 session, 95
State Medical Boards, Federation of, 913
State medical societies, relation to national association, 62
State medicine, 957; definition of, 324, 333; report of 1872 session, 84. See also *Socialized medicine*.
Steinach operation, 511
Students, medical, preliminary education, first resolution of AMA, 28
Sulfanilamide, elixir of, deaths from, 433
Sunlamps, investigations of Council on Physical Medicine, 932
Surgeon General's Catalogue, 87, 155
Surgeon General, Library of, building for, 391
Surgery, American, achievements, 142
Surgery, American Board, 907; Section on, 1094
Syphilis, address at 1874 session, 89
Syracuse University Medical Department, founding, 19

Television, health education by, 1009
Therapeutic Trials Committee of Council on Pharmacy and Chemistry, 480, 878
Thiouracil, study by Council on Pharmacy and Chemistry, 881
Tonics and Sedatives, birth of, 228
Transactions of AMA, 42; journalizing, 1880 report, 103; sale of, 848, 852
Transylvania University Medical College, founding, 19
Treasurer of AMA, office of, 846–859
Trust, medical, AMA as, 260
Trustees, Board of, 833. See also *Board of Trustees*.

Tuberculosis, Woman's Auxiliary work on, 1106

Ultraviolet radiation, report by Council on Physical Medicine, 932
University of Pennsylvania Medical School, founding, 20
Urology, American Board, 907; Section on, 1096

Venereal diseases, 229
Veterans Administration, physicians of, fellowship in AMA, 336, 392, 482
Veterans, medical service to, 399
Victory Meeting of AMA, 307, 314
Vital statistics, early work in, 997
Vitamin B enrichment of flour, 942
Vitamin C program of Council on Foods and Nutrition, 941
Vitamin D milk program of Council on Foods and Nutrition, 940
Volstead Act, 844. See also *Alcohol, therapeutic use of*.

Wagner-Murray-Dingell bill, 475, 485, 488, 970
War. See *World War I* and *World War II*.
War Medicine, 1180; first issue, 458; origin of, 457
War Participation Committee, 467
Washington, 1858 session, 66; 1868 session, 76; 1870 session, 79; 1884 session, 115; 1891 session, 148; 1927 session, 368; removal of Journal to, 144
Washington representative of AMA, 1028
Wayne County Association of Physicians and Surgeons of Osteopathic Medicine, libel suit by, 531
Wheeler-Lea bill, 405, 431
Whiskey. See *Alcohol*.
White House Conference on Child Health, 380
Wine of Cardui libel suit, 285, 495
Woman's Auxiliary to AMA, 332, 1099–1108; annual conventions, 1108; formation, 1099; health education work, 1104; objectives, 1102; past presidents, 1107; policies, 1101
Women, first representation at 1876 session, 91
Women physicians, 218; first resolution on, 77; remarks at 1871 session, 82; remarks at 1872 session, 85
World Medical Association, 490
World War I, AMA and, 298, 299, 303, 304; Board of Trustees and, 841; Journal of AMA and, 300; preparedness for, 290
World War II, AMA and, 465, 471; effect on medical education, 917; preparedness for, 452
World's Fair, Chicago, 143

X-ray technicians, educational standards for, 917